# OCCUPATIONAL THERAPY

## WITH AGING ADULTS

# OCCUPATIONAL THERAPY

## WITH AGING ADULTS

2nd EDITION

### Promoting Quality of Life Through Collaborative Practice

**Karen Frank Barney, PhD, MS, OTR, FAOTA**
Professor Emerita, AOTF Development Committee
Founder, Transformative Justice Initiative &
OT Transition and Integration Services
Chair, 2004–2013, Department of Occupational Science &
Occupational Therapy Geriatric Education Center Faculty, 1990–2013
Interim Director, Prison Education Program, 2013–2015
Saint Louis University
St. Louis, Missouri
USA

**Margaret A. Perkinson, PhD, FGSA, FAGHE, FSfAA**
Editor-in-Chief
Journal of Cross-Cultural Gerontology
Springer Nature
New York, New York;
Director (Retired)
Center on Aging
University of Hawaii at Manoa
Manoa, Hawaii
USA

**Debbie Laliberte Rudman, PhD, OT Reg. (Ont.)**
Distinguished University Professor, School of Occupational
Therapy & Graduate Program in Health and Rehabilitation Sciences,
University of Western Ontario
London, Ontario
Canada

ELSEVIER

Elsevier
3251 Riverport Lane
St. Louis, Missouri 63043

OCCUPATIONAL THERAPY WITH AGING ADULTS: PROMOTING QUALITY          ISBN: 978-0-323-87798-5
OF LIFE THROUGH COLLABORATIVE PRACTICE, SECOND EDITION

---

**Notice**

Practitioners and researchers must always rely on their own experience and knowledge in evaluating and using any information, methods, compounds or experiments described herein. Because of rapid advances in the medical sciences, in particular, independent verification of diagnoses and drug dosages should be made. To the fullest extent of the law, no responsibility is assumed by Elsevier, authors, editors or contributors for any injury and/or damage to persons or property as a matter of products liability, negligence or otherwise, or from any use or operation of any methods, products, instructions, or ideas contained in the material herein.

---

Previous edition copyrighted 2016.

*Executive Content Strategist*: Lauren Willis
*Senior Content Development Specialist*: Himanshi Chauhan
*Publishing Services Manager*: Deepthi Unni
*Project Manager*: Sheik Mohideen K
*Design Direction*: Patrick C. Ferguson

Printed in India

Last digit is the print number:   9   8   7   6   5   4   3   2   1

Working together to grow libraries in developing countries

www.elsevier.com • www.bookaid.org

My lineage includes three biological grandparents I never knew, one of whom was a half-brother to Otto Frank, Anne Frank's father. I likely owe my passion for writing to that part of my family. My granny, my mother's mother, was always a joy to be with, despite her physical frailties as she aged. Malcolm Frank, my father's first cousin, and his wife Mary were extremely supportive and adopted my sisters and me as grandparents. My loving parents, Alice and Eugene Frank, survived lengthy separations when Dad served as a Marine in World War II, and then again during the Korean Conflict. They provided inspiration and sacrifice for their four daughters to succeed in college, where I met the love of my life, Steve, my soulmate. We were married in 1965, the year that the St. Louis Arch was completed and Medicare was enacted, and have lived 58+ years together since. We have parented four children during full-time careers and graduate studies, and recently experienced aging-related changes and the best there is to be with our adult children, grandchildren, and great grandchildren.

**Karen Frank Barney**

To my friends and many relatives who have cheered me on with boundless encouragement, and to David Rockemann, my closest colleague, best friend, and spouse, who has been my constant sounding board and unending support, and whose incredible ability to keep things in perspective continues to keep me on track.

**Margaret A. Perkinson**

In loving memory of my parents, John and Eileen Laliberte, who made many sacrifices to support their children in realizing their occupational aspirations. My father's far too early departure from this world, which occurred in the midst of my doctoral work, had an immense impact on me not only as a daughter but also as a scholar—turning my attention to the social, economic, political, and cultural forces that differentially shape possibilities for health, well-being, and occupation over the life course. During the process of this book coming together, my mother experienced numerous health challenges and passed away in July 2023 at the age of 91. I have been privileged to have her in my life for such a long time and for my sons to experience her love and guidance. She has taught me much about what it means to age well and the importance of staying true to one's values.

**Debbie Laliberte Rudman**

**Karen Frank Barney, PhD, MS, OTR, FAOTA**, is a gerontological occupational therapist and advocate for aging adults globally. Having spent years providing consulting and direct services to older adults in Madison, Wisconsin, and teaching and serving as Fieldwork Coordinator for OTA students at Madison College for 6 years, her family moved to Kentucky, where she provided services to aging adults in rural areas with a home health agency and served as faculty at Eastern Kentucky University for 3 years. When her family moved to St. Louis, Missouri, she served as faculty and Fieldwork Coordinator at Washington University for 8 years, with a joint appointment with the Geriatric Education Center (GEC) at Saint Louis University, serving as gerontologic faculty in three programs. She was inducted into the Roster of Fellows of the American Occupational Therapy Association in 1998 for making a significant contribution in her field—initiating a fieldwork council in Missouri. She has served on American Occupational Therapy Association Conference national planning committees, as editor of the *Gerontology Special Interest Section Quarterly* publication, been an Editorial Board member of the *American Journal of Occupational Therapy*, and a reviewer and contributor for numerous journals. As Department Chair at Saint Louis University, she provided oversight and encouragement for all faculty to participate in the Society for the Study of Occupation (SSO), and hosted the national meeting in 2004.

Throughout her years of work with the GEC, she published many interprofessional training materials to promote injury prevention within the older adult population. Then, inspired by her younger son's incarceration, interfaced with the Saint Louis University Prison Program, she developed a model for rehabilitating incarcerated persons and founded the Transformative Justice Initiative & Occupational Therapy Transition and Integration Services (OTTIS) for persons transitioning from jail and prison to communities. She was the first faculty member on the Saint Louis University medical campus to receive The Last Lecture Award at Saint Louis University, and was awarded Professor Emerita status in 2013 in the Department of Occupational Science and Occupational Therapy, where she taught and served as department chair for 9 years. Afterwards, she served as Interim Director of the Saint Louis University Prison Education Program, which provides education to both incarcerated persons and prison staff, at Bonne Terre, Missouri, Dr. Barney has been devoted to supporting the lives of students, faculty, and aging and incarcerated adults through leadership, practice, teaching, conducting research, and interprofessional collaboration in Wisconsin, Kentucky, Missouri, Guatemala, Japan, and Korea. Her research has centered on interprofessional service models, promoting detainment prevention in younger persons, implementation of occupation-based practice, and occupation-based health-related quality of life for aging adults. With 56 years of continuing experience in practice, higher education administration, research, and service, she was honored by the St. Andrew's Charitable Foundation as one of the 2022 Ageless Remarkable Saint Louisans.

**Margaret A. Perkinson, PhD, FGSA, FAGHE, FSfAA**, is a medical anthropologist and social gerontologist with over 40 years of experience in research and applied anthropology with older adults. Dr. Perkinson's doctoral degree is in Human Development and Aging with a focus on Medical Anthropology from the University of California–San Francisco. She has conducted gerontological research in urban and rural settings across the United States and abroad. Dr. Perkinson's research interests include family caregiving of older adults, dementia care, diabetes management, residential options and service delivery for older adults, driving and dementia, participatory action research, and global aging. Her research has been supported by grants from the National Institute on Aging, the Alzheimer's Association, the AARP-Andrus Foundation, the Administration on Aging, and the National Highway Traffic Safety Administration (NHTSA). She taught aging-related courses in occupational therapy as a faculty member at Washington University in St. Louis and Saint Louis University for a total of 15 years and worked for 8 years as a senior research scientist at the Polisher Research Institute of the Philadelphia Geriatric Center, a major interprofessional research center based in a long-term care facility. With Karen Barney and colleagues Gelya Frank and others, she helped establish the National Association for the Practice of Anthropology (NAPA) Occupational Therapy (OT) Field School in Antigua, Guatemala, an international field school for occupational therapy and anthropology graduate students, and directed its gerontology component. She lived in Changzhou, China, to assist as a consultant in the development of a continuum-of-care retirement community (CCRC) for 7000 residents. Most recently, she served as the Director of the Center on Aging at University of Hawaii. She has published in numerous peer-reviewed journals, including *Human Organization, The Gerontologist, Journal of Gerontology: Social Sciences, Medical Anthropology, Mental Health and Aging, Contemporary Gerontology, Physical and Occupational Therapy in Geriatrics, Gerontology and Geriatrics Education, Practicing Anthropology, Journal of Geriatric Social Work, Journal of Intergenerational Relationships, Journal of Women and Aging*, and *Generations: Journal of the American Society on Aging*. Dr. Perkinson coedited a special issue of *Physical and Occupational Therapy in Geriatrics* that was later published as a book, *Teaching Students Geriatric Research*. She served as president of the Association for Anthropology and Gerontology (AAGE), executive board member and treasurer of the Academy for Gerontology in Higher Education (AGHE), member of the executive board of the Behavioral and Social Sciences Section of the Gerontological Society of America (GSA), and member of the Committee for Human Rights for the American Anthropological Association (AAA). She has been editor-in-chief of the *Journal of Cross-Cultural Gerontology* since 2005 and has served on the editorial boards of *Anthropology and Aging Quarterly* (charter member), *Physical and Occupational Therapy in Geriatrics, Care Management Journals, Journal of Aging Studies*, and *Occupational Therapy Journal of Research*. She is an elected Fellow of three professional organizations: Gerontological Society of America (GSA), Academy of Gerontology in Higher Education (AGHE), and Society for Applied Anthropology (SfAA). Along with Dr. Frank Barney, she was coeditor of the first edition of this textbook.

**Debbie Laliberte Rudman, PhD, OT Reg. (Ont.),** is Distinguished University Professor in the School of Occupational Therapy at the University of Western Ontario, located in London, Ontario, Canada. She is a preeminent scholar and a national and international leader within the discipline of occupational science and the profession of occupational therapy. For over two decades, Dr. Laliberte Rudman has been actively conducting research on sociopolitical determinants of occupation that centers issues of diversity, equity, and justice, with a focus on working with collectives—including older adults—facing persistent occupational inequities. Her innovative, critically informed scholarship has served as a foundation for a growing body of scholarship that has enhanced knowledge of how occupational inequities—differential possibilities to engage in occupations—are shaped and sustained through sociopolitical determinants, has informed vital shifts in both occupational science and occupational therapy, and has made significant interdisciplinary contributions in critical qualitative inquiry and social gerontology. Her scholarship, particularly the development of the concept of occupational possibilities, has been widely recognized as fostering a crucial critical turn that has pushed both occupational therapy and occupational science beyond individualistic frameworks and promoted scholarship and practices that attend to diversity and social justice, foci that are vital within contemporary societies marked by widening health, social, and occupational inequities. This recognition is evidenced by being awarded occupational science and occupational therapy lectureships in Canada, the United States, Brazil, South Africa, Japan, and several European countries. At Western University, where she has been on faculty since 2004, Dr. Rudman led the development and enactment of the Occupational Science graduate field in the Health and Rehabilitation Sciences program, creating the first Canadian program offering this specialization at the Doctoral level. Over the past decade, her scholarship has increasingly focused on advancing theoretical and methodological foundations for transformative approaches that span the knowledge generation to action continuum. She has collaborated in projects spanning this continuum with research participants, interdisciplinary colleagues, and graduate students, at local to international levels, embracing and advancing a range of participatory methodologies to address various forms of occupational inequities; in particular, in relation to seniors, these projects have addressed various forms of social exclusion, third places, ageism, and precarity. In relation to the interdisciplinary relevance and impact of her work, Dr. Laliberte Rudman's expertise in critical qualitative methodologies has been recognized across disciplines: for example, she has contributed nine invited book chapters focused on qualitative methodologies and has also been invited to bring her expertise related to critical qualitative methodologies and social gerontology to several funded projects led by Canadian gerontologists. Dr. Rudman's scholarship has been widely disseminated, including contributions to 158 peer-reviewed publications, 20 book chapters, and approximately 200 peer-reviewed conference presentations. Her work is highly collaborative and has involved partnerships with colleagues in Australia, Brazil, Canada, Chile, England, Germany, Japan, New Zealand, Norway, Scotland, Spain, Sweden, Switzerland, the Netherlands, South Africa, and the United States.

# CONTRIBUTORS

**Steven M. Albert, PhD, MS, FGSA, FAANN**
Professor
Behavioral and Community Health Sciences
University of Pittsburgh
Pittsburgh, Pennsylvania
USA

**Ganesh M. Babulal, PhD, OTD, MSCI, MOT, OTR/L, Lili Liu, PhD, MSc (OT), BSc (OT), OT Reg. (Ont.)**
Associate Professor
Department of Neurology
Washington University School of Medicine
St. Louis, Missouri
USA

**Cynthia R. Ballentine, MSOT, OTR/L**
Program Director/Professor
Occupational Therapy Assistant
St. Louis Community College
Ballwin, Missouri
USA

**Karen Frank Barney, PhD, MS, OTR, FAOTA**
Professor Emerita
AOTF Development Committee Founder Transformative Justice Initiative & OT Transition and Integration Services
Chair, 2004–2013
Department of Occupational Science & Occupational Therapy Geriatric Education Center Faculty 1990–2013
Interim Director
Prison Education Program, 2013–2015
Saint Louis University
St. Louis, Missouri
USA

**Emily Barr, OTD, MBA, OTR/L, BCG**
Executive Director
Nebraska Coalition for Patient Safety
University of Nebraska Medical Center
Omaha, Nebraska
USA

**Jane Bear-Lehman, PhD, OTR/L, FAOTA, FNAP**
Professor and Division Director
Occupational Therapy
Binghamton University
Johnson City, New York;
Adjunct Associate Professor
Psychosocial Research Unit
NYU College of Dentistry
New York City, New York
USA

**Margaret Newsham Beckley, PhD, EdD, OTD, OTR/L, SCLV, FAOTA**
Occupational Therapist, Vision Rehabilitation Specialist, and Professor
Clinical & Educational Consultants
St. Louis, Missouri
USA

**Shirley A. Blanchard, PhD, BCPR, FAOTA**
Professor
Occupational Therapy
Creighton University
Omaha, Nebraska
USA

**Pamela Block, PhD**
Professor
Anthropology
Western University
London, Ontario
Canada

**Lauren Bouchard, MS, PhD**
Senior Instructor I
Institute on Aging
Portland State University
Portland, Oregon
USA

**Erin DeFries Bouldin, PhD**
Assistant Professor
Division of Epidemiology
Department of Internal Medicine
Spencer Fox Eccles School of Medicine
University of Utah
Salt Lake City, Utah
USA

**Kathleen Brodrick, MSc, OT**
Director
Grandmothers Against Poverty and AIDS
Western Cape
South Africa

**David C. Burdick, PhD, FGSA, FAGHE**
Professor
Psychology Program
Stockton University
Galloway, New Jersey;
Director
Stockton Center on Successful Aging (SCOSA)
Stockton University
Galloway, New Jersey
USA

**Julia Buschbacher, BS**
Clinical Doctorate in Occupational Therapy Student
Division of Occupational Therapy
The Ohio State University
Columbus, Ohio
USA

**Michael Bradley Cannell, PhD**
Associate Professor
Department of Epidemiology, Human Genetics, and
    Environmental Sciences
University of Texas Health Science Center at Houston;
Adjunct Associate Professor
Department of Internal Medicine
Division of Geriatric Medicine
University of Texas Southwestern Medical Center
Dallas, Texas
USA

**Tracy Chippendale, PhD, OTR/L**
Associate Professor
Occupational Therapy
New York University
New York, New York
USA

**Susan Coppola, OTD, OT/L, FAOTA**
Clinical Professor
Division of Occupational Science and Occupational
    Therapy
University of North Carolina at Chapel Hill
Chapel Hill, North Carolina
USA

**Malcolm P. Cutchin, PhD, FGSA**
Professor
School of Occupational Therapy
Pacific Northwest University of Health Sciences
Yakima, Washington
USA

**Sue Dahl-Popolizio, DBH**
Director of Research/Associate Professor
Occupational Therapy
A.T. Still University
Mesa, Arizona
USA

**Anne E. Dickerson, PhD, OTR/L, SCDCM, FAOTA, FGSA**
Professor
Department of Occupational Therapy
East Carolina University
Greenville, North Carolina
USA

**Connie Diekman, M.Ed., RD, LD, FADA, FAND**
Food and Nutrition Consultant
CBDiekman
St. Louis, Missouri
USA

**Catherine Donnelly, PhD**
Associate Professor
School of Rehabilitation Therapy
Queen's University
Kingston, Ontario
Canada

**Sanetta Du Toit, PhD, MOT, MSc**
Senior Lecturer
Discipline of Occupational Therapy
The University of Sydney
Sydney, NSW
Australia;
Senior Research Scholar
Occupational Therapy
University of the Free State
Bloemfontein, Free State
South Africa

**Evelyne Durocher, PhD, OT Reg. (Ont.)**
Assistant Professor
Department of Occupational Therapy
School of Rehabilitation Science
Faculty of Health Sciences
McMaster University
Hamilton, Ontario
Canada

**Dorothy Farrar Edwards, PhD**
Professor
Kinesiology
Professor
Medicine
Associate Dean for Research
School of Education
University of Wisconsin–Madison
Madison, Wisconsin
USA

**Mary Geders Falcetti, EdD, OTR/L, FAOTA**
Occupational Therapist (Retired)
Mobile Rehab, LLC
Chesterfield, Missouri
USA

**Beth Fields, PhD, OTR/L, BCG**
Assistant Professor
Kinesiology
University of Wisconsin–Madison
Madison, Wisconsin
USA

**Maureen M. Fischer, MS, CCC/A**
Assistant Clinical Professor
Speech, Language and Hearing Sciences
Saint Louis University
St. Louis, Missouri
USA

**Kimberly A. Furphy, DHSc, OTR**
Associate Professor
Department of Occupational Therapy
Stockton University
Galloway, New Jersey
USA

**Julie K. Gammack, MD, CMD, FACP**
Professor of Medicine
Internal Medicine
Saint Louis University School of Medicine;
Physician
Internal Medicine
SSM Health
St. Louis, Missouri
USA

**Laura N. Gitlin, PhD, FGSA, FAAN**
Dean Emerita, Distinguished Professor
College of Nursing and Health Professions
Drexel University
Philadelphia, Pennsylvania
USA

**George Grossberg, MD**
Professor of Psychiatry
Psychiatry
St. Louis University
St. Louis, Missouri
USA

**Carri Hand, PhD**
Associate Professor
School of Occupational Therapy
University of Western Ontario
London, Ontario
Canada

**Christine Hayes Picker, MOT, OTR/L**
Adjunct Professor
Department of Occupational Science and Occupational
    Therapy
Doisy College of Health Sciences
Saint Louis University
St. Louis, Missouri
USA

**Julia Henderson-Kalb, OTD, OTR/L**
Assistant Professor and Program Director
Occupational Science and Occupational Therapy
Saint Louis University
St. Louis, Missouri
USA

**Clare Hocking, PhD, NZROT**
Professor
Occupational Science and Therapy
Auckland University of Technology
Auckland
New Zealand

**Lisa Jaegers, PhD**
Associate Professor
Occupational Science and Occupational Therapy
Saint Louis University
St. Louis, Missouri
USA

**Sarah Kantartzis, PhD, MRCOT**
Senior Lecturer
Division of Occupational Therapy and Arts Therapies
Queen Margaret University
Edinburgh
United Kingdom

**Devva Kasnitz, PhD**
Adjunct Professor
Department of Disability Studies
City University of New York–School of Professional Studies
New York, New York;
Director
Friends of Disability Justice and Culture Museum
Eureka, California
USA

**Kristen Kehl-Floberg, MSOT, OTR/L, BCG**
Graduate Student
School of Medicine and Public Health, Institute for Clinical
    and Translational Research
University of Wisconsin–Madison
Madison, Wisconsin
USA

**Helen W. Lach, PhD, RN, CNL, FGSA, FAAN**
Professor
School of Nursing
Saint Louis University
St. Louis, Missouri
USA

**Debbie Laliberte Rudman, PhD, OT Reg. (Ont.)**
Distinguished University Professor
School of Occupational Therapy & Graduate Program in
    Health and Rehabilitation Sciences
University of Western Ontario
London, Ontario
Canada

**Sarah Lamb, PhD**
Professor
Anthropology
Brandeis University
Waltham, Massachusetts
USA

**Michael Lepore, PhD**
Professor and Associate Dean for Research
Elaine Marieb College of Nursing
University of Massachusetts
Amherst, Massachusetts
USA

**Lori Letts, PhD**
Professor
School of Rehabilitation Science
McMaster University
Hamilton, Ontario
Canada

**Hedva Barenholtz Levy, PharmD, BCPS, BCGP**
Director
HbL PharmaConsulting
St. Louis, Missouri
USA

**Lili Liu, PhD, MSc (OT), BSc (OT), OT Reg. (Ont.)**
Dean
Faculty of Health
Professor
School of Public Health Sciences
University of Waterloo
Waterloo, Ontario
Canada

**Helene Lohman, OTD, OTR/L, FAOTA**
Professor
Occupational Therapy
Creighton University
Omaha, Nebraska
USA

**Lisa Luetkemeyer, JD, MHS, CCC-SLP**
Senior Counsel
Husch Blackwell LLP
Clayton, Missouri
USA

**Catherine L. Lysack, PhD, OT**
Professor and Deputy Director of the Gerontology Institute
Wayne State University
Michigan
USA

**Lydia Manning, MGS, PhD**
Adjunct Instructor
Gerontology
University of Maryland–Global Campus
Adelphi, Maryland
USA

**Jenny Martínez, OTD, OTR/L, BCG, FAOTA**
Associate Professor
Department of Occupational Therapy
Thomas Jefferson University
Philadelphia, Pennsylvania
USA

**Colleen McGrath, PhD, OT Reg. (ON)**
Associate Professor
School of Occupational Therapy
Western University
London, Ontario
Canada

**Margarita Mondaca, PhD**
Occupational Therapy
Karolinska Institutet
Stockholm
Sweden

**Thuli Mthembu, PhD, MPH, BSc OT**
Professor
Occupational Therapy
University of the Western Cape
Bellville, Western Cape
South Africa

**Keli Mu, PhD, OTR/L, FAOTA**
Professor and Chair
Department of Occupational Therapy
Associate Dean for International Relations
School of Pharmacy and Health Professions
Creighton University
Omaha, Nebraska
USA

**Raegan Muller, PT, GCS**
Regional Director of Rehabilitation
Innovate Rehab and Wellness
Hillcrest Rehab Services
Bellevue, Nebraska
USA

**Carol A. Needham, JD, MA**
Emanuel Myers Professor of Law
School of Law
Saint Louis University
St. Louis, Missouri
USA

**Denise M. Nepveux, PhD, OTR/L**
Associate Professor
Occupational Therapy Doctorate Division
Department of Orthopaedic Surgery
Duke University School of Medicine
Durham, North Carolina
USA

**Desmond O'Neill, MD, FRCPI, FGSA, AGSF**
Professor
Medical Gerontology
Trinity College Dublin
Dublin
Ireland

**Vimita Patel, MD**
Resident Physician
Psychiatry
Saint Louis University Hospital
St. Louis, Missouri
USA

**Molly M. Perkins, PhD, FGSA**
Associate Professor
Division of Geriatrics and Gerontology
Department of Medicine
Emory School of Medicine
Member of the Graduate Faculty
Sociology
Emory University
Atlanta, Georgia
USA

**Margaret A. Perkinson, PhD, FGSA, FAGHE, FSfAA**
Editor-in-Chief
Journal of Cross-Cultural Gerontology
Springer Nature
New York, New York;
Director (Retired)
Center on Aging
University of Hawaii at Manoa
Manoa, Hawaii
USA

**Michelle Perryman-Fox, PhD, MSc, BA (Hons)**
Lecturer of Occupational Therapy
Occupational Therapy and Art Therapies
Queen Margaret University
Edinburgh
United Kingdom;
Honorary Assistant Professor
Department of Occupational Therapy
University of Wisconsin–Milwaukee
Milwaukee, Wisconsin
USA

**Catherine Verrier Piersol, PhD, OTR/L, FAOTA**
Chair & Professor
Department of Occupational Therapy
Director
Jefferson Elder Care
Thomas Jefferson University
Philadelphia, Pennsylvania
USA

**Autumn L. Rebillot, MSOT, BRLS, OTR/L**
Occupational Therapist
Inpatient Therapy
Barnes-Jewish West County Hospital
St. Louis, Missouri
USA

**Kathlyn Reed, PhD, OTR, MLIS, FAOTA**
Associate Professor Emeritus
Sophie Lin School of Occupational Therapy
Texas Woman's University
Houston, Texas
USA

**David D. Rockemann, MS, NHA**
International Gerontology LTC Consultant
Honolulu, Hawaii
USA

**Miriam Rodin, MD, PhD**
Professor of Geriatric Medicine
Internal Medicine
St. Louis University School of Medicine
St. Louis, Missouri
USA

**Graham D. Rowles, PhD, FGSA, FAGHE**
Professor Emeritus
Graduate Center for Gerontology
University of Kentucky
Lexington, Kentucky
USA

**Angela Marie Sanford, MD**
Associate Professor of Internal Medicine
Internal Medicine–Geriatrics
Saint Louis University School of Medicine
St. Louis, Missouri
USA

**Michael Sarai, DO, FRCPC**
Physician
Medicine
PeaceHealth
Bellingham, Washington
USA

**Jean J. Schensul, PhD**
Senior Scientist
Department of Intervention research
Institute for Community Research
West Hartford, Connecticut;
Professor (Adjunct)
Department of Public Health Sciences
University of Connecticut Health School of Medicine
Farmington, Connecticut
USA

**Stacey L. Schepens Niemiec, PhD, OTR/L, DipACLM/
    DipIBLM**
Associate Professor of Research
Mrs. T.H. Chan Division of Occupational Science and
    Occupational Therapy
University of Southern California
Los Angeles, California
USA

**Carole A. Schwartz, MS, OTR**
Alliance for Disability in Health Care Education
Adjunct Faculty, Occupational Therapy Department
RUSH University Medical Center
Chicago, Illinois
USA

**Lauren Angela Selingo, MSOT, OTR**
PhD Candidate
College of Health Sciences
University of Wisconsin–Milwaukee
Milwaukee, Wisconsin
USA

**Virginia C. Stoffel, PhD, OT, FAOTA**
Emeritus Associate Professor
Department of Rehabilitation Sciences & Technology
University of Wisconsin–Milwaukee
Bayside, Wisconsin;
Past President (2013–2016)
American Occupational Therapy Association
Bethesda, Maryland
USA

**Donghua Tao, PhD, FA, MA, FAMIA**
Associate Dean and Associate University Librarian for
    Health Sciences
Library of Health Sciences
University of Illinois–Chicago
Chicago, Illinois
USA

**Laura H. VanPuymbrouck, PhD, OTR/L**
Associate Professor
Occupational Therapy
Rush University
Chicago, Illinois
USA

**Alexandra Wagner, PhD, OTR/L, CDP**
Clinical Assistant Professor
Department of Occupational Therapy
Yeshiva University
Bronx, New York
USA

**Selena E. Washington, PhD**
Associate Professor
Department of Occupational Science and Occupational
    Therapy
Saint Louis University
St. Louis, Missouri
USA

**Stacy West-Bruce, OTD, OTR/L**
Instructor in Occupational Therapy
Program in Occupational Therapy
Washington University in St. Louis
St. Louis, Missouri
USA

**Jenny Womack, PhD, OTR/L, FAOTA**
Professor
Department of Rehabilitation Sciences
Program in Occupational Therapy
Beaver College of Health Sciences
Appalachian State University
Boone, North Carolina
USA

# FOREWORD

Over 40 years ago, I joined Dr. Betty Yerxa and the other faculty at the Department of Occupational Therapy at the University of Southern California in Los Angeles, CA, and became part of their ongoing discussions about the past, present, and future of the field of occupational therapy. Based on the earlier work of Dr. Mary Reilly, attention had been drawn to the need to return to a focus on occupation as our central means and end of therapeutic interventions. At the same time, international pressures to be recognized as a fully professional field, with its own theories, research, and practices, were occurring. While Dr. Yerxa and our faculty strongly supported the idea of full professionalism for the practice field and the development of a research-based academic discipline, the importance of multidisciplinary, interdisciplinary, and transdisciplinary knowledge was acknowledged as well.

Our departmental focus on research in which the human participants are primarily considered to be occupational beings, not just bio psycho social beings, grew into the development of occupational science. Our first major National Institutes of Health (NIH)–funded research grant, the Well Elderly Project, exemplified this focus, testing an intervention program with community-based participants learning about, engaging in, and planning their occupational patterns in old age with resultant benefits to health and reduced health-related costs. Participant involvement in planning and interaction throughout both didactic and active elements of the program sessions respected and valued the life experience of our elderly participants. The interdisciplinary team of researchers evidenced the breadth of knowledge that was utilized. The lead article in a special issue of *JAMA* shared the results of this initial study to the widest audience yet for occupational therapy publications. A similar attitude and approach to programs for older adults were evident in other occupational therapy settings.

Dr. Karen Barney, a leading academic in occupational therapy and a hearty supporter of the discipline of occupational science whose faculty developed the Bachelor's degree in occupational science at St. Louis University, had a practice background in geriatric occupational therapy. We shared these interests, as well as our undergraduate occupational therapy education at the University of Wisconsin–Madison, and supported each other's professional interests and endeavors. I had and have the highest regard for her depth of understanding of gerontologic occupational therapy. She too saw the need for a broader perspective on aging within the field. Dr. Barney's gerontological expertise was evident in her teaching as well as in consultations for state, national, and international practice efforts. While recognized as Fellow of American Occupational Therapy Association (AOTA), she was also engaged in collaborative work with anthropologists and scholars in occupational science and occupational therapy. Dr. Barney and Dr. Perkinson developed

the interdisciplinary gerontology component of the NAPA (National Association for the Practice of Anthropology) - OT Field School in Antigua, Guatemala, founded by Dr. Gelya Frank, PhD anthropology faculty from the University of Southern California.

I met Dr. Perkinson when she was on faculty at St. Louis University and through interdisciplinary conferences and projects such as the NAPA-SIG Field School. Her interest in and efforts to strengthen interdisciplinary knowledge and research in aging were evident and appealing. As Director of the Center on Aging at the University of Hawaii, Dr. Perkinson has been a medical anthropologist and social gerontologist recognized for her research in family caregiving in dementia care, global issues of aging, and the cultural dimensions of aging. Her experience in community-based interprofessional collaboration in programming and participatory action research supports her students and colleagues as she promotes contemporary gerontological education. Dr. Perkinson promotes knowledge development and dissemination as the editor of the *Journal of Cross-Cultural Gerontology*. She has been recognized as a Fellow of the Gerontological Society of America, the Academy for Gerontology in Higher Education, and the Society for Applied Anthropology. I've been honored to consider her a colleague over the years.

Dr. Debbie Laliberte Rudman is someone I met who was then an exciting junior faculty member at Western Ontario University, with whom discussions of occupational science were wide ranging and inevitably eye-opening, as she brought a new and critical analysis to work that I had spent my career developing. Today, she is a respected and revered contributor to our understanding of the relationship of occupation and social transformation. As Distinguished Professor and Associate Director of the School of Occupational Therapy, Dr. Rudman has made an outstanding contribution to theory and research in the field through work with the international students in her Critical Occupational Science laboratory, including current projects focusing on intersection of place, occupation, and social exclusion of aging persons. Their work is currently supported by $1.5 million dollars of research grants, a major recognition of its quality. She is involved in the heart of international work through her position as Associate Editor of the *Journal of Occupational Science* and development in the Global South such as the Brazilian contribution of Social Occupational Therapy (as a member of the editorial board of the *Brazilian Journal of Occupational Therapy*).

The experience, knowledge, and expertise of these three coeditors are reflected in the book's inclusive list of topics and extensive list of authors. The authors of this book provide an outstanding sample of excellence as researchers, educators, and practitioners in gerontology as well as reading as a Who's Who list in gerontological occupational therapy. They reflect international experience and viewpoints representing concepts from the Global South as well as North. Including leaders of practice in a number of other disciplines, they offer implications for OT practice as well as models for interdisciplinary work.

This second edition of *Occupational Therapy With Aging Adults: Promoting Quality of Life Through Collaborative Practice* incorporates the best of what has gone before along with the contemporary state of the art and science. The editors and authors move the field toward the future of occupational therapy with aging people, and I look forward to joining them on this journey as I read what is bound to be the definitive publication in the field.

**Ruth Zemke, PhD, OTR (Retired), FAOTA**

# PREFACE

This second edition was developed to address requests by occupational therapy (OT) educators and individuals in other disciplines around the world for an updated comprehensive resource for OT practice with older adults, for both students and those already practicing in the field. As with the first edition, this book, commensurate with the growing emphasis on interprofessional health care and community-based practice as populations age, integrates experts and knowledge from various fields to optimally understand and address the occupational participation of older adults.

Knowledge and practices specifically addressing older adults and the communities in which they live are of utmost importance within the context of population aging. By the 2030s and beyond, demographic trends in the United States and on the global level are likely to have a profound effect on all aspects of societies, such as economic growth, global mobility, climate change, living standards, and governmental priorities and policies. Over the next several decades, as the unprecedented growth in the number of elders, along with declines in the numbers of youth, is experienced in many national contexts, the demand for services, supports, and environments to be designed and delivered in ways that facilitate the occupational participation, health, and well-being of older adults will surely increase. Incoming OT students, as well as those already in the field, have the opportunity and responsibility to equip themselves for this work by becoming familiar with the rich body of current gerontological evidence and using it to enrich their practice in health care and in communities in a wide variety of ways, spanning practices from individual to policy levels.

This book is designed to support a holistic, occupation-focused approach to practice with older adults. Physical rehabilitation textbooks typically provide comprehensive approaches for age-related conditions (e.g., arthritis, cardiovascular issues, cerebral vascular accidents, and musculoskeletal conditions) but often do not address the complex intersections of diverse environmental factors impacting functional outcomes and occupational possibilities. Additionally, in the United States, OT textbooks have tended to focus specifically on the role of OT in direct service provision with older adults, with limited commentary on global demographic issues, the role of other service providers, the systems within which services are provided, and relevant legal issues. Such textbooks are also often underpinned by a biomedical perspective and may focus only on current intervention strategies. Also, coverage of diversity, including cultural and religious positionalities, is often limited, with little attention to contexts outside of North America. To address these gaps, this textbook utilizes a global, holistic, occupation-focused, and evidence-based approach to focus on enhancing the occupational performance potentials and possibilities of older adults, and also addresses emerging and future directions for OT practice.

The overall emphases within the approaches to practice highlighted throughout this book are upon collaboration with clients (i.e., as an individual, group, agency, or community) to address the interaction of aging-related changes with physical, socioemotional, socioeconomic, political, and sociocultural environments, and to optimize occupational performance, occupational engagement, and interpersonal relationships, thus enhancing overall well-being and quality of life. *Collaboration* is a highly intentional theme throughout the textbook: the title implies that interventions are planned and executed *with* (not for) the client, whether that client represents an individual older adult and his or her support system, an aging group, or a population. The title also implies collaboration both intraprofessionally (e.g., OT, OTA) and interprofessionally (e.g., different disciplines, agencies, businesses, communities, organizations, or services), wherever relevant. Within both types of collaboration, the emphasis is on understanding, appreciating, and complementing collective perspectives to optimize efforts in providing relevant interventions and services.

Additionally, in the spirit of *collaboration*, the editors themselves represent an interprofessional approach, reflecting the emerging collaborative work of occupational therapists, anthropologists, and others working in OT, occupational science (OS), and other related areas. With their collective experience, including their own aging, they are well suited to conceptualize this textbook. All editors have extensive backgrounds working with older adults, their families, and numerous types of agencies in aging service delivery systems in the United States, Canada, and abroad within their respective disciplines.

Extending upon collaboration, many chapters are coauthored by one or more gerontological experts and one or more occupational therapists specializing in OT practice related to that chapter's topic. A wide variety of professionals in the field of gerontology contributed chapters to this text to accomplish a number of purposes. First, some provided an expanded view of the needs of older adults and a greater level of detail regarding the role of their respective disciplines in their work with older adults. Others contributed perspectives on interprofessional and intraprofessional opportunities to collaborate in service provision with older adults and their significant others. Additional contributors provided expertise to support evidence- and occupation-based practice, including international examples. The professional backgrounds of our 84 chapter authors reflect the interdisciplinary perspective of the book: anthropology, disability studies, epidemiology, geography, geriatrics, geriatric psychiatry, health services research, human development and aging, humanities and the arts, law, library science, medicine, nursing, physical therapy, pharmacology, physiology, psychology, public health, social work, sociology, and theology, in addition to OT and OS.

While most of our authors are well-established senior scholars and practitioners, renowned for their mastery and depth of knowledge in their respective fields, we also included community activists and emerging academics and professionals for expanded and diverse perspectives. Some teams of coauthors came to this project with long histories of collaboration. Other chapter coauthors were new to each other, and collaborating on the chapter afforded new insights into each other's disciplinary perspectives.

Most interprofessionally authored chapters share the same basic structure, with the intent of providing a two-pronged approach to each topic. Typically, first, the gerontological expert presents an overview of relevant, cutting-edge research on the given chapter topic. The gerontological occupational scientist or therapist then discusses how that research evidence could be incorporated into OT practice. The reader should approach each chapter for an explication of the most recent and essential research-based knowledge and scholarly resources on a given topic and for clearly stated guidelines and implications for using that knowledge to enrich their work. For the OT readers, each chapter should lead the way toward practice and research that is evidence based. For non OT readers, each chapter provides a window into the often misunderstood field of OT and guidance toward achieving informed collaborations in interprofessional gerontological work. In other chapters, occupational therapists and occupational scientists from various geopolitical contexts contribute perspectives and examples on a topic, such as age-inclusive communities or occupation-based transformative practice, as a means to diversify understandings and expand possibilities for practice.

Throughout this book, advances in the use of evidence guided by current theories and conceptual models, which include OS and OT theory, occupation-centered practice, and theories from other disciplines, are presented; each chapter is theory and evidence informed. Readers will find strategies for identifying and applying evidence relevant to practice with older adults. This information is interfaced with content related to OT processes that include screening, evaluation, intervention, and targeting of outcomes with older clients and community agencies and groups.

The impact of globalization increasingly affects many aspects of the lives of recipients of services, as well as the service providers, and requires consideration of needs, resources, and dynamics on multiple levels. To do so, the book's authors employed theoretical models from a variety of sources, proceeding from macro- to micro-level influences on practice that include (but are not limited to) the World Health Organization, international health systems, international government and public health sources, and the disciplines of OS and OT. Coverage of macro-level influences on aging and OT practice represents a unique contribution of this book. To augment our global perspective, examples of international models and approaches for service provision, within and outside health-care systems, are included within varying cultural contexts, reflecting actual or potential OT practice.

The editors selected chapter topics with the intent of providing thorough, contemporary coverage across a full range of gerontological OT practice areas with intentional inclusion of sensitivity to diversity, equity, and inclusion considerations. This process resulted in 33 chapters, divided into six sections: Conceptual Foundations, Age-Related Biological System Changes, Age-Related Psychosocial Changes, the Functional Environment of Aging Adults, Continuum of Care, and Trends and Innovations in Care With Aging Adults. In addition to coverage of traditional topics related to development and pathology in later life, this book addresses factors rarely included in aging and OT textbooks, such as ethical and legal approaches, global aging epidemiology, nutrition and oral health concerns, pharmacological issues, low vision and hearing interventions, aging with long-term disability, the integration of the humanities and arts into occupational practice, issues of occupational justice and social transformation, and community-based models of practice.

# ACKNOWLEDGMENTS

A year prior to the request to produce a second edition of this textbook, my coeditor, Margaret (Peggy) Perkinson, my close colleague as a medical cultural anthropologist, and I met to discuss content that was needed due to new gerontological and occupational science perspectives and trends, and content that could not be included in the first edition, as well as the need to mobilize occupational therapy personnel to support these needs, should we be asked for another edition. A few months later, Lauren Willis, our colleague at Elsevier, called me with the request. Excitedly, I contacted Dr. Perkinson, and we immediately agreed that we needed an outstanding younger scholar to join our team as coeditor. We both thought only of Dr. Debbie Laliberte Rudman, whose scholarship is superior, advocating in both traditional and nontraditional ways on behalf of aging adults globally, and would ably and collectively move us into the future. Her agreement to join our team of editors is therefore profoundly meaningful to us. I am also extremely appreciative of all those who have encouraged me to take on leadership, scholarship, and mentoring roles throughout my career. Also, one of my Saint Louis University faculty colleagues, Dr. Cynthia Matlock, recommended Delaney Jordan to serve as our editorial assistant for the duration of producing this textbook. Our editorial team is extremely grateful for her extraordinary support on many levels. She worked with us while practicing and finishing her OTD degree at Washington University in St. Louis, and is now a member of the Department of Occupational Science & Occupational Therapy faculty at Saint Louis University. We are grateful for all Elsevier staff support, including Lauren Willis, Lauren Klein, Himanshi Chauhan, and Sheik Mohideen K. This work is the product of 83 global interprofessional scholars and practitioners who dedicated many hours in support of our aim to reflect state-of-the-art and foreseeable future practice to support our increasing numbers of aging adults. We are so fortunate to have these contributors who are experts on their respective chapter topics. Finally, I am humbled and thrilled that Dr. Ruth Zemke agreed to write our Foreword. We are both UW-Madison BSOT graduates; she had the foresight to pursue a PhD immediately after our undergraduate days, during an era when that was not common for women, and is one of our eminent global occupational scientists.

**Karen Frank Barney**

I echo Karen's and Debbie's thanks to our many colleagues who have contributed so generously to the development of this book. I also appreciate this opportunity to acknowledge those who mentored and inspired me during the creation of this book and the path that led to it, too many to note individually. I have been blessed to have been in the right places at the right times in terms of gerontological "hot spots" throughout my career. Sincere thanks go to my professors, mentors, and colleagues; I am truly blessed to have worked with these esteemed leaders of the past and current development of the field of gerontology, and to be able to count them as close personal friends. All have contributed to my knowledge and understanding of gerontology and occupational therapy, and many have contributed directly to the writing of this book.

Special thanks go to my coeditors, colleagues, and treasured friends, Karen Frank Barney and Debbie Laliberte Rudman. They brought a wealth of knowledge, experience, and professional contacts to the making of this textbook. Their wise perspectives have been crucial to this publication.

**Margaret A. Perkinson**

Special thanks go to Karen and Peggy—contributing in an editorial role to a book was a new role for me, and the guidance of these two experienced editors was immensely valuable. I also appreciated their openness to my ideas for new chapters to add to this edition, providing a space to consider the social and political forces shaping occupational possibilities for older adults and to address emerging and potential roles for occupational therapists. Thanks also go to the many colleagues—former students, current collaborators, scholars whose work I have long admired—who readily took up invitations to contribute to chapters and generously shared their expertise and exemplary work.

**Debbie Laliberte Rudman**

# CONTENTS

CHAPTER 1

# Introduction: Gerontological Occupational Therapy

*Margaret A. Perkinson, PhD, FGSA, FAGHE, FSfAA, Karen Frank Barney, PhD, MS, OTR, FAOTA, and Debbie Laliberte Rudman, PhD, OT Reg. (Ont.)*

## CHAPTER OUTLINE

## OBJECTIVES

- Introduce historical and contemporary contextual factors that underscore the significance of the field of gerontology in general and gerontological occupational therapy in particular for understanding contemporary later life.
- Preview the scope of the book by providing brief overviews of main themes and content areas of various chapters.
- Understand how application of gerontological constructs to occupational therapy practice with aging adults varies in relation to interactions of contextual, occupational, and individual factors, at local to global scales.
- Explain how interprofessional practice, wherever indicated, is critical to holistic approaches that optimally enable occupational participation and occupational possibilities for aging adults.

These are exciting times to be a gerontologist, that is, a healthcare professional and/or researcher whose work is focused in the area of aging. Our understanding of the experience of aging and the factors influencing it is rapidly evolving. Long-held negative notions of old age are giving way to more complex, nuanced understandings of late-life experiences and processes. This book provides an introduction to these newly refined understandings, based on a growing body of aging-related research of relevance to gerontology, occupational science, and occupational therapy (OT). It is designed to inform and guide those in positions to assist aging adults in the search for an enriched later-life stage suffused, as the earlier quotes suggest, with an alive, intense state of inward beauty. Given the purview of OT, that is, "achieving health, well-being, and participation in life through engagement in occupation" (American Occupational Therapy Association [AOTA], 2020), as well as its holistic approach and emphasis on client-centered care and quality of life, occupational therapy personnel are especially well suited to benefit from and contribute to contemporary gerontological theory and practice. This book was primarily designed to prepare and support OT students and practitioners to practice in and contribute to this fulfilling and cutting-edge field. Readers in other disciplines who work with older adults should reach a better understanding of and sensitivity to issues encountered in later life and thus be better prepared to work with this population in their respective fields. Lay consumers may also find the book helpful in understanding their own aging, that of significant others, as well as the role of OT and other professions in supporting their meaningful participation and quality of life.

Guiding questions: As you read the book, its content should evoke various questions regarding aging and the role of the occupational therapy personnel in working with aging adults. Here are a few to keep in mind: What core changes do people within your contemporary sociopolitical context typically undergo in later life? How might such changes differ across time and contexts? How have perceptions of aging changed over time? What is optimal aging? What determines life satisfaction in old age?

Before presenting a brief orientation to gerontological OT, the following section frames aging in its historical and global contexts, underscoring the importance of this field. It explains why the current epoch may well be considered revolutionary in respect to old age, and why this aging-related revolution is especially relevant to the field of OT. Brief summaries of each chapter follow with glimpses of what is to come.

## The Evolution of Aging: Implications for Occupation in Later Life

### The Demographic Transition

It is no exaggeration to describe the current change in global populations as a demographic revolution. Never in the history of humankind have so many people lived so long (Crews & Gerber, 2003). To put this into perspective, physical anthropologists suggest that, on average, Neanderthals could expect to live little more than 20 years; only a small percentage reached age 40 (Crews & Gerber, 2003). Over subsequent millennia, average life expectancy barely budged. Around the turn of the twentieth century, however, conditions changed. Advances in public health in developed countries struck a blow to infectious diseases, greatly reducing infant and child mortality and allowing more people to live longer lives. (Note: The recent emergence of COVID-19 may impact this trend; Gebeyehu et al., 2022; Marois et al., 2020.) In 1900, 4% of the US population (approximately 3.1 million people) lived to age 65 or beyond. By 2040, those numbers are expected to increase to 21.6%, amounting to a total of 80.8 million older Americans (ACL, 2020). Since World War II, average life expectancy on the global level has increased from 45 years to 69.6 years. In addition, the percentage of the oldest old (those aged 80 and over) worldwide is rising rapidly and is projected to increase 233% between 2008 and 2040 (Vespa et al., 2020). As a species, we have made greater gains in average life expectancy in the past 70 years than in the previous 132,000 years!

The relatively recent global decline in birth rates represents the second major factor fueling the demographic transition. In the mid-1950s, the average number of children per woman worldwide equaled 5.0. That number has plummeted due to various social, political, and historical factors (e.g., increased education and participation in the workforce for women and transition from agricultural to industrial economies, making large families less economically appealing and feasible). The global average number of children per woman is now 2.7, with some countries experiencing birth rates below replacement levels (Ritchie et al., 2022). Decline in birth rates has a significant impact on the proportion of older adults. Globally, those aged 65 and over now outnumber children under age 5 for the first time in history (United Nations, 2022), and researchers expect the global difference in percentages between the two age groups to continue to grow. (See Chapter 3 for a more

detailed discussion of global demographic changes and their implications.)

## The Epidemiological Transition: Implications for Occupational Therapy

With the growth of older cohorts, especially the oldest old, chronic conditions are supplanting acute episodes of disease as primary health concerns, except for the recent impact of COVID-19 and other emerging infectious diseases. This epidemiologic transition will, perforce, transform health-care systems, and a greater proportion of health-care providers will, by necessity, shift primary attention from diagnosis and cure to health promotion, rehabilitation, and maintenance of function supportive of personally meaningful occupations and well-being until the end of life. Chronic illnesses, by definition, admit no cure; thus, therapeutic goals for older adults are more likely to be framed as facilitating continued participation in occupations of choice, rather than attaining a pre-disease state. (See Chapter 3 for a more detailed discussion.)

## Resulting Social Changes and Their Implications for Later-Life Occupations

It is difficult to exaggerate the effect of the global demographic and epidemiological transitions on both individual and societal levels. Life experiences and social institutions that many now take for granted in developed countries, such as retirement and empty-nest households, are modern phenomena, previously encountered by the very few (Achenbaum, 2020; Costa, 1998; Hareven, 2001). Major changes in the family, workforce, health status and health-care systems, and lifestyles interconnected with population aging also have direct effects on related and emergent occupations. For example, some occupations are changing radically, while others are newly available for older adults. With new or altered occupations come different opportunities as well as challenges to performance and participation for older adults, challenges that may be more easily met with the help of OT personnel trained in gerontology.

### Emergent Life Stages: The Role and Responsibility of Occupational Therapy

Although scholars have debated the stability and generalizability of normative constructions of the temporal ordering of the life course, policy mechanisms and social norms have constructed a structure for many aspects of life, including an expected sequence of and transitions between various roles (i.e., student, worker, spouse, parent), within various parts of the Western world (Kohli, 2007). That life structure is undergoing radical change. For example, in the context of the United States in the 1880s, the typical woman was widowed before the last child left the household, the typical man died while still employed, and very few spent their later years retired from work or from child rearing (Elder, 1977; Haber, 2006; Ruggles, 1994). However, given the demographic changes noted previously, today's growing cohorts of older adults now face a stage of later life that is relatively uncharted, lacking widely shared roles and cultural expectations (Cutler &

Hendricks, 2001). There are few widely shared roles and social expectations for a period of later life unencumbered by the demands of employment and parenthood. It is a new life era that is at once exhilarating and free, open to new possibilities and renegotiations of previous roles, and yet daunting and uncertain, with no clear guideposts in sight. As noted, never before have so many lived so long. Many current attitudes toward aging and the aged emerged from an earlier time, an era with far fewer older people and greatly differing social patterns and institutions. These outdated attitudes, and policies and systems that embed them, may impede the ability to embrace both the challenges and the opportunities of population aging in the twenty-first century. Today's older adults are in a sense reinventing the experience of aging, negotiating new later-life models in active construction and pursuit of meaningful occupations. The times cry for a cadre of OT personnel to specialize in gerontology, to use the wisdom and skills of the discipline to join in this effort to reinvent old age by identifying, supporting, and cocreating meaningful occupations in later life. Are you up to this challenge?

### Occupational Possibilities

Occupational possibilities, "the ways and types of doing that come to be viewed as ideal and possible within a specific sociohistorical context, and that come to be promoted and made available within environments" (Laliberte Rudman, 2005, 2006), would seem especially relevant to understanding and supporting optimal late life as it is defined and experienced in contemporary times. Occupational possibilities represent shared, taken-for-granted notions of what people think they can, should, and are inspired to do, notions that also become embedded in systems and structures that support what people have opportunities to do. This is precisely what today's cohort of older adults is in the throes of negotiating—occupational possibilities appropriate for a stage of life that, for the masses, is new and relatively uncharted. Because they are yet to be fully and clearly articulated, the occupational possibilities of late life remain nebulous and thus somewhat elusive, to be determined both on an individual and a collective basis. The emergent nature of late-life occupational possibilities represents an aspect of the sociocultural and political environment that, depending on the resources of the individual or associated reference group, may offer an exhilarating opportunity for creative life design or a terrifying encounter with the existential void and precarity. Assisting older individuals or groups of older adults to realize appropriate occupational possibilities in later life is the privilege and challenge of contemporary occupational therapists and OT assistants (OTAs) working with older populations.

### The Evolution of Aging as an Occupational Science and Occupational Therapy Practice Frontier

The definition of aging that guides the conception of this book represents a synthesis of current thought in gerontology, occupational science, and OT: Aging is an ongoing biopsychosocial process that is interactive, situated, and negotiated within specific sociocultural, temporal, and physical contexts (AOTA, 2020; Perkinson & Solimeo, 2014), requiring transdisciplinary approaches to both research and practice.

Predicated on the expansive body of evidence being generated within occupational science and other disciplinary spaces regarding sociopolitical determinants of health, well-being, and occupation (Laliberte Rudman et al., 2022; World Health Organization, 2021), this second edition continues and expands upon the stance of the first edition, to enlarge the vision for the field beyond medical and other health-care settings. This expansion is vital not only to aging populations but also to all generations. As you read this book, you will encounter recent understandings of optimal aging that encompass much more than the absence of or coping with medical conditions.

This edition contributes to the continuing evolution of gerontological occupational thought, recognizing the dynamic nature of aging itself, as well as the impact of micro-, meso-, and macro-level contextual changes across time. In the United States, the body of knowledge established through occupational research and practice began in 1917, with the founding of the National Society for the Promotion of Occupational Therapy in the United States (Barton, 1920; Peloquin, 1991) following World War I. The fledgling profession focused on younger age groups, without identifying the unique needs of aging adults until Naida Ackley's (1962) and Lela Llorens' (1970) lifespan-oriented Slagle lectures at American Occupational Therapy annual conferences. During the more than 50 years since their inspiration, scholars and practitioners in gerontological OT, including the authors showcased in this book, continue to further develop the field across various national contexts to prepare future practitioners, refine practice models, conduct research, and engage with various partners (i.e., interprofessional colleagues, governmental agencies, older adult advocacy groups, businesses, and communities). The goal of this ever-evolving field is to optimize the occupational participation of older adults, working with them to address individual, group, societal, and environmental factors essential to their well-being (Aiken, 1997; Barney, 1991a, 1991b, 2006, 2012; Borell, 2008; Horowitz et al., 2014; Stanley & Cheek, 2003; Turcotte et al., 2018).

### Occupational Therapy's Unique Niche in Serving and Supporting Older Adults

Occupation comprises every moment in our lives. It is central in how we individually utilize our time every day and night, and for how we participate in our families, communities, and societies. Daily occupations alter extensively from infancy through childhood to adulthood, based upon developmental needs, psycho-emotional status, self-concept and self-esteem, social roles, societal expectations and norms, available resources, and many other intersecting factors. Regardless of our circumstances, humans strive to find meaning in everyday life via a wide variety of avenues: the occupations in which we participate individually or with family or friends, events and places with special significance, cultural influences in our lives, spirituality experiences, and applying creativity uniquely to whatever we do (Hasselkus & Dickie, 2021). Occupations, or the lack thereof, are therefore driving forces that frame our participation and identity as we develop during childhood through adulthood and are key to establishing and maintaining the social fabric of our communities (Kantartzis, 2017). Moreover, meaningful occupations are central to maintaining health-related quality of life across the life course (Barney & Perkinson, 2016).

Aging adults may experience different occupational transitions as they traverse the decades, depending upon their life choices, possibilities, positionalities, changes in health, motivation, and contexts. As one example, while many older adults in Western contexts may experience transitions into retirement, when and how this transition occurs will vary according to social policies, work sectors, family situations, financial resources, gender, personal preferences, and many other factors. As well, some older adults may need to, or choose to, engage in an extended work life (Jonsson et al., 2000; Laliberte Rudman, 2013). As another example, many occupational transitions occur from middle age onward related to family relations, such as those related to widowhood, separation, or divorce or departure or reintroduction of adult children into a family home. Such transitions present opportunities and challenges, and occupation can be central in the successful negotiation of these life events (Howie & Feldman, 2004; Jonsson et al., 2000; McIntyre & Howie, 2002). For another example, see Case Study 1.1.

It is also important to think about the centrality of occupation, and the potential role of OT, in relation to adaptations that may be necessitated by lifestyle and age-related changes, particularly when such changes alter occupational choices, performance, and possibilities. For example, OT personnel may work with patients/clients who have resided in the same home environment for years, within which they transitioned from earlier family and work roles and adapted established routines and habits in ways that enable flourishing for decades. However, faced with health challenges and other age-related changes, such patients/clients may need to prioritize their occupational choices, perhaps eliminating those on which they spend little or no time, and may need to alter how and when they do occupations. They may also need to simplify their habits and routines, which likely take longer amounts of time if they experience changes in their overall health status, mentation, and/or changes in mobility. The OT role can also encompass working with older adults, as individuals and as collectives/groups, whose lives and occupations are affected by larger forces, such as climate change, wars, or forced migration, given that such changes can lead to restrictions in occupational possibilities and necessitate occupational adaptation (Huot et al., 2016; Ung et al., 2020).

OT is a discipline that works on numerous levels to enable optimal occupational possibilities and participation, spanning macro to micro levels. Diverse environmental aspects, for example, air, water, and soil quality; physical environmental features such as lighting, flooring, ambient sound, room color choices, types of doors, corridors, and other configurations of space; and social attitudes and discourses about aging, may impact occupational possibilities and participation for older adults. In addition, such environmental aspects are in continuous transaction with meso-level features, such as family relations and access to local transportation options, and micro-level features, such as physical fitness levels and cognitive skills, in ways that also shape occupation. OT personnel consider such complex transactions when supporting older adults to maintain and adapt valued occupations. Promoting meaningful occupational choices and possibilities also occurs within a range of types of settings, such as intervening with older adults who are living and working in their own homes in the community, those who continue to be engaged in workplaces elsewhere, those accessing community-based services or residing in congregate living or skilled care facilities, to those who are receiving interventions in palliative and hospice services. Increasingly, OT staff are working

## CASE STUDY 1.1

One of the coeditors of this text thrives in a fully accessible environment; however, she has lost significant height due to aging-related spinal changes and despite regular workouts, a fitness bicycle under her desk (she uses it while she writes), and daily walks has lost degrees of upper and lower extremity, as well as systemic function (cardiopulmonary, balance, coordination, endurance, grip and pinch strength, proprioception, range of motion, tactile sensation, and overall strength). She thus finds kitchen and strenuous tasks much more challenging. However, an improvement in her vision occurred following bilateral cataract surgery, enabling better vision than she has ever before experienced in her lifetime. She is also fortunate to be married to a spouse who has always contributed creative culinary talents and greatly benefits from these interests and expanded support. Thus, as an aging couple, they have experienced somewhat of a role reversal compared to their early married years when she did most of the cooking for a household of seven. She continues to manage laundry, plant care, and some in-store shopping but is fortunate to have a younger woman do regular household cleaning, one of her least favorite occupations. Since she has always loved technology, despite some challenges with personal computer changes over the more than 40 years since they were introduced, she finds publishing, online shopping, and use of state-of-the-art cell phones to be invaluable occupations. Fortunately, her passion for contributing to the profession has not been impacted! She likes to think that sharing her experiences will additionally prepare OT personnel for the varied conditions that aging adults experience and facilitate their ability to collaboratively empower individuals to adapt and maintain functional capacity to the best of their ability so that they engage in desired occupations, despite their biological system changes.

in communities and institutions with older adults who have experienced, and may continue to experience, various forms of marginalization and inequity, such as intersecting forms of discrimination tied to age, disability, ethnic, gender, racial and other social markers of difference; homelessness; immigration; incarceration; or veteran status. Chapter 33 expands upon topics related to meeting the occupational needs of individuals in marginalized groups, and other emerging areas of practice with aging adults.

In addition to a primary focus on occupation, this book contends that OT approaches with older adults are ideally person centered and based on relational practice (Restall & Egan, 2022). This means that OT staff optimally work with older adults using collaborative approaches, acknowledging that older adults have lived expertise regarding their occupations and a lifetime of experiences to draw upon in negotiating challenges to their occupational participation. This also means that they are committed to understanding older adults' perspectives and consciously work against making ageist assumptions regarding what older adults need, want, and can do (Mondaca et al., 2018; Turcotte et al., 2019; Trentham, 2019).

## The Second Edition—What's New and Different

The first edition editorial team, Drs. Frank Barney and Perkinson, welcomed an esteemed colleague and scholar in occupational science, Dr. Debbie Laliberte Rudman, in cocreating this second edition. She not only brings a critical lens to understanding aging and occupation but also increases the breadth and depth of global topics covered. Readership, queries, and translation of the first edition represented many parts of the world, prompting reflection on and expansion of relevant global and futuristic content in the second edition.

As with the first edition, chapters have integrated diverse interprofessional authors from various geographic contexts, which we consider to be a significant strength. Drs. Frank Barney (an occupational therapist health services researcher) and Perkinson (a medical anthropologist) have always thought that the textbook should be informed by the disciplines and scholars with whom occupational therapists (OTs) and OTAs work and/or have influence. Thus, in addition to OT and occupational science scholars, practicing OTs, and an OTA program director (former OTA), contributing authors span many professions and areas of expertise, such as law, ethics, epidemiology, library science, measurement, public health, physical therapy, geriatric medicine, geriatric psychiatry, nursing, ophthalmology, otolaryngology, speech and hearing, critical disability studies, nutrition science, oral health, pharmacology, neuroscience, social work, spirituality, geography, social gerontology, assistive technology, transportation, humanities and the arts, health-care administration, anthropology, and sociology. Geographically, authors represent many locations beyond North America, including Australia, Central and South America, China, Ghana, India, Ireland, New Zealand, Scotland, Sweden, and South Africa. Finally, two of the book's authors were included in

the American Occupational Therapy Association designation of the 100 most influential US OTs during the first hundred years of the discipline: Dr. Kathlyn Reed and Dr. Virginia Stoffel.

As an editorial trio, we've been very deliberate in spanning the range of topics and foundational knowledge that inform gerontological OT. For example, fundamental content related to physiological and psychological aspects of aging has been retained and updated, including current evidence on prevention of functional decline. Gaps have been addressed and new content added; as examples, hearing impairment was added to the chapter on age-related vision changes; food insecurity was added to the nutrition chapter; the limits of the dominant successful aging paradigm were more fully addressed; and more examples related to social transformation have been added. Moreover, the chapter on the family was expanded to include friends, informal supports, and social contexts; and the chapter on long-term care now offers more in-depth coverage of skilled care facilities, assisted living, and continuing care communities. New chapters cover disability in later life, humanities and the arts, primary care, and age-inclusive communities. Throughout all chapters, authors have addressed current evidence-based information and future projections regarding the needs of aging adults individually and collectively, at home within their communities and countries and regions, identifying both long-term trends as well as more recent transformations.

## Intended Audience

Based on requests for translation and inquiries from scholars and practitioners from numerous countries regarding the first edition, we expanded the overall scope and content and believe that this textbook may serve as an important resource for a number of categories of potential users, as follows:

- Occupational science and OT entry-level and graduate programs.
- OTA programs—inclusive language regarding role delineation is used throughout this edition; Chapter 30, *Intraprofessional and Interprofessional Processes in Gerontological Care*, explicates role delineation within the profession and extensively with other professions.
- Occupational therapists and OTAs in medically or community-based programs or private practice who currently serve older adults, or those considering moving into a related area of practice.
- Consulting occupational therapists and OTAs who have their own businesses that relate to aging populations.
- Interprofessional programs whose staff can benefit from this interdisciplinary resource for serving older adults.
- Scholars and practitioners from other disciplines who aim to better understand the current scope of OT practice, informed by occupational science, and how greater collaboration may support common aims regarding research and services involving aging adults.
- Scholars and practitioners from other disciplines who seek a better understanding of the field of gerontology

and the application of its theory and findings to their own work.

- Lay consumers who seek a better understanding of the experience of aging for themselves and/or who seek guidance in the occupation of cocaring for frail relatives or friends.

## Organization and Preview

This edition is organized into six sections arranged by specific content areas. Competent, effective, and ethical practice requires combining knowledge and skills both from and across these sections, given the complexity of factors to be addressed in optimizing the occupational participation of older adults. Given this, relevant chapters are cited within particular chapters, referring readers to other chapters that elaborate on particular concepts, approaches, and issues as needed.

### Section I: Conceptual Foundations of Gerontological Occupational Therapy

Chapter 1, *Gerontological Occupational Therapy: Conceptual Frameworks and Historical Contexts*, written by the editors Drs. Perkinson, Frank Barney, and Laliberte Rudman, reviews the experience of aging and later life from a historical perspective and underscores the relevance of OT for modern day elders. It introduces main emphases within the book as a whole, such as the coverage of traditional to emerging conceptual practice frameworks and approaches, and provides an introduction to each of the chapters included in the book.

Chapter 2, *Ethical and Legal Aspects of Occupational Therapy Practice with Older Adults*, was written by two lawyers: Carol Needham, based in a university law school, and Lisa Luetkemeyer, based in a professional law firm; and three faculty occupational therapists who specialize in social and occupational justice and ethical issues in health care for older adults: Evelyne Durocher, Helene Lohman, and Keli Mu. This chapter provides a comprehensive review of both ethical values and principles and legal obligations and protections pertinent to practice with elders. In step with current emphases on home and community-based practice, updated material in this chapter considers issues of patient/client safety beyond hospital settings, covering outpatient care, including ethical and legal issues surrounding health information technology.

Since health status and quality of life are central constructs in providing OT services, Chapter 3, *The Epidemiology of Health Status and Quality of Life Among Older Adults: Implications for Occupational Therapy*, written by two epidemiology scholars, Erin Bouldin and M. Bradley Cannell, and occupational therapist health services researcher Karen Frank Barney, covers a global view of determinants of health and disease, related measurements, constructs, data sources, trends that impact disability, health, and quality of life through the life course, as well as evidence-based public health prevention strategies. This foundation information provides historical and varied contextual information regarding health-related quality of life and related OT interventions.

Chapter 4, *Social Theories of Aging Relevant to Occupational Therapy*, written by two scholars in occupational science, Clare Hocking and Debbie Laliberte Rudman, provides an overview of social gerontological theories that have informed OT research and scholarship. This chapter also points to the potential contributions of critical gerontological theories, particularly for informing and expanding scholarship and practice in OT and occupational science. As a profession, we need to consider these conceptualizations, which expand our thinking beyond biomedical model interventions that are important wherever indicated, but limit our profession's views of highly relevant yet unmet occupational needs of aging adults.

An administrative university librarian, Donghua Tao, and Kathlyn Reed, an internationally recognized OT leader, contributed the comprehensive evidence-based practice, Chapter 5, *Foundations of Evidence-Based Gerontological Occupational Therapy Practice*, that will be an asset to not only practicing OTs but also researchers in any field of study. It includes a rationale for and extensive discussion of models of evidence-based practice, search and selection criteria for locating evidence-based literature in databases, guidance on critiquing and conceptually applying evidence-based literature, discussion of challenges and strategies for implementing evidence-based literature into practice, and resources for improving evidence-based practice including future application and trends.

Written by two occupational therapists specializing in geriatrics, interventions, and translational science, Jane Bear-Lehman and Tracy Chippendale, and a public health anthropologist who authored a textbook on research methods, Steven Albert, Chapter 6, *Approaches to Screening and Assessment in Gerontological Occupational Therapy*, reviews foundational approaches to screening and assessments when working with older adults. This chapter provides standards and criteria for selecting assessment tools best suited to determine quality and performance improvement within a client-centered care model.

Chapter 7, *Occupational Therapy Intervention Process with Aging Adults*, has been expanded and is authored by four OT faculty scholar practitioners, Stacy West-Bruce, Stacey Schepens Niemiec, Jenny Martinez, and Catherine Lysack, who represent diverse perspectives experientially, geographically, racially, and ethnically. They provide a comprehensive explanation of evidence-based therapeutic approaches with aging populations, including differing racial, ethnic, and gender identity groups to provide a thorough foundation for basic interventions that can be adapted, as indicated.

### Section II: Age-Related Biological System Changes and Gerontological Occupational Therapy

Chapter 8, *Musculoskeletal System Changes with Aging: Implications for Occupational Therapy*, written by OT faculty scholars Julia Henderson-Kalb, Emily Barr and Raegan Muller, a physical therapy rehabilitation director, details the implications of aging-related changes in the musculoskeletal system. This chapter addresses many aging-related changes and associated conditions that impact occupational performance and limit occupational choices, as well as intervention rationales and processes.

Angela Sanford, a geriatrician faculty scholar, and two OT faculty scholars, Laura VanPuymbrook and Carole Schwartz, wrote Chapter 9, *Physiological and Neurological System Changes with Aging and Related Occupational Therapy Interventions*, which focuses on aging-related changes, including associated cardiac, circulatory, pulmonary, and central and peripheral nervous system conditions. Understanding these changes can facilitate communication with patients/clients regarding the importance of regular medical care and adherence to physician's guidance, as well as how OT practitioners collaborate to intervene to promote optimal quality of life, despite system changes and limitations.

Chapter 10, *Occupational Therapy Interventions with Older Adults with Low Vision and/or Hearing Impairment*, is written by two private OT practitioners, Margaret Newsham Beckley and Mary Geders Falcetti, and a university clinical instructor, audiologist coordinator, Maureen M. Fischer. It covers typical and pathological changes in vision and hearing that occur with aging and provides extensive detail regarding vision and hearing therapeutic interventions. Aging adults may experience diminished capacity in one or both functional areas, affecting their motivation and ability to participate meaningfully with individuals or groups, or to participate in a wide variety of desired and meaningful occupations. When access to care is available, OT staff work with the individual, who may be reluctant to admit (or may be unaware of) their sensory changes, especially hearing limitations, but may be convinced of the merit of interprofessional intervention, with a therapeutic person-centered approach.

Chapter 11, *Disability in Later Life*, represents a new addition to the book. Its authors include two medical anthropologists, Pamela Block and Devva Kasnitz, and two occupational therapists, Denise Nepveux and Alexandra Wagner, all scholars and activists in critical disability studies. Approaching disability as a social construct, the authors review theories of disability as they relate to aging and use case studies based on ethnographic methods to explore issues of interdependence, supported autonomy, access, pride, community participation, and justice. Comparing and contrasting resources, barriers, acquired skills, and attitudes of those "aging with disability" (i.e., with life-long disabilities) to persons "aging into disability" (i.e., with disability newly acquired in later life), the authors suggest how those new to the disability experience might learn coping strategies from their more experienced peers (e.g., skills for navigating systems and situations; embracing a sense of disability rights) to achieve a resilient adaptation.

Chapter 12, *Nutrition, Food Insecurity, and Occupational Performance*, was written by a licensed dietician and national food and nutrition consultant, Connie Diekman, and an OT program director, Julia Henderson-Kalb. The chapter provides extensive coverage of age-related nutritional requirements, malnutrition, food and drug interactions, special diets for older adults with chronic conditions (e.g., diabetes), adaptive devices and therapeutic approaches to assist self-feeding and food preparation, cultural and personal meanings of food and meals, nutrition in long-term care settings and at the end of life, and social justice issues regarding food insecurity, including concerns regarding availability and access to healthy food sources.

Oral health in traditional OT practice is often limited to assessing and supporting functional toothbrushing; however, its importance extends far beyond that basic activity of daily living (BADL), impacting prevention of numerous health conditions. Chapter 13, *Oral Health for Aging Adults*, was written by an occupational therapist specializing in minority health research, Shirley Ann Blanchard, and by Jean Schensul, a medical and applied anthropologist, whose most recent research focuses on oral health outcomes in ethnically diverse and lower-income older adults. The chapter covers social determinants of oral health, including oral health disparities; age-related changes in oral physiology; medical conditions with oral health consequences; OT assessments and screening tools for oral health; oral care products and assistive technology; oral health in long-term care and at end of life; and an array of online resources.

Chapter 14, *Pharmacology, Pharmacy, and the Aging Adult: Implications for Occupational Therapy*, cowritten by Hedva Behrenolz Levy, a national leader in pharmacology, and Karen Frank Barney, is included as an extensive resource to assist OT personnel in understanding common medications that many aging adults use, including precautions; daily, weekly, and/or monthly protocol; contraindications; and the importance of close attention to communication regarding medication management directed by physicians and often assisted by pharmacists and OT personnel. Organization and timing of medications can be paramount to survival; thus, this chapter provides foundational information that will promote effective guidance for use and support by OT staff.

## Section III: Age-Related Psychosocial Changes and Gerontological Occupational Therapy

Written by a senior scholar who is an experimental geropsychologist with expertise in neuroscience, OT, and functional cognition, Dorothy Farrar Edwards, and by an occupational therapist scholar who also specializes in functional cognition, Kristen Kehl-Floberg, Chapter 15, *Neurology and Cognition in Aging and Everyday Life*, provides a comprehensive review of age-related neurological and cognitive changes in later life and the impact of those changes on complex life activities. Age-related changes to executive function, memory, and sensory-perceptual abilities are summarized, and skilled OT support strategies are provided and evaluated. The authors note the superiority of performance-based measures of executive function compared to traditional neuropsychological assessments to accurately estimate functional performance.

Chapter 16, *Cognitive Impairment, Dementia, and Occupational Therapy Interventions*, written by Ganesh Babulal, and another occupational therapist who specializes in dementia care and technology, Lili Liu, reviews the state of current knowledge in this rapidly evolving field from the perspective of a dementia specialist in both OT and health science. The chapter distinguishes between normal (nonpathological) age-related cognitive changes and cognitive impairment and reviews the different types of dementia, their prevalence rates, and clinical stages. Guidelines for dementia screening and assessment are explicated, including the more recent use of biomarkers for detection of preclinical dementia. Various interventions are discussed in depth, as well as advanced technology as it relates to dementia and eldercare.

A former national AOTA president, Virginia Stoffel, scholar/practitioner, collaborated with two OT scholars, Lauren Selingo, who specializes in mental health OT in the United States, and Michelle Perryman Fox, in Scotland, and George Grossberg, Director of Geriatric Psychiatry, in writing Chapter 17, *When Aging Adults Live with Mental Health Challenges: Barriers and Facilitators to Meaningful Occupational Engagement*. This content focuses on the varied needs of older adults with ongoing or recently diagnosed mental health conditions and related medications and functional support needs that OT personnel address to support these individuals. They stress the importance of sensitive approaches to address the often complex needs of these individuals, some of whom have been diagnosed for many years.

Chapter 18, *Spirituality and Resilience in Later Life*, written by a team of social gerontologists, Lydia Manning, Lauren Michele Bouchard, and Julia Buschbacher, and a South African occupational therapist, Thuli Mtembu, examines basic definitions and connections between spirituality and resilience. Models of integration, such as the Kawa Model, the Canadian Model of Occupational Performance and Engagement, Moody's Five Stages of the Soul, and the African concept *Ubuntu*, are reviewed as they relate to spirituality and adaptation to adversity. The connection of occupational justice to spirituality and resilience and strategies for integrating spirituality into occupational interventions are considered.

Chapter 19, entitled *Diverse Understandings of Successful Aging*, brings together two OT scholars, Debbie Laliberte Rudman and Selena E. Washington, and an anthropologist, Sarah Lamb, to outline and critically assess key characteristics of the dominant paradigm of "successful aging" that permeates many aspects of North American Society. The authors point to the importance of expanding thinking about "aging well" to ensure the relevance of OT practice with diverse older adults, providing examples of models and practices grounded in various contexts.

## Section IV: The Functional Environment of Aging Adults and Gerontological Occupational Therapy

Chapter 20, *The Physical Environment and Aging*, written by two social geographers/environmental gerontologists, Graham D. Rowles and Malcolm Cutchin, a medical anthropologist, Margaret A. Perkinson, and an occupational therapist health services researcher, Karen Frank Barney, provides updated research and practical applications to support OT personnel's understanding of the environmental barriers that aging adults may encounter, as well as ways to facilitate occupational performance at home and in the community.

A review of theories regarding the relationship of persons to their physical environments includes recent perspectives on the transactional nature of aging adults' "being in place," focusing on the situational aspects of place integration and care. Discussion of relocation in later life considers the process of making and remaking a sense of home and the role that lifelong possessions play in this process. A future agenda for a physical environment-sensitive occupational science acknowledges the impact of emerging smart home technologies in enabling occupations and the need for additional research on processes of place integration among populations of diverse ethnicities, cultural orientations, and national origins.

Chapter 21, *Driving and Transportation*, was written by two occupational therapists who specialize in driving and community mobility, Ganesh Babulal and Anne Dickerson. It provides an overview of client factors and common conditions that impact driving fitness, as well as guidelines for addressing the instrumental activities of daily living (IADLs) of driving and community mobility with older adults. Screening tools to determine levels of crash risk and general driving evaluations, including driving performance tests, are reviewed to determine the value of each in evaluating fitness to drive. Driving rehabilitation programs and alternate driving services are reviewed. New technologies to support driving behavior and improve safety are considered. Relinquishing one's driver's license in later life can be viewed as a major loss of independence; thus, plans for a nondriving future are also considered.

Chapter 22, *Assistive Technology: Supports for Aging Adults*, covers current state-of-the-art scientific knowledge on both high- and low-tech devices to assist with BADLs and IADLs, in addition to the "Fourth Wave" of technology and aging that focuses on older adults' *wants*, rather than simply needs. The chapter authors, geropsychologist David Burdick, and occupational therapist Kimberley Furphy, offer a conceptual framework of themes and issues to guide selection of client-centered technologies. New additions to the second edition focus on higher technological innovations, i.e., virtual reality, robotics, smart homes, artificial intelligence (AI), computer assistive technology, telehealth, and telemedicine, as they address the needs of aging adults. The authors also address issues of social justice in access and use of technology by aging adults.

Chapter 23, *Families, Friends, and Social Context in Later Life*, written by medical anthropologist Margaret A. Perkinson, and occupational therapist health services researcher Karen Frank Barney, explores the nature of interpersonal interactions among aging adults. Relationships between children and their parents change over time, especially as the younger generation reaches adulthood, and vary on an individual basis, from distant independence to total dependence, subject to personalities, relationships, ability to be functionally independent, financial status, and cultural norms. This chapter covers the dynamics of intergenerational relationships, the impact of genetic testing on discovering family members in later years, the evolution of friendships over time within individual and social group relationships, and dynamics of social and historical factors (e.g., migration) on family structure and relationships.

The authors of Chapter 24, *Arts, Humanities, and Occupational Therapy with Older People: An Aesthetic Lens on Practice*, note growing recognition of the positive impact of the arts and humanities on the health and well-being of aging adults and the challenges posed by aesthetic deprivation. Medical humanities geriatrician Desmond O'Neill and faculty occupational therapist Susan Coppola review community programs and performing arts interventions for aging adults across the spectrum of functional ability. By embedding aesthetics into everyday occupations, occupational therapists can incorporate arts and humanities into their practice, not only supporting clients' past or present arts-related occupations, but also using the arts to contribute to the immediate sensory environment with music, visual arts, and aromatherapy. Everyday activities may be "infused with meaning" through aesthetic choices, e.g., the selection of clothes, presentation of food in meal preparation, and home decor.

## Section V: Continuum of Care and Gerontological Occupational Therapy

Chapter 25, *Health-Care Systems and Services Overview*, written by two OT health services researchers, Beth Fields and Karen Frank Barney, and Miriam Rodin, a geriatrician and social anthropologist, provides international comparisons of health-care systems. Readers should be aware that the health-care systems within which OT staff operate may support or limit the amount of time spent with patients/clients, and that systems vary widely in their design from one country to another regarding organization, administration, policies, and reimbursable coverage for care, resources, outcomes, and guiding societal values. For example, some countries support access to health care as a basic right, while others, such as the United States, operate on a very different basis, limiting access based on medical insurance coverage or ability to pay out of pocket.

Chapter 26, *The Role of Occupational Therapy in Primary Care*, attends to existing approaches and strategies used by occupational therapists in primary care and points to priorities for research and role expansion. Written by Canadian and American OT researchers whose scholarship has had a focus on primary care, Carri Hand, Catherine Donnelly, Lori Letts, and Sue-Dahl Popolizio, this chapter addresses the key elements of primary care and emphasizes the role of occupational therapists in facilitating occupational participation and engagement within its key practice areas.

Chapter 27, *The Role of Occupational Therapy in Acute and Post-Acute Care with Aging Adults*, was written by acute care OT practitioner Autumn Gobble Rebillot, geriatrician Julie Gammack, and geriatric fellow Michael Sarai. After defining acute care, i.e., hospital inpatient medical services for short-term illnesses, and post-acute care, i.e., rehabilitation and medical care following acute care hospitalization, the chapter provides comprehensive information on interprofessional and OT-specific interventions for hospitalized, critically ill older adults, as well as both levels of care regarding infection prevention, maintaining functional status, and prevention of readmission. Once stabilized, older adults may be discharged to a post-acute care facility, a rehabilitation hospital, a skilled nursing facility, home health care, or to home without support services, based upon their medical status and level of independence.

Chapter 28, *Residential and Skilled Care*, includes scholars from health-care administration, Michael Lepore and David D. Rockemann, medical anthropology, Margaret A. Perkinson, sociology, Molly M. Perkins, and an Australian OT researcher and practitioner, Sanetta Du Toit. The chapter provides an overview of nursing homes, assisted living, and continuing care retirement communities, emphasizing the role of OT personnel for each setting. The subjective experience of life in such settings, strategies to achieve optimal adjustment, and issues of social and occupational justice for both residents and staff also are considered.

Chapter 29, *Home: An Evolving Context for Health Care*, written by scholars in social gerontology, Laura N. Gitlin, and OT, Catherine Piersol, underscores a frequent preference of aging adults to receive care at home instead of an institution. The chapter reviews funding sources for home care services, scope of practice, conceptual models that guide home care practice, the benefits of using a problem-solving approach to care, cultural considerations in providing care, and the benefits and challenges of home care for clients, family members, and practitioners.

In contrast to institutional stays, aging adults who require care may recover and eventually thrive with home care in familiar environments, where habits and routines are undisturbed by the dictates of institutional settings. At home, they may receive supportive services and also enjoy their pets and neighbors, among other advantages.

## Section VI: Trends and Innovations in Care with Aging Adults

The final section of the book addresses trends within gerontological care as well as innovations that involve occupational therapists and OTAs addressing social transformation and creating age-inclusive communities. A key trend addressed in Chapter 30, *Intraprofessional and Interprofessional Processes in Gerontological Care*, is that OT staff typically work with providers from other disciplines within institutional and community-based care settings and various types of agencies. This chapter, written by Associate Dean for Research and Nursing Helen Lach, occupational therapist health services researcher Karen Frank Barney, and the Director of an OTA program, Cynthia Ballentine, includes the disciplines that provide optimal interprofessional medical or home-based care with aging adults. However, when OT personnel work with aging adults in established neighborhoods or who are unhoused or formerly incarcerated, they may need to learn about different client needs and systems of providers.

In an attempt to foster further innovation and expansion of approaches used by occupational therapists to support the occupational participation and expand occupational possibilities for diversely positioned older adults, Chapters 31,

*Occupational Therapists, Social Change, and Social Transformation through Occupation*, encourages readers to think beyond what might be thought of as typical practice approaches. This chapter, written by OT scholars and practitioners located in different geopolitical contexts, including Debbie Laliberte Rudman, Margarita Mondaca, Kathleen Brodrick, Karen Frank Barney, Lisa Jaegers, and Christine Hayes Picker, addresses the growing call for occupational therapists to be part of social transformations addressing occupational, health, and social inequities. In addition to outlining five central characteristics of evolving practice approaches related to social transformation through occupation, three examples of initiatives are provided.

Chapter 32, *Building Age Inclusive Communities*, also challenges readers to expand OT research and practice approaches, emphasizing the importance of working with older adults, attending to diverse social positions and their intersections, engaging in dynamic processes, and generating solutions that are contextually relevant. This chapter, cowritten by OT and occupational science scholars Debbie Laliberte Rudman, Sarah Kantartzis, Colleen McGrath, Jenny Womack, and Karen Frank Barney and medical anthropologist Margaret A. Perkinson, outlines two broad models that address contextual elements central in building age-inclusive communities. It also includes attention to concepts and processes that can inform OT practice aimed at contributing to age-inclusive communities, integrating several examples of initiatives.

The concluding Chapter 33, *The Future of Gerontological Occupational Therapy*, written by the editors, provides reflections and recommendations regarding the scholarly and practice paths to be taken forward. It both considers social issues of particular relevance to the occupational participation of older adults in contemporary contexts and points to the need for continuing development of OT theory, knowledge, and practice approaches, given the dynamic nature of aging processes and older adults and their varied local and global contexts.

*The complete listing of the Bibliography and Chapter Questions and Answers are available in the accompanying enhanced eBook version included with the print purchase of this textbook. Visit Elsevier eBooks+ (eBooks.Health.Elsevier.com) to access this content.*

## CHAPTER 2

# Ethical and Legal Aspects of Occupational Therapy Practice with Older Adults

*Carol A. Needham, JD, MA, Lisa Luetkemeyer, JD, MHS, CCC-SLP, Evelyne Durocher, PhD, OT Reg. (Ont.), Helene Lohman, OTD, OTR/L, FAOTA, and Keli Mu, PhD, OTR/L, FAOTA*

## CHAPTER OUTLINE

## OBJECTIVES

- Briefly review key ethical values and principles salient in practice with older adults.
- Discuss legal obligations of occupational therapy practice.
- Describe some potential errors and potentially appropriate responses to errors made.
- Explain aspects of professional liability.
- Discuss how to address fraud and abuse in occupational therapy practice.
- Consider contextual factors shaping professional practice.

Professionals draw on a variety of sources to guide their behavior both in and out of the workplace. Past experiences, personal values, legal requirements, professional codes of conduct, role mandates, and contextual factors are but some of the influences that can inform a clinician's professional practice. The implementation of a code of ethics can help to promote the well-being of clients and maintain the high standards of the profession.

## Ethical Values and Principles

To ensure that members of the occupational therapy (OT) profession maintain high standards of behavior and client care, professional organizations across the globe publish codes of ethics to guide their members' practice. Generally, these codes include consideration of ethical values and principles as well as guidance related to confidentiality, respect for client autonomy, and informed consent.

In the United States, the American Occupational Therapy Association (AOTA) publishes the *Occupational Therapy Code of Ethics* (AOTA, 2020a). Other professional associations or regulatory bodies such as the Royal College of Occupational Therapists in the United Kingdom (Royal College of Occupational Therapists, 2021), the Occupational Therapy Australia, (Occupational Therapy Australia, 2014), College of Occupational Therapists of Ontario, Canada (College of Occupational Therapists of Ontario, 2020) publish similar codes to which their respective registered practicing OT professionals are required to adhere. These publications guide professionals to make ethical choices when interacting with clients, families, caregivers, and co-workers.

Common across many codes of ethics are values and principles relevant to professional conduct in all areas of practice and with all stakeholders. Based on these values and principles, therapists apply mindful reflection to guide their actions (AOTA, 2020a). These values and principles include:
- Nonmaleficence
- Beneficence
- Autonomy
- Confidentiality
- Justice and fairness
- Veracity, honesty, and transparency
- Fidelity and accountability

### Nonmaleficence

Nonmaleficence is the bioethical principle guiding the "*intentional avoidance* of actions that cause harm" (emphasis in original; Beauchamp & Childress, 2019, p. 157) and "obligations not to impose *risks* of harm" (emphasis in original; Beauchamp & Childress, 2019, p. 159). The principle underlies the colloquial phrase "do no harm." To act with nonmaleficence, the therapist must have adequate knowledge of the client's diagnosis, needs, abilities, wishes, and circumstances, as well as of appropriate treatment protocols. The therapist must provide the appropriate standard of care and take precautions not to cause needless injury or harm, all of which may vary based on the client's circumstances and context. The AOTA standards include the policy that occupational therapists "avoid exploiting any relationship established as an occupational therapy clinician, educator, or researcher to further one's own physical, emotional, financial, political, or business interests at the expense of recipients of services, students, research participants, employees, or colleagues" (AOTA, 2020a). An example of a possible violation of nonmaleficence would be a therapist with little experience or knowledge of shoulder injuries and related therapeutic approaches providing intervention to an older adult client having a shoulder subluxation without seeking out information about correct intervention protocols or finding an appropriate mentor to provide guidance.

## Beneficence

Beneficence is at times considered an extension of nonmaleficence, guiding action not only to prevent harm but also aimed at benefiting and helping others, or promoting their well-being (Beauchamp & Childress, 2019; Doherty & Purtilo, 2016). Beneficence underlies a professional duty to act in the best interests of the client. According to the AOTA's *Code of Ethics and Ethics Standards*, examples of application of beneficence include demonstrating concern for the well-being of those receiving OT services through referral to other health-care professionals when appropriate and providing current assessment and intervention (AOTA, 2020a). Recognizing that acts to benefit others could potentially have other consequences or implications, the principle of utility in beneficence guides practitioners to "balance benefits, risks, and costs to produce the best overall results" (Beauchamp & Childress, 2019, p. 217). An example of the application of this principle to gerontological practice could be making an extra effort to locate reasonable community services for an older adult client with a low income, which may require additional work.

## Autonomy

Autonomy refers to self-determination or self-governance. While there is debate about nuances in definitions of autonomy, traditional conceptions of autonomy generally comprise two necessary conditions: (1) liberty, that the person (or group) be free from controlling influences, and (2) agency, that the individual have the capabilities required to realize their deliberate actions (Beauchamp & Childress, 2019). Feminist notions of relational autonomy differ somewhat from more traditional perspectives to focus on individuals as inextricably linked to their social and political contexts (Mackenzie & Stoljar, 2000; Sherwin, 1998). The implications of a broader focus from an OT perspective include the idea that individuals' capabilities would therefore have been, and continue to be, shaped by their life experiences and the opportunities

offered in their contexts, and that they make decisions in relation to aspects of such contexts (for example relationships) or potential consequences of certain actions. Such premises closely align with tenets of client-centered practice, which promote both respect for and partnerships with clients, thus highlighting recognition for clients' autonomy while also seeing clients as intrinsically linked to their contexts (Law et al., 1997). AOTA guidance states that practitioners should "establish a collaborative relationship with recipients of service and relevant stakeholders, to promote shared decision making" and should "fully disclose the benefits, risks, and potential outcomes of any intervention; the personnel who will be providing the intervention; and any reasonable alternatives to the proposed intervention" (AOTA, 2020a). Respect for autonomy guides therapists to engage with clients to collaboratively identify OT goals; to inform clients of all potential options and related risks, benefits, and reasonably foreseeable outcomes; and finally, to respect the client's right to accept or refuse services (informed consent and the client's right to refuse treatment are discussed later in this chapter).

## Confidentiality

Confidentiality is maintaining as private or not disclosing, clients' personal or medical information and also following state and federal privacy laws and regulations, such as the Health Insurance Portability and Accountability Act (HIPAA) of 1996 (Centers for Disease Control and Prevention, 2022) and the Health Information Technology for Economic and Clinical Health [HITECH] Act of 2009. Confidentiality also applies to students in educational programs, such as when doing research (AOTA, 2020a).

## Justice and Fairness

The concept of justice is largely focused on fair and equitable treatment and allocation of resources (Beauchamp & Childress, 2019; Doherty & Purtilo, 2016). Multiple conceptions of justice have been delineated (distributive, procedural, restorative to name but a few), each putting into focus a particular value or aspect of justice. Conceptions more salient to occupational therapists include distributive, social, and occupational justice. Distributive justice is focused on the fair and equitable distribution of goods, services, and benefits across individuals (Beauchamp & Childress, 2019; Doherty & Purtilo, 2016). Social justice brings to light social determinants of health and requires that access to health and health-related services be equitably accessible to all regardless of race, gender, sexual orientation, socioeconomic status or any other aspect of the person or social determinants (Powers & Faden, 2006). Concepts of occupational rights, justice, and injustice promote equitable access to opportunities for engagement in occupation and are based on proposed relationships between occupation and well-being (Durocher et al., 2014; Stadnyk et al., 2010). Advocating for services for and finding different ways to meet the needs of marginalized populations who for a multitude of reasons may not have equitable access to services is an example of working toward justice in OT practice.

Procedural justice dictates that professionals have ethical and professional duties to comply with the rules and policies of their employers, the laws of the state or province and country where they are employed, and professional standards of conduct outlined by the licensing or credentialing authorities or regulatory bodies (Beauchamp & Childress, 2019). Licensing is discussed later in this chapter.

## Veracity, Honesty, and Transparency

The ethical value of veracity "refers both to timely, accurate, objective and comprehensive transmission of information and to the way the professional fosters the patient's… understanding" (Beauchamp & Childress, 2019, p. 328). Veracity thus comprises not only the duty to provide timely, relevant, and adequate information but also taking steps to maximize client understanding. Veracity is closely linked to honesty and transparency, which promote communicating truthfully using a clear process (Beauchamp & Childress, 2019). Veracity, honesty, and transparency are pervasive in all aspects of OT practice. From the comprehensive provision of information to clients, families, and staff to documentation of client care, it is ethically and legally expected that health-care professionals provide accurate and complete information. Not only could incorrect information negatively affect client care in one isolated instance, but it could also undermine the reputation of OT in the public's eye because veracity is the basis of trust. An example of violation of this principle in gerontological practice would be not providing information about all possible options for intervention or services.

## Fidelity and Accountability

Fidelity relates to being faithful to one's commitments, such as commitments to one's role and clients as an occupational therapist in a particular context (Beauchamp & Childress, 2019; Doherty & Purtilo, 2016). Having a fiduciary obligation to clients suggests that therapists have a moral obligation to act for their clients' benefit (Beauchamp & Childress, 2019). Fidelity is closely linked to accountability, which is taking responsibility for and demonstrating follow-through related to one's actions and words (Doherty & Purtilo, 2016). Examples of acting with fidelity and accountability include treating service providers, clients, and others with respect, not abandoning clients, and avoiding conflicts of interest in practice or research.

## Legal Obligations

As professionals, therapists in gerontological practice, as well as all areas of practice, are expected to adhere to not only ethical standards but also legal standards as set forth by federal and state law. Many of these legal obligations codify the ethical standards. Legal duties discussed in this chapter are standards of care and duty of care, licensure, documentation, informed consent, and confidentiality.

## Standard of Care and Duty of Care

Although there is not a medical definition for *standard of care*, the term is commonly used in medical situations (Strauss &

Thomas, 2009). Generally, standard of care refers to a diagnostic and treatment process that a prudent health care provider ought to follow for a certain type of patient, illness or clinical circumstance (Vanderpool, 2021) or in legal terms "the degree of care that a reasonable person should exercise" (Garner, 2014). Thus, standard of care is the acceptable and appropriate care that an occupational therapist provides for a client's condition.

Occupational therapists apply standard of care in practice by utilizing, as much as possible, evidenced-based practice with intervention approaches and by having practice guided by the AOTA's *Occupational Therapy Practice Framework* (AOTA, 2020b) and the standards of practice for occupational therapy (AOTA, 2021a). In the United States, standard of care may be outlined by the state licensure board by which the professional is admitted to practice. For example, to maintain a license in Pennsylvania, occupational therapists must adhere to ethical principles and standards of professional conduct outlined in the state regulations in that state. These regulations require the therapist to maintain confidentiality of client information, respect the legal rights of the client, and perform only those functions for which the therapist is trained and competent. *Duty of care* is a term more commonly found in the United Kingdom and is clearly explained in the *Professional Standards of Care for Occupational Therapy Practice, Conduct and Ethics* published by the Royal College of Occupational Therapists (2021). It states that "the duty of care exists from the moment [the therapist]…receive[s] a referral…; and/or the individual is accepted for occupational therapy or they agree and begin to receive a service… [The therapist] discharges [the] duty of care by performing [the] professional duties to the standard of a reasonably competent practitioner, in terms of [their] knowledge, skills and abilities" (Royal College of Occupational Therapists, 2021). Furthermore, duty of care has been defined as "a moral or legal obligation to ensure the safety or well-being of others" (*Oxford English Dictionary*, 2022). Thus, duty of care involves an element of concern for safety. In this chapter, the terms *standard of care* and *duty of care* are both utilized.

## Licensure

In most states, occupational therapists are required to be licensed by a state board before practicing. State boards regulating OT are generally comprised of a combination of occupational therapists, occupational therapy assistants (OTAs), and members of the general public. Some state boards may also incorporate licensed professionals from other health professions, such as licensed physicians. The board members meet on a regular basis to vote on admission of new professionals, whether they are new graduates fresh out of school or seasoned professionals who seek licensure in a new state. In addition, the board serves as the disciplinary authority, determining whether rule infractions have been committed and doling out the appropriate sanctions. Although most states have a state OT board, in some states, licensure is managed under an advisory council, the state's medical board, or another state regulatory body or department (Jacobs & McCormack, 2011).

Requirement for licensure allows states to oversee the practice of health professionals to ensure the safety and well-being of state residents. Licensing of health-care professionals is regulated by state law and regulation, and accordingly, licensure requirements vary from state to state. State-specific requirements generally include graduation from an accredited OT program, passage of the National Board for Certification in Occupational Therapy (NBCOT) examination, completion of supervised fieldwork, and payment of fees. All 50 states in the U.S. require licensure to practice as an occupational therapist (AOTA, 2023a). In states which adopt OT compact legislation, licensed occupational therapists will have the opportunity to practice in other states that also adopt the OT compact statutory language without having to obtain a new license in each additional state (AOTA, 2023b).

The purpose of professional licensure is to regulate entry into the profession to ensure that licensees have obtained a minimum level of skill and training. In addition, the applicable state regulatory body determines the scope of practice for the profession; the level of supervision required for assistants, techs, aides, and students; the amount of annual continuing education required; and the level of discipline indicated for infractions.

Occupational therapists need to understand how to comply with legal and ethical duties in the supervision of occupational therapy assistants (OTAs). As discussed, supervision guidelines can come from state licensure boards or other entities. In gerontological practice, many OTAs work in skilled nursing facilities where they are supervised by occupational therapists. As a general rule, OTAs may not perform assessments or create or alter treatment plans. In addition, it is the occupational therapist's responsibility to ensure that the OTA is properly trained to implement the delegated tasks and appropriately supervised. Supervising therapists should always review all notes from the OTA before signing them. Remember that if an error is made, the supervising therapist's license is on the line as well as the assistant's. Taking a few extra minutes to thoroughly review documentation is well worth the time and effort. By signing an assistant's notes, the therapist is asserting that the notes are truthful, accurate, and appropriate. Doing so without proper review can endanger both the client's health and the therapist's licensure.

## Documentation

Documentation involves legal and ethical obligations and is a means of communicating information to other professionals on the care team. Although face-to-face communications play an integral role in relaying information to nursing staff and physicians, documentation in the patient chart provides a lasting record. Documentation allows medical and nursing staff who may not be present to speak with the therapist the opportunity to review patient performance and progress at any time (AOTA, 2018). Thorough documentation provides vital information to the care team regarding pain management, patient functioning, and progress (AOTA, 2018; AOTA, 2022).

In addition to providing a means of communication among members of the treatment team, patient documents also serve as a legal record of patient care. Should an investigation be conducted pursuant to a lawsuit or a complaint lodged with a payor such as Medicare or a private insurer, documentation may be accessed and examined. Providing potentially fraudulent documentation may trigger a focused Medicare review (Centers for Medicare and Medicaid Services, 2020) and relates to the ethical standards of procedural justice and veracity (AOTA, 2020a). Documentation needs to be truthful and compliant with regulations and workplace policies and procedures. Therefore, all health-care providers should make an effort to ensure that documentation is clear, timely, and accurate.

Documentation standards are a product of statute, licensure regulations, facility standards, payor mandates, and professional association guidelines. The AOTA requirements, as outlined in Guidelines for Documentation of Occupational Therapy (AOTA, 2018), include documenting in a professional and legal fashion such that the contents are "complete, concise, accurate, timely, legible, clear, grammatically correct, [and] objective" (AOTA, 2018, p.2). Medicare regulations provide specific information regarding guidelines that should be reflected in documentation to justify reimbursement, such as that intervention is of a reasonable time frame and amount and appropriate for the client's condition (Centers for Medicare and Medicaid Services, 2020). In most practice arenas with older adults, payors outline specific requirements for intervention and documentation. Therapy should reflect skilled service and, as such, requires a high level of interpretation and analysis of client performance and progress. This should be reflected in the notes. In current practice, most documentation is entered into an electronic health record. Although in an electronic format, such documentation should comply with the same basic guidelines as those for written documentation (Box 2.1).

Careful and thoughtful documentation serves to protect the client, provider, and facility. The client benefits because documentation reflects provided intervention and client progress. Documentation should demonstrate consideration for client welfare through a client-centered focus. Documentation can provide justification for continuity of care. The providers benefit because documentation demonstrates evidence of an appropriate standard of care, includes the client's informed consent, and should demonstrate completion of a client-centered plan. If documentation is thorough and appropriate, it can help the professional refute charges of negligence in client care. The facility benefits because client documentation can provide a source of information for quality measurement and support for reimbursement.

## Informed Consent

All health-care professionals have the ethical and legal obligation of obtaining informed consent from their clients whether in a medical or a community setting. As stated in Principle 3 of the AOTA *Occupational Therapy Code of Ethics*, "persons have the right to make a determination regarding care decisions that directly affect their lives. In the event that a person lacks decision-making capacity, their autonomy should be respected through involvement of an authorized agent or surrogate decision maker" (AOTA, 2020a).

---

**BOX 2.1**   General Guidelines for Documentation

1. Because the patient chart is also a legal document, the therapist should carefully, accurately, and specifically record evaluations, assessments, and notes.
2. Avoid generalities with documentation. For example, if a client refuses to complete a task, the therapist should avoid simply documenting that "the client was noncompliant." Instead, note that the "client refused to complete dressing activity" or whatever task was asked of the client.
3. To maintain objectivity, document the client's own words, rather than general descriptions, if the client reports discomfort or any other concern. Instead of stating that the "client was tired," the therapist could document that the "client said she was sleepy because she did not take a nap."
4. The therapy record should contain documentation of the care provided, the client's response—including refusal to participate or noncompliance (see discussions of both later in this chapter)—and changes in medical condition.
5. Document any relevant discussions about the client made to family, caregivers, or staff as well as any teaching or education provided, whether over the phone or in person.
6. To justify reimbursement or continued authorization to treat, show clinical judgment and a plan in all documentation and avoid solely documenting observations.
7. Be objective and only include information relevant to the health and treatment of the client. Do not use ambiguous terminology (e.g., "client performed poorly"). Be specific.
8. Maintain professionalism in the chart. Do not document arguments or disagreements with other health professionals.
9. Never chart a verbal order unless one was received.
10. Only document care personally provided or observed physical findings.
11. Do not sign notes as a supervisor unless they have been reviewed for accuracy and appropriateness.
12. Do not backdate notes or alter a record. This may be considered fraudulent. If information from a prior session was accidentally omitted, document the information in a new note with the current date and write "late entry."
13. When documenting electronically, change the system password regularly and do not share it. Position the computer screen away from others and don't forget to log out.

From HPSO Risk Advisor. (2007). Document defensively: Here's how. *HPSO Risk Advisor.* Retrieved from http://www.hpso.com/pdfs/newsletters/2007/HPSO07_All.pdf; and Sames, K. M. (2005). *Documenting occupational therapy practice.* Pearson/Prentice Hall.

---

Informed consent shows respect for the client's autonomy by allowing the client to be the master of his or her own course of intervention and provides control in what the client may experience as an upsetting, out-of-control situation. Obtaining informed consent is one means to approach intervention as client-centered and in an ethical manner.

A major consideration when obtaining consent is the client's health literacy, which is the ability of the client to comprehend information provided about a specific medical procedure, condition, or intervention. Advanced age has been found to be one of the factors most highly correlated with low health literacy. (Kobayashi et.al., 2016, as cited in National Academies, 2018). In 2003, the National Assessment of Adult Literacy revealed that between 10% and 13% of all individuals between the ages of 16 and 64 have problems accessing, reading, understanding, and using health-care information (U.S. Department of Education, Institute of Education Sciences, & National Center for Education Statistics, 2003). In contrast, 29% of adults aged 65 and over demonstrate below-basic health literacy skills (U.S. Department of Education, Institute of Education Sciences, & National Center for Education Statistics, 2003). A 2007 study revealed that older adults with inadequate health literacy were more likely to die in the next 6 years than those with adequate health literacy (Baker et al., 2007).

Factors that influence health literacy include socioeconomic status, education level, cognition, and overall health. To ensure that older adults are empowered to truly make informed decisions about their course of intervention and therapy goals, occupational therapists must either informally assess their client's health literacy level through a thorough client history, chart review, and interview or by consulting other professionals on the care team, such as the speech-language pathologist or social worker. Then, client education should be tailored to that specific client's needs.

Because many adults encountered in gerontological practice settings may exhibit some sort of cognitive impairment, therapists must also consider cognition as a complicating factor of informed consent. Knowing that a person has a diagnosis of Alzheimer's disease does not provide enough information to determine whether he or she has the cognitive capacity to provide consent. It is important to critically consider the person's stage of dementia (Buckles et al., 2003) and the individual's "social and situational" context (Cole, n.d.). Buckles and colleagues examined the subjects' understanding of informed consent across the range of dementia from very mild to moderate. They found that subjects in the very mild to mild categories understood informed consent with a minimal-risk protocol. However, for subjects with moderate dementia, they suggested including a caregiver in the consent process.

Completing a simple interview may not provide enough information to determine whether a person with Alzheimer's disease has the cognitive capacity to provide informed consent. Cole suggested that to make an opinion about the person's capabilities, practitioners should consider doing a formal assessment of decision-making skills (e.g., the MacArthur Competence Assessment Tool for Clinical Research Version [MacCAT-CR]) and consider the individual aspects of the person's situation (Appelbaum & Grisso, 2001; Cole, n.d.).

Recent research considered informed consent and mild cognitive impairment (MCI), a condition that can be a precursor to dementia. A study published in *Neurology* concluded that clients with MCI demonstrated significant impairments in medical decision-making capacity compared with healthy adults (Okonkwo et al., 2007). Those clients with MCI exhibited impaired cognitive and emotional capacity, which adversely affected their ability to make decisions about whether to accept or refuse a particular medical treatment or select among intervention options.

Therapists must be sensitive to the cognitive level of their clients and either alter their communication style to ensure client understanding of education (simple language, visual or written aids, repetition of information) or consult with the physician to determine whether the client is in need of assistance in the decision-making process.

For a client to truly provide informed consent, three requirements must be met (Beauchamp & Childress, 2019):
1. Adequate information.
2. Client competency.
3. Voluntary decision making.

## Client Must Be Adequately Informed

For the client to make an informed decision, he or she must be provided with all of the information necessary to make the decision. The therapist must disclose and explain all of the following aspects:

- Diagnosis
- Nature, purpose, and probability of success of the proposed treatment
- Risks and benefits of the proposed treatment
- Any alternatives to the proposed treatment
- Risks and benefits of alternative proposals
- The risks and benefits of no treatment at all

In general, down-to-earth, everyday vocabulary should be used to describe the client's condition and plan of care. It may be best to avoid medical terminology and jargon with which the client may be unfamiliar. Information should be simplified as much as necessary and follow-up questions should be posed to the client to ensure comprehension. The client should be encouraged to ask questions or request clarification of anything that was difficult to understand. Asking the client to explain the information back to the therapist can be useful in making sure that the key points have been understood.

When providing client education, the therapist should allow adequate processing time as well as time for the client to formulate questions. With the client's permission, a family member or friend may be invited to take part in the session to provide support to the client. Most importantly, the therapist should strive to maintain an open and supportive relationship with the client. The more comfortable the client is, the more likely he or she will be to ask questions and voice concerns.

## Client Must Be Competent

If a client cannot comprehend that to which he or she is consenting, then the consent is not truly informed. Competence is a key aspect of making an informed decision. Unfortunately, there are no universally recognized criteria to determine the level of competency necessary for informed consent. Essentially, the client must be capable of understanding the risks and benefits of the proposed intervention as well as those of refusing an intervention. If there are any concerns that a client may not be competent to make medical decisions, the facility's social worker and the client's treating physician should be notified. The physician or designated members of the healthcare team may assess the client to determine whether he or she is competent to make medical decisions (Guzman-Clark et al., 2012). If the client is deemed incompetent by the physician, a surrogate decision maker must consent to treatment. Surrogate decision makers are client-designated next of kin or other appointed individuals who are expected to make the same treatment decisions as the client would if he or she was capable (Shalowitz et al., 2006). The legal right to assign a surrogate decision maker is determined by the Patient Self-Determination Act. This act addresses the ability to make decisions about health care, to formulate advance directives, and to be informed of institutional policies regarding life-sustaining treatments. The act "provides clear ethical and legal recognition of the authority of patients and surrogates in the healthcare setting by affirming the control which they have in making many decisions about their lives and what transpires in them" (Ulrich, 1999, p.11).

In the general population, circumstances under which a client may need a surrogate decision maker are most commonly the result of a sudden event resulting in brain damage such as a traumatic brain injury or cerebrovascular accident (CVA) or a progressive disease process affecting cognition. Generally, clients are considered competent to make medical decisions unless they are legally determined to be unable to do so (Leo, 1999). In those instances, a surrogate decision maker may be appointed to make those decisions if a health-care power of attorney has not already been selected by the client to make health decisions. If the client fails to select a health-care power of attorney, the physician generally makes the determination of competence at the bedside, and a surrogate decision maker is appointed. State law sets forth the persons authorized to make medical decisions on behalf of an incompetent individual absent a legal guardian or durable power of attorney. However, it is in the best interest of the client to have that decision made ahead of time and thus all clients—gerontological or not—should be encouraged to complete an advance directive and appoint a durable health-care power of attorney while still in good health.

In the gerontological population, competence becomes a more prevalent issue. Mental status is dependent on many variables, including medical diagnosis (e.g., traumatic brain injury, CVA, dementia). Disease states (e.g., urinary tract infection) and medications can alter a person's mental status (see Chapter 14). Please refer to Chapters 9, 14, 15, and 16 for additional information on aging and mental status changes. In addition, mental acuity may vary throughout the day.

A client who is coherent in the morning may exhibit diminished decision-making ability as the day progresses either due to fatigue or sundowning. Sundowning refers to the increased confusion and agitation later in the day that are often found among people with cognitive impairments. It is also possible that an injury or illness might temporarily compromise the client's competency and ability to engage in decision making (Sherwin & Winsby, 2010).

When facilitating comprehension, one should be aware of the normal changes that can be involved in the aging process. The client's senses may be less acute. Therefore, the therapist should make accommodations for known sensory deficits. If hearing is an issue, background noise should be kept to a minimum and the therapist should face the client when talking. If the client has vision problems, the therapist should use large print, ensure that the client is wearing glasses or contact lenses if needed, and provide adequate light in the environment (Hooper & Bello-Haas, 2009). (See Chapter 10 for additional information.)

### Client Decision Must Be Voluntary

Consent to medical treatment must be voluntary. Each client has the right to participate in—or refuse—therapy without pressure from medical staff. Although health-care professionals may make multiple attempts to persuade the client to participate in intervention and may even provide multiple opportunities to participate in care, it is ultimately the client's decision whether or not to participate; clients have the right to refuse treatment (*Cruzan by Cruzan v. Director,* 1990). This decision must be respected by the therapist. Under the federal Patient Self-Determination Act of 1990 (discussed earlier), every hospital, long-term care facility, hospice, and home health agency receiving Medicare and Medicaid funds must provide clients with a statement of their rights, including the right to refuse treatment.

### Autonomy

The voluntary consent requirement is merely an extension of the principle of autonomy discussed in Principle 3 of the *Occupational Therapy Code of Ethics* (AOTA, 2020a). In health care, a client's autonomy is affected by the setting. A client receiving home health services has more autonomy in the home than a client in a long-term care setting or hospital. In institutional settings, activities, meals, treatments, and even showers may be regimented and generally left to the staff to schedule, with little control left to the client. Clients are often left feeling like a cog in the machine without any control over aspects of their daily lives. In these types of settings, it is even more important to respect each client as an autonomous individual who deserves the dignity of self-determination. Because facility residents and clients may have minimal control over their environment, it is imperative to allow them as much control as possible over every aspect of care. Including clients in the planning process gives them more control and a more vested interest in their treatment. The current revision of the required screening tool for skilled nursing facilities that receive federal funding (Minimal Data Set [MDS]

3.0) includes client input through interviews (Centers for Medicare and Medicaid Services, 2020).

## Confidentiality

Confidentiality is also included in Principle 3 of the AOTA *Code of Ethics and Ethics Standards* (AOTA, 2020a). Because therapists often spend large quantities of contact time with clients, they have the unique opportunity among health professionals to learn more about the client on an intimate personal basis than many other practitioners on the care team. The large amount of contact time spent with each client on a recurring basis allows the therapist to monitor change over time and be among those serving as a first line of defense against status changes or medical complications. That said, there are limits on when and how much information may be shared with whom.

### Health Insurance Portability and Accountability Act

Although occupational therapists have been required to honor client confidentiality through the AOTA Occupational Therapy *Code of Ethics*, state licensure requirements, and internal employer policies, the HIPAA of 1996 (Garner, 2014) federally mandated this obligation (Centers for Disease Control and Prevention, 2022). HIPAA was passed to help ensure the protection of private client information, called protected health information (PHI) in the Act, in light of the increased use of emerging technologies such as the Internet and electronic databases and the security risks associated with their use. The Health Information Technology for Economic and Clinical Health Act (HITECH Act, 2009), part of the American Recovery and Reinvestment Act of 2009, widened the scope of privacy and security protections available under HIPAA. The HITECH Act also increased the legal liability of health-care professionals for noncompliance and increased enforcement (Coppersmith Gordon Schermer & Brockelman, n.d.).

Under HIPAA, health-care providers are required to maintain the confidentiality of PHI, which includes a client's medical history or diagnosis, treatment records, and billing information. PHI is protected in all forms: writings, verbal communications, and electronic records (Centers for Disease Control and Prevention, 2022; Privacy Rights Clearing House, 2013; Searson et al., 2010). Although providers are required to take measures to maintain client confidentiality, their actions are generally scalable to their size, resources, and sophistication. This notion of scalability carries with it a reasonableness approach but does not serve to completely insulate a provider from exposure to liability under HIPAA.

Most documentation is done electronically, and electronic records include those stored on computer disks, hard drives, networks, and the Internet. To safeguard electronic information, clinicians should protect their passwords and restrict access to handheld electronic devices and laptop computers. Client information may be faxed between health-care providers so long as reasonable measures have been taken to ensure protection of the information, such as confirming that the fax number is correct, putting a notice on the cover sheet to destroy the information if the fax is mistakenly misdirected, and calling to confirm receipt of the fax. If a disclosure that is not permitted by HIPAA without specific client authorization is desired, the client's written authorization is required before such disclosure takes place.

PHI must be protected for all clients, whether living or deceased, and may be disclosed only to that specific client, to other authorized individuals, or to authorized organizations; it may be used or disclosed without authorization for treatment, payment, or health-care operations (Centers for Disease Control and Prevention, 2022). In the event of an inappropriate disclosure of a client's PHI, HIPAA requires that an entity implement breach notification procedures to inform all affected individuals that their PHI may have been disclosed. The specific notification procedures required depend on how many clients are affected and whether the information is protected through encryption or some other means. If a clinician becomes aware of a breach of PHI, he or she should immediately notify a supervisor or the risk manager for the organization so that an investigation can be conducted and the appropriate actions may be taken.

Penalties for violating HIPAA (including the HITECH Act) include civil penalties of fines ranging from $100 to $50,000, with repeated violations for HIPAA beyond a one-time violation at $1,500,000 and potential criminal penalties (HIPAA, 1996). Although penalties for HIPAA violations were rarely enforced in the past, the HITECH Act increased enforcement mechanisms, and thus, health-care providers should anticipate more scrutiny in the future. In recent cases, criminal sanctions have included probation and prison time. In 2018, a former behavioral analyst at a Tennessee autism treatment center was sentenced to 30 months of imprisonment and fined nearly $15,000 for hacking into 300 patient files (United States Attorney's Office, Western District of Tennessee, 2018). In 2010, a former surgeon at the UCLA School of Medicine was sentenced to 4 months in federal prison for illegally accessing medical records (Dimick, 2010).

### Confidentiality in Practice

Although it is necessary to protect client privacy, there are many instances when the therapist needs to communicate with family members and other caregivers. Many clients need help and support from family and friends during recovery from hospitalization and acute illness. In taking on the role of caregiver, a spouse or adult child may require education regarding precautions, mobility or range of motion, transfer techniques, activities of daily living (ADLs), and adaptive equipment use. To provide information or education to family or friends, the therapist should first obtain permission from the client. Once consent is obtained, it should be documented immediately in the client's chart and necessary precautions should be taken to ensure that information is only released to those for whom the client consents (HPSO Risk Advisor, 2007). If speaking to a caregiver or family member over the phone, necessary precautions may include

requiring a password to verify that the family member is authorized to receive private information. In addition, the therapist should confirm that person's identity. Directly calling the family member provides assurance that the correct family member was contacted. Finally, all communications as well as precautions taken should be documented in the client's chart.

To ensure continuity of care and a complete assessment and appropriate intervention, client information may be disclosed to other members of the health-care team. However, only the minimum amount of information necessary for adequate assessment and intervention should be relayed. Although the client's relevant medical history and preexisting conditions may be relevant to the other therapists treating the client, knowledge of the client's personal history, however interesting, is usually not necessary for the provision of services or daily care. Be cognizant of what information is important to relay for improvement of the client's health and only provide necessary information. That said, there are some necessary exceptions to confidentiality in the cases of potential physical harm and/or abuse.

### Exceptions to Confidentiality Rules
#### *Potential Harm by the Client*
If a client appears to be a danger to self or others, the therapist has a duty to report these concerns to a supervisor, the treating physician, and possibly authorities. In addition, if a client threatens harm to another person, the therapist may be required to warn that person of the threat. In that event, the therapist should consult the risk manager of the facility for guidance on reporting requirements.

#### *Potential Harm by Others*
According to the National Center on Elder Abuse (n.d.), abuse of older adults is a hidden problem that can be difficult to monitor. Although it can be difficult to obtain specific statistics, the National Center reports an increasing trend. As health-care providers, occupational therapists are considered mandatory reporters of elder abuse in most states. Generally, if a therapist has a reasonable belief that a vulnerable adult has been abused, neglected, or exploited, this concern should be reported. Examples include a lack of basic hygiene, a verbally demeaning caregiver, a lack of adequate clothing, or inadequately explained cuts or bruises (American Medical Association, 1993). When you have a sense that something about the client's situation is just not right, find out more. Unfortunately, the most likely abusers are those closest to the abused adult: adult children, spouses, and other caregivers (Box 2.2).

If abuse is suspected, the therapist should follow company policies regarding reporting concerns in addition to calling the state's elder abuse hotline. The state-specific numbers as well as general statistics and information on elder abuse identification and prevention may be accessed at the National Center's website at www.ncea.aoa.gov (National Center on Elder Abuse).

---

**BOX 2.2**    Risk Factors and Signs of Older Adult Abuse

| Risk Factors | Signs |
| --- | --- |
| Financial or other family problems<br>Past history of abusive relationships<br>Social isolation and dependence<br>Physical, functional, or cognitive deficits in caregivers<br>Inadequate housing or unsafe conditions in the home | Depression/anxiety<br>Passive and compliant<br>Fearful<br>Socially withdrawn<br>Change in financial behavior<br>Unexplained or repeated injuries<br>Delays in seeking medical attention for an injury<br>Elusive explanations for medical conditions<br>Inconsistent laboratory findings<br>Signs of dehydration or malnutrition without a medical cause<br>Evidence of poor care (e.g., poor hygiene)<br>Muscle contractures due to restricted movement |

Data from Canadian Network for the Prevention of Elder Abuse. (n.d.). Abuse of older adults: Signs and effects. Retrieved from http://www.winnipeg.ca/police/Take-Action/elderabusefacts/FactSheet_4.pdf; and World Health Organization. (2002). Abuse of the elderly. Retrieved from http://www.who.int/violence_injury_prevention/violence/world_report/factsheets/en/elderabusefacts.pdf.

## When Errors Are Made

"To err is human" (Institute of Medicine [IOM], 1999; Pope, 1711). As with any other health-care professionals, occupational therapists do make errors (Lohman et al., 2003). In a series of research studies centered on OT practice errors (Lohman et al., 2003; Mu et al., 2006; Scheirton et al., 2007), researchers found that occupational therapists make various errors ranging from minor errors (e.g., ripping fingernails or causing client fatigue) to severe ones (e.g., rupturing tendons or leaving a hot pack on too long, resulting in burns) (Mu et al., 2006). In a study on errors in gerontological practice (Lohman et al., 2003), researchers found errors related to internal factors or external factors as well as technical and moral factors. Discussed internal factors were "poor judgment, inexperience, and lack of knowledge" (Mu et al., 2006). A typical example of an error from an internal factor was inattention resulting in an older adult falling. Discussed external factors were influences outside of the therapist's control, such as a wrongly written order regarding weight-bearing status for an older adult following hip surgery. Technical errors involved methods, skills, or approaches that led to physical harm, such as exceeding a client's limitations following a hip replacement. Moral errors related to behaviors that undermine the practitioner-client relationship or are ethically inconsistent, such as providing an unneeded service to obtain Medicare payment or being untruthful in documentation by exaggerating the level of function accomplished through therapy (Lohman et al., 2003; Mu et al., 2006). Unique to occupational therapists was the research finding of therapists being more likely to report moral errors and that therapists tended to judge moral errors as more concerning than technical ones (Lohman et al., 2003). Additionally, most practice errors occurred during the intervention phase of the OT process (Mu et al., 2006).

These research studies on OT practice errors suggest that the causes of errors are from both individual and systemic factors. Examples of individual causes are lack of experience, lack of training, lack of assertive behavior, inadequate knowledge, and misjudgment. Unrealistic productivity pressure, unclear or illegible documentation, lack of timely and effective communication, inadequate orientation to specialized equipment, and inability to access clients' medical history are among the examples of reported systemic causes of errors. In the studies focused on gerontological practice (Lohman et al., 2003; Mu et al., 2006), system causes, such as influences from regulations, contributed to some practice errors. Among all the causes, the top causes of errors, according to a national survey study, are misjudgment, inadequate preparation, lack of experience, inadequate knowledge, and miscommunication. Regardless of how errors occurred, making errors affected therapists emotionally (Mu et al., 2006).

The top causes of errors, misjudgment, lack of preparation and experience, and inadequate knowledge, are in stark contrast with the principle of beneficence of the AOTA *Code of Ethics and Ethics Standards* (AOTA, 2020a). Beneficence requires OT practitioners to take "actions (e.g., continuing education, research, supervision, training) to benefit others," as stated by the principle "occupational therapy personnel shall demonstrate concern for the well-being and safety of persons" (AOTA, 2020a).

Miscommunications among OT personnel and clients, client family members, and other health-care providers often lead to practice errors. Ensuring clear, sufficient, accurate, and concise communication (verbal, written and technology) (*HIPAA Journal*, 2014–2022) among all service providers and recipients is one key to preventing and reducing errors. Without doubt, errors are inevitable in OT practice even with the most experienced and diligent occupational therapists. The dilemma that occupational therapists face when errors happen is what to do and how to manage errors. Therapists learn from errors by gaining knowledge of safety strategies, changing practice procedures, and developing an understanding of how to morally manage errors (Scheirton et al., 2007). The ultimate goal is to create a "culture of safety" (Scheirton et al., 2007). Acceptable ways to report and disclose errors and other methods to improve error reduction are discussed next.

## Incident Reports

If a mistake by a therapist occurs and causes potential client harm, the error should be documented. Most facilities have established policies and procedures for reporting adverse events involving client care, often in the form of incident reports. These reports generally serve two purposes: (1) to protect the client by alerting management to possible safety hazards requiring investigation and correction and (2) to learn from the event and improve processes to avoid such errors in the future through quality improvement initiatives. Generally, the occupational therapist should include the specific date and time of the occurrence, any witnesses who observed the event, and who was notified after the incident occurred.

An incident report should be filed any time a client is injured. If a therapist has observed an incident, he or she should document only what was observed firsthand. The event should be described in an objective and factual manner, using direct quotes if statements made by staff, the client, or others present are relevant. Documentation should be objective and as honest as possible. Although it may be tempting to the therapist to protect himself or herself or others from blame, falsification of the records potentially violates state and/or federal law and could cause additional harm to the client if information relevant to the client's care and course of treatment is left out. Finally, the therapist should include any assessment and care that was provided before, during, and after the incident. Ultimately, ensuring client safety is paramount.

## Disclosure of Errors

One of the most important aspects of intervention and care for a client is developing a trusting relationship. This begins from the first moment the client is seen. If a mistake is made, it is necessary to apologize to the client to maintain a trusting relationship. Everyone makes mistakes, and the therapist should feel no shame in admitting an error. When an apology is warranted, the therapist should verify the employer's policy on disclosure, file an incident report, and check with the organization's risk manager. A timely and appropriate apology can deepen the relationship with client and family, and safeguard the client (Leape, 2021; Leape, 1994). Coalitions such as Sorry Works promote disclosure through apology and compensation to mitigate anger and reduce the likelihood of a lawsuit (Sorry Works, n.d.).

Even with a movement toward full disclosure of errors, for past centuries and still today, health-care providers are often trained to be perfectionists. In a perfectionism paradigm, making errors and disclosing errors to clients and families are unthinkable or irrational. Those against disclosure of errors believe such an act would diminish the trust of clients and the public in health-care providers, damage the fragile therapeutic relationship with clients, result in countless lawsuits, empower clients unnecessarily, destroy professional reputation, and result in loss of professional license. They argue that the nondisclosure is grounded firmly on the belief of therapeutic exception or therapeutic privilege. Therapeutic privilege refers to physicians withholding information that is felt to be contraindicated to share or could harm the client physically or psychologically (Bostick et al., 2006).

Proponents of disclosure of errors, however, argue that disclosure of errors is an ethical and obligated act (i.e., Principle 5, veracity, of the AOTA *Code of Ethics and Ethics Standards*). This principle includes providing thorough, honest, objective transmission of information, and as stated, therapists should "implicitly promise to be truthful and not deceptive" (AOTA, 2020a). As recipients of health-care services, patients have the right to be informed of accurate, comprehensive, and objective health-care information, including disclosure of errors. Furthermore, research findings specific to occupational therapists suggest that disclosure of errors more likely leads to "constructive coping mechanisms and changes in practice" (Mu et al., 2006), as discussed in the next section.

## Error Prevention and Reduction

As stated earlier, errors are inevitable even with the best-prepared and the most diligent OT practitioners. The encouraging news is that research literature on OT practice errors indicates that occupational therapists often use constructive strategies to prevent future errors and that OT practitioners become more vigilant in their practice after errors occur. Therapists reflected on and learned from errors, paid more attention to details, and altered their service approaches and methods (Lohman et al., 2003; Mu et al., 2006).

That said, there are strategies available to help prevent and reduce the likelihood of a practice error occurring. Specific error prevention and reduction strategies include the following measures (Mu et al., 2011).

- Strengthen departmental orientations for newly hired occupational therapists.
- Implement performance-based competency checks to improve in-service and continuing education outcomes.
- Establish new policies and programs based on collected error data.
- Capitalize on the existing infrastructures of the facility.
- Establish or improve mentorship for new employees.
- Create non-punitive cultures and environments.

### Strengthen Departmental Orientation

Strengthening on-site orientation for new therapists is an effective strategy for error prevention/reduction (Mu et al., 2011). In addition to general orientation at the worksites, providing site-specific orientations to areas that are prone to error is important. These orientations must occur and be strengthened. Identification of these error-prone areas needs to be based on data generated from the input of administrators, safety personnel, therapists, and other stakeholders through a problem-solving process.

### Implement Performance-Based Competency Checks

Outcomes-based in-service training and continuing education are effective ways to ensure professional competency of occupational therapists (Mu et al., 2011). However, *knowledge* is not the synonym of *competency*. Merely attending an in-service training or continuing education program does not guarantee competency acquisition; therapists must advocate for performance-based competency checks to ensure and improve the outcomes of training. For example, new therapists could have a competency check on safe transfer procedures. Competency checks are especially essential for infrequently used skills such as implementing physical agent modalities, or newly acquired skills such as operating recently purchased equipment.

### Establish New Policies and Programs

Establishing new safety policies and safety programs is another worksite approach to error reduction (Mu et al., 2011). Examples of such initiatives or measures include the following:
- Policies to require confirmation of signed physician orders before initiating intervention
- Committees addressing patient safety concerns, such as patient skin integrity or falls

### Capitalize on Existing Infrastructure

Existing infrastructures in treatment facilities may be used to prevent and reduce practice errors (Mu et al., 2011). Such existing infrastructures include the following examples:
- Safety committees
- Quality assurance programs that collect patient error data and enable respective programs to design and/or strengthen orientations, in-service training, health care, and patient education

The Joint Commission (TJC) plays a significant role in error reduction and patient safety improvement. For instance, several TJC standards for nursing care centers mandate that two methods must be implemented to verify the identity of patients before initiating treatment and that staff should prevent residents from falling (TJC, 2021).

### Establish a Mentorship Program for New Employees

Occupational therapists have voiced the importance of providing mentorship to new employees in research literature on practice errors in OT practice. Therapists asserted that mentors should be provided to all new graduates or to experienced occupational therapists who decide to enter a different practice area (Mu et al., 2011).

### Create a Nonpunitive Culture

The value of creating a nonpunitive culture and working environment cannot be overstated (Mu et al., 2011). Creation of such a culture or environment is essential for practitioners to share their errors with others openly, which in turn will help everyone learn to prevent/reduce errors and improve patient safety. An anonymous and voluntary reporting system for OT professionals provides an open forum for practitioners to share errors, explore prevention/reduction strategies, and ensure lessons learned for all.

## What Is New With Addressing Patient Errors

The original IOM report "To Err is Human" was published in 1999 (IOM, 1999). Since then, this IOM report has spurred many positive changes in the health-care system to enhance patient safety. Another analysis of patient safety 20 years after the original IOM report found that since then, many interventions have been put in place to address safety concerns, such as treating the wrong patient, falls, and medication safety, although responses have been variable. Looking at patient safety has expanded beyond the hospital doors to outpatient care, physician diagnostic errors, and health information technology (Bates & Singh, 2018; *HIPAA Journal,* 2014–2022). Therapists working in outpatient settings may find that there is not always as much infrastructure directed toward patient safety as in inpatient settings, where much of the original efforts were made. Like all health-care practitioners, therapists working with information technology may experience instances of concern for patient safety. Examples of such are overlooking safety alerts and system crashes (Bates & Singh, 2018). Additionally, lack of communication between systems can prevent the transfer of important therapy information.

Although no new research has taken place in the OT field since the original publications by the Mu, Lohman, Scheirton, and Cochran team (Mu et al., 2006; Scheirton et al., 2007), the findings are still relevant to today's practice environment. What is also relevant are some of the quality parameters brought about by Medicare that therapists can address, many of which are related to patient safety. For example, one of the measures for long stays in skilled nursing facilities is "application of percent of residents experiencing one or more falls with major injury" (CMS.gov, 2022). Occupational therapists have the knowledge and skills on the interprofessional team to help with this and other quality measures.

In summary, the notion of establishing a nonpunitive culture and environment needs to be fostered early in professional education. OT professional programs should be educating students that practice errors are inevitable, how to handle them when they happen, and, most importantly, to learn from errors when they occur. Therapy practitioners should stay abreast of Medicare quality parameters as they can contribute toward helping maintain a safe environment.

## Consequences for Violating Professional Obligations

Occupational therapists work in a complex, ever-changing health-care environment. Recent modifications in health-care provision in response to the Affordable Care Act resulted in new systems for gerontological care being piloted and integrated into practice, such as accountable care organizations and bundling of care. Beyond the overall macro changes to the health-care environment, therapists face day-to-day challenges in providing patient care. Sometimes, it may seem difficult to get a handle on the complexity of issues that therapists face. Therefore, it is important to refer to and apply a professional code of ethics as well as have system structures in place to help guide therapists' professional conduct in this era of increasingly complex practice. Beyond ethical standards, laws regulating health-care practice are created to protect the public's safety and to help influence actions. Laws are defined as "rule(s) of conduct or action(s) prescribed or formally recognized as binding or enforced by a controlling authority" (Mish, 2003). The next section includes a discussion of provisions in place to address violations of appropriate client care and practice.

## Violation of Standard or Duty of Care

If a client feels that a therapist has violated the standard of care, there are many avenues through which to lodge a complaint. Some clients may verbalize their dissatisfaction by reporting concerns directly to the therapist. In this instance, the therapist has the opportunity to rectify the situation before it escalates. Allowing the client or family time to voice concerns, receive validation, and suggest solutions to the problem should help the therapist resolve any issues the client may have and allow the therapist-client relationship to continue.

If the issues are not resolved to the client's satisfaction, further measures may be taken. First, the employer may be contacted and the therapist may be penalized in accordance with company policy. Another option available to clients is to file a complaint with a professional accrediting organization such as the AOTA. According to AOTA procedure, complaints against a member may be filed by anyone with knowledge of a suspected ethical violation by an association member. A signed written complaint must be filed with the Ethics Commission (EC), and EC shall make a preliminary assessment of the complaint and determine whether an investigation is warranted (AOTA, 2021b; AOTA, 2023c). If the EC determines the event does rise to the level of an ethical violation, the EC may initiate a charge. If the member is found to have committed an ethical violation, the member may be sanctioned. Any sanctions may be appealed and presented to an appeal panel, whose decision is final (AOTA, 2021b).

The NBCOT, the organization that certifies occupational therapists, may also investigate allegations of ethical misconduct. Disciplinary sanctions carried out by the NBCOT (2023) include formal written reprimand, public censure, compulsory community service, probation with conditions, suspension of certification to practice for a specified term, ineligibility for certification, or revocation of certification.

Finally, clients may also file a complaint with the state (AOTA, 2023d) in which the therapist practices. If a therapist violates any licensure requirements or a client files a complaint, the licensure board, or other entity, in the applicable state will conduct an investigation (AOTA, 2023a). If the licensee is found to be in violation, penalties may be assessed. Penalties for noncompliance vary according to state statute and regulation and degree of infraction. Sanctions may range from public reprimand, licensure suspension or revocation (e.g., Texas [40 Tex. Admin. Code §374.1]), fines (e.g., $250 to $1000 in Georgia [GA Code Ann. § 43-28-16 (2023)]), to (in extreme cases) imprisonment. Actions that violate state licensure laws may also violate federal laws; therefore, professionals may be exposed to additional liability for the same infraction.

Violating one's scope of practice and creating fraudulent documentation are two examples of issues that may be addressed by a licensure board. If a health professional acts outside the profession's scope of practice or provides fraudulent documentation, he or she may expose the client to risk of injury and expose her- or himself to civil and criminal sanctions, including licensure revocation, fines, and criminal charges.

## Reimbursement Fraud and Abuse

When dealing with reimbursement issues, therapists should document intervention codes and minutes truthfully and accurately to avoid claims of fraudulent documentation. Health-care fraud occurs when a health-care professional knowingly, willfully, and intentionally makes a false statement or claim (False Claims Act, 1863; Program Fraud Civil Remedies Act). Making false statements or documentation to obtain program benefits, such as Medicare reimbursement when a provider would otherwise not be entitled to payment, is fraudulent. For example, submitting claims for services that were not provided or billing for more minutes than were provided to increase reimbursement level are fraudulent activities.

When determining whether fraud or abuse has occurred, the government may look to whether the services were reasonable and necessary, whether the charges were appropriate and accurate, and whether documentation supports the treatment provided (Medicare Program Integrity Manual, 2022). Therefore, documentation serves as an important means for the therapist to substantiate the services provided.

## False Claims and Penalties

Unfortunately, fraud occurs in therapy practice and sometimes with rehabilitation corporations that employ therapists. In 2012, a therapist was convicted of submitting around $1.5 million in fraudulent claims to Medicaid and Medicare for therapy not provided. In 2004, the nation's largest provider of rehabilitation services agreed to pay $325 million to settle allegations that the company defrauded Medicare and other federal health-care programs (Department of Justice, 2004). The allegations included billing for physical therapy services provided by persons other than licensed physical therapists and billing for individual services when individual services were not rendered (Department of Justice, 2004).

The False Claims Act prohibits knowingly filing false or fraudulent claims against the U.S. government (False Claims Act, 1863). If an individual violates the False Claims Act by charging Medicare or Medicaid for services that were not rendered, anyone may bring a civil action on behalf of the government against that individual. Therefore, a coworker, a patient, or a patient's family member may report a violation. Under the act, fraud by a provider is considered a felony and is punishable by a fine of up to $25,000 and up to 5 years' imprisonment and civil penalty fines up to $10,000 if the provider makes a false claim, bills for services not provided, misrepresents services provided, or falsely certifies that certain services were medically necessary (18 U.S.C. § 287). If an individual is proven to have submitted false claims, he or she may be fined from $5000 to $10,000 for each false claim (False Claims Act, 1863) and the prosecutor has the discretion to triple the fine. Additional sanctions include administrative actions such as licensure suspension or revocation. Therefore, it is imperative to bill accurately and truthfully for services rendered because it could prove extremely costly financially and emotionally to submit false claims.

## Whistleblower Protections

A private citizen who becomes aware of violations of the False Claims Act may bring a civil action against the individual or company in violation of the act on behalf of the government (False Claims Act, 1863). For example, in 2008 two employees, including an occupational therapist, of a corporation that provides gerontological services filed whistleblower lawsuits alleging that excessive therapy was being provided to increase reimbursement (South, 2012). Any individual who brings such an action may share in the proceeds recovered as a result of the suit (False Claims Act, 1863). In addition, certain workplace protections are provided. An employee who lawfully reports violations, assists in such an investigation, or testifies regarding a violation may not be discharged, demoted, suspended, threatened, harassed, or discriminated against (False Claims Act, 1863). If an employer engages in any of the prohibited actions, the employee may be reinstated, receive two times the amount of lost wages, and receive compensation for any special damages sustained as a result of the discrimination, including litigation costs and reasonable attorneys' fees (Morgan & Morgan Complex Litigation Group, n.d.; False Claims Act, 1863).

## Systemic and Contextual Considerations

While ethical tensions are experienced at an individual level, it is important to consider contextual or systemic factors beyond the therapist's control that may be contributing to, or even setting up, situations of ethical or moral tension (Breslin et al., n.d.; Bushby et al., 2015; Durocher et al., 2016). Such factors shape occupational therapists' roles and mandates in

particular settings and can contribute to ethically difficult situations when practice constrained by such factors is not in alignment with personal or professional values (Durocher et al., 2016). Contextual or systemic factors identified in the literature as potentially contributing to ethical challenges in practice include, for example, being assigned large caseloads or having a lack of staff to enable practitioners adequate time to provide quality practice; working to meet predetermined lengths of stay or numbers of visits that are frequently insufficient to enable practice to meet client needs; having inadequate equipment or financial resources to inform or enable practice; or working in a context with insufficient follow-up services (Bushby et al., 2015; Carrier et al., 2010; Kassberg & Skar, 2008; Mitchell & Unsworth, 2004). Some of these factors may be long-standing issues or new ones framed as cost-containment measures intended to promote efficiency, but nonetheless reflect a shift in focus away from quality care and professional autonomy to provide and advocate for client care and toward metrics and benchmarks of performance and productivity (Clouston, 2014; Newman & Lawler, 2009; Shivji, 2009). Such constraints and shifts toward efficiency will inevitably contribute to, or even set up, situations of ethical tension for therapists who are mandated and trained to provide ethical quality practice to meet client needs.

Addressing systemic constraints can potentially seem a daunting task for individual occupational therapists. Doing so would require the attention of a multitude of stakeholders, including clients, employers, regulatory colleges, and other professional bodies, among others. Therapists might start by identifying and discussing such dimensions of practice with colleagues and mentors before deciphering the next best players to engage and how. There is a tendency to focus on individual situations and circumstances and to frame ethical tensions as a problem for an individual. Moving forward, however, it is imperative that consideration be given to systemic and contextual factors (Hocking & Townsend, 2015) and how these may be contributing or shaping the options available to therapists and circumstances that contribute to, or even set up, such ethical challenges.

## Summary

Providing intervention in today's health-care world is becoming increasingly complex, and inevitably, practice issues develop and mistakes occur. As a result, therapists need to be cognizant of ethical standards and legal protections to help guide practice. Using codes of ethics and taking time to reflect about ethical values and principles and how these apply in various scenarios to guide daily practice are paramount for good care. Furthermore, understanding the legal aspects of patient/client care helps to promote a better and safer client-care environment.

*The complete listing of the Bibliography and Chapter Questions and Answers are available in the accompanying enhanced eBook version included with the print purchase of this textbook. Visit Elsevier eBooks+ (eBooks.Health.Elsevier.com) to access this content.*

## CHAPTER 3

# The Epidemiology of Health Status and Quality of Life Among Older Adults: Implications for Occupational Therapy

*Erin DeFries Bouldin, PhD, Michael Bradley Cannell, PhD and Karen Frank Barney, PhD, MS, OTR, FAOTA*

## CHAPTER OUTLINE

## OBJECTIVES

- Understand basic concepts from public health relevant to occupational therapy practice
- Evaluate evidence generated from research studies
- Discuss historic and current occupational therapy practice trends that integrate public health and occupational therapy
- Relate relevant theoretical models applied to public health and occupational therapy practice and research
- Describe the global aging and demographic population shifts currently underway
- Compare and contrast trends in health and aging between developed and developing nations
- Define major health and quality of life topics affecting aging and lifespan
- Discuss the importance of considering the perspectives of families and caregivers in the care of aging adults
- Articulate the significance and implications of the trends and predictions regarding aging populations for occupational therapy practice, research, and service

In this chapter, we discuss some of the basic principles of epidemiology, provide examples of their application, and discuss how these principles can be used to support occupational therapy (OT) practice and research. Epidemiology is commonly defined as the study of the occurrence and distribution of health-related states or events in specified populations, including the study of the determinants influencing such states, and the application of this knowledge to control the health problems (A Dictionary of Epidemiology, 2014). In other words, epidemiologists measure who gets "sick" and why, who stays healthy and why, and how we can prevent disease and encourage health. Epidemiology is one discipline within the larger field of public health and focuses on populations rather than individuals. Nonetheless, some of epidemiology's tools and insights can be helpful to practitioners working with individuals. There are ample epidemiological and statistical techniques to allow for the investigation of health among subgroups of people or patients/clients, such as people living with limb loss, individuals who experience homelessness, or patients/clients from a specific racial or ethnic background. Epidemiological methods can also be applied to develop evidence of an intervention's effectiveness, which in turn contributes to the ability to practice evidence-based OT. Although there are clear barriers to practitioners identifying these evidence-based practices on their own, given the focus of their work on direct patient/client care (Lin et al., 2010), we describe some of the resources available in both OT and public health spaces to reduce the workload on individual practitioners seeking interventions with a strong evidence base.

This chapter also focuses on the health, function, and well-being of older adults, who make up a substantial and growing portion of the population globally. We describe the demographic patterns related to aging and discuss trends in health, function, and well-being. The diseases of older age are primarily chronic diseases. Chronic diseases also make up the bulk of conditions that historically have involved gerontological occupational therapy practitioners in medical care and community-based settings, especially those working in home health, residential care, acute and subacute care, rehabilitation centers, skilled nursing facilities, and hospice programs. Prevention is a key concept for integrating gerontological OT with public health for chronic diseases. We introduce the public health model of prevention here so that OT roles that are described later in the chapter, such as promoting wellness and quality of life, can be set into a population perspective and in clinical and other forms of OT practice. Public health thinking about preventing and treating health conditions has moved to a socioecological framework over the past decades (Institute of Medicine [US], 2002, 2003). This model of public health integrates aspects across the levels of individual, interpersonal, community, and society.

Although relatively new to public health disciplines, these concepts resonate with occupational science and OT science because, for occupational therapy personnel, intervention ideally occurs within the context of the client's environment. Prevention is considered at different levels in public health and can be considered in the context of different care delivery settings. These perspectives are especially useful in considering current health care trends and the resulting expanded practice opportunities for occupational therapists working with aging populations.

Finally, we describe methods for identifying effective interventions and implementing these widely in populations. We discuss the trends in aging in several regions of the world and the implications for care in both formal health care and community-based settings. We posit that OT practitioners are well-positioned to meet the needs of older adults as they age and discuss opportunities for intervention throughout the continuum of care to support the health and well-being of aging adults and their families.

## Public Health Concepts and an Introduction to Epidemiology

To orient the reader to the practice of epidemiology and its methods, we begin by briefly introducing the field of which it is a part: public health. While many occupational therapists may not have formal training in public health, they will likely have interacted with public health practitioners or with the public health system both as providers and as members of the community themselves.

### Public Health Foundation: Population and Prevention

Public health is a broad discipline, traditionally encompassing multiple subdisciplines, including epidemiology, biostatistics, social and behavioral sciences, environmental health, and health policy (Institute of Medicine [US], 1988). It is inherently focused on population-level health status rather than on individuals. This means that much of the work of public health is not done in one-on-one clinical settings, but instead is intended to impact groups of people simultaneously. Classic

examples of public health efforts include providing clean drinking water, requiring vaccinations for specific groups like school-age children, and prohibiting cigarette smoking in public spaces. All of these efforts are designed to prevent disease or poor health outcomes among large groups of people.

The examples above also illustrate another major focus of public health: prevention. The public health approach is one that seeks to avert negative health events and experiences but recognizes that treatment is important in mitigating the negative consequences of harm. There are three levels of prevention: primary, secondary, and tertiary (see also Chapter 25). Primary prevention seeks to stop a negative event from occurring. Therefore, vaccination and prohibitions on certain behaviors or exposures are examples of primary prevention. If implemented, these strategies stop people from contracting an infectious disease or being exposed to a substance or experience that will trigger the onset of a chronic disease or lead to an injury. Secondary prevention involves identifying disease early so that negative consequences of disease can be averted. Examples of secondary prevention include early detection or screening, like mammography to detect breast cancer or blood glucose testing to detect diabetes. Finally, when diseases and conditions are already advanced, we move to the tertiary level, where the goal is to mitigate complications and symptoms, and reduce mortality. Clinical care is perhaps the most common type of tertiary prevention and may be most familiar to occupational therapy personnel. Efforts to restore upper extremity, speech, or other functions after a stroke or brain injury, and infection control efforts following surgery to prevent surgical site infections are two examples of tertiary prevention efforts. Nonetheless, for OT practice, each of the other prevention stages is also an OT opportunity. For someone with paralysis who uses a wheelchair, primary prevention may be directed at reducing the incidence of skin ulcers, contractures, decreased strength, and potential for diminished overall quality of life. Stroke survivors could be a target group for secondary prevention if a new technique for breast self-examination were promoted to improve women's abilities in early cancer detection, for example, and occupational therapy personnel worked with clients to perform this examination manually or visually, despite the clients' sensory and/or motor deficits or hemianopsia.

Over time, public health agencies have provided more clinical services to populations. Local health departments may offer preventive services like vaccinations, nutrition services, and, particularly for those designated as federally qualified health centers, comprehensive primary and prenatal care (Institute of Medicine [US], 2012a, 2012b). As a result, public health practitioners have more closely considered prevention efforts in the context of clinical care. The resulting framework considers three "buckets" of prevention: traditional clinical prevention, innovative clinical prevention, and total population or community-wide prevention (Auerbach, 2016) (Fig. 3.1). In this conceptual model, health care delivered in a clinic or designated health-care service space would be classified as traditional clinical prevention. Innovative approaches would include those that have a similar focus as traditional clinical

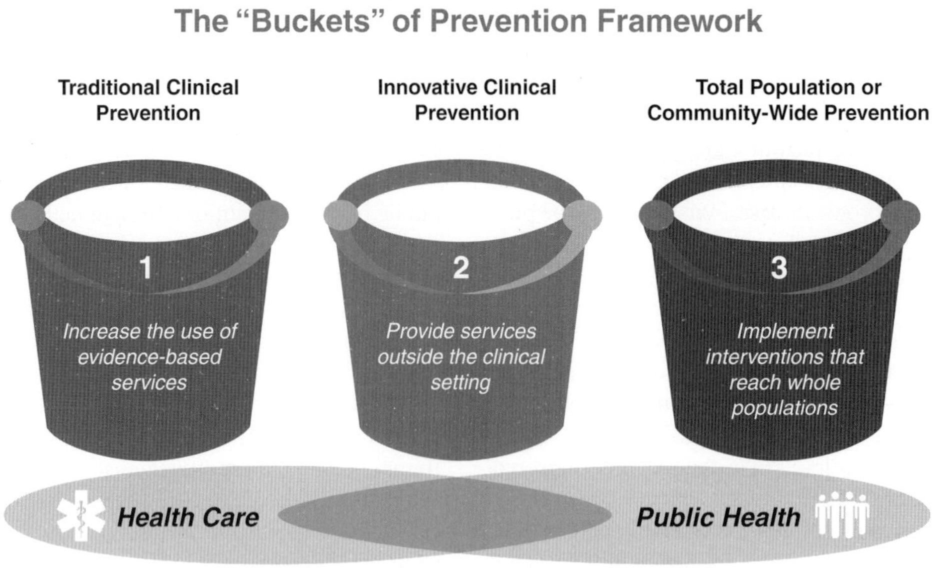

## The "Buckets" of Prevention Framework

**Traditional Clinical Prevention**

**Innovative Clinical Prevention**

**Total Population or Community-Wide Prevention**

1

*Increase the use of evidence-based services*

2

*Provide services outside the clinical setting*

3

*Implement interventions that reach whole populations*

**Health Care**                    **Public Health**

**FIGURE 3.1**    The Three Buckets of Prevention Framework.

efforts—such as blood pressure control or functional capacity—but are delivered outside of an established health-care setting. This might include home-based programs, or it might leverage peers, community health workers, or other providers not trained in a traditional health care discipline. Finally, community-wide efforts encompass those that modify the environment for an entire group of people in order to promote health or well-being, rather than addressing an individual's basic needs, basic activities or instrumental activities of daily living or activities. This framework may resonate more strongly or be more relevant than the primary, secondary, and tertiary prevention definitions for occupational therapy practitioners and others engaged in clinical or community-based service delivery. Also, many occupational therapists (OTs) and occupational therapy assistants (OTAs) already practice in settings like long-term care facilities, community-based agencies, and individual's homes, and so a clear connection exists between public health efforts and OT practice. While sometimes this link is formalized, there remain opportunities for the two disciplines to connect and collaborate in order to move toward a shared goal of improving the health and quality of life of people as they age and to structure environments in a way that supports participation and engagement.

### Social Ecological Framework

Regardless of which level of prevention or bucket of prevention is the focus of a particular public health program or effort, the social ecological framework is usually considered to underpin it. This framework recognizes that there are multiple levels of influence on health, whether the focus is the individual or the population. While different versions of the framework are used, they typically are represented by concentric circles of influence beginning with the individual, which includes demographic and personal characteristics, and moves out to consider interpersonal influences like relationships with family and friends; community and organizational influences like the characteristics of one's

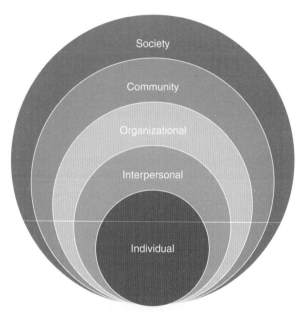

**FIGURE 3.2**    The Social-Ecological Framework.

neighborhood, school, or workplace; and societal influences including the structure of a population, cultural factors, and policies that impact large portions of the population (Fig. 3.2). One might consider the move in clinical settings to consider the social determinants of health to reflect this framework. Social determinants, those characteristics of the places we live, work, and play (Centers for Disease Control and Prevention [n.d.-a]; World Health Organization [WHO], 2022), are beyond the individual's control yet impact their access to health-related services, the likelihood of their engaging in particular behaviors that impact health, and ultimately their health outcomes.

### Evaluating Causal Evidence in Epidemiology

Epidemiology is one of the core disciplines within public health, often considered part of the foundation of public health science (Institute of Medicine [US], 1988). It is the study of the distribution and determinants of health within populations, and the application of that knowledge to control disease (A Dictionary of Epidemiology, 2014). Characterizing the distribution of health requires population-level information about the frequency of disease occurrence. Frequency is often measured in terms of **incidence** and **prevalence**. Incidence is the number of *new* cases of the outcome we are interested in. For example, approximately 610,000 people in the United States will have a stroke for the first time this year (CDC, 2022b). As of 2022, there are approximately 332 million people living in the United States (US Census Bureau, 2022). Therefore, you might hear epidemiologists describe incidence by saying something like approximately 1 out of every 544 people in the United States will have a stroke this year. Prevalence is the proportion of *existing* cases of the outcome we are interested in at a given time. For example, approximately 7.8 million people living in the United States today have ever had a stroke at some point in their life (CDC, 2022a). Therefore, you might hear epidemiologists say that the prevalence of stroke in the United States in 2022 is 2.3% (7.8 million/332 million). Notice that these two measures tell us different, but equally important, things about the outcome we are interested in. The incidence tells us about the *risk* of the outcome (e.g., "how likely is a person to have a stroke?"), and the prevalence tell us about the *burden* of the outcome (e.g., "how many people in the United States are stroke survivors, and therefore, potentially in need of stroke-related services?"). The phrase "burden of disease" is commonly used in epidemiology and other fields to encompass the total impact of a disease or health state on society (A Dictionary of Epidemiology, 2014). It is not intended to imply any negative attribute at the individual level, but to express a population-level impact of different health states.

Identifying health determinants involves identifying factors—typically called "exposures" —that caused the outcomes in which we are interested. Exposures could be anything from behaviors to environmental contaminants, to early life experiences; and outcomes similarly could range from a specific clinical state like an injury or health condition, to a measure of function, to another patient/client-important outcome like well-being. To determine whether an exposure causes an outcome, we might collect information from both exposed and unexposed groups of people and follow them for some period of time to determine whether the outcome occurs more often in the exposed or unexposed group. If there is a difference in the rate of the outcome between the two groups of people, the exposure is said to be associated with the outcome. However, as you may have heard, association is not necessarily equivalent to causation. There are several reasons for this, including the fact that the exposure and outcome may have a shared common cause that creates the illusion of a cause-and-effect relationship between the exposure and outcome in which we are interested.

Epidemiologists refer to this situation as confounding, when some variable other than the exposure of interest confuses the relationship under study. For example, imagine we want to know whether taking a particular type of medication causes people to fall. We might sample a group of people taking

the medication and another group not taking the medication then follow up with them over a year to determine the rate of falls in each group and compare them. While this would provide information about the association between medication use and fall risk, in order to determine whether the medication itself was actually causing or preventing falls, we would also want to collect more information about the reason people were taking this and perhaps other medications, whether there were differences in the age, health status, activity levels, and functional levels of people in each group, and other factors that might also influence taking the medication or fall risk.

When deciding whether there is a causal link between an exposure and an outcome using data from an observational study (one in which people's experiences and outcomes are recorded and the research team makes no effort to intervene or change their exposure), several factors in addition to confounding can be considered. First, consider whether the relationship is plausible: is there some mechanism that could explain the effect of exposure on outcome? This could be biological, as in the case of a medication causing dizziness, which could then result in a fall. Or it could be social, such as a lack of instrumental support for managing a chronic health condition results in poorer adherence to clinical recommendations or treatment. Second, consider whether the results are generally consistent across studies. If a program or practice is truly effective, it should probably be effective in multiple settings and when tested by different groups. Third, consider the design of the study, including what patients or participants were included. Was it a very specific group of people? Were they somehow very different from the general population of patients/clients you might expect to see? Was the comparison group a fair one (meaning that the unexposed or control group could have been in the exposed or treatment group)? Several guidance documents now exist to guide researchers on how to report the findings from their observational or trial results. While these guidelines were not developed to evaluate the evidence, they can be helpful in highlighting what aspects of a study a reader should consider critically. For students, they therefore provide a nice roadmap for reading an article and assessing evidence. The Strengthening Reporting of Observational Studies in Epidemiology (STROBE) guidelines (Vandenbroucke et al., 2007) are specific to observational studies, and the CONsolidated Standards of Reporting Trials (CONSORT) guidelines (Schulz et al., 2010) are for parallel group randomized controlled clinical trials and extensions thereof (see online resources for more information).

Over the past few decades, increasingly sophisticated approaches to making causal links between exposures and outcomes, or what is known as "causal inference," have developed (Hernán & Robins, 2020; Hernán et al., 2002; VanderWeele et al., 2008). These methods can be applied to data collected in a prospective manner, as described above, or to existing data such as those collected in a health record in the process of usual care. While a detailed assessment of the methods of causal inference is beyond the scope of this chapter, we do want to highlight their existence and recommend that practitioners who aim to establish causal relationships consult with a biostatistician, epidemiologist, or other data scientist with training in study design and analysis to assure the study is designed in a way that strong and accurate statements about causal relationships can be made. In order to effectively intervene to improve health, we must start with a clear understanding of what exposures actually cause health outcomes to change.

## Evidence-Based Public Health and Occupational Therapy

The final part of the definition of epidemiology involves using the information about how an outcome is distributed within a population and what exposures cause the outcome to intervene in order to improve the health of that population. While data can suggest what interventions may be best, any program, policy, or other change should be evaluated to assure it is having the intended effect and to assure that the benefits of the change are distributed equitably across the population. Evidence-based public health, like evidence-based practice in other fields, encapsulates this approach. It is the use of programs, services, or other interventions that have been shown to be effective in improving the health of the public, and using them in a way that aligns with the community's preferences (Brownson et al., 2009; Jacobs et al., 2012). Similarly, evidence-based OT involves utilizing clinical and community-based practices and strategies that have been shown to be effective (Bennett & Townsend, 2006).

Identifying evidence may include reading individual scientific journal articles that summarize the results of a study, reviews or meta-analyses that summarize or analyze data from multiple studies, or reports or evidence syntheses published by trusted sources. We will focus on this last category here, since it generally is the most accessible and the least time intensive. Evidence syntheses evaluate and summarize which interventions—either specifically or as a class—have the strongest evidence of effectiveness (impact in a controlled environment) or efficacy (impact in a real-world setting with more variation). See this chapter's online resources for examples of evidence-based practice repositories relevant to OT. Specific evidence summaries and considerations also are included throughout the rest of this textbook.

Once an intervention is identified, it may need to be adapted to fit well into the particular environment in which it will be implemented. The field of implementation science has developed in recent years to focus on the process of implementing an intervention in practice and evaluating both this process and the resulting outcomes of the intervention. Though beyond the scope of this chapter, we do want to highlight the fact that not all evidence-based interventions will translate to every setting or patient/client population. Rather than describe the methods and considerations important in implementation science, we point readers to a couple of helpful resources for learning more in the online appendix for this chapter.

## Population Demographic Shifts

Today, the older adult population, defined variously as people aged 60 or 65 years of age and over, is the largest it has ever been, and it continues to grow. The year 2018 marked the first time in recorded history when there were more older adults (people aged 65 or older) than young children (under age 5) in the world (United Nations, 2022). In 2020, these older adults represented 9% of the world's population, or 727 million people; this proportion is expected to grow to 16% by 2050, representing 1.5 billion people (United Nations & Department of Economic and Social Affairs, Population Division, 2019). Although population-level aging is occurring in every region of the globe (Table 3.1), it is not growing at the same rate in all regions (Figs. 3.3 and 3.4). Over the coming decades, the largest increases in the number of older adults are expected in Eastern and South-Eastern Asia, and the fastest rate of growth in the older adult population is projected in Northern Africa and Western Asia (United Nations & Department of Economic and Social Affairs, Population Division, 2019).

As Fig. 3.3 illustrates, the increase in the world population over age 65 is driven mostly by growth in this age group in regions designated as less developed (United Nations & Department of Economic and Social Affairs, Population Division, 2019). It is important to note that some are very

**TABLE 3.1** Number of Persons Aged 65 Years or Older by Geographic Region, 2019 and 2050

| Region | Number of Persons Aged 65 or Over in 2019 (millions) | Number of Persons Aged 65 or Over in 2050 (millions) | Percentage Change Between 2019 and 2050 |
|---|---|---|---|
| **World** | **702.9** | **1548.9** | **120%** |
| Sub-Saharan Africa | 31.9 | 101.4 | 218% |
| Northern Africa and Western Asia | 29.4 | 95.8 | 226% |
| Central and Southern Asia | 119.0 | 328.1 | 176% |
| Eastern and Southeast Asia | 260.6 | 572.5 | 120% |
| Latin America and the Caribbean | 56.4 | 144.6 | 156% |
| Australia and New Zealand | 4.8 | 8.8 | 84% |
| Oceania, excluding Australia and New Zealand | 0.5 | 1.5 | 190% |
| Europe and North America | 200.4 | 296.2 | 48% |

From World population ageing 2019, by United Nations, Department of Economic and Social Affairs, Population Division, © (2019) United Nations. Reprinted with the permission of the United Nations.

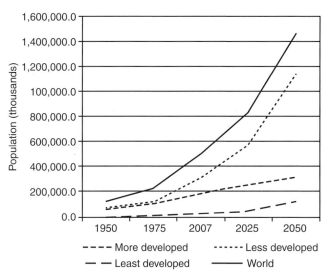

**FIGURE 3.3** Population Aged 65 or Over (Thousands) by Development Area: 1950–2050. (Data from United Nations, Department of Economic and Social Affairs, Population Division. [2007]. *World population ageing 2007.* United Nations Publications.)

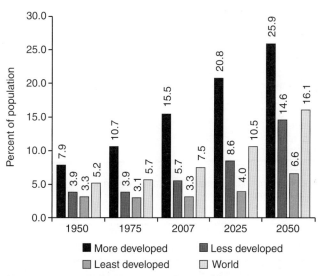

**FIGURE 3.4** Percentage of Population Aged 65 or Over by Development Area: 1950–2050. (Data from United Nations, Department of Economic and Social Affairs, Population Division. [2007]. *World population ageing 2007.* United Nations Publications.)

**TABLE 3.2** Percent of Population Aged 65 or Over, Selected Countries: 1950, 2000, 2025, 2050

| Country | 1950 | 2000 | 2025 | 2050 |
|---|---|---|---|---|
| Bolivia | 3.5% | 4.0% | 6.1% | 11.6% |
| Egypt | 3.0% | 4.1% | 7.6% | 14.5% |
| India | 3.3% | 5.0% | 8.3% | 14.8% |
| Japan | 4.9% | 17.2% | 28.9% | 36.4% |
| Mexico | 4.4% | 4.7% | 9.3% | 18.6% |
| Nigeria | 3.0% | 3.0% | 3.8% | 6.8% |
| United States | 8.3% | 12.3% | 18.5% | 21.1% |
| Poland | 5.2% | 12.1% | 20.2% | 27.9% |
| World | 5.2% | 6.9% | 10.4% | 15.6% |

From Plassman, B. L., Langa, K. M., Fisher, G. G., Heeringa, S. G., Weir, D. R., Ofstedal, M. B., et al. (2007). Prevalence of dementia in the United States: The aging, demographics, and memory study. *Neuroepidemiology, 29*(1–2), 125–132.

adult population will remain in the more developed regions of the world for the coming decades due to the much longer life expectancy of individuals in these regions.

All of the graphs and tables presented here demonstrate a concept that is central to this chapter. Population aging, simply put, is the process by which older individuals become a proportionally larger share of the total population. Generally speaking, the more developed a country is, the further along it is in the process of having an aging population.

## Population Structure: Current Characteristics and Projections

Variation in the population-aging phenomenon is also shown in Table 3.2, which notes the percentage of the population aged 65 or over for selected countries. In 1950 in most countries, older adults made up a small proportion—about 3% to 5%—of the total population. By 2000, there was significant variation in the age structures of these countries, with older adults making up 17% of the population in Japan and still just 3% in Nigeria. The difference becomes even more striking when looking at the numbers projected for 2050. Japan will have an astonishing 36.4% of its population over age 65, whereas in Nigeria, the percentage will have only increased to 6.8%. The special case of Japan is raised again later in this chapter in the context of culture, aging, and caregiving.

Another way that we can visualize the phenomenon of population aging and differences among countries is through the use of a special type of chart known as a population pyramid. Population pyramids graphically show the age and sex structure of a country. Traditionally, there is a fairly even distribution of males and females protruding laterally from the center of the graph, as well as a large base of people in the younger age groups, tapering vertically to fewer people in the oldest age groups. This structure is what gives the population pyramid its name. As we have discussed, however, the population structure is changing, and the shapes of population pyramids are changing as well.

The more traditional-looking shape is said to be expansive: There are many more young people in the population than old. Figs. 3.5 and 3.6 highlight the past, current, and projected

rapidly developing nations such as China, India, and Brazil. These three countries are still classified as less developed by the United Nations; however, their large populations and increasing average life expectancies contribute to the rapidly growing older age group in the world. The more developed nations are also increasing in numbers of older adult individuals; however, it is a much more gradual slope because much of the gain in longer life occurred decades ago. The same is true for the least developed nations, where life expectancy continues to be seriously compromised. Fig. 3.4 shows the percentage of the population that is 65 and over in comparison with the estimated total number of people. This figure shows that, although the percentage of the population constituted by older adults is growing all over the world, the nations with the largest percentage of older

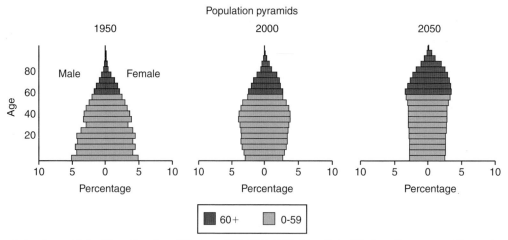

**FIGURE 3.5** Population Pyramids for More Developed Nations: 1950, 2000, 2050. (From United Nations, Department of Economic and Social Affairs, Population Division. [2007]. *World population ageing 2007.* United Nations Publications.)

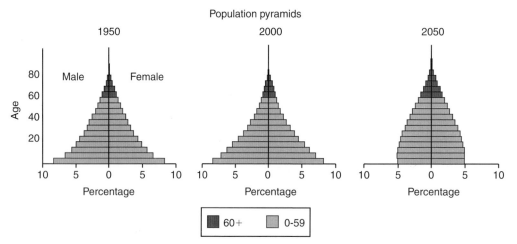

**FIGURE 3.6** Population Pyramids for Least Developed Nations: 1950, 2000, 2050. (From United Nations, Department of Economic and Social Affairs, Population Division. [2007]. *World population ageing 2007.* United Nations Publications.)

future differences in the aging structures of the more developed and less developed parts of the world. In 1950 both the more and less developed parts of the world exhibited an expansive pyramid structure; however, the more developed regions were already beginning to change. By the year 2000, there was a very clear difference between the age structures in the two areas. Whereas the less developed nations continued to exhibit the expansive structure, the more developed nations were clearly constrictive, beginning to look like a column of age groups rather than a pyramid. According to the projections for the year 2050, the more developed regions will be stationary in structure, whereas the least developed nations will begin to transition from an expansive to a constrictive structure. However, the rate of aging in the less developed regions of the globe is expected to outpace that of the more developed regions over that time period (United Nations & Department of Economic and Social Affairs, Population Division, 2013).

The health and demographic forces that lead to these different population pyramids are fertility rates, mortality rates, and longevity of older adults. As a result of decreases in the first two and increases in the latter, we see an aging of the population, on average. As shown in Fig. 3.7, life expectancy at birth has been, on average, rising steadily since 1950. Additionally,

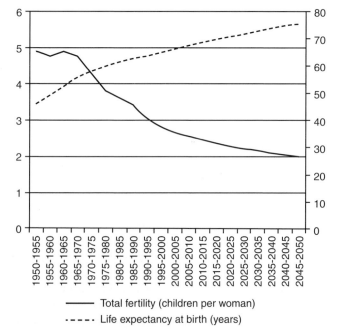

**FIGURE 3.7** World Fertility and Life Expectancy, 1950–2050. (Data from Population Division of the Department of Economic and Social Affairs of the United Nations Secretariat. *World population prospects: The 2008 revision.*)

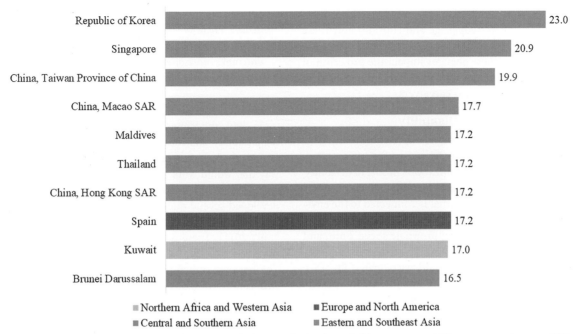

**FIGURE 3.8**   Countries or areas with the largest percentage point increase in the share of older persons aged 65 years or over between 2019 and 2050. (From World population ageing 2019, by United Nations, Department of Economic and Social Affairs, Population Division, © (2019) United Nations. Reprinted with the permission of the United Nations.)

the world fertility rate has been declining since 1950; however, the rate of decline has started to slow somewhat. Add to these trends increases in life expectancy after age 65, and the result is that a larger portion of the world's population is made up of older adults than ever before. As shown in Fig. 3.8, the highest projected increases in life expectancy after age 65 occur primarily in countries in the Eastern and Southeastern Asia region.

## Data on Population Characteristics and Population Health

Most countries collect surveillance data on the health and well-being of their populations. While individuals may be able to access these data or summaries from their own local or national public health agency, the Institute for Health Metrics and Evaluation at the University of Washington hosts a repository of much of this data, which is aggregated to form the Global Burden of Disease (GBD) study. There have been numerous publications using GBD data on a variety of topics including injuries, chronic health conditions, healthcare coverage, and population dynamics like migration and fertility.

The GBD global data repository includes information about a variety of health and health-related experiences and outcomes in a fully searchable online format. Using the GBD Compare tool, data can easily be displayed by country and, if sufficient data are collected, at the region/province/state level within countries. Data can be queried within age groups and by sex, enabling investigations into the experiences of older adults specifically. The GBD Compare tool presents data using mortality, years lived with disability, or disability-adjusted life years as the output, making it possible to understand both the causes of death and leading causes of disability

within populations. Finally, GBD data are available for about 15 years at the time of this writing, so they also are useful for understanding changes or trends over time. This information can be useful for planning programs or developing policies that will meet the current and projected needs of people within a population.

While OT practitioners may not regularly access or utilize data from the GBD or other data sources about the health and well-being of their populations, it can be useful to reference these periodically for updated information about trends and experiences that may impact the lives of clients or patients. When moving to a new practice area, it can also be a helpful starting point for understanding needs that may be common or conditions or impairments that may show up typically in the clinical or community-based practice setting. Reading published articles using GBD or similar data or engaging with an interactive tool like GBD Compare can help OT professionals be more informed and better able to anticipate the needs of the people with whom they interact in practice.

## Aging Adults: Disability, Health, and Quality of Life

The phenomenon described above, in which more people are living to older ages and there are more older adults within populations, brings with it a number of benefits and opportunities. These benefits include the accumulated wisdom of older adults and the expanded ability for older generations to exemplify continued engagement in meaningful occupations, as well as support and mentor younger generations. The opportunities include reconsidering a number of policies and services and, potentially, the expectations of society about what it means to grow older. For the purposes of this chapter, we will focus on some of the changes in disability, health status, and quality of life as people age and consider how these experiences may inform practice for occupational therapists. We also consider how these changes impact the provision of long-term care, especially as they relate to the inclusion of family and friends who serve as caregivers.

## Defining and Measuring Disability

Disability is a complex and changing experience. Many definitions of disability exist and have been used for different purposes. In the World Health Organization's model of disability, the International Classification of Functioning, Disability and Health (ICF), disability is a state that is connected to the environment in which people live (WHO, 2002). That is, given an environment in which there are appropriate social, built, and policy characteristics that accommodate a specific impairment or limitation, any person could participate fully. (See Chapter 11 for more information.) Disability is conceptually independent from health status or health conditions. As we note in the following section, there are causal links between health and disability, but not all disability is caused by a health condition and not all people living with a disability experience poor health as a result. The conceptual separation of health and disability is clearly described in the United States. *Healthy People* chapters on disability, which state:

> *Disability is a demographic descriptor rather than a health outcome. It should be used to monitor disparities in health outcomes and social participation.*
>
> **Healthy People (2010)**

> *A diagnosis of impairment or disabling condition does not define individuals, their talents and abilities, or health behaviors and health status. Consistent with the World Health*

> *Organization's (WHO) model of social determinants of health, Healthy People 2020 recognizes that what defines individuals with disabilities, their abilities, and their health outcomes more often depends on their community, including social and environmental circumstances.*
>
> **Healthy People (2020)**

In 2001, the United Nations formed the Washington Group on Disability Statistics (herein referred to as the Washington Group) to develop a set of questions to identify disability in a way that would work across cultures and enable the collection of consistent and comparable disability statistics. The group has developed several question sets designed to measure disability, including a short set that includes six items (Box 3.1) (Madans et al., 2011). These questions ask about difficulties with hearing, vision, mobility, cognition, self-care, and communication. The response options reflect the degree of difficulty one has in each area using a four-category response set: no difficulty, some difficulty, a lot of difficulty, and cannot do at all. There are also recommended cut points for defining the presence of a disability.

In addition to these questions developed for use in national surveys or censuses, the ICF has a coding scheme somewhat similar to the International Classification of Diseases (ICD) that captures information on domains of body functions (e.g., hearing functions; code b210), body structures (e.g., structure of inner ear, cochlea; code s2600) activities and participation (e.g. conversation; code d350), and environment (e.g. sound; code e250: individual attitudes of strangers; code 2445). These codes could be used by clinicians in a way that is analogous to the use of ICD codes, to document and track aspects of function and environment. For OT staff, this could include mapping therapy goals to the ICF. See the online appendix for more information about

---

| **Box 3.1** | Measuring disability using Washington Group on Disability Statistics Short Set on Functioning (the International Disability Data Collection Standard for Censuses and Surveys) |
|---|---|

**Washington Group Short Set on Functioning (WG SS)**

Preamble to the WG-SS:

Note: The purpose of the introduction is to serve as a transition from questions in the census or survey instrument that deal with other subject matters to this new area of inquiry, and to focus the respondent on difficulties they may have doing basic activities. Use of the introductory statement may not be needed in all situations, especially if including the statement may interrupt the flow of question administration.

Interviewer read: "The next questions ask about difficulties you may have doing certain activities."

1.  Do you have difficulty seeing, even if wearing glasses?
2.  Do you have difficulty hearing, even if using a hearing aid?
3.  Do you have difficulty walking or climbing stairs?
4.  Do you have difficulty remembering or concentrating?
5.  Do you have difficulty (with self-care such as) washing all over or dressing?
6.  Using your usual (customary) language, do you have difficulty communicating, for example understanding or being understood by others?

Response options are:

(1) No, no difficulty
(2) Yes, some difficulty
(3) Yes, a lot of difficulty
(4) Cannot do at all

The recommended cutoff for calculating disability is any "a lot of difficulty" or "cannot do at all/unable" response across the six functioning domains.
Source: Washington Group on Disability Statistics. (2017). *About the Washington Group.* http://www.washingtongroup-disability.com/

both the Washington Group disability measures and mapping ICF codes in practice.

## Key Health Conditions Associated With Disability

While not all disabilities are related to a specific health condition, chronic physical, mental, and emotional conditions can limit the ability of adults to perform important basic activities of daily living (ADLs) and instrumental activities of daily living (IADLs), such as working and doing everyday household chores. These activity limitations are more common among older adults than among people in younger age groups (National Center for Health Statistics [US] & Gindi, 2021). American

Community Survey data from 2020 show that among the civilian noninstitutionalized population aged 18 and older, 15.1% have a disability (calculation based on data in Table S1810, Disability Characteristics; see online appendix for direct link). Fig. 3.9 illustrates that the older a person is, the more likely they are to develop disability across each of the six domains measured. These trends together with the changing demographics described earlier in the chapter predict a future population that is more functionally limited and in need of more OT services, particularly as people reach age 75 and older.

Leading causes of death and leading causes of disability often differ from one another, illustrated in Table 3.3. While some chronic conditions may ultimately result in limitations

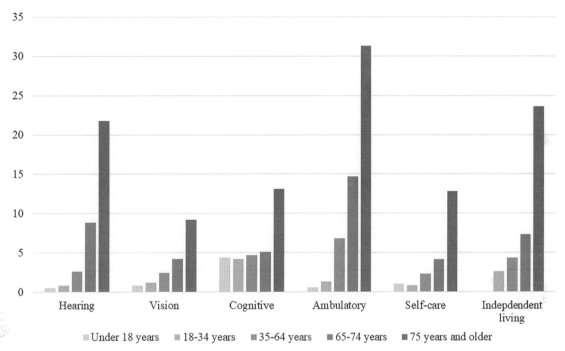

**FIGURE 3.9**    Prevalence of a disability, defined as any difficulty, by disability and age group, American Community Survey 2020. Note: Independent living disability is not asked about respondents under age 18. (Data from Table S1810, Disability Characteristics; see online appendix for direct link.)

**TABLE 3.3** Leading Causes of Mortality and Disability in the United States

| Leading Causes of Death (Deaths in 2020)[a] | Leading Causes of Disability (Estimated Population, 2005)[b] |
| --- | --- |
| Heart disease (696,962) | Arthritis or rheumatism (8,552,000) |
| Cancer (602,350) | Back or spine problems (7,589,000) |
| COVID-19 (350,831) | Heart trouble (2,988,000) |
| Unintentional injuries (200,955) | Lung or respiratory problem (2,224,000) |
| Stroke (160,264) | Mental or emotional problem (2,203,000) |
| Chronic lower respiratory diseases (152,657) | Diabetes (2,012,000) |
| Alzheimer disease (134,242) | Deafness or hearing problem (1,908,000) |
| Diabetes (102,188) | Stiffness or deformity of limbs/extremities (1,627,000) |
| Influenza and pneumonia (53,544) | Blindness or vision problem (1,460,000) |
| Kidney disease (52,547) | Stroke (1,076,000) |

[a]Source: National Center for Health Statistics (2022); see online appendix for direct link.
[b]Source: Centers for Disease Control and Prevention (2009). These are self- reported by persons in the Survey of Income and Program Participation (SIPP). Disability was defined as having difficulty with activities of daily living and instrumental activities of daily living. Centers for Disease Control and Prevention (CDC). (2009). Prevalence and most common causes of disability among adults—United States, 2005. *Morbidity and Mortality Weekly Report, 58*(16), 421–426. Note that SIPP methods have changed and more recent data are therefore not available. However, the order and classifications listed in the table are generally consistent with data from the 2019 Global Burden of Disease study data from 2019 on the years lived with disability in the United States by condition/category.

and disability, many people live without disability while having a chronic condition. Conversely, disability may arise from a condition that is unlikely to cause death, or disability may occur with no link to a diagnosed health condition.

Next, we highlight three chronic diseases with high prevalence in older adult populations and with very different needs in terms of gerontological OT. These are stroke, arthritis, and dementia. Stroke is the fifth most common cause of death in the United States, killing more than 160,000 people in 2020, the most current year for which complete data are available (National Center for Health Statistics [US] & Gindi, 2021). The American Heart Association estimates that someone in America has a stroke, on average, every 40 seconds (Virani et al., 2020). Demographic factors contribute to stroke risk. Age increases risk, as does being a member of an ethnic or racial minority (Tsao et al., 2022). Native American, multiracial, and African American groups are at higher risk of stroke compared with white and Asian Americans. In addition to mortality, there are financial, functional, and other costs to survivors, caregivers, and society.

Stroke rehabilitation needs are expansive and varied. While many people are discharged to a rehabilitation or skilled facility after being hospitalized for stroke, a substantial proportion return home directly, with or without formal home health care, and some move into palliative or hospice care (Tsao et al., 2022). Following stroke, there may be short-term complications like pneumonia or urinary tract infections, or longer-term impacts including seizure, pain, insomnia, depression, and mobility impairments (Tsao et al., 2022). Studies have shown that among those who survive stroke, physical and cognitive function declines more rapidly than among people with no history of a stroke (Tsao et al., 2022).

Another common condition that contributes to functional impairment is arthritis. Based on data from the 2016 to 2018 National Health Interview Survey (NHIS) in the United States, nearly one in four adults has arthritis and, among these, more than 40% experienced activity limitations as a result of arthritis (Theis, 2021). Arthritis-associated activity limitations were particularly high among people who were non-Hispanic American Indian or Alaska Native and people who reported multiple racial backgrounds. Based on these data, the prevalence of both arthritis and activity limitations associated with it are increasing, continuing a trend that has been observed for nearly 20 years (Theis, 2021). Other data have suggested that the prevalence of arthritis and related limitations will increase by about half in the coming decades (Hootman et al., 2016).

As with stroke, incidence of arthritis increases with age: 50% of adults aged 65 and older have been diagnosed with arthritis compared to 7% of adults aged 18 to 44 years (Theis, 2021). Risk factors for arthritis and arthritis-attributable activity limitation include obesity and physical inactivity. Other social determinants of health, including educational attainment and poverty status, have also been linked to arthritis (Theis, 2021).

Dementia is a category of diseases that shares some similar signs and symptoms and reflects damage to neurons in the brain. The most common type of dementia is Alzheimer disease, which accounts for 60% to 80% of cases (Alzheimer's Association, 2022). Dementia diagnoses increase markedly with age, with the vast majority of Alzheimer disease cases diagnosed among people aged 65 or older (Alzheimer's Association, 2022). Current estimates indicate that 6.5 million Americans are living with Alzheimer dementia, a number expected to grow to 13.8 million by 2060 without novel prevention or treatments (Alzheimer's Association, 2022). Dementia, like some other chronic health conditions, is progressive, meaning that over time more neurons will be damaged, resulting in increasing symptoms. Typically, brain regions responsible for memory, language, and thinking are affected early in the disease process while over time more regions experience damage; ultimately, movement, behavior, mood, and personality also can be changed or impaired (Alzheimer's Association, 2022).

The Aging, Demographics and Memory Study (ADAMS) has added significantly to our understanding of dementia at the population level in the United States (Plassman et al., 2007). ADAMS is a population-based study of dementia that includes individuals from all regions of the United States and aims to determine the prevalence of dementia. Based on ADAMS data (Table 3.4), 13.9% of all Americans aged 71 and older have some form of dementia. However, there is a steep increase in prevalence during the eighth and ninth decades of life, and among those 90 years old, 37.4% have some form of dementia (Plassman et al., 2007). The study found no significant difference in rate of dementia between men and women. However, because there are more women among the oldest old, there are more women living with dementia (Alzheimer's Association, 2021; Plassman et al., 2007). A few risk factors that have been consistently associated with dementia other than age are lack of physical activity,

**TABLE 3.4**  US Estimates of the Number of Individuals With Dementia or Alzheimer Disease, 2002

| Age (years) | All Dementia Number (95% CI) | Alzheimer Disease Number (95% CI) |
| --- | --- | --- |
| 71–79 | 712,000 (375,000–1,050,000) | 332,000 (181,000–483,000) |
| 80–89 | 1,996,000 (1,590,000–2,401,000) | 1,493,000 (1,111,000–1,875,000) |
| 901 | 699,000 (476,000–922,000) | 2,381,000 (1,849,000–2,913,000) |
| Total | 3,407,000 (2,793,000–4,021,000) | 2,381,000 (1,849,000–2,913,000) |

CI, Confidence interval.
Data from Plassman, B. L., Langa, K. M., Fisher, G. G., Heeringa, S. G., Weir, D. R., Ofstedal, M. B., et al. (2007). Prevalence of dementia in the United States: The aging, demographics, and memory study. *Neuroepidemiology*, 29(1–2), 125–132.

lower levels of education, and presence of the apolipoprotein E (APOE) ε4 genotype (Plassman et al., 2007).

## Family Caregivers Providing Support for Aging Adults

As the population is aging and many older adults are experiencing functional and cognitive impairments, the need for people to support and care for these older adults also is growing. Most older adults prefer to remain in their homes as they age, and in many parts of the world, there are not long-term care facilities available or accessible to all older adults with functional needs. More and more of our older adults rely on informal caregivers—those family members, friends, and neighbors who assist with everyday activities and even health care at home. When considering the effects of global aging, OT providers need to include considerations of the effects of clients on their larger social and family support systems (Boxes 3.2 and 3.3). Informal caregivers can be considered part of the environment based on the ICF model, and they can be helpful in enabling people with disabilities and health conditions to participate in daily activities and in society.

Efforts are ongoing to better involve informal caregivers in formal health-care delivery systems so that they both have the information and skills they need to provide care at home without becoming overwhelmed and to share their observations of the person for whom they are caring with the formal health-care team (Boucher et al., 2020; Shepherd-Banigan et al., 2021). One example of this effort is the Campaign for Inclusive Care funded by the Elizabeth Dole Foundation in the United States (see online appendix for link). While this training was developed for health-care professionals in the Veterans Health Administration, it was designed to be used by various practitioners, including OTs, and its principles may be applicable to other patient/client populations and settings.

## Elder Mistreatment Assessment and Best Practices

In general, elder mistreatment may be defined as any intentional, knowing, or negligent act, or failure to act, by a caregiver or another person in a relationship involving an expectation of trust, that causes harm or creates a risk of harm to an older adult (Department of Justice, 2014;

---

**Box 3.2**   Caregiving in the United States

Data from the United States provide information on informal caregiving arrangements. In the 2019, National Alliance for Caregiving (NAC) random-digit-dialed survey, caregivers were defined as individuals 18 years of age or older who provided unpaid care to a relative or friend 18 years of age or older and assistance with one or more ADLs or IADLs during the previous 12 months (National Alliance for Caregiving, 2020). The NAC estimated that there are 53 million caregivers in the United States (21% of the adult population). Among these, more than one quarter (26%) reported that they provided care for someone with Alzheimer disease, another dementia, or mental confusion; this proportion rises to one third (32%) of caregivers for people aged 65 or older. While these caregivers frequently feel the role brings positive experiences, including purpose and meaning (51%), the NAC demonstrated that caregivers who had higher levels of caregiving (measured in terms of time and activities) also had poorer outcomes, including physical, emotional, and financial strains (National Alliance for Caregiving, 2020).

The Behavioral Risk Factors Surveillance System (BRFSS) is another source of data that provides periodic reports on US caregiving Centers for Disease Control and Prevention, Alzheimer's Disease and Healthy Aging Program Home (n.d.-b). The BRFSS is an ongoing state-based telephone survey conducted by the CDC that collects information on health-related risk behaviors, chronic health conditions, and use of preventive services. In 2000, a single BRFSS question asked about caregiving of adults aged 60 and older. The prevalence of caregiving varied considerably. Nationally, 15.6% of adults reported they were caregivers for an older adult (Neugaard et al., 2008). However, there was geographic variation, with the highest levels in the southeastern states, where chronic conditions also are high (e.g., 21.2% in Missouri, and 20.4% in West Virginia), and the lowest levels in the West (e.g., Alaska, 9.9%; Hawaii, 10.5%).

Several years later, the CDC developed the Caregiver Module, a set of questions that could be added by states to the BRFSS. The new module defined caregivers as any person 18 years of age or older who provides care or assistance to a family member or friend, of any age, because of illness or disability. Based on this definition, about 20% of respondents have reported providing care (Anderson et al., 2013; Trivedi et al., 2014), though, as in the early data, there is substantial geographic variation. In these expanded inquiries, caregivers have experienced poorer health and quality of life than their non-caregiver peers. When asked about the greatest difficulties regarding caregiving, the majority of respondents reported that caregiving creates stress, leaves too little time for self or family, and creates a financial burden (Kusano et al., 2011). In combination with NAC data, these results suggest that caregiving is a common role, and that, although this role provides invaluable assistance for the recipients, it comes at a personal and perhaps societal cost.

Global estimates of the frequency of caregiving are not available, although other countries have conducted similar population-based studies, and many have found that caregivers tend to experience more stress, poor mental health, and, in some cases, poor physical health (Do et al., 2015; National Academies of Sciences, Engineering, and Medicine, 2016; Stratmann et al., 2021). It is likely that the prevalence, effects, and importance of caregiving are at least as varied globally as they are among US states. Social and cultural norms and traditions, work and family roles and expectations, geographic disbursement of families—all of these play a role in determining the likelihood that a person who ages with the need for assistance will have informal (family or neighborhood) support versus formal assistance, and the effect of providing that care on the caregivers themselves.

*ADLs*, Activities of daily living; *CDC*, Centers for Disease Control and Prevention; *IADLs*, instrumental activities of daily living.

---

### Box 3.3    Caregiving in Japan

Japan experienced dramatic increases in its older adult population following World War II. Japan has the highest proportion of older adults of any country in the world, and also the highest ratio of older adults (aged 65 and older) to working-age adults (aged 20–64): for every 100 working age adults in Japan, there are 51 older adults (United Nations & Department of Economic and Social Affairs, Population Division, 2019). Japanese culture sets care of the aged as a responsibility of the succeeding generation. These expectations are part of cultural standards related to the patrilineal extended family.

Traditionally, as a couple aged, their first son's wife was expected to fulfill all the hands-on caregiving responsibilities for her parents-in-law (Yamamoto & Wallhagen, 1997). There have been significant social changes in Japan in recent decades, including more women working outside the home and fewer homes being multi-generational, which has changed the caregiving expectations to some extent. National efforts have sought to address gaps and challenges in family caregiving. In 2000, Japan implemented a long-term care insurance system with the aim of enabling people to age in their communities without over-burdening family caregivers, emotionally or financially (Yamada & Arai, 2020). Funded by individual tax payments, government funding, premiums, and copayments, the system has been a model for other countries, but also faces fiscal challenges as the population continues to age and more people become eligible for services (Yamada & Arai, 2020). In response, Japan moved toward population-based disability prevention activities in 2015 with the aim of preventing or delaying disability for citizens as they age. While these efforts are evolving, they demonstrate the potential to integrate a public health and clinical approach to supporting people across the lifespan, including improving quality of life and enabling community living.

---

National Center on Elder Abuse, n.d.; National Research Council, 2002). However, specific legal definitions of elder mistreatment vary from state to state. Elder mistreatment is frequently categorized into six types that include physical abuse, emotional/psychological abuse, sexual abuse, neglect, financial exploitation, and self-neglect. However, it is common for multiple types of mistreatment to occur at the same time, or at different times, throughout the remaining lifespan (Williams et al., 2020). Our best estimate is that at least 11% of cognitively intact older adults (defined here as age 60+) experience elder mistreatment each year. However, because that estimate was derived from a telephone survey where people were called at random, most researchers believe that the true annual prevalence of elder mistreatment is actually higher. Further, there is evidence from smaller cross-sectional studies that as many as 30% to 50% of cognitively impaired older adults may experience elder mistreatment each year (Cooper et al., 2009; Wiglesworth et al., 2010). People who have mistreated an older adult most often fall into one of three groups that include spouses, adult children, or friends and neighbors

(Lachs & Pillemer, 2015; Pillemer & Finkelhor, 1989). Risk factors include low levels of social support, cognitive impairment, prior abuse exposure, dependence, frailty, mental health problems, substance use problems, and financial problems (Acierno et al., 2010; Dong, 2015; Lachs & Pillemer, 2015). The public health impact of elder mistreatment is considerable with elder mistreatment increasing risk for depression, functional decline, emergency room visits, hospital admissions, and all-cause mortality compared to non-maltreated older adults (Baker et al., 2009; Burnett et al., 2016; Cannell et al., 2015; Dong et al., 2012; Dong & Simon, 2013a, 2013b; Lachs et al., 1998; Mouton et al., 2010; Schofield et al., 2013). The costs associated with lost income, recovery from financial abuse, and the medical, legal, and social service intervention needed by mistreated older adults is estimated to be in the billions of dollars each year (Department of Justice, 2014).

Given the importance of elder mistreatment, it may not surprise you to learn that OT practitioners have an ethical and legal obligation to be aware of the indicators of potential elder mistreatment and to report potential elder mistreatment to the appropriate authorities. The first principle of The American Occupational Therapy Association's Code of Ethics is beneficence, which "requires taking action to benefit others—in other words, to promote good, to prevent harm, and to remove harm. Examples of beneficence include protecting and defending the rights of others, preventing harm from occurring to others, removing conditions that will cause harm to others, offering services that benefit persons with disabilities, and acting to protect and remove persons from dangerous situations" (American Occupational Therapy Association 2020 Occupational Therapy Code of Ethics, 2020). In addition to this ethical obligation, every state in the United States has laws that mandate the reporting of elder mistreatment to the authorities—typically Adult Protective Services (APS). However, if you feel your patient/client's health and safety are in immediate danger, you should also contact local law enforcement. The Elder Abuse Guide for Law Enforcement (EAGLE) website contains information about each state's specific mandated reporting laws (see online appendix for more information).

Given that OTs are mandated reporters, it is useful to be aware of some of the indicators of elder mistreatment. Table 3.5 outlines some warning signs of *potential* elder mistreatment. However, we want to emphasize that it is not your responsibility to investigate or "diagnose" elder mistreatment. That responsibility falls on Adult Protective Services (APS) and/or local law enforcement. It is only your responsibility to be aware of the indicators of elder mistreatment and report those indicators to APS if you suspect that an older adult *may* be living with elder mistreatment.

In addition to being aware of potential indicators, there are a few other best practices to keep in mind when serving patients/clients who may be living with elder mistreatment. First, remember to consider elder mistreatment as a possible factor in the older adult's presentation, and always take an older adult's self-report of mistreatment seriously. Second, make a habit of talking to older adults about mistreatment as part of their medical history. There are many reasons why

**TABLE 3.5** Some Common Indicators of Elder Mistreatment

| Type of Mistreatment | Indicators |
|---|---|
| Physical abuse | Bruises, pressure marks or sores, broken bones, abrasions, and burns |
| Emotional/psychological abuse | Withdrawal from normal activities, anxiety, depression, unusual behavior, or unease |
| Sexual abuse | Bruises or injury to the genital area which may present as difficulty moving or sitting |
| Neglect | Bedsores, unattended medical needs, poor hygiene, and unusual weight loss |
| Financial exploitation | Uncharacteristic purchases by the individual or caregiver; failure to pay bills or keep appointments; questionable behavior |

Adapted from: National Center on Elder Abuse. (2022). *What are the warning signs of elder abuse? National Center on Elder Abuse—FAQ.* Accessed March 30, 2022 (see online appendix for direct link).

people may not talk about the mistreatment they are living with if you do not ask. Third, you should typically separate the older adult and their caregiver when discussing potential mistreatment. Fourth, repeat the older adult's responses back to them. This will allow you to clarify your understanding and allow the older adult time for reflection. Finally, try to ask questions in a nonjudgmental way. Saying something like, "Caregiving is a difficult job, and many people feel angry, confused, or out of control" may help you establish rapport with the caregiver. There is even some evidence that caregivers are eager to talk to someone about mistreating an older adult if they feel as though it is safe to do so (Ahmad & Lachs, 2002).

Ultimately, if you suspect elder mistreatment *may* be occurring, you have a legal and ethical responsibility to report your suspicion to Adult Protective Services. Do not allow your suspicions or treatment/intervention plan to be influenced by misconceptions about mistreatment, including beliefs that it is rare, does not occur in "normal" families, is a private matter that you shouldn't interfere with, or that it is caused by the older adult's own actions. Discuss any suspicion of mistreatment sensitively with the older adult and explain to them that you have an obligation to contact adult protective services. The goal is not to punish anyone. Rather, the goal is to help the older adult and their caregiver get the resources they need to be safe and healthy (Ahmad & Lachs, 2002).

## Implications for Occupational Therapy Service Delivery

This epidemiologic foundation provides an understanding of changing United States and global demographics and associated current and projected effects on the incidence of disease and disability over time. The discussion specifically provides

the history and projections of aging-associated morbidity and mortality to provide a basis for reflection regarding what types of OT interventions are needed currently and will be needed in the future. Furthermore, the knowledge shared on age-related disease and disability risk factors serves to inform OT personnel in reinforcing the use of health-supporting and health-promoting interventions. This information requires us to examine our current interventions to determine whether they address the emerging needs of aging individuals, their families, and communities. In addition, the disease and disability risk data provide a roadmap for the development of new therapeutic approaches. We are called to apply continuous surveillance of both historical and new disease and disability patterns as they emerge. As holistic, quality-of-life-supporting practitioners, OT personnel are equipped to integrate this information into the changing health-care systems environment. In doing so, the profession can also serve on the forefront of meeting the changing needs of society.

Occupational therapy services have historically been predominantly provided within medical health-care delivery systems (refer also to Chapter 25 on health-care systems). Community-based services providing home health care and support systems for individuals with mental illness have been available since the 1920s in the United States; however, these have been limited in scope and capacity for reimbursement. In 1978 the WHO convened an international conference on primary health care that resulted in a declaration that health is a fundamental right of people around the globe (WHO, 2004). The influence of this declaration, the implications of the changing demographics and related disease burden reported earlier, and the evolving health-care systems globally indicate expanded opportunity for occupational therapy personnel—both OTs and OT assistants. Because demographic trajectories suggest increased numbers of aging adults and associated chronic conditions in both developed and developing countries, OT personnel are called to address health-related aging issues in health-promoting modes across the continuum of care. More than 50 years ago Leavell and Clark proposed an epidemiologic model of preventive medicine that covered the entire continuum of medical care and is well suited to the thinking of today with regard to the emphasis on health-promoting services (Leavell & Clark, 1965). Fig. 3.10, based on Leavell and Clark's model, depicts the role of occupational therapy in health promotion activities throughout the continuum of care. To align with the age-related forecasts regarding disease, disability, morbidity, and mortality, OT providers can revise their clinical reasoning processes and their orientation to the provision of services, incorporating informal caregivers into their approach. These can be expanded to "professional reasoning" and a health-promoting orientation, both of which fit all types of settings, whether clinical or community based. Furthermore, around the world and in the United States, the health-care reform era holds all providers accountable for population health—that of the communities served. Thus this adaptation is required in order to better serve the needs of individuals, communities, and other populations with whom OT personnel interact. Developed countries outside of the United States with government-funded health-care systems

| GERONTOLOGICAL OCCUPATIONAL THERAPY SERVICE OPPORTUNITIES | | | | |
|---|---|---|---|---|
| No disease or condition identified | | Disease or condition diagnosed | | |
| Health promotion interventions | Specific protection and prompt treatment | Early diagnosis and prompt treatment | Disability limitation | Rehabilitation |
| Primary prevention | | Secondary prevention | | Tertiary prevention |
| Public health practice | | Primary medical care | Secondary medical care | Long-term care/hospice |
| Community-oriented | | Individual and community orientation | | Dual emphasis |

**FIGURE 3.10**   Health Promotion Throughout the Continuum of Care. (Modified from Leavell, H. R., & Clark, E. G. [1965]. *Preventive medicine for the doctor in his community: An epidemiologic approach* [3rd ed.]. Blakiston-McGraw Hill.)

already have incorporated many of these elements and roles. Important health-promoting lessons may be learned from them, because their morbidity and mortality rates are currently better than those of the United States (Woolf, 2012). Thus, also refer to Chapter 25, which provides a health-care services overview in the United States compared with other high-income countries.

## Occupational Therapy in Community-Based Primary Prevention

Until recently in the United States, most OT providers had not participated in primary care types of services. For at least 20 years, a few entrepreneurial therapists have engaged in health-promoting and health-protecting interventions in their private practices, which have addressed the needs of individuals and communities across the lifespan. The field of occupational therapy has always been inherently holistic and can therefore address the primary health-promoting needs of aging populations (see Chapter 26).

An example of a long-term, well-established health-promoting service agency for aging adults is Independent Living, Inc. (ILI). ILI was established in 1967 by Jean Kiernat and Betty Hasselkus, OT faculty at the University of Wisconsin–Madison, and social workers in Dane County, Wisconsin; these services continue today. These OT visionaries understood the importance of occupational performance and engagement, and the social support needs of aging adults. Thus, they founded ILI to provide services so that older adults could remain living at home for as long as possible. As a non-medical agency, ILI has provided interprofessional services for approximately 3000 older adults each year. Initial OT services included home safety assessments and interventions by OTs, as well as social work support services. These later evolved so that an *OTR* and a certified occupational therapy assistant (COTA) supervised a carpenter who made grab bar installations and built chair and sofa extenders, before their commercial availability. Services were initially funded by grants or contracts, and additionally included consultations and interventions to adapt the living environments of aging residents of congregate living facilities. Adaptations included a range of modifications, including adding or adjusting

lighting, highlighting stair edges and appliances to accommodate age-related vision changes, supplying adaptive equipment for bathrooms, and educating residents on safety precautions to prevent falls and other injuries. Serving all of Dane County, Wisconsin, these services have expanded and has continued to provide health-promoting services for 55 years.

An innovative and life-enriching community-based program, Older Adult Service and Information Services (OASIS), in St. Louis, Missouri, was established by an adult educator, Marylen Mann, in consultation with Carolyn Baum, of The Program in Occupational Therapy at Washington University in 1982. OASIS initially began in a May Department Store in St. Louis. Over 40 years it expanded to sites throughout the United States and includes classes, intergenerational activities, and other health-promoting activities for adults of age 50 and over.

The Well Elderly series of randomized control trials, conducted by Florence Clark and her University of Southern California OT faculty associates, demonstrated the effectiveness and the efficacy of OT intervention with independently living aging adults. These trials have continued since findings were first published in 1997 and have provided much needed evidence to support the role of OT in health promotion and reduced morbidity among multicultural study participants (Clark, 2012; Clark et al., 1997, 2001). Overall findings have consistently demonstrated the positive effect of OT health promotion interventions on health and age-related changes, which typically result in functional decline. Their studies for the past two decades have used state-of-the-art interdisciplinary research design, including biomarker and quality-of-life measurement. Consistent results include improvement in general health and vitality, function, and quality-of-life domains (Clark, 2012; Clark et al., 1997, 2001).

The American Occupational Therapy Association collaboration with the American Automobile Association (AAA) and the American Association of Retired Persons (AARP) to develop the CarFit program is another example of a primary health promotion effort tailored for OT personnel to engage with aging adults in promoting driver, passenger, and societal safety. The program provides information and materials on resources that can enhance aging drivers' occupational performance and safety, and potentially increase their community mobility, thus positively affecting IADL function. (See also Chapters 20 and 21.)

## Occupational Therapy in Secondary Prevention Services

Occupational therapy has played a role in community programs providing secondary prevention services for the Arthritis Foundation throughout the United States for at least four decades. These have primarily consisted of classes to educate groups and individuals with arthritis diagnoses about how to manage their lives despite their disease process. Classes led by OTs teach and promote joint protection techniques, assist in organizing activities to promote energy conservation, promote arthritis-related exercise and swim programs, and coach regarding strategies to plan older adults' everyday lives to include meaningful occupational balance.

In addition, OT has been instrumental in developing programs for early intervention for aging adults with mild cognitive impairment that evolved into different forms of dementia, including Alzheimer disease. Throughout the years of increasing organizational development, occupational therapists have paired with the national and local Alzheimer's Association offices to plan and conduct numerous programs. These programs target the unique and diverse needs of those with dementia and their families and caregivers to support overall function and quality of life for all who are involved. Note that Chapter 16 offers additional information on related programs.

Occupational therapists serve on planning committees and as providers for other organizations that serve the more specific needs of those with dementia and their family and other support networks. They assist in determining and tailoring environmental and other cognitive supports for this population, including their caregivers.

## Occupational Therapy in Tertiary Care

Tertiary prevention in rehabilitation and long-term care and hospice care settings is individually oriented and tailored to the specific needs of the individual, family, and/or other supports. Historically, the profession has typically thought of this aspect of care as medical treatment. However, based upon Leavell and Clark's epidemiologic model of preventive medicine and on the public health definition of tertiary prevention, tertiary care should also be considered for health promotion interventions. Throughout the intervening years since Leavell and Clark's model was developed, as thinking about supports for quality of life and cost containment evolved, this model has stood the test of time and thus represents a "goodness of fit" with ethical, economic, and quality-of-life approaches to health care. Thus, we are challenged to view all levels of care as opportunities for health promotion, and OT is especially well aligned to meet this challenge. Hence, whether services are provided for an aging individual who sustained a hip or Colles fracture, cerebrovascular accident, or spinal cord injury, or who is certified for hospice care, a health promotion approach is optimal. Through a holistic approach in collaboration with the client, family members, informal caregivers, and the broader community, occupational therapists strive for creative problem solving and meaningful goals for each individual served.

As technological capacity has advanced and in the wake of the COVID-19 pandemic in particular, OTs, like other health professionals, have learned to utilize and leverage telehealth in the care of their clients. While many activities, like home assessments, are more challenging to do virtually, there are programs and services that can be delivered remotely in times of public health crisis or to reach people living in areas with limited access to OT services and rehabilitation care. The COVID-19 pandemic has highlighted the potential for OTs to partner with their public health colleagues who typically lead or contribute substantially to emergency preparedness at the community level. The firsthand knowledge and experience of OTs working with older adults in their homes and communities is critical to developing an effective and equitable emergency response plan (Kailes & Enders, 2007).

## SUMMARY

This chapter has introduced some of the most relevant concepts from epidemiology and public health to enable OT professionals to understand and use population-level data on demographic and health trends, and to evaluate the evidence of and intervention's effectiveness to inform their practice. As the trend toward longer lives and more older adults in populations globally continues, OTs are well-positioned to serve individuals as they age and to partner with public health agencies and colleagues to both identify the best strategies and services for older adults and to work at all levels of prevention to assure the health and quality of life of older adults is maximized, regardless of the presence of disability.

*The complete listing of the Bibliography and Chapter Questions and Answers are available in the accompanying enhanced eBook version included with the print purchase of this textbook. Visit Elsevier eBooks+ (eBooks.Health.Elsevier.com) to access this content.*

## CHAPTER 4

# Social Theories of Aging Relevant to Occupational Therapy

*Debbie Laliberte Rudman, PhD, OT Reg. (Ont.) and Clare Hocking, PhD, NZROT*

## CHAPTER OUTLINE

## OBJECTIVES

- Identify social theories and models of relevance to understanding occupation within the aging process
- Differentiate social theories and models from biomedical conceptualizations of aging
- Interpret theories and models of aging from an occupational perspective
- Explore occupational science research that draws upon and can be used to analyze the strengths and limitations of theories and models of aging
- Begin to envision possible applications of theories and models of aging to occupational therapists' gerontology-based practice

Gerontology, a discipline specifically focused on the study of aging and older adults, was founded between the late 1930s to mid-1940s. Since that time, given the complexity of the aging process, gerontology has become increasingly interdisciplinary, incorporating scholars and ideas from various biomedical, clinical, behavioral, and social sciences, as well as the arts and humanities (Bengtson et al., 2005a; Hocking & Meltzer, 2016). As a result, there are many theories that focus on different dimensions of the aging process, drawing attention to particular aspects of aging while simultaneously backgrounding other aspects (Estes et al., 2003). For example, biological theories examine cellular dimensions, psychological theories focus on cognitive and behavioral dimensions, feminist theories address gendered dimensions, geographical theories highlight spatial dimensions, and humanities theories delve into moral and existential dimensions. Aging theories also address various scales, with micro-level theories addressing aging as an individual process, meso-level theories addressing aging as an interactional process, and macro-level theories addressing aging as a socially structured process. In addition, theories exist that bring together different disciplinary perspectives and link micro-, meso-, and macro-level scales (Estes, 2005; Marcoen et al., 2007; Phillips et al., 2010a, 2010b; Skinner et al., 2018). Overall, there is no one theory that explains all of the dimensions involved in aging, but rather many theories of aging that provide ways to understand the aging process and inform how health-care professionals, governments, and other social actors move forward in designing practices, systems, and policies addressing aging and older adults (Phillips et al., 2010b). Different theories of aging provide "different lenses that can enrich our understanding of the multiple facets of ageing" (Bengtson et al., 2005a, p. 8). As such, occupational therapists need to critically consider which aging theories are appropriate and relevant to their practice contexts and the older adults with whom they are working.

Gerontological theories relevant to occupational therapy are woven through the various chapters in this book, such as Chapter 19 addressing the successful aging paradigm, Chapter 20 addressing the physical environment and aging, and Chapter 24 addressing the humanities and the arts. Given the diversity and number of theories of aging that exist, in this chapter, we have narrowed our focus to various categories of social theories of aging that attend to everyday activity as part of the aging process. Given the focus on everyday activity, these theories are relevant to occupational therapy's core construct of occupation and thus can serve to inform occupational therapy practice and research with older adults. As will be detailed below, these theories address everyday activity in various ways and at various scales, attending to its meaning and significance in the lives of older adults and various micro to macro-level factors that shape what activities older adults do and do not do as individuals and as part of a social collective.

We start this chapter by defining what we mean by "social theories" of aging and highlight the important contributions they have made in expanding perspectives in gerontology beyond a biomedical perspective. To provide an understanding of how social theories have changed over time and have contributed to increasingly complex understandings of activity and aging, we have organized the remainder of this chapter around temporal phases and corresponding theoretical strands. Using this temporal organization, it can be seen how theories have shifted from an initial focus on activity as part of individuals' successful adjustment to aging to a focus on social, economic, political, and other contextual forces that shape possibilities for activities through the aging process at individual to collective levels. Many contemporary social theories of aging attempt to link micro, meso, and macro understandings, for example, looking at how aging individuals negotiate their everyday activities in relation to broader contextual features that create both constraints and possibilities for activities. To illustrate the relevance of various theoretical perspectives, we also provide examples of knowledge produced through occupational science and occupational therapy scholarship that has been influenced by these various theoretical strands and that has contributed to deepening understanding of how older adults' occupations are experienced, negotiated, and shaped through socio-political forces.

## Expanding Beyond the Biomedicalization of Aging: Social Theories

Gerontology emerged as a discipline during an historical period in which there was a growing emphasis on how science, in the form of quantifiable, objective models aligned with the natural sciences, could advance society. In this context, "science—and most especially biomedicine—was viewed as the most influential source for tackling many of the problems and challenges associated with ageing" (Estes et al., 2003, p. 10). However, over time, it was increasingly recognized that the dominance of a biomedical perspective, while generating knowledge that informed important medical practices to address pathologies, had led to the "biomedicalization of aging" (Estes & Binney, 1989). This biomedicalization meant that aging itself had been dominantly framed as a medical problem marked by decline and decay and that aging, particularly as evidenced in the aging body and mind, was framed as a problem to be alleviated primarily through medical science (Estes et al., 2003). Moreover, the dominance of a biomedical perspective had promoted an individualistic perspective on aging; one in which problems are located within aging, individual's behaviors, bodies, attitudes and other attributes, and solutions focus on how to "fix" older adults. Critical gerontologists have raised concerns that this individualistic perspective means that the social forces and elements that shape social problems faced by older adults, like isolation or ageism, are then not addressed, or are narrowly viewed as challenges requiring individual adjustment (Estes et al., 2003; Laliberte Rudman, 2012). Although a biomedical perspective still prevails in gerontology and continues to inform important medical and rehabilitation advances, recognition of its limits has meant that other theoretical approaches to aging have also developed (Bengtson et al., 2005b; Hocking & Melzter, 2016).

Social theories of aging, based on a foundational assumption that aging is a social process, emerged partly as a response to the recognized limits of the dominant biomedical perspective (Estes & Binney, 1989; Phillipson & Baars, 2007). Over time, social theories of aging have become increasingly influential not only in gerontology but also in informing how health-care professionals, governments, and other social actors understand aging and how best to support the health and well-being of aging individuals and populations. Parallel to developments in occupational therapy and occupational science, which have increasingly recognized the need to shift beyond individualistic perspectives to understand how occupation is always situated in social, cultural, political, economic, and other contextual elements (Laliberte Rudman, 2021), social theories of aging have progressively shifted away from individualistic understandings of aging and older adults. As will be detailed below, many contemporary social theories, which draw upon sociology, psychology, anthropology, and related disciplines, attend to transactions of aging individuals and collectives with various aspects of contexts, with collectives encompassing groups of people, from small groups with intimate connections to whole groups, communities or populations who share salient characteristics. These contemporary theories propose that such transactions are essential to understanding how aging individuals and collectives experience and negotiate aging, including participation in a range of types of activities (Marcoen et al., 2007). These more complex understandings of the aging process and everyday activities of older adults can inform how occupational therapists assess and address the challenges to engagement in occupations faced by older adults, at micro to macro levels.

## Individual Adaptation to Aging Through Activity: Early Social Theories (1940s to 1960s)

Many of the earliest social theories of aging, including activity theory, disengagement theory, and continuity theory, were informed by a structural functionalist sociological paradigm and social psychology, leading to a focus on roles and individual adaptation (Phillips et al., 2010a, 2010b). While it was recognized that aging occurs in relation to social conditions, the perspective taken focused on how aging individuals should adjust to society rather than how societies should change to support the participation, health, and well-being of older adults (Phillipson & Baars, 2007). Across these theories, aging was viewed as an "individual social problem" (Phillipson & Baars, 2007), that is, an individual problem that was of increasing social concern given changing demographics and the potential social disorder that could result. Moreover, activity was proposed to be a primary means through which individuals should adapt to aging to enable life satisfaction and contribute to the desired social order (Estes et al., 2003; Phillips et al., 2010b). However, as shown in Table 4.1, the early social theories disagreed on how aging individuals should engage in activity so as to achieve optimal adaptation. For example, activity theory proposed that aging individuals should stay as socially active as possible. On the other hand, disengagement theory proposed that withdrawal from work

**TABLE 4.1** Early Social Theories of Aging: Activity, Disengagement, and Continuity Theory

|  | Activity Theory | Disengagement Theory | Continuity Theory |
|---|---|---|---|
| Key contributors | Cavan, Havighurst | Cumming, Henry | Atchley |
| When proposed | Late 1940s to early 1950s | 1960s | 1960s to 1970s |
| Key proposition regarding activity | Older adults should stay as active as possible | Aging individuals should decrease activity | Aging individuals should maintain same activities over the life course, and substitute new roles for lost roles |
| Types of activities addressed | Social activities | Work activities, social activities | Depends on activities an individual has developed over time |

Sources: Estes et al. (2003), Menec (2003), and Phillips et al. (2010b).

and social activities was beneficial for aging individuals, who naturally experienced decreasing ego energy. In addition, disengagement theory proposed such withdrawal was beneficial for society, given presumed declining productive capacities (Baars et al., 2006).

The early social theories informed a large body of research in the 1950s and 1960s that examined the relationship between various types of activities and life satisfaction among older adults (Estes et al., 2003). Another important contribution was that they were among the first theories to highlight the discontinuity in activities and roles that is often part of growing old in Western societies (Phillipson & Baars, 2007). However, for the most part, these theories have been abandoned because of their individualistic focus and failure to attend to the complexity of conditions that shape activity possibilities in the lives of older adults (Bengtson et al., 2005a; Phillips et al., 2010b). In essence, these theories focused on a one-way relationship between individuals and societies, proposing that it was up to aging individuals to adapt to society and to reduce any negative impacts they might have on the broader social order. As normative theories, they did not question social norms or structures that marginalized older adults, nor did they point to societal changes required to adapt to aging populations (Estes et al., 2003; Phillipson & Baars, 2007). Disengagement theory was particularly critiqued for having embedded ageist assumptions, such as the assumptions that aging inevitably leads to a decline in productive capacity and that it is natural for aging individuals to withdraw from social relationships (Baars et al., 2006). In addition, these early theories have been critiqued for assuming that all older adults have the power to choose and adapt their activities over time, failing to recognize diverse experiences of aging and differential choices available according to social positions tied to gender, ability status, socioeconomic status or race (Phillips et al., 2010b). However, the centrality of activity to achieving life satisfaction and well-being in later life continues to be a focus of the contemporary successful aging paradigm, which has also been critiqued for its individualistic perspective, failure to acknowledge diversity, and its normative assumptions about appropriate activities for older adults (Phillips et al., 2010b)

(see Chapter 19 for further information). These critiques of early theories informed the turn toward understanding the impact of social systems and structures on the aging process (Phillipson & Baars, 2007).

## Occupation-Focused Research Examples

Aligning with these earliest social theories of aging, the early occupational science literature includes studies based on the premise of a quantifiable relationship between life satisfaction and the ways people fill their time. Perhaps predictably, given subsequent critique of these early social theories of aging, the results were disappointing. For example, Stanley's (1995) survey of 58 elderly South Australians failed to demonstrate a correlation between time spent in valued occupations and life satisfaction scores. Nonetheless, descriptive studies have continued to pursue insights into the relationship between older adults' participation in occupation and their perceived well-being. For example, analysis of data from 2142 older adults extracted from the 2013 American Time-Use Survey (ATUS) found the association between active, balanced participation and well-being to be very small (Lee et al., 2021). Qualitative studies of older adults engaged in occupations they value, such as volunteering at a charity shop (Jones & Reynolds, 2019), might appear to lend more support to these social theories of aging. However, they are subject to the same critiques, in representing the experiences of relatively well-off, healthy older adults who are able to exercise many choices over their occupations, while neglecting those whose capacities or contexts do not support participation in such occupations. More recently, studies that uncover variability in individuals' success with adapting to the changes that accompany aging have been published, including Bertrand et al.'s (2021) narrative account of the transition from driving to driving cessation and Larsen et al.'s (2019) analysis of the process of accommodating assistive equipment such as a wheelchair into one's life. These studies zero in on transitions in occupation or adaptive demands, and acknowledge that some people are unable to negotiate particular challenges, given differential resources and conditions. In so doing, they expose the simplistic, individualistic, and privileged concept of occupation embedded in the early social theories of aging, with their one-size-fits-all assumption that particular types or arrangements of activity are a matter of choice and will necessarily promote life satisfaction in older adults.

## Structural Forces Constructing and Constraining Older Adults: Social Theories Addressing Age Strata and the Life Course (1970s to Present)

Since the 1970s, various theoretical strands in gerontology have expanded beyond an individualistic perspective. One of the earliest of these strands took a largely macro-level approach, seeking to expose how the aging process, not only for individuals but for older adults as a social stratum, was shaped through broader social structures (Estes et al., 2003; Phillips et al., 2010b). Many of these social theories, particularly those that address the life course, were developed over time and continue to inform contemporary work in gerontology (Phillipson & Baars, 2007b). As theories addressing the life course developed in gerontology, they increasingly examined how interactions of macro, meso, and micro levels shape the ways aging individuals and collectives experience and negotiate the aging process, within social structures, systems, and institutions. As displayed below, life course theories also address the implications of these structuring forces for activity engagement by older adults as a collective and have fostered research examining how they, with varying resources and social locations, negotiate their occupational possibilities (Laliberte Rudman, 2012).

Age stratification theory was one of the first macro-level gerontological theories. Proposed by Riley (1974) in the 1970s, this theory examined older adults as belonging to age strata and cohorts. Riley theorized that members of different cohorts, that is, groups of people born in the same historical time period, move through various age strata together. Riley asserted that differences between cohorts are shaped not just by age but also by their different historical experiences (Phillipson & Baars, 2007b; Riley, 1974). In turn, the values, behaviors, attitudes, activities, roles, health, and other characteristics of older adults as a collective change across time, such that, for example, there would be differences between older adults born during the Depression and older adults born during the Baby Boom. In addition, such differences are connected to changes in social structures over time. For example, the activities of older adults prior to the introduction of retirement policies would be different from the activities of older adults who had aged in a society in which retirement was a widespread social institution supported by pensions. As such, one of the main contributions of age stratification theory was to highlight how the aging process is dynamic and socially situated, serving to resist an understanding of aging as a universal, biologically driven process (Phillipson & Baars, 2007). Another important contribution of age stratification theory was that it located the challenges faced by older adults in social systems and structures, rather than solely within

individual-level changes. The concept of structural lag highlighted how social structures and systems fall behind demographic and social changes, such as changes in life expectancy, decreasing fertility rates, or rising divorce rates. These lags, in turn, create social problems, such as rising costs of public pensions or declines in family caregiving supports (Bengtson et al., 2005a; Estes et al., 2003). Overall, age stratification theory was one of the first social theories of aging that highlighted how social systems and structures shape the aging process, including what activities are deemed appropriate and socially promoted for older adults. This social theory also turned attention to considerations of how contextual elements can be designed to optimally support health and well-being for older adults. In addition, while age stratification theory has been critiqued for granting little autonomy to aging individuals and not attending to inter-cohort differences tied to gender, race, and other social identity markers, it established a foundation for subsequent life course perspectives that continue to inform contemporary research and social policies (Estes et al., 2003; Phillipson & Baars, 2007b).

Life course perspectives encompass various theories that focus on aging as a social process that begins at birth and involves moving through a series of age-linked transitions (Estes et al., 2003). One key characteristic of such theories is a shared conceptualization of the life course as structured through social institutions, such as families, schools, and social policies, and as changing across historical time. The socially constructed life course, shaped largely by dominant social forces and actors, outlines normative pathways for roles and activities; for example, marking out appropriate times for being a student or becoming a retiree (Bengtson et al., 2005a; Phillips et al., 2010b). Building from the macro-focus of age stratification theory, many life course theories aim to link macro, meso, and micro levels, seeking to understand how the socially patterned life course affects social institutions and "the way that individuals think, feel and act, as they age over time" (Bengtson et al., 2005a, p. 500). Research informed by life course theories focuses on different aspects of macro, meso, and micro interactions, including research that provides insights into how the life course shapes the occupations of older adults in a specific socio-historical context. For example, life course research that addresses linked lives focuses on the ways in which relations between generations are shaped across the life course and examines what this means in terms of which activities are socially supported for older adults and how older adults engage in such activities (Bengtson et al., 2005a). As one illustration, in their study using a life course perspective to examine how American grandparents enact their role, Silverstein and Marenco (2001) examined how occupations done by grandparents and grandchildren were shaped by family life stage in addition to geographic distance, gender, race, and educational level.

An important contribution of life course perspectives in gerontology has been that they have drawn attention to aging as a lifelong process, pointing to how understanding events, activities, relationships, and experiences in earlier life stages is important to understanding later life (Bengtson et al., 2005a).

For example, the cumulative advantage and disadvantage model has been used to examine how health and social inequities are produced across the life course, turning attention to how differences tied to axes of diversity such as race and gender, and exposure to childhood trauma can result in differential life chances that accumulate across the lifespan (Phillipson & Baars, 2007). Such differences also pertain to occupational possibilities and experiences; for example, research has examined how educational attainment in early life phases influences acquisition of various forms of resources and capital across the life course and is predictive of well-being in older adulthood (O'Rand, 2006). As such, life course perspectives have addressed key critiques of age stratification theory by examining interactions between macro, meso, and micro factors, and attending to issues of inequities and different possibilities for occupation and aging well (Laliberte Rudman, 2012).

## Occupation-Focused Research Examples

A life course perspective has informed research addressing aging and occupation carried out by occupational therapists and scientists, deepening understanding of occupation as part of aging processes and generating knowledge of relevance to occupational therapy (OT) advocacy and practice. For example, Wicks' (2005) exploration of the life course of older Australian women uncovered how historical, sociocultural, and familial contexts, along with personal factors, influenced the extent to which they felt they had been able to achieve their occupational potential. In addition to being informed by a life course perspective, research grounded in an occupational perspective adds breadth to understanding of the axes of diversity that influence differential life chances. Continuity of participation in occupations enacted in earlier life stages is an important variable. Thus, retired farmers who taper off the intensity of tasks they perform and gradually relinquish responsibility for running the farm benefit from continuity of a sense of competence, lifelong connection and identity. Similarly, older Finns who migrated to Sweden decades earlier maintain a sense of dual belonging to both countries, which supports a sense of belonging and continuity in life (Arola et al., 2018). However, grandmothers who care for grandchildren experience differential impacts depending on the extent to which other meaningful occupations and social supports are disrupted, and whether their child-rearing responsibilities are supplemental activities or necessary contributions to the wider family's functioning (Ludwig et al., 2007).

## Negotiating Aging in Context: Constructivist, Interpretivist, and Ecological Perspectives (1970s Onward)

Another strand of social theories in gerontology has focused on understanding the reciprocal influences of aging individuals and contexts. Within such theories, everyday activities are a key means through which aging individuals and collectives construct and experience meaning, identity, and

well-being within the contexts of their lives, and various aspects of context are proposed to shape the everyday activities of older adults. Theories informed by constructivism focus on understanding how social constructions of aging shape how societies and individuals understand and negotiate the aging process, while interpretivist theories attempt to deepen understanding of the ways people make meaning of aging within a particular social context (Carpenter & Suto, 2008; Phillipson & Baars, 2007). Ecological theories attend to how individual functioning and adaptation is shaped through reciprocal interactions among individuals and physical and social environmental features (Greenfield, 2011). While there are diverse aging theories informed by constructivist, interpretivist, and ecological perspectives, a shared element of such theories is that they conceptualize both aging individuals and contextual elements as ongoing active and dynamic constructions, continually reconstituted through everyday interactions and activities (Bengtson et al., 2005a).

Theories drawing upon constructivist and interpretivist sociological lenses address the reciprocal interactions of aging individuals and contextual elements from macro to micro levels (Phillipson & Baars, 2007). For example, at a macro level, there is a focus on how political, social, and economic forces influence the contexts within which individuals age and set parameters within which activities are negotiated. As one example, work informed by a constructivist perspective has investigated how ageism (Butler, 2008) is embedded within social policies and institutions in ways that create barriers for older adults, as collectives and individuals, to participate in society and achieve social inclusion. Research addressing ageism from a constructivist perspective has generated knowledge regarding constraints created through ageist environments, policies, and practices, including within health-care systems, and the detrimental implications that result when ageism is internalized by older adults (Harris et al., 2018; Palmore et al., 2005; Walsh et al, 2017). Moreover, research has explored how older adults actively seek to counteract ageism through collective and individual activity engagement (Minichiello et al., 2000; Pain et al., 2000), and has informed advocacy efforts to dismantle ageist contextual features (Kagan, 2020). As occupational therapists, it is crucial to be critically reflexive regarding how we may unintentionally reproduce ageism through our assumptions and practices and to be part of collective efforts that work with older adults to create more age-inclusive environments that support participation in diverse occupations (Trentham, 2019). For further information about the role of occupational therapy in creating age-inclusive environments, see Chapter 32. At meso and micro levels, constructivist and interpretivist theories address how the meaning of aging and everyday activities are negotiated within particular contexts, such as in the norms, relations, and physical features that exist within a long-term care facility or a particular neighborhood (Phillipson & Baars, 2007). Overall, research informed by constructivist and interpretivist perspectives provides compelling evidence for the importance of occupation, demonstrating how aging individuals not only achieve personal meaning and well-being through occupational engagement, but also actively shape the environments in which they age through their everyday occupations in ways that support collective well-being (Hand et al., 2020; Lager et al., 2019).

Ecological theories of aging are influenced by psychology, social psychology, and geography, often centering physical and spatial environmental features in addition to attending to aspects of social environments (Marcoen et al., 2007; Phillips et al., 2010a). A key foundational ecological theory of aging, Lawton's ecology of aging model, continues to influence social policies and practices related to housing and neighborhood design, as well as the development of occupational therapy models and practices that address person, environment, and occupation interactions and transactions (Hocking & Meltzer, 2016; Phillips et al., 2010a). In brief, Lawton's model focuses on how older adults can adaptively respond to environments to maintain optimal behavior, affect, and independence. According to Lawton, the best situation for adaptation involves having a good fit between environmental demands and an older adults' competencies, one that supports functioning and positive affect. However, misfit between environmental demands and competence can result in dysfunction and negative affect, for example, when environmental demands are too high for an individual's competence. This theory also proposes that as an older adult's competencies decrease, their everyday activities are increasingly determined by environmental elements. While Lawton's model has been critiqued for not attending to broader contextual forces that exist beyond an individual's immediate physical and social environments, it has provided an important foundation for the further development of more complex transactional models (Phillips et al., 2010a; Wahl et al., 1999). Given that ecological theories of aging center physical and spatial contextual elements, further detailed information on this theoretical strand is found in Chapter 20, The Physical Environment and Aging.

A final example of a theory addressing person and environment interactions, specifically Baltes' selective optimization with compensation (SOC) theory, is included here as it also has informed occupational therapy and other types of interventions with older adults (Donnellan & O'Neill, 2014; Hocking & Meltzer, 2016; Regier & Parmelee, 2021). Although SOC theory largely focuses on individual adaptation from a psychological perspective, it also proposes that individual adaptive responses are shaped within opportunity structures created within social contexts (Bengtson et al., 2005b; Freund & Baltes, 2002). The SOC theory conceptualizes individual development as a dynamic process of gains and losses occurring over the lifespan. This process consists of interrelated processes of selection, optimization, and compensation. The process of selection involves focusing on particular goals. Setting goals, in turn, organizes behavior and leads to optimization of attributes, functions, and resources tied to established goals. Compensation is required when specific strategies to achieve a goal or enact a particular function are no longer available and alternative means must be used (Macroen et al., 2007). Applied to challenges that occur in later phases of the life course, SOC examines how individuals

manage dynamics of gains and losses with age. This theory proposes that the process of selection becomes increasingly important for older adults because aging constraints and decreases in societal supports create a need to focus energy and goals on the most salient aspects of functioning. According to SOC theory, optimal adaptation and functioning in later life, sometimes framed as achieving successful aging, also requires engagement in strategies of optimization and compensation to maintain desired and essential functions, using an array of individual and environmental strategies (Bengtson et al., 2005a; Marcoen et al., 2007). For example, an older adult may prioritize the goal of maintaining adequate nutrition and, in turn, may optimize their functioning through practicing cooking skills or allocating additional time to food acquisition and preparation. If an older adult faces physical or cognitive challenges that make it difficult to carry out these activities to achieve the goal of maintaining adequate nutrition, successful adaptation would involve using compensatory strategies, such as using assistive devices, ordering meals, or asking for assistance from others. Similar to critiques of Lawton's model, the SOC theory fails to address broader contextual forces that shape if and how older adults can enact selection, optimization, and compensation. Moreover, aligned with the broader successful aging paradigm (see Chapter 19), the SOC model is underpinned by an individualistic lens that places the responsibility for aging well onto individuals, while neglecting how social power relations create differential possibilities to do so.

## Occupation-Focused Research Examples

Occupation-focused research has contributed new insights across interpretivist, constructivist and ecological perspectives of aging in context. One example of viewing aging as a process intimately entwined with context is van Nes and colleagues' (2009) sensitive interpretation of one older couple's shared occupations after the wife's stroke. In order to "keep her body alive" (p. 198), they worked together as "one body, three hands and two minds" (p. 197), with Henk, the husband, adjusting and discarding some of his own valued occupations to support Wil, the wife, to manage necessary daily activities, such as getting dressed, pursuing her handicrafts, maintaining her balance when they walked in the nearby park and supplementing her memory. While both acknowledged that "putting himself at her service" (p. 197) was hard on Henk and waiting for Henk to be free to help her was frustrating for Wil, they were learning to live their days in parallel so that each had moments of satisfaction, activity, and rest. Interpretivist approaches such as this reveal much about the meaning of occupation and aging, the centrality of identity negotiation, and the ways that couples can support each other as they age together. Constructivist approaches to occupation-focused research have uncovered ways older adults draw on occupation to create contexts in which they are valued members. For instance, older Chinese, Korean, and Indian immigrants to New Zealand, all of whom had been 55 or older on arrival, experienced language barriers and discriminatory behaviors that limited interaction with local people and with each other. Being welcomed into ethnic enclaves with co-nationals gave access to inclusive situations where their established skills and cultural practices gave meaning to their everyday lives. From that base of cultural connectedness, they sought to strengthen families, the local community and, ultimately, New Zealand society through "fulfilling one's duty" to participate in occupations that would benefit others. Whether knitting warm clothes for children admitted to the hospital, joining environmental clean-up campaigns, or joining a choir to entertain residents of aged care facilities, they gave service to pay back the support received from the host community and establish themselves as citizens (Wright-St. Clair & Nayar, 2017).

The reciprocal transactions of people and context evident in both interpretivist and constructivist studies of aging in context are more readily apparent in research taking an ecological perspective. One such example is a study of how physical and socio-demographic change in neighborhoods in Detroit came to constrain the daily occupations of long-time African-American residents. The city's slow economic decline, worsened by the economic recession and the housing crisis that followed, had led to higher rates of unemployment and criminal activity, degradation of infrastructure such as street lighting, and the closure of schools and recreational centers. As the streets became more violent and unpredictable, residents adjusted their occupational patterns, confining shopping to daylight hours, being vigilant to other people's presence when doing yard work, declining invitations to visit due to the risk of burglary if their house was vacant, and foregoing the previous practice of inviting neighbors to sit with them and talk on the porch (Fritz & Cutchin, 2017). Extending ecological models of aging that center on physical, spatial, and social features of the environment, occupational scientists have also considered the implications of aging out-of-place. In addition to the inevitable loss of meaningful occupations connected to immigrants' home country and the roles they have surrendered, such studies reveal occupation to be central to building a sense of continuity and integrating to place. In addition, such studies also reveal scarcity of interactions with members of the host society and sociopolitical forces such as immigration policies and racism that threaten possibilities for action (Wijekoon et al., 2021). Consistent with ecological models, over time older immigrants actively seek out ways to establish themselves as valued citizens in their new context (Wright-St. Clair & Nayar, 2017).

Overall, interpretivist, constructivist, and ecological theories have informed research that has deepened understanding of the meaning of aging at individual to social levels, and the complex transactions of aging individuals with social and physical contextual elements. As applied in occupational therapy and occupational science, these theoretical approaches have also served to deepen understanding of the significance of occupation within aging processes. In addition, knowledge generated through research informed by these theoretical strands can be drawn upon by occupational therapists to assess and address the complex transactions of person and environmental factors shaping occupational participation and possibilities. At the same time, theories fitting into this strand have been critiqued for inadequately attending to implications of social power relations and broader contextual elements, such as political and economic elements, for how diverse older adults negotiate their lives and occupations. Such critiques informed the next strand of theoretical development in gerontology, that is, those that fit within critical gerontology (Estes et al., 2003; Phillipson & Baars, 2007).

## Attending to Power, Inequities, and Bounded Agency: Critical Perspectives (1980s Onward)

Critical gerontology, broadly defined as approaches to the study of aging that draw upon critical social theory, emerged during the 1980s and has developed into "a distinctive voice and analytic framework for challenging power and injustice in an aging society" (Moody & Sasser, 2018, p. 35). While distinct from earlier theoretical strands in gerontology and often serving to critique assumptions of mainstream gerontology, critical gerontology itself has become increasingly diverse over time and continues to evolve in novel ways (Phillips et al., 2007b; Wellin, 2018). Critical gerontology encompasses diverse theoretical underpinnings, such as the Marxism, political economy, feminism, Foucauldian theory, postmodern theories, and queer theory, held together by a focus on understanding how social power relations shape possibilities for aging at collective to individual levels (Estes et al., 2003). While re-asserting the need to attend to structural forces identified in the 1970s, critical gerontological theories attempt to do so in ways that also acknowledge the voices and agency of older adults as collectives and individuals. As stated by Estes et al. (2003), critical gerontology seeks to fuse the "study of structural inequalities in society and personal experience of ageing, because both are essential for social action and progressive change" (p. 3). At the same time, critical gerontological theories counter an overemphasis on individualism by addressing how the individual and collective agency of older adults is always bounded within structures and systems that reflect broader power relations. As such, the possibilities for older adults to manage their everyday lives, including their occupations, and shape their contexts are always bounded in relation to various social and political forces, such as norms, ideologies, social discourses, and governing systems (Calasanti, 2002). In addition, grounded in key characteristics of critical social theory (Carpenter & Suto, 2008; Laliberte Rudman, 2012), critical gerontological theories aim to show how social power relations oppress older adults and create inequities at the intersections of age, gender, race, and other social identity markers. In addition, they embody a commitment to transform social and political elements to counter marginalization and social, health, and occupational inequities (Moody & Sasser, 2018; Phillipson & Baars, 2007). Given the diversity of theories that fit within critical gerontology, we focus on a few examples from this theoretical strand to highlight the relevance of such theories to understanding how structural and systemic forces shape everyday possibilities for diversely situated older adults, and the ways in which older adults attempt to negotiate occupation in relation to such forces.

One of the most definable and earliest theoretical approaches in critical gerontology is informed by a political economy perspective (Estes et al., 2003). The political economic approach emerged in the 1980s, when crisis constructions of the aging population were becoming dominant. Within such constructions, the aging population was increasingly framed by international bodies, national governments and within academic and popular texts as a threat to economic and social order, given concerns regarding increasing dependency ratios, unsustainable pension and health-care systems, and future labor market shortages (Phillipson & Baars, 2007). To counter these crisis constructions, which framed the "aging problem" in ways that fueled intergenerational conflict, retreat from public pensions, and individualistic discourses that framed aging individuals as problematic, political economy theory was drawn upon to demonstrate how social and political systems, particularly those aligned with capitalism, constructed dependency as well as inequities. Continuing from these origins, work in this theoretical approach focused on how the political economy, in particular historical and social contexts, shapes the roles and resources available to older adults, increasingly examining differences among subgroups of older adults (Wellin, 2018). As summarized by Estes et al. (2003), such work has demonstrated "how the state regulates and reproduces different life chances throughout the life course and how that ultimately shapes the economic and health vulnerabilities and inequalities of different subgroups of the elderly" (p. 2). For example, gerontological research informed by political economy has examined various ways pensions systems, gender inequity in the labor force, and the feminization of caregiving means that women are at higher risk for poverty in later life, how this risk is further amplified given trends such as rising divorce rates and reductions in public provisions, and how financial inequities limit possibilities for various forms of participation (Foster & Walker, 2013; Phillipson & Baars, 2007; Torres, 2014). Such work also has examined how age, gender, class, and race create intersecting axes of disadvantage within contemporary capitalistic and neoliberal contexts, further creating inequitable access to resources and conditions, as well as occupations, that support health and well-being (Laliberte Rudman, 2012; Phillipson, 2005; Walsh et al., 2017). This body of work has clearly demonstrated that the process and experience of aging is directly related to the social and political contexts in which it occurs (Estes et al., 2003).

Another key focus within critical gerontology is a commitment to "ongoing reflection and critique of how, by whom, and with what moral or political stances age and aging are rendered problematic" (Wellin, 2018, p. 12). For instance, work informed by Foucauldian, critical feminist and postmodern theories, has used critical narrative methodologies to unpack how older adults interpret and negotiate discourses of aging that mark out how older adults should age and what goals they should aspire to achieve. Such work seeks to both highlight the contradictory effects of dominant discourses, informed by broader political ideologies, in the lives of older adults, and also the complex ways older adults both take up and resist such discourses. In doing so, this strand of scholarship seeks to both critique the limits of dominant discourses of aging and the ideologies that inform them and also create spaces for the voices and perspectives of older adults (Moody & Sasser, 2018; Wellin, 2018). As one example, various studies have examined how older adults understand and negotiate their aging bodies in relation to messages conveyed through successful aging discourses (see Chapter 19 for further detail), anti-aging medicine, and consumer culture that promote engagement in an array of physical, social, dietary and other activities in order to stay fit, youthful and disease-free (Laliberte Rudman, 2006; Katz, 2010). On the one hand, while studies find that many well-resourced aging adults in North American contexts engage in such activities as a means to manage their bodies and health, they also raise concerns regarding how these same discourses create tensions for older adults whose bodies do show signs of aging and disease, lead to self-blame and blaming of others whose bodies take on signs of oldness, and fail to recognize how inequitable access to financial, social, and other resources creates barriers to many of the activities promoted (Clarke, 2018; Clarke & Kortchenko, 2011; Pack et al., 2019).

Extending out from critiques of ideologies, political forces, and other forces shaping aging, critical gerontologists have also sought to build new understandings of aging that highlight the perspectives of older adults and their ongoing contributions to society, seeking to learn from and work with older adults to resist oppressive social and political forces. For example, such work has built alternative understandings of "aging well" through engaging with diverse aging adults to understand the meanings they assign to aging, thereby moving away from normative ideals informed by political and social ideologies (Phillips et al., 2010b). More information regarding this strand of critical gerontology can be found in Chapter 24 which addresses humanities, arts, and aging, and in Chapter 19 which includes a section on alternative models of aging well. In addition, critical gerontologists have examined how older adults contribute to society and combat ageism through engagement in activism (McHugh, 2012; Trentham & Neysmith, 2018), such as through the Raging Grannies movement which seeks to challenge ageist stereotypes and empower its members to engage in lifelong learning and various forms of social participation (Narushima, 2004; Sawchuk, 2009). Participatory approaches to activist scholarship, that is, research that involves working with older adults to identify problematic situations and enact action aimed at structural and social transformation has been increasingly embraced (Benjamin-Thomas et al., 2018; Corrado et al., 2020). Such activist scholarship shifts from doing research on older adults and defining problems and solutions solely from the perspectives of academics and health-care professionals, toward doing research with older adults in ways that center their lived expertise and capacities to define problems and be part of enacting solutions. For example, critically informed participatory approaches have been used with groups of older adults to inform transformations of health-care practices, long-term care facilities, urban environments, technology design, food access, transportation systems, and community-based activity programs (Benjamin-Thomas et al., 2018; Corrado et al., 2020). For further examples of occupation-based social transformative work completed with older adults see Chapter 31.

## Occupation-Focused Research Examples

Critical social theory and critical gerontological theories have been taken up in occupational therapy and occupational science research in diverse ways. One strand has addressed the question of who has the power to define what occupations older adults should and should not do. For example, a critical discourse analysis of representations of ideal housing for retirees published in a national Canadian newspaper revealed how they are urged to be consumers and pursue physically active leisure and cultural activities, raising questions of who can access such living arrangements and lifestyles and who is excluded from them (Laliberte Rudman et al., 2009). Similar concerns were raised in relation to aging adults' use of the everyday technologies such as mobile phones and computers that are increasingly used to communicate, manage personal finances and access essential public services, including e-health. While the researchers' aim had been to track the impact of cognitive impairment on technology usage, the findings revealed systemic injustices disadvantaging sectors of the aging population with lower educational attainment in their early years and fewer financial resources (Kottorp et al., 2016). In addition to disadvantages that accumulate over a lifetime, occupational scientists applying a combination of ecological and critical perspectives can reveal current threats to aging adults' occupations. For instance, their preferences can be at odds with commercial interests, such as the tensions that may exist between owners of shopping malls, whose interests are served by high levels of retail activity, and older adults' preference for low-foot traffic, which provides safer spaces for taking a walk around the shopping mall concourse (Hart & Shank, 2016). Aligning with the move within critical gerontology of attending to the voices of aging people, Gibson et al. (2020) provide a window on the cultural obligations enacted by Elders and older Aboriginal and Torres Strait Islanders to support social and emotional well-being, but how participation in those roles, responsibilities and occupations are negatively influenced by disrespect, poor health and broken cultural connections. An additional point of connection with critical gerontology is researchers engaging in participatory work with older adults, such as Trentham and Neysmith's (2018) account of their 2-year involvement in a group of senior citizens as they engaged in advocacy to improve provision of homecare services and combat ageism.

Overall, work within gerontology, occupational therapy and occupational science that aligns with critical gerontological theories has advanced understanding of how the everyday lives of older adults are shaped through, and negotiated within, broad social and political forces. Such work has also enhanced awareness of how health, social and occupational inequities are shaped at the intersections of age, gender, race, class, and other social markers of identity (Estes et al., 2003). It has also led to an enhanced focus on the strengths and contributions of older adults, and a commitment to working with older adults to create more age-inclusive societies. This theoretical strand points to the need for ongoing critical reflexivity within occupational therapy regarding dominant assumptions, conveyed through social policies, the media, health-care systems, and other social systems, regarding what occupations older adults should and should not engage in, and an ongoing openness to understanding and supporting diverse ways of engaging in occupation in later life (Laliberte Rudman, 2012; Trentham, 2019).

## Conclusion: The Ongoing Transformation of Aging and Older Adults

Social theories of aging provide a variety of ways of understanding aging as a complex social process, one that is dynamic and diverse. As various strands have developed, these theories have highlighted that grasping the complexity of aging requires attending to it as both a lived experience and as socially and politically constructed. Social theories of aging have turned attention to the heterogeneity of older adults, raising concerns regarding the sociopolitical production of inequities and illustrating diverse possibilities for activity and well-being in later life. Research informed by these theories has generated knowledge regarding the centrality of occupation in the lives of older adults, the complexity of transactions between personal, occupational, and contextual elements, and the ways in which aging and occupation are situated within micro-, meso-, and macro-level factors. Occupational therapists can draw on these theories and related knowledge to support the occupations, health and well-being of diverse older adults at individual to societal levels. As societies continue to transform, given social trends and issues such as globalization, climate change, and technological developments, the aging process and older adults will also be transformed (Skinner et al., 2018; Wellin, 2018). As a profession, it is important that occupational therapy research and practice continues to evolve to optimize its capacity to work with and support the occupational participation of older adults.

*The complete listing of the Bibliography and Chapter Questions and Answers are available in the accompanying enhanced eBook version included with the print purchase of this textbook. Visit Elsevier eBooks+ (eBooks.Health.Elsevier.com) to access this content.*

## CHAPTER 5

# Foundations of Evidence-Based Gerontological Occupational Therapy Practice

*Kathlyn Reed, PhD, OTR, MLIS, FAOTA and Donghua Tao, PhD, FA, MA, FAMIA*

## CHAPTER OUTLINE

## OBJECTIVES

- Describe the evolution of and rationale for evidence-based practice within the occupational therapy profession and gerontological occupational therapy practice
- Describe the process for implementing evidence-based practice and the online information tools and resources for acquiring research evidence
- Identify the research designs that are appropriate for answering different types of questions in gerontological occupational therapy practice and describe the techniques for evaluating these studies
- Describe practical strategies for implementing evidence-based practice in gerontological occupational therapy
- Describe future trends in applying and implementing evidence-based practice into the occupational therapy profession and gerontological occupational therapy practice.

## Occupational Therapy with Aging Adults Rationale for the Evidence-Based Approach

Whether the term "evidence-based" is followed by the words "medicine," "practice," "rehabilitation," "client care," or "occupational therapy," the rationale or intended outcome is to bring more objective and scientific-based decision-making to the process of evaluating, planning and implementing an intervention to client care. The intent is to use the results of research studies as a major element in determining best practices in the application of knowledge to a client's problems and needs. The intended outcome is to reduce the gap between the results of research and care received by clients. Reducing the gap in occupational therapy (OT) has included challenges and barriers (Tomlin & Borgetto, 2011).

The concept of the *evidence-based* intervention appears in the official documents of the American Occupational Therapy Association (AOTA). The Vision 2025 states "Occupational therapy is evidence based, client centered, and cost-effective" (American Occupational Therapy Association [AOTA], 2021a, 2021b). The Occupational Therapy Practice Framework (American Occupational Therapy Association [AOTA], 2020a) uses the term "evidence-informed practice" (p. 6) as one of the cornerstones providing a foundation of practice. The AOTA Code of Ethics includes under the subsection of "Service Delivery" that statement "Use to the extent possible, evaluation, planning, intervention techniques, assessments, and therapeutic equipment that are evidence based, current, and within the recognized scope of occupational therapy practice" (American Occupational Therapy Association [AOTA], 2020b, p. 7, 4 C). The Accreditation Council for Occupational Therapy Standards and interpretive guide (2018) states in the Preamble "be able to plan and apply evidence-based occupational therapy interventions to address the physical, cognitive, functional cognitive, psychosocial, sensory, and other aspects of performance in a variety of contexts and environments to support engagement in everyday life activities that affect health, well-being, and quality of life, as informed by the "*Occupational Therapy Practice Framework*" (Accreditation Council for Occupational Therapy Education [ACOTE], 2018, p. 2).

Federal legislation has also included the concept of evidence-based such as the Every Student Succeeds Act (ESSA) of 2015 (Pub. L. 114-95) which replaced the No Child Left Behind Act (NCLBA) of 2001 (Pub. L. 107-110). Evidence-based is described as demonstrating a statistically significant effect on improving student outcomes based on strong, moderate, or promising evidence (S. 1177-289).

## History and Scope of Evidence-Based Practice in Occupational Therapy

### History of Evidence-Based Medicine

According to Sackett et al. (2000), the concept of evidence-based medicine was created at McMaster University in Canada as a means of describing a process of problem-based clinical teaching which required students and clinicians to search for and evaluate evidence of clinical practice. Gordon Guyatt, a faculty member at the McMaster School of Medicine, is credited with first publishing the term in an editorial entitled "Evidence-based medicine" in 1991 (Guyatt, 1991). User guides followed thereafter. Sachett and colleagues became the primary champions with their publications in 1996 and 2000 (Sackett et al., 1996, 2000).

The first mention of evidence-based practice (EBP) in the published OT literature was in an editorial entitled "Evidence-based practice for sale?" in the *British Journal of Occupational Therapy* in 1995 (Colshaw, 1995). Colshaw had attended a conference in which she reports that the concepts of EBP and randomized controlled trials (RCTs) were mentioned frequently but were not yet commonly recognized in OT practice or appeared in OT literature.

Margo Holm's Eleanor Clarke Slagle lecture in 2000 marked an increased awareness in the United States regarding the growing importance of evidence-based research to the status and recognition of OT as a profession (Holm, 2000). According to Lieberman and Scheer (2002), the AOTA began working on evidence-based projects in 1998 beginning with the Evidence-Based Literature Review Project. The *American Journal of Occupational Therapy* began publishing the Evidence-Based Practice Forum in 1999 (Tickle-Degnen, 1999). Meta-analyses had been published since 2001 (Murphy & Tickle-Degnen, 2001). The first publication out of an OT systematic review project appeared in 2008, although systematic reviews by university personnel had appeared beginning in 2002 (Hunt & Arbesman, 2008; Dolhi & Riobers, 2002). The Centennial Vision project (American Occupational Therapy Association [AOTA], 2007) includes evidence-based decision-making as one of the eight elements viewed as relevant to a shared vision of the profession and the phrase "evidence-based profession" was included in the Centennial Vision statement (Corcoran, 2007).

The first identified articles published in England include the Casson Medical Lecture by Eakin in 1997 and several articles appeared in the November 1997 issue of the *British Journal of Occupational Therapy* (Alsop, 1997; Bannigan, 1997; Lloyd-Smith, 1997; Taylor, 1997). The Canadian Journal of Occupational Therapy published a special issue with an editorial by Law and Baum (1998). The *Australian Occupational Therapy Journal* devoted a special issue to EBP in 2000 edited by Fossey (2000). Additionally, a review article appeared in the *Hong Kong Journal of Occupational Therapy* in 2002 (Leung, 2002).

Positions statements have been published by the Canadian Association of Occupational Therapists (CAOT, 1999, reviewed 2009), New Zealand Association of Occupational Therapists (NZAOT, 2002), Occupational Therapy Australia (2018), and member countries of the World Federation of Occupational Therapists (WFOT) (Serwe et al., 2021) to identify the role of each organization in promoting and supporting research, gather and evaluating evidence, and disseminating knowledge. No statements focused directly or primarily on EBP were identified for the AOTA or Royal College of Occupational Therapy.

### Definitions and Descriptions of Evidence-Based Approaches

Sackett et al. (1996, p. 71) defined evidence-based medicine as "the conscientious, explicit, and judicious use of current best evidence in making decisions about the care of individual patients. The practice of evidence-based medicine means integrating individual clinical expertise with the best available clinical evidence from systematic research." Note the definition does not address the client's needs, values, or concerns but instead focuses on translating research into practice. Lee and Miller (2001) corrected this omission by stating that "the process of evidence-based clinical decision making encourages OT professionals to include the values, knowledge, and experience of the client and other healthcare professions."

Sirkka et al. (2014) define EBP as "based on integration of knowledge from different sources such as research, theories and models of practice, the professionals' clinical experience, and experiences from clients in the local context" (p. 1). This definition is consistent with the model presented by the authors Hoffman et al. (2017), which suggests definitions for OT should include at least four elements: research evidence, therapist experience, client values, and practice context. Older definitions tend to rely on the first three elements but not include the practice context element which may provide relevant information for the successful implementation of the evidence-based intervention plan.

Law and MacDermit (2013) describe evidence-based rehabilitation as consisting of four concepts:

- Awareness: Being aware of the existence and strength of evidence in one's field
- Consultation: Collaborating with the client and other health-care professionals to determine the client's relevant problems and their clinical solutions
- Judgment: Being able to apply the best evidence to the individual with whom one is working
- Creativity: Emphasizes that EBP is not a "cookie cutter" approach, but rather the combination of art and science.

## Models Associated With Evidence-Based Practice

The first model in the OT literature is in Egan et al. (1998) called Occupational Performance Process Model outlining seven steps and two sources of evidence that are client-based versus research-based. A second model is in Bennett and Bennett (2000). The model consists of three nested boxes. The inner box is labeled Client Context and includes concepts of Person, Environment and Occupation. The middle box is labeled Occupational Therapy Treatment Process and includes concepts of Therapy Context, Information Resources, Clinical Expertise, financial Resources, and Practice Setting. The outer box lists a four-step process: Asking Clinical Questions, Literature Search, Critical Appraisal, and Use of Research Evidence which have impact or are used to influence the middle and inner boxes. A third model appears in Hamilton et al. (2014) using a pyramid to suggest how data are transformed into information, information into knowledge, and knowledge into expertise. Models associated with EBP include three major types:

- Components: Models concerned with identifying the major components, elements, or concepts involved in establishing or creating the rationale for an evidence-based approach (who, what, where, why).
- Steps: Models concerned with outlining the number of steps, processes, or sequences needed to (adequately) complete a process of initiating to completing an evidence-based approach.
- Levels: Models concerned with organizing the types of sources of research and research designs into a list of levels to facilitate the decision-making process regarding comparisons and possible "best to less" rankings.

The following descriptions are illustrations of the three types of models. Baker and Tickle-Degnen (2019) state that EBP is composed of three equal core components which act in combination with a clinician's expertise. In other words, there are actually four core components: evidence, environment, values/circumstances, and expertise stated as the following:

- The current best evidence
- The treatment/practice environment
- Each client's values and circumstances
- Clinician/practitioner's expertise

The four-core component approach (elements, concepts) is consistent with the *Occupational Therapy Practice Framework* (American Occupational Therapy Association [AOTA], 2020), which is based on the belief that the environment or context is an essential consideration in the planning and delivery of OT services. The labels change depending on the model. Evidence can be described as resources, research studies, literature, or collective knowledge. Treatment can be described as therapy, rehabilitation, or intervention. Values can be described as those of an individual, a group, a community, or an organization. Clinicians can be described as therapists (occupational therapist or occupational therapy assistant), practitioner, student trainee, end-user, researchers, or investigators.

Gitlow and DePoy (2018) state five steps in their model called Systematic Occupational Therapy Practice (SOTP). The model is defined as "the integration of critical analysis, scientific thinking, and action processes throughout all phases and domains" (Gitlow & DePoy, 2018, p. 48). The steps are:

1. Identification and clarification of the problem to be addressed by the intervention
2. Understanding of need—what is needed to resolve all or part of the problem?
3. Setting of goals and objectives to address the need
4. Reflexive intervention to achieve the goals and objectives
5. Outcome assessment

Lieberman and Scheer (2002) presented a model to organize OT outcomes research into the level of evidence based on research study design. The higher number assigned to a research study is assumed to give that study greater value or weight in the decision-making process. Additional criteria included two categories of sample size, three levels for internal validity and three levels of external validity. The model heavily favors research designs based on quantitative data using statistical methods designed to measure populations, and minimizes the potential usefulness of qualitative data based on naturalist approaches such as observation, interview, or case study.

I. Randomized control trial
II. Non-randomized control trial—two groups
III. Non-randomized control trial—one group (one treatment) pretest and posttest
IV. Single-subject design
V. NA. Narratives, case studies

Later systematic reviews and meta-analyses were added to the model at the top and the numbering reorganized.

Tomlin and Borgetto (2011, p 191) suggest a Research Pyramid for organizing OT literature that views all literature as potentially of equal value. This model contrasts with the hierarchical model focused primarily on quantitative designs presented in Lieberman and Scheer (2002). The model addresses three major categories of research design, experimental, qualitative, and outcome, and then creates a hierarchy within the three designs providing a more balanced approach to viewing the research literature for analysis and application to client-centered planning and intervention.

- Experimental research hierarchy (high to low) meta-analysis, randomized clinical trial (RCT), controlled clinical trial, single-subject study
- Qualitative research hierarchy (high to low) meta-analysis, group study with more rigor, group study with less rigor, study with an informant
- Outcome research hierarchy (high to low) meta-analysis; preexisting groups with covariates; case-control, preexisting groups; one-group pre-post study.
- Experimental and some qualitative research tend to have higher internal validity
- Outcome and some qualitative research tend to have higher external validity
- Experimental and outcome research are types of quantitative research

## Pros and Cons: What Is Useful and Not Useful

Pros or positive views of evidence-based approaches and cons or negative views have appeared in numerous articles. The following list is compiled from three major sources (Cahill et al., 2015; Upton et al., 2014; Van't Leven et al., 2011).

### Pros or Positive Views

- Practitioner can use the results of scientifically developed research studies to form the rationale for intervention as opposed to using only personal option, experience, training, or facility recommended protocols.
- Practitioner is less dependent on selecting intervention approaches based on "we or I have always done it this way."
- Practitioner has an external scientifically based explanation or answer as to why a particular intervention was selected.
- Practitioner may be able to give the client a choice of scientifically based interventions along with the pros and cons of each.
- Evidence-based approaches can provide a scientific base or rationale for a profession.
- Evidence-based approaches can provide a hierarchy for evaluating the significance or value of a research study based on the methodology of the study.
- Quantitative research tends to be stronger (less potential for bias) than qualitative studies on factors concerned with internal validity.
- Evidence-based approaches tend to be based on the philosophical and epistemological perspective of positivism that values science as a way of understanding the world. Note: These approaches can also be considered a negative.
- RCTs are the "gold standard" in choice of research design for determining potential effectiveness of intervention approaches, strategies, or techniques.

### Cons or Negative Views

- Practitioner needs to have access to research-focused database(s), which may not be available without a subscription
- Practitioner needs practice and skills (sense of competence) to search the databases and gather other relevant information
- Practitioner needs practice and skills (sense of competence) to interpret the search results from research findings, including statistical formulas, to implement intervention programs that can be implemented to real clients.
- Practitioner needs time that may not be available in a busy work setting.
- Practitioners may feel or express the option that management does not support efforts to use EBP
- The focus of EBP has been on quantitative research studies using experimental design and probability population-based statistics which may be applicable to given individual client
- Evidence-based medicine "is a bottom-up approach that integrates the best external evidence with individual clinical expertise and patient choice" (Sackett et al., 1996, p. 72). OT personnel have been encouraged to use a top-down approach.
- Qualitative and narrative based studies are either ignored or ranked as a low level of evidence, yet such studies may provide useful information in the decision making process for a particular client.
- The concepts of context and environment, values and meaning, quality of life and life satisfaction are not routinely considered in quantitative studies but are important concepts in the OT philosophy and framework.
- Quantitative research studies tend to be weak on factors concerned with external validity such as generalizability or transferability to other settings or situations such as hospital settings to home situations.
- Clinical/practice-related judgment and decision-making skills require practice to build skills.
- Often "evidence based" means "best available evidence" available from research because definitive answers are not available.
- There is no proof that one research design or methodology for conducting a research study is better than another in providing useful and relevant information for selecting and creating client intervention protocols.

## Implementation of Evidence-Based Gerontological Occupational Therapy Practice

Tomlin and Dougherty (2014) have suggested that the concept of evidence-based is not a single idea but rather a dual concept comprised of both external and internal factors and therefore should be viewed as having "separate but related purposes" called "evidence-supported practice" and "evidence-informed practice" (p. 15). They propose that the term *evidence-supported practice* (ESP) should be used to describe a "body of published research demonstrating the effectiveness of health professional services in bringing about desirable outcomes for health and quality of life." In other words, the focus is on issues related to general health and quality of life for a population in general, but not on a specific individual or identified group of individuals. In contrast, the concept labeled *evidence-informed practice* (EIP) should be used to describe all sources of evidence, internal and external, that a practitioner uses to make decisions about client care. In other words, the focus is on the decision-making process for the purpose of developing a specific client-center plan of care or intervention protocol for an individual or individuals being treated as a group, implementing that plan, and evaluating the outcome or results.

When the concept of evidence-based is viewed from the two perspectives, research studies can be organized into four groups that can be labeled as follows: Theory, Validation, Application and Monitoring. Their purpose is related to either ESP or EIP or both. *Theory*-focused research is designed to explain *why* certain interventions, protocols, treatments, or therapeutic approaches cause or result in certain client outcomes. The explanation of "why it works" provides a justification to generalize or translate external findings from one or more research studies to an individualized plan of care. In other words, theory developed as ESP can be used to support and provide a rationale for EIP. *Validation* studies are designed to develop the knowledge of the academic disciplines that support the OT profession. The focus is on justifying "why keep" the profession or allow the profession to continue to exist and provide client services that address health, wellness, and quality of life. Validating the existence of the profession is an important subject in health service delivery, but validating studies are not designed to specifically address individual clients' plans of care. Therefore, the purpose is ESP. *Application* studies are designed to directly translate external evidence (ESP) to internal informed practice (EIP). The purpose of application-based research to answer the question as to whether an existing approach to evaluation or intervention actually *works* (provides benefit to clients in terms of improving or preventing loss of health, well-being or quality of life), is generally safe and effective, and is efficient in terms of time and money. While theory research often focuses on the potential benefits to a client, validation research focuses on whether approaches already being used actually provide the intended results or outcome. Thus, the focus of application research is EIP. Finally, *monitoring* studies are designed to systematically keep track of "practitioners' local outcomes from client interventions" (p. 16). The purpose is to determine if the outcomes or results as documented by practitioners and clients are consistent with the theory studies. In other words, research studies have completed a circle from theory informing practice, to practice informing theory. Thus, EIP can enhance ESP. Enhancing theory may lead to improved or better client-centered care—and thus the circle can repeat itself along the way, validating the profession and using application studies to keep effective and efficient assessments and interventions while discontinuing those that do not meet the expected criteria.

Examples in practice may provide additional clarification. Driving assessment and intervention programs are based on the theory that continuing a client's ability to safely drive a vehicle maintains or improves the client's quality of life and sense of independence. The implementation of driving programs has been used to validate or justify the use of OT personnel in administering such service programs. Application studies may include those designed to evaluate the usefulness of a particular assessment instrument or the results of one driver training program, such as simulated driving over another, such as "on-the-road" intervention. Finally, practitioners can report based on real life experience with clients, whether quality of life and sense of independence really are observed by practitioners or reported by clients and caregivers.

The two divisions of the concept of evidence-based and the separation of research into four subgroups permit the focus of examining evidence-based sources into different groups. Suppose the question is "Why should OT personnel participate in driving programs for older adults?" The focus should be on looking for theory and theoretically based research studies addressing such concepts as improving or maintaining quality of life, independence in the community, or sense of competence and not be a burden to others by maintaining safe driving habits, or engaging in cessation of driving. Suppose the question is "Does offering and participation in driving assessment and intervention programs increase the value of occupational therapy services provided to older adults?" The focus should be on studies that address improvement in service delivery when a driving program designed for older adults is provided as part of the OT list of services. Suppose the question is "Is assessment 'ABC' reliable in measuring driving errors that reduce driver safety in older adults?" Then research studies should be identified that included the "ABC" assessment in the methodology. Finally, suppose the question is "Do occupational therapy practitioners contribute to the literature about driving programs for older adults?" The focus then should be on studies that report the success or failure of OT services that include driving assessment and intervention programs.

The following is a general guide to potential resources and type of evidence-based information that may be included:
- Textbooks: Usually provide a summary of existing theory and application up to the date of publication. Older textbooks may provide out-of-date information and may be most useful in providing a historical context.
- Monographs (books and chapters that are not textbooks): May provide original publication of a theory/model and examples of application and monitoring. The date of publication is a guide to potential usefulness. Older monographs may provide out-of-date information and may be most useful in providing a historical context.
- Academic and Research Focused Journal and Serial Articles (peer-reviewed): Usually provide the most current research for application and monitored studies if published within the past 5 to 10 years. Many provide original works on theory or model of practice or a

summary of the theory/model may be included in some application studies.

- Trade Publications or Advertising Articles (not peer-reviewed): Usually provide illustrations or case examples of application studies. Such articles may include details of assessment and intervention not covered in the peer-reviewed studies. Use with caution all information not identified as based on research studies or recognized expert opinion.
- Online Databases: Covered in the next section on search strategies
- Online Formats such as Podcasts and Webinars: Use with caution. Check the credentials of the presenter(s) for recognized expertise on the subject materials being presented.
- Popular (lay person focused) Magazine Articles (print or online): Use with caution. Information may be a summary of research studies but may also be based on personal experience or be a sales pitch designed to increase sales of a product or use of a specific service delivery program.
- Advertising Brochures and Pages (print or online): Use with caution. Information may be based in part on research studies but presented as sales pitches designed to "look good" without supporting reliable research studies to back up the claims.
- Booklets, Pamphlets, and Leaflets (print or online): Use with caution. Information may or may not be based on research studies. Interpretation of results may be different if the author is a scientist or health-care professional versus a lay person with no scientific training in anatomy, physiology, statistics, or research design. Verify all statements.
- Newspaper Articles (print or online): Use with caution. The article may be written to sell newspapers or to fit the available page limit, but not necessarily to provide factorial information to the reader based on reliable research studies. The author(s) may have no scientific training in anatomy, physiology, statistics, or research design. Verify all statements.
- Social Media (all types): Use with extreme caution. Facts have a way of getting distorted as they get passed from one person to another or are restated over time. Verify all information identified on social media with reliable research studies or recognized expert opinion.

## Searching and Selecting the Literature

### Asking a Practice-Based Question

The first step in using evidence-based literature to inform practice is to formulate a question about a specific client's problem or a problem that is common to the population of older adults. In OT the question may focus on: the efficacy of an occupation-based intervention (eating, dressing, or driving), addressing a component of an occupation-based pattern or skill (habits, hand dexterity, sense of competence), selecting the best or right assessment instrument to evaluate

| **Box 5.1** | PICO(T) Format |

P = Population/Problem/Patient (client)
I = Intervention/Independent Variable
C = Comparison/Control
O = Outcome/Objective
T = Time/Timeframe/Type of Study/Type of question (optional)

the client's problem(s), or planning an intervention program to address identified problems and goals. Straus and colleagues have suggested four elements to comprise a well-constructed practice-based question, called the PICO(T) format (Box 5.1)

The PICO(T) format is designed to help focus attention on the main characteristics of a practice-based question, such as the important client characteristics and subject (assessment, intervention, outcome) of interest and to address the limited time available to the practitioner to obtain valued information. The PICO(T) format also acts as a guide or template for choosing the search terms that will be entered into the selected online database. However, not all the words or concepts identified in the PICO(T) formatted statement may be needed to search the database. Typically, a database search begins by entering the two most important elements such as the type of client (aged, older adult, senior citizen, elderly) and the type of intervention (driving fitness, driving cessation). Then based on the number of citations retrieved, additional terms such as the expected or desired outcome can be added. For example, the question might be the efficacy of driving fitness programs provided to older adults to maintain independent living status. Rewritten in the PICO(T) format, the question might be stated as:

P—older adults living in the community (community dwelling)
I—occupational therapy intervention targeting driving fitness programs or protocols
C—compared with no intervention
O—maintain driver's license, independent living status, and ability to live at home or community
T—studies published in the last 5 years

### Acquiring the Evidence to Inform Practice

The next step is to gather resources to address the problem. Resources might include research studies published in journals with editorial staff composed of peer or colleague professionals who review manuscripts before publication (called peer-reviewed journals), authoritative up-to-date textbooks for background knowledge, professional association documents, government agency publications, and specialized online databases that synthesize and summarize research. In addition, information should be gathered from the client and from significant others, with the client's permission (family, close relatives and friends, guardian, and health providers) within the context of their everyday lives related to the problem or problems being addressed. The client is the authority on the occupations that are meaningful and purposeful to that individual, on interventions that have been successful in the past, and the outcomes that are most important to the person's well-being and quality of life. The practitioner should also evaluate the level of expertise gained from personal education and experience. Novice practitioners may want to consult with more experienced colleagues to ensure that a good decision-making process is being followed. Finally, the context should be considered. For example, is the client an inpatient or outpatient, has the client's overall health status changed recently, has the client been previously evaluated for driving fitness?

Two steps are necessary to acquire the evidenced needed to guide practice-based decision-making. The first is to identify appropriate information resources that address the question. The second is to create and execute an effective search strategy within those resources.

## Access to Information Resources for Occupational Therapy

OT practitioners have many sources of information to address practice-related questions. A useful first step is to check if practice guidelines or other resources may be available from professional associations or governmental agencies to address the question. If so, the necessary information may be readily available, and no further resources need to be gathered. If, however, the question is not answered or incompletely answered in existing guidelines, an online database or databases may be useful to search for articles published in peer-reviewed journals. Some of these databases are available to the public for free, such as PubMed or Google Scholar, while others required a paid subscription to access. In addition, searching library catalogs or e-books could find the related information as well. Consultation with a health sciences librarian is highly recommended because the librarian can identify the resources available onsite and can assist in developing an effective search strategy. Consulting with a librarian can save time and frustration. If no librarian is available at the work setting, check with a nearby OT education program for access to library assistance. Another source is the public library, although public librarians may be less familiar with health-related subjects or topics. Finally, if librarian assistance is not available, other professionals may be helpful, especially if the problem is shared with other health professionals such as client safety, improved quality of life, health promotion, or client education. Such general topics are discussed in a variety of health sciences disciplines including medicine, nursing, psychology, geriatrics, and rehabilitation. As a result, a comprehensive literature search may require the use of several online databases.

### Platforms or Hosts

Platforms or hosts are specialized software programs used to mount databases such as MEDLINE, AgeLine, or CINAHL (Cumulative Index to Nursing and Allied Health). The platform usually determines the methods which can be used to search the databases mounted on that platform. For example,

the MEDLINE database is available on several different platforms, but the methods or techniques for searching the database may be different from one platform to another because of the software system used to control how the search queries are entered on that platform. The major platforms in North America are NLM (National Library of Medicine), EBSCO, ProQuest, OVID, and Clarivate. Academic or health science libraries usually contract with at least one major platform and select the databases available to library users based on the courses of study available at that campus. Major platform vendors often package certain groups of related databases together for a set price. Thus, the databases available at one library may differ from those at another especially if the library is in an academic institution as opposed to a medical or health sciences center. Another aspect of platforms is the degree to which the architecture or code is open or closed. Open architecture allows the databases mounted on the platform to be easily accessible to other platforms. Closed architecture is proprietary and used only to mount the databases developed within or on that platform. MEDLINE, for example, resides on an open platform created by the National Library of Medicine. Therefore, the MEDLINE database can be easily mounted on other platforms and thus is available in most libraries and online. On the other hand, CINAHL is a proprietary database developed and maintained by EBSCO on the EBSCO platform. CINAHL cannot be transported or migrated to any other platform. A library must subscribe to the EBSCO platform to make CINAHL available to its users or patrons.

Two other features of platforms that are useful to know concern the degree to which the platform permits libraries to link their holdings to the database citations and the extent that to the platform allows linkage to free full-text documents on the internet. Linkage of citations to library holdings facilitates retrieval of items of interest from the search results. With a click on the link, the searcher can retrieve the item for online reviewing, printing, file saving, or reference formatting. Linkage to free full-text online documents offers the same options, plus expands the search results beyond the immediate library holdings.

### Bibliographic Citation and Full-Text Databases

Bibliographic citation databases contain citation data (author, title, and source information) and abstracts for a selected group of journal articles based on the scope or covered subjects selected by the database. Often such databases index higher standards of peer-review articles published in journals in the designed subject areas. Such databases may contain full text of some or all of the journal articles covered in the database or provide links. Some databases also include other types of publications such as book chapters, dissertations, editorials, book reviews, letters-to-the-editor, and abstracts of conference proceedings. Bibliographic citation databases are an important source of evidence-based practice. Such databases may contain the original research that provided the foundation for practice guidelines or specialized evidence-based online tools used to create such guidelines.

Within the category of bibliographic databases, there are two subtypes: general and subject specific. Both have advantages and disadvantages. General bibliographic databases cover a wider range of subjects, but the coverage may be less complete for specialized topics such as assistive technology or advanced orthotic devices. Subject-specific databases focus on fewer subjects but can cover more types of publications. The result is more detailed about fewer subjects but has less breadth of coverage. Most databases are organized based on a thesaurus or index, which is a master list of subject terms called controlled vocabulary or index terms, to organize the citations which facilitate searching the database. For example, if the thesaurus or index organizes articles under the term stroke, the searcher does not have to also search for synonyms and related terms such as cerebral vascular accident (CVA), brain attack, and apoplexy. The controlled vocabulary term "stroke" will have organized all articles related to stroke under the one subject called "stroke," thus saving time. The drawback to using or relying on thesauri and indexes is that each database has its own, so learning the controlled vocabulary for one database will not necessarily transfer to another. The databases described next start with general databases and proceed to more specialized ones.

### Biomedical Databases

MEDLINE/PubMed is the most frequently searched database for retrieving biomedical journal literature in most health-care disciplines. PubMed is the software interface (e.g., platform) to the MEDLINE database that is available to the public and can be accessed worldwide by anyone with a connection to the Internet. The database is maintained by the National Library of Medicine and is supported with taxpayer money. MEDLINE covers nine journals related to OT or edited by an occupational therapist. Since there are over 25 OT journals published worldwide, indexing only 9 journals does limit the coverage of OT. However, the scope of coverage and inclusion of most journals concerned with older adults makes searching MEDLINE/PubMed worthwhile for most search topics. In addition, true to the general database strategy most of the highly respected biomedical journals are included so the search results should contain high levels of evidence-based studies if such are available on the subject of interest. MEDLINE online is primarily a bibliographic database, but full access is available to any publication that was funded by the National Institute of Health (NIH). MEDLINE has a comprehensive thesaurus called MeSH (Medical Subject Headings) which is available online. Subjects can be limited to the controlled vocabulary by adding (mesh) to the search string. For example, to limit the search to articles indexed under the subject heading "occupational therapy," type **occupational therapy [mesh]**. Searching MEDLINE/PubMed directly online will provide the most up-to-date citations. Currency when searching through a database system within a college or university catalog depends on when the database was last updated by the database administrator in charge.

EMBASE is a second comprehensive biomedical database that is produced by Elsevier in the Netherlands in Europe and includes many foreign-language titles. Although MEDLINE does include major foreign language journals, the coverage is not as extensive as in EMBASE. Searching EMBASE requires a subscription. Medical libraries subscribe to EMBASE, but few academic libraries do so. For topics with international ramifications, EMBASE may be a good choice. The controlled vocabulary for EMBASE is called EMTREE.

### Citation Databases

Web of Science is a comprehensive subject bibliographic database maintained by Clarivate, but access requires a subscription. Most libraries in colleges and universities are subscribers but not many health-care facilities subscribe. The database indexes 13 OT journals. In addition, Web of Science includes all types of science, not just those considered biomedical. A useful feature of Web of Science is that the search results include a list of the major authors identified in the retrieved citations. Searching by author can expand the relevant journal articles with minimal additional effort.

Scopus is a second comprehensive science subject bibliographic database. Like Web of Science, access to search requires a subscription available through most colleges and universities. Coverage of OT journals is limited. Each retrieved search result does include a list of major authors.

### Subject Wide Databases

Google Scholar (scholar.google.com) is a comprehensive bibliographic subject wide database available to anyone with Internet access. It covers books, articles, theses and dissertations, conference abstracts, court opinions, and more. The search retrieval is normally sorted by relevance but can be sorted by date and limited by using the *Since Year* option to a range of years. If an item has full-text available, the link is displayed to the right of the citation. The linked item may be free or may require a subscription or fee to view or download.

Scopus covers primary documents from serial publications including journals in a wide area of subject topics. Primary documents means that the author (or authors) is identified as the researcher in charge of the research findings. Scopus does include systematic reviews and conference papers but does not cover other types of publications such as book reviews or obituaries. The Scopus database is maintained by the publisher Elsevier and is proprietary. Nine OT journals are indexed.

The Academic Search portfolio is composed of three databases: Premier, Complete, and Ultimate. The difference is the number of journals included. The Premier collection covers the smallest number while Ultimate covers the most journals and has the most expensive subscription fee. Academic Search databases cover a wide variety of topics in addition to scientific subjects. The three databases are mounted on the EBSCO platform. Like Web of Science and Scopus, a subscription is required for access. Most academic libraries subscribe and link their journal subscriptions to the indexed citations. Therefore, although the database is bibliographic, full text to some journal articles may be available to the searcher through the library's journal holdings.

Both citation databases introduced above also collect both sciences and social sciences publications.

## Nursing and Allied Health Databases

Three databases focus on nursing and allied health subjects. They are AMED (Allied and Complementary Medicine), CINAHL (Cumulative Index to Nursing and Allied Health), and ProQuest Nursing and Allied Health. AMED is produced by the Health Care Information Service of the British Library. It covers 10 OT–focused journals and is mounted on the EBSCO platform as a proprietary database.

CINAHL. There are three versions of the CINAHL database: CINAHL with Full Text, CINAHL Plus with FULL Text, and CINAHL Complete. The difference is the years of coverage, some additional features such as Evidence-Based Care Sheets, and subscription cost. CINAHL with Full Text does not include additional features. CINAHL Complete provides the most additional or expanded features. All three versions provide the most comprehensive coverage with 14 OT–focused journals and includes articles from many journals addressing health care–related issues with older adults. In addition, CINAHL includes citations to books, book chapters, and dissertations. Next to MEDLINE/PubMed, CINAHL is an important source of searching literature related to older adults and OT services. CINAHL Complete, a specialized version of CINAHL, includes full text to most journal articles indexed in the database. CINAHL and CINAHL Complete are mounted on the EBSCO platform.

ProQuest Nursing and Allied Health is available to all practitioners who maintain certification with NBCOT (National Board of Certification for Occupational Therapy). The database is proprietary to the platform ProQuest but is available at many college and university libraries and does include full-text access to many items. Like CINAHL, the database indexes 14 OT publications but some are newsletters, not journals. Subject coverage is similar to CINAHL and, depending on the search, topic may yield good results.

## Subject-Specific Databases

AgeLine is a subject-specific database focused on issues related to older adults including health sciences, economics, public policy, psychology, and social work. The database covers all the major journals concerned with the health and well-being of older adults as well as books, book chapters, and reports. AgeLine does require a subscription for access to search and therefore, is not always available. In addition, the database only indexes three OT journals (*American Journal of Occupational Therapy, Journal of Occupational Science,* and *Physical and Occupational Therapy in Geriatrics*). As a result, many relevant articles relevant to OT education and practice may not be included in the search results. AgeLine is maintained by EBSCO (www.ebsco.com/products/research-databases/ageline).

PsycInfo is a subject-specific database maintained by the American Psychological Association focused on psychological, behavioral, and mental health research. Subject coverage includes education, law, medicine, neuroscience, political science, sociology, sports and tests, and measurements. PsycInfo includes journal articles, books and book chapters, and dissertations. A controlled vocabulary is maintained in the *Thesaurus of Psychological Index Terms*. The database includes indexing of eight OT journals including *Physical and Occupational Therapy in Geriatrics*. PsycInfo does require a subscription. The database can be mounted on its own platform called APA PsycNet, but also can be mounted on the EBSCO, Ovid, or ProQuest platforms. Search guides for each platform are available on the APA main webpage (www.apa.org).

OT Search is a subject-specific database developed by the American Occupational Therapy Foundation (AOTF) but now maintained on a subscription basis by the AOTA. The advantage is that all indexed items are relevant to OT. However, only a limited number of other journals are included thus narrowing the search results. OT Search can be accessed through the AOTA main webpage (www.aota.org).

## Specialized Evidence-Based Practice Databases

Specialized databases have been developed to focus on evidence-based research studies. The items entered in the database are usually limited to systematic reviews or RCTs. Books and chapters about evidence-based research, or instruction manuals on evidence-based topics, are included but coverage is limited. The Cochrane Collaboration (www.cochrane.org) started in 1993 focuses on producing systematic reviews using the model of interprofessional collaboration. The review process is organized into review groups that focus on particular health areas such as interventions for mental health conditions and physical disorders. The reviews are produced in three formats: quick summary, summarized, and comprehensive. Coverage of OT topics is limited.

The Joanna Briggs Institute (JBI) database contains systematic reviews. Although the focus is nursing, some records do relate to OT. Searching the database requires a subscription, but the "Best Practice" information sheets can be downloaded and printed at no cost.

The Physiotherapy Evidence Database (PEDro) was developed in Australia for physical therapists, and OT Seeker was developed for occupational therapists. PEDro has continued to be funded but OT Seeker is not being updated due to lack of funds. Both use a rating scale developed for PEDro to determine which studies have higher internal validity and are less subject to bias. Both can be searched online without a subscription.

Evidence-Based Medicine Reviews (EBMR) is a database on the Ovid platform. EBMR includes the Cochrane databases plus the American College of Physicians (ACP) Journal Club, Health Technology Assessments (HTA), the Database of Abstracts of Reviews of Effectiveness (DARE), and the National Health System Economic Evaluation Database (NHS EED).

## Other Internet Resources

Internet resources can be valuable sources of evidence-based practice, such as sites maintained by professional associations including the American, Australian, British, and Canadian associations and the WFOT. All of these associations have webpages devoted to EBP. Some content may be restricted to members only, but other content is available to anyone.

Another useful internet site for finding EBP guidelines is the National Guideline Clearinghouse (NGC). NGC is maintained by the Agency for Healthcare Research and Quality (AHRQ) within the United States Department of Health and Human Services (USDHHS). National association guidelines include those of the American Geriatrics Society. Although based in the United States, practice guidelines developed in other countries are included such as those developed by the European Federation of Neurological Societies. The focus is on improving the quality and safety of health care by all health-related disciplines, but they stopped updating due to lack of funds.

A general search of the internet may yield a variety of EBP sites. The degree of trustworthiness may vary widely. Caution should be exercised. Using information from sites that are likely to be reliable, such as governmental documents or professional association guidelines, is a prudent approach. Sites maintained by individuals or local communities may address local issues that are not generalizable to other situations or clients.

## Developing a Search Strategy for Bibliographic Databases

Once the database or databases have been selected, the search strategy can be created. A search strategy is a method for efficiently finding information needed for research inquiries. It includes information resources, an organized structure of search terms and Boolean logic combinations used. Search strategy development involves continual assessment and refinement, which is an iterative process. Viewing the *Help* documentation or tutorial for each database can provide information on how the database is constructed and how to create a successful search strategy for that database. Among information sources used (e.g., books, journals, bibliographic databases), online bibliographic databases are the most frequently used resources. Most databases support multiple field searches, such as subject search (control vocabulary search and/or keyword search), author search, and the like. Often, searching multiple fields and multiple databases is needed for a comprehensive literature search.

## Useful Techniques for Database Searching

In general, there are three approaches to creating a search strategy using online databases: (1) use only controlled vocabulary terms from the thesaurus or master index, (2) use keywords only (also called text word or natural language searching), (3) use a combination of both. Box 5.2 lists terms that may be used to refer to older adults. Box 5.3 lists the names of journals that specialize in publishing articles and information about older adults.

Searching takes practice and a willingness to try more than one approach. Different databases allow or encourage different approaches. A search strategy that works well in retrieving useful citations in one database may retrieve nothing useful

### Box 5.2   Search Terms (Keyword search terms)

Old, older, oldest, oldster, oldsters
Aged, aging
Senior, seniors (in age, not academic or school rank)
Elder, elders, elderly
Geriatric, geriatrics, geriatrician
Gerontology, gerontologist,
65 plus, 65+ (or other age)
Long lived, long living
Eligible for Medicare, Eligible for Social Security or Pension

### Box 5.3   Journals on Gerontology, Geriatrics, and Aging

- *Age and Ageing*
- *Aging and Mental Health*
- *Archives of Gerontology and Geriatrics*
- *BMC Geriatrics*
- *Clinical Interventions in Aging*
- *European Geriatric Medicine*
- European Journal of Ageing
- *Gerontology*
- *Gerontology Special Interest Section Quarterly (AOTA)* closed title
- *International Journal of Geriatric Psychiatry*
- *International Psychogeriatrics*
- *Journal of Aging Research*
- *Journal of Cross-Cultural Gerontology*
- *Journal of Geriatric Oncology*
- *Journal of Gerontology: Social Sciences*
- *Journal of the American Geriatric Society (JAGS)*
- *Open Access Journal of Gerontology & Geriatric Medicine*
- *Physical & Occupational Therapy in Geriatrics (POTG)*
- *Research on Aging*
- *The Gerontologist*

in another. In general, for a quick search in which only a few citations are needed, the controlled vocabulary terms will, most likely, retrieve useful citations, if the subject or topic is indexed in the database. For a more complete search, keywords may retrieve citations not included in the controlled vocabulary alone. For a comprehensive search, both controlled vocabulary and keyword searches may be needed. In some databases such as those containing newspapers, there is no controlled vocabulary and thus, keyword searching is the only approach available. However, most other databases can be searched with both controlled vocabulary and keywords. Some pros and cons of both techniques are discussed next.

### Controlled Vocabulary (Thesaurus) Versus Keyword (Text Word) Searching

The purpose of creating subject headings into a controlled vocabulary system such as a thesaurus or master index is to organize related articles together allowing the searcher to retrieve a group of citations by entering one or two terms instead of many. A second purpose is to decrease the incidence in which a word or concept may have more than one meaning. Example: MEDLINE uses the term *Aged OR Aged 80 and over* to group articles together in which the subjects or participants were older adults. Thus one or two terms can save the searcher from having to enter all the possible terms by which older adults may be referenced. See Box 5.2.

The task of assigning the thesaurus or indexing terms to each collected publication entered into a database is performed by a person called an indexer or cataloger. Most databases employ more than one person to index or catalog items. The quality or consistency of the database depends on the skill and accuracy of the indexers to select the most accurate or best vocabulary terms from the thesaurus or indexing list and enter those terms in the individual citation record. However, entering the most accurate terms into the database is only one side of the equation. The other side depends on the skill of the searcher to identify and select the terms from the thesaurus or index that best fit the searcher's criteria. There is room for error or missed opportunity on both sides. The indexer may fail to enter all applicable terms appropriate to describe a given article or the searcher may fail to identify the best terms from the thesaurus or index to retrieve the most relevant citations.

Controlled vocabulary terms often are only applied to certain fields in the database record such as title and abstract. If the search terms appear in another database field such as the name of the institution or author's job title, the controlled vocabulary terms may not retrieve those citations into the search results. Enter the concept of keyword or natural language searching. Keywords are selected by the searcher and do not depend on an indexer for relevance. Thus, one side of the equation is eliminated. Now, however, the burden is on the searcher to identify all relevant or useful synonyms or related terms. If a term is missed, useful or important citations from the database may not be retrieved, or a second, or third search may be needed to relieve additional citations. Also, many citations may be false hits, that is, the term appears in the wrong context. For example, the term *oldest* may be used to designate the oldest child in the family, the term *senior* may refer to a senior management or a senior in college, the term *mature* may refer to a behavior such as acting mature. Eligibility to receive social security is not limited to older adults since some persons qualify due to disability or survivorship. The searcher has the burden of sifting through the citations and eliminating the false hits. Depending on the number of citations retrieved, sifting and sorting may take considerable time.

Despite the potential for false hits, keyword searching usually permits more fields in the database record to be searched automatically or by specifying the certain fields be searched. Thus, the address of the author's employment or the author's job title and position may be searchable, or the journal title and abbreviation may be added, any of which may improve the search results. Searching for OT or occupational therapist in the address or affiliation field may be the only way to retrieve citations authored by OT personnel because the abstract or text does not specifically state that OT was germane. An example might be an article in which the Lifestyle Redesign program was used in the intervention. The text includes a discussion of how the program was implemented but does not state that the program was being administered by OT personnel. The only reference to OT is in the address/affiliation field that states one of the authors is an occupational therapist at a certain hospital or clinic.

## Boolean Operators and Nesting

After selecting terms from a controlled vocabulary system or identifying keywords, the terms are connected using Boolean logic. Boolean logic is composed of mathematical formulas that designate which operations a computer will perform to identify and select citations from the database to create the search results. In bibliographic databases, the three most commonly used Boolean operators used to search are AND, OR, and NOT. The operator AND is used to connect search terms together. All terms must be present in the search results. Example: The search terms are *aged* AND *driving fitness*. All citations assigned to the term *aged* and to the phrase *driving fitness* will be retrieved from the database such as MEDLINE/PubMed. Use of the operator AND limits the search results to only those citations specified in the search string (terms entered in the search Box 5.2). The operator OR is used to connect synonyms or related concepts. Example: A simple keyword search might include older OR elderly OR senior adults. A citation must include at least one of the terms but may include two or three. Thus the search results are usually expanded and the number of citations increased. The operator NOT is used to remove or eliminate a term from the citations retrieved in the search results. Example: The search string is entered as *aged* NOT *animal*, eliminates any citation that mentions the term *animal*. The operator NOT can be tricky to use because while the intent of the searcher may be to remove animal research, articles that discuss both human and animal research will be lost. A better approach might be to search for *aged* AND *human*. Citations about animals will only be excluded from the results because there is no mention of humans. However, citations that include discussion of both human and animals will be retrieved because the search term human was stated in the search string.

A useful note is to recognize that mathematics logic performs in a manner that tends to be opposite to the language or linguistic logic. Whereas the operator AND restricts or limits retrieval the same word AND as a conjunction in the English language in mathematics would likely increase retrieval. Example: In mathematics logic entering a search strategy as *apples* AND *oranges* requires the text in the citation record to include both the words *apples* and *oranges*. Any citation that discusses apples but not oranges, or vice versa, will not be retrieved, thus limiting the retrieval. However, in the logic of language or linguistics, if a person is offered apples AND oranges the person assumes both fruits can be obtained thus the retrieval is increased. In contrast, the mathematical logic for the operator OR usually increases retrieval whereas in the logic of the English language use of the conjunction OR usually limits retrieval. Example: In mathematics logic entering a search strategy as *apples* OR *oranges* allows citations that include one or both terms to appear which generally increases the total number of citations retrieved. In the English language logic, if a person is offered apples OR oranges, the person expects to choose only one type of fruit. Finally, the mathematical operator NOT and the language conjunction NOT function in a similar style: to remove or stop access to something. However, as noted in the previous paragraph application can have unintended consequences. Example: the search strategy is entered as *apples NOT oranges*, so the retrieval should include citations that discuss apples but not oranges. However, the search system will also eliminate any article about apples even if the text simply states that oranges were not relevant to the discussion of apples. The search system does not consider context, just Boolean (mathematical) logic. Thus, any text that includes the term oranges will be eliminated, regardless of context, even if the main subject of the text is about apples. A useful principle is to review the search results carefully to determine if a revised search strategy that includes the operator NOT, actually removes unwanted items but keeps all desired items.

Other operators, often called proximity operators, exist such as adjacency (ADJ), adjacent within a certain number of words (ADJn or W/n), near (NEAR), or frequency (FREQ). Instructions for use of such operators is usually provided in the tutorial section of the database. Scopus is an example of a database that includes proximity operators. Examples: occupational ADJ therapy may decrease the retrieval of articles about the use of occupational medicine as a therapy. Using occupational W/2 therapy (within 2 words) may help retrieve articles using the phrase *occupational* and *physical therapy*. The same phrase might obtain the same results if the search string is entered as occupational NEAR therapy. The operator FREQ is designed to identify articles that use the word or phrase repeatedly in the abstract and text. The assumption is that repeated use of the word or phrase means the content of the article or resource is about the subject of interest. For example, if the phrase *occupational therapy* appears six times in an abstract or text, the chances are good the resource is about OT. Conversely, if the term occupational therapy appears only once, chances are the article is about some other topic and the term occupational therapy was mentioned to establish that occupational therapy is not germane to the subject of the article. Once again, the searcher needs to be alert to context. If the article appears in an OT–focused journal such as *Occupational Therapy International*, the authors may assume that the reader understands that the text is relevant to OT and not repeat the phrase *occupational therapy* or *occupational therapist* throughout the text.

Nesting is the technique of grouping multiple terms together in a search string, especially when two or more different Boolean operators are used. Parentheses () are most often used to nest terms. For example, a search strategy might be stated as (aged OR elder OR senior) AND (assessment or evaluation) AND driving fitness. The search results would include citations with at least one of the terms aged, elder, or senior and either assessment or evaluation and driving.

## Truncation, Wildcard, or Stemming

Truncation, wildcard, or stemming is the technique of using a symbol to standard for various letters or words in a search string. The technique is used most often in keyword searching to search for words with various endings. Example: instead of entering all of the following (old OR older OR oldest OR oldster OR oldsters), the term old is entered followed by the symbol "*," "?," "#," or "$" (asterisk, question mark, number sign, or dollar sign). A sample search might be entered as *driving fitness* AND *old\**. The search results should include all citations in which driving fitness and one of the five variations of the word *old* appear in the database MEDLINE/PubMed. Truncation can be very useful and time saving but can also lead to many false hits. Example: entering the term mass* will retrieve articles in which the word mass is used instead of tumor, but the truncation will also retrieve articles about the state of Massachusetts which may not be useful. A general rule of thumb is to limit the truncation to five letters or fewer unless the searcher is aware that false hits are unlikely. The tutorial section or tutorial of each database should state what truncation, wildcard, or stemming symbol is used by the database to substitute for letters or words when searching that database. Note that the use of truncation in the MEDLINE/PubMed database can only be applied to the last search term in the search string. In other words, only one use of the truncation symbol is allowed per search strategy and it must be the last search term. If other variations of a term are needed, the variations will have to be nested using parentheses. Other platforms and databases permit unlimited use of the truncation symbols within the same search string. Check the tutorial section of the database to determine which forms of truncation are allowed and how they are to be entered in the search string.

## Phrase Searching and Binding

Searching for phrases such as *activities of daily living* or *occupational therapy* requires understanding how the database processes a search string. Databases may permit the use of quotation marks to bind the words together to form a single string. Bind or binding in searching vocabulary refers to the process of making two or more words act within the database as though they were one. Example: without binding a database search may be interpreted as activities OR daily OR living. The result would include many false hits. Binding the phrase by added quotation marks instructs that the search to be conducted for articles that contain the phrase "activities of daily living" in that order or ADL. Binding is also useful when entering the words "occupational therapy" to avoid having the search results include all citations that mention occupational OR therapy. Note that MEDLINE/PubMed assumes ADL unless the operator NOT is used.

## Stop Words

Stop words are commonly used words such as articles, pronouns, and prepositions. Common stop words include a, an, the, in, of, on, are, be, if, into, etc. Stop words are not being indexed, but they are counted as words for proximity searching purposes. Many databases will automatically ignore common words from a search string. If a stop word must be included in a search, using quotes marks around the phrase that includes stop words is a technique. Stop words vary by database. Check the database's Help screen for a list.

## Mapping and Explode Operator

Some search engines automatically, by default, show terms that are broader (wider) or narrower (restrictive) than the term entered to provide a context. The searcher can then decide whether to use the wider term or a more restrictive concept. Mapping is based on organizing terms into an outline format. The broadest term starts with the outline followed by narrower terms. MeSH, the controlled vocabulary for the MEDLINE database, is organized in an outline format. CINAHL is another. Explode is an operator used in the MEDLINE/PubMed and CINAHL databases which is designed to take advantage of the outline format. Using EXPLODE allows the searcher to enter one command and retrieve all the concepts under the term rather than having to enter each term separately. Only databases that organize terms into an outline format allow the use of the operator EXPLODE.

## Focus Operator

The operator FOCUS in the MEDLINE/PubMed database allows the searcher to limit the documents retrieved to those that are indexed as major concepts in a citation. In a MEDLINE record, medical subject heading (MeSH) terms assigned to an article may be marked with an * or with the initials MJ (major). Both designate that the concept is considered to be a major point in the article. The operator FOCUS retrieves only those citations which are indexed with the major mark feature.

## Searching Fields

Fields are the labels given to each aspect of the citation when entered into the database. Examples include TI for title, AU for author, or AB for abstract. Most databases allow the searcher to search by the fields or limit a search to certain fields. Example: randomized controlled trial.ti would limit the search retrieval to those citations in which randomized controlled trial appeared in the title of the article. The advantage of this search strategy is that the citations retrieved are likely to be on target for requested information. The disadvantage is that many useful citations may be missed because the exact words did not appear in the title but do appear in the abstract or assigned indexing terms. The full list of search fields in PubMed can be accessed at https://pubmed.ncbi.nlm.nih.gov/help/#search-tags.

## Searching Subheadings

MEDLINE/PubMed also refines the indexing to certain subheadings designed to further classify the content. Examples include tx for treatment or st for standards. The search query can be limited to certain subheadings. For example, "Influenza in Birds/prevention and control"(Mesh) tells

PubMed/MEDLIE to retrieval articles about prevention and control of avian flu.

## Search Filters

Search filters allow a search to be limited in some manner. Search filters vary from one database to another, but some common ones allow the search to be limited to certain years, type of publication, or language. For example, in MEDLINE/PubMed a search for OT can be limited to the last 5 years, to journal articles only, and to those published in English only. Some databases display the frequently used filters to the right or left of the initial search results. The searcher can mark the filters to be applied and rerun the search strategy limiting the search results to those items that meet the search criteria.

## Search Hedges or Blocks

Search hedges or search blocks are search strategies formed by organizing a topic in advance of searching into a series of related free-text terms (words, phrases, subject headings) into a single search string. Some commonly used search hedges are published such as one for searching controlled clinical trials within the CIHAHL Plus database (Glanville et al., 2019). Search hedges are particularly useful if the searcher is interested in writing a systematic review. The length of some search hedges may be more than is needed to retrieve 95% of the literature available using the standard indexing terms already assigned such as "randomized controlled trials."

## Hand Searching

Hand searching refers to the process of examining directly the table of contents or text of articles in a resource such as a journal, book, newsletter, position paper, or other publication. The retrieval of useful information is dependent on the skill of the searcher to recognize and retrieve relevant information. Hand searching tends to be time consuming since resources must be examined individually. However, the results may identify resources not indexed in the online databases sometimes referred to as grey literature. Hand searching OT journals and newsletters that are not indexed in any database may retrieve additional useful information.

## Reviewing and Revising a Search Strategy

While planning the search strategy in advance is the preferred approach, sometimes the best plan should be revised (expanded or restricted) based on initial review of the first citation results. Scanning the abstracts may identify additional synonyms, abbreviations, or phrases that could result in more citations. Printing out a full database record for two or three articles may provide information on additional controlled vocabulary terms that were missed or not considered during the initial search. Occasionally the initial scan provides information about terms that should be avoided using the NOT operator to reduce the number of false hits.

## Appraisal Process and Tools

Not all retrieved evidence-based information is of the same level of trustworthiness (accurate, reliable, current, effective, and efficient). Before applying the evidence, all information should be reviewed to determine if the source is reliable, that is, known for telling-like-it-is for accuracy and currency. Some examples of information that usually is trustworthy are:

- Practice guidelines developed and published by government agencies and professional organizations.
- Systemic reviews and meta-analyses published in peer-reviewed scholarly journals (have an editorial board whose names are printed in an issue of the journal and published guidelines and criteria for manuscript review).
- Results of research studies that are well designed, completed, and published in peer-reviewed journals.
- Journal articles, books, and chapters written and published by recognized authorities and leaders in the field of evidence-based approaches.
- Web pages written and maintained by governmental agencies, professional organizations, or universities with accredited medical schools and health-care programs.
- Continuing education programs reviewed and approved by a professional organization or approved provider before being presented.
- Practitioners and experienced colleagues known to have implemented evidence-based approaches in their institution or facility.

Some types of evidence-based information require careful review before application because the information may be biased, misleading, out-of-date, or may contain false or inaccurate information. Such information should be checked using one or more of the reliable sources listed above before being implemented. Better to check in advance than apply techniques that may be harmful or useless. Examples of evidence-based information that requires careful review for trustworthiness before implementing in practice settings include:

- Blogs and webinars based on testimonials
- Web pages written and maintained by individual practitioners and lay persons
- Newspaper or trade journal articles
- Radio or television presentations
- Social media of all types

## Summary

A good search strategy requires knowledge of searching techniques as well as a thorough knowledge of the subject to be searched. Sometimes the search strategy must be revised after an initial review of results. To summarize the search strategy techniques, the following example is provided. Problem statement: What is the evidence for occupational therapists performing automobile driving evaluations with older adults to maintain independence?

PICO(T) Statement Example: population is older adults and synonyms. Intervention: occupational therapy, occupational therapy practitioners, and fitness-to-drive (driving fitness evaluation). Comparison: no intervention. Outcome: independence, living at home, functioning in the community.

Basic search in MEDLINE/PubMed using controlled vocabulary: aged (mesh) AND occupational therapy (mesh) AND automobile driving evaluation (mesh).

Expanded controlled vocabulary search using nesting: (aged [mesh] OR adult [mesh]) AND (occupational therapy [mesh] OR occupational therapist [mesh]) AND (automobile driver examination [mesh] OR automobile driving [mesh]).

Basic Keyword search with nesting and binding: (aged OR old*) AND ("occupational therap* OR OT) AND ("driving evaluation" OR "driving assessment"). Note: Binding is not necessary in MEDLINE/PubMed.

Expanded keyword search with truncation and nesting: (aged OR old* OR elder* OR geriatric* OR gerontology* OR senior* OR mature*) AND (driv* evaluat* OR driv* assess*) AND (occupational therap* OR OT). Note: In MEDLINE/PubMed binding is assumed so quotation marks are not needed.

Analysis of the last search results identified two issues. One, truncating the word mature (matures, maturity) resulted in too many false hits, so the term was dropped and the search was repeated before being saved. Second, three additional search phrases were identified that also addressed the PICO(T) statement. The phrases were "driving assessment," "fitness to drive," and "driving performance." Searching for these phrases resulted in additional useful citations regarding guidelines and suggested standards that did not specify age criteria but were developed to assess driving ability after the person received a certain diagnosis such as stroke or brain injury. Finally, searches by author with multiple publications added information about the development of the concepts of driving fitness and the pros and cons of different techniques for assessment such as checklists, using a driver simulator or real-time, and/or on-the-road assessment.

## Critiquing and Conceptually Applying Evidence-Based Literature to Current Practice

Once resources have been retrieved, the next step is to identify which resources are most likely to be accurate and important. Of course, the type of accuracy and level of importance depends on the purpose of the search. Working definitions of accuracy and importance of resources to assist in client care planning may be different from those useful in developing a research proposal. Regardless of the purpose, the concept of deciding on accuracy and importance of literature resources is called critical appraisal (Sackett et al., 2000). Critical appraisal involves using a systematic process of examining resources to determine their accuracy or validity (trustworthy) and importance, relevancy, or usefulness to answering the proposed question or problem. The purpose is to permit practitioners and investigators to determine whether the results of the research studies are reliable and valid in providing information that may be important, relevant, and useful to planning, implementing, and evaluating outcomes for clients or developing a research project. Critical appraisal can be subdivided into general principles and organizing models for reviewing resources and specific criteria for reviewing specific types of research design.

## General Appraisal Principles

Three general questions can be asked when reviewing any research study:

1. What is the purpose of (question to be answered by) the study, and is that purpose or question important and relevant to the problem statement for which literature is being reviewed? The purpose of a study is usually stated in the introduction section or lead paragraphs of the study.
   a. If the answer to important or relevance is "yes" the study's identifying citation information (author(s), title, and source} should be recorded for further review.
   b. If the answer is "no" the study can be disregarded from further review.
   c. If the purpose statement is unclear, and the answer to the importance of relevance
   d. If the answer to the question is "maybe," additional review may be needed to determine importance and relevance by examining the outcomes reported in the results and discussion or conclusions sections.
2. Is the study design provided in the methodology section relevant and appropriate to the research question? This question has three additional parts including:
   a. Does the study methodology address the potential sources of bias that might skew the results in one direction or another?
   b. What steps were taken to minimize the effects of bias?
   c. Can the results be considered valid or trustworthy because the effects of bias have been minimized or clearly stated so the reader can judge independently the potential impact on the proposed problem (PICOT) question?
3. Do the data or results justify the conclusions stated in the results and discussion sections of the paper? In other words:
   a. Are the results of the study important, useful, and relevant to the question or problem being asked?
   b. Is any information missing that could be important or useful? If so, identify and record the missing information.
   c. Is any information provided that does not appear to be supported by the data provided? If so, identify and record the type of missing information or data

## Research Design and Levels of Evidence

Originally models use to depict levels of evidence-based studies were organized on the assumption that research methodology using experimental design approaches which produced quantitative (numeric and statistical) data were the best sources of information, especially RCTs, cohort and case-control studies (Guyatt et al., 1995). The rationale was that experimental designs best controlled for bias, which might influence or change the study outcome. Other types of research designs were considered of lesser significance including qualitative and outcome designs such as case reports, single-subject studies, surveys, and expert opinions. For a discipline such as OT, such a narrow view of research design approaches limited the application of research to practice since many important aspects of practice are not part of experimental design protocols, including different contexts or environments and emotional variables, such as meaning or personal (client) satisfaction. A newer model proposed by Tomlin and Borgetto (2011) proposed that all research designs be considered relevant, but that the systematic reviews and meta-analyses be viewed as the best sources for application. Yet another approach is to view research studies based on whether they have been critically appraised using a process that analyzes and synthesizes the results of studies for application to practice, labeled filtered information, or are primarily reviewed for suitability to publish, labeled unfiltered information (Mitchell et al., 2012). Organizing level of evidence then changes to focus on information analysis and synthesis. Thus, the focus of evidence-based approaches shifts from viewing the research design as paramount to more reliance on review processes to sift through data and results to arrive at conclusions and recommendations applicable in practice or future research proposals. Research design based on experimental design is still important, but it becomes one of the criteria to consider when applying critical analysis techniques, not the primary consideration. Thus information from both statistical (quantitative) and narrative (qualitative) based studies is relevant to the critically appraising research studies for their potential contribution to practice settings and future research.

As stated above, the model developed by Mitchell et al. (2012) organized the evidence-based literature into two broad categories called *filtered information* and *unfiltered information*. Filtered information includes resources and techniques that appraise the quality of the research studies by persons not involved in the original research, thus is less prone to bias, using an identified protocol or guideline and often make recommendations for a particular area of practice. Filtered resources include practice guidelines, systematic reviews, scoping reviews, critically appraised topics (CATs), and critically appraised papers (CAPs). All filtered information studies are secondary resources since the authors review and summarize data from existing published studies. In other words, filtered information is based on a review process that appraises the results of primary or original resources. Unfiltered resources include most primary or original resource research designs including RCTs, cohort studies, single subject studies, case reports, and others. The advantage of the Mitchell et al. (2012) model is that it starts the process of translating research results into practical application by reviewing and summarizing data from primary resources into practice-based recommendations. A second advantage is the review process can be based on the critical appraisal of several studies to determine if similar findings are documented from more than one study. The variety and types of research designs, critically appraised criteria, and examples are described using the broad headings of filtered, unfiltered, and background headings. When recent examples of critically appraised criteria were not identified, development criteria were substituted.

## Filtered Information

### *Practice Guidelines*

Practice guidelines, clinical practice guidelines, practice standards, or practice recommendations are defined by the Institute of Medicine as "statements that include recommendations intended to optimize patient care. They are informed by a systematic view of evidence and an assessment of the benefits and harms of alternative care options" (Graham et al., 2011, p. 6). Practice guidelines may have several purposes and may be used to assist the following:

- OT practitioners in providing evidence-based interventions and communicating about the services to external audiences
- External audiences in understanding the scope of OT services; the professional education, training, and skills of OT practitioners; and determining the need for OT services
- Researchers/investigators, OT practitioners, program evaluators, and policy analysts in determining outcome measures for analyzing the effectiveness of OT intervention
- OT educators in designing curricula that incorporate evidence-based findings from the published literature
- Researchers/investigators in determining the area for future research and gathering background research on a topic of interest (AOTA, 2021a, 2021b)

Sources of practice guidelines that may be useful in OT practice include:

- AOTA www.aota.org
- Royal College of Occupational Therapists www.rcot.co.uk/publications
- EviCore Healthcare www.evicore.com
- Agency for Health Care Research and Quality www.ahrq.gov

Practice guidelines should include six major sections according to the AGREE Nest Steps Consortium (2017). The questions have been adapted from the original text

- Scope and Purpose:
  - Are the objectives of the practice guideline clearly stated?
  - Is the clinical or health question clearly stated?
  - Is the client group or health condition clearly stated for which the practice guideline is intended?
- Stakeholder Involvement
  - What professional group(s) is/are included in the guidelines?
  - Have client views and preferences been included?
  - Have the intended or targeted users (professional or lay persons) of the guideline been clearly defined?
  - Has the guideline been piloted among the intended or targeted users?
- Rigor of Development
  - What systematic methods were used to search for evidence and source materials?
  - Are the criteria clearly described for inclusion and exclusion of source materials?
  - Are the methods clearly stated that were used to formulate the recommendations?

- Is there a link that ties the recommendations to the supporting evidence?
- Are the health benefits, side effects, and risks considered in stating the recommendations?
- Were the recommendations externally reviewed by experts prior to publication?
- Is there a stated procedure for updating the guidelines?
- Clarity and Presentation
  - Are the recommendations clearly stated and not ambiguous?
  - Are different options for managing the condition clearly stated?
  - Are key (most important) recommendations clearly identifiable?
  - Are tools or suggestions clearly stated for application of the recommendations?
- Applicability
  - Have possible barriers to applying the recommendations been discussed?
  - Have potential costs been considered for implementing the recommendations?
  - Are criteria for reviewing and monitoring outcomes of the recommendations included?
- Editorial Independence
  - Is there a statement included regarding editorial independence from the funding source?
  - Have conflicts of interest been cited and recorded?

Review Criteria Checklist:

- AGREEII; Appraisal of Guidelines for Research & Evaluation II (2013). http://www.agreetrust.org
- Critical Appraisal Worksheet: Practice Guidelines. https://researchguides.dormouth.edu/id.php?context_id_48916881
- BestBet: Guidelines Checklist https://bestbet.org/ca/pdf/guideline.pdf

Example: Kaldenberg, J., & Smallfield, S. (2020). Occupational therapy practice guidelines for older adults with low vision. *American Journal of Occupational Therapy, 74*(2), 740397010p1–740397010p23. https://doi.org/10.5014/ajot.2020.742003.

### *Systematic Reviews*

A systematic review is "an analysis of the available literature (that is, evidence) and a judgment of the effectiveness or otherwise of a practice, involving a series of complex steps" that vary according to the protocol used to establish the review process (Joanna Briggs Institute, 2020). Higgins et al. (2021) define a systematic review of one that "uses explicit, systematic methods to collate and synthesize finding of studies that address a clearly formulated question". Typical protocols are the Preferred Reporting Items for Systematic Reviews and Meta-Analysis (PRISMA), (2020), Cochrane Handbook for Systematic Reviews of Intervention, (Higgins et al., 2021 or institute of Medicine, 2011). The AOTA recommends the use of the PRISMA protocol for systematic reviews submitted to the *American Journal of Occupational Therapy*. The purpose of a systematic review is to identify a specific body of literature over a designated time period and to analyze the literature using specific criteria. Page et al. (2021) suggest systematic reviews:

- Can provide syntheses of the state of knowledge in a field
- Address questions that otherwise could not be answered by individual studies
- Identify problems in primary research that should be rectified in future studies
- Generate or evaluate theories about how or why phenomena occur
  Examples of Review Criteria are:
- PRISMA guidelines. Check online for most current edition
- Guidelines for systematic reviews. AOTA.
- *Checklist for Systematic Reviews and Research Syntheses.* Joanna Briggs Institute. Check online for most current edition
- *10 questions to help make sense of a systematic review.* Critical Appraisal Skills Programme, https://casp-uk.net
  Example: Foster, E. R., Carson, L. G., Archer, J., & Hunter, E. G. (2021). Occupational therapy interventions for instrumental activities of daily living for adults with Parkinson's disease: A systematic review. *American Journal of Occupational Therapy, 75*(3), 7503190030p1–7503190030p24. https://doi.org/10.5014/ajot.2021.046581.

### Meta-Analysis Studies

Meta-analysis studies require research reports based on quantitative and experimental design such as randomized controlled studies in which statistical data are provided in the results section. Studies based on meta-analysis may be included in a systematic review study to further analyze the data from the quantitative studies or may be published separately. Meta-analysis studies usually include the statistical technique called *meta-analysis of effect estimates*, which is used "to synthesize results when study effect estimates and their variances are available, yielding a quantitative summary of results" (McKenzie & Brennan, 2019). The PRISMA 2020 Checklist states under the Results of Syntheses items that if meta-analysis is done, a summary should include the estimate and its precision (confidence/credible interval) and measure of statistical heterogeneity (PRISMA, 2020 Checklist).

Review Criteria Checklist:

- Patel, N., & Bajal, N. S. (2018). Meta-analyses: How to critically appraise them? *Journal of Nuclear Cardiology, 25*(5), 1598–1600. https://doi.org/10.1007/s12350-017-0898-8.
- Reviews and Meta-Analyses Checklist; https://bestbets.org/ca/pdf/review.pdf
  Example: Tofani, M., Ranieri, A., Fabbrini, G., Berardi, A., Pelosin, E., Valente, D., Fabbrini, A., Costanzo, M., & Galeoto, G. (2020). Efficacy of occupational therapy interventions on quality of life in patients with Parkinson's disease: A systematic review and meta-analysis. *Movement Disorders Clinical Practice, 7*(8), 891–901. https://doi.org/10.1002/mdc3.13089.

### Scoping Review

According to the authors who developed and articulated the process of scoping review, such reviews should identify the "key concepts underpinning a research area and the main sources and types of evidence available…especially where an area is complex or has not been reviewed comprehensively before" (Arksey & O'Malley, 2005, p. 21). The authors state the purpose or reasons for doing a scoping study are to:

- Examine the extent, range, and nature of (existing) research activity
- Determine the value of undertaking a full systematic review
- Summarize and disseminate research findings
- Identify research gaps in the existing literature (p. 21)

The stages for conducting a scoping study are to: identify the research question, identify relevant studies, select the studies for review, chart the data, and collate, summarize and report the results (Arksey & O'Malley, 2005). Sucharew and Macaluso (2019) provide a compare-and-contrast chart between systematic and scoping reviews. One important difference is that systematic reviews are restricted to certain study methodologies that meet the standards set by the review protocol whereas scoping reviews can include all types of research studies and nonstandard sources of information. Note: chart might be useful to copy.

Review Criteria Checklist: PRISMA-ScR Checklist. Prisma-statement.org/Extension/ScopingReviews

Example: Miranda-Duro, M. D. C, Nieto-Riveiro, L., Concheiro-Moscuso, P., Croba, B., Pousada, T., Canosa, N., & Pereira, J. (2021). Occupational therapy and the use of technology on older adult fall prevention: A scoping review. *International Journal of Environment Research and Public Health, 18*, 702. https://doi.org/10.3390/ijerph17020702.

### Critically Appraised Topics

CATs are "short summaries of the most up-to-date, high-quality available evidence that is found using thorough structure methods" (Callander et al., 2017, p. 1007). A CAT is "a method of conducting an abbreviated systematic review" (Beckers et al., 2019, p. 409). When conducting a CAT, all the rules apply as if a systematic review was being performed except that the focus can be narrowed to a specific time period, limited number of journals or specific type of intervention. A CAT may be used to determine if a systematic review could be implemented. The primary parts of a CAT are: formatting of a focused question, searching for the most relevant and high-quality evidence, critically appraising the evidence and applying the results back to the client situation (Callander et al., 2017).

Review Criteria Checklist: Lowe, R., et al., Critically Appraised Topics. (n.d.). www.physiopedia.com/Critically_Appraised_Topics

Example: American Occupational Therapy Association. (2016). *Alzheimer's disease and related disorders.* AOTA. www.aota.org

### Critically Appraised Papers

CAPs are "at-a glance summaries of the methods, findings, study limitations, and clinical implications of selected quantitative intervention-based articles" (AOTA's Evidence

Exchange, 2019). Whereas CATs review a group of articles, CAPs review one article at a time to glean useful information for practice. The AOTA has published a worksheet for performing critically apprised papers (AOTA's Evidence Exchange, 2021). A practice focused summary is stated in the section labeled "Clinical Bottomline."

Review Criteria Checklist: The CAP worksheet can be used to appraise any research article, it is most often used to appraise randomized controlled trials.

Example: Evidence Exchange (2018). AOTA Critically Appraised Paper Series: Article by Bürge, E., Berchtold, A., Maupetit, C., Bourquin, N. M., von Gunten, A., Ducraux, D., Zumbach, S., Peeters, A., & Kuhne, N. (2016). Does physical exercise improve ADL capacities in people over 65 years with moderate or serve dementia hospitalized in an acute psychiatric settings? A multisite randomized clinical trial. *International Psychogeriatrics, 29*, 323-332. https://doi.org/10.1017/s1041510216001460.

## Unfiltered Information
### Randomized Controlled Trials

RCTs are the only research design that can demonstrate whether an intervention has actually caused the outcome(s) of interest (AOTA, 2020). RCTs are based on a procedure that allocates participants or subjects to either be assigned to the intervention or control group. To qualify as an RCT study, the assignment must be "purely based on chance, not influenced by the known characteristics of the participants" (Tufanaru et al., 2020). Chance is obtained by using a printed or a computer-generated list of random numbers. In addition, the knowledge regarding allocation (who was assigned to which group) is not known to the investigators, participants, or research assistants responsible for administering the intervention(s) or evaluating the outcome(s). The purpose of concealment is to avoid potential distortion or prejudice, called bias, of the results because certain participants were assigned to the experimental or control group based on someone's opinion as to whether a participant was likely to benefit, or not benefit, from the intervention. The checklist for RCTs created by the Joanna Briggs Institute (Tufanaru et al., 2020) includes the following concepts:
- Random assignment to experimental or control group
- Concealment (blinding) of allocation to the group assignment to investigators, participants, and research associates (those administering intervention or those evaluating results and outcomes)
- Degree of similarity of participant characteristics at baseline (beginning of study)
- Degree to which experimental and control groups were treated identically (consistency) except for the intervention
- Description provided of follow-up analysis of differences between the groups
- Degree of consistency to which participants were analyzed in the group to which they were assigned
- Degree of consistency to which outcome measures were applied to the groups
- Reliability of outcomes measures

- Appropriateness of statistical analysis
- Appropriateness of research design including any deviations identified in the protocol
Review Criteria Checklist:
- Checklist for Randomized Controlled Trials. Joanna Briggs Institute https://jbi.global/sites/default/files/2020-08/Checklist_for_Cohort_Studies Check online for the most recent version.
- CASP Randomised Controlled Trial Standard Checklist. Critical Appraisal Skills Programme. www.casp-uk.net
Example: Mirz, M., Gecht-Silver, M., Keating, E., Krischer, A., Kim, H., & Kottorp, A (2020). Feasibility and preliminary efficacy of an occupational therapy intervention for older adults with chronic conditions in a primary care clinic. *American Journal of Occupational Therapy, 74*(5), 7405205030p1–7405205030p13. https://doi.org/10.5014/ajot.2020.039842.

### Non-Randomized, Cohort Studies
Cohort studies obtain data from two or more groups that have been exposed, or not exposed, to the intervention of interest. Typically, investigators attempt to match participant characteristics in the intervention group and the non intervention group (e.g., age, sex, health status). Participations are not randomly assigned because the matching process is deliberate and known to the investigators. Cohort-designed studies are useful for studying the effects of predictive risk factors on an outcome (AOTA, 2020).

Review Criteria Checklist:
- Checklist for Cohort Studies. Joanna Briggs Institute https://jbi.global/critical-appraisal-tools Check online for the most recent version.
- CASP Checklist: Cohort Study. Critical Appraisal Skills Programme. www.casp-uk.net
Example: Suzuki, Y., Tsubakino, S., & Fujii, H. (2020). Eating and grooming abilities predict outcomes in patients with early middle cerebral infarction: A retrospective cohort study. *Occupational Therapy International, 2020*, 1374527 (8 pgs). https://doi.org/10.1155/2020/1374527.

### Non-Randomized and Not Matched, Two-Group
Non-randomized and not matched studies using two groups are quasi-experimental designs that are similar to RCTs or true cohort studies but without randomization or matching of the participants. Although matching is not obtained for all characteristics considered relevant, the two groups may be matched on some characteristics being studied by virtue of the persons seen in a particular setting such as a children's hospital or senior citizen's exercise program. The control group may be selected for convenience or availability of participants. Non-randomization and lack of matching make the study easier to conduct and often less expensive but increases the risk of bias because participants are not randomized or matched. The design is useful to conduct pilot studies which may lead to RCT or cohort studies (AOTA, 2020).

Review Criteria: Checklist for cohort studies can be used but matching criteria are marked as not applicable.

Example: Okamura, T., Hayashi, A., Matsuo, S., Shinoda, K., Konishi, I, Makio, H., & Tsui, M. (2017). Prevention of falls in the elderly dementia trial: A quasi-experimental study. *Journal of Human Ergology, 47,* 37–41. https://doi.org/10.11183/jhe.47.1_37.

### Non-Randomized, One-Group (Pre-Post Design, Before-After Study)

Non-randomized, one-group studies, also called pre-post designed studies, collect baseline data (pre) on the participants, then introduce the intervention of interest, and collect the data again (post). The design is easy to administer in a clinical setting and often cost effective. The purpose of the design is to provide descriptive information on whether a change occurred in the participants (i.e., did they improve or not on the outcome of interest?). A major problem with the design is the risk of bias because there is no control group to compare to and no randomization or matching in the participant selection. Further research such as a RCT study, is usually needed to ascertain whether the intervention caused the outcome or something else caused the change (AOTA, 2020).

Review Criteria Checklist: Checklist for Quasi-Experimental Studies (Non-Randomized Experimental Studies). Joanna Briggs Institute. https://jbi.global/critical-appraisal-tools. Check online for the most current edition

Example: Renda, M., & Lape, J. E. (2018). Feasibility and effectiveness of telehealth occupational therapy home modification interventions. *International Journal of Telerehabilitation, 10*(1), 3–14. https://doi.org/10.5195/ijt.2018.6244.

### Single Subject, Single Case (ABA or ABAB)

Single-subject or single-case experimental designs. Single-subject studies are trials that focus on an individual client as the sole unit of observation in a study investigating the efficacy or side effects of different interventions to determine the optimal intervention for an individual client using objective data-driven criteria (White, 2020). Single-subject design refers to a set of experimental methods that can be used to test the efficacy of an intervention using a small number of participations and involve repeated measurements, sequential introduction of an intervention, specific data analysis and statistics (Krasny-Pacini & Evans, 2018). Single case studies are not case reports. The focus is on systematically recording and reporting on the response of a participant to an intervention over a time period and number of trials or interactions. A baseline of performance is established (A), then an intervention begins (B), next the intervention is stopped, the baseline conditions are reinitiated (A) and the results reported. In some studies, the intervention may be reinitiated (B) especially if the results are positive.

Review Criteria Checklist: Lobo, M. A., Moeyaert, M., Cunha, A. B., & Babik, I. (2017). Single-case design, analysis and quality assessment for intervention research. *Journal of Neurological Physical Therapy, 41*(3), 187–197. https://doi.org/10.1097/NPT.0000000000000187.

Example: Hayner, K. A. (2012). Effectiveness of the California tri-pull taping method for shoulder subluxation poststroke. A single-subject ABA design. *American Journal of Occupational Therapy, 66,* 727–736. https://doi.org/10.5015/ajot.2010.004663.

### Cohort Studies

A cohort study observes the effects of risk factors, incidence, and prognosis of diseases by following two or more groups of patients over a certain period of time. It answers the question of "what will happen" and is prospective. A cohort study can be a good alternative when an RCT cannot be undertaken due to reasons of cost, acceptance, ethical concerns, or other factors. The major source of bias for a cohort study is selection bias, or bias in cohort recruitment, specifically, whether all subjects were recruited in a defined time period and whether the groups had the same characteristics.

Review Criteria Checklist:
- Checklist for Cohort Studies. Joanna Briggs Institute. https://jbi.global/sites/default/files/2021-10/Checklist_for_Cohort_Studies.docx
- CASP Checklist: Case Control Study. Critical Appraisal Skills Programme. https://casp-uk.net/glossary/cohort-study/

Example: Petersson, I., Kottorp, A., Bergström, J., & Lilja, M. (2009). Longitudinal changes in everyday life after home modifications for people aging with disabilities. *Scandinavian Journal of Occupational Therapy, 16*(2), 78–87. (PubMed ID: 18821447.)

### Case-Control Study

In a case-controlled study, the investigator selects a participant group who are known to have a certain disease or experienced a certain outcome and a matching participant control group that is known not to have a certain disease or have experienced a certain outcome. Outcomes are judged based on whether the participant group changed (improved desired performance or decreased undesirable behavior, etc.) as a result of being exposed to or experiencing the intervention of interest. Case-control studies are retrospective studies, meaning the data have already been collected. The investigator analyzes the available data relative to the outcome or intervention of interest (AOTA, 2020).

Review Criteria Checklist:
- Checklist for Case Control Studies. Joanna Briggs Institute. https://jbi.global/critical-appraisal-tools. Check online for the most current edition.
- CASP Checklist: Case Control Study. Critical Appraisal Skills Programme. www.casp-uk.net

Example: Morin, L., Larrañaga, A. C., Welmer, A.-K., Rizzuto, D., Wastesson, J. W., & Johnell, K. (2019). Polypharmacy and injuries fall in older adults: a nationwide nested case-control study. *Clinical Epidemiology, 11,* 483–493.

### Cross-Sectional Studies

Cross-sectional studies are used to determine the presence or absence of disease or other health-related variables in each member of the study population or in a representative sample at one particular time. The method contracts with longitudinal studies which follow a population or sample over a period of time (Watari et al., 2022).

Review Criteria Checklist:

- Checklist for Analytical Cross-Sectional Studies. Joanna Briggs Institute https://jbi.global/critical-appraisal-tools. Check online for the current edition.
- STROBE Statement: Checklist of items that should be included in reports of cross-sectional studies. https://www.strobe-statements.org/checklists

Example: Krueger, R., Sweetman, M. M., Martin, M., & Cappaert, T. A. (2020). Occupational therapists' implementation of evidence-based practice: A cross sectional survey. *Occupational Therapy in Health Care, 34*(3), 253–276. https://doi.org/10.1080/07380577.2020.1756554.

### Single Case Study

A single case study is based on an individual client as the sole unit of observation in a study investigating the efficacy or side effects of different interventions to determine the optimal intervention for an individual client using objective data-driven criteria (White, 2020). A case study is an in-depth investigation of a single individual, family, or other entity. Multiple types of data (biographical, physiological, psychological environment) are assembled to understand an individual's background, relationship, and behavior (VandenBos, 2015).

Review Criteria Checklist: Crowe, S., Cresswell, K., Robertson, A. Huby, G., Avery, A., & Sheikh, A. (2011). The case study approach. *BMC Medical Research Methodology, 11*, 100 http://www.biomedcentral.com/1471-2288/11/100

Example: Mani, K. (2019). Occupational therapy for knee osteoarthritis: A case study. *Indian Journal of Occupational Therapy, 51*(4), 151–154. https://doi.org/10.4103/ijoth.ijoth_34_19

### Case Report

A case report is a collection of data related to a person's medical or psychological condition (VandenBos, 2015). The focus is on the medical history, diagnosis, prognosis, previous interventions, past and current diagnostic test results, medications, and the person's response to current intervention including positive results and adverse events.

Review Criteria Checklist: Checklist for Case Reports. Joanna Briggs Institute. https://jbi.global/critical-appraisal-tools. Check online for the most current edition.

Example: Wilcox, J., Peterson, K. S., Lewis, C. M., & Margetis, J. L. (2021). Occupational therapy during COVID-19-Related critical illness: A case report. *American Journal of Occupational Therapy, 75*(Suppl. 1), 7511210010p1–7511210010p7. https://doi.org/10.5014/ajot.2021.049196.

### Case Series

Case series studies consist of reporting on the treatment of several individual participants with the same condition or multiple reports on a single participant. Case series are used to illustrate an aspect of a condition, successful intervention, or adverse reaction to intervention. Case series studies can be useful in deciding what intervention may be appropriate or assist in establishing a diagnosis (AOTA, 2020).

Review Criteria Checklist: Checklist for Case Series. Joanna Briggs Institute https://jbi.global/critical-appraisal-tools. Check online for the most current edition.

Example: Cunningham, R., & Valesek, S. Occupational therapy interventions for urinary dysfunction in primary care: A case series. *American Journal of Occupational Therapy, 73*(5), 7305185050. https://doi.org/10.5014/ajot.2019.038356.

### Qualitative Studies

Qualitative studies use descriptive (non-numerical) data collection systems such as observation of behavior or personal accounts of experiences. A variety of techniques include content analyses of narrative, in-depth interviews, focus groups, participant observation, and case studies that may be conducted in naturalistic settings (VandenBos, 2015).

Review Criteria Checklist:

- Checklist for Qualitative Research. Joanna Briggs Institute. https://jbi.global/critical-appraisal-tools. Check online for the most current edition.
- CASP Checklist: Qualitative research. Critical Appraisal Skills Programme. www.casp-uk.net.

Example: Minami, S., & Kobayaski, R. (2019). A qualitative study of the practice structure of home-based occupational therapy for the realization of daily living activities in the elderly: Promoting co-operative construction of the life performance. *Asian Journal of Occupational Therapy, 15*, 19–25.

### Survey Research

### Survey: Quantitative

A survey as a quantitative research method is used to collect information describing the characteristics of a large sample of individuals (Ponto, 2015). Common survey data collection methods are printed or online questionnaires and person-to-person interviews via technology or face to face are conducted. Surveys can be used to collect information about a subject or subjects quickly and often at minimal cost, especially when posted online. Outcomes of surveys use descriptive statistics such as the number of responses and percentages. Usually, there is no control group and there is significant potential for bias. The wording of questions may lead the participants to answer in a manner designed to please the interviewer or organization.

Review Criteria Checklist:

- Roever, L. (2015). Critical Appraisal of a Questionnaire Study. *Evidence Based Medicine and Practice, 1*, 1. e110. https://doi.org/10.4172/EBMP.1000e110.
- BestBets: Survey Checklist—https://bestbets.org/ca/pdf/survey.pdf

Example: Cunningham, C., & O'Sullivan, R. (2021). Healthcare professionals' promotion of physical activity with older adults: A survey of knowledge and routine practice. *International Journal of Environmental Research and Public Health, 18*, 6064. https://doi.org/10.3390/ijerph18116064.

### Survey: Qualitative

A survey as a qualitative method is used to collect information about one or more topics of interest from a group of participants. The survey usually is composed of open-ended questions on behaviors or preferences and be self-administered or administered by a professional to one person at a time or to a group (Ponto, 2015). Answers may be written, typed, or recorded. The information is usually reported by organizing the data into themes with examples from various participants to provide illustrations.

Review Criteria: Critical appraisal of a questionnaire study, Roever, 2015.

Example: Park, K. -H., & Park, J. -H. (2020). Development of an elderly lifestyle profile: A Delphi survey of multidisciplinary health-care experts. *PLoS One, 15*(6), e0233565. https://doi.org/10.1371/journal.pone.0233565.

### Economic Evaluation or Cost Factor Analysis

"An economic evaluation examines the impact of occupational therapy in relation to financial costs of providing a service" (World Federation of Occupational Therapists, 2021, p. 3). The analysis compares the costs of OT with an alternate (control) intervention to determine if OT is more beneficial than the control intervention in attaining desired outcomes such as improved functional performance or quality of life.

Review Criteria Checklist:

- Checklist for Economic Evaluation. Joanna Briggs Institute https://jbi.global/sites/default/files/2020-08/Checklist_for_Cohort_Studies. Check online for the most recent version.
- CASP Checklist: Economic Evaluation. Critical Appraisal Skills Programme. www.casp-uk.net.

Example: Wales, K., Salkeld, G., Clemson, L., Lannin, N. Gitlin, L., Rubenstin, L., Howard, K., Howell, M., & Cameron, I. D. (2018). A trial based economic evaluation of occupational therapy discharge planning for older adults: the HME randomized trial. *Clinical Rehabilitation, 32*(7), 919–929. https://doi.org/10.1177/0269215518764249.

### Psychometric, Measurement, Instrument Study

The purpose of psychometric, measurement, or instrument studies is to establish the reliability and validity of an assessment or test instrument(s) to measure the concept or constructs accurately and consistently. An additional purpose may be to determine if the assessment provides sensitivity (persons with a disorder test positive) and specificity (persons without the same disorder test negative) results with a certain type or population of clients labeled with a medical diagnosis or group of characteristics. In the medical literature, such studies are called diagnostic test studies (Sackett et al., 2000).

Review Criteria Checklist

- Australian Skills Quality Authority, Guide to developing assessment tools, 2015
- Checklist for diagnostic test accuracy studies. Joanna Briggs Institute, 2020
- Critical Appraisal Skills Program. 12 questions to help you make sense of a Diagnostic Test study, 2018

Example: De Vriendt, P., Cornelis, E., Cools, W., & Gorus, E. (2021). The usefulness of evaluating performance of activities in daily living in the diagnosis of mild cognitive disorders. *International Journal of Environmental Research and Public Health, 18*, 11623. https://doi.org/10.3390/ijerph182111623.

### Ecological Study

Ecological studies are observation studies that analyze data of a population or group, rather than at the individual level. Such studies may be used to measure the prevalence and incidence of a disease, availability of resources such as the number of OT personnel, or other entity (AOTA, 2020).

Review Criteria: No current criteria form identified.

Example: Jesus, T. S., Landry, M. D., Hoenig, H., Dussault, G., Koh, G. C., & Franteira, I. (2020). Is physical rehabilitation need associated with the rehabilitation workforce supply? An ecological study across 35 high-income countries. *International Journal of Health Policy Management, 11*(4), 434–442 (9 pgs). https://www.strobe-statements.org/checklists.

### Observational Study/Participant Observation Study

Research in which the experimenter observes the behavior of the participants without any attempt to intervention or manipulation of the behaviors being observed. Such studies typically involve observation of cases under naturalistic conditions rather than the random assignment of participations to experimental conditions (VandenBos, 2015).

Review Criteria Checklist: STROBE Statement- checklist of items to include in reports of observational studies. https://www.strobe-statements.org/checklists.

Example: Pimouguet, C., Le Goff, M., Wittwer, J., Dartigues, J.-F., & Helmer, C. (2017). Benefits of occupational therapy in dementia patients: Findings from a real-world observational study. *Journal of Alzheimer's Disease, 56*, 509–517. https://doi.org/10.3233/JAD-160820.

### Mixed Methods

Mixed-methods research design includes procedures from both quantitative and qualitative research methods into a single study to collect and analyze data.

Review Criteria Checklist: Mixed Methods Appraisal Tool version 2018. http://mixedmethodappraisaltoolpublic.pbwork.com.

Example: Takashima, R., Inoue, T., Yoshida, Y., Sakaue, M. Suzuki, T., & Ogasawara, K. (2020). Effects of color narrative in community-dwelling older adults: A mixed methods study. *Scandinavian Journal of Occupational Therapy, 29*(7), 542–554. https://doi.org/10.1080/11038128.2020.1849395.

### Literature Review

Works about published materials that provide an examination of recent or current literature. The articles can cover a wide range of subject matter at various levels of completeness and comprehensiveness based upon analysis of literature that may include research findings (Watari et al., 2022).

Review Criteria: Reviewing the literature, Smith & Noble, 2016.

Example: Kirsh, B., Martin, L., Hultqvist, J., & Eklund, M. (2019). Occupational therapy interventions in mental health: A literature review in search of evidence. *Occupational Therapy in Mental Health, 35*(2), 109–156. https://doi.org/10.1080/0164212X.2019.158832.

### Narrative Review

It may be a synonym for a literature review or may be a focused review in which a select number of articles are chosen by limiting the subject review to articles published within a certain time period such as the last 5 years or to only those articles published by a certain author or type of journal. Narrative reviews summarize literature and published studies, but the criteria are developed by the author or by the instructor if the narrative review is a course assignment (Baethge, et al., 2019).

Review Criteria Checklist: SANRA—a scale for the quality assessment of narrative review articles. Baethge et al. (2019).

Example: Furlong, B., Vas, A. K., & Luedtke, A. (2020). Physical activity and cognition: A narrative review. *Indian Journal of Physiotherapy and Occupational Therapy, 14*(3), 56–61. doi: https://doi.org/10.37506/ijpot.v14i3.9667.

## Background Materials

### Position Statements

Position papers, statements, briefs, or white papers are documents prepared by organizations to state the group's expert or expressed opinion on a subject of interest to the organization but can also be a course assignment. Most position papers cite the studies reviewed in preparing the position paper, so they may qualify as filtered information but are not currently listed in the models or diagrams of evidence-based filtered and unfiltered literature. One caution regarding the use of position papers is to note the date of issue. Position papers tend to be time limited in their usefulness, since the studies cited may have been rendered out-of-date by subsequent studies or the opinions of an organization may have changed.

Review Criteria Checklist: Position statement template. Occupational therapy Australia.

Example: Perglotti, M., Battisti, N. M. L., Padgett, L., Sleight, A., Abdallah, M., Newman, R., & Van Dyk, N. K. (2020). Embracing the complexity: Older adults with cancer-related cognitive decline – A Young International Society of Geriatric Oncology position paper. *Journal of Geriatric Oncology, 11*(2), 237–243. https://doi.org/10.1016/j.jgo.2019.09.002.

### Consensus Statements

Consensus statements are public statements on a particular aspect of knowledge that is generally agreed upon by a representative group of experts (De Boeck et al., 2014). The objective is to provide the best possible and acceptable way to address a particular decision-making area for evaluation, planning, and intervention. Consensus statements reflect opinions drafted by content experts to identify areas of agreement and disagreement (Rosenfeld et al., 2015). Consensus statements often synthesize new information from recent or ongoing research that

may have implications for ongoing practice issues (De Boeck et al., 2014). The same caution applies to consensus statements as for position papers. The date of publication should be noted, and possible updates should be sought.

Review Criteria Checklist: The criteria may vary according to journals.

Example: Nicholson, C., Edwards, M. J., Carson, A. J., Gardiner, P., Golder, D., Hayward, K., Humblestone, S., Jinadu, H., Lumsden, C., MacLean, J., Main, L., Macgregor, L., Nielsen, G., Oakley, L., Price, J., Ranford, J., Ranu, J., Sum, E., & Stone, J. (2020). Occupational therapy consensus recommendations for functional neurological disorder. *Journal of Neurology, Neurosurgery and Psychiatry 91*, 1037–1045. https://doi.org/10.1136/jnnp-2019-322281.

### Editorials

An editorial consists of a statement of the opinions, beliefs, or policy of the journal or newsletter editor usually on current matters of medical or scientific significance to the medical community or society at large. The editorials published by the editors of journals representing the official society or organization are generally substantive (Watari et al., 2022).

Review Criteria Checklist: The criteria may vary according to journals.

Example: Laver, K. E. (2021). Editorial: Occupational therapy and the language of healthy ageing. *Australian Occupational Therapy Journal, 68*, 285–286. https://doi.org/10.1111/1440-1630.12745.

### Expert Opinion

A statement prepared by one or more persons recognized as having specific knowledge and/or skill (authority) on a particular subject (no specific source).

Review Criteria Checklist: Checklist for Text and Opinion. https://jbi.global/critical-appraisal-tools.

Example: Chazen, L. -A., & Franzsen, D. (2016). Expert opinion on splinting adult patients with neurological injuries. *South African Journal of Occupational Therapy, 46*(2), 4–9. https://doi.org/10.17159/2310-3833/2016/v46n2a2.

## Research Design and Types of Practice Questions

Different types of practice questions can be best answered by different research designs (methodology) to address the issues or problems. Below are the more common research designs (Methodologies) for each type of clinical question (Kapoor, 2016).

- Assessment/Evaluation: Randomized controlled trial (RCT), meta-analysis
- Therapy/Treatment/Intervention: Randomized controlled trial (RCT), meta-analysis
- Prognosis/Outcome/Results: Cohort study, case series, outcomes research
- Etiology/Cause: Randomized controlled trial (RCT), meta-analysis, cohort study, case-series
- Diagnosis/Symptom Identification: Randomized controlled trial (RCT), cohort study, case-controlled study

- Prevention/Health Maintenance: Randomized controlled trail (RCT) meta-analysis, pre-post/prospective study, cohort study, case-controlled study
- Cost/Economic: Cost analysis study, audit, outcomes research
- Meaning/Purpose (living with a disability, life in general): Qualitative study (interview, questionnaire, journaling or photo-journaling, story-telling, narrative review)

## Conceptually Applying Evidence

Through the critical appraisal process, research evidence that is relevant to the current practice question, with a valid research design and clinically important study findings, is distilled from the numbers of the retrieved literature. The next step is to consider whether or not the valid and potentially useful evidence can be applied to current practice.

Based on Straus et al. (2005, p. 1), evidence-based practice requires "the integration of the best research evidence with our clinical expertise and our patient's unique values and circumstances." In the OT profession, this traditional evidence-based practice definition may need to be expanded. Application and integration of evidence into an OT clinical decision need to consider both client context (preferences and values, occupation, and environment) and therapy context (clinical expertise, practice setting, information resources, financial resources, and other resources available to the therapist) (Bennett, 2005; Bennett & Bennett, 2000). Both clients and their families or caregivers should be included in the decision-making process. Due to this highly context-driven practice characteristic, three factors should be considered for the application of evidence into the current practice: appropriateness, acceptability, and feasibility.

Appropriateness of evidence refers to the applicability of study results to patients/clients in the current practice. Attention needs to be paid to the variations among a study population and the patients/clients in question. Patients' values and preferences, age, gender, socioeconomic status, ethnicity, occupation history, severity of disease, and the environment in which they live are some of the factors that may affect the application of the study results to the current patients (Tickle-Degnen, 1999, 2000b). In addition, client-centered practice in OT is deeply concerned with patients'/client's needs and goals for treatment (Tse et al., 2000), which is also a very important consideration when an intervention or a clinical practice guideline, proven effective by research, is applied to the current practice. When the study population carries important differences in the aforementioned aspects from the patients in question, applying the treatment or intervention concluded in the study may result in a very different outcome. Questions like "Do the results apply to my clients?," "What differences do my clients have from those in the study?," and "Does the intervention fit in with my clients' values, preferences, and their special needs?" should be asked to analyze the applicability of the evidence to the current practice (Bennett & Bennett, 2000).

After considering the patient context for identifying the appropriateness of the evidence, the context of therapy also needs to be analyzed. Acceptability and feasibility of the evidence for the current practice are determined by the answers to such questions as "Will occupational therapists and staff accept the evidence?," "Will patients/clients accept the intervention?," and "Is it feasible to implement the intervention considering the cost, equipment, and other resources in the current practice setting?" (Tickle-Degnen, 2000a).

Many clinical questions in OT deal with general patterns and individual variation in occupation and occupational performance, methods for assessing occupation and occupational performance, and planning and implementing the most effective intervention that satisfies patients' general well-being (Lopez et al., 2008; Tse, et al., 2000). Traditional evidence that is dominated by quantitative methods is not appropriate for answering all of these types of clinical questions. For example, an RCT masks individual variations among study subjects in its use of the group-comparison design, which loses the "art" of OT (Tse, et al., 2000). In RCTs, random allocation of individuals to intervention and control groups is conducted from the perspective of research design rather than considering individual choice and the environmental context. Therefore, the intervention focused on in the RCT study may not be effective for all of the patients/clients because the intervention is potentially irrelevant to some individual patients within their own environmental contexts. However, the "art" of OT requires consideration of client preferences, along with analysis of the occupation and environment that is relevant to each individual, and the design of an individualized intervention plan. To engage in "meaningful occupation" (Tse, et al, 2000), the therapist should consider both client-generated evidence and retrieved research evidence.

Therefore, occupational therapists recognize multiple types of evidence, which include not only research literature, but also daily influences such as clinical expertise, consultation with experts and colleagues, and practice-based experience (Rappolt, 2003). It has been suggested that the best available evidence should be applied from "a variety of designs based on the 'goodness of fit' to the research question" (Bartlett, 2008, p. 106), and be integrated with patients'/client's choices and needs and clinician expertise.

Evidence-based practice is a toolbox of methods to "integrate research study evidence into the clinical reasoning process" (Tickle-Degnen, 1999, p. 537). It must serve the patient's/client's needs. Sometimes no evidence can be found to answer specific clinical questions due to insufficient research or due to novel situations. In such cases, clinical expertise and practice experience play important roles. Often available evidence may not provide the exact answers for the clinical questions or may provide conflicting results (Hilton et al., 2009; Lopez, et al., 2008). In such cases, critically appraising multiple types of evidence, applying the best available evidence and advising patients/clients of the bias and limitations inherent in the evidence in a straightforward manner, and encouraging patients/clients to participate in the decision-making process are the strategies to achieve the optimal outcome (Bennett & Bennett, 2000; Tickle-Degnen, 2000a, 2000c).

## Summary

Different research designs were developed to answer different types of issues and questions. Each has a place or niche in the world of published literature. Quantitative research designs such as Randomized Controlled Trials (RCTs) tend to excel in answering questions based on numbers and statistical analysis. Qualitative research designs tend to excel at answering questions based on narrative and linguistic explanation. One study often leads to another. For example, a case study report is often the initial description of a condition. Once the symptoms and characteristics are identified through one case report, other cases may be identified. When a group of cases are identified, quantitative studies can provide numeric data. In contrast, unusual numeric data, sometimes called outliers, may require narrative explanation; and thus the interaction between quantitative and qualitative design is continued. Mixed-methods designs are an attempt to combine the best aspects of quantitative and qualitative designs into one project. Critically appraising studies require an understanding of research design because different research designs provide different data or information. Practice-based questions can best be answered by examining studies that produce data and information consistent with the purpose of the question. Questions that can be answered best by numeric processes (statistical analysis) should be directed to experimentally designed studies. Questions that can be answered best by narrative processes (text or words) should be directed to qualitative studies. The development of hierarchies in which quantitative studies were given a higher ranking than qualitative studies may be of little use to OT personnel. Numbers are not inherently better than text or words, they are different. Each serves a different purpose. The concepts of filtered and unfiltered provide a method to critically appraise studies for their potential to provide information relevant to practice questions and proposed research studies. The best answers to practice questions may require both numbers and words or text.

## Implementing Evidence-Based Practice

OT personnel have generally reported a positive attitude toward evidence-based research, but also have identified challenges or barriers to implementing evidence-based results into their practice settings (Reifenberg & Heinekamp, 2018; Samuelsson & Wressle, 2015; Thomas et al., 2021). The challenges and strategies to meet the challenges can be examined in three levels: individual, institutional, and professional organizations.

### Challenges and Strategies at the Individual Level

According to the survey conducted by Samuelsson and Wriessle (2015), statements by respondents could be grouped into three major categories: OT personnel lacked time to read the evidence-based research studies, they had difficulty understanding statistical analyses, and facilities were inadequately prepared to implement the evidence-based practice concept or process. Lack of time may be the result of lack of skills or a scheduling problem. Lack of skills reduces efficiency and scheduling problems interfere with effectiveness. Increasing skill level may include:

- Learning to use the PICO(T) question based on issues or problems experienced in the practice setting
- Identifying print and online resources related to the client population seen in practice (books, chapters, journals, articles, webpages, databases, organizations, conferences)
- Developing a system to tract new or revised resources
- Increasing skill in searching databases to locate relevant studies
- Increasing skill in critically appraising research studies
- Discussing with colleagues and team members how to implement evidence-based findings into care plans
- Attending or providing instruction of in-service and continuing education program content related to increasing and improving translation of evidence-based research into practice.
- Working with management and administrators to identify changes in facility systems that could facilitate implementation of evidence-based findings
- Contacting educational institutions, especially OT educational programs and university-based librarians, for help to identify resources, and increase knowledge and skills

### Challenges and Strategies at the Organizational Level

The challenge for facilities and institutions can be summarized in four approaches according to Lucian et al. (2019): data, resources, goals, and preferences. The approach labeled data means understanding the relevance of the evidence-based data to the local context. Resources should be examined in terms of making substitutes within the organization without compromising results. Goals involve identifying what they are and how they can be met. Preferences involve identifying what adoptions and changes are most comfortable for the facility to make. Facilities and institutions may need to review policies and procedures to determine if they are consistent with the concepts of evidence-based processes. For example, do productivity standards require time utilization criteria that preclude time for identifying and incorporating new methods or techniques into clients' plans of care? Is there time and opportunity to consider change and improvements? Are resources available for practitioners to improve or increase their skills?

### Challenges and Strategies at the Disciplinary and Professional Level

The challenge for professional OT organizations include: (1) summarizing evidence-based studies to support the claim that OT is of value to society as a professional discipline, (2) providing evidence-based advocacy at the local, state, or higher governing bodies levels, and (3) providing evidence-based resources to support members as practitioners, educators, and investigators. Organizations may find the resources to address a topic when the topic is new to the awareness of members but may find maintaining available resources difficult over time when the newness wears off and is replaced by other topics. Personnel in organizations can provide access to and identification of resources that may be less accessible at the local level. Maintaining a webpage listing evidence-based resources and methods can be a project for professional organizations. Resources could include publications, podcasts, listservs, and links to other online resources.

## Actions and Activities to Increase Knowledge and Skills and Share Expertise

- Retrieve copies of practice guidelines developed by OT associations and supplement with guidelines developed by other organizations associated with the conditions seen in the practice setting
- Consult secondary resources for systematic reviews, scoping reviews, and CATs or papers of recognized diagnoses or cluster of symptoms, assessments, plans of care, interventions, outcomes and service delivery programs
- Set up search hedges or alerts in databases frequency used to simplify the search process to identify and retrieve up-to-date publications for conditions seen in the practice setting
- Join online groups that discuss topics or post materials related to conditions seen in practice
- Create or attend a journal club to review articles of interest and discuss relevance to OT professionals and other team members.
- Develop a recording system (database, notebooks, file drawer, etc.) of relevant materials that is organized by topics related to practice issues and questions.
- Provide or participate in in-service or continuing education courses on topics related to conditions seen in the practice setting or to improving health-care services.
- Contact OT educational programs to be a guest lecturer regarding implementation of evidence-based practice in practice settings.
- Assist OT educators in preparing evidence-based content in the OT curriculum

## Sample Practice-Related Questions

Sometimes the hardest part of implementing an evidence-based project is stating a coherent PICO(T) question. Some examples of questions may be useful to act as "starters" for defining an issue in preparation for formulating a PICO(T) statement and search strategy.

Diagnosis or Label Questions:
- Is there a role (purpose, goal, level of function, program description) identified in the literature for occupational therapy services for older/elderly/aged adults diagnosed/labeled with _____ (name of disease/disorder/deficiency/condition/type or group of symptoms) called _____ or _____? If so, what is the role?
- Are there theories, practice models, or frameworks available to support occupational therapy intervention

or guide practice for older/elderly/aged adults diagnosed/labeled with _____ (name of disease/disorder/deficiency/condition/type or group of symptoms) called _____ or _____? If so, what are the theories, practice models, or frameworks?
- Is there currently published evidence-based research studies (last 5 years) on the use (implementation) of occupational therapy services for clients diagnosed/labeled with _____ (name of disease/disorder/deficiency/condition/type or group of symptoms) called _____? If so, what is the role and how is that role described?
- Is there a new or evolving role for occupational therapy services that does not appear to be fully addressed in the published literature? Should a scoping review be considered?
- Is there a group or team of professionals with whom occupational therapy personnel are expected to interface in performing the occupational therapy role(s) related to _____ (name of disease/disorder/deficiency/condition/type or group of symptoms?

*Assessment or Evaluation Questions*
- What assessment instruments are available to assess _____ (name of disease/disorder, deficiency, condition, or type or group of symptoms or life circumstances)?
- Is there research on the validity and reliability of an assessment instrument by the name of _____?
- Is there a "gold standard" (considered best) assessment instrument to be used with this _____ (name of disease/disorder/deficiency/condition/type or group of symptoms/life circumstances)?
- What is the current version or revision of the assessment instrument named _____ and where or how can it be obtained?

*Intervention or Treatment Questions*
- What is the best evidence available to support the use of occupational therapy services with _____ (disease/disorder/deficiency/condition/type or group of symptoms or life circumstances)?
- What is the best evidence available to discontinue using certain methods and modalities because they are ineffective or harmful? (See AOTA, 2021a, 2021b.)
- What occupational therapy focused interventions and goals (priorities) are recommended in practice guidelines or expert statements for clients with _____ (name of disease/disorder/deficiency/condition/type or group of symptoms or life circumstances)?
- What evidence is available to support the use of _____ (name of technique, method, medium, approach, theory, model) with older/elderly/aged adults with _____ (name of disease/disorder/deficiency/condition/type or group of symptoms)?
- Is there evidence that occupational therapy can assist in primary care prevention for a given population
- What is the usual total number of intervention sessions (treatment units) for clients with _____ (name of

disease/disorder/deficiency/ condition/type or group of symptoms/life circumstances)?

- What is the frequency (number of intervention sessions) per unit of time (day, week, month, year, or grading period)?
- In what locations can intervention occur (in-patient, out-patient, community, home, face-to-face, telerehabilitation, telehealth, or teleconference)?

*Outcomes or Results Questions*

- What evidence is available to demonstrate the value of occupational therapy services (specific or general) in meeting stated outcomes/results/goals?
- Are there examples of effective intervention programs using occupational therapy services to obtain stated outcomes/results/goals?
- What is the expected or documented financial cost of providing occupational therapy services for clients with _____ (disease/disorder/deficiency/condition/type or group of symptoms/ life circumstances)?
- What other costs are incurred (time away from a job, transportation, client/family education, equipment, remodeling home or living space, etc.)?
- What non-tangible costs are incurred by caregivers (grief, stress, depression, strain on relationships, loss of valued leisure activities etc.)

## Models of Intervention

Models of interventions have been summarized into three types: research-based practitioner or individual model, embedded research model, and organizational excellence model (Ilott, 2012). The *research-based practitioner* or individual model places responsibility for applying the evidence-based process on the practitioner or individual to write the PICO(T) question, identify potential resources, search the database literature, retrieve relevant documents, critically appraise the documents, translate and apply findings to the PICO(T) question, and evaluate the outcomes. Ilott (2012) states the model was not successful in implementing the evidence-based process because of the complexity of changing professional behavior as opposed to simply asking a colleague for advice. The second model, *embedded research*, involved the development of clinical guidelines and audit programs which required managers and policymakers to play a key role. The assumption of the model is based on the belief that creating and packaging guidelines will automatically lead to implementation. Studies showed that implementing evidence-based research into practice required planning changes in service delivery at the individual, team, organizational, and system levels. Without facility support and acceptance resulting in service delivery changes, the existence of evidence-based recommendations did not reach the client's plan of care. The third model, *organization excellence*, expands the process of implementing evidence-based research by including collaboration between health-care service programs and educational institutions such as universities to adapt research findings to fit the needs in local contexts and environments. The research findings are customized and combined with the knowledge from research studies and local practitioners to address the problems identified in the community.

Combining the objectives of the three models identifies the challenge of implementing evidence-based research into practical application. The individual professional must have the knowledge, skills, and attitudes summarized in five As: *assess* the evidence base, *ask* an answerable question, *acquire* relevant evidence, *appraise* the relevance and scientific rigor, and *apply* in practice (Ilott, 2012). The facility and/or system must be an active participant, accept the use of evidence-based research as a tenet of its mission statement, and facilitate changes in organization structure to implement the process of translating research findings to practice, including devoting resources needed to support staff development. Support from health-care systems and educational institutions at the local, state, and national levels can provide external resources to local facilities by expanding the resources.

## Understanding Negative Views of Evidence-Based Practice and Programs

All models, methods, strategies, techniques, approaches, and programs have supports and detractions. EBP is no exception (Ilott, 2012). Some examples are as follows:

- EBP is one of many ideas and tools to improve client care and health-care service delivery through OT. Holism (treating the client as a whole) and client-centered care existed in the OT literature long before EBP entered the picture.
- EBP has the same fault as other practice models and methods. There continues to be lack of carry-over or impact of teaching evidence-based practice in educational programs to implementation in client care. Translating results of research into applications for practice continues to be a challenge (Thomas et al., 2021).
- Expert opinion based on experience should be given high value in the evidence-based levels or hierarchy of evidence. Learning from experienced practitioners has been an excepted teaching method since the evidence-based approach was published
- EBP has not demonstrated that outcomes are better than establishing regulations and codes of practice adopted by health-care service providers and reimbursement systems.
- The mindset of the practitioners is more important than the model or method. Practitioners who want to improve their knowledge and skills will do so regardless of what model or method is sought or implemented.
- Scientific evidence and clinical research are not more important than practitioner decision-making skills and client choice. Evidence from research is one criterion, not the only or best criterion.
- The answers are not there. The available evidence-based studies may not provide the answers practitioners are hoping to find, especially to complex problems in clients with multiple diagnoses (comorbidities) and mixed environments (living alone, staying with adult children

or relatives, moving in and out of hospitals or nursing homes). Practitioners may have to seek other sources of information to aid in the decision-making process such as colleagues, team members, or social service coordinators.

## Why Evidence Does Not Match Practice—and Possible Solutions

- The rules of conducting an experimental research study require that all variables be controlled or eliminated except the one or more being studied so the results can be determined to be caused, or not caused, by the variable(s) being studied. In practice settings, controlling variables (comorbidities, living arrangements, social support, financial resources, therapy location, therapy instructions, etc.) of clients is often not possible and must be taken into consideration in implementing the method or modality. Possible solution: look for studies using research designs that address multiple variables, such as qualitative designs, and very large quantitative datasets with permission. For example, the VA, health-care systems, or the longitudinal Framingham Heart Health study.
- Research study protocols are often carried out for several weeks, months, or even years. Practitioners rarely have the luxury of working with a client for extended periods of time. The results of the research study demonstrate positive change over time. The same or similar results might be obtained by the client if the time and provision of services are available. Getting the same results in less time does not seem to be possible. Possible solution: Could the time and service provision be accomplished if family members or caregivers were trained to carry out the protocol? Could the client learn to carry out the protocol? Could teleconference follow-up be added?
- Research studies have a budget that includes acquiring equipment considered necessary to conduct the research protocol. Practitioners may not have access to the same amount of money or access to the same equipment used in the research study. Money and equipment may not be available. Equipment may have been specially built for the study, or the equipment cannot be imported into the country where the client and practitioner reside. Possible solution: Could equivalent equipment be made using less expensive materials? Could equivalent equipment be made locally?
- Research studies, especially experimental designed studies, are best conducted in a consistent setting since the environment or location is one of the variables to be controlled. Practitioners may not be able to ensure that a consistent setting or environmental conditions can be achieved or maintained in their work setting. Possible solution: to the extent feasible, set up environmental conditions that simulate where the client will be living. Consider how the protocol could be implemented when the client goes home or to another living environment.
- The protocol in a research study may require special education and training to achieve proficiency in administration. Such education and training (leave time and continuing education funds) may not be available to train the practitioner or to train family or caregivers. Possible solution: Are instructional videos or classes available online? Could an instructional video be made or an instructional manual be provided, to which family members or caregivers could refer?
- Assessment instruments developed within a research project may require numerous special items (equipment, tools) to administer the assessment. Obtaining all the items, keeping them together and in working order (not lost or broken) may be a challenge in the practitioner's workplace. Possible solutions: keep replacements available for items that tend to disappear or break. Consider if another assessment that requires fewer pieces but can provide similar information is available.
- The details of how the protocol (assessment, plan of care, implementation strategy) was conducted in the research study is summarized but important details are not stated. When the practitioner tries to implement the protocol, missing details may become evident or may result in failure or unsatisfactory results. Possible solutions: contact the author or principal investigator for a copy of the protocol or ask for specific details that appear to be missing.

## Generalizability, Applicability, and Transferability

Finally, each research study should be reviewed to determine if it contains useful information. In other words, is there information that can be generalized, that is applicable, and that can be transferable to the practitioner's service program or individual client? Fossum et al. (2019) suggest the following questions that may help to determine the answer:

- Would my client have met the inclusion criteria for the research study? If the answer is yes, reading the study may be worth the time and effort to look for potential useful results. If the answer is no, the study may contain little or no relevant information.
- Are the results of the research study applicable and transmittable to clients other than those in the original study? If the answer is yes, could the results be applied to my client? If no, the study is unlikely to provide relevant information.
- Are there reasons to suspect that my client would not achieve the results presented in the research study? If so, are those reasons major obstacles to generalization, applicability or transferability? If major obstacles exist, the study results may be limited or of no use.
- Do the study results cover all relevant aspects of my client's situation or concerns? If so, information may provide useful solutions. If no, other resources need to be sought to provide information on those aspects not covered by the immediate study.
- Do the advantages of incorporating the research findings into my client's plan of care, outweigh any potential side-effects, complications, or costs?

In addition to the suggestions offered by Fossum et al. (2019), OT practitioners, educators, and investigators should keep in mind that certain types of inventions used historically in OT practice have been identified and flagged by members of an AOTA committee, Choosing Wisely, as questionable approaches to initiating OT intervention, and recommend the techniques not be used. The first five were presented and discussed in an article by Gillen et al. (2019) and the second five were added to a handout on the webpage in 2021 (AOTA, 2021a, 2021b). Although three of the items apply primarily to children and youth, the other seven statements are relevant to older adults. They are summarized as follows and include avoiding the use of:

- Intervention activities that are non-purposeful (not occupation-based, no relevance to occupational performance tasks) such as stacking cones, placing and removing pegs in holes, using shoulder arc or arm bike equipment
- Physical agent modalities (PAMs) without also providing purposeful and occupation-based intervention activities
- Overhead pulleys for individuals with a hemiplegic shoulder
- Cognitive-based interventions, such as paper-and-pencil tasks, table-top tasks, cognitive training software, without direct application to occupational performance
- Any interventions without first completing the client's occupational profile and setting collaborative goals
- Slings for individuals with a hemiplegic arm that place the arm in a flexor pattern for extended periods of time
- Ambulation or gait training interventions that do not directly link to functional mobility

## Summary

Implementing the results of evidence-based studies and research into practice is a process involving several steps. Each step has a learning curve from beginner to expert and each step can be facilitated or derailed depending on available resources. Gathering resources requires more than pulling together literature and publications. People, professionals, patients/clients, politics, policies, and procedures need to be supportive of the evidence-to-practice continuum. Time, or more precisely, the lack of time seems to frequently derail the process or act as a barrier. Figuring out how to best manage the time dimension is a major step in moving from evidence to practice. The second barrier is resolving the perceived or real lack of knowledge and skills. Figuring out how to obtain the knowledge and master the skills is a goal to be achieved within the evidence-to-practice continuum. The third barrier is overcoming the roadblocks raised by the politics, policies, and procedures of the facility, workplace, or system. Figuring out how to move from the primary outcome of creating billable units to other measurable outcomes is another potential barrier. Financial returns and/or costs to the facility or governmental systems should be balanced with the concepts of improving client care and satisfaction while increasing professional competence and proficiency to provide the best service delivery. Ideas to facilitate the process of translating research evidence into practice application may require implementing several

strategies, including better searching techniques and more sharing of findings with colleagues. Professional organizations can help by identifying and providing printed and online resources.

## Resources for Implementation of Evidence-Based Practice

The results of studies have pinpointed resources that are needed to implement evidence-based data into practice at the individual, facility, and professional organization level. Although the general aim or purpose of implementing evidence-based data is consistent across the three levels, differences in requirements exist to improve the quality of care by increasing the reliability of the intervention strategies and processes (Camargo et al., 2017). The resources have been identified in the nursing literature but can be translated into OT practice, education, and research.

### At the Individual Level

Individual practitioners, educators, and investigators require specific education and training to develop competencies needed to participate effectively in evidence-based projects (Camargo et al., 2017). The educational and training needs have been identified as:

- Knowledgeable about methodological approaches and different types of research
- Skilled in critical analysis/appraisal of publications (primary studies)
- Ability to use methods of synthesizing the results of primary studies (systematic review)

The authors state that education and training received during courses may not develop the necessary competencies (knowledge, skills, and attitudes) in sufficient detail to translate into a practice setting. Johnson et al. (2020) found that classwork assignments during basic education were also not sufficient to develop needed competencies and that additional practice during a fieldwork assignment and clinical placement settings was considered essential. Melnyk et al. (2022) compiled 13 competencies every nurse should be able to perform. The competency statements have been revised to better fit OT concepts and terminology. The practitioner will:

- Question the OT process for the purpose of improving quality of client care (based on current edition of OT practice framework).
- Describe problems identified within the process based on details existing in the work setting such as client assessment, intervention technique, outcome management, or quality improvement.
- Participate in the formation of the search question or statement using the PICO or PICO(T) format.
- Search for external evidence from research studies.
- Participate in critical appraisal of filtered (pre-appraised) evidence such as practice guidelines, CATs, systematic reviews, evidence-based position papers (policies and procedures), other evidence syntheses.

- Participate in the critical appraisal of published research studies to determine strength and applicability to OT process.
- Participate in the evaluation and synthesis of a body of evidence gathered to determine its strength and applicability to a client population and practice setting.
- Collect practice data (e.g., individual client data, quality improvement data) systematically as internal evidence for decision making in the care of individual clients, groups, and populations.
- Integrate evidence gathered from external and internal sources to plan EBP changes.
- Implement practice changes based on evidence and practitioner expertise and client preferences to improve client-center care and outcomes.
- Evaluate outcomes of evidence-based decisions and practice changes for individual clients, groups, and population to determine best practices.
- Disseminate best practice supported by evidence to improve quality of care and client outcomes.
- Participate in strategies to sustain an EBP culture within the work setting and professional organization culture.

### At the Facility Level

From a facility perspective, Camargo et al. (2017) and Melnyk et al. (2022) state that the essential elements of a facility that supports evidence-based practice should include:
- Statements appear in the mission and vision statements, role expectations and job descriptions, and governance charts that address the process of EBP.
- Supports for all staff, managers, and workers (care team members) to engage in evidence-based research activities.
- Processes are documented to monitor and evaluate evidence-based programs and disseminate results.
- Teaching-service integration between researchers/investigators and facility personnel exist and can be identified.
- Educational and skills building programs are available to support attainment of the evidence-based competencies.
- Competency statements are expected of all employees related to EBP.
- Support for the development of mentors/champions who meet or exceed the EBP competencies.
- Questions about evidence-based competencies are included in the job interview process.
- Information about evidence-based programs is included during orientation period for all new employees.
- Review of evidence-based program competencies is included during performance reviews or appraisals.
- Imbedded evidence-based program competencies appear in practice policy and guideline development processes.

### At the Professional Organizations Level

Literature on the services professional organizations should provide is limited. A review of resources offered by OT associations can be grouped into five categories:

- Identify existing external and internal resources: people (experts), databases, agencies, books, journals, websites, videos, podcasts, and journal clubs focused on evidence-based topics and activities.
- Creating resources tailored to individual or group member needs: how OT can benefit from and incorporate evidence-based results/findings into OT practice.
- Distributing resources: evidence-based products available in multiple formats for sale or free.
- Providing educational opportunities: sponsor or co-sponsor continuing education and professional development programs in individual or group formats.
- Support research and dissemination of results: provide grant funds, assistance in grant preparation, publish results.

### Future Applications and Trends in Evidence-Based Practice

The future may rest on OT personnel, and their team members, coping successfully with three interrelated concepts: being aware of the "data pile," determining "what works," and having "application sense." The "data pile" refers to the constantly increasing number of ideas and amount of evidence presented in multiple formats on a variety of platforms. Just being aware of what is "out there" can be a time-consuming task. Dealing with the inconsistent use of terminology (words and phrases) and multiple terms for the same subject is another. "What works" refers to being able to glean or sort from the "data pile" the evidence which has been found "to work" in some settings or under certain conditions and should be considered for implementation into the OT work setting. Many potentially useful ideas exist but not all good ideas or evidence can be incorporated effectively and successfully into a given OT work setting. Selecting the best of "what works" requires careful analysis and consideration of the factors that exist in any given OT work setting. "Application sense" is the ability to translate the ideas presented in the information sources into a plan of action that can be applied to the OT work setting. The best of "what works" is useless if the ideas cannot be arranged into a plan that translates knowledge into action statements/plans to be implemented and sustained over time in the OT work setting. And then, the whole process starts over again as more new ideas are added to the "data pile" to be sorted for "what works" and may require "application sense" to distill, adapt, and incorporate relevant information from research studies into an OT work setting and/or client care. Problems related to dealing with the "data pile" have been addressed through the development of computerized databases which organize materials into a consistent outline format that can be searched by entering controlled vocabulary terms or keywords. Databases are available in a wide variety of subject areas and formats which include topics of interest to OT personnel. Access to the databases does vary from totally free to subscription only, and search skills do require practice to improve and perfect. In addition, not all databases and entries in the databases are of equal value in terms of authority, accuracy, or truthfulness. The searcher needs to be aware of levels of authority and be able to spot inaccuracies or falsehoods. The problem of selecting the best search terms and synonyms is partially addressed by the development of thesauri and master index files. However, not all terms are listed and working definitions provided. Keyword searching may identify terms not listed in the thesauri or index list. Working definitions or descriptions may have to be developed by the searcher. Pettersson and Iwarsson (2017) provide an example. Their review question was based on the concept of re-ablement, a term used in Europe and Australia to describe home-based programs, but not widely used in the United States. The authors used keyword searches to identify related terms such as *restoration* or *rehabilitation*. According to the search strategy listed in the article, the authors did not use the terms *independent living* or *community dwelling*, but such use of terms might have increased the retrieval of relevant studies. Searching for "what works" is aided (and complicated) by the wide variety of information available. Useful information is attainable within the print and online publications and formats. However, OT personnel do need to be able to discern quality from quantity. Formats for reviewing the research literature for "what works" have been created including practice guidelines, systematic reviews, meta-analyses, critical appraised topics and papers, and scoping review.

The major problem is translating the results of published studies into everyday application including implementation into practice, teaching and education, and conducting better research studies. "Application sense" has many names and models including knowledge translation, knowledge exchange, knowledge transfer, knowledge integration, and research utilization. Camargo et al. (2017) reviewed 16 different models. Thus, the lack of consistent terminology and definition has hindered the process of translating and transferring the results of science research publications into application settings. Recently, the term *implementation science* has been advanced. Eccles and Mittman (2006, para. 2) define *implementation science* as the "scientific study of methods to promote the systematic uptake of research findings and other EBPs into routine practice, and hence, to improve the quality and effectiveness of health services." The techniques or processes used to apply research findings are called *implementation strategies* defined as "techniques used to promote the adoption of EBPs into a real practice setting (Juckett et al., 2019). According to Juckett et al. (2019) implementation strategies reported in the OT literature include chart audits, coaching, educational workshops, fidelity vignettes, follow-up consultations, and standardized or manualized training modules.

Dougherty and Conway (2008) described a three-block model for translating research into practice. The Translation 1 (T1) block focuses on studies designed to test what works by translating basic biomedical science knowledge into clinical (applied) efficacy research. The T2 block focuses on activities to test who benefits from the applied research by performing studies designed to compare effectiveness, achieve certain outcomes, or improve health-care services, and the T3 block focuses on activities to test how to deliver high-quality care

reliably in all settings by conducting studies on the implementation of intervention methods, the scaling and spread (adoption) of effective interventions and the measurement and accountability of health-care quality. Glasdam et al. (2021) refers to T3 studies as "practice development projects." An example is the literature on the Well Elderly Study and Lifestyle Redesign intervention module developed at the University of Southern California. A T1 study, The Well Elderly Study conducted from 1994 to 1996 focused on translating the biopsychological-based concepts of influencing successful aging by promoting health through occupation. Occupation being defined as "regularly performed activities such as grooming, exercising, and shopping" (Clark et al., 1997, p. 1322). The findings demonstrated that participation in occupation could have a positive impact on individual patterns of personally satisfying and health-promoting occupations. As a result, a T2 project was undertaken to develop an intervention program based on the framework of the Well Elderly Program and the model of occupational science called Lifestyle Redesign and published in a manual (Mandel et al., 1999), revised in 2015 (Clark et al., 2015). The first published T3 practice development project, which did not include authors from the Well Elderly project, was published in 2004 (Horowitz & Chang, 2004). The methodology for the project reportedly followed the Lifestyle Redesign protocol. However, different outcome assessments were used. Nevertheless, the experimental group participants in an adult day program showed favorable results in promoting well-being and engagement in life activities. Note the gap in years between the original T1 project is seven and between the T2 project is 5 years. The gap in years between T1 and T3 projects is an ongoing challenge to bring research results to the practice (or educational) setting.

Rapport et al. (2018) have suggested five categories of (steps to) implementation science: diffusion, dissemination, implementation, adoption, and sustainability. *Diffusion* is described as the spread of ideas, behaviors, and practices over time. *Dissemination* is the spread of evidence to target audiences. *Implementation* includes capturing the idea(s) or ideal from the research evidence and applying or translating the idea to a practice endeavor. *Adoption* is the taking up or accepting the new idea(s), behaviors, practices, or organization structure. *Sustainability* involves the extent to which the intervention becomes firmly entrenched within a service delivery system. The categories are not linear but rather circular so as new ideas, behaviors, and practices become known, the cycle of categories or steps starts again. Therefore, practice is a dynamic process that changes as new ideas, behaviors, and practices evolve. The challenge is to recognize and embrace the cycle of implementation science and apply its categories to the application arenas including client-focused practice, education and training, and investigative and research settings.

Proctor et al. (2011) are credited with suggesting that there are three interrelated types of outcome levels for implementation research which are labeled *implementation outcomes*, service outcomes, and *client outcomes*. Implementation outcomes are defined as the "effects of deliberate and purposive actions to implement new treatment, practices, and services" (Proctor et al., 2011, p. 65). The taxonomy consists of eight implementation outcomes: adoption, acceptability, appropriateness, costs, feasibility, fidelity, penetration (reach), and sustainability. Proctor et al. (2011) suggests that implementation outcomes research usually precedes service and client outcome research and mostly attempts to answer "what" questions such as what is acceptable, what can be adopted, what is appropriate, what are the costs, what is feasible, what fidelity standard is required, what penetration (adoption) can be obtained and what sustainability is possible. The "what" questions tend to focus on the social, ethical, and cultural issues regarding perspectives on health, well-being, and quality of life. If the answers to the "what" questions are positive (socially, ethically, and culturally acceptable), they provide the general framework for examining the six service outcomes outlined by the Institute of Medicine (2011): effectiveness, efficiency, equity, patient-centeredness, safety, and timeliness. Service outcomes address issues related to health-care delivery such as: Is the proposed service program effective? is it efficient? is it equitable? is it patient (client) focused? is it safe? and can it be administered in a timely manner? Service outcome questions address the overall question of "Can the proposed program be implemented in a given service setting and is the program worth the effort to implement?" Proctor et al. (2011) suggests that service outcomes research is designed to address population-level issues rather than those at the individual client level. If the answers to the service outcomes are favorable the third set of outcomes can be addressed regarding, client satisfaction, client gain in function and reduction in client symptomatology. Client outcomes are addressed through specific developmental programs answering how the objectives and goals will be targeted and obtained. Examples include guidelines, manuals, videos, and other formats that demonstrate how to implement intervention strategies, methods, approaches, and techniques to and with the individual client or group. Proctor et al. (2013) in a subsequent article stress that authors should clearly identify in the reporting what level or type of outcomes research is being studied and reported. The implication is that implementation and outcomes research need to occur in an orderly transition. Although the timeline is not fixed, attempting to implement a client-focus outcome program before service outcomes and implementation outcomes have been studied, may negatively impact the success of the practice development program. In setting OT research agenda for the future, Proctor et al. (2013) discuss ideas about outcome levels may be useful to consider.

Other considerations for the future of implementation science have been observed in the literature. Once again, the studies based on the Well Elderly Study and Lifestyle Redesign provide examples. The Well Elderly Studies methodology and Lifestyle Redesign protocol were envisioned and conducted in the United States specifically in southern California. As Glasdam et al. (2021) points out the sociocultural conditions identified in other countries such as Denmark, can differ from those in the United States. The Well Elderly Studies were based on the theory that successful aging (in the United States) depended on the

"do it for yourself" approach to independent living associated with cultural norms in the United States. The modules in the Lifestyle Redesign manual draw heavily on the cultural attitudes and behaviors expected of elders and older adults in the United States—namely maintaining independence from, and non-reliance on, others and an "I can do it myself, for and by myself" motto. Societies where intergenerational interdependence is the accepted and expected norm, find the "independent mindset" difficult to understand and even more difficult to translate into OT interventions and sustainable practices. OT literature covers a wide range of societies and cultures. One size or set of publications does not fit all. Practitioners, educators, and investigators have the responsibility of studying the socioeconomic culture in which OT is being practiced and identifying what OT literature can best in implemented to improve the health, well-being, and quality of life for older adults in their living environment. The article by Proctor et al. (2013) provides an illustration of how to proceed in developing outcomes research, if little or none is currently available.

Another consideration is to follow consistently one theory, model, or framework at a time in translating research to practice. A *theory* is a "set of analytical principles or statements designed to structure out observation, understanding and explanation of the world" (Nilsen & Bernhardsson, 2019, p. 2). Theories clarify phenomena and assist in developing and testing hypotheses (Rapport et al., 2018). Theories lead to new knowledge to explain implementation outcomes. A model is a "deliberate simplification of a phenomenon or specific aspect of a phenomenon" (Nilsen & Bernhardsson, 2019). Models are "designed to enable specific assumptions to be made about a set of parameters or variables that can then be tested on outcomes" (Rapport et al., 2018, p. 120). A *model* is primarily descriptive, whereas a theory is explanatory and descriptive. Models lead to dissemination or implementation strategies. A *framework* usually "denotes a structure, overview, outline, system or plan consisting of various descriptive categories, e.g., concepts, constructs or variables, and relations between them that are presumed to account for a phenomenon" (Nilsen & Bernhardsson, 2019, p. 2). Frameworks help to define variables and the relations between them leading to evaluations of the determinants of success or failure of implementation outcomes (Rapport et al., 2018). The Well Elderly Studies were based in the evolving theory of Occupational Science (OS) (Yerxa, 1990). Although the original Well Elderly Study publication (Clark et al., 1997+ does not mention occupational science, a subsequent publication in 1998 states that the "Well Elderly Treatment Program was designed through the explicit application of occupational science theory and research" (Jackson et al., 1998, p. 327). Mixing different theories together in one research project muddies the waters regarding the use of models or frameworks unless the authors are very deliberate in clarifying which models or frameworks are based on or came from what theory. For example, the Johansson and Björklund (2016) study states that the "present intervention study is inspired by the LR (Lifestyle Redesign) program adapted to a local context and

Swedish culture with support from Norwegian and English research findings" (p. 208) yet the abstract states that Model of Occupational Adaptation was used in performing content analysis. Occupational Adaptation (OA) (Schkade & Schultz, 1992) is a separate theory and model from Occupational Science (OS), the theory on which Lifestyle Redesign program is based. The major focus of OA is the desire for relative mastery and adaptive capacity of the person (Schkade & Schultz, 1992), whereas the major focus of OS is the transformative, meaningful, and personal identifying properties of occupation (Clark et al., 2015). Mixing theories, models, and frameworks runs the risk of canceling out the qualities and values of either. According to the Johansson and Björklund (2016) study there were no statistically significant differences between the intervention and control groups. The rationale stated in the study is that the two groups were not fully matched. Another reason could be that the intervention program was based on a different theory (OS) than the rationale for the study (OA) and therefore the intervention program did not actually translate the theory of OA into a practice project. Furthermore, the Johansson and Björklund (2016) study used the data collection tools identified in the Well Elderly Studies but did not use the Relative Mastery Measurement Scale developed for OA (George et al., 2004). A similar mismatch between OS and another theory and model occurred in two studies on stroke except the theory-model was the Canadian Model of Occupational Performance and Engagement (CMOP-E). Once again, the results of the study found no statistically significant difference (Lund et al., 2011, 2012). Statistical analysis "crunches numbers," but does not automatically sort the therapeutic effects or outcomes of one theory from another. Outcome measures are created for specific purposes. If the outcome measure is not designed for the outcome(s) specified in the theory, the results of analysis may be misinterpreted as non-significant, not because the theory is wrong but because the measurement system is inappropriate. While expecting all theories to be of value and useful may be wishful thinking, finding the ones that are valuable and useful is a major objective of EBP.

The final question for the future is: Can we become better consumers of resources in implementation science topics to advance EBP in OT? Based on Proctor et al. (2013) a possible generalized critique format follows:

- Name it: Is the theory, model, framework or outcome program named and is it unique? "To be measured, an implementation strategy must first be named or labelled" (Proctor et al, 2013, p. 3). And the name or label must be described and differentiated in terms that address homonymy (multiple meanings for the same term), synonymy (different terms for the same or overlapping, meanings) and instability (unpredictable changes in the previous two items).
- Define it: Is the implementation strategy defined as a concept? A general sense of what the strategy involves or includes should be defined. If more than one strategy is involved, each strategy should be individually described,

and the findings separated and organized to address each strategy.
- Specify it: Seven specifications should be identifiable in the resource:
  - The Actor: Is the actor clearly stated? The resource should Identify who enacts the strategy (clients, consumers, therapists/providers, teachers, family members, administrators, payers, advocates, etc.). If more than one actor is expected to enact the strategy, each actor should be clearly identified.
  - The Actions: Are the actions clearly stated that the actor is expected to perform? Actions should be written using active verb statements to specify the specific actions, steps, or processes that need to be enacted by the actor. If more than one actor is involved the actions for each actor should be stated separately.
  - Action Target: Are the targets specified according to the conceptual model(s) of implementation? Is the unit of analysis for measuring implementation outcomes identified (level of occupational performance, degree of satisfaction, criterion measurement on a standardized test, etc.)? Intervention strategies should be consistent with the proposed model. Unit or units of analysis should be stated (number of repetitions, range of motion, number of correct responses, weights lifted, steps taken, items of clothing put on/taken off, tasks completed (bathe, dress, eat breakfast, brush teeth) etc.
  - Temporality: Is the temporality specified? Temporality may be stated as time of day, week, month, relation to another task etc. (morning, afternoon, evening, weekly, monthly, seasonal, before work/school, after work/school).
  - Dose: is the dosage specified? Is the dosage stated in amount and frequency? Dosage can be stated in amount of time per session, number of interactions, or frequency of sessions (once per day, twice a week, every other day, every month, every grading period etc.)
  - Implementation Outcome Affected: is the outcome measure or measures identified and named for each implementation strategy? Assessment instruments and types of equipment should be stated, and the purpose of each described, in terms of measurement criteria (quantity or quality) for each implementation strategy.
  - Justification: Is the empirical, theoretical, or pragmatic justification provided for the choice of implementation strategies? The rationale or purpose for each implementation strategy should be stated and described.

If any of the items of information is missing, analysis of the implementation will be impaired, and the results may be different than stated in the resource. Contacting the authors or institution may provide answers to missing information or contacting persons who have already implemented the programs may be helpful. Reading other works by the same author(s) may also provide additional information because full descriptions may appear in one publication but summarized in another with reference to the publication with more complete description.

## SUMMARY

The purpose of this chapter is to provide the reader with an introduction to obtaining and planning the implementation of evidence-based resources. Planning ahead and having a clearly stated purpose and objectives can facilitate the search for evidence-based resources and the analysis of which

evidence-based resources are most likely to be useful. Many potential evidence-based resources are available. The challenge is to select the best ones consistent with the purpose and objectives. Some strategies have been included to help meet the challenge.

*The complete listing of the Bibliography and Chapter Questions and Answers are available in the accompanying enhanced eBook version included with the print purchase of this textbook. Visit Elsevier eBooks+ (eBooks.Health.Elsevier.com) to access this content.*

## CHAPTER 6

# Approaches to Screening and Assessment in Gerontological Occupational Therapy

*Jane Bear-Lehman, PhD, OTR/L, FAOTA, FNAP, Tracy Chippendale, PhD, OTR/L, and Steven M. Albert, PhD, MS, FGSA, FAAN*

## CHAPTER OUTLINE

## OBJECTIVES

- Describe selection of assessment tools that suit quality assessment and performance improvement concepts within an evidence-based, client-centered care model
- Identify the methods, challenges, and uses of assessment in gerontological occupational therapy
- Describe considerations in assessment instrument selection for good practice, including the utility of standardized and non-standardized instruments, determination of reliability and validity, and suitability for a client sample

The overriding aim of gerontological occupational therapy (OT) is to improve the ability of older adults to attain satisfactory and successful achievement of their occupations, including completion of daily life task performance, and fulfillment of roles and responsibilities in their home and community that may have become or have the potential to become difficult because of age-related changes, onset of disease, or the development of disability (Bear-Lehman & Miller, 2006; Chippendale & Bear-Lehman, 2011). Human occupation and client-centered care are the two main concepts that direct the OT evaluation process. *Occupation* is an important component of the OT assessment of health and performance, and for the determination of an older adult's ability to interact effectively with his or her living environment to complete tasks and gain satisfaction through these transactions. Thus, the OT evaluation is designed to measure how the client's strengths, skills, weaknesses, and limitations affect functioning in a specific personal environment. In a *client-centered evaluation*, the client is considered an essential part of the evaluation process in that the evaluation will determine what the occupational therapist will do in partnership with the client and what occupational goals are appropriate. The gerontologic OT assessment identifies goals of performance just as the geriatric clinical evaluation elicits goals of care.

The specific OT evaluation is carefully selected to assess the client in the client's environment. In selecting the assessment tools for the evaluation, the occupational therapist determines the need for the assessment, the intended uses for the assessment, and the purpose of the assessment. An OT evaluation is initiated once a physician—or, in some states, a nurse practitioner—writes a referral directly to the OT or rehabilitation team. (Medical referrals are not required for some primary and secondary care OT services, e.g., community education programs and home safety assessments.) Occupational therapists often work as integral members of an interdisciplinary team that may include the client, physicians, nurses, physical therapy practitioners, speech-language pathologists, psychologists, and social workers. Team consultation can help determine which team members can best meet the client's needs and help the client accomplish goals.

The selection and application of assessments for the OT evaluation are influenced by the occupational therapist's knowledge, skills, and clinical/professional reasoning, and are selected to be in accordance with both the needs of the client population and the requirements of the practice setting. But occupational therapists must also choose from among a great many assessments. These differ in quality, suitability for clients or assessment environments, and complexity, and in the kinds of information they produce. In this chapter, we review some of the factors occupational therapists must consider when choosing or designing assessment tools.

## Measurement and Assessment

### Types of Measures

An initial important distinction is the source of assessment information. Does the assessment yield reports of performance from a client or the client's designated representative (when a client is unable to respond to questions), or does the assessment directly assess performance? Self-reports introduce a number of biases, even when these reports are elicited by occupational therapists or trained research assistants. An older adult may deny or exaggerate deficits consciously, or not report accurately because of loss of insight related to cognitive deficit. Surrogates may not report accurately because of similar biases, or because they themselves are overwhelmed by caregiving challenges and cannot perceive older adult competencies accurately. Still, for some older adults self-reported function is perhaps more accurate than performance-based assessments. For these older adults, self-reports involve appraisals of habitual behaviors that cannot always be captured well in a single, short-term assessment of performance.

In considering performance-based assessments, it is important to distinguish between fully standardized tests (e.g., donning a prespecified blouse or making change in a simulated shopping transaction) and assessments of ecologically valid tasks, such as a task habitually performed by an older adult in his or her home environment. The former offers the advantage of greater standardization and reliability (see discussion of reliability later in this chapter), and perhaps greater likelihood of access to population or clinical norms. But the latter is likely to offer greater validity—that is, a more accurate assessment of functional ability (see discussion of validity later in this chapter). Assessing daily activities actually performed by an older adult in his or her home environment is likely to give a truer picture of needs or competencies.

A second consideration is the degree of intrusiveness of assessments. Does the assessment require great investment of attention or effort by older adults? Or can it be performed simply in the normal course of an older adult's daily activity? The first offers the advantage of stress or challenge that may reveal deficits, but this sort of assessment also demands great motivation from clients. The second captures a baseline level of daily activity but may underestimate occupational competencies if older adults have unnecessarily restricted their activity.

Finally, a third consideration is the complexity of the assessment. Assessments range from simple checklists or score sheets (a simple global rating of bathing ability, for example) to quite complex multidimensional assessments that require ratings of each ergonomic and cognitive element of a task.

The best assessment is the one that yields the most accurate information with the least intrusiveness and the most flexibility in administration. Of course, such an assessment is not always available. Hence the development of instruments and assessment technologies to overcome these trade-offs remains a major research concern for OT.

### Levels of Data

A further consideration is what kinds of data an assessment produces. Are these data *nominal*, that is, simply categorical, denoting a type or kind of attribute, such as type of residence, without any true numerical significance? Or are the data *ordinal*, implying a rank ordering as, for example, in the following three grades of independence: "able to live independently," "able to live independently with supervision," and "not able to live independently?" Or, finally, are the data *interval*, with constant differences between values? For example, an interval measure would allow the investigator to say one older adult is able to live independently across 80% of his or her activities and another across only 40%, suggesting that the second older adult is twice as impaired as the first. Each type of data allows different levels of sophistication in analysis. *Ratio* levels of data, where an indicator has a meaningful zero value, were traditionally unavailable for OT measures, but new measurement approaches, such as Rasch models (see below), now allow this level of precision in assessment data.

Many OT functional assessments involve the summing of nominal or ordinal data to create an index of the client's functional ability (Fisher, 1993). For clinical purposes, this level of sophistication in data may seem reasonable and customary. However, many rehabilitation professionals now question the validity of assessments that simply total all of the nominal and ordinal data to determine an aggregate functional outcome score regardless of the type of metric or construct validity of the tool and its components. Rehabilitation professionals are now calling for the application of Rasch modeling in the design of the functional tools. Rasch modeling relies on item response theory (IRT) to improve the level of the data and permit *ratio* levels of data (measures that allow a true zero value) (Fisher, 1993; Rasch, 1960).

### Evaluating Assessment Tools

An assessment tool is obviously not useful if it gives a different result with repeated administration to the same client unless the client has truly changed in functional status. In this case we say it is *unreliable*. An assessment is also not useful if what it measures does not provide information about what we are trying to measure. In this case we say the assessment is *invalid*. Tests may be good at identifying a case (e.g., dementia or a balance disorder), in which case we say the assessment is *sensitive*. But the same test may also identify many noncases as cases, giving the test poor *specificity*. Finally, a test or assessment may be efficient in each of these domains but still fare badly in tracking change in a client over time. In this case we say the assessment is *nonresponsive*.

In choosing an OT assessment, it is important to consider each of these elements. Often, an assessment will be strong in one area but weaker in another, requiring the OT to decide which element is more important for the clinical task at hand.

## Reliability

Reliability is the extent to which a measurement instrument yields consistent results when repeated multiple times over a short interval where change is unlikely. Think of getting on a scale several times in a row: Does the scale always read the same value? If so, that scale is reliable. Reliability is relatively easy to determine, and, in general, is assessed as a correlation between repeated administrations (test-retest reliability), multiple raters (interrater reliability), or related content or ability areas (internal reliability). Unreliable assessments introduce error that makes it difficult to see true relationships between the assessment and underlying clinical conditions.

## Validity

Validity is the extent to which an assessment reflects the concept or quantity that it is intended to measure. The assessment should be considered a surrogate or proxy for the entity we really want to understand. If that surrogate or proxy is a good indicator of the underlying entity, then the assessment is valid. A measure can be reliable but not valid, but a valid assessment must always be reliable. Otherwise, error from the assessment itself (i.e., poor reliability) will make it difficult to gauge how well the assessment measures the clinical condition or concept in question.

Just as reliability takes many forms, so too does validity. Face (or content) validity suggests that a measure includes a reasonable set of indicators to assess the concept or clinical condition we seek to measure. Construct (or convergent) validity indicates that an assessment is highly correlated with other indicators of the underlying clinical condition. Divergent validity is indicated by a low or absent correlation between the assessment and indicators *not* hypothesized to be related to the underlying condition. Criterion validity assesses the extent to which a measure correlates with another indicator of some underlying true value. External validity, or generalizability, suggests that an assessment may be useful across different client or clinical settings.

As an example, think of the occupational therapist–elicited report of activities of daily living (ADLs), originally developed by Katz et al. (1963). The ADL assessment identifies the individual's ability to perform competencies considered essential for personal self-maintenance. Older adults self-report their degree of difficulty with bathing, dressing, personal grooming, transfer, continence, and use of the toilet. The underlying measurement quantity or concept is "personal self-maintenance competency," and the assessment is a count of the number of ADL tasks older adults report they have difficulty performing. The measure has face or content validity in that it elicits the degree of difficulty in performing a wide range of basic adult competencies. The tasks are not gender specific, optional, or subject to variation in lifestyle. The measure has construct validity in that people reporting

ADL disability are likely to have motor, cognitive, or psychiatric conditions that compromise a person's ability to perform self-maintenance activities without difficulty; indeed, ADL disability is correlated with severity of these disease conditions. The measure has criterion validity to the extent that ADL disability increases the risk of mortality, hospitalization, and nursing home placement. Finally, the ADL measure has external validity in that the measure correlates with these indicators both in community and long-term care populations (Katz et al., 1963).

The ADL measure yields ordinal data. That is, ADL tasks can be numerically ranked. The tasks differ in levels of complexity and in motor and cognitive demand. As a result, ADL competencies appear to be gained and lost in a generally consistent (but not necessarily fixed) order. Early on, Katz et al. (1963) suggested that the order in which ADL tasks are acquired in childhood development (first, feeding and transfer; later, toileting and dressing; last, bathing) is the reverse of the order in which they are lost in chronic disease (so that the first lost is bathing, the most complex of the tasks). He noted as well that the order in which they are regained in recovery from stroke or brain injury repeats the sequence for childhood development (so that the last competency reacquired is again bathing).

Katz's early research showed that the disability status of almost all older adults in a skilled care setting adhered to this rough hierarchy of preservation and loss of task ability. That is, people who were unable to do just one task from this set of tasks almost always had lost the ability to bathe. People who could perform only one task independently from the set of ADLs were likely to have retained the ability to feed themselves. The ability to group tasks according to complexity suggests a particular approach to scale development, with meaningful thresholds. It is no accident that variants of the ADL measure have become standard in gerontological assessment.

## Sensitivity and Specificity

It is important to know the *sensitivity* and the *specificity* of an assessment for its capacity to detect the presence or the absence of a given characteristic among those who have a disease or condition. Sensitivity tells us how likely it is that the assessment will detect the presence of a characteristic among those who have the disease or condition, whereas specificity shows how likely it is for the assessment to detect the absence of a characteristic in someone known not to have the disease or the condition. A related concept is positive predictive value, which gives the probability that a person screening positive (i.e., with a value on the assessment indicating disease) truly has the disease. Sensitivity and specificity tell us about the validity of a test. Positive predictive value tells us how important a test is likely to be for investment in prevention activities for a population.

Assessments can also lead us to wrongly categorize a healthy person as either diseased or having a characteristic of a disease or a condition. This error is captured by the *specificity* of the assessment. Among those without the disease, what proportion is wrongly identified as a case? Specificity tells us whether a test goes too far and identifies people as having the disease when they really do not.

Very rarely is an assessment both highly sensitive and specific. Consider an assessment with a threshold score to define disability. If we lower this score, we will capture all cases, making the test maximally sensitive, but we will increase the likelihood of netting non-cases and falsely labeling them as such (decreasing specificity). In practice, it is perhaps best to err on the side of increasing sensitivity to identify cases and offer treatment. False positives can be assessed with more sensitive tools and reclassified as non-cases in follow-up assessments if these are not too intrusive.

## Responsiveness

If a client's status has changed, assessments should be able to detect this change over repeated assessments. Responsiveness is a measure of how well an assessment captures such change in clients. Thus, in a client with declining cognitive ability, a good assessment will register slower performance, or perhaps a greater number of errors, in a performance test of cooking or cleaning, relative to baseline values. The "minimal clinically significant difference" is the degree of change in an assessment associated with a change in performance or status perceived to be meaningful to a client or occupational therapist.

## Selection of Assessment Instruments and Type of Practice Setting

Occupational therapists need to be aware of the following specific, real-world factors when selecting and using assessments for the specific practice setting.

### Reimbursement as a Driver

Reimbursement for OT services may drive the selection of screening tools and assessments. For example, in skilled nursing facilities in the United States, staff must complete the Minimum Data Set (MDS), an assessment tool required by the Center for Medicare and Medicaid Services (CMS) (Centers for Medicare & Medicaid Services, 2021). Occupational therapists are often responsible for completing the GG section of the MDS, which includes an assessment of the client's level of functional performance in ADLs (e.g., eating, toilet hygiene) and functional mobility (e.g., toilet transfers). In some facilities, it is also the occupational therapist who completes the Brief Interview for Mental Status (BIMS) cognitive screening, another component of the MDS. Consistent with CMS guidelines, occupational therapists must also assess and document the level of complexity of the evaluation process. Using these guidelines, the occupational therapist will determine if the assessment involves low, moderate, or high complexity. In home care, the OASIS, a standardized assessment used to plan care, measure quality, and determine reimbursement, is required (O'Connor & Davitt, 2012). The OASIS includes, among other components, an assessment of ADL and IADL function (e.g., dressing, grooming, bathing, medication

management), functional cognition, and mobility (Centers for Medicare & Medicaid Services, 2021).

State Medicaid programs in the United States, which fund in-home personal assistance services, also use functional assessments to determine eligibility. For example, in the Pennsylvania Medicaid waiver program, eligibility depends on having health-related care and service needs that may be less complex than those typically met by skilled nursing or rehabilitation, but which at one time were only provided through institutional facilities. This statutory guidance defines "nursing home clinically eligible" (NFCE) but leaves the definition of care and service needs open. Pennsylvania uses the Functional Eligibility Determination (FED) for this purpose, which is based on a subset of items from the InterRAI-Home Care (PA Department of Human Services). In the FED, a geriatric social worker or nurse conducts a standardized assessment of cognitive skills, behavioral or psychiatric symptoms, ADL, mobility, medication management, and continence to establish NFCE. Partial deficits (need for some help) in any three domains or full deficit (need for complete assistance) in one or more basic domains (cognition, continence, mobility, more than half of ADL tasks) establishes NFCE and eligibility. A subsequent administration of the InterRAI-Home Care tool confirms results from the brief FED screening and establishes weekly hours of personal assistance services provided to people meeting criteria for NFCE.

### Length of Administration

The amount of time available and the goals of the practice setting need to be considered in the selection of the tool. Opportunities to conduct assessments may depend on how long clients are in a particular setting, which in turn depends on the setting of health-care delivery, residential arrangements associated with each type of facility, and Medicare guidelines.

### Diversity and Cultural Humility

The population of older adults in the United States is increasingly diverse. Occupational therapists must strive for cultural humility in the assessment and treatment of the clients they serve (Bonder et al., 2004; Krefting & Krefting, 1991). Cultural humility is an approach that includes lifelong learning as well as a recognition of the power dynamics in health care. The occupational therapist who embraces cultural humility recognizes that a client's cultural perspectives are as valid as their own (Agner, 2020). Fundamental to cultural humility is continuous self-reflection regarding one's own values and beliefs, and the recognition of personal biases. Critical reflection is needed regarding the selection of practice models and frames of reference used to inform OT assessment and treatment, given that many are informed by the dominant culture (Hammell, 2013; Sterman & Njelesani, 2021). Assessments should be selected based on a client-centered approach, including performance of occupations that an older adult client needs or wants to do. Following a thorough review of the client's medical record, the next step in the assessment process is for the occupational therapist to use their interview and observation skills to complete the occupational profile (American Occupational Therapy Association, 2020). The selection of appropriate follow-up screening tools and assessments should be done collaboratively with the client. During the selection process, the occupational therapist should also be mindful of the origins of standardized assessments, including the content and cultures being represented (Sterman & Njelesani, 2021). For example, the clock draw, an element of the Mini-Cog, may not be appropriate for clients from cultural communities that ordinarily do not mark time intervals with the precision expected in the test.

## Training of Occupational Therapists and Recertification

Licensed occupational clinician/practitioners have an earned master's or clinical professional doctoral degree, although some practicing OTs still have bachelor's degrees. Certified OT assistants (COTAs) have an associate's degree and some hold a bachelor's. Registered and Certified assistants hold a state license. Occupational clinician/practitioners conduct the initial evaluations, design the interventions, and supervise the COTAs, who implement interventions and may contribute to the evaluation or reevaluation process if permitted by state guidelines and pending demonstration of competency (AOTA on State Licensure, retrieved November 27, 2021).

In addition, some assessments require the practicing occupational therapist to acquire advanced training or certification in the assessment. For example, occupational therapists require advanced training to use the Functional Independence Measure (FIM), which is designed to document the severity of client disability and measure outcomes of medical rehabilitation in a uniform way. Occupational therapists also must satisfactorily complete certification requirements to evaluate ADL task performance using the Assessment of Motor and Process Skills (AMPS) (Fisher, 1993; Hamilton et al., 1994).

## Quality Assurance and Performance Improvement

Some evaluations conducted by occupational therapists are not focused on a specific client or patient but rather on the services provided by the OT department or facility as a whole. The Center for Medicare and Medicaid services (CMS, 2021) requires nursing homes to implement Quality Assurance and Performance Improvement (QAPI) programs. In order to develop a written QAPI plan and put in place a comprehensive QAPI program, an evaluation of existing programs and services is needed. Data from local and national sources are used to establish benchmarks, that is, to compare the performance of a rehabilitation department or nursing home with others in the area. Examples of evaluation tools that may be used to establish a QAPI program and plan include a review of medical records and interviews or questionnaires conducted with staff members, residents, family members, and other employees regarding satisfaction with programs and services. Facilities must have a system in place to determine when in-depth analysis of a problem and its causes are needed. Examples of potential problems that may warrant

analyses and follow-up attention include falls that occur in the facility, staff turnover, adverse events, and rehospitalization rates. Occupational therapists involved with the QAPI program must also be able to conduct root cause analysis (RCA) to uncover how problems may be caused or exacerbated in order to take appropriate action for performance improvement (CMS, 2021).

## Assistive Technologies

Since OT helps the older individual maintain daily life performance tasks (including basic and instrumental activities) and maintain familiar social roles and activities while encouraging new ones, the OT must often consider use of assistive technologies in assessments as a way to compensate for a change in functional capacity to increase learning, facilitate social exchange with family and friends, and to gain access to care services. With the accelerated development of digital technologies during the coronavirus pandemic, telehealth became an essential rehabilitation and habilitation delivery model to alleviate social isolation and to address functional performance components (American Occupational Therapy Association Position Paper, 2018; Oh-Park et al., 2021). Thus, the OT role includes assessment of the person's performance to use computer-related occupations to manage daily life skills (Fischl et al., 2021). At this time, knowledge about the management technology is just developing as is the ability to reliably assess it. The META (Management of Everyday Technology Assessment) is one example of a method aimed to measure and to validate this capacity (Malinowsky et al., 2011).

## Practical Considerations in Selecting Assessment Tools

In addition to type of practice setting, there are several specific practical considerations regarding assessment that should be considered when selecting assessment instruments (Box 6.1).

### Assessments in the Public Domain

Some assessments are in the public domain, which means that they can be obtained at no cost to the user, such as the Katz ADL Index mentioned earlier. Some instruments may have originally been in the public domain but were later removed, such as the Mini Mental Status Exam (MMSE), the Montreal Cognitive Assessment (MOCA), and the semi-structured, client-centered Assessment of Awareness of Disability (AAD). The MMSE, a widely used instrument to detect dementia, can only be obtained through Psychological Assessment Resources (PAR) (Crum et al., 1993); the AAD requires credentialing from the Karolinska Institute in Stockholm before use (Tariq et al., 2006); and the MOCA is now licensed through Neurosearch Developments Inc. Occupational therapists may consider the Saint Louis University Mental Status scale (SLUMS), which is designed for early detection of mild dementia in its 11-item questionnaire; SLUMS demonstrates validity with the MMSE and is available in the public domain (Tariq et al., 2006). A scientific review of the utility and the

| BOX 6.1 | List of Instruments Reviewed |
| --- | --- |

AAD: Assessment of Awareness of Disability (Malinowsky et al., 2011)

AMPS: Assessment of Motor and Processing Skills (Chisholm et al., 2014)

Beck Depression Inventory (American Occupational Therapy Association Position Paper, 2018)

Braden Risk Assessment (Baum & Edwards, 1993)

CDC's home fall prevention checklist for older adults (http://www.cdc.gov/homeandrecreationalsafety/falls/adultfalls.html)

COPM: Canadian Occupational Performance Measure (Hammell, 2013)

Dynavision Performance Battery (Fisher, 1993)

FIM: Functional Independence Measure (Classen et al., 2018)

Fitness to Drive Screening Measure (FTDS)

FPS: Faces Pain Scale (http://www.geriatricpain.org/Content/Assessment/Intact/Pages/FACESPainScale.aspx)

FM: Functional Reach (Chippendale & Bear-Lehman, 2011)

GDS: Geriatric Depression Scale (Oh-Park et al., 2021)

GUG: Get Up and Go (Katz et al., 1963)

Hamilton Rating Scale for Depression (Crum et al., 1993)

I-HOPE: In-Home Occupational Performance Evaluation (Law et al., 2005)

Katz ADL (Fischl et al., 2021)

KTA: Kitchen Task Assessment (American Occupational Therapy Association, 2020)

MMSE: Mini-Mental Status Exam (Chippendale & Bear-Lehman, 2010)

Mini-Cog (Bohannon et al., 2007)

Occupational Profile (Agner, 2020)

PAINAD: Pain Assessment in Advanced Dementia (O'Connor & Davitt, 2012)

Patient Health Questionnaire-9 (PHQ-9)

Performance Assessment of Self-Care Skills (PASS)

SLUMS: Saint Louis University Mental Status (Mahmood et al., 2020)

Stakeholders' Walkability/Wheelability Audit in Neighborhood (SWAN)

Timed Up and Go (Kroenke et al., 2001)

VAS/NRS: Visual analog scale/numeric rating scale (Bonder et al., 2004)

validity of the tests and measures will provide the necessary determination for suitability and access.

## Changes in Normative Values

As the population of older adults has grown in size and there is noteworthy increased longevity, it is important to consider whether the scores on standardized assessments suit those who are to be measured. Only recently, age-specific impairment scores for 5-year increments above the age of 70 years have been published for a number of measures, such as hand strength (Bohannon et al., 2007).

## Suitability for Setting

The format of the assessment may call upon the occupational therapist to direct observation of an individual or a group of individuals, or administer a performance-based measure, or elicit reports using a written or oral questionnaire. The suitability of a given assessment format depends on features of the client population, for example, whether clients can complete a paper-and-pencil or electronic questionnaire on their own.

## Goodness of Fit

In reviewing the assessment, it is important to determine whether the construct in the assessment tool is standardized on a population similar to the one in the practice setting, and whether the items on the assessment are good representations of the underlying construct and sensitive enough to detect the level of function or change in function that is desired to be measured (Fisher, 1993). Moreover, it is critical that the assessment is well suited for the demographic characteristics, cultural group, and clinical or community-based needs of the population to be assessed.

## Cost

Some instruments, particularly those with standardized protocols and normative data tables, may have a cost for the assessment manual, tools, and data-collection sheets, whereas others may require a specific training course or credentialing.

## Human Resources

The occupational therapist needs to meet the training requirements for the selected assessments and determine whether the format of the assessment is conducive for the practice setting. If the assessment is a self-report questionnaire, it may seem that many clients could complete the assessment on their own. However, if there are clients who require assistance in manual skills to complete the form, or who require cognitive cues to appreciate the question being asked, then additional staff time will be required to complete the assessment.

## Computerized Assessments

In addition, the assessments that the occupational therapist administers may require specific computer technology or software during the test administration. For example, the Assessment of Motor and Process Skills (AMPS; http://www.innovativeotsolutions.com/content/amps) requires physical setup for the occupational therapist to observe the client completing carefully selected routine daily life tasks (such as making a sandwich or sweeping the floor), as well as specific computer software to score test results (Fisher, 1993). Alternatively, occupational therapists conducting off-the-road driving assessments require the use of simulators and computerized programs, such as DriveABLE (http://www.driveable.com) or Dynavision Performance Battery, during the assessment process (Klavora et al., 1995).

## Client Considerations

### Client-Centered Evaluation

Before choosing an assessment, there are a number of factors to consider. First, based on the client's diagnosis and medical history, it is imperative to take into consideration appropriate precautions. For example, in the case of someone with a recent orthopedic injury, the occupational therapist needs to consider weight-bearing status and range-of-motion restrictions before initiating further assessment. In the case of a client with a cardiopulmonary condition, the occupational therapist must determine any activity restrictions or surgical precautions. *Pain levels* should also be noted before administering any assessment. For performance-based assessments in particular, it is important to time the assessment with a client's pain medication. In addition to pain levels and precautions, the client's *cognitive status* should be considered, as this will affect the client's ability to follow directions, as well as the client's safety, during performance-based assessments. *Sensory impairments* including vision and hearing loss should also be considered. In some instances, hearing loss is misconstrued as cognitive impairment when a client provides inappropriate responses to questions because they were not heard clearly. Or a client may struggle with a pen-and-paper assessment because of vision loss. For some performance-based assessments and home safety assessments, a client's *mobility status* and use of an assisted device should be noted. For example, a client going home in a wheelchair will require different home safety considerations than someone who uses a cane or rolling walker.

Sociodemographic factors need to be considered as well. *Language skills* are important for most assessments, but for accurate cognitive assessment in particular. Therefore, assessments should be administered in the client's native language whenever possible. Some standardized assessment tools, such as the MMSE, have been translated into many languages (Crum et al., 1993). *Education level* can also affect the results of cognitive assessments. In these cases, assessments identify low levels of education rather than true cognitive loss.

Finally, *practice setting* will influence assessment choice. An occupational therapist working in home care will encounter clients at a different functional level and in a very different context than an occupational therapist working in subacute or acute care. For example, an occupational therapist who works in a subacute care center may be concerned with kitchen safety and administer a standardized assessment, such as the Kitchen Task Assessment (KTA), to assist with discharge planning. In the acute care setting, this type of assessment may be inappropriate due to a client's limited strength, mobility, and activity tolerance at this stage of the client's recovery (Baum & Edwards, 1993).

### Client-Centered Practice

Client-centered practice is a philosophy of practice that emphasizes client autonomy, client choice in decision making, respect for the individual, partnership with the client, and a need to ensure services are accessible and fit the client's context

(Law et al., 2005). It includes a therapeutic relationship rooted in strong communication and trust. Therefore, client centeredness affects the quality of interactions between clients and occupational therapists. This being the case, a client-centered approach affects not just the assessments chosen but the way in which they are administered. Occupational therapists who are client centered engage the client as an active participant in the therapy process. Specifically, they discuss with the client the assessment tools to be used, the purpose of the assessment, and the assessment findings.

In a client-centered evaluation, the occupational therapist helps the client prioritize activities and occupations that the client may want or need help with because of current or anticipated age-related functional decline. Clients are evaluated for the full spectrum of functional performance capacities; occupational therapists often use the Occupational Profile to begin assessment of cognitive and functional status to identify the limitations in occupation that can be improved from interventions and to determine strengths that can be used to compensate for weaknesses (American Occupational Therapy Association, 2020, 2021). Often, age-related changes may produce functional limitations that can be remediated through intervention or compensatory strategies to improve achievement in the desired activity performance or occupation.

In addition to the occupational therapist's interaction with a client, some assessment tools themselves are client-centered with regard to the types of information they gather. Client-centered assessment tools involve exploring a client's values and preferences, beliefs, hopes, ways of dealing with adversity, and sense of what is important. A client-centered assessment takes into consideration information about the client's family and other contextual data (Classen et al., 2018). It also allows for the recording of a client's goals and treatment/intervention preferences. Examples of client-centered assessment tools include the Assessment of Motor and Process Skills (AMPS) and the Canadian Occupational Performance Measure (COPM). The AMPS allows the client or a family member to select a specific ADL or an instrumental ADL (IADL) task to be used during the assessment. This translates into an assessment that is relevant to the client's life and cultural background. The COPM includes a client rating of importance for areas of occupation that are identified as problematic. This aspect of the assessment tool facilitates collaborative goal setting between the client and occupational therapist.

There are a number of documented benefits to a client-centered approach. These include improved care and quality of life, reduced depression and anxiety for the client, and a means to address ethnic and socioeconomic disparities. Moreover, this approach is ethically and morally superior to purely occupational therapist–driven approaches (Epstein et al., 2010).

### Quality Assessment From Outside Agencies

Assessment of quality of care can also be carried out by outside agencies. In other words, individuals who are not employed by the facility or health-care organization itself review quality standards. For example, the state sends a team of health-care professionals annually to evaluate the overall quality of care provided at each health-care institution. This includes both a thorough examination of medical records as well as on-site observations of care.

The Joint Commission on Accreditation of Healthcare Organizations (JCAHO) is an independent, nonprofit organization that provides accreditation to facilities and organizations that achieve quality standards. Health-care organizations that contract their services are provided with education and advice to help achieve these standards. JCAHO provides accreditation of organizations and certification for specific programs across the health-care continuum, including hospitals, nursing homes, and home health agencies (Joint Commission on Accreditation of Healthcare Organizations, 2015).

## Applying Assessment Tools: A Case Study

To see how occupational therapists make assessment tool decisions, consider Case Example 6.1.

---

**CASE EXAMPLE 6.1**    Mr. Gomez

### Social Background

Mr. Gomez is a 92-year-old bilingual Spanish- and English-speaking widower who has been residing in an assisted living environment for the past 3 years. He and his wife moved into the assisted living center due to Mrs. Gomez's declining medical and functional status. Mrs. Gomez passed away 2 years ago, and Mr. Gomez continued to reside in the apartment they shared together in the center. He retired from being a jeweler when he was 85 to be home full time for his wife, whose health had begun to decline. Mr. Gomez speaks with his daughter daily and enjoys the ability to connect with his grandchildren on the Internet. His daughter visits 2–3 weekends each month and always wants to move Mr. Gomez to an assistive living center near her home, but Mr. Gomez enjoys being close to his friends in the center and those few friends who still reside in that town.

Mr. Gomez limits his driving to daytime and maintains a car in the assisted living center garage. The assisted living center provides housekeeping, two meals a day, and a network of friends. Mr. Gomez enjoys playing bridge, collecting coins, singing in the assisted living center's choir, and acting in the center's theater group. He and his group of friends enjoy music and museum outings that are sponsored by the center.

### Medical History

Mr. Gomez was first admitted to the local acute care hospital following a fall incurred while stumbling over a sidewalk crack. He was treated for his hip fracture with open reduction internal fixation; a joint replacement was not needed. Three days after surgery, he was transferred to the subacute rehabilitation skilled nursing facility adjoining his place of residence.

His past medical history is significant for hearing loss in both ears, right more than left; heart attack 10 years ago; history of elevated blood pressure and cholesterol; and an old left shoulder rotator cuff football injury.

### Assessment Upon Admission to the Subacute Rehabilitation Facility

Mr. Gomez is very determined to return to his apartment in the assisted living center, reunite with his friends, and restore his usual and customary activities as soon as possible. Using a client-centered approach, selection of screening tools and assessments is done collaboratively with Mr. Gomez. Further, findings will be shared with Mr. Gomez and discussed immediately.

The occupational therapist interviews the client to clarify the medical and social history from his perspective and to understand his living context. First, the occupational therapist needs to verify surgical or medical precautions related to his precipitating hip injury and his past cardiac-related diagnoses.

The occupational therapist should assess self-reported pain at the outset of the assessment. Since this Spanish-/English-speaking client does not have a diagnosis indicating dementia, a visual analog scale (VAS) rating for pain (0–10, where 0 is no pain and 10 is the worst pain experienced) is selected (Fig. 6.1). There are a number of reliable and valid pain scales to choose from had there been noted issues about language or severe cognitive impairment. In that case, other tools, such as the self-report Faces Pain Scale or the clinician-/practitioner-administered ***Pain Assessment in Advanced Dementia Scale*** (PAINAD), could be considered (O'Connor & Davitt, 2012). The Faces Pain Scale provides a visual facial expression associated with numeric values commonly used on the Visual Analog Scale that can help guide a client to anchor a pain level with a numeric level by a facial expression (Fig. 6.2) (Carlsson, 1983). The PAINAD is specifically designed for the clinician/practitioner to assess pain in older adults who are unable to communicate their pain experiences or responses reliably due to cognitive impairments associated with Dementia (Warden et al., 2003).

Even though Mr. Gomez's fall was caused by stumbling over a crack in the sidewalk, a hazardous environmental condition, the occupational therapist should be mindful to observe for safety and awareness during the functional assessments.

In order for Mr. Gomez to return to his own apartment at the center, it will be necessary for him to be independent in ADL tasks; he will need to ambulate with either a straight cane or a walker, not a wheelchair (Fig. 6.3). Therefore, the assessment will address:

- physical measures of range of motion, strength, and sensation, recognizing that the left shoulder will be compromised from the old football injury
- bed mobility assessment for rolling, supine to sit, sit to supine
- transfer from the wheelchair to bed, toilet, and chair, with the goal to increase standing tolerance

*Continued*

and balance to engage in ADL without need for a wheelchair

Due to the cardiac history, vital signs need to be monitored at rest, during, and following activities. They must also ensure monitoring of vital signs during the early standing, mobility, and balance program.

The goal is to increase functional mobility over all surfaces (e.g., carpeted, uncarpeted, uneven surfaces), improve balance, and foster self-confidence and independence to safely complete ADL and IADL tasks using only a straight cane or walker. The larger personal goal is to return Mr. Gomez to his active lifestyle. Achievement of this goal can be measured by ADL, IADL, and fall risk measures.

The occupational therapist needs to note clinical signs that could be interrupting performance during the assessment process. For example, Mr. Gomez appears to have difficulty following verbal directions during the physical performance assessment and requires physical cues. The occupational therapist may question whether his need for physical cues indicates an undetected cognitive deficit or an unaddressed problem with hearing.

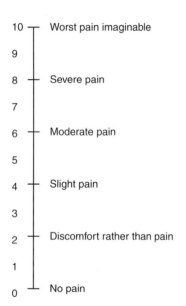

**FIGURE 6.1**    Visual Analog Scale for Pain.
(Adapted from O'Brien, P. D., Fitzpatrick, P., & Power, W. [2005]. Patient pain during stretching of small pupils in phacoemulsification performed using topical anesthesia. *Journal of Cataract & Refractive Surgery, 31*[9], 1760–1763.)

A cognitive screening is first performed to determine whether further assessment of cognition is indicated. The occupational therapist considers two reliable and valid cognitive screening tools: the Folstein MMSE and the Mini-Cog (Borson et al., 2003). However, the occupational therapist uses the Mini-Cog because of its specificity and sensitivity and because it can be administered quickly (in about 5 min). The Mini-Cog tool is readily accessible; it is in the public domain. The occupational therapist observes for how Mr. Gomez responds to verbal cues and questions during the course of the ongoing assessments to determine whether to make a recommendation for a hearing assessment.

After the preliminary OT assessment, the occupational therapist schedules a bedside ADL to assess Mr. Gomez's self-care tasks when they are usually performed in the morning along with help from the nursing staff. The occupational therapist assesses level of assistance, independence, and safety in personal ADL performance of bathing, dressing, grooming, and toileting; and the occupational therapist completes the corresponding section of the FIM related to personal care. The FIM is a multidisciplinary tool that requires certification and training for use.

Given Medicare requirements for sub-acute rehabilitation facilities, the OT also completes the Brief Interview for Mental Status (BIMS), the GG section of the MDS pertaining to ADLs, and assigns a complexity rating for the OT evaluation as a whole.

### Assessment After 2 Weeks in the Subacute Rehabilitation Facility

Based on comments made by Mr. Gomez during OT treatment, the occupational therapist is concerned about his mental health. After a discussion with Mr. Gomez, the occupational therapist and client mutually agree that a screening for depressive symptoms is warranted. There are a number of assessments to identify depression, including the Hamilton Rating Scale (Hamilton, 1960), Patient Health Questionnaire-9 (PHQ-9) (Kroenke et al., 2001), Beck Depression Inventory (Beck et al., 1988), and Geriatric Depression Scale (GDS) (Yesavage et al., 1983). The GDS is selected because it was designed and developed specifically for use with older adults. It is also in the public domain. Mr. Gomez scores in the mildly depressed range on the GDS and likes the idea of a referral to psychiatry for further assessment.

The occupational therapist and client discuss fall risk and decide that further assessment is warranted. There are a

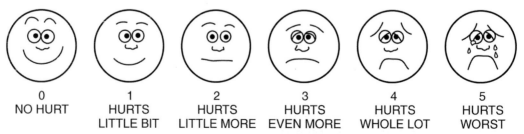

**FIGURE 6.2**    Faces Pain Scale. (Adapted from Hockenberry, M. [2014]. *Wong's nursing care of infants and children* [10th ed.]. Elsevier.)

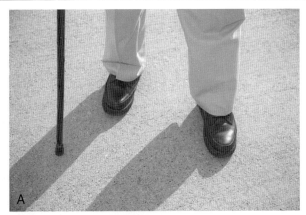

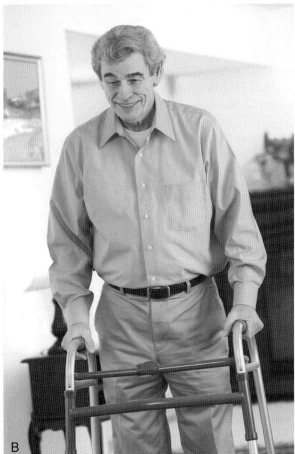

**FIGURE 6.3** (A) Using a straight cane. (B) Using a walker. (Photos © istock.com.)

number of assessment tools available, including the Functional Reach Test and the Timed Up and Go (TUG) (Shumway-Cook et al., 2000). Both measures are used, and goals are set based on the results to improve Mr. Gomez's balance and mobility so that he will be in a low-risk fall category.

The client no longer requires the wheelchair for indoor mobility within the subacute rehabilitation facility and relies only on a straight cane to complete mobility-related personal ADL tasks independently and safely. Furthermore, he ambulates within the facility for scheduled appointments and to visit his friends.

The client expresses concern with regard to his ability to return to the same apartment in the assisted living center and to complete instrumental tasks safely. Specifically, he mentions the ability to make his own lunch, which is not provided at the center. Although a number of tools can be used to assess meal preparation and other IADLs, such as the Kitchen Task Assessment (KTA) and the Assessment of Motor and Process Skills (AMPS), the clinician/practitioner chooses the Performance Assessment of Self-Care Skills (PASS) because it is a reliable and valid performance-based measure of ADLs and IADLs, and because it does not require specialized software to use.

### Assessment at the Assisted Living Center

Prior to Mr. Gomez's return home, the OT completes a home safety assessment to ensure there are no environmental risk factors. The occupational therapist has the option of an environmental checklist such as the one developed by the Centers for Disease Control (CDC), "Check for Safety: A Home Fall Prevention Checklist for Older Adults" (http://www.cdc.gov/homeandrecreationalsafety/falls/adultfalls.html). This type of assessment requires the occupational therapist to conduct a survey of the physical home environment only (Chippendale and Bear-Lehman, 2010). The OT adds the In-Home Occupational Performance Evaluation (I-HOPE), a more comprehensive client-centered option, to observe the client complete ADL and IADL tasks in the natural environment.

Mr. Gomez returns to his apartment in the assisted living center with a raised toilet seat and a bathtub seat. The assisted living center occupational therapist incorporated these into the I-HOPE assessment (Stark et al., 2010). Based on the assessment, the occupational therapist also discusses with the client other options to decrease fall risk within his apartment.

Given that Mr. Gomez was independent in community mobility and shopping prior to his hospitalization, the OT will evaluate Mr. Gomez's ability to navigate curbs and environmental obstacles safely. His ability to cross the street safely with the traffic light will also be assessed. Mr. Gomez's activity tolerance and the number of rest breaks he needs to make the return trip to his local grocery store will be determined. Goals are set to increase safety awareness for outdoor environmental hazards and to increase activity tolerance and independence with shopping.

During another therapy visit, Mr. Gomez and the OT complete an audit of personally relevant street segments in his neighborhood using the Stakeholders' Walkability/Wheelability Audit in Neighborhood (SWAN) (Mahmood et al., 2020). The SWAN requires the permission of the developer to use, which was obtained. The results of the audit are used for safe route planning and to advocate for correction of safety hazards by reporting them to the city.

Goals are also set to increase standing and activity tolerance for the purpose of returning to the theatre group.

A physical therapist continues to work with the resident on his gait, balance, and endurance, and collaborates with the occupational therapist to help the client meet his goals without duplicating services. In collaboration with the client, the OT and PT set up his smart watch so that it can

*Continued*

detect a fall and can allow him to call emergency services if needed.

Shortly after Mr. Gomez's return home, the client's daughter approaches the residence staff with regard to her concerns about her father's driving. She is encouraged by the care coordinator to talk to the occupational therapist. The occupational therapist begins a conversation with Mr. Gomez and his daughter about driving fitness. The OT encourages the daughter to use the online Fitness to Drive Screening (FTDS) (Classen et al., 2018) available on the AOTA website, which can be helpful in detecting older drivers at risk. The occupational therapist also plans to assess the client for any underlying deficits that could potentially affect driving health.

These include visual acuity and visual scanning ability; visual field screening; visual perception; reaction time; cognitive skills, including attention, memory, insight, and judgment; and potential musculoskeletal changes, such as upper extremity, lower extremity, and neck range of motion (ROM). Depending on the results, the occupational therapist may suggest that the client be referred to a driving specialist for a more detailed assessment, including an on-road assessment. See Chapter 21 for more information regarding driving assessments.

Once these goals have been met and the client is satisfied with his performance on his ADLs, IADLs, and leisure activities, or he has reached his highest level of functioning, the client is discharged from the OT service.

## SUMMARY

In this chapter, we identify the methods, challenges, and uses of assessment in gerontological OT. We provide criteria to aid occupational therapists in the selection of assessments for their clients. A case example is presented with the intention to illuminate the decision-making process for the selection of assessments at three stages in the continuum of OT service provision. The chapter defines the standards and criteria for determining quality assessment and performance improvement within a client-centered care model. Suggestions are made to help the occupational therapist select assessments relative to availability of standardized and non-standardized instruments, determination of reliability and validity, and suitability for client samples across care levels during the trajectory of disease and rehabilitation.

*The complete listing of the Bibliography and Chapter Questions and Answers are available in the accompanying enhanced eBook version included with the print purchase of this textbook. Visit Elsevier eBooks+ (eBooks.Health.Elsevier.com) to access this content.*

CHAPTER 7

# Occupational Therapy Intervention Process With Aging Adults

*Stacy West-Bruce, OTD, OTR/L, Stacey L. Schepens Niemiec, PhD, OTR/L, DipACLM/ DipIBLM, Jenny Martínez, OTD, OTR/L, BCG, FAOTA, and Catherine L. Lysack, PhD, OT*

## CHAPTER OUTLINE

## OBJECTIVES

- Discuss the similarities and differences of environmentally focused models relevant to the occupational therapy intervention process in later life
- Discuss important considerations for the occupational therapy intervention process relevant to older adults
- Explain the major steps in the occupational therapy intervention process
- Discuss what comprises successful occupational therapy interventions with older adults
- Provide examples of intervention process components embedded within the *¡Vivir Mi Vida!* lifestyle intervention

## Introduction and Chapter Overview

From its inception, occupational therapy (OT) has been a profession that uses engagement in occupation as the therapeutic medium to address clients' holistic needs. Clients of OT may be individuals, groups with a common purpose or interest, or populations of people who have shared characteristics or contexts (AOTA, 2020a). When clients are referred to OT, regardless of their age, condition, setting in which they present, or group/population to which they belong, the occupational therapist begins by critically analyzing the presenting problem and the activities the client needs and wants to do. The successful therapist will find a way to maximize the abilities of the client and modify and strengthen other influential contexts (e.g., the built environment), so that necessary and desired activities can be achieved.

Think for a moment about an older person discharged from the hospital in a wheelchair after a debilitating stroke. They will be eager to return home, likely apprehensive about their ability to manage tasks or for other reasons, but also looking forward to "getting back to normal" and resuming what they like to do, whatever that happens to be. What kind of intervention plan can the therapist develop that considers the client's abilities and optimizes the environment to support these activities while also placing the most meaningful life roles and passions this person enjoys at the forefront of the intervention? The therapist may include an occupational therapy assistant in this process, work as a team, and make recommendations for simple modifications to the bathroom, kitchen, bedroom, and laundry room with the aim of improving the safety and desired level of independence when performing self-care and other household activities for the older adult client.

Chisholm and Schell (2019) write: The OT process "provides a structure for practitioners to employ therapeutic professional reasoning based on evidence in order to address the client's health-related problems" (p. 352). They stress that problem-solving and competency in reading and interpreting evidence-based indicators that can lead practitioners along the best route for intervention are essential. In addition, it is vital for OT practitioners to consider that every older adult lives in a wider context that includes the physical environment (e.g., home, neighborhood), which may be more or less accessible, and a social environment (e.g., friends, family, co-workers, the public), which may hold more or less positive attitudes and be more or less supportive. The overarching goal of OT is to find ways to facilitate a client's return to the specific kind of daily life they would like to have, or an adapted version that is agreeable and meets their needs. This means putting the meaningful occupations of clients at the center of intervention efforts.

It follows, then, that the goal-setting process must be a genuine collaborative partnership between the therapist or therapy team (OT & OTA) and client, where trust is built, power is shared, and the rights people have for self-determination are respected (Restall & Egan, 2021). If an intervention is designed correctly, it will provide the "just-right challenge" to a client because it optimizes the best of what the client can do within the client's unique, multifaceted context. OT interventions must be particularly attentive to identifying the most meaningful activities and occupations in clients' lives, working intentionally to integrate them into the intervention process.

Think again about the client discharged home after a stroke. Therapeutic activities during inpatient rehabilitation aimed at improving the functioning of their affected arm and hand could include repotting houseplants, for example, if gardening is a favorite activity. If swimming has been a fun recreational interest, then a water aerobics class and return to the pool might also be recommended. If the therapeutic intervention focuses on what is most important to the client, then the intervention will be much more interesting, engaging, and motivating. When the client's wishes and choices are well-integrated into the therapeutic process, there is a greater chance that positive outcomes will be achieved.

This chapter explores the OT process within the context of later life with a focus on OT intervention and is organized into four main sections:

1. Use of environmentally focused models to guide occupation-based intervention with older adult clients
2. Important considerations for intervention in later life
3. Overview of the OT intervention process to promote positive aging and optimal outcomes
4. Evidence-based OT intervention with older people

In the first section, the chapter provides an overview of three environmentally focused models and theoretical frameworks—(1) the International Classification of Functioning, Disability, and Health (commonly referred to as the ICF); (2) Bronfenbrenner's ecological system's theory; and (3) person-environment-occupation performance (PEOP) model—that can serve as useful guides for intervention with older adult individuals and collectives. In the second section, the chapter presents key considerations when intervening with older adults, groups, and populations with diverse backgrounds, contexts, and experiences. It describes selected factors relevant to older people that should be considered as a part of an OT evaluation and influential intervention, such as common changes in one's social roles in older adulthood and social drivers that can affect later life health and occupation. The third section details OT intervention as a multilayer step within the overall OT process, particularly through the use of the OT practice framework-4 (OTPF-4) from the United States (AOTA, 2020a), complemented with a population health lens focused on social determinants of health. The final section describes an exemplar OT intervention that has been implemented in a community of late-midlife people and that embodies best practices and successful approaches to addressing the needs of clients in later life. The overall goal of this chapter is to provide timely and highly useful knowledge about the OT intervention process to practitioners to promote high-quality OT care with the older population across a range of practice settings.

## Use of Environmentally Focused Models to Guide Occupation-Based Intervention With Older Adults

The design of interventions and treatments for older adults is aided by theoretical frameworks or models that organize key concepts and knowledge. There are many models that guide practice in OT, as noted in Chapter 4; therapists need to be familiar with them. The models discussed next are important to OT because they include a strong emphasis on the environments in which clients work, play, and live. These models provide a "big-picture" view and remind the practitioner that an older adult's personal situation and broader environment exert a significant influence on the older adult's occupational performance.

### The International Classification of Functioning, Disability, and Health

A useful model to consider when intervening with older adults is the World Health Organization's (WHO) International Classification of Functioning, Disability and Health (commonly referred to as the ICF) (WHO, 2001). The ICF model views a person's functioning as a dynamic interaction between health conditions and contextual factors. In this model, contextual factors are divided into personal and environmental factors. Personal factors are internal influences on functioning, such as age and gender, for example. Environmental factors are external influences on functioning that include features of the physical, social, and attitudinal world. Thus, in the ICF model, disability is viewed as an interaction between features of the person and the overall context in which the person lives. This contrasts with the more traditional medical model—in which disability is viewed as a feature of the person, directly caused by disease that requires medical care—and aligns more closely with the social model of disability, which identifies limitations on participation as a societal failure to respond appropriately to the needs of those living with a disability (Oliver, 2013). The ICF model provides valuable guidance to OT practitioners because it underscores the role that personal and environmental factors play in shaping a client's participation in activities and life situations. The ICF model is also a universal model, reminding us that everyone has a range of functional abilities, regardless of the presence of disability. Furthermore, the model can be seen to empower persons with functional needs because it underscores the right all human beings have to participate in society. Under the ICF model, people are not defined as "dis-abled." Instead, they are viewed as having a basic human right to participate in the activities and life situations they choose.

## Bronfenbrenner's Ecological Systems Theory

Another useful model to guide intervention approaches with older adults is Bronfenbrenner's ecological systems theory. Originally developed in the 1970s to focus on the development of children, this theory is now used to broadly explore development across the lifespan (Bronfenbrenner, 1977; Rigby et al., 2019). Bronfenbrenner's ecological systems theory examines the interplay of the client (who is at the center of the model) with the ever-expanding environmental and social contexts in which they live (Bettis et al., 2020; Rigby et al., 2019). There are five systems within Bronfenbrenner's theory, the first comprises the microsystem that encompasses a client's immediate environment (e.g., friends, family, health services) (Bronfenbrenner, 1977; Rigby et al., 2019). The client will have the most direct interaction with this system. The second is the mesosystem, which involves the interaction of the microsystems and their impact on the client (Bronfenbrenner, 1977). Think, for example, of an older adult whose family members are involved in their health care and engage in regular communication with their health-care provider with the client's permission. The older adult is not directly involved but most likely will be affected either positively or negatively by the interactions of their health-care provider and family members. Third, the exosystem involves a broadening of the mesosystem to include social structures that may not interact directly with the client but have an impact on them (e.g., social services, government policies) (Bronfenbrenner, 1977; Rigby et al., 2019). The fourth system, the macrosystem, is what ultimately produces the outcomes that we see in the micro-, meso-, and exosystems (Bettis et al., 2020; Bronfenbrenner, 1977). The exosystem encompasses the overarching culture and values of an environment, such as how older adults are viewed and treated in a society and what social programs are supported in helping to care for older adults (Bronfenbrenner, 1977; Rigby et al., 2019). The fifth and final system in Bronfenbrenner's theory is the chronosystem. This system considers the effect of change in the social context in which one lives and engages, based on time and history (Rigby et al., 2019). The holistic view of Bronfenbrenner's ecological systems theory is useful during intervention because it considers not only the client but also the context in which the client performs occupations and the effect of that context on occupational engagement.

## Person-Environment-Occupation Performance Model

One widely used model specific to OT is the PEOP model. The PEOP is a client-centered model developed in 1991 by Charles Christiansen and Carolyn Baum (Bass et al., 2015). This model provides a structure with which to examine the complex relationships between the person and environmental factors of the client and the effects of this interplay on occupational performance and participation (Murly et al., 2017; Cole & Tufano, 2020). The PEOP process involves a client narrative, assessment/evaluation, intervention, and outcomes. The intervention component of the PEOP process is useful as a means to explore the needs and goals of the client (Bass et al., 2015). Contained within this step are many of the same intervention approaches as those listed in the OTPF-4 and include *create/promote*, *establish/restore*, *maintain/habituate*, *modify/compensate*, and *prevent*, along with the additional approaches of *educate*, *consult*, and *advocate* (Bass et al., 2015; AOTA, 2020a). Interventions using the PEOP model also elevate certain principles to guide the intervention process, such as the use of evidence-based practice, the consideration of culture, therapeutic use of self, and communication (Bass et al., 2015).

Regardless of the model or framework selected to guide one's approach to OT intervention with older adults, meaningful occupation and full participation in life should serve as the central foundation for overall health and well-being.

## Important Considerations for Intervention in Later Life

OT interventions with older adults have much in common with interventions designed for younger adults, yet there are important considerations that should be made for intervening in later life. Certain factors and experiences are uniquely linked to older adulthood or only arise if one has lived for many years and there has been enough time for various events to occur. Additionally, older adulthood has unique societal implications based on social and political views and practices regarding aging. All hold the potential to affect the OT intervention process, positively or negatively. Older adults, by virtue of their advanced years, bring an expertise about living life that young adults, including many occupational therapists newly entering the workforce, simply may not possess (Ledgerd & World Federation of Occupational Therapists, 2020). Such experience with major life events exerts an enormous influence on the therapeutic environment.

### Aging in Place and Residential Relocation

OT practitioners who work in the field of aging will be familiar with the phrase "aging in place." The US Center for Disease Control and Prevention (CDC) has defined aging in place as, "the ability to live in one's own home and community safely, independently, and comfortably, regardless of age, income, or ability level" (CDC, 2009). Gerontology research has demonstrated the strength of "place attachment" in older people's lives (Afshar et al., 2017). (Chapter 20 covers the role of the environment in age-related well-being and quality of life.) A national survey undertaken in the United States for the American Association of Retired Persons (AARP) found that nearly 80% of Americans age 50 and older wished to remain in their current homes as long as possible (Binette & Vasold, 2019). Interestingly, the desire to age in place within their current residence or community remains high among the older adult population; however, the intensity of this preference has somewhat lessened since 2010 (Binette & Vasold, 2019).

Influencers of residential relocation have been categorized as "push" or "pull" factors: push factors drive or force an older adult from their home, whereas pull factors are attractive and draw them to relocate (Franco et al., 2021). For instance, some older adults may be pushed to make a community-based move to downsize the space in which they live because housework and upkeep of the home are no longer manageable (Tyvimaa & Kemp, 2011). Others undertake residential moves because relocation is enticing, such as having the ability to be closer to family or proffering access to new activities among people of a similar age as would be available in a retirement village. Although residential mobility rates vary widely, on the whole, older adults do not actually relocate very much (Sergeant et al., 2008). When they do move, key reasons are because of limitations in ADL functioning (van der Pers et al., 2018) or an unexpected health "shock," resulting in health decline (Bloem et al., 2008; Sergeant & Ekerdt, 2008). Sudden relocations and unwelcome relocations are stressful and can even result in "relocation stress syndrome," which is a nursing diagnosis used to describe symptoms of anxiety, confusion, and loneliness often experienced by older adults transitioning from their private homes to long-term care or assisted living facilities (Walker et al., 2007). Not only would the individual (or couple, or family) be dealing with what triggered the need for relocation, such as serious health problems, but the individual must also adjust to losing a much-loved familiar home at the same time. All this would happen while the older adult would be trying to reorient to new habits and routines in a new setting with new people (Diaz Moore & Ekerdt, 2011). Residential moves may also require significant "downsizing" of possessions, which can be surprisingly difficult, especially when those possessions may represent one's family history or legacy (Luborsky et al., 2011). Another complication is learning how to manage downsizing decisions within the wider sphere of family life and cultural expectations (Luborsky et al., 2011). In Case Example 7.1, Alenush is considering downsizing from a two-bedroom house to an apartment to

be closer to her daughter (a pull factor). Her attachment to place is simultaneously apparent as she expresses reluctance to move due to the sentimental memories made in her current home. The most challenging move situations of all, however, are the so-called "last moves." Here, an older adult may have to leave independent living in their longstanding home and transition to a more supported environment, such as an assisted living facility or nursing home, where they are dependent on others for care.

As a part of the intervention process, therapists may work with older clients and their families to modify and renovate spaces in the home so older adults can remain independent at home as long as possible (see Chapters 20 and 29 for more detailed information). If residential relocation is needed, occupational therapy personnel can assist older clients and their family members by providing comprehensive assessment data about the client's function so that the best possible decisions about relocation can be made. What type of facility would be best? Will the client receive the needed care? Will the environment and other residents provide social and occupational enrichment? What steps can be taken to make the residential move easier for an individual who is relocating and who may be faced with leaving significant others behind? occupational therapy practitioners can play an integral role in finding clients optimal housing that fits their needs and managing the residential transition. Assessment is part of the equation, but so is up-to-date knowledge about the range of community services and assistance (paid and unpaid) available. (Chapter 32 covers a wide range of OT services that relate to community services.)

## Aging With Disability

Older adults, on average, have poorer health and more chronic conditions than younger adults (Violan et al., 2014). In part

---

**CASE EXAMPLE 7.1    Alenush**

Alenush Heydari is a 78-year-old Iranian-Briton who lives alone in a two-bedroom bungalow with her two cats in London, England. In her 20s, she had immigrated from Iran to England with her life partner and husband. They were married for 55 years and had one daughter, Maryam. Three years ago, Alenush's husband passed away after a decade-long battle with cancer. During that time, Alenush was her husband's primary care partner. Alenush is generally healthy. She takes no prescription medications, and she rides her bicycle for an hour each day on a neighborhood trail. Alenush is independent in all her housework and most of her outdoor yard work, although she relies on a handyperson for heavier chores like cleaning the gutters each fall and washing the windows each spring. Alenush drives only when necessary—her husband used to do the nighttime and long-distance driving. She has had three minor car accidents in the past year. No one was hurt in these collisions, but they were distressing to Alenush and her adult daughter, Maryam. Alenush has decided to ride with a friend to the mosque for Friday afternoon prayers

and to Wednesday night book club now, instead of driving herself.

Although Alenush describes herself as "doing better than many others my age," Maryam sees a different picture. Maryam believes her mother "hasn't been the same" since her father died. Maryam is also concerned to see her mother lose interest in drawing, something she has loved to do throughout her life. She reports that Alenush's social network is small, with only a few close friends from the mosque. Alenush's neighbors are mostly young families native to England. Alenush has stopped hosting family dinners, too. Several times when Maryam would visit, she noticed how little food was in the fridge, and days can go by without Alenush driving anywhere or talking to anyone. Alenush has been considering moving into an apartment to be closer to Maryam but feels that her current home holds too many memories. She has admitted to feeling "a little sad," but Maryam thinks her mother may be depressed. Maryam wants her mother to be more forthcoming about her health and well-being issues so together they can find solutions.

this is due to normal aging, which brings with it some declines in various bodily systems, such as the sensory systems with reduced vision and hearing and the musculoskeletal system with decreased range of motion and strength. (Chapters 8, 9, 10, and 11 are additional resources for these and related topics.) Age-related changes are not the same thing as pathological aging—that is, when a disease process is involved. Even with normal aging, older adults may experience declines in their capacity to participate and perform daily tasks to their satisfaction. Imagine, then, an older adult client referred to OT following surgery for a hip fracture. The intervention process could be quite straightforward and no different from the approach taken for the same client who is 20 years younger. In later life, however, the chance of comorbidities rises considerably, and this implies a more complicated assessment and intervention process. Although the older client may have been referred following a hip fracture, if the client was also simultaneously managing diabetes, then the OT intervention must account for the impact of this condition. Wound healing may be delayed, for instance, therefore elongating standard protocols for hip fracture rehabilitation.

It is also highly probable that older clients are taking medications for some or all of their health conditions. A study across Europe showed that 32% of older adults were taking five or more daily medications (Midão et al., 2018). The prevalence of hyperpolypharmacy in older adults in India is even more startling: 31% of older adults from south India are taking 10 or more medications (Bhagavathula et al., 2021). Therapists need to be attuned to the expected therapeutic effects of the medications on their clients, but also how side effects of medications can adversely affect function. For more on this issue, see Chapter 14, which covers medication side effects and medication management in detail. Taking multiple medications also places an older adult at increased risk of an injurious fall (Xue et al., 2021). The occupational therapist must be prepared to assess fall risk using the best evidence-based tools available (see Chapter 6) and then use the data gathered from the assessment to make necessary adjustments to the treatment/intervention plan.

## Late-Life Social Role Changes

In many health-care settings, the physical diagnosis of an older client becomes the exclusive focus of the OT intervention. Therapists must remember that the client's social context, which includes their personal history and current life circumstances, exerts an enormous influence, too. Some key social role changes that may occur in later life that are important to consider with occupation-based intervention with older adults are discussed below (also see Chapter 23 on these topics).

### Work-Related Routines and Retirement

The experience of retirement can vary widely from individual to individual. For instance, a teacher or a government employee might retire at age 65 because they are working in a state with mandatory retirement or they are eligible for a full pension at this age, or both. However, a lawyer or a doctor might work for many years beyond 65 and never retire. On the other end of the spectrum are those who have had prolonged periods of unemployment and those who retire earlier than age 65 for health or other reasons. Additionally, ageism can also affect the retirement plans of older adults and force them into retirement before they are ready. The WHO defines ageism as "the stereotypes (how we think), prejudices (how we feel), and discrimination (how we act) toward others based on their age" (WHO, 2021, para. 1). Forced retirement can be problematic; retirees' mental health is better protected when retirement is perceived as voluntary and includes a pension (Fernández-Niño et al., 2018). Experiences of retirement can also vary depending on culture and environment because retirement, as it is often discussed, is a Western construct that is not duplicated in many parts of the world (Luborsky & Leblanc, 2003; Matuska & Barrett, 2015). For instance, individuals who are situated in family-oriented societies may be more apt to spend time care partnering for aging family members or grandchildren, while older people who belong to labor market-oriented societies might have a strong desire to re-enter the workforce shortly after retiring.

The transition to retirement is often a process that takes place over time and can bring with it changes in financial and psychological well-being, social networks, identity, self-efficacy, and time use (Bordia et al., 2020; HRS, 2017; Olds et al., 2018). There are also many styles or paths to retirement, including those who continue to work on a part-time basis, those who continue to work as a means of exploring new interests, and those who retreat from employment-related occupations and social contexts (HRS, 2017; Scaffa & Reitz, 2020). All of these factors affect not only one's experience of retirement but also the timeline toward retirement. Consider, for example, the different experiences of retirement for two individuals. Both are 70 years old and have decided they are ready to enter retirement. The first individual has worked for 40 years at the same factory job. This person has qualified for government-funded assistance at a designated age, has a sizeable pension saved, and has adult children who live independently with their families. They have the means to engage in travel, spend more social time with family and peers, and are considering part-time work within animal rescue, as this has always been a personal passion. The second individual has also worked full-time for the past 30 years but has had multiple jobs earning minimum wage. This person also qualifies for government assistance at age 65 but does not have a pension or significant savings. Additionally, the second individual is part of a multi-generational household where they are the primary caretakers for their two grandchildren. For this reason, they must maintain at least part-time employment in order to support their family. Their retirement resources will not allow for extras such as travel and interest exploration in the same way that the first individual is experiencing retirement. It is important, therefore, when engaging in intervention with the retired older adult to be client-centered and to consider the personal and environmental factors that have an effect on their occupational participation, physical and mental health, and well-being.

## Care Partnering and Caregiving

Informal caregiving—whether that means care partnering in a dyad with an adult child, lifelong partner, or medical professional, or caregiving for grandchildren—is a common feature of older adults' late-life experiences. The informal "caregiving career" typically commences when a care recipient first experiences symptoms, illness, or debilitation and continues along a pathway until that care recipient recovers, their disease remits, or they die (Larkin & Milne, 2017). In Alenush's case, she was the primary care partner for her husband, who had cancer—she held this role for nearly a decade. Per the OTPF-4 (AOTA, 2020a), care partnering is an instrumental ADL (IADL) and can entail a variety of tasks, including assisting someone with the completion of ADL (e.g., bathing, dressing) and additional IADL (e.g., home management, shopping, meal preparation). Providing assistance and care for someone, under even the most ideal circumstances, can be exhausting and stressful. If not properly addressed, a sense of "caregiver burden" and a growing sense of loneliness and social isolation can emerge. However, caregiving can also carry certain benefits with it, such as delaying undesired residential relocation, helping older adults stay active, the sharing of knowledge and ideas among care partners, and a certain sense of reward (Bennett et al., 2017). Care partnering and caregiving are also grounded in culture and social context and, depending on the cultural and social contexts, may look different depending on definitions of family, subscribed gender roles, and the availability of support services. Fortunately, through the use of valid and reliable screening and assessment tools, the occupational therapy practitioner is uniquely positioned to identify the strengths and limitations of the care partnering relationship by exploring such topics as leisure interests, meaningful life roles, and depression. (Chapter 6 covers screening approaches in gerontological OT.) The outcomes of the screenings and assessments coupled with a client and culturally centered approach can help strengthen the occupational therapy practitioner's intervention approaches, ultimately enhancing the care-partnering experience.

## Social Isolation and Grief

Although the physical impacts of aging regularly receive attention, too often mental health problems go unrecognized in later life. (Chapter 17 covers age-related mental health conditions and challenges.) Late-life depression is one of them. Depression in community-dwelling older adults is underrecognized and undertreated (Allan et al., 2014; Morichi et al., 2015), even by rehabilitation practitioners who work closely with older clients (Vieira et al., 2014).

Living until older adulthood means that one has likely had innumerable life experiences that have forged valuable connections, perspectives, and resiliency factors. Such qualities often position older adults as valued and knowledgeable members of the community; however, they can also place older adults at risk for isolation and grief when facing the loss of valued roles and loved ones. Per the CDC (2021), social isolation among older adults is a serious public health issue experienced by a third of adults 65 and older and is associated with undesirable health conditions such as dementia, heart disease, loneliness, and depression. Experiences of social isolation can also be amplified for immigrants and members of the lesbian, gay, bisexual, and transgender (LGBT*) community of older adults due to societally imposed challenges with social integration, language barriers, discrimination, and stigma (CDC, 2021). Most recently, the issue of social isolation was magnified worldwide with the onset and persistence of the COVID-19 pandemic. Early on, older adults were strongly encouraged (if not forced) to isolate due to a higher chance of severe illness and mortality from COVID-19 (Chong et al., 2020; Vahia et al., 2020).

Grief, although a normal and expected response to loss, is something practitioners should be aware of when working with older people. Over the span of a lifetime, older adults are likely to have faced a multitude of losses, including the loss of loved ones, previously held roles, habits and routines, and possibly independence. Two types of grief that may be experienced by older adults are anticipatory and complicated grief. Anticipatory grief is an emotional response that can happen in advance of a loss that has not yet occurred, such as the impending death of a family member with a terminal illness (Aldrich, 1974). Complicated grief, also known as persistent complicated bereavement disorder, describes persistent and severe grief that affects quality of life and functioning (Perng & Renz, 2018). Occupational therapy practitioners have the responsibility, when developing plans of care and intervention approaches with older adults, to consider the physical, mental, and emotional factors of clients who are experiencing social isolation and various forms of grief. In revisiting Alenush's case, she may still be feeling the loss of her husband. It may be true that her grief could be contributing to her isolative behaviors and lack of interest in occupations that previously brought her joy. Aligned with her daughter's concern, the occupational therapy practitioner needs to be alert to the signs of depression Alenush seems to be showing.

## Diversity in Aging Experiences

Longevity and an increase in life expectancy have prompted calls for a paradigm shift that normalizes aging and avoids treating old age as a problem to be fixed (Calasanti & King, 2020). Such a perspective requires embracing the aging process and older adults while simultaneously battling common stereotypes and misconceptions about aging. As the population of older adults expands across the globe, the scope and urgency of addressing this issue are also expected to grow.

## Ageism and Stereotypes

Ageism is defined as the stereotyping, prejudice, and discrimination against persons based on their age (Burnes et al., 2019). Ageism can be seen in society's negative attitudes or stereotypes, individual acts, and systems (e.g., structures, programs, services) that fail to consider the needs of older adults. Ageism directed at older adults has serious psychological, social, and economic impacts and directly impacts personal well-being.

Because it can be so deeply embedded into everyday systems, cultures, and actions, it can often be missed or overlooked (Gendron et al., 2016). For example, many older adults report ageist experiences (Gendron et al., 2016; Perron, 2018) such as:

- Others assuming memory problems or physical impairments simply because of older age
- Hearing jokes that make fun of aging and older people
- Not being taken seriously due to one's older age
- Experiencing ageist remarks that appear as compliments (e.g., being addressed as "young lady" or as 86 years "young")
- Being spoken about in an infantilizing way (e.g., "cute," "adorable," "sweet")
- Not being taken seriously by health-care providers or even being denied medical treatment
- Denied employment or promotion

Health-care providers are not immune to ageism. Health-care providers may view older adults as inflexible and unable to change their ways, or they may overlook and undertreat health concerns by instead attributing them to old age. Although research indicates that OT practitioners may have more positive biases in favor of older adults (i.e., positive ageism) than other allied health professionals (Giles et al., 2002), negative ageism is still prevalent. Friedman and VanPuymbrouck (2021) found that 70% of OT students held implicit negative biases about older adults, with the majority moderately to strongly preferring younger people.

### Intersectionality

The aforementioned experiences of ageism may further differ based on the many aspects of older adults' personal and social identities. In fact, the interconnected nature of social categorizations (e.g., age, class, gender, sex) creates overlapping and interdependent systems of discrimination or disadvantage. The framework of intersectionality helps elucidate the complexity of prejudices persons face from this perspective. To this end, some groups of older adults may experience unique barriers because of their age, combined with aspects of their identity such as their gender, disability, sexual orientation, race/ethnicity, religion, culture, or language (Box 7.1).

Occupational therapy practitioners must work to dispel common stereotypes and misperceptions about aging. At a systems level, practitioners can be effective advocates for inclusive planning, design, and collaboration with older adults. Occupational therapy practitioners must also recognize that aging and the aging experience are highly individualized.

It is impossible to understand a person solely based on one aspect of their identity, age included. Further, occupational therapy practitioners must understand the complex, dynamic interplay between the intersectionality of a person's identities and their respective privileges or disadvantages. This reflection extends to the practitioner themselves, is part of a life-long reflective practice, and should not be devoid of action to reduce age-related discrimination.

## Overview of the Occupational Therapy Intervention Process to Promote Positive Aging and Optimal Outcomes

### Occupational Therapy Intervention According to the Occupational Therapy Practice Framework-4

The OT process, as outlined in the OTPF-4 widely used in the United States (AOTA, 2020a), encompasses the three steps of evaluation, intervention, and review as the typical course of OT services with clients (i.e., persons, groups, and populations). The second step of the OT process, intervention, is highlighted in this chapter as a means to promote positive aging. Positive aging, a concept that emerged to counteract ageism, aims in part to dissociate aging with a decline in health and instead focus on positive aspects of aging that are achievable through activity, personal responsibility, health, and well-being (Laliberte Rudman, 2006; Webster et al., 2021). Intervention in OT to the purposeful, directed actions taken by the occupational therapy professional to put plans into action. As presented in Fig. 7.1, there are three steps to the intervention process: (1) intervention planning, (2) intervention implementation, and (3) intervention review. For the remainder of this section, we will review the three steps of the intervention process in more detail and discuss how they can be leveraged to promote positive aging in work with older adults.

### Occupational Therapy Intervention Process With Older Adult Clients
#### Intervention Planning

As with any aspect of OT services, the intervention plan should be client centered. The plan should be developed in partnership with the older adult client with recognition of the client as a human being with a lifetime of experiences and occupational needs that have individual and contextual meaning (Gretschel et al., 2017; WFOT, 2010). The intervention plan begins following the completion of the client evaluation or assessment and entails a detailed plan of care that includes meaningful

---

**Box 7.1    Applying Concepts of Intersectionality**

Islamophobia is a growing global phenomenon, particularly in white-dominant, Christian-majority countries of the West, and that has a major negative impact on Muslims' physical and mental health and access to resources (Samari et al., 2018). Return to Case Example 7.1. It is noted that she is living in London, where she is actively practicing her religion (i.e., going "to mosque for Friday afternoon prayers"), and in a community with young families who are not immigrants. The mental health issues she is experiencing with bereavement may be exacerbated by social discriminations—whether overt or covert—she is likely to encounter as an Iranian, Muslim woman living in a predominantly white, Christian region and may deter her from seeking help from health-care providers.

**Intervention Plan**

- Develop plan
- Consider potential discharge needs
- Make recommendations or referrals

**Intervention Implementation**

- Select and carryout the intervention(s)
- Monitor through evaluation and re-evaluation

**Intervention Review**

- Re-evaluate the plan
- Modify as needed
- Continue or discontinue therapy

**FIGURE. 7.1**   OT Practice Framework-4 (OTPF-4) Occupational Therapy Intervention Process.

activities and approaches to meet client goals. It is driven by the client's occupational needs, values, discharge plan, and the best available evidence while being created in consideration of the client's health, well-being, and occupational performance needs (AOTA, 2020a). The occupational therapy staff uses a combination of art and science to design the intervention plan, including clinical reasoning skills informed by evaluation and assessment results, clinical/practice experience, professional judgment, and client goals. Also critical to the intervention plan is the occupational therapist's incorporation and knowledge of the occupational therapy Code of Ethics and Standards for Professional Behavior (AOTA, 2020b). The intervention plan should result in specific activities, approaches, and methods to meet the client's goals and abilities, with consideration of the client's specific discharge context.

While all interventions are aimed at the promotion of occupational participation, there are five types of occupations or activity interventions to consider during intervention planning: (1) those to support occupational engagement, (2) interventions for education and training, (3) advocacy-related interventions, (4) group interventions, and (5) virtual interventions (AOTA, 2020a). Interventions to support occupational engagement are often categorized by performance factors related to ADL, such as bathing, dressing, eating, or IADL related to life management, such as paying bills, home management, safety, and shopping. Interventions focused on occupational engagement recognize the significance of participation in occupations of necessity and meaning as being critical to the health, well-being, and social participation of all people, including older adults (Scott & Foley, 2020; Smallfield & Molitor, 2018; Turcotte et al., 2015). Here, the occupational therapy practitioner will also use knowledge about therapeutic communication modes, such as empathy, therapeutic use of self, collaborating, and problem-solving, to engage the older adult in the intervention plan. The next type of intervention—education and training—involves clients but may also include family members,

other members of a care team, and caregivers. With this type of intervention, the occupational therapy practitioner uses education and training around a specific topic relative to the client's health and well-being, as well as participation in occupations. The third type of intervention approach includes advocacy-related interventions. These interventions involve raising consciousness of an occupational injustice or occupational rights issue and the promotion of self-advocacy often related to barriers to occupational participation for clients (AOTA, 2020a). For older adult clients, there may be occupational injustices related to ageism, racism, religious discrimination, or physical barriers to participate in meaningful and health-promoting occupations.

**Intervention Implementation**

Intervention implementation is the second step in the intervention process, in which the OT practitioner selects and executes the intervention plan (AOTA, 2020a). Prioritizing which aspects of the intervention plan to implement at what time will depend on client needs, priorities, and setting, and may involve one or several aspects of the OT domain (AOTA, 2020a). After initiating the intervention implementation, the practitioner must monitor client progress and provide reassessment as needed (AOTA, 2020a). This ongoing monitoring and assessment of the intervention implementation allows practitioners to modify the plan, if needed, to more optimally address the older adult client's needs. Monitoring and reassessment also highlight the importance of communication and collaboration between occupational therapists and occupational therapy assistants (OTAs), who are working together to meet a client's needs. For example, imagine a situation in which an occupational therapist performs the initial evaluation and develops an intervention plan with the client before passing the evaluation results and intervention plan on to the occupational therapy assistant. In order for the plan to be executed well and to the benefit of the client, it is critical that the supervising occupational therapist and the occupational therapy assistant have effective and regular communication. The occupational therapy assistant may notice during intervention implementation that the client's priorities have changed or that an intervention thought to be suitable is not. The occupational therapist must be open to collaboration and discussion to optimize the intervention implementations in order for the client to meet their goals.

**Intervention Review**

The third and final step of the intervention process is intervention review. This step continues to incorporate re-evaluation along with the added step of review to ensure the intervention plan is effective in supporting the client's goals (AOTA, 2020a). Intervention review requires the practitioner to consult with the client to review progress and make changes as needed to optimize the intervention plan. For example, the occupational therapy staff practitioner and client review may lead to changes in client goals, the context in which interventions are performed, and the priority in which goals are addressed. This highlights the intervention process and plan as a dynamic one that can be modified as appropriate. Finally, during the intervention review, the practitioner compares re-evaluation outcomes to the initial evaluation and subsequent assessments. The practitioner uses clinical reasoning and discharge planning to determine if further OT is warranted or if it is appropriate to discontinue therapy and refer to other services (AOTA, 2020a; Chisholm & Schell, 2019). It is also important to consider additional factors such as insurance coverage and therapy setting as influencing the timing of discharge from OT services. While the occupational therapist's discharge recommendations should always be client centered and driven by clinical reasoning, there are times when the discharge recommendations of the practitioner are not possible. For example, think of an older adult client who is admitted to a skilled nursing unit after a hip replacement. The client's insurance provider may cap the amount of OT sessions the client may have. On the other hand, a community-based occupational therapy practitioner may not receive direct reimbursement based on OT visits and, therefore, have more flexibility on the frequency and duration of sessions for the older adult client. Whatever the circumstances of discharge, if the occupational therapy practitioner has been practicing interprofessionally, the referral to additional services should be a collaborative and empowering process among the practitioner, older adult client, and interdisciplinary team members.

## Evidence-Based Occupational Therapy Intervention With Older People

There are a myriad of evidence-based interventions that can be used when working with older adult clients. For instance, the CAPABLE Program (mentioned in Chapter 19) is an intervention involving an occupational therapist, nurse, and handy worker developed to support the community-dwelling older adult to continue aging safely in their home (Szanton et al., 2021). The Lifestyle-integrated Functional Exercise (LiFE) program, developed through collaboration of OT and physical therapy, integrates balance and strength training into older adults' daily routines to improve functional capacity and prevent falls (Clemson et al., 2012). As is true for each of these interventions, the OT intervention processes identified through the OTPF-4 can be implemented with older adult clients based on their occupational performance needs and goals. To further understand how the OT intervention process can be integrated into contemporary evidence-based interventions, highlighted below is a culturally specific program for Latino older people entitled ¡Vivir Mi Vida! (Lee et al., 2022; Schepens Niemiec et al., 2015, 2018, 2019, 2021). Follow along to learn more about this intervention and how it aligns with the intervention process as outlined in the OTPF-4. Keep an eye toward important considerations influential to intervention in later life, as discussed throughout this chapter.

## Application of the Occupational Therapy Intervention Process Through the Lens of the ¡Vivir Mi Vida! Lifestyle Program

The Latino community is the second fastest-growing racial/ethnic group in the United States and the largest in rural areas, making this an important population for OT intervention

(Figueroa et al., 2021; Flores, 2017). Drawn by perceived employment options and connections with others, Latinos are a major driver of expansion in rural regions (Stone et al., 2022). Although the growth of Latino communities in rural areas proffers many socioeconomic opportunities, health disparities in the Latino population seem to be exacerbated by rural living. For example, rural-dwelling Latinos have limited access to health-care services, poorer health (e.g., physical, mental, behavioral), and significant psychosocial stressors linked to their immigration experiences (Figueroa et al., 2021; Schminkey et al., 2019; Stone et al., 2022).

¡Vivir Mi Vida! (¡VMV!) is an occupation-centric lifestyle intervention designed to address the aforementioned health inequities frequently experienced by rural-dwelling Latino communities, concentrating on health and well-being in late-midlife (50- to 64-year-olds) (Lee et al., 2022; Schepens Niemiec et al., 2015, 2018, 2019, 2021). ¡VMV! supports clients via a unique, interprofessional approach where OTs or COTAs partner with promotores de salud—trusted individuals who empower peers through education and connections to health-promoting resources in Latino communities (MHP Salud, n.d.)—to deliver in-home care linked to clients' safety-net primary care services. Extended details of the intervention methods can be found in Schepens Niemiec et al. (2019). Circling back to the environmentally focused models presented earlier in this chapter, ¡VMV! aligns well with Bronfenbrenner's ecological systems theory. The program attends to older Latinos' needs at multiple levels, from clients' immediate environment (e.g., microsystem of family dynamics in the home as it relates to their personal health), all the way to the policy level (e.g., exosystem of governmental policies relevant to home-based health services), and cultural context (e.g., macrosystem of shared values and health beliefs of the Latino community). Below is a description of how the OT intervention processes were integrated into this evidence-based program.

### Intervention Planning in ¡Vivir Mi Vida!

Intervention planning took place in multiple stages, starting with conceptualization of the ¡VMV! program. To ensure the meaningfulness, effectiveness, life-stage appropriateness, and cultural responsivity of the intervention, ¡VMV! was developed using an iterative, community-participatory process involving key stakeholders (e.g., older Latino safety-net patients, occupational therapists, promotores de salud, community advocates) (Schepens Niemiec et al., 2015). Stakeholders provided guidance on the intervention's content, tone, and cultural relevance. For instance, they emphasized the need for a celebratory, strengths-based tone and the importance of inviting the client's family or friends to join sessions and share what they learned with others. These recommendations were incorporated as core features of ¡VMV!.

Alongside intervention conceptualization, the research team was taking dedicated steps to build trust and rapport with the community, working to establish the necessary partnerships and gather key resources that would make intervention implementation possible (Lee et al., 2022). Identifying a Spanish-English bilingual occupational therapist skilled in lifestyle intervention and *promotores de salud* who had experience working in the targeted rural community were just two of many logistics the team tackled early during the intervention planning stages. Once the intervention had been established, the occupational therapist and *promotores de salud* participated together in a week-long training workshop about *¡VMV!*. The training focused on understanding the OT-*promotor de salud* partnership along with becoming familiar with the *¡VMV!* Intervention's content and delivery.

Intervention planning took place again once clients enrolled in the program. The *¡VMV!* intervention was tailored to each person through the development of a health action plan. Important background health information was pulled from clients' medical records in advance and prefilled at the top of the plan. The remaining health action plan content was generated during the first visit, where the *promotor de salud* joined in person and the occupational therapist took part via telehealth. The action plan guided the client in developing health-related priorities and taking an initial inventory of barriers and facilitators to achieving said goals. The occupational therapist and *promotor de salud* met after this session to review the client's goals and develop a treatment plan that would direct intervention implementation.

### Intervention Implementation in ¡Vivir Mi Vida!

Clients engaged approximately weekly with a *promotor de salud* over the 16-week *¡VMV!* program. This involved seven one-on-one home sessions, two group sessions at a local community center, and two phone check-ins. During each visit, the *promotor de salud's* process was guided by a structured intervener's manual. The *promotor de salud* presented health educational content in the client's preferred language, using conversational strategies, a picture-based flip-over booklet, and demonstration tools. The content addressed multiple dimensions of health. Different topics were covered at each visit, ranging from nutrition and financial wellness to physical activity and grief. The discussions were tied back to the client's goals at the conclusion of each session.

Complementing the work the *promotor de salud* was doing with the client, an occupational therapist provided direct coaching to the individual via two telehealth visits. These sessions provided a focused, personalized exploration of the link between wellness and participation in meaningful habits, roles, and routines. The occupational therapist used multiple techniques to promote behavior change and progress toward the personalized health action plan, including goal-setting and tracking, building social support and self-efficacy, providing health education, and encouraging clients to play an active role in their own health self-management. The occupational therapist also met with each *promotor de salud* weekly to review individual client cases and emphasize the use of behavior change techniques to help the clients achieve their health goals. During these meetings, *promotores de salud* were also able to obtain peer support from other *promotores de salud* and discuss questions about individual cases. Additionally, these meetings served as a way to maintain the rapport built between the occupational therapist, *promotores de salud*, and participating clinical facilities, reinforcing that this community-based intervention was a collaboration between all stakeholders.

### Intervention Review in ¡Vivir Mi Vida!

Much like the intervention planning, the intervention review happened at different levels for *¡VMV!*. During the OT visits, which happened less frequently than those with the *promotor de salud*, the occupational therapist consulted with the clients to review progress on and satisfaction with their health action plans. The intervention plan was adjusted as needed.

At a programmatic level, the *¡VMV!* research team reviewed the intervention using both qualitative feedback and quantitative data. Clients described wanting to join *¡VMV!* because they were interested in managing their health, improving the health of their family, and finding support to live a healthier lifestyle (Lee et al., 2022). Through their participation in *¡VMV!*, clients described forging new social bonds with the *promotores de salud*, the OT, and other peers. Clients also described important health-relevant outcomes such as improved diet and physical activity behaviors, better quality sleep, stress reduction, and confidence in communicating with providers (Lee et al., 2022).

Through analysis of self-report questionnaires and clients' clinical health indicators taken before and after the intervention, results suggested potential health benefits relevant to lifestyle behaviors (e.g., sodium intake), subjective health (e.g., symptom severity), and cardiometabolic health (e.g., systolic blood pressure) (Schepens Niemiec et al., 2018). Further, a 12-month long-term follow-up study demonstrated that those significant psychosocial and clinical improvements observed immediately post-intervention were maintained long after the intervention conclusion (Schepens Niemiec et al., 2021). The research team continues to work with *¡VMV!* community collaborators to identify funding sources to conduct a large-scale study and avenues that could support iterative intervention review and provision of this important program beyond the research context. *¡VMV!* serves as a unique example of the OT intervention process applied in later life and how OT intervention has the potential to lead to positive health and lifestyle changes in hard-to-reach, under-resourced communities.

*The complete listing of the Bibliography and Chapter Questions and Answers are available in the accompanying enhanced eBook version included with the print purchase of this textbook. Visit Elsevier eBooks+ (eBooks.Health.Elsevier.com) to access this content.*

CHAPTER 8

# Musculoskeletal System Changes With Aging: Implications for Occupational Therapy

*Julia Henderson-Kalb, OTD OTR/L, Emily Barr, OTD, MBA, OTR/L, BCG and Raegan Muller, PT, GCS*

## CHAPTER OUTLINE

## OBJECTIVES

- Describe how the aging process changes each of the musculoskeletal structures as it relates to functional task performance
- Describe common musculoskeletal disorders in the older aging adult, particularly osteoarthritis, rheumatoid arthritis, osteoporosis, fractures, back pain, lumbar spinal stenosis, and degenerative lumbar spondylolisthesis
- Identify different joint arthroplasties and describe treatment protocols to maintain precautions and facilitate compensatory strategy training
- Discuss principles of joint protection and explain adjunct interventions involved in the management of rheumatoid arthritis
- Identify the three stages of rheumatoid arthritis and treatment goals associated with each stage
- Describe the treatment choices that occupational therapists have for clients with lumbar spinal stenosis and degenerative lumbar spondylolisthesis
- Describe the management, considerations and precautions, and importance of exercise to facilitate occupational engagement and performance
- Describe the effects of changes that occur in the mobility of aging adults
- List and describe the factors causing falls in aging adults and the effects of musculoskeletal changes
- Select balance and mobility assessments that can be applied to the aging adult to measure fall risk and occupational performance
- Describe occupation-based interventions in the management of musculoskeletal conditions
- Discuss the psychological effects of mobility impairments in older adults
- Distinguish the roles of the interprofessional team in relation to evaluating and treating aging adults with musculoskeletal conditions

## Introduction

Through every developmental stage in life, changes occur and affect our abilities to perform functional activities. For older adults these changes can lead to a decline in functional status and increased risk for injury. Musculoskeletal disorders are one of the most debilitating and costly disorders that affect older adults around the globe. As one ages, musculoskeletal tissue changes include decreased bone strength, decreased articular cartilage resiliency, reduced elasticity, and loss of muscular strength. When working with older adults in therapy, it is likely that a musculoskeletal issue will need to be considered and addressed as either a primary or secondary condition for treatment.

## Variations in Structure and the Normal Aging Process

### Bone

Bones are organs that move, protect, and support the body. More specifically, the functions of bones involve mechanical, synthetic, and metabolic purposes. Mechanical functions involve protecting the brain and other internal organs, giving shape and support to the body, and working with the muscles and nerves to provide movement (Fig. 8.1). The synthetic function involves production of blood in the bone marrow. Bones serve various metabolic functions: mineral storage, growth factor storage, fat storage, acid–base balance (by absorbing or releasing alkaline salts), and detoxification (removing heavy metals from the blood). Bone also acts as an endocrine organ through the release of the hormone osteocalcin, which contributes to the regulation of glucose (Lee et al., 2007).

In both sexes, aging bones lose calcium and become more brittle. This affects the strength of the bone. Bone density reaches its peak during the 20 s and is higher in males. Healthy individuals, who have had a diet rich in calcium from childhood on and have been physically active, have the best prognosis for maintaining strong bones. Weight-bearing activities and muscle contraction stimulate bone density (Karinkanta et al., 2009; Kukuljan et al., 2009; Stuck et al., 1999).

Bones changes take place throughout life in a process called *remodeling*. In this process osteoclasts reabsorb bone and osteoblasts lay down new bone. Remodeling is influenced by how much mechanical stress was placed on the bone; the levels of calcium, phosphate, and vitamin D; and the levels of certain hormones, such as parathyroid hormone, calcitonin, cortisol, growth hormone, thyroid hormone, and sex hormones (Downey & Siegel, 2006). With age, some bones can change shape. For example, the femur may become wider in diameter, and the mandible and maxilla may shrink. Because of changes in cartilage, the length and breadth of the nose and ears may increase.

Trabeculae comprise spongy cancellous bone. Trabecular patterns are important within the femoral neck and greater trochanter areas of the femur because they form a type of bone organization that helps the bone to absorb compressive, loading, and shear-bending forces directed through the femoral neck. Where the bundles cross there is an increase in bone strength, but where there is little or no crossing there is an inherent weakness in the bone and a susceptibility for a fracture (Hertling & Kessler, 2005).

### Muscles

Muscles are groups of contractile fibers that connect to bones, producing stability and movement in the body. There are three different types of muscle in the body: smooth, skeletal (striated), and cardiac. Muscle functions vary depending on the type of muscle (see Fig. 8.1). The musculoskeletal system is composed of "skeletal" or "striated" muscle. For the purposes of this chapter, the following discussion will refer to skeletal muscle.

Skeletal muscles are typically spindle shaped and consist of a central portion called the muscle belly. The ends of the muscle have attaching sites with tendons that connect to bone. "The more stationary attachment to bone is called the origin; the more movable attachment is the insertion" (Lieber & Bodine Fowler, 1993). Skeletal muscle produces strength and movement of the connecting bones.

Muscle strength, like bone strength, peaks in the 20s. Muscle fibers are composed of fast twitch, type II (which generate energy mostly through anaerobic metabolism and produce rapid, quick, powerful contractions), and slow twitch, type I (which generate energy through aerobic metabolism and produce slow, sustained contractions recruited in postural activities).

Older adults experience a greater loss in type II fibers (Rudy et al., 2007; Venes, 2013). This may be associated with nonuse and also genetic influences. Important, also, is type of use. For example, older marathon runners may not show the typical age declines in strength in their lower extremities and lower abdominals but may show these in their upper trunk and upper extremities.

Sarcopenia is a condition characterized by loss of skeletal muscle mass and function. Sarcopenia is mainly diagnosed in the elderly; its development may be associated with conditions that are not exclusively seen in older persons. Sarcopenia is a syndrome characterized by progressive and generalized loss of skeletal muscle mass and strength and it is correlated with physical disability, poor quality of life, and death. Women experience greater loss of muscle mass than men. The decline in both sexes is greater after 70 years. The loss in muscle mass may be associated with increased body fat. Despite normal weight there is marked weakness; this is a condition called sarcopenic obesity. There is an important correlation between inactivity and losses of muscle mass and strength; this suggests that physical activity should be a protective factor for the prevention but also the management of sarcopenia.

Besides muscle strength, declines in muscle power (ability to generate force at a fast speed) and muscle endurance (ability to sustain a muscle contraction) play a significant role in aging. An older adult may slip because of the inability to produce a quick muscle contraction to avoid losing balance, or an older adult may have trouble standing for prolonged periods of time due to fatigue in the lower extremity and trunk muscles.

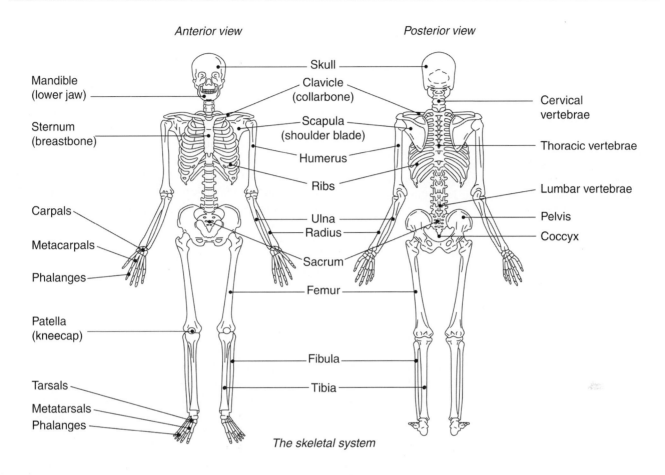

*Anterior view*    *Posterior view*

*The skeletal system*

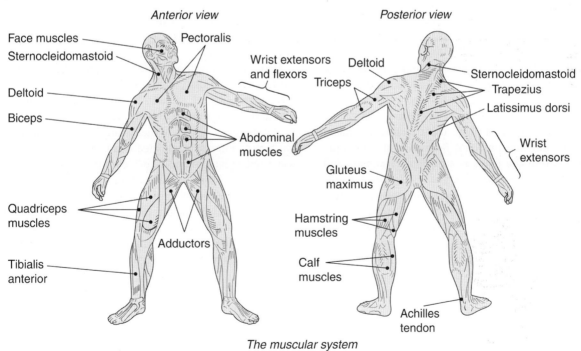

*Anterior view*    *Posterior view*

*The muscular system*

**FIGURE 8.1**    Muscles and the Skeletal System. (From Hechtman, L. [2011]. *Clinical naturopathic medicine.* Churchill Livingstone.)

## Joints

A joint, or place of articulation, is the location in the body where two or more bones make contact. Joints are constructed to allow movement and provide mechanical support, and they are classified based on their structure and function. For example, there are fibrous or immobile joints and there are cartilaginous joints. These are joints where the articular surfaces of the bones forming the joints are attached to each

**Box 8.1** Characteristics of Synovial Joints

- The joint cavity is filled with synovial fluid.
- The synovial fluid provides nutrition and lubrication to the articular cartilage that covers the ends of the articulating bones.
- The joint is enclosed by a connective tissue that forms the articular capsule.
- The articular capsule is composed of two distinct layers and reduces friction at the joint.
- The internal layer consists of a thin synovial membrane, which secretes synovial fluid into the synovial cavity and lubricates the joint.
- The external layer is a fibrous layer composed of dense connective tissue that supports and/or controls specific motions in the joint (e.g., dislocation of the joint during normal movement).
- The joint capsule is supplied with blood vessels, sensory nerves, and pain and proprioception receptors.

other by means of white fibrocartilaginous discs and ligaments. These joints allow only a limited degree of movement. The most common type of joint in the body is the synovial joint. These joints allow for the greatest degree of mobility in the joint. See Box 8.1 for a list of characteristics of synovial joints.

Synovial joints can be further classified by the joint's function into different types based upon their movement. For example, there are gliding, hinge, ball-and-socket, pivot, and compound joints.

Degeneration in joints begins early in life, even in the teen years. Articular cartilage consists of collagen fibers and does not have a direct blood supply. It responds to mechanical stimulation (exposure to compressive and decompressive forces) by thickening. Too much or not enough stimulation can damage this. With age, articular cartilage can erode, lose tissue compliance, and become more brittle and less able to cope with stresses. Aging cartilage also contains less water, making it even more noncompliant. Formation of bone spurs (osteophytes) within the joints is common. Ligaments and tendons also become less extensible. The results are joint stiffening and limited range of motion (ROM). Finally, joint proprioception declines with age, especially at the knee and ankle (Dieppe & Tobias, 1998; Pai et al., 1997; Rudy et al., 2007).

## Common Musculoskeletal Disorders in Older Adults

### Osteoarthritis

Osteoarthritis (OA) is a nonsystemic musculoskeletal condition that includes the progressive deterioration of articular cartilage and its underlying bone (commonly referred to as subchondral sclerosis), as well as an overgrowth of periarticular bone that forms osteophytes at the margins of the joint. OA is the most common form of arthritis. Before the age of 50, the prevalence of OA is higher in men than women, but after 50 years of age, women are more likely to be affected, especially in the hand, foot, and knee (Fig. 8.2) (Goodman, 2009).

The disease exhibits progressive worsening with age, rising two- to tenfold in people from 30 to 65 years of age (Felson et al., 2000). When it occurs in middle age with no known cause (i.e., degenerative joint disease [DJD]), it is classified as being idiopathic. OA can also be classified as secondary if it occurs in response to an injury, deformity, or a disease process. Traumatic OA can occur due to a single macrotraumatic injury or it can be caused by cumulative microtrauma. The incidence and prevalence of OA in different regions of the body vary depending on how they are defined—either by clinical symptoms, radiologic findings, or by a combination of the two—as well as factors such as gender, age, and genetics. OA has a substantial impact on society due to its disabling symptoms. Growing evidence is showing OA as a complex process involving interactions between multiple organ systems. The mechanical, biological and structural elements of the disease require a comprehensive multidisciplinary approach. OA of the hip and knee are two of the most significant causes of pain and physical disability in community dwelling adults.

Several risk factors have been identified for OA, and the relative importance of these risk factors can vary depending on the joint that is involved, the stage of the disease, and whether the disease has been classified by radiographs or by symptoms (Zhang et al., 2010). In addition, risk factors are considered to be modifiable or nonmodifiable. Modifiable risk factors are those that can be changed; nonmodifiable factors are those that are out of an individual's control. Regarding nonmodifiable risk factors, besides age and gender, heredity appears to play a major role in the development of generalized OA; a gene for the disease has been identified. In addition, the prevalence of OA and the joints it affects vary among racial and ethnic groups.

There are many modifiable risk factors that need to be considered when discussing the etiology of OA. As early as 1997 Slemenda et al. (Sinaki, 2003) reported that decreased muscle strength, relative to body weight, could play a role in the development of OA. In their study of individuals without a history of knee pain, isolated quad weakness was strongly associated with radiographic evidence of OA of the knee. This study suggested that decreasing body fat and increasing muscle strength may assist in the prevention of OA; if nothing else, the intervention could be an effective tool for decreasing pain and improving function. Since Slemenda et al.'s initial work, multiple other studies have supported the idea of muscle weakness playing a role in the development and progression of OA. It should be noted, however, that at least one study has acknowledged that although strength increases seem to have a protective effect in healthy joints, increased strengthening may possibly encourage OA progression in mal-aligned joints secondary to the increased joint reaction forces sustained across the articulating surfaces (Sharma et al., 2003).

Decreased joint proprioception has also been cited as a possible risk factor because it has been linked to joint instability and decreased shock absorption, both of which can lead to muscle weakness, and therefore possibly OA (Sharma et al., 1997). However, in the case of proprioception, there

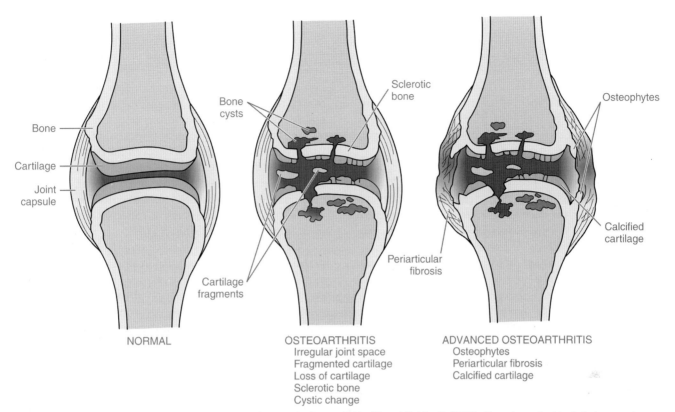

**FIGURE 8.2**   Schematic Presentation of the Pathologic Changes in Osteoarthritis. (From Ulbricht, C. [2010]. *Natural standard herbal pharmacotherapy.* Mosby.)

is no consensus on whether decreased proprioception is the cause or the result of the OA (Sharma et al., 1997), and some recent literature suggests that the link between OA and deficits in proprioception may not be as strong as previously thought.

Obesity has also been shown to play a role in the development of OA, possibly due to the excessive loading on the joint surfaces of the lower extremities that increases the biomechanical stresses across the articulating surfaces. An association has been shown to exist between obesity and the progression of knee OA (Belo et al., 2007; Chapple et al., 2011; Neogi & Zhang, 2011). Body mass index (BMI), waist circumference, waist to hip ratio, weight, and body fat percentage are all associated with higher incidence of knee OA. The incidence of hip OA has a smaller but still significant correlation with increased weight.

A history of joint trauma, such as a transarticular fracture or meniscal tear, and the presence of a bony deformity, such as developmental dysplasia of the hip, are also modifiable risk factors for the development of OA (Blagojevic et al., 2010; Englund et al., 2008; The Ottawa Panel, 2005). In all these situations, mechanical forces seem to be the underlying cause, but not necessarily because they directly damage the joint. Instead, it is hypothesized that these physical forces stimulate mechanical receptors in the chondrocytes that produce cytokines and enzymes that degrade the cartilage and surrounding joint tissues in an attempt to repair the damaged tissue (Middleton et al., 2011).

In addition to mechanical forces, congruency of the articulating surfaces seems to play a role in the development of OA; the more incongruently the joints are aligned, the greater the chance that OA will develop. For example, developmental hip dysplasias are associated with the development of hip OA in young adults (Baker-LePain & Lane, 2010; Reijman et al., 2005). Recent studies have started looking at whether femoroacetabular impingement might be a risk factor for the development and progression of hip OA (Reid et al., 2010). There is evidence to support that malalignment of the knee joint is a risk factor for progression of knee OA due to the fact that the malalignment changes the load distribution over the joint surfaces (Swezey, 1997). Leg-length inequalities are also associated with knee OA, but it is unclear as to whether they are a cause or consequence.

Moderate amounts of recreational physical activity, including jogging, do not appear to increase the risk of OA, but strenuous physical activity and/or intense competitive activity throughout life may contribute to OA development. In addition, participating in active occupations, such as farming, and those that require heavy lifting has been associated with hip OA (Jensen et al., 2008). The risk of developing knee OA in individuals whose occupations require squatting or kneeling is even higher in those individuals who are overweight, so it appears there is a summative effect with risk factors (Reijman et al., 2007). Aging does not cause OA, but due to the summative impact of risk factors over time, it is one of the strongest risk factors for the disease (Lawrence et al., 2010). It has been obvious for a number of years that just because we age, it does not necessarily mean that we are going to develop OA; however, aging does play a role in the progression of the pathology and should be considered in relation to our past experiences and activities, as well as comorbidities. This statement is supported by multiple examples of older individuals who experience OA in only one joint of the body as well as the young individual who experiences OA at a joint secondary to multiple orthopedic injuries. In summary, then, if we take all risk factors into account, it should be stated that there is no single predisposing factor for OA; rather, it is a disease process to which there are a multitude of contributors.

OA is the result of tissue damage to a joint and the immune reaction that occurs as a result of that damage. Initially, swelling of the cartilage is seen as the chondrocytes attempt to repair the damage by increasing the production of proteoglycans. As the disease process continues, there is a decrease in the level of proteoglycans, a reduction in the thickness of the joint surface, and a loss of elasticity in the cartilage that contributes to its softening and ultimate deterioration.

The common clinical presentation of OA is joint pain, stiffness, joint swelling, a feeling of "bone on bone" grating, or joint instability. Clinicians can quantify decreased ROM, crepitus, joint malalignment, postural abnormalities, joint laxity, and joint effusion.

Chronic pain, functional decline, and dependency are not necessarily inevitable consequences of aging with joint disease. In developing intervention plans for clients with OA, the first approach should be to understand the modifiable risk factors of OA, identifying them early in clients, to reduce or eliminate them. The next step of intervention is to reduce pain and improve function by individualizing the specific needs of the client based on his or her impairments. Postural and joint alignment, quality of movement, and avoiding exacerbation of pain are priorities in exercise prescription. Increasing the level of physical activity in clients with OA helps to reduce pain and morbidity. In determining intervention plans, the goals remain the same for any level of client: control pain, increase flexibility, and improve muscle strength using client education principles, modalities, and exercise.

The body of evidence for practice continues to grow. Groups, including the American Physical Therapy Association (APTA), American College of Rheumatology, Arthritis Association, Osteoarthritis Research Society International (OARSI), and the American Academy of Orthopedic Surgeons (AAOS) work independently and in conjunction to publish Clinical Practice Guidelines. All the guidelines and criteria have been, and will continue to be, reviewed and updated as more evidence becomes available. In developing these guidelines, the panel of experts summarize the level of evidence that supports these interventions, the extent of consensus of agreement for each recommendation, and the strength of recommendation for each proposition. Allied health clinicians should find these guidelines extremely useful in developing intervention plans for their clients with OA. Clinicians should interpret guidelines considering the individual impairments, goals, and expectations of their client population.

## Rheumatoid Arthritis

Rheumatoid arthritis (RA) is a systemic autoimmune disease process that exhibits both articular and periarticular impairments that include, but are not limited to, joint pain and stiffness. Although some of the impairments might be reversed over time, others cannot be, and these impairments ultimately interfere with the performance of functional activities and can lead to joint deformity (Fig. 8.3). In comparing RA with OA, the main difference between the two is that RA is a systemic disease and OA is not. In other words, with RA, all systems of the body (e.g., visual, cardiovascular, integumentary, renal, etc.) can be affected by the disease process, not just the musculoskeletal system. RA affects women more than men. Smoking and family history of RA are also risk factors.

Diagnosis of RA is made based on inflammatory arthritis in two or more large joints, inflammatory arthritis in smaller joints, positive biomarker tests, elevated inflammation markers, and symptoms lasting longer than 6 weeks. The most common biomarker tests include anticitrullinated protein antibody (ACPA) and rheumatoid factor (RF). Inflammation markers used most often are C-reactive protein (CRP) and erythrocyte sedimentation rate (ESR). In 2010, the ACR and the European League against Rheumatism (EULAR) collaboratively developed a new classification scheme focused upon early features of the disease process rather than later ones (Aletaha et al., 2010). The revised classification sought to identify individuals earlier in their disease process to provide effective disease-suppressing drug therapies sooner, thereby encouraging more successful outcomes. The most recent set of criteria for classifying RA includes the presence of synovitis (swelling) in at least one joint, the absence of a better diagnosis for the synovitis, and a total score of 6 or greater (out of a possible 10) in four areas: number and site of involved joints, serologic abnormality (RF and/or ACPA), elevated inflammatory markers (CRP and/or ESR), and symptom duration. As allied health practitioners are frequently the individuals initially recognizing the signs and symptoms of RA and referring clients to rheumatologists for further workup, diagnosis, and medical management, they should be aware of these new classification criteria.

RA is classified into three primary types: seropositive, seronegative, and overlapping. The type of RA will guide the

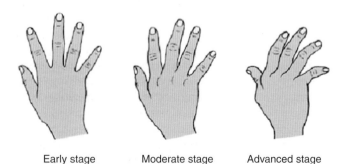

Early stage          Moderate stage          Advanced stage

**FIGURE 8.3**   Rheumatoid Arthritis. (From Jonas, W. [2005]. *Mosby's dictionary of complementary and alternative medicine.* Mosby.)

medical treatment prescribed. The ACR revised the functional classification system in 1992 to better describe the global functional consequences of RA regarding disability. Class I reflects completely able to perform usual activities of daily living (ADLs) including self-care, vocational and avocational activities. Class II demonstrates the ability to perform usual self-care and vocational activities, but limitations in avocational activities. Class III individuals can perform usual self-care activities but are limited in vocational and avocational activities. Finally, Class IV persons are limited in ability to perform usual self-care, vocational and avocational activities. By using this classification system, health-care professionals can understand how a client is functioning because everyone is using the same language.

Although it is understandable that clients will never be "cured" of their RA, it is possible that their health and functional status will improve, and even go into remission. The ACR Criteria for Evaluating Clinical Improvement in RA defines the specific criteria that must occur for this designation including remission. The ACR has also defined factors resulting in a "poor" prognosis for a client with RA: earlier age at onset of disease, high titer of RF, an elevated ESR, swelling in more than 20 joints, and extraarticular manifestations. An awareness of these classifications and prognostic characteristics is important for therapists as they determine intervention plans for their clients. Therapists should consider initial classification of RA as well on ongoing classification to adjust intervention plans appropriately.

## Osteoporosis

Osteoporosis is a disease of bone in which the bone mineral density (BMD) is reduced, bone microarchitecture is disrupted, and the amount and variety of proteins in bone are altered. These consequences can result in fragile, porous bones, placing individuals with osteoporosis at a higher risk for bone fractures.

The rate of calcium loss accelerates during the first 5 years after menopause in women. By the age of 80 years women lose 30% compared with men losing 20%. The World Health Organization has classified bone density as normal, low, osteoporotic, and severe osteoporotic as measured using dual x-ray absorptiometry (DXA). Those in the last two categories are at risk for fractures, especially in the vertebrae, hip, and wrist (National Osteoporosis Foundation, 2008). Bone fractures depend on bone strength (density) and bone quality (microarchitecture, bone vitality, ability of bone to repair itself) ("NIH Consensus Development Panel on Osteoporosis Prevention, Diagnosis, and Therapy", 2001).

Osteoporosis affects both genders, but the incidence is higher in women; an estimated 10 million in the United States have osteoporosis. Individuals at greater risk are those who are older, inactive, and of slight build, and those who have a history of a previous fracture. Individuals may have a history of adverse health practices (such as use of alcohol, cigarettes, and caffeine; diet low in calcium and vitamin D). Other risk factors can include prolonged use of medications (such as

corticosteroids) and certain medical conditions, such as renal disease (National Osteoporosis Foundation, 2008).

Preventive treatment includes calcium (1500 mg/day), vitamin D (800 to 1000 IU/day), exercise, and, in certain individuals, hormones. Vitamin D has taken on increased significance today as older adults have difficulty absorbing calcium and need vitamin D to induce the calcium-binding protein to move calcium across the cell membrane and encourage absorption of calcium in the small intestine. Weight-bearing and resistive exercises are important, but exercise should stress those skeletal sites most at risk for fractures (National Osteoporosis Foundation, 2008; Suominen, 1993; Swezey, 1996). Current research suggests that the best exercise for bone metabolism and decreasing the risk of falls involves impact forces (Kort et al., 2009).

Medical treatment includes taking medications to inhibit the action of osteoclasts and their effect on bone resorption (bisphosphonates) or taking parathyroid hormone (to stimulate bone formation). As with prevention, daily intake of vitamin D and of calcium is important, as is exercise.

Therapists should be aware of osteoporosis and the relationship between bone health, fall risk, and risk for fracture. Therapists can assist clients in understanding their disease process and engage in both exercise and activity modifications to increase safety and reduce fracture risk.

## Fractures

A fracture is defined as a break in bone or cartilage and can occur anywhere in the body where these tissues reside (Stamm et al., 2004). One of the most common fractures that occur in the geriatric client is a hip fracture, which is defined as a break in the upper quarter of the femur; a fracture of the acetabulum or hip socket itself is not considered a hip fracture.

## Epidemiology of Hip Fractures

Hip fracture has been recognized as the most serious consequence of osteoporosis. In 1990, it was estimated that there were 1.66 million hip fractures worldwide; it is projected that this number will rise to 6.26 million by 2050 (Cooper et al., 1992; Zhang & Jordan, 2010). This increase is believed to be due to the increased aging of the population, but also due to an increase in the incidence of osteoporosis, diminished overall muscle volume, and decreased neuromuscular responses to physical challenges (Raaymakers, 2006). In addition, with the rise of aging populations globally, there are a greater number of medical comorbidities that complicate the aging individual's health status, such as cardiopulmonary diagnoses and dementia. Because fracture care and intervention has evolved and improved in the past decades, opportunities for individuals to sustain second fractures are becoming more commonplace.

In general, women have a greater incidence of hip fracture than men, and the highest rates have been reported in predominantly white populations in the Northern Hemisphere. There appear to be two main risk factors for hip fractures: decreased bone strength that can occur with pathologies such as osteoporosis and cancer and/or occurrence of fall-related trauma (Cummings et al., 1997).

Hip fractures are typically classified by orthopedic surgeons according to the area of the femur that is involved. In the case of an intracapsular hip fracture, the head and neck of the femur are involved. About one-half of all hip fractures involve the femoral neck and necessitate opening the femoral joint capsule during surgery, which increases the risk of infection. An increased rate of infection can complicate the postoperative course of events for individuals who may already be at risk due to their possibly frail health status. Not all fractures are intracapsular; intertrochanteric and subtrochanteric fractures are considered extracapsular and do not require that the capsule be opened during fixation. An intertrochanteric fracture occurs between the femoral neck and the lesser trochanter, and a subtrochanteric fracture occurs within an area approximately 2.5 inches inferior to the lesser trochanter.

For rehabilitation professionals involved in the postoperative care of clients with hip fractures, hip fracture classification is usually dependent on the surgical approach used, the soft tissue involved, and the client's potential for rehabilitation. In this classification system, hip fractures are categorized as being in one of the following five categories: nondisplaced/minimally displaced femoral neck fractures, displaced neck fractures, stable intertrochanteric fractures, unstable intertrochanteric fractures, and subtrochanteric fractures. Hip fractures may be repaired surgically through an open reduction internal fixation (ORIF), total hip arthroplasty, or partial hip arthroplasty. If a client with a hip fracture does not have a surgical repair, it is usually because of comorbidities that prevent it or due to the client being nonambulatory before injury (Beaupre et al., 2005; Maxey & Magnusson, 2013).

However, Raaymakers (2006) encouraged physicians to consider nonsurgical early mobilization for clients with impacted femoral neck fractures as long as they are healthy, which is considered to be any individual under the age of 70 with one or less comorbidity. Most intertrochanteric fractures are managed by the surgeon using either a compression hip screw or an intramedullary nail. Both will allow for impaction at the fracture site in order that the fracture will heal, so the decision to use one type of fixation over another is typically based on the surgeon's preference and his or her expertise with using the hardware. Subtrochanteric fractures are usually fixated with a long intramedullary nail and screw or the use of screws alone. Occasionally, a plate may be used rather than a nail.

Regardless of the age of the individual, one of the most important elements to consider in the case of a hip fracture is whether there has been compromise to the femoral head's blood supply. If the blood supply was disrupted, the cartilage and underlying bone in the area may have not received an adequate blood supply, and avascular necrosis, or tissue death due to lack of blood supply, may occur. Vascular necrosis can result in the loss of the spherical shape of the femoral head, leading to incongruency of the hip joint. Over time, this incongruency can result in arthritis of the hip joint, as evidenced by an antalgic gait and impaired hip joint ROM. Eventually, a total hip arthroplasty may be needed. Intracapsular fractures are more likely to lead to avascular necrosis of the femoral head because the femoral neck has a thin periosteum and minimal amount of cancellous bone. Subtrochanteric fractures tend to require some type of implant device, such as a long intramedullary nail, plate, rod, or screws. With a mechanical device in place, along with the high stresses endured by this part of the femur, there is an increased tendency for the implant to ultimately fail. Stability of the hip is proportional to the severity of the fracture, the quality of the bone, and the expertise of the surgeon, but the client's functional success is most dependent on his or her premorbid physical and mental abilities.

Therapists must understand the surgical or nonsurgical approach chosen for hip fracture due to the impact on the rehabilitation process. Clients may have restricted weight bearing or precautions based on surgery and surgical approach.

## Vertebral Compression Fractures

Vertebral compression fracture (VCF) occurs when a vertebral body of the spine collapses. This collapse results in pain, deformity, and loss of vertebral height. Clients with severe osteoporosis can sustain a VCF during simple daily movements such as stepping off a curb or sneezing forcefully. Clients with moderate osteoporosis may sustain a VCF during a fall or lifting a heavy object. VCFs present as a sudden onset of pain, worsened by standing or upright posture and improved when laying flat. Surgery options include vertebroplasty and kyphoplasty. Both involve injecting surgical bone cement into recently fractured vertebra. The results of surgery show good pain reduction and return to function (McGirt et al., 2009).

## Back Pain

Although lower back pain (LBP) is a common complaint of the population in general, it is the most frequently reported musculoskeletal problem among older adults and their most frequently reported symptom (Hicks et al., 2009). Of all the visits that are made to a physician for LBP, 20% are made by individuals over 65 years of age. In a study by Weiner and colleagues in 2003, 42% of the community-dwelling older adults who participated in the study reported at least one incident of LBP in the previous year (Weigl et al., 2007) However, despite the fact that many older individuals suffer from it, little research has been done to try to delineate the pathoanatomic cause(s) of LBP in the adult population over 65 years of age (Bressler et al., 1999). The most common diagnosis made in the senior population is "degenerative spinal disease," which could encompass a number of specific pathologies (e.g., spinal stenosis, degenerative disc disease [DDD], spondylolisthesis, degenerative facet disease [DFD], etc.). Why is specific diagnosis so difficult? First, DDD is commonly found at all spinal levels in older adults, regardless of the specificity of the imaging technique used, and there is poor predictive validity for pain in adults between 53 and 70 years of age (Jarvik et al., 2001).

Second, both DDD and DFD (which are included in the degenerative spinal disease category) have been associated with LBP, but there is disagreement as to the relationship between these pathologies and spinal pain. Also, it is felt that psychological factors may play a role in pain pathogenesis, a concept that is supported by Hicks, who in a 2009 study found that the severity of disc and facet disease was indeed associated with chronic LBP, but not with the pain complaints self-reported by those with chronic LBP (Hicks et al., 2009).

The breakdown of client diagnoses for a typical internal medicine clinic that sees primarily adult clients consists of compression fractures (4%), spondylolisthesis (3%), malignancies (0.7%), ankylosing spondylitis (0.3%), and vertebral osteomyelitis (0.1%) (Lazaro & Quinet, 1994). For clinics seeing predominately older adults, the percentages for compression fractures and malignancies are slightly higher. Therefore, when examining older adult clients with LBP, it is critical to consider concomitant contributions such as medical comorbidities, nutritional status, BMD, and activity levels. It has become apparent in health care that the older adult client's well-being is influenced not only by the status of the body's individual systems (such as the cardiac, pulmonary, and renal systems), but also by the interactions between these systems. Because of the complexity of these interactions, it is beneficial for clinicians to follow recommendations for the diagnosis and treatment of LBP, such as those suggested by the American College of Physicians and the American Pain Society, not only for their geriatric clients, but for any of their clients with general LBP (Belo et al., 2007).

## Lumbar Spinal Stenosis

Degenerative spinal stenosis is an acquired condition with an insidious onset that is commonly diagnosed in the older adult population. Spinal stenosis is defined as OA of the intervertebral discs and facet joints along with hypertrophy of the ligamentum flavum. Most commonly, it begins between the disc and the vertebral bodies, but it can also start at the level of the facet joint. It is a cycle of degeneration; as the degeneration worsens, there is osteophyte formation at the level of the facet joint and disc, and calcification/hypertrophy of the ligamentum flavum. Because these degenerative changes decrease the amount of room available for lumbar nerve roots in the central canal, lateral recess, and neural foramina, classic symptoms such as neurogenic claudication are experienced. It is believed that the pain that is experienced by the client occurs due to mechanical compression on the nerve roots and its resultant compromise to the neural blood supply (Hart et al., 2012). It is interesting to note that the prevalence of DDD increases with caudal progression from the T12/L1 level to the L4/L5 level, with a mild decrease of the disease process noted at the L5/S1 level. This makes sense when correlating these findings with the progressively higher compressive loads that the spine must endure at those levels. At the level of L5/S1, shearing forces are the predominant load sustained by the joint, and therefore the degenerative effect on that joint level is different from the effect at the more cranial lumbar joints.

The neurogenic claudication that occurs with spinal stenosis can occur unilaterally or bilaterally, but it is almost always asymmetric and brought on by functional activity or extension of the lumbar spine.

## Degenerative Lumbar Spondylolisthesis

Lumbar spondylolisthesis is defined by *Stedman's Concise Medical Dictionary* as a forward movement of the body of a lumbar vertebra on the vertebra, or sacrum, below it (Stamm et al., 2004). In the case of adults older than 50 years of age, spondylolisthesis is primarily degenerative in nature, differing from the spondylitic spondylolisthesis seen in younger populations. In spondylitic spondylolisthesis, there is a pars interarticularis defect, most commonly seen as a fracture, but in degenerative spondylolisthesis, the pars is intact and the vertebrae as a whole slips forward secondary to OA of the facet joints and insufficient ligamentous support. Degenerative spondylolisthesis occurs most frequently at the L4/L5 level (compared with the spondylitic type, which occurs most often at L5/S1) and results in similar symptoms as spinal stenosis, because both include compromise of the vertebral canal. Although x-rays can often determine the nature of the spondylolisthesis and the grade of the slippage, magnetic resonance imaging (MRI) or computed tomography (CT) with myelogram can help evaluate any associated compression of the neural elements, as well as screen for differential diagnoses of LBP, such as VCFs.

## Occupational Therapy Interventions for Musculoskeletal Conditions in the Aging Adult

Occupational therapy (OT) intervention should be guided by the client's disease process and by the identified problems or deficits noted during the evaluation. The client's perception and understanding of the disease process and correlating limitations should also be considered when designing interventions for the client. It is also relevant to consider the client's current adaptation or adjustment to those limitations in relation to participation, engagement, and satisfaction with meaningful occupations. Therapists must understand kinesiological and physiological concepts of the musculoskeletal system to appropriately analyze functional activity and performance. Using these concepts and professional judgment, therapists can identify relevant assessments, interpret findings, and create a collaborative intervention plan with the client.

The intervention process brings together OT practitioners and clients to facilitate engagement in occupation related to health, well-being, and achievement of established goals (American Occupational Therapy Association [AOTA], 2020). Interventions should integrate information regarding the client's musculoskeletal status, along with other client factors, contexts, personal factors, performance patterns, and skills. To design an intervention plan with clients experiencing acute and chronic musculoskeletal conditions, an occupational therapist needs to consider the client's goals and occupational needs, overall health and well-being, and use best available evidence to guide clinical decisions. The OT professional should consider using the biomechanical frame of reference to guide and facilitate an occupation-based intervention design approach.

## Conditions in the Older Adult

Musculoskeletal conditions in the older adult covered in the next sections include OA, RA, osteoporosis, lumbar spinal stenosis, and degenerative lumbar spondylolisthesis. OT assessment and intervention strategies are discussed to assist in creating meaningful, client-centered plans of care for those musculoskeletal conditions.

## Client and Caregiver Education

Intervention should always include ongoing client and caregiver education throughout the entirety of the therapeutic relationship. Information gathered from the initial evaluation, including assessment measurements and analysis of findings, should be communicated to the client and caregivers. Findings should be presented to the client and caregivers to provide clarity and to begin the collaborative process of designing occupation-based goals and intervention strategies. Communication and education should involve all relevant caregivers to ensure appropriate carry-over strategies and recommendations. Education should focus on the disease process itself, the anticipated healing process, specific intervention strategies targeting occupation-based activities, safety precautions, environmental adaptations, and any follow-up recommendations. Musculoskeletal conditions are often chronic in nature and may require psychological adaptations along with physical adaptations. Occupational therapists must be prepared to address mental health concerns that may arise during the intervention process related to trauma, depression, and anxiety, among others. OT practitioners should also consider how working with older adults with cognitive impairment may influence the intervention process for musculoskeletal conditions. Therapists and assistants should provide clients and caregivers with the necessary knowledge to promote healing, health, and overall well-being during and after the intervention process.

## Osteoarthritis

OA is a common joint disease that most often affects middle-age to elderly people (Arthritis Foundation, 2022). OA is a musculoskeletal disease of an entire joint, including the cartilage, joint lining, ligaments, and bone. Breakdown of the cartilage, deterioration of tendons and ligaments, and inflammation of the joint lining can all contribute to the severity of OA. OA typically occurs in the hand, spine, hips, knees, and great toes. Symptoms of OA include joint pain and stiffness, decreased function at the affected joint(s), swelling at the affected joint(s), and a cracking or grinding sound with movement. Currently, there is no treatment that can reverse the damage caused by OA; however, occupational therapists are equipped to integrate appropriate intervention strategies to lessen the burden of this musculoskeletal condition.

For management of OA affecting the hand, practitioners should evaluate the client's ability to perform functional activities, recommend assistive devices to help perform meaningful ADL and IADL tasks, provide education on joint protection techniques, and provide thermal modalities and orthotic devices as needed. OA of the hand most commonly affects the trapeziometacarpal (TMC) and carpometacarpal (CMC) joints of the thumb, and distal (DIP) and proximal (PIP) interphalangeal joints of the other digits (Arthritis Foundation, 2022). For management of OT affecting the knee and hip, practitioners should incorporate intervention to include cardiovascular and/or resistance exercise programs and encourage clients to be an active participant in self-management programs. Interventions such as aquatic exercise or tai chi may prove to be beneficial to clients, based on individual preference of participating. Other self-management programs may include joint protection during functional ADL and IADL performance, use of adaptive equipment and assistive devices, energy conservation techniques, and mobility devices as recommended by physical therapy.

Joint protection techniques are a main intervention strategy to incorporate with clients with OA. Education to the client and caregivers on integrating these techniques into daily routines and activity throughout the day may prevent further joint deterioration, and promote overall comfort and higher levels of function. Clinicians must have an understanding of the joint's anatomy and mechanics in order to incorporate effective joint protection techniques. General education for the client experiencing OA includes (1) maintain the ROM around the joint, (2) increase the strength of the muscles around the joint, (3) reduce excessive loading on the involved joint(s), (4) acknowledge and avoid pain in the joint(s) during activity performance, (5) avoid keeping the joint in one position for prolonged periods of time, and (6) balance activity and rest throughout the day.

### Managing Joint Range of Motion

ROM is the degree of movement that occurs at a joint. Maintaining joint ROM involves sustaining the length of the agonist and antagonist muscles around the joint and maintaining full mechanical motion of the articulating bony surfaces in the joint. Maintaining joint ROM is important to sustain use of the joint to allow for participation in meaningful and functional activities. Joint ROM is also important to prevent the development of or decrease the severity of joint contractures.

### Muscle Strength

Functional muscle strength is the use of muscles in a smooth and coordinated manner during functional activities (Rybski, 2019). Factors including age, gender, pain, cognition, psychological/psychosocial, and environmental can all influence an individual's muscle strength capacity. Muscles around a joint can provide stabilization and protection during a sustained lengthening force (isometric contraction). When external forces are placed upon a joint, the strength of the muscles is also important to protect that joint while in motion. If muscles are weak, there is an increased risk for damage to the joint and the possibility of more stress on other supporting joint structures. The joint structure may also be vulnerable to damage or injury during sudden and unexpected movement, such as a fall.

Weakness in lower limb muscles (particularly the quadriceps) influences knee joint load, which is believed to be a major contributor to knee OA. Impairments such as weakness and altered movement patterns are commonly associated with individuals with OA. Practitioners will typically integrate therapeutic exercise into the management of knee OA. Management of OA with any joint should include performance of daily activities and exercise within the range of a client's acceptable range of pain to prevent muscle disuse atrophy and to continue to strengthen muscles.

### Adaptations and Environmental Modifications

Adaptations and environmental modifications can positively influence engagement, performance, and satisfaction with meaningful occupations for individuals living with OA, as well as enhancing a client's level of independence and safety while performing everyday tasks. Assistive devices, such as reachers (Fig. 8.4A), jar openers (Fig. 8.4B), sock aides, long-handled shoehorns, dressing sticks, buttons hooks, or elastic shoelaces (Fig. 8.4C), may be recommended by the OT practitioner, particularly when the condition is chronic or progressive. When possible, it is best practice to evaluate a client in their actual home and other meaningful and relevant environments. Practitioners working in the home health setting have an ideal opportunity to make significant interventions in this area based on individualized needs of the client in each relevant environment or context. OT practitioners can evaluate clients with OA in their homes and other relevant

environments to analyze client performance that may be limiting due to pain or other contributing symptoms of OA, to recommend activity and environmental modification while performing tasks in client's actual environments.

### Joint Protection Education

Joint protection education will be discussed further to explore environmental modifications, activity modifications, and adaptive and assistive devices to maintain joint integrity. Principles of joint protection and intervention strategies will be outlined to manage symptoms associated with OA and RA.

### Joint Protection Education Through Activity Performance

Activity pacing is a plan for balancing periods of rest and activity to alleviate symptoms associated with OA, such as flares of inflammation that often cause prolonged periods of rest (Murphy et al., 2012). Activity pacing is intended to break the cycle of increased periods by incorporating short periods of rest that are scheduled throughout activity before the symptoms of flaring and inflammation occur. Further investigation suggests that the practitioner must understand the client's physical activity patterns in order to understand how instruction and incorporation of activity pacing can be effectively used for symptom management of OA. OT professionals need to address the physical aspects of activity (weakness, joint protection, body mechanics) in addition to the environmental and behavioral barriers involved with activity performance. The importance of exercise in individuals with OA continues to be recognized across health-care disciplines. A study conducted by Kjeken et al. (2015) demonstrated the effectiveness of utilizing evidence-based exercise protocols

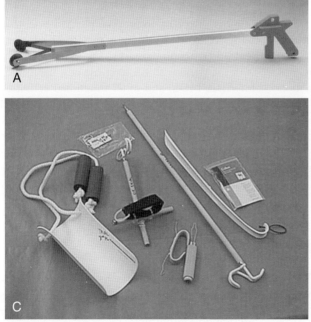
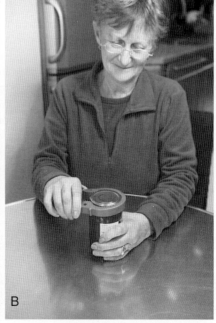

**FIGURE 8.4**  Assistive Devices. (A) Extended-handle reacher. (B) Jar opener. (C) Adaptive equipment used for dressing includes sock aid, adapted dressing stick, button aids, dressing stick, shoehorn, and elastic laces. (A, From Early, M. B. [2013]. *Physical dysfunction practice skills for the occupational therapy assistant* [3rd ed.]. Elsevier. B, Photo from istock.com. C, From Sisto, S. A. [2009]. *Spinal cord injuries.* Mosby.)

for individuals with hand OA, with tailored exercises used to also enhance strength and stability of the shoulder, arm and wrist muscles, grip strength, and finger joint stability. The study also concluded that individuals that are given clear and consistent education on the therapeutic exercise regimen were more likely to follow through with continued completion of the exercises.

## Rheumatoid Arthritis

According to the American College of Rheumatology, RA is the most common type of autoimmune arthritis, affecting more than 1.3 million Americans. RA causes pain, swelling, joint stiffness, and decreased movement of the joints. Small joints of the hand and feet are most commonly affected. OT interventions should always include improving or restoring function and well-being, with specific interventions for RA to include (1) decreasing pain, (2) preventing and/or control joint damage, and (3) decreasing the extraarticular manifestations of the disease. Pharmacological and surgical intervention may be warranted, with OT intervention focusing on lifestyle modifications. Intervention decisions are made in collaboration with the client, and consideration of the degree of joint synovitis, deformity, pain levels, and overall lifestyle. Goals for each client are dependent on the stage of the disease process.

### Active Disease

If an individual is experiencing a flare-up of their RA, it is considered to be in an "active" disease stage. Goals during the active stage of the disease include reducing joint pain, energy conservation, and maintaining functional ROM. Modalities may be used to treat pain and inflammation as well. Those in the active disease stage should be encouraged to maintain joints in a neutral position with potential use of a splint/orthotic device to maintain joint integrity. Prolonged inactivity, however, should be avoided as this can lead to other negative outcomes, such as decreased muscle strength and activity tolerance. Joint protection techniques and energy conservation strategies are relevant intervention techniques during the active disease stage. Gentle active range of motion (AROM) or active-assistive range of motion (AAROM) may also be beneficial to maintain joint motion and avoid soft tissue constriction. Passive ROM should be avoided during this stage. Isometric exercises can be incorporated to prevent muscle atrophy; however, there is minimal evidence to support intensive exercise at this stage.

### Subacute Disease

After acute disease flare-ups resolve, the individual moves into the subacute stage. Intervention strategies in the subacute stage focus on preventing deconditioning and maximizing functional capacities. The occupational therapist must use clinical judgment during interventions to prevent regression of the disease process. Modalities are used to heat tissues before performing passive ROM and stretching exercises. AROM is performed at a higher frequency with increased sets and repetitions of isometric exercises. Progressive resistance training may also be used at this stage, along with aerobic exercise such as a bicycle ergometer or aquatic therapy to reduce the stress on weight-bearing joints. Tai chi and dance therapy may also be used as a way for clients to adhere to an exercise regimen.

### Inactive Disease

The American College of Rheumatology recommends strengthening and aerobic exercise for clients at the inactive stage of their RA. Improving muscle strength, joint mobility, flexibility, and activity tolerance are also important intervention strategies during the inactive disease stage. Joint protection and self-management techniques of RA continue to be relevant during this stage. Physical activity has demonstrated to have other benefits at the stage including improvements with cardiovascular health, body composition, functional ability, and psychological well-being (Tan et al., 2019). Tan et al. conducted a study that explored the barriers to engaging in physical activity with individuals with RA, including physical limitations, pain, joint stiffness, fatigue, and lack of arthritis-specific interventions as the most common. The study showed that participants preferred low-intensity exercises that can be completed independently, with walking rated as the most preferred form of physical activity (Tan et al., 2019). Understanding an individual's perception of physical activity along with perceived barriers to activity is important for clinicians to consider when working toward lifestyle modifications. Although there are benefits from both cardiovascular and neuromuscular exercise, caution needs to be taken for clients with significant joint damage. For those with significant joint damage, exercises that unload weight-bearing joints, and low-intensity physical activity should be used. Education regarding the disease process and symptoms is important to incorporate into the intervention process, including demonstration and reinforcement of techniques in actual performance of ADLs and other functional tasks. The OT professional can work with the client with RA to create new habits of performance for ADL, IADL, and other functional activities. A systematic review titled, "A Systematic Review for Educational Interventions for Rheumatoid Arthritis," concluded that OT practitioners that incorporated educational approaches to increase coping skills for pain, fatigue, and energy conservation were effective in increase joint protection behaviors with clients (Carandang et al., 2016). The study also showed that creating client-centered interventions for each individual may increase likelihood of applying these strategies toward everyday behavior and functioning.

### Joint Protection Education

Joint protection strategies have shown to be beneficial in managing RA. OT practitioners can integrate the following joint protection techniques as part of a self-management program to enhance overall function and performance with clients with RA (Box 8.2, Principles of Joint Protection).

| **Box 8.2**    Principles of Joint Protection |
| --- |
| • Respect pain.<br>• Maintain muscle strength and range of motion.<br>• Use each joint in its most stable anatomic and functional plane.<br>• Avoid positions of deformity and forces in their direction.<br>• Use the largest, strongest joints available for the job.<br>• Ensure correct patterns of movement.<br>• Avoid staying in one position for long periods.<br>• Pace activities—energy conservation.<br>• Balance rest and activity. |

From Trombly, C. A., & Radomski, M. V. (2002). *Occupational therapy for physical dysfunction* (p. 1009). Lippincott Williams & Wilkins.

## Respecting Pain

Joint pain during the inflammatory stage of RA is common and should be seen as the body's way of alerting to potential stressors that may damage the joint structure. Joint capsules are weaker during the inflammatory stage and may be prone to deformity. Clients should be educated to acknowledge the pain and eliminate or modify activities that cause repeated and/or prolonged pain to the joints during periods of inflammation.

## Maintain Muscle Strength and Range of Motion

Muscles surrounding a joint provide the stability and protection to allow for movement. In order for appropriate joint mechanics, there needs to be a balance between the agonist and antagonist muscles. Imbalances in strength place the joints at greater risk for injury to the capsule, ligaments, and cartilage. When acute inflammation is present, gentle and pain-free ROM exercise can be incorporated to protect the joint. Practitioners must practice caution here to avoid excessive ROM, to decrease risk of further pain and inflammation.

## Avoid Positions of Deformity and Forces in Their Directions

Clients should be taught to avoid external loads and internal forces that can cause deformity. For example, opening container lids places an ulnar force on the digits and can lead to ulnar drift of the metacarpophalangeal (MCP) joints. Modification of techniques to everyday tasks can help with new patterns of behavior and performance with clients that can positively contribute to independence with these daily tasks.

## Use the Largest, Strongest Joints Available for the Job

Using a larger joint to complete a task can prevent unnecessary force and exertion on smaller joints that are more vulnerable to damage and deformity. An everyday example of this is carrying a bag over the shoulder instead of holding the bag over the smaller joints of the fingers. OT professionals should observe and analyze tasks that the client performs daily to identify opportunities for modifications or adaptations to integrate this protection technique.

## Ensure Correct Patterns of Movement

Proper joint alignment during task performance, particularly resistive activities, can alleviate symptoms of pain, tenosynovitis, and potential deformities of the joint capsules.

## Avoid Staying in One Position for Long Periods

Prolonged static positions can lead to muscle fatigue and instability to the involved joint. Instability can lead to overall imbalances of the muscles and surrounding structures.

## Pace Activities—Energy Conservation

For individuals living with RA, OT intervention should include analyzing and modifying as needed the pace at which activities are completed. Energy conservation techniques can be incorporated in daily routines to help clients avoid excessive fatigue to ultimately complete more meaningful activities throughout the day. Clients should avoid starting activities that cannot be interrupted or stopped.

## Balance Rest and Activity

Another energy conservation and activity pacing technique is balancing periods of rest and activity. Individuals with RA generally fatigue more easily and need more rest. Education on balance can help clients anticipate fatigue and plan their daily schedules to balance activity appropriately, allowing individuals to prioritize and accomplish more throughout the day.

## Modifications and Adaptations

OT professionals should make recommendations for environmental modifications, adaptive equipment, and assistive devices that may prevent injury and fatigue and increase overall independence with daily tasks. This could include modifications such as changing surface heights, changing round doorknobs to levers, or built-up handles on commonly used tools to place less stress on smaller joints and weakened muscles.

## Splinting and Orthoses for Joint Protection and Pain Reduction

Hand and wrist orthotics are commonly used for individuals with RA. Joint rest by immobilization may reduce inflammation during the inflammatory process. Orthotics can provide support and reduce pain to unstable joints during functional performance. For example, an MCP ulnar deviation orthosis can prevent misalignment of joints and overstretching during occupational performance, and can be used to prevent ulnar deviation. To prevent hyperextension of the finger proximal interphalangeal (PIP) joints (swan-neck deformity), a three-point, or "ring," splint may be used to allow for flexion of the PIP joint while preventing hyperextension. Dynamic splinting with finger extension outriggers may often be used after finger MCP implant arthroplasty.

## Osteoporosis and Fractures

Osteoporosis, typically, does not lead to impaired functional performance unless a fracture of a bone occurs. Osteoporosis alone usually does not require the intervention of OT; however, it is a common comorbid condition that should be considered for precaution and safety recommendations. Osteoporosis is a common condition seen by therapists in adult and geriatric populations in areas of wellness and rehabilitation. It is imperative that clients have an understanding of the effects of the condition and how to make lifestyle choices and potential changes to reduce risks that are associated with osteoporosis.

### Vertebral Fractures

Interventions for individuals who have sustained an osteoporotic fracture include reducing pain, healing in appropriate alignment, reducing risk of further fractures, and maintaining/improving function. Vertebral fractures are common in the older adult population. Education on spine decompression exercises is an appropriate intervention strategy to implement in the acute phases following vertebral fractures. Decompression exercises can be done by lying in the supine position on a firm mattress with hips and knees flexed. Clients can also be taught to "lengthen" each leg as another decompression exercise. During the acute phases following vertebral fractures, clients are also taught how to complete log rolling for bed mobility, use adaptive devices for ADL completion, how to sit supporting their backs in straight-backed chairs, how to "hinge at the hips" when standing and reaching forward, and how to avoid movements that twist the trunk. Following spinal surgery, a client will be on spinal precautions. This includes no bending or twisting the spine and no lifting greater than 10 pounds. In the acute stage, muscle strengthening may be limited to isometric contractions (such as lying supine and pressing the head and shoulders into the mattress).

Individuals that progress to the post-acute stage of vertebral fractures may be referred to physical therapy to perform an evaluation of height and of thoracic and lumbar curves. Postural examinations can be completed at this stage within the interdisciplinary team, to assess trunk and leg strength, protruding abdomen, and forward head. The space between the lower ribs and pelvic rim is also measured to account for potential loss in vertebral height.

Functional assessment and intervention should also address transfer training, ROM and strength, and cardiopulmonary response to physical activity. Often women with kyphotic spinal deformities from vertebral fractures show a decrease in lung capacity, resulting in difficulty breathing. Education at this stage should also include body mechanics training for positions of sitting, lying, standing, walking, bending, and lifting. OT professionals should incorporate spinal protection strategies when coughing or sneezing, and modifications for activities that require bending, lifting, and twisting (such as standing to shower, or carrying groceries).

Mobility following a vertebral fracture involves protecting the spine during any activity and working on standing with a neutral spine posture, avoiding flexion of the upper spine. Avoiding activities that place compressive loads on the back should be discussed with clients, as well as activities to promote strengthening of back muscles. Weight-bearing activities such as walking, going down stairs, and higher-

impact activities such as jumping or hopping, are options for maintaining bone health. Therapists should work with their clients following vertebral fractures to safely incorporate these intervention strategies into their plans of care.

### Hip Fractures

In addition to vertebral fractures, hip fractures are common with the older adult population. The primary goal for OT intervention at any stage during a hip fracture is to return the individual to previous levels of function. The treating practitioner should be aware of the type of surgical procedure that was performed on the client, the client's previous health and medical history, and precautions set forth by the surgeon. Risk factors for clients should be taken into consideration for clients who have sustained hip fractures. According to a literature review conducted by Lee et al. (2020), there has been increased focus on proper rehabilitation following hip fractures in the older adult population, as a means to shorten hospital stays and improve overall clinical outcomes. The literature review also notes that by the year 2050, it is anticipated that the number of hip fractures will increase to about 4.5 million per year (Lee et al., 2020). Even with successful surgery, risk of permanent disability and even mortality remain high in older adults who have sustained a hip fracture. Important factors to consider for optimizing post-surgical hip fracture rehabilitation include the fracture type, localization of other injuries, and the mode of fixation (Lee et al., 2020).

Occupational and physical therapy services are also initiated in the acute phase (I) following hip fracture surgery. Early mobilization is imperative for clients following surgical treatment for hip fractures. This includes functional mobility interventions of bed mobility, transfers, and ambulation with an assistive device. Weight bearing is typically allowed during the early mobilization phase, unless it has been indicated otherwise by the surgeon. Early mobilization is associated with more likelihood of discharging to the home setting instead of continuing rehabilitation in a facility-based setting. OT and physical therapy professionals will collaborate in the acute phase following surgery to recommend appropriate therapeutic exercises, assistive devices, and compensatory strategies for daily tasks. Therapists will also implement assessments to gauge ROM, strength, ambulation, balance, and completion of ADL and IADL tasks such as through the Timed Up and Go test. Further OT intervention will address functional transfers, particularly with bed and toilet transfers, and recommendation and training of adaptive equipment to perform ADL tasks safely, such as lower body dressing.

In phase II of the rehabilitation process, typically 2 to 4 weeks after hip surgery, more progressive exercises will be introduced, along with further safety techniques and education regarding ADLs, IADLs, and car transfers. OT professionals can include upper body resistive exercises here as the client may be more dependent on upper body strength if using an assistive mobility device. If no other significant comorbidities exist, typically clients return to independence in self-care ADLs and functional transfers at the end of this 2- to 4-week time period. Further education following hip fracture surgery should include integration of mental health interventions, fall prevention in the home and other environments, and further musculoskeletal condition(s) management, such as osteoporosis management.

Another consideration is working with older adult clients that have a form of cognitive impairment, following hip fracture surgery. Approximately 19% of all older adults with hip fractures have dementia, and approximately 40% have some form of cognitive impairment (Lee et al., 2020). OT professionals must incorporate appropriate assessment tools and intervention strategies to ensure that individuals with cognitive impairment have a safe recovery process.

## Back Pain

Clients experiencing acute muscular back pain are typically prescribed a period of activity modification and medication from their physician to decrease pain and inflammation to the area. Following the initial acute phase of back pain, light activity may be beneficial in the healing process. In a study titled "Correlation between Postural Stability and Functional Disability in Patients with Chronic Low Back Pain," it was noted that postural stability decreases with an increase in disability noted with chronic low back pain, indicating that balance assessments and training should be incorporated in the rehabilitation process with those experiencing back pain (Desar et al., 2021). Therapists can assess using various assessments, including the Oswestry Disability Index, Timed Up and Go, and BERG Balance. Assessment of functional movement, posture, balance, and positioning during completion of ADL and other functional tasks to recommend techniques can help control the pain and limit future reinjury. Lifestyle changes, such as weight loss and activity modifications, can be discussed as a means of preventing further injury to the back. Typically, clients with acute back pain are referred to physical therapy to work toward muscle stretches and strengthening exercises. OT professionals can work collaboratively with the team to focus intervention on body mechanics during daily task completion, such as proper lifting techniques. Further interventions for two common musculoskeletal conditions that commonly cause back pain are discussed further in the next sections.

## Posture

Posture is relevant to assess when examining back pain, stability, and occupational performance. Poor posture stems from asymmetry and/or imbalances in the tissues of the body. Standing and sitting posture should be considered during an assessment. Individuals experiencing musculoskeletal conditions of lumbar spinal stenosis and degenerative lumbar spondylolisthesis may present with poor posture, which can contribute to long-term pain and decreased occupational performance. Assessment of the client's head position, upper body, trunk control and stability, and pelvic positioning and control are relevant when assessing posture and its effect on musculoskeletal conditions of the back. Therapists can assess sitting and standing balance, with or without support, posture, and body movements during functional bed mobility

and transfers as a means to gauge how postural abnormalities may alter occupational performance or contribute to pain.

## Lumbar Spinal Stenosis

Lumbar spinal stenosis is a narrowing of the spinal canal in the lumbar region of the spine and is the most common site of stenosis. The narrowing of the spine can cause symptoms of pressure on the spinal cord or nerves, which may lead to pain or numbness in the legs, which can cause difficulty walking and completing daily tasks. The most common cause of lumbar spinal stenosis is OA, but it can also be caused by injury to the spine, certain bone diseases, past surgical intervention, and/or RA. Symptoms of lumbar spinal stenosis include pain in the back, pain that radiates down through the buttocks and legs, numbness or tingling, sensation loss in the feet, "foot drop," sexual abilities, and in more severe cases, loss of bowel or bladder control. Lumbar spinal stenosis is typically diagnosed by a physician through x-rays, CT scan, or MRI.

The health-care practitioner must distinguish if the pain brought on by the stenosis is due to neurogenic versus vascular claudication, as they are treated with different protocols. Distinction can be determined through assessing pulses in the lower extremities, as clients with vascular claudication will exhibit diminished pulses. Any type of ambulation will exacerbate pain in the lower extremities if vascular claudication is present. Pain symptoms in neurogenic claudication are present with extension of the spine as this decreases the diameter of the spinal canal, therefore, pain can be relieved/eliminated by flexion of the spine. A thorough neurological assessment must be performed as well, because compromised autonomic innervation of the lower extremities may inhibit a vasodilation response. If no neurological deficits are noted through the diagnostic imaging process, common interventions include use of nonsteroidal antiinflammatory drugs (NSAIDs), and therapy services. Exercises including spinal flexion are integrated, with therapists working to reach the least amount of lumbar flexion that eliminates the pain, in order to prevent poor positioning. OT professionals will work toward environmental and task modification strategies to increase independence with meaningful ADLs and IADLs. In some cases, spinal surgery is completed, with spinal decompression being the most common surgical intervention, with spinal fusion as another surgical intervention that is used with clients experiencing lumbar spinal stenosis (Hayes et al., 2016). Recent literature has compared use of decompression and spinal fusion surgical approaches. In a study completed by Taiji et al. (2021), investigators explored the effects of decompression surgery, and if it can be used as a standalone treatment for some lumbar spinal stenosis patients that experience low back pain. Further studies need to be conducted to continue to evaluate decompression and fusion surgical techniques in alleviating symptoms associated with lumbar spinal stenosis and pain.

## Degenerative Lumbar Spondylolisthesis

Non-operative interventions for degenerative lumbar spondylolisthesis should be utilized first prior to surgical intervention consideration. Surgical treatment may be warranted if persistent low back pain, neurological deficits, and/or bowel and bladder symptoms arise. Surgical interventions include decompression as a standalone intervention, or decompression with a fusion. Continued studies need to be conducted to determine the most optimal treatment protocol for those with degenerative lumbar spondylolisthesis. The use of NSAIDs, aerobic conditioning, body-weight reduction, and medical management also may be beneficial in managing this condition. Physical therapy is often incorporated to restore ROM and flexibility, increase muscle strength, alleviate pain, and improve mobility and spinal stability. OT professionals may work with this client population with environmental and activity modifications. In a study titled "Evaluation of Occupational Performance and Pain Intensity: Before and After Back Surgery and Rehabilitation," participants were provided with OT interventions focusing on performance with physically involved occupations, with encouragement of participation in meaningful social activities (Perneros et al., 2014). This study showed good results at the 6-month and 12-month follow-up for improvements in occupational performance and pain intensity; however, the study could not conclude if this was a result of surgery or postoperative rehabilitation and evaluations.

## Occupational and Functional Performance Deficits

Functional performance is defined as "the ability to conduct a specific task that could be related to daily living activities" (Stamm et al., 2004, p. 919). Occupational performance can be defined as "The accomplishment of the selected occupation resulting from the dynamic transaction among the client, their context, and the occupation" (AOTA, 2020, p. 88). Although these words are often used interchangeably, it is important to note that functional performance refers to a person's ability to complete a task in a standardized environment while occupational performance is what the individual is able to do in their current environment. Aging persons experiencing musculoskeletal changes often experience a decline in their abilities to perform functional activities. By many accounts, these limitations are referred to as *functional performance deficits*. However, given the above differentiation, it seems that referring to such issues would better be described as *occupational performance deficits*. These occupational performance deficits may be experienced gradually with the normal progression of muscle deterioration with age, from a chronic condition such as DJD, or from an acute injury or illness that results in an accelerated loss of motion and/or muscle wasting. With any of the above reasons, musculoskeletal degradation will be accelerated with immobility and bed rest. Kehler et al. (2019) found that as humans age, even short-term bed rest can cause declines in strength and volume of musculature as well as impacting the muscle's ability to regenerate and recover. Prolonged bed rest can also contribute to bone loss and bone density, as well as cardiovascular decline.

From a physical perspective on the musculoskeletal system, occupational and functional performance may be affected in aging adults by loss of muscle mass, decreased muscle strength, decreased flexibility, limited joint ROM, and/or joint/muscle pain. However, other areas also need to be considered. Lifestyle factors such as levels of physical activity and individual nutritional status are important. Psychosocial factors, including (but not limited to) fear of falling, loneliness, psychological resiliency, and self-efficacy, can have direct and indirect relationships to skeletal muscle performance in the aging adult (Tieland et al., 2018). Regardless of the speed of onset or the factors that contribute to musculoskeletal loss, many aging adults will experience the transition from independence to requiring varying levels of assistance with functional tasks.

## Decline in Mobility With Aging

The loss of skeletal muscle mass (also referred to as sarcopenia) in aging adults can directly affect mobility. Tasks such as walking speed, stooping, crouching, kneeling, or standing up from a chair can be affected by sarcopenia (Janssen et al., 2002; Tieland et al., 2018) J. Use of a cane or walker and a history of falling is also directly related to sarcopenia (Baumgartner et al., 1998). Declines in these mobility tasks can reduce a person's ability to safely complete functional mobility that require multitasking, such as carrying on a conversation with another person or carrying items like a glass of water. Furthermore, decreased walking speed and poor performance on functional mobility increases a person's risk for falls (Faulkner et al., 2007).

Poor muscle endurance limits the distance an aging person can travel. As a result, many find it difficult or impossible to complete personally meaningful tasks: walking outdoors for pleasure, hiking, or even walking the distance required from a parked car to a store, house of worship, or other significant locations.

## Basic and Instrumental Activities of Daily Living

Occupational performance is a key concept when considering ADLs. ADLs, a term originally coined by Dr. Sidney Katz in the 1950s (Katz, 1983), has been an integral part of OT practice since its inception. The physical as well as psychological benefits of performing everyday life activities is rooted in the philosophy and foundation of the profession. According to the Occupational Therapy Practice Framework: Domain and Process (OTPF), ADLs refer to "activities that are oriented toward taking care of oneself" (AOTA, 2020, p. 83). Such activities may also be referred to as basic activities of daily living (BADLs) and personal activities of daily living (PADLs) (Box 8.3). Instrumental activities of daily living (IADLs) are "Activities that support daily life within the home and community" (AOTA, 2020, p. 87). IADLs are usually considered more complex interactions than what is required in standard ADL activity (Box 8.4).

The ability to perform ADLs has been found to be a significant predictor for admission to nursing homes, use of paid home care, need for alternative living arrangements, and hospitalization admissions (Guidet et al., 2020; Costenoble et al., 2021). In addition to these factors, determining functional status and limitations is now required for the Centers for Medicare and Medicaid Services (CMS) reimbursement

<table>
<tr><td>

**Box 8.3**   **Examples of Basic or Personal Activities of Daily Living**

- Bathing, showering
- Bowel and bladder management
- Dressing/grooming
- Eating
- Feeding
- Personal hygiene
- Functional mobility
- Sexual activity
- Sleep/rest
- Toilet hygiene

</td></tr>
</table>

**Box 8.4**   **Examples of Instrumental Activities of Daily Living**

Care of others (including selecting and supervising caregivers)
Care of pets
Childrearing
Communication device use
Community mobility
Financial management
Health management and maintenance
Home establishment and management
Meal preparation and cleanup
Safety procedures and emergency responses
Shopping

**Box 8.5**   **Activity-Specific Activities of Daily Living Instruments**

Canadian Occupational Performance Measure (COPM)[a]
Patient Specific Functional Scale (PSFS)[a]
Arnadottir OT-ADL Neurobehavior Evaluation (A-ONE)
Arthritis Impact Measurement Scales (AIMS2)
Barthel Index (BI)
Functional Autonomy Measurement System (SMAF)[b]
Functional Independence Measure (FIM)
Health Assessment Questionnaire (HAQ)
Katz Index of Activities of Daily Living
Melville Nelson Self Care Assessment[b]
Physical Self-Maintenance Scale (PSMS)[b]

[a] Activity of daily living (ADL) instruments that address client-identified ADL activities.
[b] Instruments designed specifically for older adults.
Modified from Letts, L., & Bosch, J. (2005). Measuring occupational performance in basic activities of daily living. *Measuring occupational performance: Supporting best practice in occupational therapy.* Slack.

While the Functional Independence Measure (FIM) was used for over 20 years as a common tool for measuring functional outcomes (Ottenbacher et al., 1996), Centers for Medicare and Medicaid Services (2018) guidelines have replaced this with Section GG: Functional Abilities and Goals (GG). The passage of the Improving Post-Acute Care Transformation Act mandated a switch to one functional assessment measure across all post-acute care providers in an effort to streamline communication between these entities. Since then, GG has become a part of the Minimum Data Set (MDS) for Skilled Nursing Facilities (SNF), the Inpatient Rehabilitation Facility Patient Assessment Instrument (IRF-PAI), and the Long-Term Care Hospital (LTCH) Continuity Assessment Record and Evaluation (CARE) Data Set for LTCHs. GG includes eight self-care items and 15 to 17 mobility items that are coded on a six-level rating scale. Though GG is a required measurement, it does not replace standardized functional assessments that occur during OT evaluations.

## Occupation-Based Intervention

### Management of Musculoskeletal Conditions

Managing musculoskeletal conditions is critical to reduce symptoms and improve daily life for the aging adult. Although several approaches are listed in the OT Practice Framework (AOTA, 2020), primary approaches for musculoskeletal conditions include remediation/restoration and compensation/adaptation. For chronic diseases, such as RA, a maintenance approach might also be appropriate. As noted previously in the discussion of specific musculoskeletal conditions, intervention will also include client and caregiver education on several aspects of personal function and environmental modifications.

### Considerations and Precautions

Whenever an aging adult requires intervention for a musculoskeletal condition, it is important to be aware of any active precautions involved with the diagnosis. Skeletal fractures and any subsequent surgeries, along with elective joint

(Centers for Medicare and Medicaid Services, 2019). For these reasons, determining one's ability to complete ADL activities has become standard practice.

## Assessments of Activities of Daily Living

While observation of ADL tasks is still an appropriate way to assess function, standardized assessments are important to use to quantify levels of independence and to identify occupational performance deficits. From these assessments, intervention approaches take shape in the form of remediation/restoration, adaptation/compensation, health promotion, health maintenance, or disability prevention (AOTA, 2020).

Several assessment tools are available to assist with evaluating an aging adult's ability to complete ADLs. These instruments can involve self/caregiver-reporting, direct observation, or a combination of the two. Although self-reporting tools have been found to be the least accurate assessment of function (Daltroy et al., 1999), they can be important in understanding a client's perception of independence and quality of life. Each assessment has its advantages and disadvantages. They vary in cost (from free to several hundred dollars), training, and administration time. Box 8.5 provides a well-rounded (although not thorough) list of assessments that can be used for evaluating ADL and IADL independence in aging adults. It includes how information is disseminated, cost, time to administer, and training required. Several assessments specific to certain disease processes are not included in the table.

replacement surgeries, often involve restrictions in movement and weight-bearing status. For the patient's physical safety, including safe performance of functional activities, it is important to be aware of any restrictions/precautions through review of the medical chart. Furthermore, although there are generalized precautions for several specific surgeries, surgeons vary in what they recommend in relation to these precautions. Open communication with the operating surgeon is critical to ensure appropriate follow through and continuity of care.

Another consideration with the aging adult is the possibility of comorbidities. Other conditions, including but not limited to diabetes, cardiopulmonary diseases, dehydration, malnutrition, and cancer can affect what can and cannot be included in the intervention process. To holistically treat aging adults for musculoskeletal issues, one must be aware of not just what affects them externally in the form of environment and culture, but also what affects them internally by means of their past medical history.

## Restoration of Function

According to the OTPF (AOTA, 2020), using the intervention approach of establish/restore (remediation/restoration) includes restoring a skill or ability that has been impaired. This can be completed by both biomechanical and occupational means.

## Importance of Exercise in Musculoskeletal Intervention

For a growing number of older adults, physical exercise has become a routine and meaningful occupation during their adult lives. According to the International Health, Racquet, and Sportsclub Association (IHRSA) 2021 Health Club Trend Report, 7.88 million Americans over the age of 65 are health club members, up from 5.88 million in 2010—an increase of 34.16%. Further, the report states that 69% of people between the ages of 56 and 75 report wanting to be more active. For individuals who routinely exercise, this can be considered an important occupation and is an appropriate goal for OT. For adults who do not consider routine physical exercise to be meaningful, exercise might still be used as a preparatory intervention and/or incorporated into the overall intervention plan, since physical exercise and activity are considered important parts of the aging adult's musculoskeletal health and conditioning. Multiple studies have shown that exercise and physical activity can significantly reduce or sometimes even prevent decline in muscle metabolism and function (Clarke, 2004; Peterson & Gordon, 2011; Distefano & Goodpaster, 2018). Meta-analytic evidence supports the effectiveness of progressive resistance exercises to improve both strength and lean body mass in aging adults (Peterson & Gordon, 2011).

Based on the above and other studies, the Centers for Disease Control and Prevention (CDC), the American College of Sports Medicine, and the World Health Organization (WHO) currently recommend that every aging adult who is physically able should participate in 150 minutes of moderate-intensity aerobic activity each week (or 75 minutes of vigorous-intensity aerobic activity or some equivalent mix

of the two) combined with two or more days of muscle-strengthening activities. Examples of this type of aerobic activity can be 30 minutes per day, 5 days per week at a moderate-intensity (such as walking briskly on a treadmill or riding a bicycle) or 15 minutes per day, 5 days per week of a more intense activity such as jogging. Muscle strengthening should focus on all major muscle groups. Further, increasing aerobic activity by up to 60 minutes of moderate intensity activity or 30 minutes of vigorous-intensity activity daily can further increases health benefits. It is also encouraged that if an individual cannot comply with these recommendations for whatever reason, they still should be as physically active as their abilities and/or conditions allow (Centers for Disease Control and Prevention, 2021; World Health Organization, 2020). In OT practice, when considering exercise prescription as part of the restorative process, it is important to consider (among other things) the individual's current and former strength level, their comorbidities, what forms of exercise are the most interesting to the individual, and what might be available to them after discharge from your services. Depending on the musculoskeletal condition, treatments that have been found to be effective in the biomechanical area of OT practice include joint mobilization, supported ROM exercises, resistive exercises, and a wide range of modalities (Marik & Roll, 2017; Poole & Siegel, 2017).

Whether the aging adult enjoyed physical exercise prior to OT intervention, encouraging the continuation of it after treatment is complete can be beneficial in maintaining gains made during therapy. Some individuals have access to gyms or workout equipment within their homes, others have it available within their communities (such as independent or assistive living facilities or senior communities). Silver Sneakers is a health and fitness program that is designed specifically for aging adults and is often covered by insurance. This program provides free gym memberships in many parts of the country and has online classes and a free app for phones that provide digital exercise opportunities (Walker, 2021).

## Using Occupation as Intervention

A person's occupations are what make them unique. People attribute meaning to their occupations, and those meanings change over time. Occupations make up one's sense of identity and increase engagement Furthermore, a focus on occupation is what gives OT its distinct value as a profession. When creating client-centered interventions to improve musculoskeletal issues such as strengthening, balance, flexibility, and endurance, it is important to consider occupations that are meaningful to the individual and how those occupations can be used to target performance skills.

In a study of community dwelling, physically frail aging adults, interventions that were client-centered, tailor-made, and activity-oriented were created by a trained OT. They were compared to a control group who received standard treatment that was organized by community care services. Participants in the intervention group improved significantly in basic activities of daily living. Bodily pain also decreased significantly. Improvements were also found in physical functioning, physical role functioning, and vitality, although these improvements were not significant (De Vriendt et al., 2016) Wong et al. (2018) also found value in occupation-based interventions. Participants in the study valued occupation-based intervention and allowing for client-centered care in which the clients share in decision-making leads to improved health service use and health outcomes.

Physical activity, including gardening, light housework, and physical recreational activities, has been demonstrated to affect positive functional outcomes. Other examples of therapeutic activities that have been shown to provide musculoskeletal benefits include swimming, water aerobics, yoga, and tai chi (Pool & Siegel, 2017; Siegel et al., 2017). Weigl et al. (2007) suggest that using recreational activities while rehabilitating musculoskeletal conditions can have a positive effect on body perception, expand skills, improve general conditioning, and increase social support, all of which may enhance participation and carryover.

When designing an occupation-based intervention plan, the occupational therapist needs to consider the specific musculoskeletal limitations that are affecting functional performance in relation to the goals identified by the client. Intervention programs should then be designed that can aid in the remediation of the identified limitations. For example, an upper body dressing activity can address limitations in shoulder ROM and strength. To improve or maintain the muscle condition of smaller musculoskeletal structures that affect fine motor skills, occupation-based intervention can include playing the piano, playing board games, sewing, or cooking. Appropriate ROM and resistance is determined by the therapist. Furthermore, grading any of these activities can be used to target functional endurance during intervention. Occupational therapists should incorporate physical or verbal feedback during these interventions to educate the client regarding appropriate movements or avoiding compensation; manual assistance may also be needed to provide optimal stretch to muscle fibers.

## Compensation/Adaptation

Modification (including compensation and adaptation) includes finding ways to change a person's context or activity demands to support performance in the natural setting (AOTA, 2020) and is another OT approach that can be used alone or in conjunction with remediation. For chronic musculoskeletal conditions, such as arthritis or DJD, compensation strategies and/or modified environments can permanently allow aging adults to complete the activities that they need, want, and have to do with less or no assistance while helping to prevent pain and/or further joint deterioration. For acute musculoskeletal issues, such as a hip fracture or recent shoulder arthroplasty, modifying tasks or environments can be used in a more short-term capacity to allow the aging adult to complete important occupations while regaining strength and function to return to their prior performance patterns. Examples of adaptive equipment were discussed earlier in

this chapter. It can be important to consider if the diagnosis is chronic or acute when recommending modifications for several reasons. It is important to remember that although AE can be extremely helpful, it can also be costly and is not normally covered by insurance. An aging adult with a chronic condition might think that the cost is worth the benefit, while the individual with an acute condition might want to look at ways to modify the tasks without purchasing equipment. Further, if a modification reduces the ROM or the amount of energy needed to complete an activity, does it also eliminate the opportunity to improve these skills? The benefits should be weighed and integrated into the overall therapeutic intervention and discharge plans.

As musculoskeletal conditions relate to falls, as will be discussed in the following section, modifications of the aging adult's environment are also an important consideration. Please see Chapter 29 for more information on this topic.

## Falls in Older Adults

A fall can be defined as an unintentional coming to rest on the ground, floor, or other lower level (Nevitt et al., 1989). More than 25% of adults 65 years and older experience falls each year resulting in an estimated 2.8 million ER visits per year. Falls result in diagnoses ranging from hip fractures to traumatic brain injuries and cause a decreased ability to complete ADLs independently (Centers for Disease Control and Prevention, 2016). Although many falls do not produce a serious injury, they are still the sixth leading cause of death in the aging population (Hotchkiss et al., 2004).

Factors that influence falls include behavioral, extrinsic, and intrinsic factors (Dirette & Gutman, 2021). Behavioral factors involve the way a person acts, such as participating in risky activities or a sedentary lifestyle. Extrinsic factors include the environments that interact with the person and can include throw rugs on the floor or cracks in the sidewalk. Intrinsic factors relate to the individual person. The musculoskeletal issues discussed in this chapter are included in this factor and can greatly affect a person's fall risk (Dirette & Gutman, 2021).

### Effects of Musculoskeletal Changes as They Contribute to Falls

As discussed earlier in the chapter, musculoskeletal changes occur naturally during the aging process. These changes are part of the intrinsic factors that contribute to fall risk. This includes systemic muscle weaknesses and general lower body. Other intrinsic factors include pain, especially chronic pain and decreased ROM. Specific pathologies, such as osteoporosis and Parkinson disease, are also strong contributing factors to the increased possibility of falls (Larson & Bergmann, 2008). Increased variability in walking patterns can also be associated with falls (Barak et al., 2006).

### Assessments and Measurements of Fall Risk

The OT can use certain assessments to determine an aging adult's individual fall risk. This can include the Timed-Up-

and-Go (TUG), which requires standing up from a chair, walking forward 3 m (10 feet) at a comfortable pace, turning around, walking back to the chair, and sitting down (Podsiadlo & Richardson, 1991). If an individual takes longer than 13.5 seconds to complete the TUG, that person is at an increased risk for falls. Since poor balance is often associated with falls, the Tinetti Falls Efficacy Scale (Tinetti et al., 1990) or the Berg Balance Scale (Berg et al., 1992) are other options for a standardized way to assess fall risk potential.

Other questionnaires, such as the Activities-specific Balance Confidence (ABC) Scale, the Falls Efficacy Scale (FES), and the Survey of Activities and Fear of Falling in the Elderly (SAFE), have been found to measure fear of falling in the aging adult (Hotchkiss et al., 2004). Fear of falling can be both a cause for falls in the future or an effect of previous falls. It can limit a person's willingness to participate in daily activities, which can once again have both physical and psychological effects on the aging adult.

Whether due to the physical or emotional toll that they can have on a person, falls will ultimately restrict mobility as individuals seek to be safe in their environment and no longer challenge their potential. This then begins a downward spiral of hypokinesis. Therefore, preventing falls is of utmost importance. Studies completed in both inpatient rehab (Haines et al., 2007) and home health (Robertson et al., 2001) determined that aging adults who participated in exercise programs had a statistically significant decreased incidence of falls. In a study by Iwamoto et al. (2009), an exercise training that consisted of calisthenics, balance training, strength training, and walking ability training 3 days/week reduced the incidence of falls when compared with a control group.

## Psychological Effects of Mobility Impairments in Older Adults

It is impossible to separate the physical and psychological effects that mobility impairments have on aging adults. Personal well-being, including both emotional and somatic well-being, has been found to be decreased in aging adults with lower body limitation (Freedman et al., 2017). Studies have shown that there is an association between the effects of musculoskeletal disorders (such as pain and physical disability) and depression/reduced quality of life Karp & Reynolds, 2009). Major depressive disorder (MDD) is not only common with aging adults, but it can intensify disability, accelerate cognitive and functional decline, increase risk of hospitalization, and reduce quality of life (Karp & Reynolds, 2009). As previously discussed, the loss of physical mobility is linked to functional independence. This loss of independence can mean a loss of personal identity and can at times cause depression and even despair. According to the National Council on Aging (2021), loneliness due to being homebound (and living on their own) as well as the loss of self-sufficiency are two of the top reasons that aging adults commit suicide in the United States.

Less alarming but still important, depression can reduce participation in rehabilitation treatment, which impacts the potential benefits therein. Because this can become a vicious cycle, it is important that the occupational therapist acknowledge and address a client's psychosocial stressors, anxiety, and depression to improve compliance and fully engage the client in treatment.

## Interprofessional Interventions

Patient-centered care (PCC) is the concept that individual patient preferences, needs, and values are considered and guide all intervention decisions (New England Journal of Medicine, 2017). The health-care industry has been expanding the use and implementation of PCC in recent years. Interprofessional collaboration of clinicians providing care within their respective health-care fields is the foundation to achieving PCC. The general idea of an interprofessional approach is that different perspectives from different areas of expertise improve the intervention and provide a more holistic approach to an individual's areas of concern. Regarding musculoskeletal conditions, the interprofessional team can include (but is not limited to) individuals from physical medicine (possibly rheumatology and/or orthopedics), OT, physical therapy, social work, and clinical psychology. Not only is the trend of interprofessional collaboration growing, but there is also an increasing amount of literature that analyzes the benefits of multidisciplinary treatment interventions for musculoskeletal disorders.

In a literature review of 10 randomized, controlled trials to assess the effectiveness of intensive (>100 hours of therapy) multidisciplinary approaches in clients with chronic LBP, Guzman et al. (2001) concluded that there was strong evidence that such a multidisciplinary approach improved function when compared with non-multidisciplinary rehabilitation. There was also moderate evidence that such an approach reduced pain.

## SUMMARY

Musculoskeletal conditions are one of the most debilitating and costly conditions that affect older adults, resulting in the need for occupation-based interventions and further preventative measures to decrease further risk of injury. Skilled OT professionals require understanding of the complexities of the physiologic and kinesiologic factors of the musculoskeletal system in order to integrate meaningful interventions and further client and caregiver education. Collaboration with the interprofessional team can further enhance the client's clinical outcomes and transitions across different care settings. Successful implementation and management of exercise programs, joint protection, pain regulation, mobility and fall prevention strategies can assist the older adult population with maximizing their functional status and quality of life.

*The complete listing of the Bibliography and Chapter Questions and Answers are available in the accompanying enhanced eBook version included with the print purchase of this textbook. Visit Elsevier eBooks+ (eBooks.Health.Elsevier.com) to access this content.*

# Physiological and Neurological System Changes With Aging and Related Occupational Therapy Interventions

*Angela Marie Sanford, MD, Laura H. VanPuymbrouck, PhD, OTR/L, and Carole A. Schwartz, MS, OTR*

## CHAPTER OUTLINE

## OBJECTIVES

- Describe how the aging process changes physiologic and neurologic functions relative to performance of, and participation in functional activities
- Discuss considerations that an occupational therapy (OT) must make that to attend to factors beyond the client's individual capacity that might additionally impact the occupational performance and participation of individuals throughout the aging continuum
- Describe common physiologic and neurologic disorders in older adults, particularly within the cardiovascular and pulmonary, respiratory, genitourinary, gastrointestinal, endocrine, integumentary, muscular, and neurologic systems; their sequelae; and implications for OT assessment and intervention
- Discuss how use of OT interventions support aging adults with physiological and neurological conditions that include loss or reduced performance in cognition and or communication and use of a collaborative, interprofessional approach to assessment and intervention
- Describe occupational-based interventions in the management of falls in the presence of physiologic and neurologic conditions

## Introduction

### Overarching Framework and Strategies to Support the Function of Aging Adults and Applying Best Practice Approaches

The population growth rate of adults 65 years of age and older has tripled during the 20th century. For the first time in world history, year 2035 is projected as the transition point marker where adults over age 65 will outnumber persons age 18 (Arigoni, 2018). Improving and optimizing older adult function require knowledge of the science behind the range of functional changes in each aging bodily organ. This chapter presents aging as a heterogeneous/individual process that is impacted by physiologic, neurological, and pathologic factors, and the intersectionality with sociocultural, environmental, and lifestyle factors. Patient/client-centric health-care professionals will learn from older adults by recognizing their strengths and using person-appropriate communication that considers cultural, health literacy, and cognitive factors when assessing their physiologic and neurological conditions with the goal of supporting a clients' functional status.

Current medical advances, including prevention guidelines in the areas of nutrition (Kalache et al., 2019), regular exercise (Daskalopoulou et al., 2017), stress reduction (Acevedo et al., 2016), and regular and routine health screenings (Edelman et al., 2021) have enabled extended health and longevity. See the resource section for more resources on extending health and longevity.

The fundamental physiologic and neurologic changes during life maturation are discussed in this chapter, including the individual variance in these changes (e.g., prior lifestyle, genetic profile) during the aging process. This chapter highlights changes that may affect occupational performance and participation, thus influencing overall health and well-being. Occupational therapy (OT) can mitigate the effects of age-related changes by optimizing success in achieving client-driven goals with interventions supporting individual and group activities, occupations, education, training, advocacy, group interventions, and virtual interventions to maximize participation, health and well-being in life. Further detailed aging-related physiologic and neurologic information sources include *Pathy's Principles and Practice of Geriatric Medicine* (Sinclair & Morley, 2012) as well as the *Oxford Textbook of Geriatric Medicine (3rd ed.)* (Michel et al., 2017). Additionally, Table 9.1 provides relevant abbreviations.

**TABLE 9.1** Terms Associated With Aging-Related Physiological or Neurological Changes and Interventions

| Term | Definition | Term | Definition |
|------|-----------|------|-----------|
| AAA | Abdominal aortic aneurysm | CS | Carotid stenosis |
| AAROM | Active assistive range of motion | CSF | Cerebrospinal fluid |
| ADL | Activities of daily living | CT scan | Computed axial tomography (type of x-ray that shows 2-dimensional images of the parts of the body) |
| A.Fib. | Atrial fibrillation (cardiac arrhythmia) | | |
| AICD | Automatic implantable cardio-defibrillator (pacemaker) | CVA | Cerebrovascular accident (stroke) |
| ALS | Amyotrophic lateral sclerosis | CXR | Chest x-ray |
| AMA | Against medical advice | DM | Diabetes mellitus |
| Amyloid | Abnormal protein usually produced in bone marrow and can be deposited in any tissue or organ | DME | Durable medical equipment |
| | | DNR | Do not resuscitate |
| | | DOB | Date of birth |
| A/P | Anterior-posterior | DOE | Dyspnea on exertion |
| AROM | Active range of motion | Dx | Diagnosis |
| AVR | Aortic valve replacement | ED | Emergency department |
| B | Bilateral (both sides) | EEG | Electroencephalogram |
| BM | Bowel movement | EKG | Electrocardiogram |
| BP | Blood pressure | ENT | Ear, nose, and throat |
| BPH | Benign prostatic hypertrophy | ESRD | End stage renal disease |
| CA | Cancer | FTT | Failure to thrive |
| CABG | Coronary artery bypass graft | f/u | Follow-up |
| CAD | Coronary artery disease | Fx | Fracture |
| CHF | Congestive heart failure | GAD | Generalized anxiety disorder |
| CN | Cranial nerves (there are twelve) | GCS | Glasgow coma scale |
| COPD | Chronic obstructive pulmonary disease | GERD | Gastroesophageal reflux |
| COTA | Certified occupational therapy assistant | GYN | Gynecology |
| CPAP | Continuous positive airway pressure | HA | Headache |
| CPR | Cardiopulmonary resuscitation | HD | Hemodialysis |
| CRF or CKD | Chronic renal failure or chronic kidney disease | HEENT | Head, eyes, ear, nose, throat |

**TABLE 9.1**  Terms Associated With Aging-Related Physiological or Neurological Changes and Interventions —cont'd

| Term | Definition | Term | Definition |
|------|------------|------|------------|
| h/o | History of | PET | Positron emission tomography (used for cancer screenings and follow-up) |
| HR | Heart rate | | |
| HTN | Hypertension (high blood pressure) | PFM | Pelvic floor muscle rehabilitation |
| IADL | Instrumental activities of daily living | PID | Pelvic inflammatory disease |
| ICP | Intracranial pressure | PMH | Past medical history |
| ICU | Intensive care unit | PRBC | Packed red blood cells (used for a blood transfusion) |
| IDDM | Insulin-dependent diabetes mellitus | | |
| I&O | Intake and output | PRN | As often as necessary |
| IVC | Inferior vena cava | PROM | Passive range of motion |
| L | Left | PT | Physical therapy |
| LE | Lower extremity | PTCA | Percutaneous transvenous coronary angioplasty (balloon angioplasty) |
| LBP | Low back pain | | |
| LLQ | Left lower quadrant | | |
| LOC | Loss of consciousness | PUD | Peptic ulcer disease |
| LOS | Length of stay | PVD | Peripheral vascular disease |
| LUQ | Left upper quadrant | R | Right |
| MCA | Middle cerebral artery | RA | Rheumatoid arthritis |
| MD | Medical Doctor | RBC | Red blood cells |
| MET | Metabolic equivalent | RCA | Right coronary artery |
| MI | Myocardial infarction | REM | Rapid eye movement |
| MRI | Magnetic resonance imaging | RLQ | Right lower quadrant |
| MS | Multiple sclerosis | RN | Registered nurse |
| MSW | Master of Social Work | ROM | Range of motion |
| MVP | Mitral valve prolapse | RPE | Rate of perceived exertions |
| MVR | Mitral valve replacement | RT | Respiratory therapy |
| NIDDM | Noninsulin-dependent diabetes mellitus | RUQ | Right upper quadrant |
| NKA | No known allergies | SCI | Spinal cord injury |
| NOS | Not otherwise specified | SDH | Subdural hematoma |
| NPO | Nothing by mouth | SLP | Speech-language pathology or pathologist |
| NREM | Nonrapid eye movement | SOAP | Subjective, objective, assessment, plan |
| N & V | Nausea and vomiting | SOB | Shortness of breath |
| NWB | Non-weight, bearing | s/p | Status post (following a procedure) |
| $O_2$ | Oxygen | ST | Speech therapy |
| OA | Osteoarthritis | STD | Sexually transmitted disease |
| OB/GYN | Obstetric and gynecology | SW | Social worker |
| OOB | Out of bed | sx | Symptoms |
| OR | Operating room | TAH | Total abdominal hysterectomy |
| ORIF | Open reduction internal fixation (typically used in orthopedic patients; may consist of screws and nails to correct a bone fracture) | TB | Tuberculosis |
| | | TBI | Traumatic brain injury |
| | | THA | Total hip arthroplasty |
| | | THR | Total hip replacement |
| OT | Occupational therapy | TIA | Transient ischemic attack |
| PA | Physician's assistant | TKR | Total knee replacement |
| PAM | Physical agent modality | TMJ | Temporomandibular joint |
| PE | Pulmonary embolism (blood clot in the lung) | TURP | Transurethral resection of the prostate |
| PEG | Percutaneous endoscopic gastrostomy (typically put in patients if adequate nutritional intake not being obtained due to malnourishment or dysphagia) | UI | Urinary incontinence |
| | | UTI | Urinary tract infection |
| | | WBC | White blood cells |

## Assessment and Intervention Design Grounded in Models of Occupation, Theories, and the Occupational Therapy Practice Framework

The Occupational Therapy Practice Framework (OTPF) (American Occupational Therapy Association [AOTA], 2020a) directs an OT to integrate information from the OT evaluation with "theory, [occupation-based] practice models, frames of reference, and research evidence" (p. 28). Readers can refer to Chapter 4 Theoretical Models Relevant to Gerontological OT Practice for further information.

When working with older adults, OTs must use data-informed decisions, driven by evidence-based practice models to achieve optimal participation for their client. The growing body of literature points to how OT interventions support aging in place and continued well-being for the older adult (Clark et al., 2001; Fields et al., 2021; Leland et al., 2012). However, it is essential that OTs are also informed by theories from gerontology, about successful aging, and productive aging, to adapt interventions for this population. More research is needed on older adult outcomes that are based on occupation and participation, self-care, productivity (work and volunteer), and/or leisure with interventions targeting environmental, physical, socio-economic, cultural, psycho-emotional, and/or cognitive-neurological that reflect client factors (Law & McColl, 2010).

## Best Practices: Developing Therapeutic Rapport Using Approaches Such as Motivational Interviewing, Action-Planning, as a Means to Ensure Client-Centered Care

Using evidence-based treatment to guide clinical reasoning and decision-making framed by occupational-based practice models is vital for effective OT practice (AOTA, 2020a). Equally as critical, is the OT practitioner's (OTP's) understanding of how to support a client throughout the therapy process via therapeutic use of self, evidence-based methods to support client goal identification and achievement, and methods of collaborative client communication. The Intentional Relationship Model describes therapeutic use of self as "the extent to which one applies empathy and intentionality to an interpersonal knowledge base and corresponding skill set that can be applied thoughtfully" during interactions with clients (Taylor, 2020, p. 2). For older adults, empathy and rapport through a therapeutic use of self support open communication and collaboration with the OTP (AOTA, 2020a). This can help ensure that identified and prioritized goals are developed to achieve higher functional abilities and participation in meaningful daily activities.

Therapeutic interventions directed at aging in place or health management may require collaborating and identifying lifestyle changes. One evidence-based method an OT can use to collaboratively promote client behavior change is motivational interviewing (Hettema et al., 2005). Motivational interviewing can include action planning for clients with chronic conditions to achieve a lifestyle modification. Action planning (Lorig & Holman, 1993) is a strategy OTs can incorporate when working with older adult clients to adopt and maintain health behaviors into their daily routines. Action planning focuses on an intended action in terms of when, where, and how to act (Lorig & Holman, 1993). This technique is grounded in developing client self-efficacy for changing their health behaviors (Bandura et al., 1999). Action planning has strong evidence for supporting older adults in managing chronic conditions and adopting health management strategies (Ory et al., 2013). See further resources in the online resource section.

When working with older adults, therapeutic use of self and developing client self-efficacy through strategies of motivational interviewing are examples of how an OT can work to both strengthen the therapeutic relationship and achieve client-identified and prioritized goals. Readers may refer to Chapter 6; Approaches to Screening and Assessment in Gerontological Occupational Therapy and/or Chapter 15; Neurology and Cognition in Aging and Everyday Life, for further information.

## Considerations for Identifying and Addressing Sensory, Cognition, and Communication Impairments and Use of Health Literacy Assessment and Teach-Back Techniques

Importantly, for an older adult, impairments in cognition, receptive or expressive communication, or sensory function (e.g., hearing) can impact quality of care due to assessment errors and intervention barriers (Hemsley et al., 2012). Overarching each of the physiological and neurological conditions that older adults present with is the need to begin by assessing the individual's sensory, cognition, and communication status. The knowledge from each of these combined assessment data contributes to the development of best practice interprofessional interventions (Lande & Wanlass, 2015).

Populations with sensory, cognitive, and/or communication impairments require a multimodal approach. One of these is the use of Teach-Back. The Teach-Back, an evidence-based approach, matches client capacity with the delivery of important health information, allowing the person empowerment, comfort, and success in communicating with their OTP (Abrams et al., 2012). Teach-Back (see online resources) asks the client to recall information by restating information back to the health-care provider in their own words. This confirms the client's understanding of the OTP's communication and attends to issues of health literacy as well as cognitive and communication impairments (Abrams et al., 2012). The American Occupational Therapy Association recognizes that attending to a client's health literacy is critical to supporting their success in performing health-related activities of daily living (AOTA, 2020b). Maximizing comprehension of provider information further maximizes the client's ability for participation and shared decision-making (Jin, 2022).

## Understanding and Addressing the Impact of Environment, Context, and Social Determinants of Health Associated With Aging-Related Physiological and Neurological Function

There is a growing awareness of how social determinants of health (SDOH) impact physical and psychological health as either a support or a barrier to processes of healthy aging and impact function and quality-of-life outcomes producing many social inequities (Pega et al., 2017). Social inequities include economic, educational, health-care access, housing status, living environment, and social community context (Pega et al., 2017). Advanced medical treatments are allowing once-fatal diseases to be eliminated or managed, resulting in longer lifespans; however, this is not true for all due to factors related to SDOH (Artiga et al., 2020). For a more in-depth examination of these concerns, readers can refer to Chapters 2, 11, 12, 25, and 31.

## Integrating Interprofessional Collaboration and Communication for Best Practice Care and Improved Person-Centered Care Outcomes

There is indication of positive outcomes for interprofessional collaboration in treating older adults, but further studies are needed (Tsakitzidis et al., 2016). For example, while literature highlights the need for interprofessional collaboration, there is a scarcity of literature for interprofessional, collaboratively designed, validated and published, patient/client cognitive, communication and/or sensory assessments and interventions. Nash and Foidel (2019) state:

> By creating a holistic and interprofessional assessment system, care plans can be created that directly address individual ability and increase staff coordination of care. In addition, opportunities for regular staff education to increase understanding of cognitive domains and the impact impairment has on function can increase the quality of care. (p. 88)

For example, a patient/client's assessed need for mode and level of communication if initiated by the OT can then be strengthened by collaborating with the speech language pathologist (SLP) to consider additional assessment data (including a collaborative plan of care). A best practice example of interprofessional collaboration is presented in Case Example 9.1.

## The Physiological and Neurological Systems and Aging-Related Changes

### Cardiovascular and Cardiopulmonary System

Cardiac changes can be significant for the older adult and demand close attention by the OTP. Cardiac output typically decreases by 1% each year after age 50. Results of the physiological aging process include the following changes in the cardiovascular system:

- Cardiac muscles are more resistant to hormonal control, resulting in myocardial stiffness and reduced relaxation of the heart. This can lead to impairment in the cardiac

ventricle's ability to fill with blood during each cardiac cycle, reducing the amount of blood pumped effectively (and thus oxygen delivery) throughout the cardiovascular system.
- The prevalence of hypertension (HTN) increases the risk of cerebrovascular accident (CVA), coronary artery disease (CAD), and congestive heart failure (CHF). Each of these conditions can lead to increased morbidity and mortality in the aging adult.
- With aging, the presence of lipid-rich cholesterol plaque deposition in the blood vessels increases, resulting in atherosclerosis. These plaques lead to a thickening of the blood vessel walls, resulting in inflammation and obstructing blood flow and reducing oxygen delivery to surrounding tissues (Fig. 9.1).
- Aging increases the risk of amyloid protein deposition in the heart. This causes increased cardiac stiffness and inability for the ventricles to fill and results in CHF.

## Occupational Therapy Interventions Related to Cardiovascular and Cardiopulmonary Disease and Optimization of Cardiovascular and Cardiopulmonary Function

The differing aging-related cardiovascular disease sequelae include the psychological, physical, and functional effects that can be further complicated by loss or reduced functional cognition (Greaves et al., 2019) and/or communication and can greatly affect older adults' everyday living. Traditional OT cardiac interventions include conditioning programs and lifestyle management, such as energy conservation and work simplification that meet the patient/client-centric needs of these interventions (e.g., accounting for cultural differences, health literacy, and communication with and without cognitive impairment needs). However, research points to the need for clinicians to understand the many factors that may affect a client's quality of life (QOL), especially for their older patient/clients with CHF (Hopp et al., 2010) or other cardiovascular deficits. The findings suggest that psychosocial aspects and patient/client uncertainty about their prognosis are important components of QOL among CHF patients/clients (Hopp et al., 2010). Careful attention to contextual factors such as cultural values and beliefs, spirituality, temporal issues, family and other relationships, and feelings regarding work or avocational-related losses should be a component of the OT's collaborative treatment plan with the patient/client, in addition to traditional treatment approaches. Overarching each of the conditions that older adults present with is the need to begin by assessing the patient/client's sensory, cognition, and communication status. There are a number of interventions that OTs may use during treatment sessions to instruct the older adult who has cardiovascular disease and other conditions, as described in the next section. Interventions should match the patient/client's assessed sensory, cognitive, communication, and literacy/health-care literacy levels.

**CASE EXAMPLE 9.1**    Considerations for Identifying and Addressing Cognition and Communication

A 72-year-old African American woman post stroke was transferred to an inpatient rehabilitation facility with orders for OT and physical therapy (PT) evaluation and treatment. Patient/client presented with left upper extremity and lower limb weakness and apparent cognition and communication impairments. The master in social worker/ discharge planner gathered social/family/work history and discharge planning information to prepare the team. The discharge planner reported the patient/client lived alone but had frequent family visitors in a high-crime, extremely low socioeconomic area that limited independent mobility in her neighborhood. Patient/client completed a 6th grade education with a career history, primarily as a housekeeper. The hospital's standards of practice included clinician training on cultural competency and self-recognizing and self-correcting the impact of implicit bias as a means to support equitable clinical decision-making throughout the patient/client's course of care. This would include matching patient/client literacy levels during provider communication.

After the OT completed a full chart review and patient/client screening, she recommended medical doctor (MD) orders for a speech language pathologist (SLP), dietician, and pharmacist for further assessment and treatment. This interprofessional (collaborative) plan was used to better meet patient/client centric care. The SLP, OT, PT, and masters of social work (MSW) discussed initial patient/client sensory, cognitive, receptive, expressive, social communication, and literacy/health literacy assessments and further discussed cultural factors (e.g., use of assessments standardized to be inclusive of patient/client's culture, and ensuring cultural preferences were recognized and honored). Clinician recommendations and collaborative input were completed and decisions were finalized, for which members were to complete which of the ranges of assessments discussed. Each discipline's assessments and recommendations were well documented in the patient/client's chart. Intervention approaches at follow-up team huddles were completed early in the patient/client's stay and in subsequent team rounds.

Further functional assessments of patient/client physical deficits as related to function were included. All interventions were to include external cognitive cues. Further SLP input for collaboration and additional areas of cognitive and communication impairment were identified and discussed to further understand how interventions could better impact positive outcomes for the patient/client's functional activity. Interventions for patient/client safety and maximizing function were prioritized by patient/client input for occupational preferences. These tasks were reinforced by each discipline and patient/ client family education was completed by each discipline that reinforced external verbal and non-verbal cues for the patient/ client's performance and safety. The team ensured all communication during treatment and encounters with the patient/ client, matched her needs (e.g., sensory [hearing impairment; loudly speaking]) literacy (simple communications and confirming comprehension using teach-back methods), cognitive and communication levels (one to two step simply stated brief instructions, facilitative problem solving, visual and memory cues, chunking information, patient/client's return demonstration). The patient/client's needs were well documented for all care staff to read in the patient/client's chart and shared in team meetings. Use of patient/client return demonstration of comprehension both verbally and in all physical function tasks were emphasized to ensure that clinicians were meeting the patient's sensory, cognitive, communication, literacy, and physical function needs.

Further into the patient/client's stay when it was determined that the patient/client could return home with 24-hour family supervision, additional functional assessments were added by the OT, for example, medication management. After this assessment, the OT collaborated with the pharmacist in simplifying medication scheduling, medication packaging, and literacy needs for patient medication information strategies and needs. Patient/client family education began as soon as the patient's discharge destination was confirmed. Patient-family education included all strategies used by clinical teams to maximize patient function and ability to meet the complex sensory, cognitive, communication, literacy, and physical needs of the patient/client.

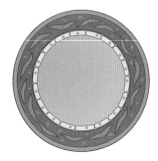

Normal arterial
lumen

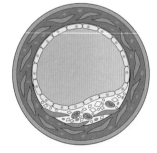

Atherosclerotic
plaque deposit

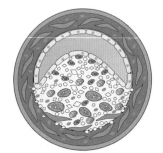

Advanced arterial
atherosclerotic
disease

**FIGURE 9.1**    Vascular Arterial Changes Associated With Aging. (From Frazier, M. S., & Drzymkowski, J. W. [2013]. *Essentials of human diseases and conditions* [5th ed.]. Elsevier.)

## Specific Client Focused Interventions

### Energy Conservation

Energy conservation involves the deliberate, planned management of one's energy through balancing rest and activity during times of high fatigue so that valued activities and goals can be maintained (Dreiling, 2009; Matuska et al., 2007). Basic energy conservation strategies incorporate scheduled rest, principles of ergonomics, and home and activity modifications. Educating clients to adjust their priorities by choosing how to spend energy, simplify activities so they require less energy, plan a balance of work and rest times, and change the time of day to do an activity are all part of the energy conservation approach used in OT (Dreiling, 2009). This approach requires close collaboration between the client and the therapist or OT assistant and detailed activity analysis (Fig. 9.2A and B).

### Work Simplification

Evidence-based practice has demonstrated that when affected clients combine work simplification with energy conservation approaches, there is greater benefit to the client (Matuska et al., 2007). Work simplification objectives aim to minimize waste of labor, increase the effectiveness of each activity, eliminate duplication, and prevent fatigue. Examples of work simplification strategies that can be incorporated into intervention approaches for clients with cardiovascular or cardiopulmonary disease include the following:

* Prioritize patient /client preference for activities or sports to determine recommended modifications or adaptations to meet patient/client occupational preferences.
* Replace heavy items with light ones (e.g., place larger quantity food goods into smaller and lighter containers, use lightweight cookware).
* Eliminate unnecessary motions (e.g., fold items in two rather than fourths).
* Use adaptive equipment to assist in activities (e.g., electric can opener, electric citrus juicer).
* Store supplies at the location where the task is performed (e.g., place often used dishware above/near dishwasher to ease return to cabinet shelf).
* Arrange the environment to minimize fatigue or extraneous motions (e.g., replace standing with sitting while performing tasks).
* Carefully plan necessary and desired weekly tasks to ensure that difficult tasks are not all done on the same day or successive days.

### Physical Conditioning

Conditioning programs focus on increasing strength and endurance. Many facilities have cardiac conditioning rehabilitation programs for patients/clients with any diagnosis of cardiopulmonary disease (Austermiller, 2012). Based on the evaluation of a patient/client's various risk factors, an OT can work with other professionals to help customize the appropriate program of exercise intensity. Home programs developed by the therapist need to consider the patient/client-centric needs for comprehending interventions that

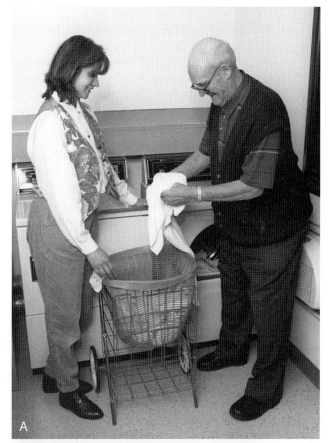

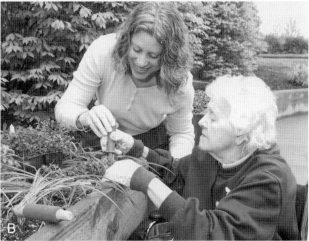

**FIGURE 9.2**   An occupational therapist observes elders practicing energy conservation (A) while doing laundry and (B) while gardening. (A, From Padilla, R., Byers-Connon, S., & Lohman, H. [2012]. *Occupational therapy with elders.* Mosby. B, From Byers-Connon, S., Lohman, H., & Padilla, R. [2004]. *Occupational therapy with elders.* Strategies for the COTA. [2nd ed.]. St. Louis: Mosby.)

reflect patient goals. Attending to health literacy concerns, therapeutic interventions need to be presented verbally and in written form that recognize the patient/client's needs in communication styles for patients/clients with and without cognitive impairment. Home programs may vary in complexity and include focusing on teaching clients to assess their physical response to exercise using the Borg Rate of Perceived Exertions Scale (RPE), (AOTA, 2020a; Williams,

2017) as well as heart-rate monitoring. As patients/clients increase their strength and functional endurance, their ability to perform functional tasks at higher values of metabolic equivalency (MET) is expected to increase. This increased functional capacity, in addition to lifestyle modifications, can provide increased physical participation potential for a patient/client with a cardiovascular or cardiopulmonary condition.

In summary, OTs should collaborate with the client to arrive at mutually agreed-upon goals that will work to improve performance of activities of daily living (ADLs) and instrumental activities of daily living (IADLs). The most common interventions used for patient/clients with cardiovascular or cardiopulmonary conditions include work simplification, energy conservation methods, stress management, and increased awareness of cardiopulmonary distress symptoms that are based upon the individual's medical status and risk factors (Hand et al., 2011; Štefanac, 2011). If unmet psychological needs of the patient/client, spouse/partner, or caregiver are identified during therapy, these should also be addressed by the OT, who may also refer to other providers for professional assistance. Refer to Chapter 17, Mental Health and Common Psychiatric Disorders Associated With Aging.

## Respiratory System

After age 20 when lung function peaks, age-related changes begin to occur in the respiratory system, resulting in a moderate, progressive decline in pulmonary function to varying individual degrees. Typical changes affect all aspects of the respiratory system, including the thoracic cavity, muscles of respiration, lung tissue, large and small airways, alveoli, pulmonary blood flow, and immune response (Fig. 9.3).

- After lung function peaks in early adulthood, vital capacity, the total volume of air that can be forcefully expelled from the lungs, decreases by an average of 26 mL/yr for men and 22 mL/yr for women. Total lung capacity, the volume of air that the lungs can hold during maximum inspiration typically stays the same throughout adulthood, whereas functional residual capacity (the amount of air left in the lungs after passive expiration) and residual volume (the amount of air left in the lungs after forceful expiration) typically increase with age. These changes, while they occur in a progressive nature during the physiologic aging process, are much more pronounced in lung conditions such as chronic obstructive pulmonary disease (COPD) (Cho & Stout-Delgado, 2020).
- Changes in the thoracic cavity structure that impact respiratory status include narrowing of the intervertebral disk spaces, causing kyphosis and curvature of the spine (Bartynski et al., 2005). Kyphosis results in a decreased anteroposterior diameter of the chest and overall smaller thoracic cavity. There is also an increased ossification of rib cartilage, resulting in less ability for movement of the thoracic cavity with inspiration and expiration. These changes lead to an overall less mobile and compliant chest wall and

can result in more difficulty moving air in and out of the lungs quickly (Lowery et al., 2013).

- Reduction in respiratory muscle fibers (accessory, anterior abdominal, diaphragm, and intercostals) results in diminished inspiratory and expiratory capacity and also impacts the ability to forcefully cough. These changes result in the individual's greater use of all respiratory muscles, especially the diaphragm, because breathing is more difficult. Greater reliance on the diaphragm fosters heightened sensitivity to changes in body position or comfort following a large meal. Decreased respiratory muscle strength when coupled with the thoracic cavity bony changes detailed above can also make it more difficult for clearance of foreign bodies or mucous from the airways and predispose to higher rates of infections, such as pneumonia (Lowery et al., 2013). Additionally, lack of respiratory muscle endurance can make it more challenging to meet oxygen needs during times of increased respiratory demand (e.g., exercise).
- Although bronchial structures are generally unchanged in the aging process, mucus production, necessary for coating the airways of the lungs, is reduced with aging. This adds to challenges in foreign body clearance and protection from virus and bacteria particles (Svartengran et al., 2005).
- The alveoli and underlying capillary network are responsible for gas exchange in the lungs and do not decrease in number with aging. However, changes in alveolar structure appear microscopically similar to the changes that occur in emphysema, and are known as "senile lung." Optimal gas exchange relies highly on elastic recoil of the alveoli and these become stiffer with less ability to recoil, resulting in closure of smaller airways during normal breathing and less surface area for gas exchange. Fortunately, an individual may lose a maximum of 20% of the alveolar surface area without resulting effects on respiratory function (Sinclair & Morley, 2012).
- Risk for aspiration increases with age, largely secondary to reduced cough reflex from diminished muscle strength and impairment in swallowing (e.g., dysphagia). This coupled with reduced mucous production and clearance of particles from the airway can result in aspiration pneumonia, which in some individuals, can be a recurring process.
- Respiratory infections (viral, bronchial, aspiration) may also increase in older adults due to decreases in immune system function in the airways. Poor oral hygiene can contribute to a decrease in the flow of saliva and promote the production of gram-negative bacilli in the oral cavity. These conditions foster greater susceptibility to lower respiratory tract infections such as bronchitis and pneumonia. Readers may refer to Chapter 13, Oral Health for Aging Adults, for further information.
- Antioxidant defenses in the respiratory system decrease with age and increase susceptibility to environmental toxins such as cigarette smoke and pollution (Sharma et al., 2009). Often these exposures are repeated throughout the lifecycle and repetitious exposure can lead to accumulated lung damage over time.

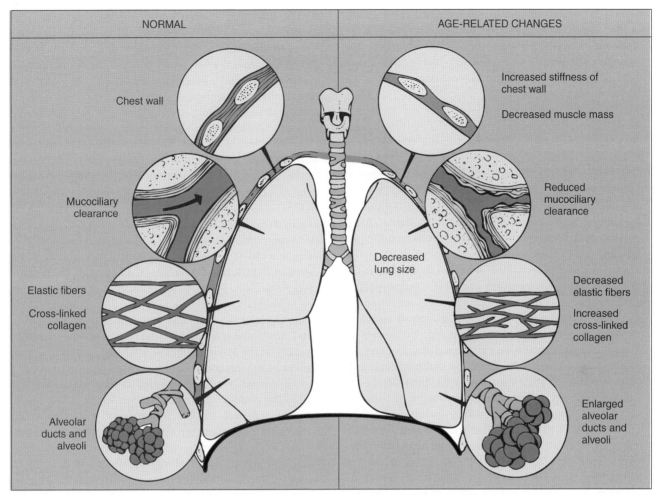

**FIGURE 9.3**  Respiratory System Changes Associated With Aging. (From Urden, L. D., Stacy, K. M., & Lough, M. E. [2015]. *Priorities in critical care nursing* [7th ed.]. Elsevier.)

- Causes that may additionally limit lung function include asthma, COPD with emphysema, chronic bronchitis, bronchiectasis, pulmonary fibrosis, immobility due to bed rest, obesity, smoking, and surgical procedures that include anesthesia and/or postoperative complications.

## Occupational Therapy Interventions Related to Respiratory System Dysfunction and Optimization of Respiratory Function

The role of OT in working with aging adults with pulmonary conditions will vary with the treatment setting, depending on individualized protocols. The following steps describe the basic process for assessment and intervention:

1. First, the OT should review the chart to determine with which pulmonary disease(s) the client has been diagnosed. This will determine: the most recent oxygen requirement including if oxygen is needed (note, these orders can frequently change due to improvement or decline in oxygenation ability); note other ongoing treatments that may impact therapy tolerance and endurance (e.g., radiation, chemotherapy, dialysis); and contraindications in particular activities (e.g., lying position precautions) (degrees of upright sitting may be required to discourage aspiration or difficulty breathing), ADL sessions that include showering (due to steam) or range of motion (ROM) (e.g., UE full extension and/or sustained above the head UE movements). Also important is attention to scheduling coordination with other therapies to maximize patient/client tolerance/participation and a review of medications and administration times that may impact therapy.

2. Next, overarching the conditions that older adults present with is the need to begin by assessing the patient/client's sensory, cognition, and communication status. Interventions should match the patient/client's sensory, cognitive, communication, as well as literacy/health-care literacy levels. The patient/client can be interviewed with the goal of understanding preferences and difficulties in activities performed at home and outside the home. It should be determined with the medical team/discharge planner if the patient/client will be using oxygen at home, and if so, what type of portable oxygen device is to be used. Intervention activities may include energy conservation instructions and demonstrations, where indicated, with expected $O_2$ equipment use; problem solving mobility-related issues for anticipated home activities; precautions for

$O_2$ use in the kitchen and bathroom; and fall prevention with $O_2$ use. If $O_2$ tubing will be used, to prevent falls determine length of tubing line and the need for visual enhancement (e.g., bright $O_2$ line/tube colors or color-taped stripes onto tube/line, especially for patients/clients with visual impairments).

3. Vital signs are very important to monitor, especially oxygen saturation and respiratory rate. The delivery modality of oxygen is also of concern, because this relates to the severity of the client's pulmonary disease and has a direct effect on the patient's cardiovascular and respiratory systems. Determination of the patient/client's severity depends on the presence of a ventilator, tracheostomy collar, oxygen mask, and nasal cannula—in that order. Blood pressure and heart rate are also important to monitor, particularly if the patient/client is under any stress.

4. Upper extremities should be evaluated for limitations in strength, endurance, sensation, and ROM. Communication with a pulmonologist and the patient/client are important to determine if UE upper range of motion or sustained elevated UE positions are contraindicated.

5. Patient-caregiver education on proper oral hygiene can reduce patient/client risk of infection that may contribute to production of gram-negative bacilli, fostering potential susceptibility to pneumonia, aspiration pneumonia, COPD, and lung cancer (especially in individuals who smoke tobacco), as was stated earlier. Compensatory techniques or adaptive equipment may facilitate patient/client effective self-care. This is especially important for persons whose long-term NPO (nothing by mouth, e.g., no liquids, no foods, no medication; thus, other means of nutrition, hydration, and medication administration are provided) status increases susceptibility to aspiration pneumonia. Patients/caregivers (in and out of hospital caregivers) need precautionary care instructions (e.g., avoiding too much liquid in the oral cavity during hygiene, removing residual oral liquid). Interprofessional collaboration with SLP (e.g., for beneficial positioning and community referrals and dental follow-up in further oral hygiene techniques may benefit the patient/client).

6. Reduce steam during showering by turning on an exhaust fan, opening the bathroom window, opening the bathroom door (if possible), taking brief showers, and using less hot water. Use a bath seat during showers to conserve energy and ensure that a shower caddy is within easy reach for shampoo, soap, and bathing accessories to reduce the risk of falls in standing.

7. OTs should observe clients in their typical activities, including walking, carrying capacity, ADL, and I/ADL. The client's symptoms are the most important indicator of pulmonary distress; therefore, always observe for shortness of breath (SOB), use of chest accessory muscles, cyanosis, respiratory rate, and depth of breathing before, during, and after therapy activities.

In pulmonary rehabilitation, the role of the OT is to assess and treat activity limitations associated with symptoms of COPD, including dyspnea and/or other similar pulmonary conditions (Anderson & Hennen, 2010). Goals are established to maximize the aging client's ability to participate in ADLs and IADLs, leisure activities, and vocational pursuits (Lorenzi et al., 2004; Maekura et al., 2015). Additional treatment areas focus on upper extremity strengthening, evaluation and need for adaptive equipment or modifications of activities, and education in stress management and relaxation techniques including deep breathing techniques. Moreover, work simplification and energy conservation, as described in the cardiopulmonary section, are also common components of a comprehensive treatment approach for clients with COPD.

Clients with pulmonary diseases often require supplemental oxygen during activity, and in more extreme conditions, there is a constant need for supplementation and close vigilance in monitoring this need, on the part of the therapist (Fig. 9.4). The OT should be aware of this need and monitor $O_2$ saturation levels via a pulse oximeter intermittently or during activities (Fig. 9.5). It is critical to be aware of the effect functional tasks have on the client's oxygen saturation; typically, if the levels fall below 90%, the activity is considered to be too strenuous for the client to perform. Educating the client and practicing controlled breathing techniques within the context of physical activity exertion is a recommended approach to OT intervention with clients who have COPD (Maekura et al., 2015). Controlled breathing techniques recognized as especially beneficial are diaphragmatic and pursed-lip breathing (Fig. 9.6A and B, Boxes 9.1 and 9.2). These techniques improve ventilation by releasing air that is trapped in the lungs, keeping the airways open longer, decreasing breathing demands, slowing the rate of breathing, relieving SOB, and fostering client relaxation (Yang et al., 2020).

A third technique that can improve ventilation, particularly in times of increased demand, is lower rib breathing. This is achieved by having the client apply her or his own hands on either side of the lower section of the rib cage during breathing. With each expiration, this applied force provides some tactile resistance that allows the ribs to expand during inspiration. Finally, relaxation techniques, such as progressive muscle relaxation, can be performed via a series of isometric contractions that are held for 7 to 10 seconds, followed by relaxation for 20 to 40 seconds.

Upper extremity muscle wasting also may accompany pulmonary diseases, resulting from disuse and the effects of prolonged steroid utilization (Cielen et al., 2014). A meta-analysis of randomized control trials on unsupported upper extremity exercise (UUEE) and its effect on dyspnea concluded that "UUEE can relieve dyspnea and arm fatigue in clients with COPD during ADLs." Pan et al. (2012) found that "unsupported upper extremity exercise can improve dyspnea and arm fatigue during ADL in patients/clients with COPD and should be included in physical rehabilitation programs" (p. 1524). Traditional OT approaches might incorporate upper extremity exercise through the use of

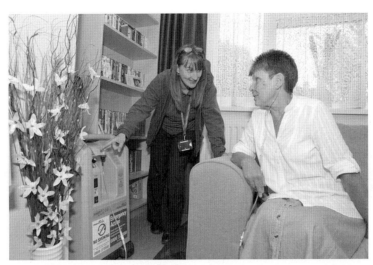

**FIGURE 9.4**   A Patient With Chronic Obstructive Pulmonary Disease at Home With Oxygen. (From Quint, M., Thomas, S., & Twose, P. [Eds.]. [2012]. *Cardiorespiratory assessment of the adult patient: A clinician's guide.* Churchill Livingstone.)

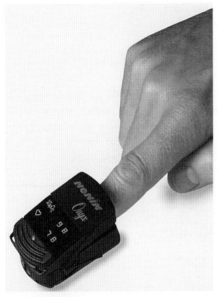

**FIGURE 9.5**   Pulse Oximeter Monitoring $O_2$ Saturation Levels. (Courtesy Nonin Medical, Plymouth, MN.)

free weights. Alternatively, the use of weights wrapped and attached to more distal joints (e.g., forearm) can be used if held weights due to stressing hand/wrist joint or tendons are contraindicated. TheraBand or other forms of progressive resistive exercises can be used, and again, adjustments for placement to reduce stress on distal joints may be indicated. This approach would require careful attention to the patient/ client's blood pressure, heart rate, breathing rate, and oxygen saturation levels, and if within the physician-prescribed parameters, upper extremity exercise is recommended and beneficial.

Energy conservation and work simplification strategies, as discussed in the cardiovascular section, are critical components of interventions with clients with COPD. Part of this approach would include evaluation of work sites, including the client's home, to determine the need for adaptive

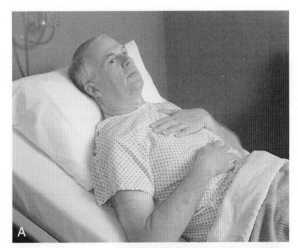

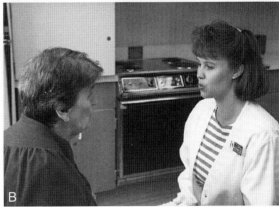

**FIGURE 9.6**   (A) Client practicing diaphragmatic breathing. (B) OT teaching pursed lip breathing. (From DeWit, S. C., & Williams, P. A. [2013]. *Fundamental concepts and skills for nursing* [4th ed.]. Saunders.)

equipment or environmental modifications. Finally, clients with COPD may benefit from stress management in conjunction with breathing technique instruction (Cafarella et al., 2012; Volpato et al., 2015). Using these techniques can help

---

**BOX 9.1** Steps in Teaching Diaphragmatic Breathing

Belly breathing, also called diaphragmatic breathing, is a breathing technique that helps individuals living with asthma or COPD when they experience shortness of breath.

- This technique helps to slow down your breathing so you can catch your breath and use less energy to breathe.
- When you feel short of breath, belly breathing helps get more oxygen into your lungs and calms you down so you can better control your breath.

To practice belly breathing, sit down in a comfortable chair, sit up straight and put your hands on your belly or if it's more comfortable you can lay down.

- Close your mouth and take a slow, deep breath in through your nose.
- When you breathe in, you want your belly to fill with air and get bigger like a balloon.
- Blow all of the air out slowly and gently through pursed lips as if you were blowing bubbles.

- Concentrate on your breathing as you continue to breathe in through your nose and out through your mouth.
- Repeat belly breathing for five to ten minutes and relax.
- Just remember to keep your hands on your belly, as it helps you to concentrate on the air going in and out.

The more you practice, the easier it will be to calm down and breathe more freely.

If you continue to be short of breath, call 911 and seek immediate medical attention.

For more breathing techniques and information on living with COPD, asthma, and other lung diseases visit the American Lung Association's website at Lung.org.

To watch a video on these instructions go to: https://www.lung.org/lung-health-diseases/lung-disease-lookup/copd/resource-library/belly-breathing-video

Adapted from Take a Deep Breath. (2009). Retrieved from http://www.health.harvard.edu/staying-healthy/take-a-deep-breath.

---

**BOX 9.2** Steps in Teaching Pursed Lip Breathing

Encourage the client to use this technique during parts of any strenuous activity (e.g., bending, lifting, stair climbing, walking more briskly, etc.), and instruct as follows:

- First, find a comfortable sitting position and relax your neck and shoulder muscles.
- Breathing normally, inhale slowly through your nose for two counts, keeping your mouth closed. It may help to count to yourself: inhale, one, two.

- Pucker (purse) your lips as if you were going to whistle or gently blow at a candle flame.
- Breathe out slowly and gently (exhale) through your pursed lips while counting to four. It may help to count to yourself: exhale, one, two, three, four.
- Practice this technique four to five times a day at first so you can get the correct breathing pattern; with regular practice, this breathing technique will seem natural to you.

Adapted from Asthma. (2015). Retrieved from http://www.lung.org/associations/states/minnesota/events-programs/mn-copd-coalition/patient-toolkit/coughingand-breathing.pdf and What to expect during pulmonary rehabilitation. (2015). Retrieved from http://www.nhlbi.nih.gov/health/health-topics/topics/pulreh/during.

---

the client relax and better manage the physical and physiologic changes that can occur during a stressful situation.

As for cardiovascular conditions, OT interventions with respiratory conditions should also generally include work simplification, energy conservation, and body mechanics strategies, such as the following:

1. Balance rest and work by allowing time to complete a task before becoming fatigued, and take frequent rest periods during activities.
2. Ensure adequate ventilation at home by turning on the exhaust fan when cooking, having windows open, and using portable fans during the summer in homes without air conditioning.
3. Prioritize all tasks to reduce demands on the respiratory muscles. Whenever possible, do not carry heavy objects; instead, slide them across the table or counter, use a multipocket apron, work in a sitting position, and have a cart on wheels to carry multiple items.
4. Shop by phone or online and use the related delivery services.
5. Avoid reaching or extended reaching and overhead movements by pre-arranging items that are frequently needed (e.g., arrange lighter objects in high cabinets).
6. Use equipment with long handles for dustpans, sponges, squeegees, or any home care product (but avoid use of long handles that require overhead, sustained positioning of the upper extremities).
7. Reduce steam during showering by turning on an exhaust fan, opening the bathroom window, opening the bathroom door (if possible), taking short showers, using cooler water as tolerated, and running cold water before the hot water is turned on.
8. Use a bath seat during showers to conserve energy and a shower caddy within easy reach for shampoo, soap, and accessories (Fig. 9.7).
9. Avoid spray cleaners or powdered harsh chemicals, which may irritate bronchial airways (avoid cleaning personnel use of these as well, for example, steam in shower will cause breathing in of these evaporating chemicals if used on floor and walls of shower).

10. To support lung function, exhale when bending or flexing at the trunk. This includes avoiding holding one's breath upon exertion or exercising.
11. Wear loose clothes that allow the chest and abdomen to expand, and dress legs and feet first, because this requires the most energy.
12. Use long-handled dressing equipment, such as a dressing stick, long-handle shoehorn, and/or long-handle reacher, to conserve energy and prevent exhaustion during an activity/ADL (Fig. 9.8).
13. Keep one's hairstyle simple to reduce energy expenditure. Rest elbow on higher counter surface when brushing hair or using a hairdryer to support upper extremity and lessen workload.

All of these recommendations clarify a number of ways that aging clients can be taught to simplify their lifestyle when they have respiratory diseases.

## Genitourinary System

As the proportion of older adults in the population increases, there has been an increase in the number of age-related renal impairment diagnosis (Hommos et al., 2017). This is additionally true of other diseases of the genitourinary system, which compromises the kidneys, ureters, bladder, urethra, and genital organs. The following list describes normal aging-related changes in genitourinary system structures and functions:

- Kidneys decrease in volume, size, and develop diminished adaptability to injury and toxicities. There is also an increased propensity to develop renal cysts, which disturb the architecture of the kidney surface (Hommos et al., 2017).

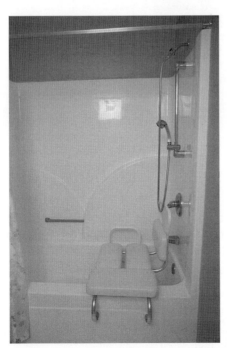

**FIGURE 9.7**  Shower bench, handheld shower head, and grab bar assist the weak patient. (From Monahan, F. D., Sands, J. K., Neighbors, M., Marek, J. F., & Green, C. J. [2007]. *Phipps' medical-surgical nursing: Health and illness perspectives* [8th ed.]. Mosby.)

- Nephrons and tubules, which are the basic filtering unit in the kidney, decrease in number, size, and function, and the concentrating and diluting abilities of the kidneys are reduced (O'Sullivan et al., 2017). These changes may promote renal failure, especially in older adults with hypertension, diabetes mellitus, and dehydration. The reduced filtering capabilities also can result in reduced ability to filter out toxins or medication byproducts from the blood, leading to an increase in potential medication adverse side effects.
- The prevalence of chronic kidney disease (CKD) markedly increases with age and nearly 50% of those over 70 years of age meet the criteria of CKD. The majority of these cases represent the slow decline in renal function seen with "healthy" aging and do not represent pathologic disease (Coresh et al., 2007).
- The bladder muscle weakens, and holding urine for an extended time without voiding becomes more difficult. Younger individuals have an average bladder capacity of 500 to 600 mL, while those older than 65 have a reduced bladder capacity as small as 250 mL. Typically, younger adults have a sensation to void when the bladder is more than half full, but older adults may have a reduced fullness sensation, resulting in sensing the bladder much later when the bladder is nearly full, or not sensing fullness at all, leading to unexpected incontinence.
- Nocturia, defined as the need to get up out of bed overnight to urinate, is often one of the most bothersome of the urinary symptoms that can occur with age. One in three older adults urinate overnight at least twice, causing significant disturbances in sleep, reduced quality of life, and putting them at risk for nocturnal falls (Leslie et al., 2021).
- Many older adults experience symptoms related to overactive bladder syndrome (OAB). These symptoms include heightened urinary urgency and frequency, nocturia, and urge incontinence. The etiology of OAB is often multifactorial, resulting from changes in the bladder or pelvic floor muscles and nervous system innervating the genitourinary system with contributions from comorbidities such as diabetes mellitus, congestive heart failure, and lower extremity edema. Medications used to manage these chronic conditions may also predispose to incontinence (e.g., diuretics).
- Stress incontinence is the involuntary leakage of urine associated with coughing, sneezing, or physical exertion. Two mechanisms are thought to be responsible for symptoms in this condition. The first is loss of bladder neck and urethral support from surrounding pelvic floor musculature and the second is weakness of the urinary sphincter itself (Aoki et al., 2017).
- While in women, pelvic floor and bladder musculature dysfunction causes the majority of urinary incontinence, in men, incontinence is typically related to prostatic enlargement or treatment of prostate cancer. The prostate, which is a gland surrounding the urethra in males, frequently enlarges with age, causing urethral and bladder

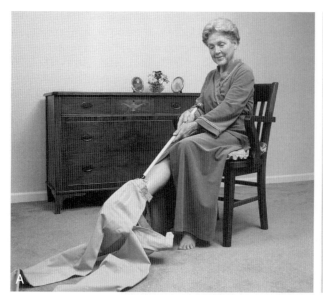
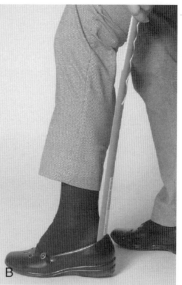
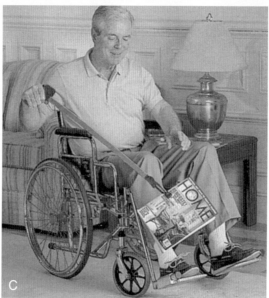

**FIGURE 9.8**    Collapsible dressing stick (A), long shoe horn (B), and long-handled reacher (C). (A, Courtesy North Coast Medical Inc., B, From Daley, T., Cristian, A., & Fitzpatrick, M. The role of occupational therapy in the care of the older adult. *Clinics in Geriatric Medicine*, 22[2], 281–290. C, From Monahan, F. D., Sands, J. K., Neighbors, M., Marek, J. F., & Green, C. J. [2007]. *Phipps' medical-surgical nursing: Health and illness perspectives* [8th ed.]. Mosby.)

outlet compression. This may lead to urinary retention and overflow incontinence from elevated pressures in the bladder. Men aged 80 and over have a more than 90% chance of developing benign prostatic hyperplasia (BPH). In those who had been treated for prostate cancer, the frequency of incontinence is high owing to either the absence of the prostate gland (prostatectomy) or shrinkage/scarring of the gland (radiation therapy).

- With age, the external and internal genitalia atrophy in males and females leading to:
  - Diminished vaginal secretions and lubrication, thinning, more friable vaginal tissue, delayed sexual arousal, and more difficulty with orgasm in females.
  - Males can experience delay in achieving erection, difficulty maintaining erection, and delayed ejaculation.

- Both sexes may additionally experience changes (usually a decrease) in libido with age.

## Occupational Therapy Interventions Related to Genitourinary System Dysfunction and Optimization of Genitourinary Function

Overarching each of the conditions that older adults present with is the need to begin by assessing the patient/client's sensory, cognition, and communication status. Recall from earlier discussion that interventions need to match the patient/client's sensory, cognitive, communication, as well as literacy/health-care literacy levels. During initial evaluations with older adult clients, OTs should routinely include sexuality/sexual function and participation within an ADL/IADL assessment. Inclusion of this topic will allow for timely discussion, should the aging adult have questions or concerns. As with any other adult age group, OTs can discreetly adapt client sexual participation approaches according to individual physical abilities and preferences. The patient/client's cultural, psychological, and personal preferences in comfort level of discussing sexuality with same sex or non-same sex OTs should be considered to meet the patient/client's preferences. Clinicians who may be untrained in this area should seek additional training to adopt effective strategies with older adults to provide a supportive environment that minimizes anxiety or discomfort for optimal OT strategies to meet their patient/clients' needs (Bauer et al., 2016).

The myth that incontinence is a part of normal aging can prevent older adults from seeking treatment for this treatable condition (Horrocks et al., 2004). OTs who have specialized or advanced training in evaluating and providing interventions for urinary incontinence and pelvic floor disorders are valuable in addressing these treatable diagnoses. The occupational therapist provides a functional assessment and interviews the client or caregiver about the habits, routines, and behaviors of the client to analyze what factors may contribute to the etiology of the incontinence. The context in which the incontinence occurs is examined, as well as activity demands, to facilitate thorough inclusion of essential factors for a client-centered approach and a comprehensive evaluation. Occupational therapists with advanced training may be able to carry out a physician's order for a pelvic floor muscle (PFM) assessment to determine the cause of the incontinence.

A physician-ordered assessment of the strength, tone, isolation, and coordination of the pelvic floor muscles may be conducted. If ordered and indicated, the OT instructs the client in strength, endurance, and PFM coordination and relaxation as well as inhibition of problematic motor responses. Another technique that may be included is electromyography (EMG), or biofeedback, in addition to a home exercise program, if the individual is seen as an outpatient. For successful continence, the client can be instructed to concentrate on decreasing times between toileting, thus using behavioral skills to avoid rushing to the toilet. Bladder training has been documented to reduce incontinence by at least 50%. These techniques may include increasing bladder storage capacity and changing behaviors or habits to extend the client's ability to resist voiding immediately, spreading the demand over a longer period. Other individuals may need to be educated to void more often, due to a larger-than-normal bladder, through the use of timed toileting techniques (self-cuing methods to ensure the toilet is used at specific intervals during waking hours) (Balk et al., 2019; Erderm & Chu, 2006; Neuman et al., 2009; Shamliyan et al., 2008). Case Example 9.2 demonstrates an OT approach to urinary incontinence/overactive bladder.

## Gastrointestinal System

As with other body systems, changes in the gastrointestinal (GI) system are common within the physiologic aging continuum. These include alterations in esophageal and colonic motility, nutrient absorption, GI immunity, and changes in the oral cavity (Bhutto & Morley, 2008). The following are typical aging-related changes:

- Changes in the oral cavity, including the teeth, soft tissues, salivary glands, mandible, and taste buds, can affect physical appearance, appetite, nutritional intake, and swallowing function. One of the most common complaints regarding the oral cavity is dry mouth due to decreased saliva production. This can be exacerbated by common medications, particularly those with anticholinergic effects (Nagler & Hershkovich, 2005). Tooth decay and loss and/or ill-fitting dentures can result in impairment in mastication and decreased oral intake. Dietary modification, i.e., pureed or soft foods, may promote more comfortable and improved nutritional intake. (Readers may refer to Chapter 13, Oral Health for Aging Adults for further information)
- Dysgeusia, (altered taste), and ageusia, (lack of taste) are not uncommon in older adults and can cause a diminished appetite and weight loss. These are often secondary to medication side effects and may resolve when the offending medication is stopped (Jain & Pitchumoni, 2009).
- Oropharyngeal dysphagia, which is difficulty swallowing, becomes more common with age and certain comorbidities (i.e., Parkinson disease, stroke, dementia). It may result in difficulty initiating the swallowing reflex or the sensation that food is stuck in the throat or esophagus and increases the risk of malnutrition, dehydration, aspiration, and aspiration pneumonia (Wirth et al., 2016).
- The aging process can lead to decreased peristalsis within the musculature of the esophagus and diminished esophageal sphincter tone, resulting in delayed esophageal emptying and increased propensity for gastroesophageal reflux and aspiration of stomach contents (Grande et al., 1991)
- In the stomach, diminished acid production caused by atrophic gastritis can lead to anemia, malabsorption of essential nutrients (i.e., impaired calcium absorption and subsequent osteoporosis), and increased risk of gastric cancer (Dumic et al., 2019). Older adults are often more susceptible to the development of peptic ulcer disease and ulcer formation because of sub-par gastric and intestinal mucosal repair mechanisms and also medications (i.e., nonsteroidal antiinflammatory drugs) (Lanas & Chang, 2017).
- In the small intestine, there are few differences in nutrient absorption and small bowel motility between the younger and older age groups. However, certain diseases such as celiac disease, an autoimmune disorder that affects absorption and causes sensitivity to the dietary protein gluten, and diseases that affect blood flow to the bowels (i.e., mesenteric ischemia caused by atherosclerosis) are more likely to occur in older adults (Karkkainen et al., 2015). Older adults are also more likely to experience bleeding from their GI tract, usually resulting from angiodysplasias in the intestines (Lewis, 2000).
- Changes in the large intestine include a slower transit rate, decreased anal sphincter tone and strength, and

**CASE EXAMPLE 9.2**    Urinary Incontinence/Overactive Bladder

Irene is a 72-year-old woman who was referred to occupational therapy for bladder urgency, urinary frequency, and urinary incontinence (UI). In the months before her referral her symptoms had gradually worsened, and her fear of having an incontinent episode in public had caused her to become homebound. Irene also had constipation, which affected her quality of life and contributed to her UI. The occupational therapist assessed the patient/client's cognitive and communication status to determine how best to meet the patient/client's literacy/health literacy, cognitive and communication needs during the occupational therapist's (OT's) interventions. The therapist educated Irene on the role of diet's impact on incontinence by using simple words and pictures (to match the assessed needs of the patient/client) resulting in evident patient/client comprehension. The OT suggested that she reduce her caffeine intake to reduce involuntary bladder contractions/urges and increase her dietary fiber to avoid episodes of constipation. It was also recommended that she keep a daily chart to better recall success or need for further adjustment of this intervention. Pelvic floor muscle reeducation was provided using teach-back verification of the patient/client's comprehension. Irene noticed that by reducing the amount of caffeine her urgency to void urine decreased. Also, as Irene gained better control of her pelvic floor muscles, she was taught how to inhibit bladder urges, particularly when she was out in the community when shopping, socializing with friends, attending church, or participating in other activities. Irene was encouraged to set her cellular phone alarm to facilitate her recall when using timed toileting to ensure she did not over fill her bladder. Irene was instructed to prior to outings, locate "public toilets" or businesses where the use of a public toilet was acceptable to compliment her timed toileting schedule. She was also taught how to relax her pelvic floor muscles during a bowel movement. Over the course of therapy, Irene's bowel patterns became more regular and she was able to control her bladder urges, significantly reducing her urinary frequency and incontinence. As Irene's bladder control improved, she had the confidence to resume public speaking engagements, volunteer work, social visiting, and shopping on a more regular basis and engage in other activities that were meaningful to her quality of life. Also important to her overall health status and well-being, she was able to resume her twice-weekly exercise group without urinary leakage.

less rectal compliance. These factors may lead to chronic constipation and diverticulosis, which is characterized by outpouchings in the colonic wall. Diverticulitis can occur if fecal material becomes trapped in these pouches and causes a risk of severe infection, abscess formation, and bowel perforation. Constipation is a common complaint in older individuals and can have a prevalence of up to 40% (Talley et al., 1996). Risk factors include reduced mobility, cognitive impairment, dietary changes, poor hydration, and polypharmacy (particularly anticholinergic and opioid medications) used to treat multiple medical comorbidities. Fecal incontinence may also occur because of diminished rectal sensation and tone and is one of the most psychologically traumatic experiences in older adults.

- Changes are seen in the pancreas, liver, and gallbladder throughout the physiologic aging continuum. In general, organ weights decline with age due to fatty and fibrous tissue infiltration and this can often result in an overall decline in organ function (Sawabe et al., 2006). In the pancreas, this can manifest as a reduction in the number of insulin-producing cells and lead to the development of diabetes mellitus (Matsuda, 2018). In the liver, there is less recovery with exposures to toxins (i.e., alcohol), and increased susceptibility to fatty deposits (i.e., fatty liver) and scaring (i.e., liver fibrosis); all of which can reduce the liver's ability to metabolize drugs, produce bile, and synthesize necessary proteins (Durazzo et al., 2019).
- The prevalence of cancers of the GI tract—esophageal, gastric, colon, rectal, pancreatic, and gallbladder all increase with age.

## Occupational Therapy Interventions Related to Gastrointestinal System Dysfunction and Optimization of Gastrointestinal Function

Overarching each of the conditions that older adults present with is the need to begin by assessing the patient/client's sensory, cognition, and communication status. OTs may use a similar approach with patient/clients with GI dysfunction as for individuals with symptoms of bowel incontinence as for patient/clients with urinary incontinence (see earlier example), always individualizing the approach to meet the individual patient/client's needs matching the patient/client's sensory, cognitive, communication, as well as literacy/health-care literacy levels.

Interprofessional collaboration (e.g., SLP and/or dietician) can meet the goals of the patient/client via training that facilitates safe eating and swallowing needs for verbal cuing (e.g., chin tuck when swallowing) and oversight of food and liquid consistency during meal preparations. If common comorbidities (e.g., Parkinson disease, stroke, dementia) affect cognition and communication, then caregiver training in safe food is indicated.

## Endocrine System

The basic function of the endocrine system, comprising both endocrine and exocrine glands, is to produce and secrete hormones. Endocrine glands secrete hormones directly into the bloodstream and include the hypothalamus, pituitary, pineal, adrenals, thyroid, parathyroid, ovaries, testicles, and pancreas. Exocrine glands secrete their products through a duct and include salivary, sweat, mammary, lacrimal, sebaceous, and prostate glands. The liver and pancreas function as both endocrine and exocrine glands, as they secrete some substances directly into the bloodstream and some into the GI tract via a ductal system. In general, the endocrine system is regulated by a series of complex hormone feedback loops. Most of these feedback loops originate in the hypothalamus and/or pituitary gland. Within the aging continuum in general, there is diminished secretion of hormones from glands as well as decreased responsiveness to the hormones secreted. Many endocrine functions are so intertwined that reduced function in one gland greatly affects another. Aging-related changes also include the following:

- Diabetes mellitus (DM): DM results from diminished pancreatic insulin production or peripheral insulin insensitivity. It is highly prevalent in the aging population and occurs in approximately 33% of adults over age 65 (Menke et al., 2015).
- Growth hormone (GH): GH is released by the pituitary gland in response to growth hormone releasing hormone (GnRH) secreted by the hypothalamus and binds to receptors in bone, muscle, adipose tissue and liver to stimulate cellular growth, reproduction and regeneration (Bartke et al., 2021). There is a rapid increase in GH during puberty, leading to a period of rapid growth and sexual maturation. After age 30, GH production declines by approximately 15% per decade, termed "somatopause." This decline results in decreased lean body mass and bone density and increased fat mass (Cummings & Merriam, 1999).
- Thyroid-stimulating hormone (TSH): TSH is produced by the pituitary gland in response to thyrotropin-releasing hormone (TRH) secreted by the hypothalamus and stimulates the thyroid gland to release thyroid hormones. Hyperthyroidism occurs when too much thyroid hormone is released into the blood, whereas hypothyroidism occurs when too little thyroid hormone is released. The incidence of hypo and hyperthyroidism increases with age and can result in other comorbidities (i.e., atrial fibrillation, elevated cholesterol, cardiovascular disease, and osteoporosis) when left untreated (Gauthier et al., 2020).
- Gonadotrophic hormones: These hormones are considered to be "sex hormones" and regulate ovarian and testicular function. GnRH is secreted by the hypothalamus and binds to receptors on the pituitary, resulting in the release of follicle stimulating hormone (FSH) and luteinizing hormone (LH). LH and FSH act on the ovaries and testes to regulate the production of estrogen and testosterone. While we think often of estrogen as a purely female hormone and testosterone as a purely male hormone, it is important to note that both of these hormones are produced in both sexes and can be affected by the aging continuum. Decreased levels of testosterone, also known as "andropause," can result in an increase in body fat mass, depression, erectile dysfunction, loss of libido, and higher risks of adverse cardiovascular events. Diminished estrogen production, also termed "menopause," can lead to a decline in skeletal mass and density (osteoporosis), atrophy of vaginal and surrounding tissues, loss of libido, and can increase the risk of skeletal fractures and adverse cardiovascular events (Chahal & Drake, 2007).

Steroid hormones: These include mineralocorticoids, glucocorticoids, and androgens, which are secreted by the adrenal glands in response to signals from the pituitary and hypothalamus. The main mineralocorticoid is aldosterone, and this regulates blood pressure and electrolyte balance. Glucocorticoid hormones include cortisone and cortisol, and these are primarily involved in the body's stress response and metabolism regulation. They are released in a cyclical manner throughout the day, also playing a role in the regulation of the body's natural circadian rhythm (Yiallouris et al., 2019). Additionally, the adrenal glands produce small amounts of sex hormones in concert with the ovaries and testes. Physiological aging produces small changes in steroid hormone secretion. There is often an increase in cortisol levels which may have an impact on the body's response to stress and also may have adverse effects on cognition (Ennis et al., 2017). Aging tends to result in a decrease in the production of adrenal sex hormones.

## Occupational Therapy Interventions Related to Endocrine System Dysfunction and Optimization of Endocrine Function

Overarching each of the conditions that older adults present with is the need to begin by assessing the patient/client's sensory, cognition, and communication status. When working with patients/clients with diabetes, OT personnel should be aware of the symptoms of hypoglycemia (low blood sugar level) and hyperglycemia (high blood sugar level).

*Hypoglycemia* can present with confusion, headache, lassitude, drowsiness, shallow respirations, tremulousness, anger, and nausea. To raise the blood sugar level, as soon as possible the individual should be given orange juice, candy, soda, a teaspoon of honey, or one ampule of D50 or glucagon, if seen in a hospital setting. *Hyperglycemia* can present with fast and deep breathing, heartburn, excessive thirst and urination, nausea, headaches, blurred vision, constipation, and abdominal pain, and coma in diabetic ketoacidosis. If OT personnel observe symptoms of either hypoglycemia or hyperglycemia during a therapy session, these should be orally reported to the medical team, so that appropriate and immediate action can be taken.

While working with persons who are diabetic, it is important to avoid any likelihood of injuries, because individuals with this diagnosis are more prone to infection and ulcers. For those who receive insulin injections at sites where they are receiving OT, the insulin may metabolize faster and the patient/client can develop hyperglycemia. Patient/clients with diabetes can also develop hypoglycemia after a therapy session if all the glucose is utilized during the session. OT staff should review each patient/client's chart for the values of a patient/client's recent blood-glucose level (accuchecks) and times of insulin or relevant medication administration (Box 9.3). It is also important to note the time of the patient/client's last meal or snack, as a missed meal may lead to hypoglycemia during an OT session.

Finally, as previously indicated, OTPs, by matching the patient/client's sensory, cognitive, communication, as well as literacy/health-care literacy levels, can educate on energy conservation, work simplification, and time management, based upon the individual's priority activities. Note, further information is available in Chapter 7, Occupational Therapy Intervention Process With Aging Adults.

## Integumentary System

The skin is the largest organ system in the human body. Composed of three layers (epidermis, dermis, and hypodermis), it serves as a barrier to the outside environment, including microorganisms, water, sun, and chemical or physical trauma. It is also crucial for temperature regulation and has both endocrine and exocrine functions. Generally, more than any other organ system, the skin reflects the aging process. Changes in the hair, skin, and nails are typically apparent in aging adults. In general, in the skin, there is wrinkling, loss of elasticity, laxity and an overall rougher skin texture (Zhang & Duan, 2018). There are several intrinsic and extrinsic factors that influence the rate and degrees of skin changes that occur within each individual. Intrinsic factors reflect genetic influences on aging and are often less modifiable, whereas extrinsic factors reflect environmental influences (i.e., sun exposure) and lifestyle habits (i.e., smoking). *Photoaging* is a term referring to changes in the skin seen from cumulative effects of sun exposure and is perhaps the most modifiable factor determining the degree to which the skin ages (Baumann, 2007). Interestingly, 80% of facial aging is thought to be secondary to chronic sun exposure (Uitto, 1997). The following list is a summary of aging-related skin changes that may influence occupational performance and overall well-being.

Epidermis: This is the outermost layer of the skin and provides the majority of protection against the outside environment.
- Keratinocytes, which are the most prominent cells in the epidermis, atrophy with age. This can lead to excess water loss from the skin, resulting in dryer skin and potentially contributing to the increased susceptibility to dehydration that is seen in older adults (Wilhelm et al., 1991).
- The overall turnover rate of epidermal cells declines 30% to 50% by age 80, which results in slower and less efficient wound healing (Yaar & Gilchrest, 1999).

Dermis: This is the middle layer in the skin and is sandwiched between the epidermis and hypodermis. The dermis contains blood vessels, nerves, glands, hair follicles, and connective tissues such as collagen. This layer thins with age due primarily to reduced collagen production, fostering fine and coarse wrinkles, and reduced skin elasticity.

Glands: These represent the exocrine function of the skin and are necessary for the production of sweat and sebaceous material. During the physiologic aging process, production from these glands decreases. Diminished sweat production alters thermoregulation and makes it more difficult to dissipate heat when overheating occurs.

---

**BOX 9.3    Intervention Tips for Clients With Diabetes Mellitus**

1. Encourage the client to monitor his or her blood sugar before and after exercise or any strenuous activity. If there are any symptoms of hyperglycemia or hypoglycemia, the client should check his or her blood sugar or obtain medical assistance.
2. Assist in insulin regulation and glucose control by increasing the client's strength, endurance, range of motion, and activity tolerance.
3. Provide aerobic exercise programming and graded upper extremity occupation-based activities that are meaningful to the client.
4. A client with a below-the-knee amputation as a result of diabetes should be reassured that she or he will receive a posterior knee conformer as soon as possible to minimize potential joint contractures.
5. Teach clients the importance of personal monitoring of the following:
   a. Check for sensory problems (e.g., changes in/decreased sensation), especially in the lower extremities.
   b. Inspect feet daily with a mirror; any cuts, abrasions, or openings should be reported for immediate medical attention. Until the client sees a health-care provider, the client should apply triple antibiotic ointment and dry dressings.
   c. Wash feet daily in warm water, do not walk barefooted, use socks with no holes, and change socks daily.
   d. Keep toenails trimmed straight across; do not cut calluses or corns.
6. Clients may benefit from specially made shoes to prevent diabetic ulcers. Clients should wear wide-fitted shoes, and break in new shoes slowly.
7. Clients should be taught diabetic-related safety factors regarding the use of a stove and the importance of maintaining the water temperature not higher than 110 degrees, to prevent burns.
8. Ensure that any diet-related instructions are provided to client.

From Millsap, P. (2007). Neurological system. In A. Linton & H. Lach (Eds.), *Matteson & McConnell's gerontological nursing: Concepts and practice* (pp. 406–412). Saunders Elsevier.

Hypodermis: The hypodermis is the innermost layer of skin and comprises subcutaneous tissues, primarily adipose tissues, as well as some hair follicles, neurons, and blood vessels (Yousef et al., 2022). This adipose tissue thins markedly with age and antimicrobial protection by the adipose layer is significantly reduced. A thinner adipose layer also contributes to more difficulty with thermoregulation.

Hair: During the aging process, hair follicles become less dense and smaller in size, resulting in an overall thinner appearance (Williams et al., 2021). A reduction in the function and number of pigment producing cells in the hair follicles (melanocytes) leads to loss of color and the hair shafts turn gray or white (Tobin, 2008).

Nails: With aging, nail growth tends to slow and nails become more brittle, leading to splitting or fissuring along the length of the nail. The color of the nail plate changes and can result in yellowing or grayish nails (Abdullah & Obbas, 2011). Fungal infections of the nail, known as onychomycosis, are common in older adults and can exacerbate physiologic nail changes and result in nail disfiguration.

## Occupational Therapy Interventions Related to Integumentary System Dysfunction and Optimization of Integumentary Function

OT staff working with aging adults can encourage their patients/clients to take measures to alleviate skin-related problems. Overarching each of the conditions that older adults present with is the need to begin by assessing the patient/client's sensory, cognition, and communication status.

Patients/clients with diabetes are especially at risk for consequences of skin integrity issues. Strategies to improve skin dryness and itching include patient/caregiver education for reducing frequency of bathing (except genital areas and feet), if indicated (identification of harsh soap products causing excess dryness), using non-irritating lotions and emollients, applying lubricants to moisten lips, and taking protective measures when environmental exposure is likely (e.g., excessive home heating, inadequate humidity [Payne, 2020]). Use of adaptive equipment (e.g., long handled sponge) may be indicated to improve access to the lower body. Finally, if encouraging hydration is not contraindicated due to other medical conditions, then patient/caregiver education may include aging effects in lack of thirst. Interventions may include achieving adequate fluid intake with visual reminders (e.g., setting up a daily pitcher of water in the morning to visually remind and gauge water consumed).

## Musculoskeletal System

The extent to which the musculoskeletal system ages, either pathologically or physiologically, can greatly impact function, mobility, and quality of life (Roberts et al., 2016). The following is a list of aging-related changes that occur in bones, muscle, and cartilage, and the impact these changes may have on the older adult.

Bone: Throughout the normal lifecycle, the bony skeleton is constantly being broken down and remodeled by osteoclasts and osteoblasts (i.e., the basic cells responsible for bone remodeling). During the aging process, this delicate balance can shift toward more bone breakdown by osteoclasts and less bone formation by osteoblasts, resulting in osteoporosis (Armas et al., 2012). Bone remodeling is highly influenced by several different hormones produced from the endocrine system (see section above). Estrogen in particular has a significant impact on bone turnover and diminished estrogen production after menopause results in over-stimulation of osteoclastic activity and bone breakdown, while it has less effect on stimulating osteoblastic activity and bone formation. Reduced bone mass and strength predisposes a person to an increased risk of fractures, and fractures at older ages contribute to high rates of morbidity and mortality. For example, hip fractures are independently linked to increased rates of loss of function, loss of mobility, institutionalization, depression, and overall decreased quality of life. (Gilboa et al., 2022). The 1-year mortality of a hip fracture in older adults is as high as 25% in women and 35% in men (Brauer et al., 2009) with even higher rates of loss of independence post-fracture. Healthy bone aging is essential for preservation of independence and quality of life throughout the aging continuum.

Muscle: Sarcopenia, which refers to low muscle mass and loss of muscle function, is quite common in older adults (Bauer et al., 2019). It can be physiologic and associated with the normal aging process or pathologic and accelerated due to chronic comorbidities and/or low activity level. At the cellular level, muscle loss occurs because there is a decrease in muscle protein synthesis, reduced muscle cell repair/regeneration and damage to the small blood vessels that supply oxygen to muscles as well as damage to small fiber neurons that innervate muscles to contract. With age, endurance and strength typically decline, but it is important to note that resistance training and aerobic fitness can improve strength and endurance even at extreme ages (Siparsky et al., 2014).

Cartilage: Loss of cartilage in large synovial joints such as the hip, knees, and shoulders can result in osteoarthritis (OA). In these joints, cartilage facilitates bone movement, allowing bones to glide past one another. When cartilage loss occurs, there is loss of lubrication and more friction within the joint, resulting in diminished or painful range of motion (i.e., OA).

Note that Chapter 8, Musculoskeletal System Changes With Aging: Implications for Occupational Therapy, provides a comprehensive discussion of aging-related changes in the musculoskeletal system and related OT interventions. This chapter provides a supplemental discussion of topics that are pertinent to understanding physiologic aspects of aging in a comprehensive way.

## Occupational Therapy Interventions Related to Musculoskeletal System Dysfunction and Optimization of Musculoskeletal Function

Traditionally, OT will begin interventions for patients/clients with orthopedic issues with a comprehensive OT evaluation.

This would include an occupational profile and assessment of ROM, strength, hand and wrist function, skin changes, and the effects of any of these factors on performance of ADL/IADL. Overarching each of the conditions that older adults present with is the need to begin by assessing the patient/client's sensory, cognition and communication status, matching the patient/client's sensory, cognitive, communication status, as well as literacy/health-care literacy levels when educating the patient/caregiver.

In addition, special considerations should be taken during the initial session with the patient/client. These might include discussion and documentation of morning stiffness, if present, and its effects; percentages of "good days to bad days"; fatigue; and pain, both with and without activity and also with and without medication management. Initial documentation of the patient/client's reports in each of these areas can be useful in determining the effectiveness of intervention strategies and improvement or decline in quality of life. Other areas that should be discussed or visually evaluated by the therapist or assistant with the patient/client include:

- Body and extremity positioning at night and during leisure/work activities (e.g., placing a bed pillow between the patient/client's knees and ankles can better align hips, knees and decrease stress on the lower back); ergonomic assessment of the patient/client's "work station" can improve postural alignment
- Use and height of seats in typically used spaces at home and work (if this applies) to increase ease of sit-to-stand transfers using furniture feet blocks to elevate furniture, or using blankets or other material to elevate seat cushions, when indicated
- Amount of stair climbing required to access typically used environments (e.g., home, work; if this applies, and medical appointments)
- Typical use and heights of work surfaces to reduce neck, shoulder, back strain
- Quality of mattress and pillow (e.g., various conditions require different levels of mattress firmness that can be informed via interprofessional collaboration and patient/client preference; pillow(s) height need to be assessed for the patient/client's sleeping position preferences, shoulder/neck/head alignment for side lying versus back lying; also, hip alignment with or without a pillow between the patient/client's knees when side lying)
- Need for and access to public versus private transportation with interventions (e.g., prompting cards to inform and ease wayfinding) problem solving with the patient/client using local disability transportation options (if applicable)
- Current adaptive equipment and how it is being utilized

Immediate intervention strategies will be different within each realm of occupation for the patient/client, depending on the stage or process that the individual is currently experiencing. If the patient/client is in an inflammatory stage of arthritis, for example, he or she will present with swollen and painful periarticular or extra articular joints, making the need to reduce edema a priority (Fig. 9.9). Reduction of stressors and proper positioning during ADL/IADL participation

through incorporating adaptive strategies can help reduce pain and potential deformity development. Typically, orthotic management is a useful intervention at this stage. Orthoses for OA and rheumatoid arthritis (RA) are frequently used to decrease pain, minimize deformities, decrease inflammation, decrease stress to the joints, provide support for increased function, and assist with joint stability (Beasley, 2012).

Use of orthotics for reducing inflammation and protecting unstable joints during occupational performance is one method for eliminating joint stress; however, joint protection strategies should also be introduced and incorporated into the intervention process. "Joint protection and energy conservation tie in with basic science by understanding the process that occurs at the joint cartilage when joints are under prolonged stress" (Beasley, 2012, p. 165). Both for patients/clients with OA and those with RA, the stressors of performing everyday tasks in the usual way may aggravate the processes and hasten the destruction of joints. Evaluating the approach a patient/client uses to open containers, carry items, and perform basic ADLs and IADLs can facilitate collaboration in adapting these daily tasks to protect the joints, eliminate pain, and increase independence (Fig. 9.10).

Therapeutic exercise programs for aging adults with OA and RA must always consider the amount of joint stability, muscle atrophy, and inflammation, if present (Beasley, 2012). Exercise recommendations and use of physical agent modalities (PAMs) in the treatment of arthritic conditions are common in OT practice. Because many patient/clients with RA and OA report that beginning their day with a warm shower or bath results in temporary neuromuscular effects that decrease pain and muscle tension, the OT or assistant may recommend bathing before engaging in exercise (Beasley, 2012). Traditionally, exercise includes gentle active ROM (AROM), gentle progressive resistive exercises, and no- or low-impact aerobic activities (including fall prevention tips). Careful attention to all symptoms and disease processes and individualization of program development are suggested for effective incorporation of exercise programs into the

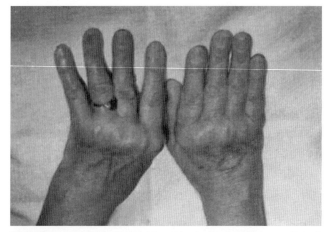

**FIGURE 9.9**    Rheumatoid Arthritis of Hands. (From Christensen, B. L., & Kockrow, E. O. [2010]. *Adult health nursing* [6th ed.]. Mosby.)

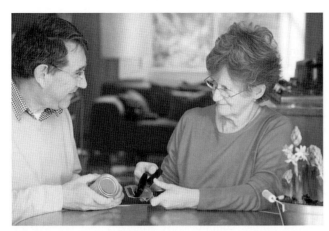

**FIGURE 9.10**  The occupational therapy practitioner shows a woman, who has arthritis, how to protect her joints while opening a can. (Photo © istock.com)

intervention of patient/clients with arthritic conditions. Additionally, OT staff should ensure that their recommendations for exercise are balanced with the desired meaningful occupations that the individual pursues on a regular basis, to support optimal patient/client quality of life. Arthritis is a chronic condition that can benefit from the self-management strategies suggested earlier in this chapter (Lorig & Holman, 1993). Successful OT intervention with patients/clients who have been diagnosed with an arthritic condition should include exposure to traditional OT approaches and incorporation of a self-management program for long-term benefits and increased participation in occupation.

## Neurological System

The neurological system, comprised of the peripheral nervous system (PNS) and central nervous system (CNS), is the command center for the body, controlling muscle movements, bodily functions, and thought processes. It is the major link between the brain and the remainder of the body, and also drives how our body responds to both internal and external stimuli. The following list details several aging-related changes that occur within the neurological system:

- Central nervous system: The CNS encompasses the brain and spinal cord. In general, physiologic aging results in the gradual loss of neurons and their supportive cells. These cells typically do not regenerate and once cellular death occurs, they are not replaced. This can lead to subtle changes in cognition that do not typically interfere with activities of ADLs, such as an overall slower processing speed, difficulty with dual and multi-tasking, difficulty with learning new concepts, and delayed recall. Refer to Chapters 15 and 16 for a comprehensive review of age-related changes of cognitive function and neurodegenerative diseases.
- Peripheral nervous system: The PNS consists of nerves that exit the spinal cord and travel to peripheral sites

in the body. It is responsible for conveying signals from the brain to muscle fibers, organs, and the skin, and also relaying information from the body and the outside environment back to the CNS. With age, changes in the myelin sheath surrounding nerve cells results in delayed conduction of peripheral nerve impulses (Verdu et al., 2000). This can lead to reduced or altered sensation (i.e., neuropathy) and impaired motor function (i.e., muscle weakness and gait unsteadiness), both of which increase the risk of falls. Changes in the PNS can also result in an overall slower muscle reaction time and create challenges for safe driving.

### Occupational Therapy Interventions Related to Neurological System Dysfunction and Optimization of Neurological Function

Changes in both the central and peripheral neurological system can progress slowly over time such as with dementia, or nerve impingement, or acutely as in the case of a cerebral vascular accident. The sequelae that accompany these different scenarios will dictate much different approaches of assessment and intervention design by the occupational therapist. Overarching each of the conditions with which older adults present is the need to begin by assessing the patient/client's sensory, cognition, and communication status. Given the multitude of different neurological diagnoses, OTPs must examine current evidence from OT literature to determine best practice approaches for a patient/client. Additionally, as with all other interventions the OTP will also be informed by the patient/client's specific wants and needs. Frames of reference can include biomechanical restorative approaches that target remediation of functional loss, as well as rehabilitative frames of reference focusing on education and modification or adapting the patient/client's environment or the way a given ADL or I/ADL is performed. For a detailed description of OT interventions for neurological dysfunction, refer to Chapters 15 and 16 of this text.

### Challenges Occurring in Self-Management of Physiological and Neurological Conditions That Can Impact Performance and Satisfaction in Occupational Participation

Physiologic and neurological changes that are more frequently observed in older adults may cause impairments in occupational performance that result in a physician's referral for a patient/client to see an occupational therapist in a number of types of settings. An increase in symptoms may cause the client to be admitted to an acute care facility, or the combination of these symptoms in conjunction with another disease process may require the patient/client to have extended inpatient, outpatient, or home-based therapy. These changes and chronic components of the disease process demand that the therapist incorporate self-management strategies into the treatment to promote optimal quality of life for the patient/client. Interventions are matched with the patient/client's assessed sensory, cognitive, communication, and literacy/health-care literacy levels. Self-management of chronic illness implies that the patient/client is monitoring and managing symptoms, adhering to treatment regimens, keeping a healthy lifestyle, and managing the effects of the illness on daily functioning, emotions, and social relationships (Lorig & Holman, 1993, 2003).

The traditional approach of health-care providers treating patient/clients with chronic illness, although well intentioned, fails to afford optimal clinical care or meet patient/clients' needs to be effective self-managers of their illness. For example, the traditional approach for working with a patient/client with HTN consists of prescription and explanation of secondary prevention medication, explanation of stroke and risk factors, and possibly a discussion of lifestyle modification (Santos-Parker et al., 2014). Gillham and Endacott (2010) suggest that addressing lifestyle change has not been routinely and consistently implemented by health-care providers, with discussion of lifestyle recorded in only 37% of consultations, and with questionable effectiveness in improving self-reported lifestyle-related risk factors. The health-care provider working with patients/clients with chronic conditions such as those described in this chapter must act as a teacher and collaborator in defining how to work with the patient/client to control the condition while optimizing the potential for participation in activities and occupations that are relevant and meaningful. The crux of appropriate care for chronic disease is a partnership between patients/clients and health professionals in management over a period of time (Clark et al., 2001).

### Additional Intervention Approaches to Optimize Patient/Client Satisfaction With Performance and Improving Occupational Participation

Each section of this chapter highlights the increasing challenges that individuals must address for healthy aging. Despite the variance in degree of older adults' declines in a variety of capacity areas, OT interventions can provide methods for patients/clients to continue functioning in all meaningful life roles. However subtle, cumulative decline can increase the risk for devastating interruption of the ability to participate in meaningful occupations. For example, approximately 30% of people over 65 years of age living in the community fall each year (Clemson et al., 2019). This concern is highlighted here, and more information may be found in Chapter 27, The Role of Occupational Therapy in Acute and Subacute Care with Aging Adults. Falls in nursing care facilities and hospitals are common events that cause considerable morbidity and mortality for older people (Cameron et al., 2018). New recommendations for fall prevention by the American Geriatrics Society (AGS) and the British Geriatrics Society (BGS) were released in 2010. Recommendations included ADL assessment, fear of falling, and the person's perception of their function.

Additional assessment of safety in the patient/client's home and community environment is indicated. Interventions for improving ambulation, balance (including appropriate footwear) and strength via exercise, and medication management may be indicated (Kontou et al., 2021). For a closer review of OT interventions, readers can refer to other chapters of this text focusing on successful aging (see Chapter 19) and the role of the physical environment (see Chapter 20).

The National Council on Aging (2018) is a useful resource for OTPs and for patients/clients and family members. An example of one resource is "6 Steps to Protect your Older Loved One from a Fall." This consumer-friendly resource outlines simple, commonsense strategies that OT personnel can review with a patient/client and use as an adjunct within treatment. The guest editors of the special edition of the *American Journal of Occupational Therapy* dedicated to fall prevention, mentioned earlier, states: "In the context of fall prevention, the importance of developing, using, and evaluating diverse approaches to intervention (e.g., remediation, maintenance, compensation, disability preventions) described in the Occupational Therapy Practice Framework: Domain and Process (AOTA, 2020a) cannot be overstated" (Peterson et al., 2012, p. 128). An OT intervention with any older patient/client should consider the patient/client's functional capacities and environments for assessment of fall risk and prevention.

## SUMMARY

The human body is comprised of a complex integration of multiple systems that work together for humans to survive and hopefully thrive. Aging is a heterogeneous process where each individual does not follow the same "schedule" of each organ's decline as we become older. There are many factors that influence the individual's health. As discussed, social inequities greatly impact physical and psychological health, and thus functioning. These compounded inequities are especially health impactful for older adults' quality of life. Targeting patient/client interventions and patient/caregiver education are essential. An OT and/or assistant can utilize best practice principles to support the aging patient/client's decline in function. Patient/client interventions and caregiver education must reflect the client/caregiver needs that can be best understood from thorough functional assessments that consider how the patient/client's physiological and neurological conditions have impacted patient/client function. Further, the inclusion of the patient/client's sensory, cognitive, communication abilities, and literacy/health-care literacy abilities is vital. Intervention approaches must be informed by these assessments and the consideration of cultural preference, as well as environmental and socioeconomic factors, as this approach can better meet the collaborative patient/client goals. These interventions support and/or improve performance in activities of daily living with exercise and other forms of training driven by patient/client informed preferences to increase activity tolerance. Strategies in energy conservation and work simplification are provided to support the aging adult's participation in her or his preferred activities. Furthermore, coping strategies, such as stress management and relaxation techniques, and home safety assessments are incorporated, as indicated. Whenever appropriate, family members/caregivers are educated about the interventions and practitioners should consider the family/caregiver's sensory (e.g., hearing, vision), cognitive, communication, and literacy/health-care needs using teach-back techniques to determine how best to accomplish this training. Caregiver training can improve and support the patient/client's status, with an overall aim of supporting the individual's well-being, their ability to participate, and quality of life.

*The complete listing of the Bibliography and Chapter Questions and Answers are available in the accompanying enhanced eBook version included with the print purchase of this textbook. Visit Elsevier eBooks+ (eBooks.Health.Elsevier.com) to access this content.*

## CHAPTER 10

# Occupational Therapy Interventions for Older Adults With Low Vision or Hearing Impairment

*Margaret Newsham Beckley, PhD, EdD, OTD, OTR/L, SCLV, FAOTA, Mary Geders Falcetti, EdD, OTR/L, FAOTA, and Maureen M. Fischer, MS, CCC/A*

## CHAPTER OUTLINE

## OBJECTIVES

- Describe the impact of low vision and hearing loss in older adulthood.
- Define low vision.
- Identify the diseases and conditions associated with low vision in older adults.
- Distinguish low vision from the typical vision changes associated with aging.
- Understand the function and components of vision.
- Identify the components of low vision evaluation.
- Understand how lighting, magnification, contrast, and working distance affect function.
- Identify strategies to improve the use of remaining vision for everyday tasks and occupations.
- Be familiar with referral sources to support older adults with low vision.
- Describe the opportunities available for professional development for low vision practice.
- Describe the differences between age-related hearing loss and other hearing loss.
- Identify the conditions and diseases that contribute to hearing loss in older adults.
- Understand the anatomical components involved in hearing.
- Identify the preferred components of hearing loss evaluation.
- Articulate strategies to compensate for hearing loss in older adults.
- Understand how to use hearing aids, cochlear implants, and assistive listening devices effecting function.
- Recognize opportunities for professional development practice for age-related hearing loss with older adults.
- Be familiar with reputable referral and community resources available for older adults dealing with hearing loss.

Low vision has been found to have an adverse effect on people's ability to participate in their everyday occupations (Beckley & Greg, 2019; Smallfield & Kaldenberg, 2020). An older adult with low vision may have difficulty with reading, writing, activities of daily living (ADLs), instrumental activities of daily living (IADLs), functional and community mobility, social, leisure, spectator activities, and vocational tasks. As a result, the individual experiences a loss of independence, safety, life roles, and an increased potential for isolation and depression.

The incidence of low vision disorders among older adults is on the rise; they make up two-thirds of those diagnosed with a visual impairment (Prevent Blindness America, 2017). In 2000, the number of older adults (65+ years old) in the United States was 35 million, an increase of 3.7 million (11%) since 1990 (Administration on Aging [AOA], 2002). Of these older adults, approximately 1.3 million (4%) had a low vision impairment (Massof, 2002). In 2008, the National Center for Health Statistics (NCHS) reported that 6.5 million older adults (65+ years old) reported experiencing significant vision loss

(Pleis & Lucas, 2009). By 2030, experts in the field predict the rates of severe vision loss will double as the US aging population increases (Prevent Blindness America, 2017). These numbers do not include older adults in institutionalized living environments, such as skilled nursing facilities.

In addition, the prevalence of older adults with low vision and a cooccurring hearing impairment is reported to be 8.6% of the US population over 70 years of age (Crews & Campbell, 2004). This population with co-occurring conditions are more likely to experience an increase in falls (3 times more) and a broken a hip (2 times more), report having hypertension (1.5 times more), report having heart disease (2.4 times greater), and/or experience a stroke (3.6 times) compared to the same age group without low vision or a hearing impairment (Crews & Campbell, 2004). Due to the "invisible" nature of low vision and hearing loss, often a lack of screening for these conditions can lead to a misdiagnosis of dementia among older adults. Knowing the importance of screening and intervening for low vision and hearing loss allow for modifying the risk factors for dementia (Kuo et al., 2021).

## Dual Sensory Impairment in Older Adults

Low vision and hearing loss can occur independently or together in older adulthood. Yet occupational therapists have not historically been prepared to screen for these types of sensory losses during their educational programs (Wittich et al., 2016). A Canadian Association of Occupational Therapy study on this topic identified a gap between academic preparation and the needs of the aging population in the areas of sensory screening. Occupational therapy (OT) practitioners are well positioned to identify vision and hearing losses during the evaluation process. This chapter will provide practitioners the tools to identify problems by raising an awareness of aging adult sensory needs. While low vision and hearing impairment may cooccur, this chapter will address each functional loss separately, leaving the OT practitioner to assess and intervene based on the needs of their patients/clients.

## Functional Performance and Low Vision

Combined with the other physical changes associated with aging, the development of a low vision impairment further challenges the functional performance and safety of those 65 and older (Beckley, 2016). Furthermore, the psychological impact from the physical changes accompanying aging is compounded for those with a low vision impairment (Teitelman & Copollilo, 2005).

Low vision can be described as impaired visual perception due to visual acuity that is less than 70/200 or limited visual fields of 20 degrees or less, and results in limitations in a person's ability to participate in daily activities and occupations (Beckley, 2016). It occurs as the result of a chronic visual disorder that cannot be corrected medically, surgically, or with conventional eyeglasses (Massof, 1995). Low vision is different from typical vision changes associated with aging, and most often results in a disability. The four most common

eye diseases leading to low vision impairments are glaucoma, age-related macular degeneration (ARMD), diabetic retinopathy, and cataracts (Centers for Disease Control and Prevention [CDC], 2020; National Eye Institute [NEI], 2004).

Low vision also impacts a person's safety. For those with low vision impairment, there is an increased risk of falls and fractures. This usually results in admission into a hospital or nursing home and thus an older adult can run the risk of becoming disabled or die prematurely (CDC, 2001). With low vision, there is also an increased risk of related depression. Older people with vision impairments have a 57.2% risk of mild or moderate depression, compared to 43.5% of those without vision loss (American Foundation for the Blind [AFB Press], 2017). Another safety issue for someone with low vision is having difficulty identifying medications. Misidentification of medications can lead to drug-related errors that affect the health of older adults. These types of errors have become the fifth leading cause of death among seniors. Forty percent of seniors take five or more prescription drugs a week and 12% take more than 10 (Gleckman, 2003)—increasing the chance even more for misidentifying medications. Please refer to Chapter 14 for more information on pharmacology and aging adults.

## Low Vision Versus Age-Related Changes in Vision

Due to typical vision changes associated with aging, low vision disorders may be dismissed as normal changes. Low vision disorders are not the same as the normal vision changes that occur with aging. The typical age-related vision changes result from alterations in the cornea, pupil, lens, aqueous (liquid between the cornea and the pupil) and vitreous (semiliquid that fills the globe of the eye), and macular pigment over time (Rubin, 2000) See Fig. 10.1 for typical structures of the eye.

As a result, visual acuity gradually decreases, making it difficult to read fine print. Contrast sensitivity, the eye's ability to detect subtle changes in light and dark objects, decreases and may result in reduced reading speed or facial discrimination when looking at photographs. There is an increased discomfort experienced with glare and a greater glare recovery time—the speed with which the visual system regains function following exposure to bright light. In addition, color discrimination decreases with age, causing for some colors to appear more muted, particularly those along the blue-yellow axis (Rubin, 2000). Low contrast, low lighting levels, and the presence of glare have been shown to reduce older adults' acuity levels as a result of aging changes (Haegerstrom-Portnoy et al., 1999). These typical changes associated with aging can be further compounded by a low vision impairment that develops in later life, leading to greater functional impairment.

Due to the potential of a low vision impairment being present with or without an older adult client's knowledge, it is important to ask the client about his or her visual health and history. In addition, it is important to screen for the presence of a visual field deficit or visual impairment. This can be done with functional types of reading or identification

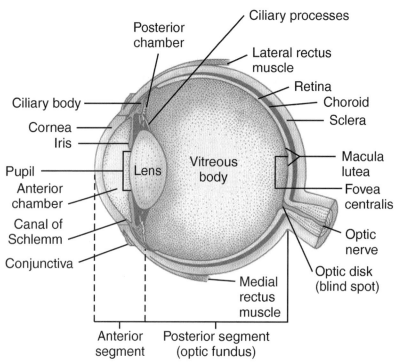

**FIGURE 10.1**    Anatomy of the eye. (From the National Eye Institute, National Institutes of Health, Ref. NEA05.)

tasks at various distances or with a low vision quiz from the NEI (2010). Questions from the NEI quiz (see Appendix A) are concerned with a person's performance on typical daily activities with or without the use of prescription glasses. The questions for the client include recognizing faces of family and friends, doing things that require the person to see well up close, like reading, cooking, sewing, or fixing things around the house, being able to pick out and match the color of clothes, doing things at work or home in which lights seem dimmer than formerly, and being able to read street and bus signs or the names of stores.

Older adults who develop low vision and mistakenly think it is a normal part of aging may not seek support services or be aware that services are available. In addition, older adults with low vision, more often than not, have a myriad of symptoms, conditions, and related impairments. Interdisciplinary services that address the many areas impacted by low vision have been found to improve the quality of life of older adults (Hinds et al., 2003; Lovie-Kitchin et al., 2001). Whether service is direct intervention, team treatment, or a referral to another service provider, the various needs of an older adult client with low vision has a greater chance of being met through an interdisciplinary approach. The 5-year National Plan for Eye and Vision Research (NEI, 2004) identified interdisciplinary collaboration in low vision treatment as a program goal. Related to this, *Healthy People 2030* also specifies objectives to increase the use of the various rehabilitation services by people with low vision, and to increase the use of assorted visual and adaptive devices (US Department of Health and Human Services, 2020). To this end, occupational therapists and OT

assistants need to work in collaboration with other health and social service providers to ensure that older adults with low vision receive necessary services and intervention.

An examination by an optometrist or ophthalmologist who specializes in low vision therapy is usually the first step in the process. In addition to OT professionals, a certified low vision therapist (CLVT) or a certified vision rehabilitation therapist (CVRT), formerly known as a rehabilitation teacher, can assist with many of the challenges one may face with ADLs and IADLs. Physical therapists can provide intervention with ambulation, transfers, safety, and balance. A certified orientation and mobility specialist (COMS) can also assist with managing safe mobility in the home, in addition to providing instruction for traveling safely and efficiently in the community. Additional services from members of the team can be provided by skilled nursing, a diabetic educator, a social worker or psychologist, and a family practice physician or geriatrician. The members of the low vision rehabilitation team may vary depending upon the service environment and funding sources. Occupational therapists and OT assistants need to be aware of the different service environments, delivery models, funding sources, and community resources associated with low vision rehabilitation in order to provide effective client-centered care.

## Function and Conditions of the Eye

### Physiology of Vision

To see words, objects, faces, or landscapes, their reflections are carried by light through the eye to the retina. Light enters the eye through the cornea, passes through the aqueous, pupil, then lens.

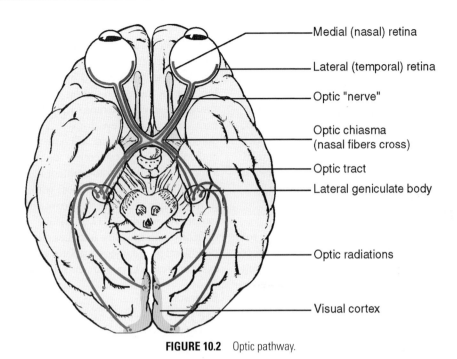

- Medial (nasal) retina
- Lateral (temporal) retina
- Optic "nerve"
- Optic chiasma (nasal fibers cross)
- Optic tract
- Lateral geniculate body
- Optic radiations
- Visual cortex

**FIGURE 10.2**   Optic pathway.

Light then continues to travel posteriorly through the vitreous to the first layer of the retina. The layers of the retina, from anterior to posterior, are (1) the internal limiting membrane, (2) axons, (3) ganglion cells, (4) inner plexiform layer, (5) inner nuclear layer, (6) outer plexiform layer, (7) outer nuclear layer (rod and cone cell bodies), (8) external limiting membrane, (9) photoreceptors, and (10) pigmented epithelium. Light is attracted to the internal limiting membrane and enters through the membrane onto the axons, ganglion cells, inner plexiform layer, and then the inner nuclear layer. At the outer plexiform layer, light is converted into chemical energy. This energy then stimulates the rods and cones to become hyperpolarized, creating an electrical impulse. The electrical impulse is carried posteriorly through the external limiting membrane to photoreceptors and the pigmented epithelium. At this point, the collection of nerve fibers from the retina, known as the optic nerve, carries electrical impulse information from the retina, exiting the eye, to the optic tract (after chiasm), which then proceeds eventually to the visual cortex of the brain in the occipital lobe (Fig. 10.2).

Pressure within the globe of the eye needs to be maintained for accurate transmission of light, chemical, and electrical energy. The average range of intraocular pressure (IOP) is 10–22 mmHg. Abnormally low IOP is when the pressure measures below 10 mmHg. An abnormally high IOP is a measure of 30 mmHg or higher, and very high IOP is considered to be 40–60 mmHg. Abnormally high IOP results in glaucoma.

## Pathology of Low Vision Impairment

Low vision impairments occur when there is a chronic deteriorating condition or an acute trauma that causes damage to the structures of the eye or the pathway from the retina to the visual cortex. In addition to the identification of glaucoma, ARMD, diabetic retinopathy, and cataracts as the four most common eye diseases leading to low vision impairments for older adults (CDC, 2020; NEI, 2004), visual field deficits due to cerebral vascular accidents (CVAs) or trauma are responsible for visual impairments in older adults as well. A gradual loss of vision can occur with chronic conditions such as diabetic retinopathy or macular degeneration. An acute loss of vision can occur as the result of a sudden traumatic event such as stroke near the optic chiasm or visual cortex. For older adults, adjustment to acquired vision loss has been found to be more difficult than adjustment to congenital vision loss. In addition, adjustment to an acute loss of vision is more challenging than adjustment to a gradual loss of vision.

Vision loss is an individualized condition; two clients with the same diagnosis, of the same age, and the same gender may have very different impairments. Additionally, vision is multidimensional. When working with older adults with an acquired vision loss, OT practitioners need to be aware of the five components of vision: visual acuity, visual field, contrast sensitivity, light modulation, and visual perception and interpretation (Mogk, 2011). The descriptions of the vision components provided by Mogk (2011) can enhance the Occupational Therapist's comprehension of clients' needs during both evaluation and intervention. Visual acuity refers to the level of detail in perceiving objects, and the visual field encompasses the entire area visible in a single glance without the need to shift the head or eyes. Additionally, the visual field can be categorized into the central visual field, which includes the immediate surroundings of the focal point, and the peripheral visual field, which extends beyond and around the central field (Mogk, 2011). Contrast sensitivity is the ability to differentiate between similar shades of light and dark, as well as to discern similar colors. Light modulation involves the capacity to regulate light, manage glare, and adapt to changes in lighting conditions, transitioning from light to dark or vice versa.

Lastly, visual perception and interpretation entail the accurate processing and understanding of the information received by the brain from the eyes (Mogk, 2011).

## Conditions Causing Low Vision Impairment

The four most common conditions causing low vision impairments in older adults include macular degeneration, diabetic retinopathy, glaucoma, and cataracts (https://www.nei.nih.gov/, 2021). Since older adults are more prone to a CVA, or stroke, than younger populations, acquired field loss due to stroke is another visual impairment that can impact this population.

### Macular Degeneration

The most common eye condition that leads to low vision for older adults is macular degeneration and it is found more frequently in White populations. ARMD occurs as a result of degeneration of the macula—the area of the retina that is responsible for central vision and much of color vision (Orr, 1998). When degeneration alone occurs, this is considered to be dry ARMD. For some people with ARMD, abnormal new blood vessels can form under the macula and leak (Flom, 2004b) and is referred to as wet ARMD. Macular degeneration usually progresses for several years, resulting in central scotomas. A person with ARMD will have reduced contrast sensitivity and color vision, with a preference for bright task lighting and a high sensitivity to ambient lighting (Flom, 2004b). Since the macula is responsible for central vision, ARMD impairs vision needed for activities such as reading, fine motor tasks, seeing faces in social situations, viewing pictures, or completing hobbies and leisure activities.

### Diabetic Retinopathy

Another leading cause of low vision in older adults is diabetic retinopathy. Diabetic retinopathy is found more frequently among Black, Latinx, and Native American populations. Diabetic retinopathy is associated with diabetes and occurs when small blood vessels in the retina stop functioning properly (Orr, 1998). Laser treatment or surgery may be used to stop the small vessel leakage and stabilize the condition (Flom, 2004b). Vision may fluctuate based on dysregulated glucose levels, and the field of view that is impacted depends upon the areas of the retina that are damaged (Flom, 2004b). Someone with diabetic retinopathy has reduced contrast sensitivity and color vision, a preference for moderate task lighting, and a moderate sensitivity to ambient lighting (Flom, 2004b). In early stages of the disease, the small blood vessels in the retina may leak fluid into the retina with the risk of impairing the entire retina, including the macula, and the vitreous, leading to distorted vision (Orr, 1998). The degree of visual impairment can range from mild to total blindness. Depending upon the location and amount of damage to the retina, someone with diabetic retinopathy can have difficulty with near, midrange, or distant activities.

### Glaucoma

Glaucoma is another common cause of low vision in older adults and is found to run in families. The risk of developing glaucoma is six times greater in Blacks compared to Whites, and the rate for a visual impairment that results in blindness is 16 times greater for Blacks than it is for Whites (Siegfried et al., 2011). Glaucoma is caused by an increase in IOP due to fluid build-up in the eye, resulting in compression and damage to the optic nerve. Glaucoma can be treated successfully, if found early enough, using eye drops that decrease IOP (Mogk, 2011). Someone with glaucoma will have reduced contrast sensitivity and color vision, a preference for moderate task lighting, and a moderate sensitivity to ambient lighting (Flom, 2004b). The distinctive pattern of vision loss with glaucoma is initial loss is in the midperipheral field, progressing toward the center and periphery (Mogk, 2011). Someone with glaucoma will have difficulty with mobility activities due to the midperipheral and peripheral field damage and later with near activities if the disease progresses to impair central vision.

### Cataracts

The fourth common cause of low vision in older adults is cataracts. Cataracts cause clouding over the lens of the eye, decreasing light from passing through the lens and limiting vision (Orr, 1998). The most common form of cataracts affects distant vision, then near vision, eventually causing blurriness and muted colors throughout the entire visual field (Mogk, 2011). Cataracts develop as a result of aging. Surgical removal of the lens is a viable option for most older adults and vision becomes clear again with a replacement lens. For someone with an advanced cataract, visual acuity and details for distant, intermediate, and eventually near activities will be impaired.

### Stroke

Visual field cuts that may result from stroke are not one of the common low vision conditions; however, due to the impact on older adults who experience a field cut as the result of a stroke, it is frequently included in discussions of low vision impairments in older adults. Visual field cuts that result from a stroke may involve one side of the visual field, known as homonymous hemianopsia, or a quadrant of the visual field, sometimes referred to as quadrantanopsia. As shown in Fig. 10.3, the location of the damage along the optic pathway determines the type of visual field deficit that may occur. If a lesion occurs along the optic tract or along the entire width of optic radiations to the visual cortex, a contralateral hemianopsia will occur (Fig. 10.3D–G). For lesions at the optic chiasm, preventing temporal field information from crossing to the contralateral optic tract, a bitemporal hemianopsia will occur (Fig. 10.3C). A lesion occurring along the upper radiations of the optic tract that lead to the visual cortex will cause a lower quadrant contralateral field loss (Fig. 10.3F). In the first several months following a stroke, vision may improve. After this point, vision can be considered stable (Flom, 2004b) and will not deteriorate any further due to the stroke. Visual field losses from stroke frequently cause difficulties with reading, finding items in a kitchen drawer, or bumping into objects in the environment as a result of not seeing the entire near, intermediate, or distant visual field (Figs. 10.4 to 10.11).

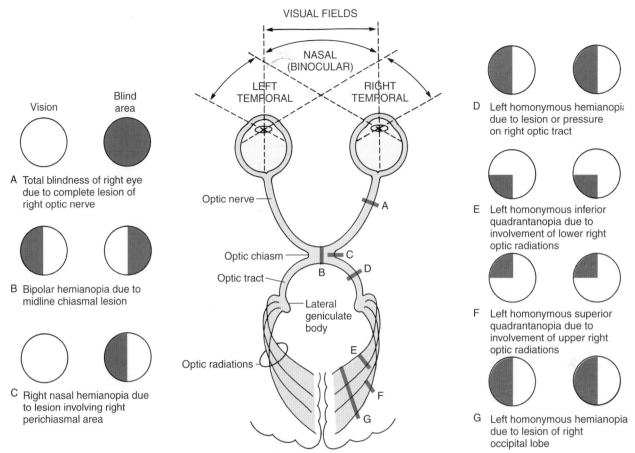

**FIGURE 10.3**   Lesions along the optic pathway. Diagram showing the effects on the fields of vision produced by lesions at various points along the optic pathway: (A) Complete blindness in the left eye; (B) the usual effect is a left junction scotoma in association with a right upper quadrantanopia. The later results from interruption of right retinal nasal fibers that project into the base of the left optic nerve (Wilbrand's knee). A left nasal hemianopia could occur from a lesion at this point but is exceedingly rare; (C) bitemporal hemianopia; (D) right homonymous hemianopia; (E and F) right upper and lower quadrant hemianopia; and (G) right homonymous hemianopia. (From Victor, M., & Ropper, A.H. [2008]. *Adam & Victor's Manual of Neurology*, 7th ed., New York: McGraw-Hill Companies.)

## Occupational Therapy Assessment and Intervention

The Centers for Medicare & Medicaid Services (CMS) in the United States considers consumers with a low vision diagnosis to have reduced physical functioning and, therefore, are covered for OT and physical therapy services related to mobility, ADLs, and other medically necessary goals. In 2002, CMS authorized payment for physician-prescribed low vision rehabilitation services provided by an occupational therapist (Table 10.1) or a physical therapist. And, for consumers with a low vision diagnosis, optometrists (OD) are considered physicians with the authority to prescribe for low vision rehab services.

Due to the large number of older adults currently with low vision and projections for an increase in that number through 2030 (Prevent Blindness America, 2017), it is important for OT professionals to screen their clients for low vision conditions and refer to an ophthalmologist or optometrist with a specialty in low vision for a full low vision evaluation, as needed.

When a client is referred for low vision rehabilitation, it is necessary to review the report from the optometrist or ophthalmologist as part of the initial evaluation process. The content of a typical eye report includes ocular history, visual acuity with and without glasses, eye muscle function, IOP reading, contrast sensitivity, color vision, visual field test, pupillary response, presence of photophobia, prescription, and prognosis. The eye report information is helpful in the assessment process in many ways. For instance, the visual acuity information can indicate the amount of magnification needed with optical devices, determines the degree of residual vision, and provides documentation to qualify a client for services (Brilliant, 1999).

On the other hand, the occupational therapist needs to realize that the eye exam is completed in a controlled environment, without the lighting changes or distractions that are present in natural and everyday environments. In addition, the information from the eye report will not indicate how well a client with low vision can perform functional tasks. To determine the client's occupational performance skills and

**TABLE 10.1**  Occupational Therapy Procedures for Low Vision Rehabilitation

| CPT Code | Description |
| --- | --- |
| 97165 | Occupational therapy evaluation—low |
| 97166 | Occupational therapy evaluation—moderate |
| 97167 | Occupational therapy evaluation—high |
| 97168 | Occupational therapy reevaluation |
| 97110 | Therapeutic activities (eccentric viewing training) |
| 97533 | Sensory integrative techniques for enhanced sensory processing |
| 97535 | Self-care/home management training. Activities of daily living (meal preparation, safety, use of adaptive equipment) |
| 97537 | Community/work integration (shopping, transportation, money management) |

barriers to participation, the occupational therapist needs to assess the client in different environments and under various conditions. The results of the OT evaluation will help to identify intervention strategies, adaptive equipment and low vision devices, and other professional low vision services and community resources needed to improve a person's ability to complete daily activities and occupations.

## Occupational Therapy Assessment

An important aspect of the low vision evaluation is for it to be a positive experience for the client and that they are exposed to a success-oriented atmosphere related to their potential. Doing so can relieve the client of some of the limitations and fears associated with vision loss and motivate him or her to accomplish their goals. The OT low vision assessment includes four components: (1) the occupational profile, (2) evaluation of visual factors, (3) evaluation of environmental factors, and (4) evaluation of occupational performance (Whittaker et al., 2016).

### Occupational Profile

The occupational profile can be obtained through interview, questionnaire, and previous medical, vision, and social history. The occupational profile will help guide the development of intervention strategies and goals based on the client's priorities and interests. It may also reveal the need for referral to other professionals, based on the client's needs. Gathering information for the occupational profile can be completed with, but not limited to, the Occupational Therapy Practice Framework, 4th ed. (American Occupational Therapy Association [AOTA] 2020), the NEI Visual Functioning Questionnaire-25 (VFQ-25), version 2000 (see Appendix B), The Geriatric Depression Scale, short version (Sheikh & Yesavage, 1986) (see Appendix D), or any other formal or informal data collection tools (e.g., Table 10.2) that will provide a thorough appraisal of the client's occupational performance history.

## Evaluation of Visual Factors

The second component for low vision assessment is evaluation of visual factors. This part of the assessment may vary, depending upon the amount of information received from a client's optometrist or ophthalmologist. If the information from the eye doctor's clinical low vision assessment is limited, evaluation of visual factors can be completed as part of the functional low vision assessment. Evaluation of the client's visual factors includes assessing visual acuity at a distance, reading acuity for near, peripheral visual field, contrast sensitivity, scotoma assessment, and reading assessment for reading speed (Whittaker et al., 2017).

### Assessment of Visual Acuity at a Distance

Testing visual acuity at a distance can be completed with the Feinbloom Distance Test Chart which is easily portable, or the ETDRS Chart (Fig. 10.12), which is not as portable and can be illuminated.

### Assessment of Reading Acuity for Near Vision

Reading acuity near testing can be completed using the Minnesota Low Vision Reading Test, also known as the MN Read Card. The MN Read Card has black print on a white background and printed sentences change in incremental sizes (see Appendix G). It is important to have proper task lighting on the MN Read Card and to position it so the client is reading at a 90-degree angle.

### Peripheral Field Testing

The third assessment of visual factors is peripheral field testing. Functional peripheral field testing can be completed with converging and/or dynamic activities to determine if the client can detect an object or movement near and around them, and at what point. One method for testing for functional peripheral field loss is to have the client focus on a target or object straight ahead, while seated or standing, with their back to the occupational therapist. The client keeps their eyes and head facing forward. The occupational therapist stands next to the client's shoulder and proceeds to walk forward, parallel to the client's line of sight. The client indicates the point at which any part of the OT is visible. This process is repeated on the client's other side as well (Geruschat & Smith, 2010). The distances from where the OT started and the points at which the OT came into the client's field of view is the measure of the client's restricted functional peripheral field for each side. There are other commonly used peripheral field testing procedures (Meyers & Wilcox, 2011; Whittaker et al., 2017). The selection of the testing procedure may be determined by the client's potential and goals. Peripheral vision testing is important, as it is part of a client's early warning system, informing the client that something in their environment is moving, changing, or coming into their pathway. Being able to detect these changes is necessary for many functional activities whether the client is sitting at a table, using a wheelchair, walking, or driving.

### Contrast Sensitivity

Contrast sensitivity is the ability to detect grayness and background (Orr, 1998) or distinguish between similar shades of

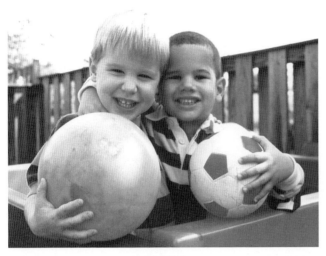

Normal Vision

**FIGURE 10.4**    Normal vision. (Courtesy: National Eye Institute, National Institutes of Health (NEI/NIH)

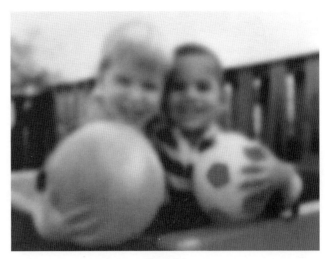

Cataract

**FIGURE 10.6**    A scene as it might be viewed by a person with cataract. (Courtesy: National Eye Institute, National Institutes of Health (NEI/NIH)

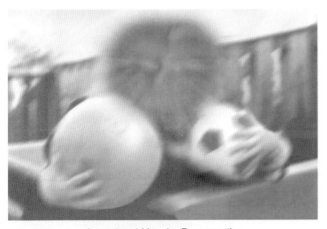

Age-related Macular Degeneration

**FIGURE 10.5**    A scene as it might be viewed by a person with age-related macular degeneration. (Courtesy: National Eye Institute, National Institutes of Health (NEI/NIH).

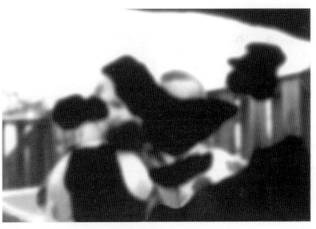

Diabetic Retinopathy

**FIGURE 10.7**    A scene as it might be viewed by a person with diabetic retinopathy. (Courtesy: National Eye Institute, National Institutes of Health (NEI/NIH).

light and dark (Mogk, 2011). There are a variety of testing charts for contrast sensitivity. Some are used for distance testing, such as the low contrast ETDRS chart or the Mars Letter Contrast Sensitivity Test, and others are used for near contrast sensitivity testing, such as Lea Numbers Low-Contrast Flip Chart or the Eschenbach Continuous Text Low Contrast Chart. Whether testing for distance or near contrast sensitivity, the client reads or names the objects on the chart as the contrast of the objects is progressively reduced. The client will continue down the chart until they are unable to distinguish the letters, numbers, words, or figures from the background of the chart. Reduced contrast sensitivity may cause difficulties reading, recognizing faces, or seeing a pedestrian in the crosswalk when driving on a rainy day.

Associated with the contrast sensitivity is the need for adequate lighting. The low vision assessment needs to include evaluation of a person's ability to discern the absence or presence of light, their sensitivity to the degree of brightness of light, and the need to decrease or increase illumination (Koenig et al., 2000). Considerations regarding lighting as it relates to assessment include the types of light, the position of the light, a client's ability to adapt to light and dark, and glare (Zimmerman, 1996). The occupational therapist should observe the client under various lighting conditions and determine the client's preferences for lighting during visual factor assessments. It is necessary to assess the client's lighting needs during various functional tasks. Therefore, assessment should include how well the client performs functional activities indoors and outdoors, determining how well the client manages the transition of moving into and out of bright lighting, and identifying the client's preference for light-absorbing lenses, shields, contrast lenses,

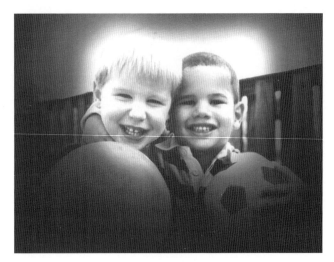

Glaucoma

**FIGURE 10.8**    A scene as it might be viewed by a person with glaucoma. (Courtesy: National Eye Institute, National Institutes of Health (NEI/NIH)

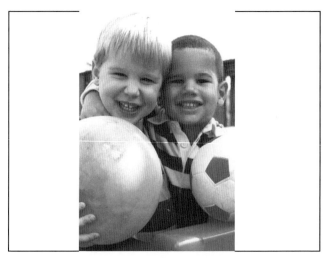

**FIGURE 10.10**    Simulated bitemporal hemianopsia following stroke—alteration added. (Courtesy: National Eye Institute, National Institutes of Health (NEI/NIH)

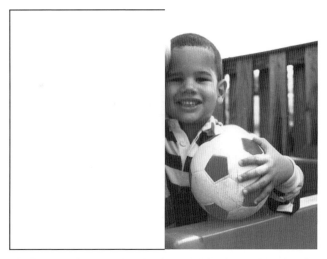

**FIGURE 10.9**    Simulated right hemianopsia following stroke—alteration added. (Courtesy: National Eye Institute, National Institutes of Health (NEI/NIH).

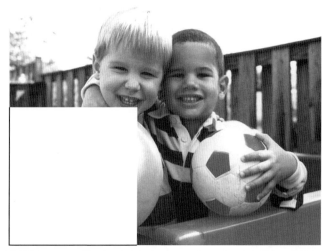

**FIGURE 10.11**    Simulated right lower quadrant visual field loss following stroke—alteration added. (Courtesy: National Eye Institute, National Institutes of Health (NEI/NIH).

dark lenses, and visors or and hats (Koenig et al., 2000). In addition, a person with a greater need for light should be assessed in various situations such as a dimly lit room, at dusk, a cloudy day, with the provision of additional light (Koenig et al., 2000), and should be allowed time for his/her eyes to adapt when moving from a bright environment to a darker environment or vice versa (Carter, 1983).

While assessment of lighting can be completed informally by changing lighting conditions and using glare-reducing devices as needed, there are specific lighting assessments available to the occupational therapist. Some of the specific assessment tools related to lighting include the Cone Adaptation Test, developed by Lea Hyvärinen, MD; The Farnswroth D-15 Color Panel Test, developed by D. Farnsworth; the Foot-Candle Reading Monitors, which measure the amount of light luminating from a surface;

and the Home Environment Lighting Assessment (HELA) developed by Perlmutter et al. (2013) for near-tasks in the home. These types of assessment tools produce valuable information, although in and of themselves, do not give an indication of a client's overall functional performance. It is therefore important to remember that two clients with similar low vision diagnoses may have different functional performance levels. As such, the occupational therapist needs to consider all aspects of lighting in the assessment process to develop accurate and thorough baseline information on which to build the intervention plan.

### Scotoma Assessment

Scotoma testing completed by an optometrist or ophthalmologist gives very precise information about the size and location of a scotoma. A scotoma is the name given to the dense

**TABLE 10.2** Adapted Questions From AWARE—Center for Vision Loss

Reading and near vision activities:
- What size print can you now read?
- Do you want to continue reading newspapers?
- Can you read your bills?
- Do you want to read the TV Guide?
- Do you "spot" read more than you read novels or other books?
- Have you had low vision devices, such as magnifiers, in the past? If so, do you still use them? If not, why not?

Everyday activities:
- Can you see to use a checkbook?
- Can you read your watch?
- Can you do regular household tasks, such as cleaning and laundry?
- Can you care for your personal grooming needs, such as shaving or applying makeup?
- Can you see to use a computer, tablet, and/or cellphone?
- Are you able to continue your hobbies?
- Can you watch television?
- Can you travel independently and safely?
- What difficulties are you having when traveling in your community?
- Are you still driving? If so, do you still feel safe driving?
- Does bright sunlight bother you?
- Has your vision problem affected your employment or educational studies?
- If you have diabetes, can you see to fill your insulin syringes?
- Can you differentiate between your medications?

American Foundation for the Blind.

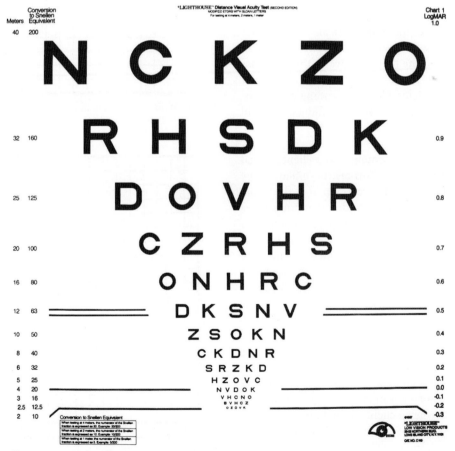

**FIGURE 10.12** ETDRS chart.

and localized visual field defect that creates a blind spot in the client's vision (Flom, 2004a). When a person has a scotoma near or in the central visual field, reading and fine motor activities are difficult to complete. If information on the presence of a scotoma on a client's eye report is not available, there are functional assessments that can be used to determine if a client has difficulty seeing in a particular area of the visual field.

## Amsler Grid

The Amsler grid (Fig. 10.13) is a tool used to measure the central 10 degrees of vision. Often, it is this part of the visual field that we rely on to do close meticulous work, such as placing tiny screws in a jewelry box. The Amsler grid is a 10-cm × 10-cm one-dimensional square made up of many smaller boxes. Most frequently, it is a white background with black lines making up the boxes and square; however, the contrast of the grid can be increased by using a black background and white lines. It is used to identify the presence of scotomas in a person's visual field—indicating changes in the macula. The test is completed with one eye at a time and with glasses if the client normally wears them. The grid is held 28–30 cm away and the client is asked to look at the dot in the center of the grid. If the client does not see the dot in the center of the grid, it could be indicative of a scotoma. Then, the client is asked to look at all four corners of the square and to report if the corners are present or not. If the client does not see a corner, this response could be indicative of the presence of a scotoma. And last, the client is asked to report whether the squares are all the same size and if any of the lines look wavy. If the squares do not all look equal or if some of the lines look wavy, this response may indicate changes in the macula (Fig. 10.14). The Amsler grid is not sensitive for clients with longstanding visual loss, which may be due the client unconsciously filling in the grid so it appears completely normal (Greer, 2004).

## Tangent Screen Test

Another test that can indicate scotomas in a client's visual field is the Tangent Screen Test. This test is similar to the Amsler grid in that it measures the central part of the visual field. It is different from the Amsler grid in that it measures a larger field of view: 20–30 degrees. This part of the field of view is used while reading. The tangent screen test is completed with a large black felt screen mounted on the wall. Testing on the Tangent Screen is completed with one eye at a time and with glasses if the client wears them. The client is seated facing the screen at a distance of 1 m. The client is told to focus on the white X in the middle while the OT moves a target in and out of the client's field of view to random locations. If a target is placed within the meridians on the Tangent Screen that correlate up to 30 degrees of central vision and the client does not report seeing it, this response could be an indication of a scotoma. This type of testing is a good method to use when a client has had difficulty reading. If the client indicates having a blind spot to the right of the fixation mark, this response may indicate a scotoma that is preventing the client from reading through a line of text (Greer, 2004).

## Clock Face Test

A third method to test for the possible presence of a scotoma is the clock face test. This method of testing is completed with one eye at a time and with glasses, if the client wears them. The client is seated facing the clock at eye level at a distance of approximately 2 feet. Using a clock face drawn on a white paper and a center focal point (see Fig. 10.15), the client is told to focus on the center. If the client cannot see the center, there is probably a scotoma directly in the client's central vision. If while looking at the center focal point, the client reports being able to see the focal point, but is unable to see one of the numbers on the face of the clock, the location of the

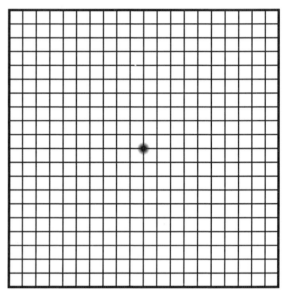

**FIGURE 10.13**    Amsler grid. (Courtesy: National Eye Institute, National Institutes of Health (NEI/NIH).

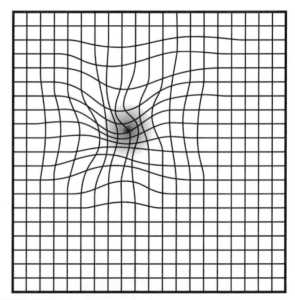

**FIGURE 10.14**    Amsler grid as it might appear to someone with age-related macular degeneration. (Courtesy: National Eye Institute, National Institutes of Health (NEI/NIH).

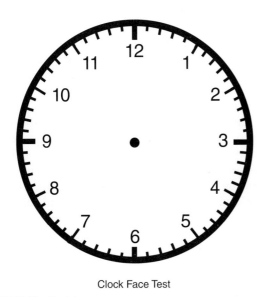

Clock Face Test

**FIGURE 10.15**   Clock face.

number that is not visible to the client could be indicative of the location of a scotoma.

For example, if the client reports not being able to see the number 3, ask the client if focusing on the number 9 caused the middle focal point to disappear. If so, there is a good chance the client has a scotoma in the right middle quadrant of their visual field. In addition, it may also indicate that the client is a candidate for eccentric viewing as a compensatory strategy. Eccentric viewing will be discussed later as an intervention technique.

### Reading Assessment for Reading Speed

The final visual factor testing is a reading assessment for reading speed. The Pepper Visual Skills for Reading Test (Pepper VSRT) is an evaluation available for use by occupational therapists to obtain a measure of reading speed and errors made while reading a series of unrelated letters and words. This evaluation tests vision regarding word recognition ability, rapid eye movement control, return-sweep eye movement control, and scotoma placement while reading (Watson et al., 1990). The Pepper VSRT scoring instructions suggest guidelines that will help the occupational therapist determine if the client's reading performance would be described as *inaccurately and slowly, accurately but slowly*, or *with both speed and accuracy* (Watson et al., 1990). Another evaluation that can be used for reading assessment and reading speed is the Minnesota Low Vision Reading Test (MN Read Test) discussed earlier. Assessment of reading skills is important for reasons other than reading abilities and comprehension. The act of reading may also be an indicator of how a client with low vision performs with other near activities such as bilateral fine motor tasks, writing, or needle point.

### Evaluation of Environmental Factors

The third component of an OT low vision assessment is evaluation of environmental factors (Whittaker et al., 2017). Consideration of environmental factors is important as this can make the difference in the low vision client being able to

complete a task successfully in one environment, yet failing to complete the same task when performed in another environment with different features. A difference in successful task completion can depend upon the time of day and the amount of available light in a particular environment. It may be that a client is able to read at the kitchen table that sits next to an east-facing window in the early morning with only the use of a magnifier. However, by late morning, the kitchen may be flooded with light, causing too much glare for the client to see the words on the page.

In assessing the environment, the occupational therapist should evaluate (1) the available sources of light and glare; (2) possible positions for task lights, reading stands, and tables; (3) organization systems; (4) access to low vision devices; (5) ergonomics of task performance; and (6) emergency response procedures (Whittaker et al., 2017). Identifying environmental features that impair a client's performance may provide direction to a relatively simple solution that can mitigate or eliminate the problem. Consideration of all environments a client uses is important. Environments may vary greatly for some clients and may include, but are not limited to, various rooms of the home, various outdoor venues in different types of weather conditions, grocery stores, senior centers, shopping malls, museums, churches, medical office buildings, and restaurants. Asking a client to go through their schedule of a typical weekday and weekend day with you is one way to determine the different types of environments that may need to be considered in your evaluation.

### Evaluation of Occupational Performance

The fourth component of the OT low vision assessment is evaluation of the client's occupational performance (Whittaker et al., 2016). Occupational performance is the ability to carry out activities of daily life, which includes areas of occupation. Areas of occupation include basic and personal ADLs, IADLs, education, work, play, leisure, and social participation. In the evaluation of a client's occupational performance, performance skills and patterns used in performance are identified, along with the other features that influence performance such as client factors, activity demands, and context(s) (AOTA, 2020). Therefore, in evaluating the occupational performance of the client with low vision, multiple methods of assessment in relevant environments are necessary. Considering the assessment information that has already been discussed, the occupational therapist will have a direction as to the assessments that need to be completed with the client to determine the impact low vision has on the client's performance.

Some assessments that may be chosen by the OT are those that are used with various populations, and include tasks and activities that are found to be challenges for clients with low vision. Other assessments are designed more specifically for problems encountered by clients with low vision. In any case, it is important to consider the client factors, activity demands, and context(s) during the assessment of the client's performance in the various areas of occupation. As discussed previously, two clients with the same low vision condition may have very different experiences and challenges. Also, the same client with low vision may be able to perform an activity well, but when the context of the activity changes, the ability to succeed may change as well.

Assessments frequently used in the evaluation of the occupational performance of a client with low vision include the survey and observation of typical activities. Some of those assessments may include, but are not limited to, the Canadian Occupational Performance Measure (COPM), the Barthel Index, and the Performance Assessment of Self-Care Skills (PASS). Activities that are particularly challenging and require routine assessment for clients with low vision include reading labels on medicine bottles and food containers, reading the newspaper and mail, pouring liquid, and using the microwave (Whittaker et al., 2017). Depending upon the facility, organization, or environment where an occupational therapist practices, other observational assessments may include basic and personal ADLs and IADLs, including education, work, play, leisure, and social participation.

A standardized assessment of ADLs and IADLs developed specifically for occupational therapists' evaluation of the client with low vision is the Self-Report Assessment of Functional and Visual Performance (SRAFVP) (Warren et al., 2008). This assessment is made up of a 38-item self-report questionnaire and a 7-item observational assessment. The self-report questionnaire is the client's assessment of their performance of vision-dependent tasks and the observation activities are an opportunity for the OT to confirm the client's reported visual abilities (Gilbert & Baker, 2011).

As part of a comprehensive occupational performance evaluation, it is also important to consider the output of effort and energy on the part of the low vision client (Whittaker et al., 2017). Many times, older adults with low vision are considered independent with ADLs; however, they require a significant amount of mental and physical effort on their part. This independence is achieved with an uncertain level of safety and little margin for error. As a result, the client is performing ADLs with maximal effort and has little to no reserve for other activities (Warren & Lampert, 1999).

During the evaluation process, the occupational therapist is developing and reviewing data that will be used to develop the client's goals and intervention plan. As part of the process, the OT must also assess the client's rehabilitation potential. For the client with low vision, the process of determining rehabilitation potential needs to consider the visual, movement, environmental, and cognitive components of tasks (Whittaker et al., 2017). The goals and intervention plan need to be meaningful, achievable, and developed to promote the client's ability to complete necessary and desired activities.

## Intervention

The process of intervention consists of three components—intervention plan, intervention process, and intervention review—and leads to the client's outcome, which is engagement in occupation to support participation (AOTA, 2020). The *intervention plan* will guide actions taken and is developed in collaboration with the client. It is based on selected theories, frames of reference, and evidence and confirms the

targeted outcomes for the client. *Intervention implementation* includes the ongoing actions taken to influence and support improved client performance. Interventions are directed at identified client outcomes and the client's response is monitored and documented. The *intervention review* is a review of the implementation plan and process as well as its progress toward targeted client outcomes (AOTA, 2020). The occupational therapist and OT assistant do not follow the components of the intervention process as linear steps, rather OT practitioners continually reassess the intervention process based on how the client is responding, the impact of the environment, and the availability of resources, and adjustments are made as needed. The intervention process for the client with low vision allows the client to attain the desired outcome, as the OT practitioner guides and adjusts the intervention process along the way.

The approach to intervention for the client with low vision will vary from one practice environment to another; however, there are components that should be included in any comprehensive OT plan. In addition, it is important to refer to other low vision rehabilitation professionals to support the client's overall function, safety, and health as needed.

One approach to intervention is a seven-step sequential treatment plan developed by Whittaker et al. (2017). This approach includes the course of intervention strategies that follow: (1) Education—including the nature of the eye disease, the outlook for the future, and expectations of vision rehabilitation; (2) Therapeutic Activities—including eccentric viewing, scanning, and reading skills; (3) Environmental Modifications—including lighting contrast and glare; (4) Nonoptical Assistive Devices—including visual, tactile, and auditory; (5) Optical Magnification; (6) Computer Technology in Low Vision Rehabilitation; and (7) Resources and Handouts. This approach is comprehensive in nature and provides specific areas to include in an OT low vision intervention plan. This is not to say it is the only approach, as there are many others to consider (e.g., Warren, 2011). Whatever approach the OT practitioner chooses to use with low vision clients, it should be one that provides clients with strategies, resources, support, and confidence to successfully overcome the challenges of living with a low vision impairment.

There are many aspects to occupational low vision intervention —too many to be covered in this chapter alone. A general overview of the areas the OT practitioner needs to address includes patient and family education, the use of optical and nonoptical devices, and application of low vision rehabilitation strategies. This overview provides fundamental information for general practice OT professionals and students. For more extensive learning on the practice of OT in low vision rehabilitation, further professional development is encouraged.

### Patient and Family Education

Initial OT sessions for the client with low vision may require a fair degree of patient and family education. Low vision clients have many questions and concerns about their eye condition, the prognosis regarding whether they will be able to drive, read, care for children, socialize with family and friends, travel, work, or continue in particular roles and leisure activities, and whether they will go blind. It is helpful for the OT practitioner to be prepared for these types of questions ahead of time, giving the client general information about the disease process, what they may be able to accomplish through low vision rehabilitation services, and referring more specific diagnostic and prognostic questions to their physician. The OT practitioner can prepare handouts on various topics to distribute to low vision clients as needed (see Appendix E, Tips for Making Print More Readable). Helpful topics for handouts may include (1) OT Services in Low Vision Rehabilitation (see Appendix F); (2) Tips for Talking to the Doctor (see Appendix C); (3) Information on Conditions—Low Vision, Glaucoma, Macular Degeneration, Diabetic Retinopathy, and Cataract (see NEI's brochure and fact sheet site, https://www.nei.nih.gov/learn-about-eye-health/outreach-campaigns-and-resources/eye-health-among-african-americans/write-vision-resources/resources-type/fact-sheets); (4) National Resources and Support Organizations (see national resources listed at the end of this chapter); and (5) Local Community Resources and Organizations. Since OT sessions are limited in time, some of these resources may help the low vision client and family pursue local opportunities on their own time; however, it is still the role of the OT practitioner to educate the client and family on the impact of low vision on occupational performance and how OT services may be able to reduce barriers to the client's engagement in occupation and support the client's participation.

## Use of Optical and Nonoptical Devices

Low vision clients frequently require devices to support the use of their remaining vision. Devices are usually categorized as optical or nonoptical devices. Optical devices are magnifiers used to enlarge printed materials, medication labels, photographs, street signs, or any other items a client has difficulty seeing Even so, it is important to remember fundamental facts about optical devices (Nowakowski, 2011). First, an optical device serves as a functional aid rather than a remedy, offering improved functionality with the remaining vision of the user rather than restoring lost vision. Second, while an optical device does not provide clear vision to individuals with visual impairments, it can enhance object visibility by making them appear larger. However, it cannot enhance clarity when disease or trauma has compromised the eye's ability for clear vision. Third, the low vision physician prescribes optical devices in a specific manner tailored to an individual's needs and tasks. Allowing clients to self-prescribe or choose through trial and error is counterproductive and does not yield optimal results. And lastly, for effective use of the prescribed device, practitioners must have a precise understanding of its functionality and how it aligns with the individual's needs. Clear communication between the prescribing low vision physician and the practitioner is crucial to ensure the therapy's effectiveness, preventing frustration and potential failure associated with incorrect device usage (Nowakowski, 2011). Nonoptical devices are small adaptive equipment items or materials that do not incorporate the use of a lens, and function to improve a client's ability to access visual information in the environment.

Optical and nonoptical devices are usually not covered by insurance carriers; however, in the United States, most states have funds available through Title VII of the Rehabilitation Act of 1973 to support the independence of older adults with visual impairments. Often, these funds are discretionary and can be used, in part, to pay for low vision devices (Orr, 1998). The OT practitioner would benefit from exploring the many devices and adaptive equipment items available to low vision clients (see https://cdn.shopify.com/s/files/1/0003/2391/1741/files/Optelec_for_Professionals_Product_Catalog_Rev_8-2021.pdf?v=1629486010). For devices and adaptive equipment items with which the OT practitioner is less familiar, s/he may gain skills and knowledge in pursuing hands-on training opportunities.

### Application of Low Vision Rehabilitation Strategies

There are many strategies available to the OT practitioner to overcome barriers that result from low vision conditions. Some of those strategies are identified here as they pertain to specific visual deficits. A discussion of the use of those strategies follows.

For the low vision client with a restricted field due to a *peripheral field loss*, strategies to improve function include (1) increasing lighting, (2) teaching scanning in vertical and horizontal planes, (3) increasing contrast, and (4) teaching functional mobility skills to improve safety with mobility. For the client with peripheral field loss, it is better to refer them to a COMS for more complicated mobility tasks such as multilane street crossings. Clients with *central field loss*, such as the those with macular degeneration, can overcome some of the challenges they face by (1) increasing lighting, (2) teaching eccentric viewing skills, (3) increasing contrast, and (4) instruction in the use of magnifiers for smaller printed items and dials. A client with *decreased acuity* that cannot be corrected with eyeglasses would benefit from some of the same strategies. The impact of decreased visual acuity may be lessened by (1) increasing lighting, (2) increasing contrast, (3) instructing them in the use of magnifiers, and (4) enlarging dials on appliances and numbers on cell phones.

### *Lighting Strategies*

To address lighting issues, the OT practitioner needs to consider the environment and the task at hand. There are circumstances in which a client would benefit from more light, which may be remedied with a task lamp, or would benefit from reduced light, which may be accomplished with a dimmer switch. At times, clients may need a *portable* light source. A small high-powered LCD flashlight improves readability of a menu in a dark restaurant or helps with mobility when directed to the floor or sidewalk in low light or dark environments.

For indoor environments, lighting may include overhead fluorescent sources or incandescent, halogen, and or combination bulbs typically found in lamps or ceiling fixtures in the home. In addition, natural light from the sun may enter through windows. Natural light can be an asset in the home or office when it is controlled with shears, shades, or blinds on the windows. Outdoors, natural light is more helpful in early or late parts of the day. Frequently, the use of a visor, sunglasses, or colored sun lenses will improve a client's vision. The OT practitioner needs to determine the best type of lighting and the best position for the light source to allow the low vision client to be successful with everyday tasks.

When there is too much light in an environment, the low vision client will likely experience glare. Glare can occur for several reasons, including reflected sunlight in an outdoor environment or reflected light indoors from surfaces such as floors, counters, and walls It is important for the OT practitioner to be aware of sources of glare for low vision clients as it can be discomforting at best and disabling at its worst.

### Contrast Strategies

To increase contrast, the OT practitioner needs to consider adapting a client's environment with high-contrast colors and introduce nonoptical devices that will improve contrast while performing tasks. For instance, a simple use of colored electrician's tape along a door jamb, the edge of a step, a countertop, or along the edge of the bathtub can provide the low vision client enough visual information to judge the depth, distance, or presence of an object. Other examples to improve contrast with reading and writing activities include the use of a gel sheet, bold underlining for reading and writing, a writing guide, and a dark, thick felt pen (e.g., Sanford 20/20 Easy to Read Pen)

### Scanning Strategies

Scanning is an effective technique to use with clients with visual field loss who have difficulty finding a landmark, the door to a business, or the edge of a page. When a client is outdoors, horizontal and vertical scanning techniques are effective in helping a client orient to their environment and locate an address, business, or doorknob. The client is instructed to systematically view the environment starting at the top and scanning right to left, then left to right until the object of interest comes into their visual field. The same technique can be used by scanning vertically, moving from top to bottom and bottom to top, working across the designated environment until they find what they are looking for. In applying scanning techniques to near tasks, a client with a left field deficit and the goal of reading effectively can benefit from the placement of a high-contrast border along the left margin of the reading material. The client would be instructed to scan into the left until the border comes into their line of sight. After reading the line of print, the client would be reminded to look for the border on the left to continue the reading process. Scanning techniques can be applied to many situations, allowing a client to orient and locate distant targets, while aligning their visual field appropriately for near and intermediate tasks as well.

### Functional Mobility Strategies

Supporting the client with low vision in functional mobility skills is, in part, the responsibility of the OT practitioner. The client may need instruction for proper transfers in the bathroom, bedroom, living room, office, and car, to name a few. The client needs to be encouraged to keep pathways and furniture clear of clutter to avoid a fall or injury. Appropriate lighting and contrast in any given environment will aid the low vision client in judging depth and distance during functional mobility tasks. The OT practitioner may also choose to instruct the client and caregiver in the use of sighted guide techniques. These techniques will increase the client's safety in crowded or unfamiliar environments and areas that have poor lighting and uneven walking surfaces.

Functional mobility also includes the topic of transportation. For low vision clients who have been driving for most of their adult lives, being faced with the prospect of not being able to drive can be difficult. Fortunately, a person with low vision can drive safely under the right circumstances (Peli & Peli, 2002). There is not one isolated visual skill that can be associated with determining if a person with low vision is fit to drive (Huss & Corn, 2004). It is best to refer low vision clients who want to continue to drive to an occupational therapist who is also a certified driving rehabilitation specialist (CDRS) Association of Driver Rehabilitation Specialists. These specialists are equipped with the knowledge and resources to intervene with the low vision client interested in driving. For those clients who will not be driving, the OT practitioner can assist them in finding and using alternative transportation resources. Being familiar with public, private, and community transportation services in the local area will allow the OT practitioner to help the low vision client make this transition with greater ease.

### Eccentric Viewing Strategies

For clients with central field loss due to conditions such as macular degeneration, eccentric viewing is a strategy used to help them "look around" the blind spot in their field of view. With eccentric viewing, the client looks slightly away from their intended target, to bring it into view of the peripheral visual field. Once the client has determined the location of the scotoma or blind spot in their central visual field (as described earlier with the clock face test method), training in looking around the scotoma is necessary to help develop eccentric viewing skills. The clock face, along with other visual tools, can also be used to further develop a client's eccentric viewing skills.

When using the clock face for eccentric viewing activities, the client with a scotoma in the center of the visual field is instructed to direct the scotoma to the right (toward the number three) to locate the center focal point. Then the client returns the scotoma to the center and is instructed to direct the scotoma upwards (toward the number 12) to again locate the center focal point. This method of eccentric viewing training continues until the client is able to look around the scotoma with ease. Once a client has mastered the clock face, they can progress to read lines of individual letters, then individual words, then lines of text, and finally to view pictures. Although some clients may have developed an eccentric viewing method subconsciously, for others, it takes quite a bit of practice. Both the client and OT practitioner need to be patient with the process.

### Magnification Strategies

Many times, clients with low vision benefit from magnification; however, it is not an intervention strategy that solves all low vision problems (Nowakowski, 2011). When used properly, it can improve a client's functional visual abilities. There are several strategies for achieving magnification, which include (1) use of a magnifier, (2) relative size magnification, (3) relative distance magnification, (4) angular magnification, and (5) projection magnification (Whittaker et al., 2017)

Magnifiers are optical devices that use lenses to enlarge text and other materials. Magnifiers come in different powers and are measured in diopters (D). It is important to note that the stronger the power of a magnifier, the smaller the field of view; therefore, the higher-powered magnifiers will have smaller viewing windows. Magnifiers can be illuminated or nonilluminated and are available in different designs, such as stand magnifiers or handheld magnifiers. All these features should be considered to meet the needs of individual clients.

Relative size magnification is the process of increasing the size of an object to make it more visible. Simply put, relative size magnification is an enlargement process (Whittaker et al., 2017). This can easily be achieved for client handouts by using font change features on the computer (see Appendix E, Tips for Making Print More Readable). Another method to achieve magnification is by decreasing the distance between the client and the object. This is known as relative distance magnification. The closer the client is to an object, the larger the image becomes that is projected onto the retina (Whittaker et al., 2017).

Angular magnification is achieved using an optical device: the telescope. The use of a telescope allows an enlarged image of an object at a distance to be projected onto the retina (Whittaker et al., 2017). This is very valuable to clients with low vision who need to read street signs, locate addresses, or identify a person from a distance. Another type of magnification is projection magnification. This type of magnification enlarges an image of an object by projecting it onto a screen (Whittaker et al., 2017). This method is used in overhead projectors, closed circuit televisions (CCTVs), and portable electronic magnifiers.

The magnification devices and systems identified here are only a few of those that are available. It would be helpful to the OT practitioner to not only find hands-on training opportunities, but to also learn about the costs, and possible funding sources in the local community. Some of the devices and systems may be cost-prohibitive. However, many of the clients who require the more expensive items may be able to qualify for funding from a local agency. In addition, as with any type of adaptive equipment, if a client doesn't know how to use the magnifying devices and systems properly, they will not be used. It is important for the OT practitioner to do all they can to make the most out of client education opportunities when it comes to the use of magnifiers. The client has much to gain if they're able to use the magnifiers efficiently and effectively.

## Professional Development in Low Vision

As the field of low vision OT grows and expands, more skills are necessary to meet the needs of the low vision OT client. As a result, occupational therapists and OT assistants can benefit from pursuing professional development opportunities in the area of low vision.

Professional development opportunities for low vision practitioners include professional certification programs, graduate education with a focus in low vision rehabilitation, face-to-face seminars, and online continuing education opportunities. The AOTA's Board and Specialty Certification program provides an avenue for recognition in low vision practice for occupational therapists (SCLV) and OT assistants (SCLV-A). Obtaining professional credentials indicative of advanced knowledge, skills, and experience in low vision provides the OT practitioner the opportunity to have their expertise recognized by consumers, third-party payers, and professional peers.

## SUMMARY

The OT practitioner who works to improve the occupational performance of older adults with low vision is providing them the opportunity to return to the roles and activities that give their lives meaning. It is an area of OT that has been growing and should continue to grow for the next several decades, based on the projected increases in the older adult population.

### Functional Performance and Hearing Loss

Hearing loss is a common problem among aging adults. The National Institute on Aging states approximately one in three persons between the ages of 65 and 74 in the United States have a hearing loss (NIA, n.d.). Some hearing losses can be remediated with medical assessment and intervention, but this is not the typical case for age related hearing loss. When medical intervention cannot restore a patient's normal function, they will live with a loss of hearing sensitivity that typically causes ongoing deficits. Interventions used with this population are hearing aids, cochlear implants, and other amplification devices coupled with rehabilitation. Even with the best evidence-based treatment, this population will, in many cases, still live with some deficits related to their hearing loss.

The most notable effect of adult hearing loss is impaired communications, which can adversely affect all aspects of interpersonal relationships with others and create problems in the workplace for aging adults (Cunningham & Tucci, 2017; Davis & Hoffman, 2019). In addition, recent studies have shown us that individuals with hearing loss also experience increased rates of depression, social isolation, and cognitive decline (Cosh et al., 2019; Gopinath et al., 2012; Lawrence et al., 2020; Lin et al., 2011; Lisan et al., 2019; World Health Organization, 2019). Hearing loss can be so insidious that persons do not even realize they are experiencing hearing loss, making it even more difficult to recognize (Wittich & Simcock, 2019) and treat.

More men than women are affected by hearing loss between the ages 45 and over, but the prevalence increases dramatically for men as the population ages increase (ages 45–64) from 8.9% to 19.2% (ages 65 and older) in men, compared to

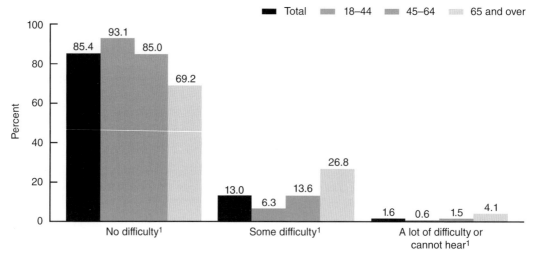

**FIGURE 10.16**    Percentage of adults aged 18 and over with difficulty hearing even when using a hearing aid, by age group: United States, 2019. [1]Significant quadratic trend by age ($p < 0.05$). Notes: Hearing limitation is based on responses to the survey question, "Do you have difficulty hearing, even when using a hearing aid? Would you say no difficulty, some difficulty, a lot of difficulty, or you cannot do this at all?" Estimates are based on household interviews of a sample of the US civilian noninstitutionalized population. (From the National Center for Health Statistics, National Health Interview Survey, 2019.)

5.4% for women (ages 45–64) to 10.6% for women (at ages 65 and over) (Fig. 10.16; NCHS et al., 2021). There are also ethnic differences in hearing loss (Fig. 10.17; NCHS et al., 2021). Non-Latinx Whites aged 45–64 (16.4%) have the highest incidence of difficulty hearing even when using a hearing aid, followed by non-Latinx Black adults (7.7%), then Latinx adults (8.6%), and finally non-Latinx Asian adults (5.7%). The percentages only increase for each ethnic group for 65 years and older. It was estimated that persons suffering with hearing loss wait an average of 10 years before seeking any help, perhaps because hearing loss associated with aging is unrecognized and therefore undertreated (Walling & Dickson, 2012). Walling and Dickson (2012) estimated that 20% of persons 65 years or older with a moderate to profound hearing loss did not consider themselves hearing impaired.

According to the Occupational Therapy Practice Framework and Domain ("Occupational Therapy Practice Framework," 2020). OT practitioners should include hearing concerns and maintenance of hearing devices in our consideration for assessment of ADL training. The Global Burden of Disease (GBD) study estimated that persons with mild and unilateral hearing loss increased from 1.2 billion (17.2%) in 2008 to 1.4 billion (18.7%) in 2017 (GBD, n.d.). The increases in hearing loss have been touted as a public health crisis.

Recent efforts by some members of Congress are considering covering hearing aids as part of changes to Medicare. Other efforts by legislators are looking at making some amplification devices as over-the-counter, bypassing the medical necessity requirement altogether. No matter what type of hearing loss an individual is experiencing, OTs are uniquely positioned to work with clients to lessen the disability associated with the hearing loss. We discuss types of hearing losses subsequently in this chapter to provide a basis for making

educated recommendations to patients/clients as to which path is best for their needs and finances.

## Age-Related Hearing Loss

Hearing loss can strike suddenly or gradually and at any age. In this discussion, we focus on **presbycusis** or the progressive hearing loss related to aging. In the past, presbycusis was accepted as a normal part of aging and many times, unfortunately, not treated. It is true that one in three individuals over the age of 65 will have some type of hearing loss, so it is a common or "normal" part of the aging process, but we now have tools that when used properly can alleviate some of the typical consequences of untreated hearing loss, such as depression, social isolation, increased rate of cognitive decline, and lower quality of life.

### Slow Progression of Age-Related Hearing Loss

Presbycusis is not something that one wakes up with in the morning after going to sleep with normal hearing. It typically occurs over the span of many years and will not create a functional impairment until a client's communication needs put enough stress on the auditory system that a disability or functional impairment is noted. This is one reason why the application of person-centered care and tools like the COSI are essential in evaluation, as they allow the clinician to consider community needs of the client when making treatment decisions. The COSI (Client Oriented Scale for Improvement by National Acoustic Lab--a division of Australian Hearing) is a self-scoring client-centered tool that they fill in and the clinician grades, regarding how much the hearing aid (or devices) helped them in functional situations. The COSI is easily found on the internet (https://www.nal.gov.au/nal_products/cosi/).

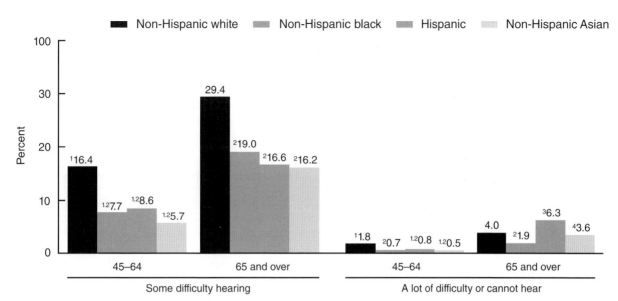

**FIGURE 10.17**   Percentage of adults aged 45 and over with difficulty hearing even when using a hearing aid, by age group and race and Latinx origin: United States, 2019. [1]Significantly different from age group 65 and over ($p < 0.05$). [2]Significantly different from non-Latinx white ($p < 0.05$). [3]Significantly different from non-Latinx black ($p < 0.05$). [4]Relative confidence interval width is greater than 130% (actual value = 182%). Notes: Hearing limitation is based on responses to the survey question, "Do you have difficulty hearing, even when using a hearing aid? Would you say no difficulty, some difficulty, a lot of difficulty, or you cannot do this at all?" Estimates are based on household interviews of a sample of the US civilian noninstitutionalized population. (From the National Center for Health Statistics, National Health Interview Survey, 2019.)

Screening for hearing loss, referral to a hearing health care provider, and counseling around the issue of hearing loss are essential measures for maintenance of quality of life in the population experiencing presbycusis. Occupational therapists working with individuals who may be experiencing presbycusis are uniquely positioned to take on some of these functions.

## Function and Conditions of the Ear

### Anatomy and Physiology of Hearing (See Appendix B)

#### Outer, Middle, and Inner Ear

The structures that carry sound from the environment to the brain for processing are commonly referred to as the ear, and are divided into three sections—**outer ear, middle ear, and inner ear**. The outer ear consists of the **pinna** and **ear canal**, and sound travels from the pinna down the ear canal and into the next structure, the eardrum or **tympanic membrane**. The tympanic membrane serves as the border between the outer and middle ear, and begins to vibrate due to the sound energy hitting it. These vibrations are carried by the smallest bones in the body, the **ossicles**, from the tympanic membrane to the first part of the inner ear, a membrane covered opening that serves as sound energy's entrance to the cochlea, called the **oval window**. The cochlea is part of the inner ear and is filled with fluid. The movement of the oval window pushing into the cochlea causes the cochlear fluids to move. The movement of the cochlear fluids causes the **auditory neurons** in the inner ear to be simulated, and these neurons are able to send information to cranial nerve VIII (CNVIII) and then to the brain for processing.

### Central Auditory Nervous System (CANS)

The CANS is the pathway of neurons, nuclei, and synapses that takes the information from CNVIII to the auditory association areas in the brain for final processing. It should be noted that these structures run from the brainstem all the way up to the cortex of the temporal lobe and take an active role in signal processing—essentially translating the sound coming in into a message that the listener can understand. This process is not fully understood and is an area of active research.

### Pathology of Hearing Loss

When any problem occurs with the outer, middle, or inner ear or CANS, there is a possibility of hearing loss. The location of the problem within the auditory system makes a difference in the prognosis and treatment recommendations.

#### Conductive, Sensorineural, and Mixed Hearing Loss

When problems arise within the outer or middle ear, and cause hearing loss, the loss is referred to as a conductive hearing loss. Conductive hearing losses typically require medical treatment and will often resolve with that treatment. When problems arise within the inner ear and CANS, and cause hearing loss, the loss is referred to as a sensorineural hearing loss. Sensorineural hearing losses typically do not require medical treatment, as they are permanent in nature. This is where the provision of hearing aids, cochlear implants, or other assistive devices by an audiologist is typically the recommended treatment. Presbycusis is one type of hearing loss that is sensorineural in nature.

## Conditions Causing Hearing Impairments

### Presbycusis, Age Related

As discussed earlier, presbycusis is a slowly progressing sensorineural hearing loss that many individuals over the age of 65 will experience. These age-related changes can occur in the inner ear, the CANS, or in a combination of both of these areas. It is typically bilateral, and symmetrical, meaning that the loss occurs in both ears, and both ears have the same severity of hearing loss.

### Genetic Causes

Hearing loss can be caused by an individual's genetic code. Many of these losses are sensorineural, and the patient/client deals with the effects of the hearing loss throughout their life. It may be the case that a patient/client over the age of 65 who has been living with a hearing loss for most of their life will have interventions in place that work for them. However, discussion of the interventions being used may be warranted depending on the individual's deficits from the hearing loss and their personal communication goals.

### *Syndromic*

Hearing loss can occur in conjunction with other abnormalities. Syndromes have distinguishing clinical features in addition to hearing loss and are more easily clinically recognized than nonsyndromic genetic hearing loss. Examples of genetic conditions related to hearing loss include Waardenburg's syndrome and Crouzon's disease.

### *Nonsyndromic*

Most hereditary hearing loss is not related to a particular syndrome. There is much variation in the presentation of these hearing losses. The loss can differ in its severity and progression, affect one or both ears, and affect different parts of the ear, resulting in loss at different pitches. Identifying the genes involved has been difficult to date.

There have been autosomal dominant forms of hearing loss, autosomal recessive, and x linked recessive types found. Mutations in a particular gene, called connexin 26, have been found to be responsible for a significant proportion of childhood genetic deafness (Survey of Audiology: Fundamentals for Audiologists and Health Professionals, 3rd Edition, 2020).

### Noise-Induced Hearing Loss (NIHL)

In most cases, NIHL takes place gradually, over a long period of time. The severity of the hearing loss depends on several factors, including the duration of exposure, the level of the noise, and individual susceptibility ("Survey of Audiology: Fundamentals for Audiologists and Health Professionals, 3rd Edition," 2020). Some sounds, such as a gunshot or a rocket launch, are so loud that they can cause hearing damage after only one exposure.

### Meniere's Disease

This is a condition that affects the inner ear. There is a characteristic group of symptoms that include hearing loss, tinnitus, and vertigo. The individual with Meniere's disease may have any combination of the previous symptoms. The patient/client also has symptom free periods, and the hearing loss can fluctuate. Over time, the hearing loss may become permanent.

### Otosclerosis

This condition is due to a build-up of spongy bone around the stapes footplate that causes a decrease in movement of the ossicles, and a subsequent hearing loss. The bone can harden, or invade the cochlea, worsening the effects.

## Occupational Therapy Assessments

Any OT assessment should begin with the elements in the *AOTA Occupational Profile Template*. Depending upon the work setting and the amount of time available for data gathering, that may dictate the assessment the OT chooses to use. After obtaining the initial patient/client information, the occupational therapist has several quick-tests available for an assessment of hearing loss. Of course, there is no substitute for working with other health professionals who specialize in hearing loss and treatment. The OT practitioner will need to assess the patient's/client's ability to follow the instructions for testing. The most practical and immediate method is through direct observation. The *One Question screener* simply asks the patient/client, "Do you believe you have a hearing problem/loss?" If your patients/clients are asking you to repeat your questions, especially if they are not looking at you (or vice versa), that is an obvious clue that they may be lip reading and not even realize it. With the onset of COVID-19 and all the variants to come, wearing facial masks has made communication with older adults even more difficult. This chapter will not go into the merits or disadvantages of one type of mask over another, but be aware of how some masks can protect the therapist and still allow your voice to be less muffled by the mask.

The *Whisper Test* is a simple test and can be found on the internet (Pirozzo et al., 2003). The patient/client is seated and the tester is about an arms-length (2 feet) behind them. The tester instructs the patient/client to cover the ear not being tested. The tester takes a deep breath and exhales fully before giving a number-letter-number combination. Have the patient/client repeat what they hear. If the response is correct, move on to the other ear. If the subject is unsuccessful, reattempt testing with a different number-letter-number combination. If they get three total letters and/or numbers correct after a second attempt, that is considered a pass.

Two high-frequency hearing loss tests for the bedside are the *Finger Rub* and *Ticking Watch Tests* (Torres-Russotto et al., 2009). The tester rubs two fingers together and records how far away from the ear the subject can still hear. This method fails if the OT thinks the subject pretends to hear. The same method is used for an analog watch (with audible "ticking"). The same caveat is true for this method.

The *Hearing Handicap Inventory in the Elderly* (Ventry & Weinstein, 1982) is the best method for a self-reported tool and easily scored by the practitioner. There are two versions available: one is a modified version of 10 questions; the original version includes 25 questions, both with stated norming scoring scales. The patient/client would need to hear or read the questions, and answer them honestly. This inventory takes a relatively short time to administer. Both versions include some environmental questions that can be useful in setting patient-oriented goals for treatment.

What are the client's priorities for their hearing performance and needs? For older adult clients, especially if they are still in the workforce, this may be exceedingly important to the OT plan of care. There are at least two tools that can help the OT and the client prioritize their hearing goals. One is the National Acoustic Laboratories (NAL; division of Australian Hearing) *Client Oriented Scale of Improvement (COSI)* and the *COPM*. The COSI was designed to be performed by an audiologist to determine the degree of improvement before and after being issued a hearing aid (see addendum for copy of COSI). The *COPM* is a well-established self-scoring tool for therapists and clients to help prioritize importance of tasks. It includes three areas of classification: self-care, work, and leisure pursuits. This test can take upwards of 20 plus minutes to administer, at least initially, but can be used for additional updating of scores for subsequent visits.

Along with any assessment of the client's hearing should be an assessment of their immediate environment, either in-person or virtual. This is best if done through a home visit, but can be accomplished virtually if the OT asks the right questions. It is important to ascertain what mitigation to one's environment can improve an individual's ability to hear better, especially if they are not reaching their communication goals. This would have to be established by a hearing/audiology professional. Questions to ask may include:

- Can you reduce the acoustics of your environment, i.e., using noise-absorbing materials like pillows, carpets, heavy curtains, pillows, or plants?
- Does your TV have closed captioning capability?
- Would you consider using infrared (Bluetooth) headphones to reduce TV volume in consideration of others in the room?
- Do you have caller ID?
- Can you get visual transcripts of your voice messages on your phone?
- Do you have any visual alerting devices at home, i.e., fire alarm or alarm clock?

There are other compensatory strategies to improve conversational speech and understanding conversations one-on-one. These are listed as part of Table 10.3 under *Compensatory Strategies*.

## Medication Considerations

This next section deals with medication considerations that occupational therapists should be aware of that may affect hearing in adults. Also note that Chapter 14 on Pharmacology is another resource. The following medications can be considered potentially detrimental to adult hearing:

- **Aspirin**—in large doses (>8 to 12 pills a daily); adult dose can be buffered or not. They should be individually set by a physician but will vary if prescribed for various types of arthritis, lupus, pain, fever, myocardial infarction (prophylactically), revascularization procedures (prophylactically), just to name a few.

- **Nonsteroidal antiinflammatory** (NSAIDs) (Ibuprofen and Naproxen)—is an over-the-counter (OTC) pain reliever. These pain relievers can also place individuals at risk if dosage is incorrect for kidney or stomach issues. It is recommended that individuals take the smallest amount effective and for the shortest time possible.

- **Certain antibiotics**—especially aminoglycosides (i.e., gentamicin, streptomycin, and neomycin). These antibiotics (ABX) have been known to cause hearing loss.

- **Loop diuretics** used to treat high blood pressure, liver disease, kidney disease, or edema due to congestive heart failure (Lasix, Furosemide, Bumetanide). These drugs work by making the kidneys pass out more fluids. They do this by interfering with the transport of salt and water across certain cells in the kidneys. Known side effects that are shared with other medications include: dizziness, headaches, dehydration, hyponatremia, hypokalemia, and gastrointestinal upset.

- **Cancer treatment medications** (Cyclophosphamide, Cisplatin, and Bleomycin)—chemotherapy drugs can be *ototoxic* meaning it is harmful to hearing. About half of the individuals who receive Cisplatin develop hearing loss, tinnitus, or vertigo *(Healthy Hearing, September 20, 2021). All three of these drugs have potential to affect hearing depending upon where the cancer is located.*

## Occupational Therapy Intervention

There are many great suggestions listed by Kristen Marie-Weber Chang (Chang, 2020) in Table 10.4 that were completed as part of her dissertation document. She has done an excellent job of organizing potential interventions for OT practitioners in a relatively comprehensive list.

Occupational therapists and OT assistants cannot nor should not treat clients with hearing loss in a vacuum. Interprofessional collaboration is necessary when addressing the full scope and needs of the problem and whether or not it is correctable. Consider a referral to other appropriate disciplines as part of the intervention.

### Referrals to Other Disciplines

In general, it is important to refer individuals to an audiologist for further testing if the patient or caregiver notes any concern about hearing, or if the OT practitioner finds an issue while administering any of the tests mentioned earlier. It should be noted that the whisper test, finger rub, and watch tick tests are still mentioned in the literature and used for referral, but if the patient reports difficulty hearing and is willing to consult a hearing health-care provider, referral is appropriate. When you determine your patient is in need for referral due to a hearing loss, you have several options for referral location. Your goal is to find a hearing health-care provider who is qualified to diagnose and treat all types of hearing loss, and will focus on patient centered care, as well as have a billing model that works for the patient.

Typically, referring to a hospital ear, nose, and throat (EN-T) department, sometimes called otolaryngology, is a good place to

**TABLE 10.3** Alternative Hearing-Related Intervention

| **Hearing Assistive Technology (HAT)** | | |
|---|---|---|
| **Television** | **Telephone, Cell Phone** | **Alerting Devices (i.e., Doorbells, Alarm Clocks, Fire Alarms, Kitchen Timer)** |
| • Turn on closed captioning<br>• Use wireless infrared headphones<br>• Amplify treble<br>• Turn off audio enhancements | • Caller ID<br>• Hearing aid compatibility<br>• Phone noise cancellation<br>• LED flash/vibrating ringtone<br>• Visual voicemail<br>• Captioned telephone<br>• Video calling (Facetime/Facebook Messenger chat) | Modified by:<br>• Vibration<br>• LED flashing<br>• Visual cue |

**Acoustic environmental modifications**

- Reduce noise by furnishing home with noise-absorbing material (e.g., carpeting, pillows, heavy curtains, bookshelves, ceiling tiles, plants)
- Block external noise through soundproofing windows and doors
- Minimize background noise (e.g., remove source, turn down volume, wear slippers in home, use bumper pads for cabinets/drawers)
- Use decibel-measuring app to monitor noise

**Compensatory strategies**

- Maintain eye contact and face the individual
- Ensure good lighting
- Increase physical gestures and facial expressions
- Add more pauses and enunciate
- Avoid mint/gum/toothpick in mouth
- Repeat in a different way
- Avoid dismissive comments (e.g., "Never mind," "Forget it," "I'll tell you later")
- Wear clear face masks

*LED*, Light-emitting diode.

Reprinted with permission from Chang, K. (2021, August 2). *Hearing Loss and Older Adults: Supporting Quality of Life, Function, and Well-Being.* Retrieved from https://www.aota.org/Publications-News/otp/Archive/2021/Hearing-Loss-and-Older-Adults.aspx.

begin. A not-for-profit audiology clinic, such as one operating within a university setting, or a standalone not-for-profit clinic supported by reputable nongovernmental agencies is another good referral choice. Many audiologists also work in private practice settings, and these clinics can be wonderful places to refer your patients; however, due to the large variation in service models, license requirements for practice and service cost in the hearing health care industry, you are encouraged to be very familiar with a private practice and their outcomes providers and billing practices before referring to that type of facility.

## Audiology

### The Audiogram

Once a suitable provider has been identified, your patient/client will be administered a battery of diagnostic tests. The following is a description of the tests most likely to be performed, and some tools to help the OT practitioner understand how to talk with your patient about the results.

The most common diagnostic test for hearing loss given is the pure tone audiogram. The results are recorded on a form (Fig. 10.18). From top to bottom (the y axis), sounds go from very soft (quieter than a whisper) to extremely loud (train rushing by). The loudness of sounds on the audiogram is measured in a unit called decibel hearing level, or dBHL.

This will be shortened to dB on many audiograms. From left to right (the x axis), you will find sound go from low pitch to high pitch. The range of pitches tested correlates with the pitch of the sounds in the English language. We test from around the pitch of the lowest sound in English—the "J"—to the highest—the "th." This diagram is also useful to see the average loudness of the sounds in the English language.

The audiologist will record the softest sound the patient can hear at each frequency or pitch, in each ear while wearing headphones over the ears or small headphones inserted into the ears. These are called "thresholds," and are marked on the audiogram. The right ear thresholds are recorded with a circle, and the left ear thresholds are recorded with an "x."

In the diagram (Fig. 10.19), you can see that the softest level the patient/client can hear is different in each ear. Now, with a hearing loss shown with speech sounds on the same images, you can see any sound above the thresholds, marked as a circle or an x the patient cannot detect. These data are based on conversational speech at a typical speaking level, at 6 feet away from the speaker (Fig. 10.20).

- Type, degree, and recommendation for HL
  - Hearing loss can be conductive, meaning that the source of the loss is in the outer and/or middle ear (see ear diagram). Many of these hearing losses can be

**TABLE 10.4** IADLs and Leisure Interventions for Older Adults With Hearing Loss

**IADL Interventions**

***Communication management***
- Telephone/cell phone
- Caller ID

***Hearing aid compatibility***
- Phone noise cancellation
- LED flash/vibrating ringtone
- Visual voicemail
- Captioned telephone
- Video calling (Facetime/Facebook Messenger Chat)

***Driving***
- Turn off radio
- Install emergency vehicle warning system
- Constantly scan rearview and side windows
- Look for emergency strobe lights on top of traffic signal

***Meal preparation***
- Tea kettle (modified through haptic/visual cue)
- Kitchen timer (modified through haptic/visual cue)

***Religious expression***
- Sit at the front near the speakers
- Request written copy of the sermon

***Safety and emergency maintenance***
- Fire alarm/weather alert (modified through haptic/visual cue)
- Doorbell (modified through haptic/visual cue)

***Shopping***
- Go at less busy times
- Look at till for price display
- Pay with credit card
- Use self-check-out

**Leisure Participation**

***Television***
- Closed captioning
- Infrared and RF headphones
- Amplify treble

***Podcasts music radio***
- Use noise-reducing headphones
- Amplify treble
- Choose hosts with deeper voices

***Movie***
- Closed captioning viewings
- Request an assistive listening device

***Appointments***
- Text-based booking systems
- Call ahead of time to explain your needs

***Eating out***
- Choose places with sound-absorbing materials (i.e., tablecloths, carpeting)
- Sit in a high back booth or with back to the wall or corner
- Sit away from speakers, entrances, and heavily trafficked pathways
- Request background music be turned off or down
- Frequent quieter times
- Use decibel app to monitor background noise

*IADLs,* Instrumental activities of daily living; *LED,* light-emitting diode; *RF,* radiofrequency.
Reprinted with permission from Chang, K. (2021, August 2). *Hearing Loss and Older Adults: Supporting Quality of Life, Function, and Well-Being.* Retrieved from https://www.aota.org/Publications-News/otp/Archive/2021/Hearing-Loss-and-Older-Adults.aspx.

treated medically, and the patient/client will not have ongoing disability related to the problem. An example of this would be a cerumen "wax" blockage of the ear canal. The wax can act as a plug and cause a significant hearing loss. Once the plug is removed, which can be done safely by a trained medical provider with the right equipment, the hearing will return to normal.

- Speech Perception Score
  - While many diagnostics tests used in audiology are designed to determine the softest sound or word a patient/client can hear, the Speech Perception Score is aimed at determining the ability to understand words when they are turned up in volume to a comfortable level. This can be compared to turning up the television or radio loud enough for the patient/client to hear it. This essentially takes all the speech sounds and increases their volume, making as many as sounds as possible audible to the individual. It may seem that this would be a surefire way to have them score 100% on the test. Unfortunately, this is not the case. It is the nature of hearing loss that even with increased volume, the patient/client experiences distortion of sounds, making it difficult to understand. The speech perception score is an estimate of their ability to understand words if all the sounds are loud enough to be heard. A score of 96%–100% is considered "excellent" and is what we would expect for a patient/client with normal hearing. Some people with hearing loss will score in this excellent range as well. A score of below 70% is considered poor and the individual will typically have a significant amount of disability resulting from the hearing loss, even with well-fitted hearing aids. These patients/clients can be considered for cochlear implant evaluations. The audiologist working with the individual will determine if referral for cochlear implantation evaluation is the right option for them.

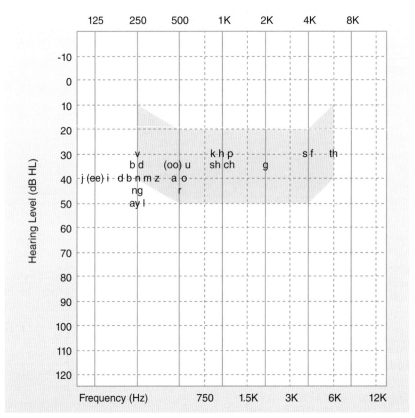

**FIGURE 10.18**    Long-Term Average Speech Spectrum (LTASS) plotted on a standard audiogram.

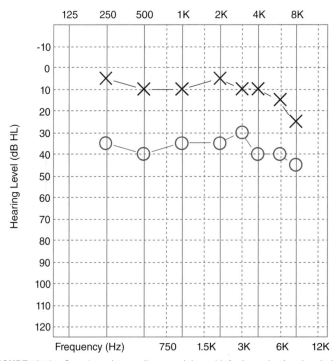

**FIGURE 10.19**    Sample patient audiogram: right and left air conduction thresholds.

- Selection and fitting of appropriate hearing devices
  - The audiologist will use a full battery of diagnostic tests, as well as patient/client factors, to decide the best treatment for each person. If hearing aids are an appropriate treatment option, the audiologist will, together with the patient/client, select the size and

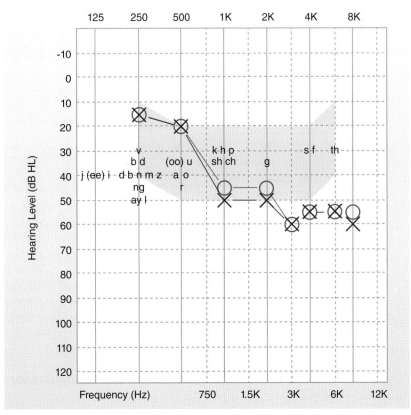

**FIGURE 10.20**   Sample patient audiogram, right and left air conduction with thresholds, with loudness and pitch information for English sounds included.

type of hearing aid. The fitting is done by the audiologist and includes customizing both the sound and the physical fit to the patient/client. Counseling on use and care is also part of the fitting process. The patient/client will see the audiologist a few times to get the hearing aids set correctly and will follow up with them on a continual basis for maintenance of devices as well as monitoring of hearing thresholds.

## Client and Family Education

Whenever possible, the treating practitioner should include handouts that give patients/clients and their family members the options and resources for improving hearing outcomes. Patients/clients or family members can be overwhelmed with too much information at once, so handouts can be beneficial for recall of education. As previously mentioned, some persons are unaware of their own hearing loss. The OT, therefore, must approach the subject carefully if s/he feels that is the case.

The implications for IADLs are varied and comprehensive in the preceding Table 10.4. The suggestions cover both IADLs (general communication, driving, meal preparation, religious expressions, safety and emergency maintenance, shopping) and leisure activities (television viewing, leisure listening activities (podcasts/music/radio, movies, appointments, and

dining out). As OT practitioners, we are experts at problem solving with our patients/clients to optimize function and minimize risks when possible.

Driving cessation can be a very sensitive subject with many older adults, and therefore, the subject must be approached cautiously. The hearing-impaired older adult has additional challenges to overcome when on the road. Driving is the ultimate multisensory and complex IADL anyone performs. A study conducted by Hickson et al. (2010) concluded that older adults in the presence of auditory and/or visual distractors were more likely to have trouble driving and be involved in more multivehicle crashes in complex traffic conditions at intersections. The AOTA sponsors the *Car-Fit* program in conjunction with the American Association of Retired Persons (AARP) and the American Auto Association (AAA). The program is another excellent way for a standardized assessment of aspects of driving skills for older adults (Car-Fit, n.d.). The Car-Fit programs are sponsored all over the country by individuals who have a specialty certification in the Car-Fit assessment. An occupational therapist can find the nearest program to them by contacting https://www.car-fit.org/.

## Hearing Aid Management—Service Models

As stated previously, helping the patient/client to properly use or maintain their hearing devices is considered within the OT practitioner scope of practice ("Occupational Therapy Practice Framework," 2020). One should understand the care standards and best method to maintain hearing devices from the hearing professional who issued the device to ensure the training is appropriate and comprehensive.

- Hearing aid management
  - Frequently, hearing aids are not used correctly or at all by patients who are fit with them. Problems such as clogging of the aids with wax, poor physical fit of the aids, improper insertions, and lack of full-time use are common. As OT practitioners, you are uniquely positioned to alleviate some of these issues, as your scope of practice allows.
- A few tips for supporting successful hearing aid use include:
  **Encourage and support full time use.** Hearing aids should be worn during all waking hours. The hearing aids should not be removed except for sleeping and any activity where they may become wet (showering, swimming). If the patient is unable to tolerate full-time use, the audiologist can often scaffold them into successful full-time use or adjust communication goals. The OT can consult with the fitting audiologist on how to best support full time use with their patient.

  **Facilitate correct insertion of the hearing aids.** Many individuals struggle with putting the hearing aids in the ear correctly. If the aids are not inserted correctly in the ear, they will not deliver the appropriate amount of sound for the patient/client, which will affect their ability to successfully reach their communication goals. If the individual is unable to insert the aids, the audiologist can reinstruct the patient/client and caregivers on proper insertion. If properly trained, the OT practitioner can facilitate proper insertion as well.

  **Verify that the patient/client and/or caregivers are knowledgeable on general maintenance of hearing aids, including cleaning and ensuring proper power supply.** Hearing aids can become clogged with wax or debris easily, and there are many ways to clean them depending on the type of aid. The power for the hearing aid can come from disposable or rechargeable batteries, and batteries and chargers come in many shapes and sizes. The OT practitioner can determine if the patient and caregiver are familiar with maintenance and power on their specific hearing aid and refer back to the fitting audiologist for training if the patient is unable to maintain and/or power their hearing aid.

- Cochlear implant management
  **Encourage and support full-time use.** Cochlear implants should be worn during all waking hours. The implants should not be removed except for sleeping and any activity where they may become wet (showering, swimming). If the patient is unable to tolerate full-time use, their audiologist can often scaffold them into successful full-time use or adjust communication goals. The OT can consult with the fitting audiologist on how to best support full time use with their patient/client.

  - Verify the patient and/or caregivers are knowledgeable on general maintenance of cochlear implants.
  **Implants come in many shapes and sizes.** The OT practitioner can determine if the patient and caregiver are familiar with maintenance and power on their specific implant, and back to the fitting

**TABLE 10.5** Occupational Therapy Intervention Codes for Hearing Loss

| CPT Code | Description |
| --- | --- |
| 97530 | Therapeutic activities |
| 97533 | Sensory integrative techniques for enhanced sensory processing |
| 97535 | Self-care/home management training activities of daily living, meal preparation, safety, use of adaptive equipment |

audiologist for training if the patient is unable to maintain and/or power their hearing aid.

- Assistive listening devices management/resources
  There are many options for devices that may "turn up" the sound, but that are not hearing aids. The most common are TV amplifiers, as well as basic microphone/amplifier/headphone systems. Typically, they are used when the patient is not successful with hearing aids or is not yet ready to try hearing aids. An audiologist can work with your patient/client to determine if these devices are a good fit.

## Compensatory Strategies for Hearing Loss

There are limits to how effective compensation strategies can be with persons with hearing impairment.

The OT practitioner must know when to refer to a hearing specialist. The main focus should be to help the individual recognize that they have a hearing deficit, and then support them on a solution as appropriate (Table 10.5).

## HEARING IMPAIRMENT SUMMARY

The reimbursement table earlier suggests CPT codes that can be used by OT practitioner to cover their billable time with patients/clients where appropriate in your work setting. OT practitioners are well positioned to identify and help patients/clients navigate hearing deficits and solutions. This chapter has discussed several quick tests, concerns, and considerations to help detect or confirm hearing issues with your patients/clients and incorporate the hearing loss into the care plan. Include education as an intervention for individuals and their families. Refer to a hearing specialist who can further provide assistance for this important problem if feasible. Loss of hearing can lead to other mental health problems including depression, isolation, and perhaps an increased risk for cognitive decline. OT practitioners are uniquely positioned to assist persons with sensory issues, to improve access to resources and to build competency with tools improving these deficits, resulting in improved quality of life for both aging adults and their caregivers.

*The complete listing of the Bibliography, Appendices, and Chapter Questions and Answers are available in the accompanying enhanced eBook version included with the print purchase of this textbook. Visit Elsevier eBooks+ (eBooks.Health.Elsevier.com) to access this content.*

## CHAPTER 11

# Aging Disgracefully: Perspectives on Disability Experience and Activism From Disability Studies and Anthropology

*Denise M. Nepveux, PhD, OTR/L, Alexandra Wagner, PhD, OTR/L, CDP,*
*Pamela Block, PhD, and Devva Kasnitz, PhD*

## CHAPTER OUTLINE

## OBJECTIVES

- Identify the value of interdisciplinary collaboration in practice, theory, and research
- Identify meanings of aging and disability from a social perspective
- Understand how place and community interact with disability and aging
- Articulate the importance of mutual, active engagement between occupational therapy (OT) and older adult and disability community groups in order to assure full societal participation of adults aging with or into disability
- Compare and contrast aging with disability and aging into disability
- Identify potential skills and aptitudes produced by and emergent from experiences of aging with disability
- Critically explore how disability studies and anthropology concepts such as life course, disabling barriers, and accommodation may apply to occupational science (OS) and OT practice, theory, research, and community development with older adults

It has been said that we will all experience disability "if [we] live long enough" (McRuer, 2006, p. 304). What do you think about when you read this statement? Whatever your initial answer, we hope that reading this chapter will expand and complicate your perspective on how aging and disability are related.

This chapter results from an interdisciplinary collaboration between two occupational therapy (OT) educators (authors Nepveux and Wagner) with doctoral training in disability studies and two anthropologists, one (author Block) who taught in an OT Master's program for 14 years and one (author Kasnitz) who is 72 and disabled from childhood, teaches in a disability studies graduate program and has directed independent living centers (ILCs). All four authors utilize ethnography, the signature research method of anthropology, to articulate an understanding of aging and disability experiences through the lens of disability studies across social, cultural, and temporal variations.

Dialogue between OT and disability studies has deepened over the past 20 years. Nick Pollard, Dikaios Sakellariou, Frank Kronenberg and colleagues have published the *Occupational Therapies Without Borders* series, which—along with their other work—brings OT, disability studies, and development studies into close dialogue, showcasing the vast potential of a global politically, culturally, and economically informed practice of OT (Block et al., 2016; Lopez & Block, 2011). Two special issues of the *American Journal of Occupational Therapy*—59(5) in 2005 and 75(4) in 2021—have focused on disability studies. A 2008 special issue of Practicing Anthropology, co-edited by author Block, focused on "Anthropology, Occupational Therapy, and Disability Studies Collaborations and Prospects." More recently, initiatives such as OT + DS on Twitter (@otdsnetwork) and Access Health Activist (AHA, n.d.) Moments are available as examples. Anthropology, gerontology/aging studies, and disability studies have also enjoyed an increasingly intense and productive engagement.

In the 2016 book, *Occupying Disability: Critical Approaches to Community, Justice, and Decolonizing Disability*, Block, Kasnitz, Nishida, and Pollard outlined ways that substantive conversation among people who often have multiple identities as clinicians, interdisciplinary scholars, and disabled activists can transform disability policy and practice in numerous geographic and cultural spaces. This chapter extends that conversation to address how the phenomenon of disability interacts with aging. It explores the knowledge and, perhaps more importantly, the questions that emerge from interdisciplinary and multiple identity dialogue and collaboration among our target fields of OT, anthropology, aging studies, and disability studies and activism.

This chapter explores these intersections while emphasizing how interdisciplinary engagement contributes to OT research and practice. The chapter provides different and meaningful perspectives about aging and disability. It explores the differences between "aging with disability and aging into disability" (Kasnitz, 2001; Putnam & Bigby, 2021; Verbrugge & Jette, 1994). It also unearths questions that need further discussion and exploration in new research. An interdisciplinary ethnographic approach to these questions leads not just to theoretical innovations but also provides research substantiation of new directions for practice, policy, and more research.

## Collaboration in Practice, Theory, and Research

OT embraces collaboration as a strategy for fulfilling commitments to uphold client values, priorities, and autonomy. Occupational therapists (OTs) collaborate with "clients" to identify occupational issues to be addressed, learn more about them, and intervene to promote occupational engagement. (We find "clients" a problematic term but better than "patients.") Collaboration with clients and within systems is a pillar of the American Occupational Therapy Association's (AOTA's) vision that OT will "[maximize] health, well-being, and quality of life for all people, populations, and communities…" (AOTA Board Expands Vision 2025, 2019, p. 1). Collaboration is one of the 10 skills included in the Canadian Model of Client-Centered Enablement (Townsend & Polatajko, 2007).

Collaborative interprofessional practice "happens when multiple health workers from different professional backgrounds work together with patients, families, carers and communities to deliver the highest quality of care" (World Health Organization, 2010, p. 7). Interprofessional collaboration in health care is part of what OTs imply when speaking of collaborative practice. (See also Chapter 30.)

A significant shortcoming of interprofessional practice and education models is that they rarely require the inclusion of client or community perspectives. Further, they seldom include dialogue and collaboration with scholars working outside health care. This leaves community members, activists, and scholars uncertain of how and in what spaces to translate their relevant expertise to practitioners (Warren et al., 2018).

Research and theory development are related areas where collaboration is vital to OT. It does occur but is perhaps less documented in publications commonly read by practitioners. Interdisciplinary research entails learning from, and often

with, other academic disciplines. Interdisciplinary research has been described as

> … a mode of research by teams or individuals that integrates information, data, techniques, tools, perspectives, concepts, and/or theories from two or more disciplines or bodies of specialized knowledge to advance fundamental understanding or to solve problems whose solutions are beyond the scope of a single discipline or area of research practice.
>
> **Institute of Medicine (2005, p. 26)**

Interdisciplinary research has been necessary for the growth of OT from the beginning and continues today. For example, Jean Ayres' sensory integration theory was built upon her intensive study of neuroscience, psychology, and the social sciences (Kielhofner, 2004), as well as postdoctoral research training among neurophysiologists at the University of California, Los Angeles (Gorman & Kashani, 2017).

As we see in this chapter, a crucial part of OT's interdisciplinary research engagement must involve learning from, being in dialogue with, and collaborating with fields, such as medical anthropology, aging studies, and disability studies that approach medicine, health, and other "caring" practices with a critical eye or that make these practices themselves a focus of study. Such fields bring in the voice and perspective of lived experience—even (or perhaps especially) when these voices may raise uncomfortable issues that challenge practice (Block et al., 2005; Pollard & Block, 2017).

Understanding disability experience across the life course (Kasnitz, 2001) from the perspective of disabled people, particularly those who typically have the least power and voice, is central to evidence-based practice. This chapter argues that this crucial knowledge may be manifested in practice through dialogue and collaboration among activists, practitioners, and academics of various scholarly disciplines. Such cooperation is often challenging because of differences in methodology, values, priorities, and how we evaluate and express ideas. While the academics, practitioners, and community leaders may work hard to have meaningful collaboration, fully including the student, the patient, the client, and the community members with the most at stake and the least power is even more complicated. Histories of power inequities also contribute to making dialogue difficult. Communities of color, indigenous peoples, migrants and refugees, women, and people considered disabled have experienced betrayal and exploitation by the powerful medical establishment (e.g., Tuskeegee) and thus may understandably hesitate to collaborate or enter into dialogue with Certified Occupational Therapy Assistants (COTAs), whom they are likely (and understandably) to see as part of this medical industry establishment.

OT emphasizes its role and potential with groups, communities, and populations. As OT broadens its scope, we need to broaden interdisciplinary and public policy engagement. Multidisciplinary teams are likely to craft interdisciplinary work that considers context and challenges each other's biases.

We join in interdisciplinary collaboration in this book because we believe that OT/science is the health field most concerned with context: individual, group, and societal. We are also convinced that authentic mutual interdisciplinary engagement is necessary in order to accomplish the crucial work of both OT/OS and disability studies.

## Knowing Aging, Knowing Disability: Interdisciplinary Approaches

Before we explore some questions about the distinctions, overlaps, and intersections between disability and aging, we must clarify how we approach these complex constructs.

Aging is both a process that human beings (and other beings) experience over time and an effect of the passage of time. We may understand aging from the perspectives of "lifespan" and "life course." (See Box 11.1 on lifespan and life course.) OT practitioners may refer to lifespan research to learn what is generally expected based on a client's age; this is especially common when working with children and has application in later years of life. For example, the age-delineated stages "young-old," "middle-old," and "old-old" are used to generalize and predict biological, psychological, and social tendencies and needs. However, a life course perspective is more relevant in this chapter. It acknowledges and takes an interest in how contexts drive vast variations of human experience. Life history evaluation tools such as the Occupational Performance History Interview II (Kielhofner et al., 2001) utilize a life-course perspective. An OT practitioner guided by a life-course view will delve into how past patterns of contextualized group and individual experiences and future hopes inform current needs and priorities.

In this chapter, as in disability studies, disability is foregrounded as the core subject, the core idea. This chapter utilizes a social-relational understanding of disability (Thomas, 1999). (See Box 11.2 on disability definitions.) Within this

core idea of disability are many experiences. Disability is social, political, economic and cultural, among other facets. And disability intersects with age, gender, race, ethnicity, sexual identity, and many other identity categories essential to power differentials in complex, dynamic, and compounding ways. Meaningful change is made *by* and *with the leadership of* and not *for* people who experience disability. At a minimum, our perspective as practitioners builds upon knowledge borrowed from the efforts and accomplishments of people who experience disability, and we acknowledge sources.

## Disability Studies

Disability Studies is one of several scholarly fields that emerged out of a desire for self-determination by groups of people who had previously been studied from the outside and in ways that diminished their power. Other examples are women's and gender studies and African American and diaspora studies. Founding disabled scholars in disability studies broke off from general medical sociology and anthropology and rehabilitation research associations in 1980 with Irving K. Zola in the lead in the US. Disabled people began to theorize and formulate research questions that reflected their own lived experiences of disability both within and beyond any medical context. Activist collectives such as the Union of the Physically Impaired Against Segregation (1976) in the United Kingdom developed some of the founding ideas of the disability studies field, particularly the differences between medical and social models of disability. (See Box 11.3 on models.) In the ensuing decades and even today, the term "disability studies" was used by programs and efforts that did not embrace a social perspective. This appropriation was evidence of the field's growing presence and voice, but it muddied the field, threatening to obscure its critical voice. Disabled scholars and their allies then felt a need to articulate that not everything

---

**BOX 11.1**  Two Aging Perspectives: Lifespan and Life Course

The "**lifespan**," a conceptual lens often used in developmental psychology, refers to how long people live and the experiences to be expected by all people at each stage in life: our commonalities, which are often described statistically in terms of probabilities and norms. Lifespan approaches are likely to track changes in particular variables over time.

In this chapter, we primarily consider aging from a "**life course**" perspective (Priestly, 2001). Life course is a concept developed in sociology. When we look at the life course of individuals, groups, and even things longitudinally, we are

looking for patterns, events, or other changes that are not necessarily common to all people, and we consider how people or our issues of concern are shaped by contexts throughout lifetimes. Researchers engage in life course research via extensive interviewing, utilizing historical data, and in some cases following a person's life in real-time into the future. For example, Kasnitz (2001) charts the life course experiences of disabled leaders to see what early events impacted change and led to their assumptions of disability identity and involvement in political advocacy.

---

**BOX 11.2**  Definitions: Power, Environments, Bodies and Minds

Disability has many definitions. Throughout this chapter and in international scholarship, disability is explored and understood socially and relationally, rather than as a characteristic of a person (Ginsburg & Rapp, 2020). Disability is a relationship between bodies and minds or "bodyminds" (Price, 2015; Schalk, 2018) and environments (political,

social, historical, natural, and built). This relationship involves power. Contexts powerfully facilitate or hinder bodyminds' abilities to access, engage, and find meaning in different spaces. Disability may thus be defined as a socially imposed restriction (Thomas, 1999, p. 29) of opportunity to access, engage, and find meaning in occupation.

## BOX 11.3    The Social Model of Disability

The social model of disability was first developed by activists in the Union of the Physically Impaired Against Segregation (Union of Physically Impaired Against Segregation [UPIAS], 1976) and further developed by UK scholars Michael Oliver and others to redefine disability as a form of unjust exclusion and inequality caused by inaccessible and unaccommodating environments. This shift of focus from the body to the environment involved a powerful change of consciousness for people who identified with disability. It was meant as a direct challenge to existing medical and rehabilitation research, practice, and policy approaches that viewed disability as a direct result of bodily injury or difference, and that allocated research funding and rehabilitative interventions toward healing and repairing the body rather than making environments equitably inclusive.

about disability is disability studies, a corollary to "nothing about us without us" (Charlton, 2000). Since then, some (not all) disability studies scholars have taken up the term "critical disability studies."

With emerging theoretical ideas and new intersectional coalition building, disability studies is growing and shifting rapidly. Relevant to this chapter, even basic vocabulary around aging and disability is still not consistent (Kasnitz, 2020), but aging and media studies scholars such as Chivers (2019, 2021) and disability studies scholars such as Yoshizaki-Gibbons (2018) have been leading the way in exploring intersections between disability and aging.

### Ethnography and Disability

The authors of this chapter argue that ethnography—the primary research method of anthropology—is a precious tool for learning about the lived experience of individuals, groups, and communities (Block et al., 2008). Ethnographic methods are built on participation, observation, studying artifacts, taking notes and other memory aids, and then putting this data all together so that your focus is wholly contextualized. Reflexivity concerning one's relationship to the people and topic is another crucial element, along with checking your conclusions with other participant observers and the people who are your focus. Often through ethnography, we learn that the way people's experience is portrayed in medical texts or news media is different from how it plays out on the ground or from their perspective. We gain a deeper understanding of the relationships between concepts and theories and how lives are lived. For example, anthropological studies have shown us how complex and culturally driven "disability" is, in the sense that each sociocultural context may label different experiences of bodyminds' interaction with the environment in various ways, including (but not limited to) "normal," "illness," "impairment," and "disability" (Kasnitz & Shuttleworth, 2001). Similarly, the anthropology of aging and the life course shows us a diversity of ways people are seen in relation to perceived age and stage of life. Labels and categories powerfully shape the social roles and opportunities people are and are not afforded, and how people see themselves.

### A Word About Language

As disability studies scholars and activists, we write about "disability" rather than "disabilities." This is a way of asserting that we are talking about a common core of human dynamics and experience rather than a variety of medical diagnoses or impairments. Disability studies is "disability" studies (rather than disabilities studies) because it examines an essential core idea common to all of disability's manifestations.

As part of their professional education, OT students learn to adapt their core skill of enabling occupation for working with people experiencing a diversity of medically categorized conditions and impairments, which may often be referred to collectively as "disabilities." Although there are multiple experiences of impairment or human variation for which most people use the plural "disabilities," some activists and scholars regard this term as divisive because it invites discussion of the plurality, often diagnosis-related, and often without defining the core commonalities that constitute disability.

You may also be aware of a debate between the language use of "disabled person" and "person with a disability." These usages are also called "identity first" versus "people first" language. We encourage readers to think beyond this contested binary, in that each approach has merits rooted in history and values. In preparing this chapter, we have found language we all agree with. Practitioners must do the same, inquiring about and respecting the language choices of individuals and groups, which may change over time.

### Is Disability for Everybody Sometime? Unresolved Distinctions and Overlaps

Here we return to our opening comment on the oft-heard statement that *everyone experiences disability if they live long enough*. It is all too easy to trivialize disability by saying this, even though the phrase is often used to engage people when arguing for better disability policy. Divisions between disability experience and aging experience, disability identity and aging identity, and even disability and ill identity are complex and unresolved. Much is in the eye of the beholder. For example, in contemporary US culture, a 94-year-old woman who walks with a cane may be seen as old and perhaps "frail"—another loaded term—but not as disabled, an elusive social condition residing ultimately in the mind. She may not be disabled any more than she was as an infant before she walked or while leaning on the midwife while giving birth. Assisted walking is generally perceived as an inherent part of specific moments in a person's life course.

Some disability scholars argue that a significant facet of disability experience is "crip time," or the disruption of normative expectations concerning time and the life course (Kafer, 2013). Ellen Samuels reflects that,

> Crip time is time travel. Disability and illness have the power to extract us from linear, progressive time with its normative life stages and cast us into a wormhole of backward and forward acceleration, jerky stops and starts, tedious intervals and abrupt endings. Some of us contend with the impairments of old age while still young; some of us are treated like children no matter how old we get.

**Samuels (2017, quoted in Ljuslinder et al., 2020)**

Here, Samuels points out that "crip time" and the disability experience know no age: they do not honor the lifespan predictions of epidemiologists. As discussed, disability is a social construct and a contested, changing one. This is not to say that illness and impairment are not real, but we experience them in a social context that includes categories and expectations concerning what is to come. Some disability scholars disagree with the assertion that everyone will, one day, experience disability because it implies that disability is a specific, concrete, bodily experience rather than one that is socially defined. While bodyminds change over time, new impairments may arise over a typical lifespan, and social definitions of normality vary over time and place. Individuals will not inevitably embrace disability, be perceived by others as disabled, experience environmental barriers that hinder their participation or be regarded as disabled under policy or law.

The matter of expectation is crucial; all cultures designate some embodied changes as expected parts of aging (or human variation or the life course) and not a sign of disability (Kasnitz, 2020). Yet many older adults do age into disability experience, and often without benefitting from the insights, community, pride, and even the fundamental rights for which many disabled people of all ages have fought long and hard. Internalized ableism, discrimination based on presumed inability due to disability, is one barrier to identifying one's own experience as disability or even making or accepting accommodations to suit changing bodily needs. Older adults may (often reasonably) fear that the way they are regarded and treated by strangers and intimates alike, and even the autonomy they are allowed in decisions, will change once they take on trappings of disability. After all, isolation, disregard, and disempowerment do happen to disabled people. Despite the complexities discussed here, disability advocates stress that we can design in a way that supports all people. Universal Design is meant to bridge gaps. (See Box 11.4)

Likewise, ageism is a powerful thread throughout our culture, including in older adult social spaces and services. Ageism is also likely to be common and unconfronted in disability rights and independent living communities as well as among scholars of disability. They (and we) may be reluctant to extend disability solidarity to older people who are newly experiencing disability (Yoshizaki-Gibbons, 2018), especially those who shrink from identifying as disabled. Understanding how ageism and ableism intersect, negatively impact us, and may be internalized over time is critical to individual and group well-being (Gibbons, 2016). There is much to learn and do on scholarship and advocacy fronts.

## Aging *With* Disability: Pride, Skills, Attitudes, Knowledge

This section draws especially upon the lived and community experiences of author Kasnitz. In the 1950s, when the Baby Boom generation was in its infancy in the United States, disability segregation was commonplace and legal. Disabled people and allies in the disability rights and independent living movements fought for access to transportation, education, and public places. Funding from the Rehabilitation Act of 1973 helped create a national system of ILCs to enable the autonomy, freedom, and full participation of people with disabilities by offering peer-run services, referrals, skills training, and mutual support as alternatives to institutional care systems controlled by nondisabled professionals. These made it possible for many formerly institutionalized young disabled people to move back into their communities and helped many to avoid institutionalization. Although this has changed as these "peer-run" services have professionalized, thanks to decades of committed organizing and advocacy, there is now a cohort of people who "claimed disability" early in life, reaching their 60s to 80s. People aging *with* plenty of disability experience approach disability differently than those who age *into* disability, that is, newly experience disability late in life. Of course, there is a gray area between the two groups and perhaps other variations that we do not address here. But we find the distinction between aging with and aging into disability helpful in the sense that we notice that people who become disabled early in life may have opportunities to develop skills for navigating systems and situations. These skills may serve them well in their older adulthood.

People who age with disability may have valuable sets of knowledge that people aging into disability lack. For example,

---

**BOX 11.4** Accessibility and Universal Design

Older adults and people with disabilities often benefit from similar accommodations but without much discussion about why this is so. Universal design (Mace, 1998) and accessibility features such as curb cuts benefit a considerable percentage of people, including those who move with bicycles, strollers, walkers, and carts and those who, for other reasons, need graded adjustments of surfaces rather than steps. Designated seats on public transportation, which are required under the Americans with Disabilities Act, often identify several prioritized populations, including people who are pregnant, disabled, or "elderly." The socially recognized identity distinctions are retained while shared accommodations are appreciated when provided. Universal Design was never intended to collapse aging and disability.

they may have a sense of disability justice and rights and be able to recognize instances of environmental barriers and ableism. They may also have experience calling out such instances and advocating for change. People aging into disability, depending on many factors in their personal history, may rarely resist ageist and ableist exclusion or negotiate for access. Instead, they accept such instances as natural or inevitable responses to their changing bodymind and its mismatch with customary arrangements.

Many people gain insight through disabled life that the need for care and support is not a source of shame. Indeed, it is "inherent to being human" (Kittay, 2011, p. 54). Nondisabled adults and those aging into disability often fear eventually needing assistance with activities of daily living because such a transition may seem to threaten one's "independence," interpreted to mean dignity and control over one's life choices. Yet reliable assistance at home is a powerful resource. Knowledge of the kinds of help one needs and access to that help are sources of freedom. ILCs/Centers for Independent Living (CILs) are now beginning to shift their focus to meaningful "interdependent living" in recognition that "independence," in the sense of adequate support and freedom from control, is not an end in itself but simply a baseline situation enabling people to fully and joyfully engage in their community lives. Adults aging into disability can learn from disabled people that we are all interdependent and that interdependent life is meaningful. Rather than viewing changes in function over time as signaling loss of dignity or personhood, they may be understood as necessitating a shift in networks of interdependence.

Another valuable insight from life with disability, specifically the Independent Living movement, is the importance of consumer direction of services and supports. Aging services have traditionally been designed to take away power and choice from the individual, compensating with care and protection. Nursing homes and home care agencies are examples of this paternalistic model. People who age with disability are less likely to accept such trade-offs as necessary and inevitable because, as a group, they have struggled for and won battles for the right to control their own services and use of funds.

Disabled people learn to be early adopters of technological adaptations and strategies, including mobility equipment, audiobooks, speech input and output, and technology for remote participation. Technology is seen not as a threat to personhood but as something that enables participation. In April 2020, when many scholarly conferences in the United States were canceled due to the Covid-19 pandemic, the Society for Disability Studies successfully transformed a 400-person conference—including a dance celebration—from in-person to online. This was possible because its members had been early adopters of remote technology (see Piepzna-Samarasinha, 2018 for an explanation of bed-space activism) and were accustomed to practicing mutual support and technical assistance roles. Mutual support capacity was also dramatically demonstrated in how disabled people in the San Francisco Bay Area quickly and effectively organized mutual support networks early in the pandemic lockdowns.

Systems navigation, planning and literacy skills are vital to avoiding institutionalization. People aging with disability may have acquired these skills by necessity through years of struggle and practice. In contrast, people aging into disability may not know how to access government housing and home help support.

Those who age with disability may be better at planning for multiple contingencies than nondisabled people who assume that an "able-bodied norm" will follow them into old age. More research is needed to explore these hypotheses. Having experienced and navigated power inequities throughout their lives, disabled people may also be appropriately cautious about financial arrangements and signing over power (e.g., power of attorney) to others. They may be wary of taking actions that may heighten their vulnerability to financial and other forms of abuse.

People who age with disability also encounter an array of difficulties. They may encounter unfamiliar problems to treat as illnesses or tackle as disability. As their bodies and circumstances change, accustomed strategies, accommodations, and technologies may no longer work, and they may or may not find that they have the resources to adapt. They may be forced to navigate different systems that afford (or are used to affording) less choice and control. For example, as they are required to transition from "disability" to "aging" services, they are allowed much less control over these services. Where previously they may have hired, supervised, and paid personal assistants through government disability programs, they now face home care agencies who gatekeep requests and absorb much of the cost of disability accommodations in the name of fiscal control. They also may be impacted emotionally by the exacerbated condescension they experience that they could better deflect when disabled but not old. Particularly in the absence of a supportive community and a sense of mutuality, it may be hard to hold on to hard-won pride in disability identity.

We hope that practitioners and all people aging into disability will benefit from what we have learned from people aging with disability and their ways of living. More research is needed to confirm and share this knowledge, as well as to explore the myriad subtle contrasts between aging with and into disability that, in reality, complicate this rhetorical binary.

## Examples From the Authors' Ethnography and Lived Experience: Identity, Communication, and Community

As professionals and as allies or disabled ourselves (Carey et al., 2019), we want to give readers a few simple but powerful ethnographic examples of how we both derived our perspective from what we learned from our "consumer" constituency and our own lives, and how we apply these ideas to our practice and hope to see them in new research and social program development.

The examples we choose are straightforward. First, we think about identity. Identity is always contextual. For instance, while Pam and Devva identify as Jewish, that identity surfaces most often when we find ourselves among others who also identify as Jews or when we are the only Jew or the only Ukrainian Jew in a group. Despite the added possibilities of remote interaction to counter the effects of migration and diaspora, chosen for "a better life" or imposed by danger, most people become identified with a place, want to communicate colloquially without undue effort, and live in a community, either known or entirely self-made/chosen.

Next, we address the complexities of aging in place. This concept goes far beyond physical safety within the home and requires a complete understanding of the existing supports and barriers within that geographic space and the local human community. (See also Chapter 20 on the physical environment and Chapter 32 on age-inclusive communities.) To support aging in place requires the ability and commitment to track the larger environmental, socioeconomic and policy dynamics that may dramatically alter that landscape. Following this, we look at human communication, without which we cannot thrive. This topic, too, goes beyond its immediate associations with literacy, speech, and even language. We address communication first in the specific case of cognitive changes with aging. Finally, we consider community. We present a case study of how place, presence, and co-occupation over time create community and how resilient community can be when faced with the cannibalism of many neoliberal forces of "development" that destroy the existing community rather than using it as a foundation.

## Claiming and Disclaiming Disability: Matters of Identity

Meanings of identities and terms attached to them change over time and with the influence of social movements. For many, disability is now a powerful identity, not one from which "disabled people" seek to distance themselves. Over 20 years ago, Linton (1998) wrote the influential book, *Claiming Disability*. Disability studies scholars and activists claimed disability and still do so as an act of resistance and solidarity. Through multiple disciplinary and interdisciplinary approaches, disability

studies inquire about how different possible identities interact with disability, both within an individual's consciousness and experience and as perceived by others. Age and cohort/ generation are parts of this intersection, as are gender, race, education, nationality, sexuality, health and illness, and many others.

Of course, "disabled" or "nondisabled" are not the only identities available to bodyminds who encounter barriers to participation in everyday life activities. Many people who experience long-term, chronic or intermittent health conditions may embrace disability as part of their identity. However, the more involvement one has had with medicine, the more robust an illness identity may be, and the more difficult or unlikely it may be to envision one's situation as (also) disability. This imaginative transition is problematic for younger adults with nonapparent chronic illness, for example, type 1 diabetes or chronic fatigue syndrome, but many are beginning to see where a disability identity, and a focus on rights and justice, are valid and valuable—for instance, in shifting one's expectations concerning access and accommodations.

Linton (1998) has taught us to claim disability and affirm that disability is a valued perspective and can be a thing of beauty. Several mostly disabled or mixed ability professional dance troupes have thrived for decades, and we see more disability as knowledgeable and beautiful on stage and screen. (See Case Study 11.1.)

With the increasing strength and visibility of the disability activist movements and arts across their lifetimes, older adults now have more options for how they see themselves and each other. Whereas older adults may have eschewed identifying as "handicapped" when that term was commonly used, disability is arguably not as stigmatized an identity. Insights and strategies trickle over to older age groups as those aging into disability interact with and learn from people aging with disability—including, in some cases, their children. (See Case Study 11.2.)

Claiming disability identity and demanding equitable access and accommodations have been powerful strategies

---

**CASE STUDY 11.1**   Katherine Sherwood

**Katherine Sherwood**, a renown painter teaching at UC Berkeley, was always interested in anatomy. A stroke at a young age impacted her mobility and speech. She incorporated a disability identity and disability studies perspective in her artwork. She began painting her own "Brain Flowers" (https://www.katherinesherwood.com/#/brain-flower-2/), recasting MRI images of her own brain as images of organic beauty. Sherwood's work—like that of Sins Invalid, Petra Kuppers, Riva Lehrer, Neil Marcus, Sunaura Taylor, AXIS, Infinite Flow Dance, Alice Shepperd, Antoine Hunter, and many others—addresses imaginative, political, and aesthetic questions people face as they make sense of life lived through a changing bodymind, encounters with and struggles to access services and problematic interactions with environments, all of which impact one's sense of identity. (All of these artists have a web presence.)

---

**CASE STUDY 11.2**   Harold

**Harold**, my father, had a massive stroke at 82. In the hospital he grabbed the arm of the tall, strong male physical therapist beside me and told us, "Go buy me the best power chair and a van with a lift and take me home." Gesturing to the PT, he said, "You come work for me as my personal assistant." I thought to myself, "How many 82-year-olds have that vocabulary?" Well, he had been watching me, his 58-year-old daughter, age (gracefully) with disability (Kasnitz autoethnographic notes, 2009).

for many disabled from an early age. It has enabled them to experience a sense of community and solidarity with other disabled people, including those whose bodily or lived experiences and the barriers they face may differ from their own. But people who are aging into disability without such a supportive community may experience the painful combination of ageism and ableism they encounter within their communities as normal or to be expected. (See Case Study 11.3.) Without solidarity and consciousness-raising, we are likely to experience instances of ableism and ageism as personal— evidence of personal failings, individualized rejection or sidelining, or simply a "natural" evolution of devaluation—rather than part of a larger political dynamic that merits resistance. (See Case Study 11.4.) Even with raised consciousness, such instances remain painful, but our response strategies and avenues for solidarity multiply and strengthen.

## Aging in Place and Community

**Helena** has the information and skills necessary to navigate systems. (See Case Study 11.5.) She has planned well and made informed choices. Although a change for her, her mobility problems at 93 are not pushing her or anyone else to suggest she identify as disabled if she would prefer not, nor should she relinquish control over her housing. However, her mobility impairments make her eligible for "disability" services commonly understood as available for the "frail elderly." How common or uncommon is Helena's situation?

Like younger adults with disabilities, older adults generally aspire to live unrestricted lives in communities of their choice.

Younger and older adults may fear needing to transition to an institutional setting, with good reason (Riedl et al., 2012). As we see in **Colleen's** story, disabled adults are increasingly vulnerable to the pressures of institutional settings over time, especially if they do not have experience and assistance with planning and navigating systems. (See Case Study 11.6.)

Many adults aspire to remain in their homes and communities throughout their lives. According to a 2018 American Association of Retired Persons (AARP) survey, three-fourths of Americans wish to do so, but many fewer believe they will be able to. The Centers for Disease Control and Prevention (CDC, 2009) defines aging in place as "the ability to live in one's own home and community safely, independently, and comfortably, regardless of age, income, or ability level." The idea of aging in place and community is compelling to OT practitioners from the standpoint of maintaining autonomy and full participation in family and community life. However, it requires a critical contextual analysis. Aging in place is often discussed as a freely made choice. About 9% of US adults aged 65 and older live in poverty (Bureau of Labor Statistics, 2020). For many, financial constraints make aging in place impossible (Carder et al., 2016; Wagner, 2021). Economic factors, including personal finances, government support, and housing affordability, strongly influence older adults' opportunities to remain at home and in the community. Fixed incomes are incompatible with escalating housing costs, which may take up a disproportionate share of older adults' resources and make it difficult or impossible to cover food and other basic needs (Lopez, 2017).

---

**CASE STUDY 11.3**   Mary

**Mary**, a church musician and liturgist, joined a church choir after her retirement. Soon, however, she lost valued song-leading roles. The director said that Mary now walked too slowly to the lectern, which also was difficult for her to climb. This distracted from the mass. Apparently, no thought was given to physical or procedural accommodations. Mary was disappointed but saw this as an appropriate decision and for the good of the congregation (Nepveux, autoethnographic notes, 2008).

---

**CASE STUDY 11.4**   Henry

**Henry** belonged to a shooting club for years before his stroke and subsequent diagnosis of vascular dementia. Sally, his daughter, became his primary care partner and worked tirelessly to support him. Although Henry was no longer able to shoot, he still enjoyed visiting and chatting with friends in the snack area outside the range. Sally would drive him there to see his old friends, but she described the experience as increasingly difficult and unwelcoming. She said his friends did not seem to know how to interact with Henry, who now used a wheelchair and sometimes lost the thread of conversations. After a few visits, Sally was told that Henry's use of a wheelchair presented a liability; they were asked not to return (Wagner, 2020, p. 127).

---

**CASE STUDY 11.5**   Helena

**Helena**, a 93-year-old woman, lived in Florida in subsidized housing with a live-in paid assistant. Her daughter lived nearby. After her daughter passed away, Helena was able to move to be near her other daughter in California. She was able to continue her subsidized rent and her 100 hours per month live-in PAS assistant benefits in California without mishap or interruption, but it took months of family premove planning (Kasnitz, 2022, ongoing unpublished research).

## CASE STUDY 11.6    Colleen

**Colleen**, a 64-year-old woman, lived with two roommates in supportive housing for people with chronic mental health conditions. Recently she had been experiencing cognitive changes. Seeking relief from the squalid conditions of her apartment and a hostile, unpredictable roommate, Colleen asked if she could move in with her daughter's family. This met with resistance, which Colleen struggled to come to terms with. "…She has this big, beautiful house and…I don't know. I always think kids should take care of their parents when they are older." Colleen went on to say, "but [my daughter] thinks…I'm too much." When we met 2 weeks later, Colleen said she had begun "praying I could go into a nursing home." She reasoned that at a nursing home she could move about freely rather than hiding away in her room, and help would be available when she needed it. Also, she was barely making rent. She worried that if her Social Security payments were ever reduced, she could become homeless (Wagner, 2020 p. 130).

## BOX 11.5    A Comparison of Home Care and Personal Assistant Services

**Home Care** comes out of a nursing tradition, focused on ensuring the safety of the individual and providing support identified by society as necessary to ensure maintenance of physician-recommended regimes of care. The US system is tied to Medicare, private health insurance, and other public and private benefits. Medicare pays for only short-term support following hospitalization. Medicaid covers home-based long-term care in some states for people over age 65 under the Home and Community Based Waiver system. Medicaid eligibility is income and asset based. The Medicaid application is complex, and the application process is difficult for many. (See Case Study 11.7.) Denials and the need for appeals are common. People with less education and poorer health tend to have greater difficulty with the application and face more barriers than others (Stuber & Bradley, 2005).

Disabled people, depending on various factors, may qualify for paid and more consumer-directed **Personal Assistant Services** (PAS), which vary greatly state by state. States determine if PAS is offered within the Medicaid Waiver system, how, and from where providers are chosen, who determines what the workers do, and whether they contract through a for-profit, supervising agency. In one of the best examples of PAS, it is common in California for a low-income resident to qualify for 100 or more hours of PAS per month or for a live-in attendant. Providers are paid $15.50/h in 2022 and the supply of providers is growing. Younger disabled people usually prefer this model, depending upon their state's regulations, because it is more transparent, less bureaucratic, and more consumer directed. Taking the PAS model into old age without consumer prior experience is not easy but is entirely possible. However, the process and costs of hiring providers are burdensome on older adults with limited finances who do not qualify—or do not know that they are eligible—for government-paid assistance.

Further, aging in place implies that home and neighborhood already support one's needs, including security, safety, and comfort. Sadly, in the US today, these home and community experiences are increasingly out of reach to people and families who lack substantial financial resources (Granbom et al., 2021). Economic inequality, housing market trends and policies, and relative financial means throughout the life course shape what one's "own home" is: where people can own or rent, and the relative accessibility, autonomy, security, and permanency of these situations. Older housing stock tends to have external and internal staircases, narrow doorways, small bathrooms, and other features that make it difficult and expensive to retrofit. Low-income disabled adults encounter financial and policy barriers to moving to a more physically accessible home or adapting their home to increase its accessibility, thus creating a situation of being "stuck in place" or even trapped indoors rather than aging in place.

Family members provide the bulk of home-based assistance that older adults receive (Janus & Ermisch, 2015). About a quarter of older adults who do not live with family members, and 18% who do, receive some form of paid care (Kaye et al., 2010, cited in Janus & Ermisch, 2015). Only about 28% of the care that older adults receive at home is provided through public programs, and the rest through personal finances (Janus & Ermisch, 2015). We describe two different avenues to support at home, namely home care and personal assistant services. *(See Text Box 11.5 on personal assistance services.)* The support that assistance workers provide allows disabled younger and older adults to maintain autonomy and manage responsibilities toward themselves, their homes, and family members. Assistants also provide a source of friendship and family-like relationships when family support is not present (Piercy, 2000). Individuals can be lost in this bureaucratic morass. (See Case Study 11.7.)

The existence, accessibility, and salience of government supports inequitably impact aging in the community. Often people who most need support that would enable them to age in the community encounter the most barriers to receiving them. For instance, states with the largest impoverished populations are less likely to have exercised the federal Medicaid waivers that fund home-based support programs known as Home and Community-Based Services. Disability, race and gender inequities compound the financial restrictions that older adults face; African American women with insufficient financial means to age in place have been identified as the most vulnerable group (Johnson & Lian, 2018).

**CASE STUDY 11.7**    Henry

> **Henry**, diagnosed with vascular dementia, and his daughter Sally worked on his application for Medicaid. They hoped it would enable him to receive home care services for daily support so he could continue to live at home even if his cognitive changes progressed. The approval process took 8 months, even with help from an elder law attorney and Henry's other daughter. Sally explained that the paperwork demands were extensive: "We had to go through documents. We had to provide medical history or financial history—copies of mortgages, copies of tax bills, copies of his veteran's status…copies of insurance, homeowner's insurance, medical insurance, copies of utility bills to see what his monthly status is going to be going forward.…" After Henry received approval for Medicaid, Sally and her father sat down with eight different home health-care companies, who interviewed her father about his functional status and his needs. The answers he gave would determine the monthly hours of care he was eligible to receive (Wagner, 2020, p. 122).

As discussed above, planning is also a factor. Nondisabled adults, even those of economic means and ample formal education, often do not plan for disability. When environmental and personal situations are uncertain, future planning requires anticipating and preparing for potential changes in support needs, openness to different ways of living life, and self-advocacy skills. In Janice's case, the unpredictable human factor made aging into a simple mobility disability, a trigger for the unraveling of plans that never anticipated disability. (See Case Study 11.8.) Janice's planning choices, which preserved her savings for the next generation, made her vulnerable to economic elder abuse. Further, the individual can only compensate so much for public systems that are inadequate and underfunded. Becoming unable to drive, for example, is a significant loss for many older people that no public system fully addresses.

Support services rely upon a well-supported service-providing workforce. This is not the case currently. Workers' rights and physical and emotional health and well-being are overlooked and underprotected (Franzosa et al., 2019). Direct care workers are predominantly women. Almost one in four direct care workers is an immigrant. Most are persons of color; in terms of race and ethnicity, direct care workers identify themselves as Hispanic, non-Hispanic and Asian, or non-Hispanic and Black (Zallman et al., 2019). Racial discrimination is common; about 23% of Black home care workers report experiences of racial discrimination (Lee et al., 2016). Justice in Aging and the Domestic Workers Alliance advocate for better pay, protections, and working conditions for direct care workers. It is in the whole community's interest to ensure that a future of aging in communities with disability is possible; it will be possible only with a well-supported workforce whose rights are protected.

## Navigating Age-Related Cognitive Changes

The uncertainties of aging can lead to fear of embodied changes that may dramatically alter one's way of interacting in the world. In particular, many people fear developing dementia (Yun & Maxfield, 2020). Dementia is one of the most stigmatized disability experiences, given its fraught associations in the popular imagination with caregiver burden, "loss of self" and even "living death" (George, 2010, p. 586). The term, dementia, originates in the Latin "demens," meaning to lose one's mind (Jellinger, 2010). Medical literature tends to portray dementia and Alzheimer disease as adverse events with bleak prognoses (DiZazzo-Miller & Pociask, 2015). Media representations portray dementia through a lens of tragedy (Milligan & Thomas, 2016). Campaigns for research dollars have often used war metaphors, characterizing those with Alzheimer disease as "victims" under "attack" (George, 2010, p. 586). These representations add to the associated stigma (Milligan & Thomas, 2016).

Reframing and destigmatizing this category of experience may begin with naming (George, 2010). Since 2013, dementia—which is a syndrome or cluster of impairments caused by several disorders rather than a single condition (Jellinger, 2010)—has been renamed major neurocognitive disorder in International Classification of Disease (ICD) codes as well as the Diagnostic and Statistical Manual, Version Five (DSM V). This renaming was an attempt to move away from the tremendous social stigma attached to Alzheimer disease and related conditions. "Age-related cognitive changes" (Wagner, 2020, p. 5) is another term preferred by author Wagner to descriptively name rather than label and diagnose a broad array of human experiences, many of which impact daily functioning. This is similar to the use of "deeply forgetful" rather than dementia. "Deeply forgetful" (Post, 2013) acknowledges the shared humanity of forgetfulness. There are varying degrees of forgetfulness that everyone experiences; some experience forgetfulness to a greater extent than others. Dementia continues to be used in common parlance, however, thus we do use it intermittently here.

Engaging with research and first-person narratives that document the lived experience of progressive cognitive changes may help practitioners more fully recognize the capability and enduring humanity of people experiencing them. For instance, Eugenia Zukerman's (2019) book, "Like Falling Through a Cloud: A Lyrical Memoir," poetically chronicles her experiences of uncertainty, struggle, hope, meaning and purpose following a diagnosis of dementia. People living with cognitive differences do report "rough spots" throughout their life and require "new and innovative types of interaction" (Beard et al., 2009, p. 234). However, there remains the possibility of joy, fun, and pleasure (Driessen, 2018). Disabling barriers (Shakespeare et al., 2019) that isolate and exclude must be replaced by efforts to understand, support, celebrate and include people with cognitive differences through making spaces, activity events, and communications accessible.

## CASE STUDY 11.8   Janice

**Janice** is 85 and has aged into mobility impairments after a long career as a teacher in California. Janice thought she had planned well for her retirement by focusing on acquiring assets—large houses in Pennsylvania and California—rather than a larger pension. In her 70s, as she began to experience mobility impairments, she divided her assets between her two daughters to avoid inheritance tax and qualify for government disability programs including rent relief and over 100 hours per month of home help in California, more than she used. She planned to occupy a studio within the California house, which she had given to one of her daughters. However, her plan to age in place was foiled when her daughter rented out the entire house, forcing Janice to move out on her own. She barely subsisted; her pension was inadequate to cover even subsidized rent for an accessible apartment along with her other bills. Janice's other daughter had sold the Pennsylvania home she had given to her and moved to Hawaii. Janice hesitated, but eventually told her other daughter about her plight, and was invited to move in with her. When we last spoke, she was moving soon, but it was unclear to Janice whether the programs she had depended on in California existed in Hawaii (Kasnitz, ethnographic notes 2022).

## CASE STUDY 11.9   Richard

**Richard's** wife, Marie, had Alzheimer disease. As her cognition changed, he recognized that he needed to adapt. He adjusted his style of communication, presence, and interaction to suit her needs. As a result of his flexibility and patience he learned to work with his wife and change with her. He explained, "…if I'm impatient or imperious or demanding or something like that, immediately Marie pick[s] up on that. When I shift into gentle and loving mode, you know, things go beautifully. But if I get selfish or irritated or something like that, you know, Marie is just a wall of resistance. And it makes sense. You know, …it's a refinement of a spiritual practice because a lot of that's in our heads" (Wagner, 2020, p. 127).

## Connecting: Communication and Advocacy

**Richard** narrates his efforts to adjust his communication style to meet his wife Marie's needs. (See Case Study 11.9.) His wife, with whom he shares a home, has been diagnosed with Alzheimer disease. As he describes, adjusting his behavior and modes of communication requires awareness, new ways of communicating, and practice. He relates these needed shifts to his spiritual practice, recognizing that what is needed is not performance, but a way of being, both within himself and in relation to his beloved. Adults with dementia, like other people, respond not only to the words said to them but to the whole interaction. The emotional tone influences their response. For example, communication in a tense, controlling style has been correlated with resistance to help (Williams & Herman, 2011).

Adjustments are also needed in how nondisabled people attend to those living with dementia. Often how people with dementia communicate their feelings and needs is misunderstood or not perceived as communication. In medical literature, behaviors typically associated with dementia include aggression, agitation, and resistance to care. These are often considered disease symptoms. However, when these "symptoms" of dementia are contextualized, they may be understood as meaningful modes of communication. For example, a person experiencing dementia might not be able to say, "please don't touch me" or "I would like some space" when feeling intruded upon. Instead, they may express their discomfort with unwanted approaches or physical touch with emotional intensity. Regrettably, such expression may be misread simply as aggressive behavioral symptoms (Ryden et al., 1991), and thus the underlying needs and desires they express are likely to be ignored and overruled.

Frequently, people with dementia are spoken to in elderspeak: a style involving a high-pitched voice with short, abbreviated sentences. Elderspeak is analogous to baby talk, that is, how people often talk to infants (Williams & Herman, 2011). People with speech/language impairments are also frequent targets of elderspeak and similarly condescending speech patterns. Older adults—including those with age-related cognitive changes—have perceived this style as disrespectful, unprofessional, and patronizing (Balsis & Carpenter, 2006; Williams & Herman, 2011). When "elder spoken" to, people are more likely to decline help or interaction (Cunningham & Williams, 2007; Williams & Herman, 2011). More respectful and effective strategies include using a natural tone of speech, active and reflective listening, and matching your pace to your conversational partner's. Keeping the focus on the present moment also accommodates the person's cognitive orientation.

Communication is vital to OT practice. The collaborative relationship tends to rely upon, by default, verbal communication. However, it is the therapist's responsibility to meet the client's communication needs. The therapeutic relationship may break down if the therapist is not attentive, flexible, and skilled in holistic communication, recognizing that people with (and indeed without) dementia communicate and exercise agency in multiple ways. As with the example of the husband-wife team above, OT's commitment to collaborative practice that enables occupation (Townsend & Polatajko, 2007) requires mindfulness, attention to these various forms of communication, self-awareness, openness to learning new ways to communicate, willingness to shift, and practice.

People with age-related cognitive changes are also seen as candidates for interventions typically applied to children, people with autism, and people with intellectual disabilities. Many consider these interventions intrusive and traumatizing when inflicted without consent. Applied Behavior Analysis researchers and practitioners (Buchanan et al., 2011) are marketing their intervention as a treatment for people with cognitive differences. Applied Behavior Analysis attempts to change behaviors through structured repetition and reward. It is expensive and time-consuming, and many who have experienced it report it as unpleasant and even harmful (Gibson & Douglas, 2018). However, it is marketed as a way to "Address Behavior Problems Associated with Alzheimer's and Dementia" (appliedbehavioranalysisedu.org, n.d.). As always, interventions should only be considered if the person wishes them. People with dementia retain various ways to communicate unhappiness even when language ability is absent. Ethical practice requires that we value and attend to such cues.

Many technological interventions have brought joy to the lives of people with age-related cognitive changes, for example, playing recorded music that targets meaningful and joyful memories (Moreno-Morales et al., 2020). However, technology has just as much potential to cause distress and even trauma if misused.

Technology is often seen as a cost-saving solution when staffing (whether in institutions or the community) can be scarce. Telehealth has been deployed extensively during the Covid-19 pandemic, and although it did, in some cases, solve access issues, make lives easier, and allow effective clinical treatment, in other cases, it led to disastrous consequences for the mental and physical health of elders needing health services (Chang et al., 2021). Robots have also been pitched as therapeutic and surveillance tools, companions, and comfort objects for disabled and aging populations (Seelman, 2016; Williams, 2021). Consider how the economies of efficiency and nursing home management influence how technologies are used on people, perhaps without offering choice or confirming consent. How does technological surveillance impact desires for privacy, already a scarce commodity in institutional settings? To hug a robotic stuffed seal may seem innocuous enough but substituting inhuman objects for companionship and skilled nursing is unlikely to improve quality of life. On the other hand, there are many easily available and relatively inexpensive technologies that could be offered to nursing home residents even in a rotating lending library. An iPad, Kindle, or other communication and entertainment device can be a wonderful interface with the world beyond the home or facility. Though such access may be given in extreme situations (e.g., giving loved ones the chance to say goodbye when pandemic protocols do not allow visits), we argue that it should be routinely available along with any adaptive software, apps, or positioning equipment that might make it easily useable with minimal help from staff. The days of $3,000 "medical" Augmentative and Alternative Communication devices rationed by "service providers" are thankfully numbered.

Advocacy can address some of the barriers that people with age-related cognitive changes face, including the stigma associated with the disease. Advocacy efforts bring attention to the neglect of this group's rights. Placing dementia under the disability umbrella can allow people to be their own advocates and "help provide an enabling identity" (Shakespeare et al., 2019, p. 2). A new research and advocacy group, *Communication First* (https://communicationfirst.org) advocates for the needs and rights of people who experience communication barriers in relation to a variety of impairments and conditions, including dementia.

Self-advocacy provides people with a sense of purpose and a means to combat stigma and discrimination (Seetharaman & Chaudhury, 2020). People with age-related cognitive changes can participate in advocacy efforts with proper attention to temporal aspects (Bartlett, 2014). There may be periods of time when individuals can share their ideas more readily than others; at such times, they can express and document what they wish to be respected in the event that they become less lucid. Often individuals with dementia who participate in advocacy are in the earlier stages of the condition. There is a risk that those who have more advanced cognitive changes, limited verbal skills, or mobility, for example, may encounter enhanced discrimination due to their apparent challenges to participation in advocacy (Bartlett, 2014). With their creativity and commitment to promoting inclusion and engagement, OTs can skillfully help promote the self-advocacy of older adults with age-related cognitive changes.

## A Community in Exile: Devalued Elders, Distancing From Disability, and Artful Protest

This section explores the experience of a community of lower-income older adults within a city that was undergoing gentrification. It is included here as a case study that brings together several themes from this chapter, including identity, disability, community, intersections, and advocacy. All of the quotations derive from author Nepveux's (2016) chapter and fieldnotes.

The Ida Benderson Senior Citizens Center occupied a rented space in the center of Syracuse, New York. Managed by the city Parks Department for 26 years, it was especially popular among lower-income elders and those who used public transit. Members described the center as a "second home" where they experienced "real love and respect" from others in similar situations. One described a "freshness" of encountering new and old friends, contrasted with the "dullness" of staying home. Some volunteered or held paid jobs at the center. Some were insecurely housed, staying with friends or extended family because they could no longer afford rent.

When the city announced in September 2011 that the center would close in a little over a month to be replaced by a Salvation Army Day Program in another location, center participants spoke out through street marches, speeches, songs of the Civil Rights Movement, and even staging a faux sidewalk barber shop where women members voluntarily had their heads shaved in protest. At these events and in Council hearings, participants expressed heartbreak and outrage about the closure and how they were overruled by the city—their concerns portrayed as mere foolishness and age-related rigidity (Nepveux, 2016).

Contrary to this portrayal, center participants "expresse[d] a demand for dignity and the right to participate in city life and decisions affecting [their] community" (Nepveux, 2016, p. 180). Most were long-time Syracuse residents who had lived through the "urban renewal" project that destroyed hundreds of homes in the 15th Ward, a historically Black and working-class neighborhood, to make way for a freeway, hospitals, and other large public institutions. This decision had resonance for them in that they were informed and persuaded, but not consulted.

City officials justified their decision to close the center partly on unsubstantiated claims of "six to eight" ambulance calls per month by center staff. They insisted that participants would be better served at a service center that included on-site nursing care. Indeed, part of the reluctance that many felt to accept the city's offer to participate at the Salvation Army's Social Day Program was in relation to a shared perception that such a program was designed for disabled people—whatever disability meant. Disabled, to those Ida participants I (Denise) spoke with, meant frail or incompetent, in need of direction or supervision. In contrast, they experienced themselves as vital, self-directing, interdependent members of this small, imperfect community. One garnered appreciative laughter at a press conference when he quipped, "The mayor says we are frail. Do I look frail?" (Nepveux, 2016, pp. 186–187). While he and a few others traveled by bicycle, others moved on and off city buses using wheelchairs or walkers. Some had experience with the mental health system and adult protective services. Yet few, if any, identified themselves as disabled. Some found a place to continue to experience this via the action group, which continued to meet weekly for several years after the closure. One member of the action group said this: "[The group] gave me hope. Ida had been an oasis for me. I'm frustrated that people say it's over. And I say no! Our building has closed, but we are remnants of Ida. We are meeting, and we are continuing. … we are not Salvation Army. We are not people in a nursing home" (Nepveux, 2013).

As discussed previously, escalating economic inequality marginalizes lower-income older adults and their families through housing unaffordability. However, in the case of the Ida Benderson closure, ageism intersected with neoliberal governance when the city chose to promote its downtown as a center of youthful consumerism at the expense of spaces and services for older adults and multigenerational families. Members distanced themselves from allegations of frailty and neediness—and thus from "disability"—as part of attempting to reclaim their dignity, value, and belonging in the city. What would our communities look like, and what could they become if dignity, worth and belonging were not contingent on youth, strength, and productivity? What if age and disability could mean many things but not a loss of human value? (For more discussion of productive aging frameworks and age-inclusive communities, please see Chapters 19 and 32).

## Recommendations for Practice and Research

When examining disability in its relation to aging, it is essential to consider how disability experience differs from the experiences of aging while recognizing that there is also a critical overlap, especially with regard to service provision and access needs. However, each group experiences different sociocultural perceptions and treatment; these must be considered while always utilizing an intersectional lens.

Some key concepts from this chapter include disability studies and anthropological approaches to life courses, accommodation, and contextualized knowledge. Readers should understand and value these contributions and consider how they might apply to OT practice with older adults. Readers should understand and celebrate that aging with disability experience differs from aging into disability experience and that those who experience each of these may profit from working together and learning from one another. Both groups benefit from thinking in a life course rather than a lifespan perspective and looking creatively at environmental supports and accommodations to enable them to remain healthy and fulfillingly occupied as part of communities: Interdependence, not independence. This change reinforces OTs' need for interdisciplinary and public policy engagement in partnership with relevant equity-seeking groups.

OTs have broad expertise in supporting aging in place and often work to promote older disabled adults' ability to remain in their homes by focusing on home modification, occupational adaptation, and improving functional skills to promote aging in place (see Chapters 19, 20, and 32). However, OTs need to expand their approach to addressing aging in place by attending to the structural factors that impact older adults' opportunities to age in their homes and communities. When working with both younger and older adults, OTs need to consider and discuss the economic and policy factors that impact our clients' prospects for continuing to dwell safely and interdependently in their communities throughout their life course. By working in solidarity with disabled and older adults and at the systems level, OTs may proactively effect change to enable equitable access to aging in community. (See also Chapter 31, OTs as Change Agents.)

OTs can include arts-based practice as articulated by disabled and aging artists as opportunities to explore meaning, identity transition, and unpack and push back against false, oppressive, and restrictive identity categories (see also Chapter 24). OTs need to understand the many models of home supports and their funding streams and pass that knowledge on to their client communities, at a minimum, referring them to local actors well versed in these systems that vary by state and local agencies (see Chapter 29). OTs can work with and refer people to ILC/CIL, with disability movement policy folk, as well as disability justice mutual support communities who can provide support beyond the scope of OT practice. Disability "services" still support huge gatekeeping autocracies. It is essential to train professional gatekeepers to work with the disability community, not against it.

We strongly advocate for understanding age-related cognitive changes (Wagner, 2020) by infusing different approaches from outside the medical model to promote full participation and engagement. OT should join in efforts to encourage communication access and self-advocacy of older adults with dementia. (See Chapters 15 and 16.)

Directions for future research include seeking a better understanding of how the experience of disability varies among people who age into disability. Age at disability onset, time passed since onset, and the timing of various life course changes are still significant and understudied variables. Other aspects needing further study include experiences of intermittent impairment and chronic illness.

## Conclusion

In this chapter, we have used anthropological ethnography and disability studies methodologies to evaluate how elders experience aging into disability versus aging with disability. Our critical theoretical and methodological approach emerges from disability and antiageist activism, especially as articulated by groups who experience multiple marginalizations related to disability, aging, gender, class, and racial discrimination. We fully engage and invite OTs, COTAs, and other health professionals to partner with community activists to ensure that experiences of disability and aging, and the wishes and goals of the people most primarily concerned—those living these identities and experiences—are respected and represented.

*The complete listing of the Bibliography and Chapter Questions and Answers are available in the accompanying enhanced eBook version included with the print purchase of this textbook. Visit Elsevier eBooks+ (eBooks.Health.Elsevier.com) to access this content.*

## CHAPTER 12

# Nutrition, Food Insecurity, and Occupational Performance

*Julia Henderson-Kalb, OTD, OTR/L and Connie Diekman, M.Ed., RD, LD, FADA, FAND*

## CHAPTER OUTLINE

## OBJECTIVES

- Understand how malnutrition can lead to poor overall health outcomes in aging adults
- Outline the impact of food security on health and quality of life
- List three common nutritional deficiencies in aging adults
- Understand the role nutrition plays in chronic disease
- Recognize that foods can often interact with commonly used drugs
- Describe appropriate occupational therapy interventions to assist older adults who have feeding problems, including interventions targeting food preparation
- List and explain the use of adaptive devices that can assist aging adults with self-feeding and food preparation
- Discuss factors that might impede eating and swallowing and related intervention approaches
- Summarize feeding techniques that caregivers should know to optimally assist an aging adult with feeding problems
- Consider how occupational justice can affect nutrition in the aging adult
- Understand the relevance of social, cultural, and personal meanings of food and eating in the everyday lives of aging adults
- Discuss the meaning of food and eating in later life in relation to different cultures, contexts, and genders

## Nutritional Requirements in Aging Adults

In 2019, the Administration on Aging reported that there were 54.1 million persons in the United States over the age of 65, a 36% increase since 2009. This number represents 30 million women and 24.1 million men. Projections for growth in this group indicate that by 2050, in the United States, there will be about 80 million people 65 and older, and globally that number could reach two billion (Administration on Community Living, 2020; Shilisky et al., 2017). Aging triggers many changes in the body, changes that impact nutrition. Whether it is decreased appetite, lack of interest in cooking or eating, medications, finances, or a variety of other reasons, the outcome is often the same—malnutrition.

According to the *2020–2025 Dietary Guidelines for Americans* (US Department of Agriculture and US Department of Health and Human Service), aging adults should use the dietary patterns recommended for the general population. The major difference for the aging adult is in terms of calories. Calorie needs for the aging adult range from 1600 to 2200 for women, and 2000 to 2600 for men (US Department of Agriculture [USDA] & the US Department of Health and Human Services [HHS], 2020). While the aging adult population is consuming a better-quality diet than any other age group, they are missing the mark on some food groups. Aging adults are not consuming the recommended intake for fruits, vegetables, dairy, and protein foods, except for men meeting the protein recommendation. One way for aging adults to meet the recommended food group intakes is to focus on choosing more nutrient dense foods, rather than foods that contain calories with little nutrition. In addition to following the dietary patterns outlined in the *2020–2025 Dietary Guidelines for Americans*, aging adults need to focus on fluid and fiber intake.

The aging body has less fluid volume than a younger body. Sixty percent of a younger person's body weight is water, but as we age this drops to about 50% of body weight. (Stephenson et al., 2022). Along with this change in fluid volume, the perception of thirst declines with age, and kidney function can less effectively conserve fluids, leading to an increased need to urinate. If mobility is an issue for the aging adult, these two factors can cause the aging adult to consume fewer fluids. The lack of fluids can lead to dehydration, weakness, confusion, and constipation. The Institute of Medicine recommends that women over the age of 50 consume at least 91 ounces of fluid from water-based beverages, foods and drinking water. Men over the age of 50 should consume at least 128 ounces of fluid (National Academies of Science, 2005).

At the same time, the aging adult often limits fiber intake. Although this is a problem for most age groups in the United States, for the aging adult, constipation can be a more frequent problem, and poor fiber intake can increase the problem. The Institute of Medicine recommends that women over the age of 50 consume 21 g of fiber per day, and that men consume 21 g/day (Quagliani et al., 2017). Including more fruits, vegetables, whole grains, and beans, which also help the aging adult meet other nutrient needs, is an effective way to boost fiber intake. There are two types of fiber, soluble and insoluble. While insoluble fiber aids in preventing constipation, soluble fiber can help with reduction of the risk of some types of cancer and the incidence of heart disease. Aging adults should focus first on boosting fiber intake by consuming more of the food groups that

many are missing, and then work with a Registered Dietitian to determine how much of their fiber intake should come from insoluble versus soluble.

As is true for all population groups, the aging adult needs to reduce intake of added sugars, saturated fat, and sodium, points that will be discussed later in this chapter.

This chapter will review the key aspects of nutrition and the aging adult as well as ways that health-care professionals can help the aging adult, and their caregiver, meet their nutritional needs.

## The Malnourished Aging Adult

Malnutrition is when the body is not receiving the nutrients it needs for proper functioning. Malnutrition is often viewed as only a state of undernutrition or weight loss, but in fact malnutrition can reflect the overconsumption of calories without adequate nutrient content. While undernutrition is the more commonly addressed form of malnutrition, the growing incidence of overnutrition in the aging adult is important and will be addressed in this chapter.

Estimates as to the percentage of aging adults who are malnourished vary, since many aging adults are not seen by a health-care professional, who can provide quantification of numbers. In 2018, the Academy of Nutrition and Dietetics estimated that up to one-half of people in the United States over the age of 65 may be malnourished or at risk for malnutrition (Academy of Nutrition and Dietetics, 2018a). The impacts of malnutrition range from cost to the health-care system, decreased quality of life, and risk for increased mortality. In addressing these potential risks, the Academy of Nutrition and Dietetics identified that the economic burden of diseases associated with malnutrition could be over $50 billion. At the same time, the malnourished adult is five times more likely to die during hospitalization and has a higher rate of readmittance than the well-nourished aging adult (Academy of Nutrition and Dietetics, 2018a). In light of this fact, the Centers for Medicare and Medicaid Services has approved the inclusion of the Global Malnutrition Composite Score into its Hospital Inpatient Quality Reporting Program effective in the fiscal year 2023 budget and the full implementation by hospitals in 2024 (Valladares et al., 2022). This new system will allow hospitals to improve their malnutrition care by offering another means to track those who come in malnourished and the impact of their care in the hospital. While malnutrition often is a singular factor, it is more common to see it occur in combination with other chronic diseases or lifestyle risks (Table 12.1). Chronic diseases and lifestyle risks can impact eating, whether by impacting taste, or due to medications or other treatments that affect appetite. These factors call for regular screening of nutrition to avoid missing early stages of malnutrition.

In their paper "Malnutrition in the elderly: Underrecognized and increasing in prevalence," Haines et. al looked at the growing incidence of malnutrition in aging adults. The paper addressed the importance of recognition of malnutrition in inpatient and outpatient aging adults. To help health-care

**TABLE 12.1**  Impacts of Malnutrition

| Risks for Malnutrition | Impacts |
|---|---|
| Dentition | Elimination of hard to chew foods > decreased nutrient intake |
| Disease | CVD, DM, COPD, Cancer, and other diseases > changed diet and meds which can impact nutrient intake and absorption |
| Mental health | Anxiety, depression, OCD, and other mental health issues > decreased nutrient intake |
| Income level | Finances can impact the foods purchased often > lower nutrient intake |
| Social issues | Living alone often > eating a smaller variety of foods > missed nutrients |

*CVD*, Cardiovascular disease, which includes hypertension and stroke; *COPD*, chronic obstructive pulmonary disease; *DM*, diabetes mellitus; *OCD*, obsessive compulsive disorder.

professionals recognize malnutrition, they proposed the use of the nine Ds of malnutrition (Haines et al., 2020)

- Dementia
- Dysgeusia
- Diarrhea
- Depression
- Dysphagia
- Disease
- Dentition
- Drugs
- Dysfunction

These nine categories will be reviewed a bit more in this chapter, as well as other chapters. The categories are important flags to prompt screening. Screening hospitalized patients for malnutrition has been required by The Joint Commission since 1995, but it is not standard in aging adults seen in community settings (Patel et al., 2014).

The Academy of Nutrition and Dietetics, in their Evidence Analysis Library, includes a policy recommendation on unintended weight loss. In this document, they recommend that registered dietitians work with other health-care professionals, administrators, and policy makers to ensure that all aging adults are screened for any changes in weight (Academy of Nutrition and Dietetics, 2009). The Malnutrition Quality Improvement Initiative (MQII) is a process that allows all health-care team members to understand how to assess malnutrition and how to identify their role in the assessment and management process (Malnutrition Quality Improvement Initiative, 2021).

Several tools exist for malnutrition screening, but the accuracy of the tools vary, leading to a call for a standardization of a malnutrition screening tool. In 2019, the Academy of Nutrition and Dietetics conducted a systematic review of validation studies for malnutrition screening tools. This review resulted in a classification of screening tools and indicated

that the Malnutrition Screening Tool (MST) had a moderate degree of validity, agreement, and inter-rater reliability in identifying malnutrition risk. In addition to these factors, it was the only test to yield a Grade 1 in terms of strength of evidence. The other reviewed tests included the MUST, MNA-SF, SNAQ, MNA-Sf-BMI, and the NRS-2002 (Academy of Nutrition and Dietetics, 2019). Many of these rated well in some categories, but they all only achieved a Grade 2 in the category of strength of evidence.

Traditionally, it has been recommended that serum albumin and prealbumin be used to provide insight into nutritional status. In 2020, the American Society for Parenteral and Enteral Nutrition (ASPEN) issued a position paper on the use of albumin and prealbumin in assessing malnutrition (Evans et al., 2020). In this paper, the authors discuss the role of serum albumin and prealbumin as measures of inflammation and their role in assessing nutritional status but not as markers of inflammation. As the authors state, illness and infection are connected to inflammation in the body. While inflammation can trigger malabsorption leading to malnutrition, the cause is not the lowered levels of albumin and prealbumin, but the inflammation caused by the illness and or infection. When health-care professionals are assessing nutritional status, it is important to recognize that serum levels of albumin and prealbumin are one part of the assessment and not indicators of malnutrition.

## Common Reversible Medical Causes of Malnutrition

Malnutrition is when the body fails to get enough of the nutrients needed for the body to perform. Malnutrition impacts all body organs, generating lack of energy that can lead into some of, or even all the 9 Ds identified by Haines et al. While not all causes of malnutrition can be reversed, with early intervention several can be changed. Common medical causes include certain medications, depression, chronic health conditions that impact diet or mobility, economic status, and mental or social disabilities.

Since many aging adults have health problems, many are taking medications for those problems. Food and drug interactions can impact nutrition by changing the foods people choose or changing the absorption of the medication. Health-care professionals should assess medications' impact on food intake and adjust prescriptions to avoid possible food-drug interactions.

Impaired mobility can lead to avoidance of preparing meals or shopping. It can also result in inability to open containers, often causing people to skip eating rather than deal with the frustration and challenge of opening containers. When it comes to mobility and shopping, helping the aging adult shift their shopping to online services or even participate in meal programs like Meals on Wheels or Congregate Dining Sites may be desirable.

For many aging adults, finances are an issue, and the ability to purchase a variety of produce and adequate protein-rich foods, along with whole grains, is a challenge. In addition, if the choice is medication or food, it is not uncommon for people to choose their needed medications at the expense of a well-balanced diet. Once again meal or food programs available in the community can often help close this gap. Healthcare professionals need to have lists of available options to help their clients find the food necessary for health.

For aging adults who are struggling with depression, dementia, or Alzheimer disease, shopping and meal preparation can be difficult. People with these conditions will benefit from help from family members, a caregiver, or again community programs. Ensuring that adequate nutrition is available for people who are dealing with cognition issues will not only prevent malnutrition but help decrease some of the cognitive challenges.

## Consequences of Under and Over Nourishment

As addressed in the beginning of the chapter, malnutrition is often viewed as lack of nutrition or the starving population. In fact, it is possible to be overnourished and still have malnutrition. Over consumption of calories, leading to overweight and obesity, does not immediately imply adequate nutrition. The diet of many aging adults tends to mimic that of the population, consuming too much saturated fat and not enough fiber, fruits, vegetables, and dairy, leading to gaps in vitamin and minerals, even in the presence of adequate or excess calories. It is important to provide the aging adult with proper guidance on choosing nutrient-dense foods instead of energy-dense choices. It has been estimated that inadequacies in vitamin and mineral intake could be as high as 35% for those over the age of 65 (Amarya et al., 2015). Referrals to a registered dietitian can help the aging adult learn how to meet nutrient and energy needs within their budget.

Overnutrition can lead to increased risk of excess body weight. While conversations continue on advantages versus disadvantages to excess weight in the aging adult, it is known that excess body fat increases the risk for hypertension, diabetes, heart disease, certain types of cancer, and potential mobility issues. According to the Centers for Disease Control and Prevention the prevalence of obesity in those over the age of 60 is 42.8% (Centers for Disease Control and Prevention, 2021b).

## Nutritional Supplements

Nutritional supplements can be in pill, capsule, powder, or liquid form, and they encompass daily multivitamins and minerals, protein supplements, herbal supplements, antioxidants, fiber, amino acids, and even enzymes. When eating food becomes difficult or when medical conditions impact digestion and absorption, some nutritional supplements may be the only way to meet nutritional needs. Aging adults should always consult with their physician and, if possible, a registered dietitian, to determine which supplements are needed to improve nutritional status (National Institute on Aging, 2021).

As will be discussed later in this chapter, certain vitamins and minerals are required in higher amounts in aging adults, possibly making it difficult to consume enough through foods. Vitamins $B_{12}$, $B_6$, folate, calcium, and vitamin D are a few nutrients that can be more difficult to meet the higher

needs of those over the age of 50, making supplements helpful. Efforts should always be to boost nutrient intake through food first, but if chewing, lack of appetite, or chronic conditions that impact digestion and absorption exist, supplementation is an option.

When swallowing is a problem, or if an aging adult can chew but just cannot eat enough to meet nutrient needs, a liquid meal supplement can help. When choosing a liquid supplement, a registered dietitian should be consulted to ensure that the macro- and micronutrients are properly provided.

## Dietary and Herbal Supplements

Another category of supplementation is single nutrient supplements. These might be antioxidants, herbals, or even essential amino acids. Antioxidant supplements are promoted as disease preventers, but the body of evidence on their effectiveness is limited, so they should not be relied on for disease prevention. Herbal supplements may provide some health benefits, but the body of evidence is mixed, and herbals need to be assessed in terms of usage related to other medications the individual might be taking, since the potential for nutrient interaction is high.

Herbals are plant compounds that have a chemical structure just like medication, so interactions can occur. Once again, consultation with a registered dietitian is recommended. Essential amino acids, especially leucine, are important to muscle strength, but whether they can restore muscle mass without regular physical activity is not clear. If an assessment is made that indicates a need to boost muscle mass, the treatment plan should be food first, then the addition of protein powder or shakes, especially those made from whey protein, and both done in balance with allowable activity (Feeding America, 2019).

## Poor Dentition and Oral Health

Losing teeth as we age is not uncommon, even though the percent of aging adults who have lost one or more teeth is declining from the numbers found in the early 70s. The National Institute of Dental and Craniofacial research estimates that 27.7% of aging adults have no teeth remaining, and that adults over the age of 65 have, on average, 18.9 remaining teeth (National Institute of Dental and Craniofacial Research, 2018). The loss of teeth is due to a variety of factors, but one identified factor is the existence of other chronic diseases. Data from NHANES has identified that the more chronic diseases an individual has, the higher the risk for dental loss. NHANES data found that for those over the age of 50 having even just one chronic condition increased the risk of tooth loss (Centers for Disease control and Prevention, 2020). The data did indicate that from the 1999–2004 assessment to the 2011–2016 assessment, the percent of aging adults with lost teeth decreased. Since Medicare Parts A and B do not cover routine dental care, monitoring dental health is something health-care professionals should add to their list of questions related to food and ability to eat.

In addition to tooth loss, periodontal disease affects 70.1% of those over the age of 65, according to the CDC (Centers for

Disease Control and Prevention, 2013). Periodontal disease can cause infection in the gums leading to tenderness that can make it difficult to chew, resulting in a need to eat soft or even pureed foods to meet nutritional needs.

Finally, dry mouth, which can be a natural outcome of aging or the result of certain medications, x-rays, or chemotherapy of the head and neck area, can also contribute to difficulties eating. With diminished saliva, mastication and the swallowing of food is more difficult, often leading to an avoidance of drier foods, meats, and grain foods. Diminished saliva can also impact the digestion of carbohydrates, since the normal process begins in the mouth with the release of salivary amylase. Artificial saliva can help with dry mouth, and not only make eating easier but can help increase the digestion and absorption of carbohydrates (see also Chapter 13).

## Refeeding Syndrome

One of the potential consequences of beginning to feed someone when they are malnourished is refeeding syndrome. When the body has been deprived of needed nutrients, it shifts how it provides fuel for the body from using the glucose from carbohydrates to using stored fat and protein. The process of reestablishing a nutritional balance needs to be done with care and in a well-planned manner. Providing nutrients to a malnourished body can trigger an imbalance in electrolytes and fluid balance, due to the body's response to more carbohydrates, leading to more insulin and to shifts in the cells of glucose and electrolytes. Most commonly these electrolytes are phosphate, potassium, magnesium, and sodium. The imbalance is a lowering of phosphate, magnesium, and potassium while fluid levels increase, due to the kidney's retention of sodium. These consequences can cause organ damage, and if not caught quickly, death.

Before refeeding a malnourished person, whether that feeding is oral, enteral, or parenteral, a risk assessment should be completed. The first step in assessing is using the MST screening tool or, if not available, any of the other validated, though lower grade in strength, of evidence tools. Existence of one or more chronic diseases is also an indicator for the potential for refeeding syndrome, as is severe underweight or recent rapid weight loss (World Health Organization, 2020). Since so many factors can impact risk, the potential for it to occur can often be missed. Any malnourished aging adult should be monitored by a nutrition support team to ensure that refeeding syndrome is avoided or at least caught within the first 72 hours of refeeding (Aubry et al., 2018).

## Common Nutritional Problems in Aging Adults

Population projections suggest that by 2050 the number of people over the age of 60 will be close to two billion, a doubling of the current number. Given that people are living longer, the percentage of the population who will be over age 80 could approach 392 million (Academy of Nutrition and Dietetics, 2009). The concern with these numbers is that aging changes every cell in the body, impacting all body functions including digestion, metabolism, and absorption. (See also

Chapter 9.) Changes in digestion, metabolism, and absorption lead to nutritional changes, as well. At the same time, projections continue to predict a higher number of aging adults who are overweight and obese, but malnourished at the same time. A few of the nutrients that are of concern to the aging adult population are discussed here, but more information can be found in Table 12.2.

### Calcium and Vitamin D Deficiency

Vitamin D deficiency is a global health problem with close to one billion people, worldwide, being deficient (Sizer et al., 2021). The aging adult is at higher risk for deficiency due to decreased ability of the skin to convert the inactive form of the active form, the decreased ability of the liver and kidneys to convert vitamin D to calcitriol, and the intestines' decreased ability to absorb vitamin D. In addition to these metabolic changes, many aging adults do not spend enough time in the sun to even reap the benefit of sun activation of D in the skin. Due to these factors, the RDA for vitamin D for those over the age of 70 increases from $15\mu$ or 600 IU/day to $20\mu$ or 800 IU. There are studies looking at higher amounts of vitamin D and clearly high amounts might be needed by some people, but the RDA reflects the current body of evidence. Achieving these increased amounts requires close attention to intake of vitamin D–rich foods and regular assessment of vitamin D levels to determine need for supplementation. These changes to vitamin D absorption impact calcium as well. Vitamin D status is important to calcium absorption. When vitamin D levels are low, the intestines absorb less of the calcium provided by the diet. Vitamin D is also essential to bone cell development of calcium phosphate. Without adequate vitamin D, the bone formation process is compromised. Like vitamin D, calcium needs for those over the age of 70 are higher. The RDA for calcium is 1200 mg/day.

Most adults, of any age, do not meet their calcium needs through food. Calcium supplementation is common in adults, including the aging adult.

### Iron Deficiency/Anemia

Iron deficiency, defined as lowered levels of hemoglobin, is common in the aging adult. Deficiency occurs due to a variety of factors including, poor dietary intake, medication interactions, chronic disease, hormone imbalance, and GI malabsorption. The 2016 National Health and Nutrition Examination Survey (NHANES) reported that 14.1% of men over age 65 and 10.2% of women over age 65 are iron deficient (Seitz et al., 2018). Iron deficiency anemia occurs in 2% to 5% of the US adult population. Current recommendation for iron intake is 8 mg/day for both men and women 51 years and older. Consuming enough iron from one's diet gets harder as people age, because the main food sources of iron are meat and enriched or fortified grain foods. While the aging adult can easily consume grain foods, the iron in grain foods is not as well absorbed, making meat the preferred source of heme-iron. Since dentition often is an issue for the aging adult, meat intake often declines with age, thus reducing heme-iron intake. Iron supplementation is an option, and obviously

**TABLE 12.2** Common Nutritional Deficiencies, Consequences, and Interventions

| Nutrient | Consequences | Intervention |
|---|---|---|
| Vitamin D | Increased fall risk<br>Increased hip fracture risk<br>Increased risk of mortality<br>Increased risk of osteoporosis<br>Functional deterioration | Screening for vitamin D deficiency<br>Replacement if necessary<br>Prophylactic vitamin D supplements for older adults in institutionalized settings |
| Iron | Anemia—fatigue, exercise intolerance | Screening for anemia<br>Screening for possible causes of bleeding<br>Replacement if necessary |
| Vitamin $B_{12}$ | Poor cognition<br>Loss of balance<br>Megaloblastic anemia<br>Increased risk of vascular disease<br>Increased risk of depression<br>Possible increased risk of age-related macular degeneration | Screening for vitamin B12 deficiency, especially in those with history of abdominal surgery<br>Replacement if necessary<br>Prophylactic supplements for older adults with history of gastrectomy or terminal ileectomy |
| Vitamin $B_6$ | Increased risk of vascular disease<br>Increased risk of cognitive decline<br>Anemia<br>Increased risk of depression<br>Possible increased risk of age-related macular degeneration | Usually borderline deficiency in older adults<br>Improve diet<br>Replacement with supplements if necessary |
| Folate | Poor cognition<br>Megaloblastic anemia<br>Increased risk of vascular disease<br>Increased risk of depression<br>Possible increased risk of age-related macular degeneration | Screening for folate deficiency<br>Replacement if necessary |
| Calcium | Osteoporosis | Prophylactic vitamin D and calcium intake in the form of foods or supplements |
| Zinc | Loss of taste, mental lethargy, compromised immune system, weight loss | Boost intake of protein foods from animal and/or plant sources |
| Omega-3 | Increased risk of CVD, decreased cognition | Fatty fish, walnuts, canola oil, and supplements if coordinated with the physician and registered dietitian |
| Magnesium | Weakness | Encourage intake of dark leafy greens, legumes, nuts, and whole grains |
| Potassium | Muscle cramps and weakness | Boost intake of fruits and vegetables, monitor use of diuretics, supplementation may be needed if malnutrition and dehydration are prolonged |

*CVD,* Cardiovascular disease.

From Kaiser, M., Bandinelli, S., & Lunenfeld, B. (2010). Frailty and the role of nutrition in older people. A review of the current literature. *Acta Biomedica, 81*(Suppl. 1), 37–45; and Rohde, L. E., Silva de Assis, M. C., & Rabelo, E. R. (2007). Dietary vitamin K intake and anticoagulation in elderly patients. *Current Opinion in Clinical Nutrition and Metabolic Care, 10,* 1–5.

needs to be considered when the aging adult has iron deficiency anemia, but close monitoring of gastrointestinal issues is important since supplements can irritate the stomach and cause nausea and/or constipation. In addition, iron, calcium, and zinc all compete for the same absorption sites, so supplementation of the three must be carefully balanced. Iron absorption is enhanced when iron is consumed along with an acidic food like oranges, lemons, lime, and other foods rich in vitamin C. Taken in the presence of antacids, iron absorption will be negatively impacted.

## Vitamin $B_{12}$/Folate (Vitamin $B_9$) Deficiency

Vitamin $B_{12}$ and folate, also referred to as vitamin $B_9$, are often deficient in the aging adult due inadequate intake. Vitamin $B_{12}$ is also deficient because of poor absorption, due either to a lack of the intrinsic factor in the stomach or due to incomplete absorption in the intestines. Vitamin $B_{12}$ and folate, along with vitamin $B_6$, are important to cognition and may help in the prevention of Alzheimer disease and dementia. The process by which they help with cognition is associated with their role in keeping homocysteine levels down. Elevated homocysteine appears to be connected to changes in cognition, and adequate levels of vitamins $B_{12}$ and $B_6$, along with folate, help prevent elevations in homocysteine levels (USDA & HHS, 2020). $B_{12}$ is only available in animal foods, so intake can often be low given some of the limitations that occur with aging – due to chewing, cost, preparation, and taste changes. $B_{12}$ supplements provide the form of $B_{12}$ that is easier to absorb, they do not rely on the intrinsic factor, so encouraging the aging adult to add a $B_{12}$ supplement is helpful. Folate is found in leafy green vegetables, broccoli, orange juice, and some fortified foods. Since fortification of grain foods, folate deficiency is rare, with less than 1% of the US population showing a deficiency. Folate is important to red blood cell formation, and a deficiency can lead to megaloblastic anemia. Folate and $B_{12}$ deficiencies can each demonstrate as megaloblastic anemia, so it is important to always check both vitamins with a diagnosis of megaloblastic anemia. As referenced previously, folate deficiencies can lead to elevated blood homocysteine, a key risk factor for cardiovascular disease (CVD) and possibly a marker for Alzheimer disease (Stephenson et al., 2022). Supplementation with folate can help prevent deficiencies, but they should be kept below the upper limit (UL) of safety of 1000 μ/day to avoid masking a $B_{12}$ deficiency.

## Protein

Adequate protein is essential for muscle development and maintenance of body muscle. Adequate muscle mass helps the aging adult with movement, balance, bone, and overall health. According to the 2020–2025 Dietary Guidelines for Americans, the average protein intake for those over the age of 71 is lower than those aged 60 to 70 (USDA & HHS, 2020). Overall, 50% of women and 30% of men over the age of 71 are consuming less protein than recommended. Age changes the ability of the body to maintain muscle mass and along with lowered protein intake increases the risk for sarcopenia in the aging adult. Recommendations suggest that 25 to 30 g of high-quality protein at each meal can facilitate adequate intake of protein and especially the essential amino acid leucine (Kaur et al., 2019).

## Omega-3

Omega3 fatty acids eicosapentaenoic acid (EPA) and docosahexaenoic acid (DHA) have been researched in terms of their role in the prevention of CVD and maintenance of healthy cognition. While research is still evolving, the average intake of these fatty acids by most adults, including the aging adult, is below the recommended intake level. A 2018 prospective study found that higher intakes of omega-3s from seafood consumption was associated with a higher likelihood of healthy aging (Lai et al., 2018). The study followed subjects for more than 20 years and assessed healthy aging based on chronic disease occurrence, cognitive and physical assessments, and medical records. The recommendation from the study supports the 2020–2025 Dietary Guidelines recommendation of eight to ten ounces of seafood per week for those 60 and older (USDA & HHS, 2020).

## Magnesium

The mineral magnesium is not one that is often viewed as a mineral that is consumed below recommended levels; however in the aging adult, intake and poor absorption can often cause deficiency. Magnesium plays a role in over 300 metabolic functions, including muscle and nerve function, blood pressure, and blood glucose regulation. As we age, the body absorbs less of the magnesium we consume in the diet. In addition, losses in the urine increase with aging. On top of these two metabolic impacts, for aging adults who take diuretics, magnesium deficiency grows more likely. Magnesium deficiency can trigger weakness, which for the aging adult, can increase risk of falls. Magnesium is found in all plant foods, so developing eating plans around the core recommendations of the Dietary Guidelines can help meet magnesium needs.

## Potassium

Potassium and sodium are key nutrients in the regulation of blood pressure. While most people know about sodium food sources and consumption levels that often exceed recommendations, few know the importance of potassium. While the general intake of sodium exceeds recommended amounts, the intake of potassium is less than recommended. This imbalance is significant, given that 65% of those over the age of 60 have hypertension (Stephenson et al., 2022). The 2020–2025 Dietary Guidelines list five nutrients of concern, all of which are issues for aging adults. Nutrients of concern are nutrients that are not consumed at adequate levels by the population. Given the incidence of hypertension in the aging adult population, along with the use of potassium-wasting diuretics, focusing on more potassium is a key step.

## Nutrition in Special Client Populations

The Dietary Guidelines for Americans provide the foundation for meeting nutrient needs, but certain populations require adjustments to their eating plans. Aging adults with chronic conditions will need to make some adjustments to ensure maintenance of their health. However, it is important for all health-care providers to remember that quality of life, appetite, cognition, and ability to chew are all factors that should be weighed before telling an individual what they should be eating. Eating plans that restrict favorite foods or eliminate ingredients that make food more enjoyable can often cause the aging adult to skip meals. Collaborating with a registered dietitian can help develop eating plans that meet health and nutrient needs while keeping meals enjoyable for the individual.

## Diabetes

Estimates indicate that 33% of adults over the age of 65 have diabetes. In addition, an estimated 26,000,000 adults over the age of 65 have prediabetes. Metabolic changes due to age puts the aging adult with diabetes at a higher risk of developing hypoglycemia than younger adults (Endocrine Society, 2022). For many aging adults, diabetes is just one of the chronic conditions they might be dealing with, so assessing A1C levels, in terms of acceptable levels, is often more liberal than in those who are younger. Poor blood sugar control can contribute to falls, cognitive dysfunction, and damage to small blood vessels, so while diet might be liberalized, the importance of monitoring blood glucose levels and A1C levels cannot be ignored.

CVD is the number one cause of death in those with diabetes. Working to keep diet as well-balanced as possible along with regular activity can help keep blood glucose levels within an acceptable range. While heart healthful eating plans may restrict some food choices, working with the aging adult to identify likes and dislikes can often result in an eating plan that manages blood glucose while meeting their nutritional needs and their food preferences. Getting the aging adult to eat regularly is especially important to blood glucose control. Flexibility in meal planning can help provide food when the aging adult is hungry or when they will eat better while still managing A1C levels. As with any chronic condition that involves diet changes, working with a registered dietitian is a good idea.

### Cardiovascular Disease

Cardiovascular disease (CVD), which includes coronary heart disease, cerebral vascular disease, peripheral arterial disease, rheumatic heart disease, congenital heart disease, deep vein thrombosis, and pulmonary embolism, affects more than 77% of males and more than 75% of females over the age of 60 (USDA & HHS, 2020). In addition, hypertension impacts between 64% and 78.5% of those over the age of 65 (Academy of Nutrition and Dietetics, 2018b).

The guidance for the management of CVD is grounded in the Dietary Guidelines for Americans but includes some modification to address issues related to hypertension and lipid elevations.

For those with hypertension, the DASH diet has been found to help reduce blood pressure levels in a manner that is equal to or better than medications alone. The DASH diet is a diet high in fruits, vegetables, whole grains, fatty fish, nuts, seeds, low-fat dairy, and vegetable oils. The intake of other animal products is significantly limited. The concept behind the diet is that the high intake of potassium, calcium, and magnesium rich foods, along with foods rich in omega-3 fatty acids, aids in blood pressure control. The DASH diet encourages a sodium level of 2300 mg/day. The DASH diet is also effective with lower sodium levels. For the aging adult, reducing sodium below the 2300 mg/day may trigger dehydration and loss of appetite, so focusing on that level with a strong push to consume the food groups that make up the DASH diet is a better approach.

When it comes to management of lipid elevations, the focus of care should depend on the aging adults' overall health and other risk factors. Relying on medications to lower lipid levels should be preferred over severe restrictions in diet.

### Congestive Heart Failure

Congestive heart failure (CHF) or heart failure (HF) affects more than 7% of males and 3% of females between the ages of 60 and 79 years of age. For those 80 years of age and older, the incidence jumps to more than 9% of men and 11% of women. HF is managed through medications, but adjustments to diet also help. Lowering sodium intake is one aspect, as is limiting fluid intake. Given the increased incidence of dehydration in the aging adult, it is important to monitor fluid intake to avoid both over and under consumption.

When it comes to sodium intake, the current Dietary Guidelines for Americans recommend a daily intake of 2300 mg/day, with a reduction to 1500 mg/day for those over the age of 51 (Academy of Nutrition and Dietetics, 2018b). This guidance is appropriate for those with HF in that it reduces sodium intake but allows for enough to provide flavor to meals. Obviously, these recommendations should be adjusted based on the individual's appetite and degree of failure. Fluid intake will depend on the individual, the degree of HF, and medications they consume, but guidelines suggest a level of 2000 mL of fluid per day (Stephenson et al., 2022).

### Osteoporosis

Osteoporosis affects more than 12% of adults over the age of 50 and close to 18% of those over the age of 65, with women making up a larger percentage of the risk (Centers for Disease Control and Prevention, 2021a). Once an individual has been diagnosed with osteoporosis, the main concerns for care are watching for and preventing fall triggers, strengthening muscle mass to provide bone support, and consuming a diet that offers enough vitamin D and calcium. The use of medications to maintain bone mass is a frequent part of care for osteoporosis, with medications adjusted to the individual's ability to swallow pills, avoid gastrointestinal distress, and adhere to a consistent medication routine.

Vitamin D and calcium from food sources should be adjunct to other treatments. The previous section on Calcium and Vitamin D Deficiency discusses the RDAs for both nutrients.

### Nutrition in Dementia

As the body ages, so does the brain. Neurons decrease with age, leading to changes in memory, language, and other cognitive functions. While dementia is often associated with the aging adult, it is not a normal part of the aging process. Decline in neurons does not mean an automatic loss of cognitive functions. Dementia can be viewed in two ways, reversible and irreversible. Nutrition can play a role in both types, but its impact will be more significant in the reversible type. Cognition is impacted by several of the B vitamins, so focusing on adequate intake of vitamins $B_{12}$, $B_6$, and folate may provide some benefit and will help overall nutrition. Consumption of too much saturated fat is connected to an increased risk for CVD, which will impact blood vessels in the brain as well as throughout the body, so limitation of their intake may serve a benefit. The goal with nutrition might vary with the type of dementia, but the overall goal is to provide a well-balanced eating plan that addresses overall nutrition.

## Reversible Dementia

Reversible dementia can be a consequence of poor diet, medications, or imbalances in the body. Common dietary factors include deficiencies of thiamin, vitamin $B_{12}$, or dehydration. The B vitamin thiamin is found in whole grains, legumes, and nuts—foods that the aging adult may not include in their eating plans either due to dislike, difficulty chewing, or hesitation to prepare legumes.

Vitamin $B_{12}$ is found only in animal foods, so if the aging adult avoids these foods either due to dislike and/or inability to adequately chew or digest these foods, supplementation may be needed. In addition to failure to eat these foods, many medications can change the environment in the stomach, resulting in lowered levels or complete loss of production of the intrinsic factor compromising absorption of $B_{12}$.

## Nutrition and Prevention of Dementia

Even though a few nutrients play a bigger role in brain health, maintenance of cognition is like maintaining overall body health—one should consume a well-balanced diet. Maximize cognition by focusing on more plant foods, especially those that are darkly colored or strongly flavored. These foods contain more phytonutrients, many of which function as antioxidants. Antioxidants help avoid oxidation, the process that contributes to aging of cells. Adding more fruits, vegetables, and even nuts can help provide the body with nutrients and antioxidants. The use of supplements has not been clearly shown to provide benefits, so focus on food first.

Another area of nutrition that can impact brain health is the types of fat contained in the diet.

Saturated fat, found in animal foods and coconut and palm oils, has been found to contribute to the clogging of arteries, leading to blockages. If these blockages are in the brain, besides being potential triggers for stroke, they can cause cognitive impairment. Shifting fat intake to plant-based fats and adding omega-3 fats are two ways to help reduce this risk. Omega-3 fats are found predominantly in oily fish like salmon, tuna, sardines, herring, etc.

## Nutrition in Aging Adults Diagnosed With Dementia

Alzheimer disease, vascular dementia, and Parkinson disease are the three most common causes of dementia. Alzheimer disease affects more than 6 million Americans, and projections indicate this number might reach 14 million by the year 2050 (American Heart Association, 2021). Vascular dementia, caused by a series of small strokes, is the second most common form of dementia. Parkinson disease affects 10 million people worldwide, and progression of the disease can lead to dementia.

With all types of dementia, the challenges to nutrition include difficulties with mobility, impacting grocery shopping, inability to prepare food, forgetting to take time to eat, difficulty chewing and swallowing, and failure to consume adequate nutrition. Educating caregivers on programs that can provide access to food, or tools to aid individuals with eating is one step. As dementia progresses, the consistency of food will need to shift from regular to soft to pureed and possibly to nutrition support with enteral or parenteral feeding. One of the goals, at all stages of feeding, is focusing on healthier fats, adequate fruits, vegetables, and whole grains along with low-fat dairy.

## Nutrition in Long-Term Care Communities

Nutrition in long-term care can vary depending on the level of care. If the aging adult is receiving home health care, this care may include an in-home aide who can help with meal preparation or even monitoring of meals. This service may be limited for many aging adults due to cost, but in some short-term cases Medicare may provide some coverage.

For the aging adult who is in an independent living facility, the option of still preparing meals or dining in the common dining area might be desirable. This ability to choose helps as the aging adult transitions from living on their own to depending on others for their care. In assisted living facilities, the aging adult might improve their eating since the burden of shopping and cooking is removed. As the level of care moves to skilled nursing, the aging adult may require more help with eating meals.

An important aspect of nutrition in long-term care communities is working with the aging adult to assess their food likes and dislikes, along with nutritional needs. Facilities that offer a more restaurant-like option for their residents while recognizing the need for therapeutic diets can make the dining experience more enjoyable for the aging adult. (See also Chapter 28.)

Given the fact that estimates indicate that one-half of those over the age of 65 may be malnourished or at the risk of malnutrition, it is important that all risk factors are assessed before developing a meal care plan for the aging adult (Academy of Nutrition and Dietetics, 2018a,b). If the aging adult is malnourished or at risk of malnutrition, the option of nutritional supplementation should be assessed. As addressed earlier in this chapter, supplementation can provide the nutrients that are missing due to poor appetite, difficulty chewing or swallowing, or even lack of appetite due to depression or dementia. In addition to supplementation, using oral supplements as small meals or snacks can make it easier to consume needed calories without overwhelming the aging adult.

## Nutrition in End-of-Life Care

Nutrition during the end of life is one of many challenges. Nutritional support is thought to be essential for terminal patients to ensure the dignity and value of a human being until the end of life (Kang et al., 2018). During this time, family and friends may feel the tug to feed their loved one and health-care professionals work through how to keep the individual comfortable, how to assess when food and hydration are wanted by the individual, and when to shift feeding and hydration to compassionate care. As death approaches, the digestive system slows and signals for eating and drinking decline. This change is a part of the process of avoiding energy expenditure when the body is slowing down. In some cases, nutrition support can be a desirable choice during this time, but its use must be based on the wishes of the patient, if they can express them or have written directives, along with discussion with the medical team, the shared decision-making process is still important in the decision of how to feed. While the end-of-life process is never clear in terms of timeframe, the best approach to nutritional care is to monitor blood pressure, heart rate, respiration, and other functions to assess when to shift the offering of food or drink to only what is done to provide comfort to the individual. It is also important that health-care professionals know the legal requirements within their state and the rules covering their facility.

## Food and Drug Interactions

Food and drug interactions are well known. Whether it is an interaction that changes drug or nutrient absorption, metabolism, or elimination, the impact of food on drugs, and drugs on nutrient absorption, can be positive or negative (Koziolek et al., 2019). Food and drug interactions are especially concerning in the aging adult since many are consuming one or more drugs, or may have impaired digestion and absorption due to age or previous disease conditions. According to Merck Manual, 90% of older adults take at least one prescription drug, 80% regularly take at least two, and 36% regularly take at least five prescription drugs (Merck Manual, Consumer Version, 2021).

### The Role of Food in Drug Metabolism

During the process of digestion, food changes the environment within the gastrointestinal tract. This change in environment can impact the pharmacokinetic properties of drugs, affecting rate of drug release, absorption, metabolism, and elimination. These effects will vary with the food consumed and the drugs, but they can enhance or inhibit absorption. In addition to the interaction of food and drug, the overall health of the microbiome plays a role in drug availability just as it impacts nutrient availability. Food can also change the pH of urine, leading to changes in the pharmacokinetics as the drug is eliminated by the kidney (Koziolek et al., 2019).

### Common Drug-Food Interactions

Foods are chemical substances that require enzymes, hormones, and other digestive compounds to help the food release the macro and micronutrients. The changes that occur in the digestive tract during the process of digestion, metabolism, and absorption not only facilitate absorption of nutrients but can generate a change in the environment that then changes drug absorption. Some foods are well known for their drug interactions, with grapefruit juice being one of the most studied and well understood. Grapefruit juice interacts with almost all drugs by changing how the body metabolizes the drug or how it affects the liver as it moves the drug through the body. Some other foods that can interfere with medications include black licorice, cranberry juice, milk, and

alcohol. Table 12.3 provides some examples of potential food and drug interactions.

## Nutrition Security and the Aging Adult

Nutrition security may be a new term for many, but likely food insecurity is a bit more familiar. *Food insecurity* is defined as "Limited or uncertain availability of nutritionally adequate and safe foods or limited or uncertain ability to acquire acceptable foods in socially acceptable ways" (Bickel et al., 2000, p. 6). This translates to inadequate nutrition. In some cases, people have access to food, just not to nutrient-dense food, thus the need to focus on *nutrition security*. For the aging adult, who has a higher risk of malnutrition, nutrition security is a major concern. It is worth noting that the World Health Organization has identified that the number of people worldwide who are overweight and malnourished equals the number of people who are underweight and malnourished, making detection of nutrition security a bit more challenging (Ponzon et al., 2021).

### Food Insecurity

Feeding America has tracked the level of food insecurity and hunger in America for over 20 years. The trend in terms of those who are food insecure jumped significantly in the early part of this decade with a peak occurring in years 2011–2015 (Feeding America, 2019). In 2019, 4 million adults aged 50–59 and 5.2 million adults over the age of 60 were food insecure (Feeding America, 2019). Food insecurity does vary by race and ethnicity, by income, by housing, and by overall health. BIPOC (Black, Indigenous, People of Color) elders have a higher incidence of food insecurity across all age groups, so the aging adult does not escape this issue. Obviously, income level is a major factor. According to Feeding American, 32.1% of those who live below the poverty line are food insecure (Feeding America, 2019). In addition to impacting nutrition, for those who require regular medication for chronic health conditions, low income can lead to making choices between purchasing food or medications.

Living conditions can also impact nutrition. If the aging adult lives alone, they may not want to prepare meals, and they may limit expenditures for food to allocate funds to other needs. and if the aging adult is living with others, especially children, the aging adult may skip eating to ensure that children are fed. Chronic health conditions impact food and nutrition security due to medication costs, medications that may interfere with certain foods, or even an inability to shop due to physical limitations.

In looking at the impact of food insecurity on health and nutrition for those aged 50 to 59, Feeding America found that intake of vitamin A was 14.9%, vitamin C was 12.9%, and iron was 7.1% lower than those aged 50 to 59 who were food secure. In those over the age of 60, iron was 13.3% and calcium was 9.7% lower than comparable aged adults who were food secure (USDA & HHS, 2020). The Food Research and Action Center (FRAC) has reported that food/nutrition insecurity is a key predictor of health-care services utilization

**TABLE 12.3** Common Drug-Food Reactions

| Drug | Clinical Use | Effect With Food |
|---|---|---|
| Acetaminophen | Analgesia | Slower absorption and later onset of analgesia |
| Captopril | Hypertension Heart failure | Decreased absorption with food |
| Ciprofloxacin | Antibiotic, often used for urinary tract infections | Substantially decreased absorption when taken with cations (calcium, zinc, iron, magnesium) |
| Digoxin | Heart failure | Decreased absorption with high-fiber food |
| Levodopa/carbidopa | Parkinson disease | Decreased absorption, especially with high-protein meals |
| Metformin | Type 2 diabetes management | Decreased absorption, especially with high-fiber food |
| Warfarin | Anticoagulation | Decreased absorption vitamin K effects |
| Aspirin | Anticoagulation Heart disease prevention | Increased absorption |
| Hydrochlorothiazide | Hypertension | Increased absorption with food |
| Simvastatin | Cholesterol management | Increased absorption with food |
| Tricyclic antidepressants (nortriptyline, amitriptyline, imipramine) | Depression, not recommended in older adults Neurologic pain | High-tyramine-containing foods such as cheese, alcohol, and liver can cause hypertensive crisis |
| Lovastatin | Cholesterol reduction | Food intake enhances absorption and availability |
| Rosuvastatin | Anti-lipemic | Food intakes decrease absorption |
| NSAIDs | Analgesia | Can irritate stomach, take with food |
| Cimetidine, Fexofenadine, Loratadine | Antihistamines | Consume on an empty stomach to increase absorption |

*NSAIDs*, Nonsteroidal antiinflammatory drugs.
From Bressler, R. (2006, November). Grapefruit juice and prescription drug interactions. Exploring mechanisms of this interaction and potential toxicity for certain drugs. *Geriatrics, 61*(11):12–18.

(Food Research & Action Center, 2019). In 2014, the last year that data were reported, the direct and indirect cost of health-related care due to hunger and food insecurity was $160 billion (Food Research & Action Center, 2019).

## Nutrition Programs

In an attempt to provide access to food for aging adults, the USDA and the HHS have six programs designed to help the low-income, aging adult (Seitz et al., 2018). Table 12.4 provides a summary of the programs.

Supplemental Nutrition Assistance Program (SNAP) serves over 36 million people each month, with approximately 5 million or 24% of the total, being over the age of 60 (Food Research & Action Center, 2019). While this is a positive note, this is only 48% of those who qualify for SNAP. Health-care professionals should make sure that when assessing hunger and food access that they provide information on the SNAP program. SNAP benefits allow the aging adult, based on income guidelines, to purchase food using an electronic benefit transfer (EBT) card. Studies show that use of the SNAP reduces malnutrition, hospitalization, nursing home admissions, and the incidence of depression.

Congregate Nutrition Programs and Home-Delivered Nutrition program are two programs under the HHS that are available to those over the age of 60. These programs are available to all over the age of 60, but they are limited in

terms of the funds that are available. Estimates indicate that only about 10% of low-income adults over 60 take advantage of congregate or home-delivered meals. Congregate meals can have limitations for aging adults who have mobility or transportation issues, but for those who can use this service the food provided, as well as the socialization, are great assets. Home-delivered meals can provide not only food for those who cannot get to congregate settings, but they also provide a chance for someone to check-in on the aging adult.

The Commodity Supplemental Food Program (CSFP) provides food to supplement the diets of low-income aging adults monthly. The program will not provide adequate nutrition but will offer USDA foods that can supplement the foods the aging adult might be buying on their own or through other food and nutrition programs. CSFP works with local organizations to coordinate distribution of the food.

Senior Farmers Market Nutrition Program (SFMNP) is a community program that provides locally grown fruits, vegetables, honey, and herbs to low-income adults. The Child and Adult Care Food Program (CACFP) provides reimbursement for meals and snacks those aging adults receive when participating in an adult daycare program. Adult day care programs can work with their state agencies to determine how to receive reimbursement of meals and snacks provided to adults over the age of 60, in their programs.

**TABLE 12.4** Community Food and Nutrition Programs

| Program | Service | Eligibility | Contact |
|---|---|---|---|
| SNAP | An EBT card to allow for purchase of foods and beverages | Those over the age of 60 and who meet income guidelines. | https://www.fns.usda.gov/snap/supplemental-nutrition-assistance-program |
| Congregate Nutrition Services | Healthy meals in a community setting for those over the age of 60 | Those over the age of 60 and their spouses, no matter their age | https://www.mealsonwheelsamerica.org/docs/default-source/advocacy/oaa-nutrition-program-title-iii-c-overview.pdf?sfvrsn=b104bf3b_4 |
| Home-Delivered Nutrition Services | Home delivered meals for those who are frail, have health issues or conditions that make it difficult to leave home. | Those over the age of 60 and their spouse, no matter their age. | https://www.mealsonwheelsamerica.org/docs/default-source/advocacy/oaa-nutrition-program-title-iii-c-overview.pdf?sfvrsn=b104bf3b_4 |
| Commodity Supplemental Food Program (CSFP) | Monthly packages of USDA foods. | Low-income adults over the age of 60 | https://www.fns.usda.gov/csfp/csfp-fact-sheet |
| Senior Farmers Market Nutrition Program (SFMP) | Access to locally grown fruits, vegetables, honey, and herbs | Low-income adults over the age of 60 with a household income of not more than 185% of the federal poverty level. | https://www.fns.usda.gov/sfmnp/senior-farmers-market-nutrition-program |
| Child and Adult Care Food Program (CACFP) | Reimbursement to adult daycare programs for nutritious meals and snacks | Those over the age of 60 who attend adult daycare | https://www.fns.usda.gov/cacfp |

*EBT*, Electronic benefit transfer; *SNAP*, Supplemental Nutrition Assistance Program.

These six programs offer some means by which aging adults can get access to nutritious food, helping to reduce the amount of money they must spend on food. Health-care professionals who work with the aging adult should use Table 12.4 as a quick reference as they work to provide nutrition security for their clients.

## Occupational Therapy Evaluations for Feeding and Nutrition

As with any area of occupational therapy (OT) practice, it is important to complete a thorough assessment prior to intervention related to feeding and/or nutrition. Oftentimes, nonstandardized observation and assessment occurs in this situation. The therapist observes the client through an entire meal and assesses body structures and function, sitting position, environmental influences (e.g., lighting or noise), and dinnerware or adaptive equipment used.

A few standardized assessments are also available specifically for feeding or nutrition. The Edinburgh Feeding Evaluation Questionnaire (EdFED-Q) is a free measure that can be used to quantify the level of assistance someone might need while eating as well as mealtime interactions with caregivers (Watson et al., 2001). It is completed during observation of mealtime performance. Created for aging adults with dementia, this 11-item assessment has also been used with other neurocognitive disorders and the general aging adult population. The McGill Ingestive Skills

Assessment (MISA) is another option for a feeding evaluation via observation of mealtime routine (Lambert et al., 2003). This measure quantifies a person's ability to consume various food and liquid textures. Developed for the aging adult population, the MISA includes 43 items that address positioning, self-feeding skills, liquid ingestion, solid ingestion, and texture management.

Two options to assess malnutrition risks available to occupational therapists include the Mini Nutritional Assessment-Short Form (MNA-SF) and the Minimal-Eating Observation Form-Version II (MEOF-II). The MNA-SF is a free, six-item questionnaire that screens for both malnutrition and risk of malnutrition (Rubenstein et al., 2001). The MEOF-II is also free but is completed via meal observation (Vallen et al., 2011). This measure is composed of three domains: ingestion, deglutition, and energy/appetite. It gauges malnutrition risk.

## Occupational Therapy Interventions for Feeding Disorders and the Aging Adult

Treatment options for feeding issues with aging adults are vast and are often similar to those for the general adult population. As with all treatment in OT, the type of intervention used will depend on the person's diagnosis and functional level. The following sections list several options for intervention, and possible diagnoses that relate to these interventions.

## Grocery Shopping

Grocery shopping is often an overlooked but absolutely necessary part of food preparation and feeding. The aging adult's ability to participate in this instrumental activity of daily living (IADL) may be impacted by income level and/or distance to grocery stores. Additionally, if an aging adult has low vision, mobility issues, or low activity tolerance, grocery shopping might be a difficult activity to complete independently. The scope of this discussion will focus on the act of shopping and not the physical act of getting to the grocery store but note that many options do exist for transportation. Once at a grocery store, there are options for the aging adult to make the shopping experience easier. Simply having a grocery cart to steady oneself can often be the only assistance an aging adult needs.

However, if an individual is unable to walk distances within the grocery store due to decreased activity tolerance, loss of balance, or weakness, most stores provide motorized scooters with baskets to allow for greater mobility. Upon exiting the store, the aging adult can ask for assistance from an employee to load heavy bags of groceries into a car.

If an aging adult has difficulty getting around the grocery store or is unable to use transportation for one reason or another, there are still options for grocery shopping, depending on where the person lives. Some stores provide services for home delivery or in-store/curbside pick-up. These services allow a person to call in or go online and place a grocery order, and the grocery store will collect the chosen items. The food is then either delivered to the home or a person can go to the store and collect the order (Kempiak and Fox, 2002). There are also companies that hire shoppers to complete shopping for a person if the grocery store does not already provide such a service. A person can go online and place their order on these company's websites, and a hired shopper will collect all of the requested items. Most of these services will either provide home delivery or curbside at the store, whichever is preferred by the customer (Good Housekeeping, 2022). Most of the time there are fees associated with these services, but they can be invaluable for a person who needs them to live independently.

There are also food delivery services that are available to deliver groceries and already-prepared heat-and-serve meals or measured ingredients to prepare the meals in the home. With these companies, a person can receive a catalog of available food options and order them online or over the phone. Then the food is delivered to the home. Such items can be heated and served or stored in a freezer for future use. Researching the options for the area in which a person lives can be a helpful reference for any aging adult.

## Food Preparation

For many in the aging population, women especially, food preparation (cooking) can foster feelings of nostalgia. Giard (1998) noted that "doing-cooking is the medium for a basic, humble, and persistent practice that is repeated in time and space, rooted in the fabric of relationships to others and to one's self, marked by the 'family saga' and the history of each, bound to childhood memory just like rhythms and seasons" (p. 157). Because of this, it is necessary to consider food preparation as an important occupation that must occur before feeding itself.

First consider the environment in which food is prepared: the kitchen space itself. Many adaptations can be made to the physical environment to make food preparation easier for the aging adult.

### Adaptations for an Aging Adult in a Wheelchair

It is typically necessary to make special adaptations to the kitchen when an individual is in a wheelchair. The minimum turning radius for a wheelchair is 5 feet by 5 feet, so that amount of space is necessary to make a kitchen accessible for a wheelchair. If the space is not accessible via the wheelchair, most of the prep work can be done at a table outside of the kitchen. From a wheelchair level, it is easiest to complete kitchen tasks with lowered cabinets and knee space beneath counters and the sink (Fig. 12.1) (ADA Compliance, 2010).

If lowering the cabinets is cost-prohibitive, removing the cabinet doors below the sink and a few cupboards can allow for an individual in a wheelchair to be in closer proximity to the countertops. If this is the chosen option, it is recommended that the hot water pipes either be removed or insulated with foam rubber or other protective material to prevent scalding. The garbage disposal might also need to be insulated (ADA Compliance, 2010).

Adaptive equipment can also be used to make food preparation easier from a wheelchair level. To see what is being prepared on the stovetop burners, an oven-stove mirror may be installed. It is easiest for an individual who is in a wheelchair to use a stovetop with knobs on the front of the stove versus rear-mounted knobs (Fig. 12.2). However, if rear-mounted knobs are the only option, a long stove knob turner may be used to reach the knobs. (See also Chapter 22 for more information on adaptive technology.)

### Adaptations for an Aging Adult With Low Vision

For aging adults who have difficulty with low vision, food preparation can be a difficult and dangerous task. Adapting the environment may be imperative for these individuals.

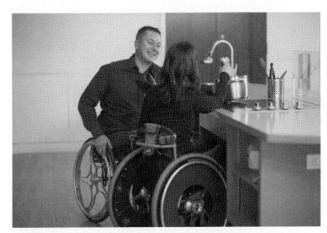

**FIGURE 12.1**   Space Under the Sink for a Wheelchair.

Lighting in the kitchen can be helpful or harmful for an aging adult with low-vision deficits. Lighting levels for an aging adult should be at least two or three times brighter than those comfortable for younger people. Fluorescent or halogen lights are often a better alternative to incandescent light bulbs. Painting the kitchen a light color also increases the amount of light reflected in the room (Figueiro, 2001).

There are also options to reduce the glare that some lighting creates. Using shades or sheers to filter natural light from windows can help reduce glare. It has been found that opaque or translucent light shades or covers reduce glare, so avoiding clear-glass light fixtures is recommended. Shiny surfaces, such as linoleum tile or Formica countertops, can also cause glare. Matte-finish surfaces reduce glare, as does changing the position of the light source relative to the normal line of sight (Figueiro, 2001). Wearing sunglasses or hats can reduce glare without changing the environment.

Using contrasting colors in food preparation can be helpful. A dark cutting board for light-colored foods and a light or white cutting board for dark-colored foods can allow an individual to more easily see the food being cut. Other types of adaptive equipment are also available, such as a large-digit timer that can be easier to see for people with visual impairments. Also, liquid filling indicators are small gadgets that can be placed on any container and will make a buzzing sound when liquid has reached about 1 inch from the top of the container, to avoid overflow or spilling.

## Adaptations for Energy Conservation

Preparing a meal takes energy. If the aging adult has decreased endurance, meal preparation can be challenging. Multiple adaptations can be made to decrease the amount of energy it takes to prepare a meal. A general rule of thumb is to place the most-used kitchen items between eye and waist level to decrease the amount of stooping and reaching that an individual will need to do. A rolling cart can be used to move heavy items from one area of the kitchen to another, and sitting versus standing to prepare food will also conserve energy. Microwaves and toaster ovens are often easier to manage than standard ovens that are part of a stove, especially if located at counter height. Crockpots, air fryers, and food processors can also make cooking more manageable for an individual with limited activity tolerance. Instructing aging adults on energy conservation techniques is also important so that meal preparation can be completed with little to no fatigue (Box 12.1).

## Adaptive Equipment for Food Preparation

Many other pieces of adaptive equipment can be used for general food preparation. A nonslip material called Dycem, for example, can be used for a multitude of purposes, including but not limited to holding items in place while cutting and preparing food and providing additional grip when opening jars. A paring board may have several adaptations, including corner guards to support items being cut, prongs to hold items in place, and/or nonskid bases to prevent the paring board from sliding (Fig. 12.3) (Healthy Products for You, 2022).

For aging adults with decreased strength, a bowl and beverage holder/tipper can hold large bowls or 1- to 2-gallon jugs and make tipping them over and pouring out their contents easier. For decreased grip strength, jar openers with long, nonslip handles can be useful to open jars, and long-handled levers on faucets can make it easier to turn on water (Healthy Products for You, 2022).

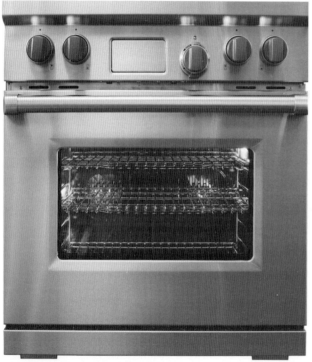

**FIGURE 12.2**    Stove With Knobs on the Front.

---

**Box 12.1**    Meal Preparation Techniques to Minimize Fatigue

- Plan ahead. Have all ingredients and utensils out before beginning a cooking task.
- Pace yourself. Rest while food is baking or items are boiling.
- Have a place to sit in the cooking area in case a rest break is needed.
- Sit while dicing, mixing, etc.
- Kitchen gadgets often save energy. Use a food chopper to dice food rather than manually completing the task. Use a blender or a food processor to blend food.

- If a kitchen is overly warm, prepare the majority of the food just outside of the kitchen. Excessive heat can decrease activity tolerance.
- Use a handled trivet on wheels to move a filled pot or pan along a countertop without having to carry it. Use a rolling utility cart to move heavy items from countertop to table.
- Allow dishes to air dry.
- Cook multiple meals at one time and freeze them in single-portion servings for future use.

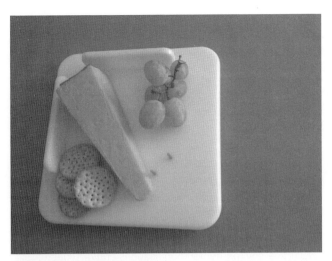

**FIGURE 12.3**   Nonslip cutting board.

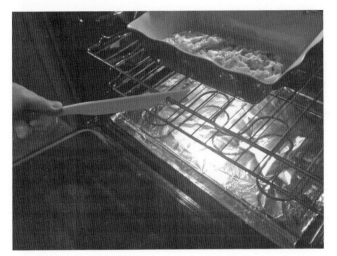

**FIGURE 12.4**   Push-Pull Helper.

For the aging adult who is having difficulty reaching items in a cabinet, reachers with circular rubber tips can be used to retrieve items. A push-pull helper may be used to retrieve or push in oven racks or hot dishes (Fig. 12.4) (Healthy Products for You, 2022).

Therapists can review adaptive equipment catalogs and select the appropriate pieces on an individual need or benefit basis. It is important to note that not every aging adult will want or need a certain adaptation. Sometimes when an aging adult is not familiar with a piece of adaptive equipment, it can be more confusing than beneficial. Introduce each item to the individual, and supervise the person using the equipment before approving it for independent usage. This approach can ensure appropriate use and adherence, as well as cost effectiveness.

### Other Food Preparation Options

If preparing a meal becomes too difficult, there are other options for an aging adult to obtain meals ensuring good nutrition. Meals on Wheels is a US-based national organization that provides fully cooked, ready-to-eat meals for aging adults who are, for one reason or another, in need of

them (Meals on Wheels America, 2022). The cost of these programs varies, but the expense is usually very minimal. There are more than 5000 of these nutrition centers throughout the country. Some programs serve meals at a specific location, whereas others deliver meals directly to a person's home. These programs usually deliver a meal at lunchtime, providing the aging adult with at least one nutritional, hot meal each day (Meals on Wheels America, 2022). Frequently, aging adults report that the meals are of large enough portions that they can make two meals out of each one, providing food for lunch and dinner. If an aging adult lives in a community that does not have a Meals on Wheels program, there is likely some similar service through a local church, temple, or senior center.

Case Example 12.1 describes an aging adult struggling with food preparation.

### Feeding

Once food is prepared, it is necessary to look at any issues the aging adult might have with self-feeding. There are multiple reasons why a person may struggle with self-feeding. The issue may be neuromuscular, such as decreased grip strength following a stroke, or tremors in Parkinson disease; or it could be cognitive, such as a person diagnosed with Alzheimer disease who cannot cognitively initiate or continuously carry out the feeding process (Marcus & Berry, 1998). Regardless of the reason, it is important to help the aging adult maintain self-feeding independence for as long as possible, and in such a way that is dignified for that particular individual. The following paragraphs discuss, and Table 12.5 summarizes, multiple adaptations that can be made so that a person can complete this task. (See also Chapter 13.)

### Utensils

For impaired grip, plastic utensils with built-up handles can be useful (Fig. 12.5). Lightweight cylindrical foam padding can be purchased by the yard and can be cut to fit any utensil or food preparation item as well as pens, pencils, or anything that the aging adult might be having trouble gripping. For those who are unable to grasp at all, a universal cuff (Fig. 12.6) or a utensil holder (with or without wrist support) will allow the individual to self-feed without gripping a utensil. For people who have limited upper extremity movement or control, curved (angled) utensils (Fig. 12.7) and extension utensils allow for food to be brought to the mouth with less upper extremity range of motion required. A person who experiences tremors might benefit from a weighted utensil or simply wrapping a wrist weight around the wrist at mealtimes. Research has demonstrated that weighted wrist cuffs, ranging from 1/5 to 4 pounds, decrease intention tremors. The amount of weight that is beneficial, however, is variable and specific to each individual person (McGruder et al., 2003). For those people who want to cut their own food for self-feeding or meal preparation but have limited wrist movement or grip strength, a rocker knife might be helpful.

## CASE EXAMPLE 12.1 Aging Adult Struggling With Food Preparation

Melba is an 85-year-old female who lives alone in a senior apartment complex across the street from her church. Approximately 2 years ago she was in a car accident that killed her husband and left her with several broken vertebrae in her cervical and thoracic spine. She had a history of osteoarthritis (OA) before the accident, and over the past 2 years has begun to demonstrate moderate to severe weakness in her neck and shoulders. She wears a neck brace most of the time to compensate.

After leaving her home of over 50 years and moving into the apartment, Melba was very determined to remain independent and maintain her ability to cook, a task that was always a central part of her life. But recently, she has begun to struggle with some of the more involved aspects of cooking. This is only known because her daughter, who lives nearby, has observed her struggles and reported them to her physician, who wrote an order for an OT home health evaluation.

Through verbal report from her daughter and grudging agreement from Melba, it is reported that she has, on more than one occasion, dropped a plate or bowl when retrieving it from the cabinets. During the home health evaluation, it is noted that she has difficulties getting her pots and pans out from underneath the stove, where they are stored. She also becomes slightly short of breath with approximately

5 min of kitchen activity. Melba uses no assistive device for mobility, but she is observed holding onto the kitchen countertop, the kitchen table, or the refrigerator handle with one hand when carrying a pot in the other hand. When asked how she feels during the activity, Melba reports "I feel just fine—no complaints!"

Melba has a difficult time admitting that she is having any problems in the kitchen. She makes the comment, "I really miss my husband. Being in the kitchen is something that I can still do that I love. It reminds me of him a little bit."

### Case Study Questions

1. What other questions might you ask Melba? What else would you like to observe during the evaluation?
2. List five environmental modifications and/or types of adaptive equipment that might be appropriate in this situation.
3. Would you recommend that Melba needs an assistive device for walking? If so, why and what type? If not, why not?
4. Are there any outside programs to which Melba could be referred?
5. List two short-term goals and one long-term goal for Melba.

## TABLE 12.5 Impairments and Adaptations for Self-Feeding

| Impairment | Adaptation | Comments |
|---|---|---|
| Impaired grip | Plastic built-up utensils<br>Easy-grip cups with either one or two handles<br>Bilateral glass holder | Lightweight cylindrical foam padding can be purchased by the yard and can be cut to fit any utensil or food preparation item as well as pens, pencils, or anything that the older adult might be having trouble gripping.<br>Glass holders can slip onto glasses of any size and are an excellent way to maintain independence with self-drinking. |
| Absent grip | Universal cuff<br>Utensil holder (with or without support) | These devices will allow the individual to self-feed without gripping a utensil. |
| Limited upper extremity movement or control | Curved (angled) utensils<br>Extension utensils | These utensils allow for food to be brought to the mouth with less upper extremity range of motion required. |
| Tremors | Weighted utensil<br>Wrist weight<br>Weighted cup with a lid | Research has demonstrated that weighted wrist cuffs, ranging from 1/5 to 4 pounds, decrease intention tremors.<br>The amount of weight that is beneficial is variable and specific to each individual person. |
| Limited wrist movement or grip strength | Rocker knife | The utensil allows individuals to cut their own food and can assist in meal preparation activities. |
| Visual impairment | Dishes in a contrasting color to the food | Using a plate that is the opposite color of the food being served can help the individual to visualize the food on the plate.<br>A dark-colored plate for lighter items, such as pasta or rice, can allow the person to see the food more clearly. |

**TABLE 12.5** Impairments and Adaptations for Self-Feeding—Cont'd

| Impairment | Adaptation | Comments |
|---|---|---|
| Difficulty scooping food | High-sided dishes Compartment plates<br>Clip-on food guards | Scoop dishes have a high side and a low side, allowing a person to use the side for easier scooping while still being able to move the feeding arm in at a lower, more natural angle.<br>Clip-on guards are good for older adults who prefer to use existing dishware. They clip on to any standard plate and can be used like a scoop dish.<br>When using a scoop dish or a clip-on food guard, it is important to remember to angle the plate so that the high side is opposite of the individual's feeding extremity. For example, if a person wants to feed himself with his right hand, the high side of the plate should be placed on the person's left. This allows the right hand to push the food across the body in a natural motion and use the high side of the plate as a scoop at the end of the motion. |
| Only has use of one hand | Easy-cut plate<br>Suction cups or nonskid mats | An easy-cut plate that has stainless steel pins to stabilize food can make it possible to cut food with one hand.<br>Suction cups or nonskid material on the bottom of dinnerware can prevent plates or bowls from moving while the person is trying to eat. |
| Difficulty in tipping the head<br>Needs to maintain neutral head alignment | Nosey cups<br>Straws<br>Cup with a built-in straw | Nosey Cups have a cutout in the cup that allows the individual to drink without extending the neck.<br>If the individual has difficulty using straws because the straws are difficult to control in the cup, a cup with a built-in straw or a straw holder might be the answer.<br>Some straws have one-way valves that stay filled with fluid, eliminating the possibility of sucking in too much air when drinking. |
| Taking too large of a sip | Regulating drinking cups (with or without straws) | Regulating drinking cups allow for a certain measured amount of fluid to be released from the cup with any given sip. Sometimes these are controlled by a caregiver pressing and releasing a regulator trigger; other times the cup simply will only release a specific measured amount, such as 5 or 10 cc of fluid. |

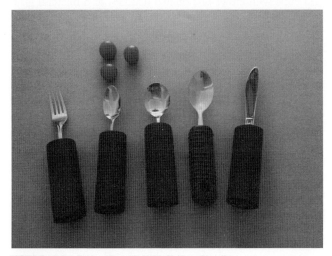

**FIGURE 12.5**  Eating Utensils With Built-up Handles.

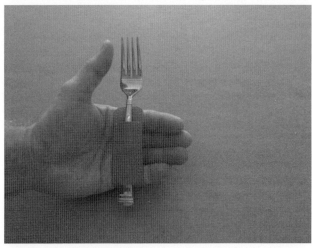

**FIGURE 12.6**  Universal Cuff.

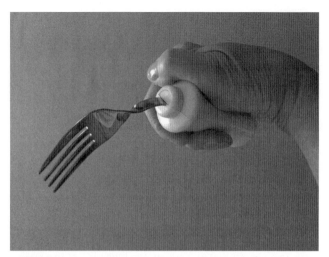

**FIGURE 12.7**    Bendable Fork.

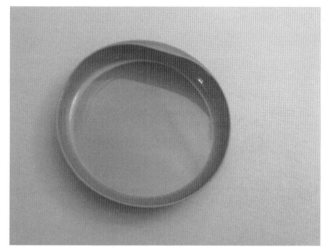

**FIGURE 12.9**    Scoop Dish.

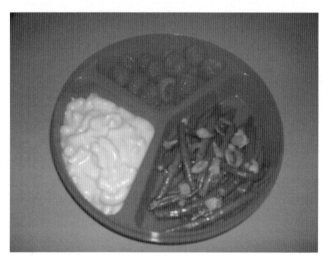

**FIGURE 12.8**    Compartment Plate With Lid.

## Plates and Bowls

Frequently, aging adults have difficulty seeing food on their plates due to multiple visual impairments. Using a plate that is the opposite color of the food being served can be helpful in visualizing food on a plate. For example, a dark-colored plate for lighter items, such as pasta or rice, can allow the person to see the food more clearly, due to the contrasting colors.

There are multiple diagnoses that can cause a person to have difficulty scooping food onto a utensil or cause problems in pushing food off the plate in an effort to put the food on the spoon or fork. High-sided dishes or a compartment plate can make scooping food onto a spoon or fork much easier (Fig. 12.8). Scoop dishes have a high side and a low side, allowing a person to use the side for easier scooping while still being able to move the feeding arm in at a lower, normal angle (Fig. 12.9). If a person does not want to commit to a new plate, a clip-on food guard is a possibility. These clip on to any standard plate and can be used like a scoop dish. When using a scoop dish or a clip-on food guard, it is important to remember to angle the plate so that the high side is opposite of the individual's feeding extremity. For example, if a person wants to feed himself

with his right hand, the high side of the plate should be placed on the person's left. This allows the right hand to push the food across the body in a natural motion and use the high side of the plate as a scoop at the end of the motion.

An easy-cut plate that has stainless steel pins to stabilize food can make it possible to cut food with one hand. Suction cups or nonskid material on the bottom of dinnerware can prevent plates or bowls from moving while the person is trying to eat.

### Beverage Containers

Sometimes drinking liquids can be difficult for the aging adult, causing frustration and possibly leading to decreased fluid intake. Inadequate fluid intake can often lead to dehydration (Bernstein and Luggen, 2009). For those individuals who simply have a problem with successfully bringing a cup to the mouth, there are many types of adaptive equipment that can help.

For individuals who have decreased grip strength, easy-grip cups with either one or two handles, or a bilateral glass holder that can slip onto a glass of any size, are excellent adaptations to maintain independence with self-drinking. If tremors are an issue, a weighted cup with a lid or once again simply using wrist weights (as stated in the utensils discussion of this chapter) would be an appropriate intervention.

If the aging adult has difficulty tipping the head back to drink, or if he or she simply needs to maintain a neutral head alignment, Nosey cups have a cutout in the cup that allows the individual to drink without extending the neck (Fig. 12.10). A straw might also be used in this instance. If the individual has difficulty using straws because the straws are difficult to control in the cup, a cup with a built-in straw might be the answer. There are also straws that have one-way valves that stay filled with fluid, eliminating the possibility of sucking in too much air when drinking.

Many aging adults have problems with taking too large of a drink at any one time, which can result in coughing or aspiration. Regulating drinking cups, either with or without straws, only allow for a certain measured amount of fluid to

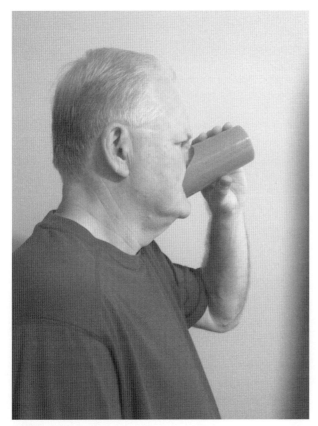

**FIGURE 12.10**    Nosey Cup.

- Although use of restraints is generally not encouraged, lap belts can be used to position the pelvis as close to midline as possible (Trefler & Taylor, 1991)
- A solid seat or back insert can help maintain good posture and reduce the possibility of skin breakdown (Goodman, 2012).
- Lateral supports can prevent the aging adult from leaning to either side.
- Several seat cushions may be used, including a pommel (abductor) cushion to prevent hip adduction and a wedge cushion to discourage forward leaning.
- There are also multiple head supports to maintain the head in a neutral alignment.

When choosing a positioning device for an aging adult, whether it is to increase independence in feeding or for any other reason, it is important to remember to select devices that will fit the unique needs of that individual (Goodman, 2012).

## Eating and Swallowing

"Feeding, eating, and swallowing are interdependent activities" (Clark et al., 2007, p. 686), and therefore it is necessary for an occupational therapist to have the skills necessary to assess and intervene in all of these areas. Feeding, which is defined as "the process of setting up, arranging, and bringing food [or fluid] from the plate or cup to the mouth" (p. 686), has already been discussed. However, occupational therapists are also able to address eating and swallowing.

Eating, which is defined as "the ability to keep and manipulate food or fluid in the mouth and swallow it" (p. 686), and swallowing, defined as the "complicated act in which food, fluid, medication, or saliva is moved from the mouth through the pharynx and esophagus into the stomach" (p. 686), are both areas that are well within the occupational therapist's scope of practice.

As there are multiple issues that can cause feeding difficulties, there are also multiple issues that can affect eating and swallowing. Box 12.2 lists common eating and swallowing challenges that an occupational therapist might encounter, and Box 12.3 discusses different techniques that might be used to treat these issues. (See also Chapter 13.)

## Routine

Warde and Hetherington noted, "For some people, what and where they eat is a very conscious expression of their personal identities and style of life" (Warde & Hetherington, 1994, p. 769). Often when a person has been sick, becomes disabled, or has moved to a new location, routines are interrupted. This is true for mealtime routines. If it is possible to allow an individual to follow his or her normal mealtime routine, that person might consume more and perform the feeding task better. For example, if an aging adult woman has moved to a skilled nursing facility and seems distracted during meals, an attempt could be made to allow the woman to eat in her room or a quiet office. It might very well be that she is used

be released from the cup with any given drink. Sometimes these are controlled by a caregiver pressing and releasing a regulator trigger. Other times the cup simply will only release a specific measured amount, such as 5 or 10 cc of fluid.

## Positioning Options

The position in which a person is seated, either in a chair or a wheelchair, is an integral part of successful independent feeding. While eating, the ideal sitting posture is for the hips, knees, and feet to be at 90 degrees, with weight evenly distributed to both sides of the body (West and Redstone, 2004). The head should be upright and tilted slightly forward. It should be possible for the individual to move closer to the table so that his or her mouth can be 10 to 15 inches from the plate (Litchford, 2005).

Frequently, when an aging adult with small stature is positioned correctly, he or she is in a shorter wheelchair (hemi-height). These wheelchairs normally have a seat-to-floor height of 17 to 18 inches, as opposed to a standard wheelchair, whose seat-to-floor height is 19 to 21 inches. The height of a standard dining table is 28 to 30 inches. Therefore, when a person requires a hemi-sized wheelchair, standard tables are too tall. Using an adjustable-height bed/chair table or a desk might be more useful.

It is important for a person to sit at a 90-degree angle when eating to facilitate proper digestion. Multiple positioning devices can be used for this:

---

**Box 12.2**  Common Eating and Swallowing Issues

- Aspiration: The entry of secretions, fluids, food, or any foreign substance below the vocal cords and into the lungs; may result in aspiration pneumonia.
- Dysphagia: Difficulty with any stage of swallowing (oral, pharyngeal, esophageal); dysfunction in any stage or process of eating; includes any difficulty in the passage of food, liquid, or medicine during any stage of swallowing that impairs the client's ability to swallow independently or safely.

- Pocketing: Retention of food between the teeth and cheek.
- Reflux: Reflux of food, medication, liquids, and gastric juice from the stomach into the esophagus; also called gastroesophageal reflux disease (GERD).
- Silent aspiration: Aspiration that occurs without coughing or overt choking; indication of motor and/or sensory deficits (if present) that inhibit protective responses.

---

**Box 12.3**  Common Swallowing Intervention Techniques

- Chin tuck: A strategy in which the head is flexed (chin tucked downward toward the chest) during the swallow, allowing the anterior structures of the pharynx posteriorly, resulting in a smaller entrance to the larynx; this strategy reduces the chance of food or liquid to fall into the airway.
- Clearing techniques: Strategies used to clear the mouth or pharynx of food or liquid residue.
- Diet liberalization: The relaxation of standards of accepted diets as ways to treat illness or decrease symptoms related to dysphagia.
- Double/multiple swallows: A swallow strategy whereby two or more attempts are used to swallow the food, medication, or liquid.
- Food consistencies: There are four levels of semisolid/solid foods proposed in the National Dysphagia Diet (NDD):
    - Regular: Normal food consistency
    - NDD Level 3 (i.e., Advanced): Soft foods that require more chewing ability
    - NDD Level 2 (i.e., Mechanical Altered): Cohesive, moist, semisolid foods, requiring some chewing
    - NDD Level 1 (i.e., Pureed): Homogenous, very cohesive, pudding-like, requiring very little chewing ability
- Liquid consistencies: There are four levels of liquid

viscosity (i.e., thickness or resistance to flow):
- Thin: Normal fluid viscosity
- Nectar-like: Fluid viscosity that is slightly thicker than water
- Honey-like: Fluid viscosity that is approximately that of honey
- Spoon-thick: a.k.a. "pudding-like"; fluid viscosity that is approximately that of pudding
- Mendelsohn maneuver: A swallowing technique to facilitate prolonged laryngeal elevation during the swallow; results in keeping the upper esophageal sphincter open longer to allow passage of the bolus.
- Therapeutic feedings: Controlled delivery of food, medication, or liquid used to facilitate therapeutic outcomes to improve feeding, eating, and swallowing ability; not used as a primary source of nutrition or hydration.
- Thickening agent: Substance used to increase the viscosity of liquids.
- VitalStim: A method cleared by the Food and Drug Administration (FDA) to promote swallowing through the application of neuromuscular electrical stimulation to the swallowing muscles to strengthen and reeducate muscles and to facilitate motor control/function of the swallowing mechanism.

From Clark, G. F., Avery-Smith, W., Wold, L. S., Anthony, P., Holm, S. E., Eating and Feeding Task Force, & Commission on Practice. (2007). Specialized knowledge and skills in feeding, eating, and swallowing for occupational therapy practice. *The American Journal of Occupational Therapy, 61*(6), 686–700.

---

to eating in a quiet location, and the noise of a dining room is too distracting (Hasselkus, 2006)

### Caregiver Education

Many aging adults depend on a caregiver to assist them in at least some aspect of the feeding process. Whether it is to help with purchasing groceries, cutting up food, or bringing a utensil to the mouth, caregivers can play an integral role in ensuring that aging adults receive the proper amount of nutrition, calories, and fluids (Chang & Roberts, 2008). The amount and quality of care that an aging individual receives might influence the intake of food and thus the individual's weight (Berkhout et al., 1998). To maximize carryover from OT treatment to daily feeding activities, occupational therapists should educate the caregivers on any adaptive equipment

or alternative feeding techniques that are being used with the aging adult. It has been noted that ongoing caregiver education, rather than a 1- or 2-day education just before discharge, is more beneficial to everyone involved in the process. Ongoing caregiver education allows for improved follow-through and better relations between caregivers and therapists due to the collaborative effort required by all parties (Elliott, 1997).

A caregiver should be educated on any special techniques (e.g., energy conservation techniques used during cooking or a chin-tuck strategy during meals) or any adaptive equipment (e.g., a Nosey Cup or a divided plate) that are being used on a regular basis. They should also be made aware of any safety issues that the occupational therapist has noted. Besides some of the other areas discussed in this chapter, general feeding techniques might also be taught. Box 12.4 gives examples of feeding techniques on which an occupational therapist might want to instruct a caregiver.

Case Example 12.2 describes the feeding problems of a resident in a skilled nursing facility.

## Occupational Therapy: A Holistic Approach

It is important to remember that every aging adult is an individual with a unique life story, not simply a client

whom we are treating for a feeding issue. As Hasselkus (2006) so eloquently mentioned in her Eleanor Clarke Slagle Lecture:

*And what does this all mean for the older woman who becomes disabled? As OTs, we might be advising her to no longer do much cooking, to take shortcuts, to use more prepared foods, to let some other member of the family do most of the*

---

**Box 12.4    Caregiver Instructions for Feeding Techniques**

- Keep distractions to a minimum; turn off the television and radio. If someone is easily distracted, eating alone might be better than eating with a group.
- Make sure that the individual is positioned properly; the ideal sitting posture is for the hips, knees, and feet to be at 90 degrees, with weight evenly distributed to both sides of the body.
- Try to prevent soiling of clothing; use a bib, an apron, towel, or one to two full-size napkins to cover clothing if an individual is at risk for spilling food. Have a box of moist, disposable washcloths nearby to clean off the hands and face. Remember that although many individuals can benefit from a clothing protector (i.e., bib or apron), some people might object to using one.

Work with the individual to decide what is best for him or her.
- Give verbal cues as needed; using one-step commands, instruct the individual in each area that is needed. Speak in a calm, soothing voice and use words that are appropriate for adults. Remember that cues may need to be repeated.
- Give physical cues as needed; use hand-over-hand assistance to allow the individual to go through the motion of eating. Use verbal cues at the same time as the physical cues to reinforce the steps in feeding. Do not provide more assistance than is needed.
- Give praise freely and recognize even the smallest steps toward independent eating.

Adapted from Litchford, M. (2005). Feeding instructions for caregivers. *Adult day care resource manual for the USDA Child and Adult Care Food Program.* National Food Service Management Institute. University of Mississippi. https://agcacfp.mwg.state.nj.us/webdocs/AG_CACFP/RESOURCE%20LIBRARY/4.%20%20USDA%20PUBLICATIONS/ADULT%20DAY%20CARE%20RESOURCE%20MANUAL.PDF.

---

**CASE EXAMPLE 12.2    Resident in a Skilled Nursing Facility**

Jim is an 89-year-old male who entered a skilled nursing facility (SNF) approximately 15 months ago after falling at home and sustaining a right hip fracture. He underwent an open reduction–internal fixation (ORIF) procedure and came to the SNF for skilled therapy. Although he improved physically and was able to walk with a walker throughout the facility, his family decided that his diagnosis of mild Parkinson disease along with his recent falls at home made for an unsafe living environment. They had a long talk with Jim, and it was decided that it was in his best interest to remain at the SNF for long-term care.

Since that time, Jim has become depressed. Although he understands that he needs to remain at the facility, he misses his home. He developed the flu last winter, and it caused his Parkinson's to become more progressed. He has begun to experience moderate intention tremors and has also begun to demonstrate mild dementia.

To ensure that the residents are not gaining or losing weight in an abnormal fashion, the facility performs monthly weight measures on all residents. When they weighed him, it was noted that Jim had an 8-pound weight loss in the last month. He completed a barium swallow diagnostic procedure, which came back negative for any swallowing issues. He has been referred to skilled OT for evaluation and treatment as indicated for feeding difficulties.

As the occupational therapist, you arrive for lunch in the assistive-feeding dining room where Jim has recently been

placed. He is sitting slightly slumped forward in a wheelchair and there is a nursing assistant at the table with him, along with two other residents. The other two residents, both males, are falling asleep at the table. The nursing assistant is busy trying to wake them up and open up all of the containers on all of the trays. You observe Jim attempting to drink from a full juice glass. His tremors are such that the drink spills some onto his lap and Jim curses under his breath. He is able to eat a fish stick using his fingers but struggles in using utensils to eat his green beans and gelatin. Within approximately 10 min of beginning to eat, Jim throws down his fork in frustration and stares at the wall. Shortly thereafter, the nursing assistant begins to put food on a spoon and feed it to Jim, who grudgingly eats it.

**Case Study Questions**
1. What do you believe is the most important issue to address with Jim, and why?
2. List five separate adaptations that you could try with Jim to make his self-feeding more independent.
3. How might you address his sitting position during meals?
4. Do the caregivers at this facility need to be educated on feeding issues? If so, how would you educate them? If not, why not?
5. Write two short-term goals and one long-term goal for Jim.

*work now, to give up some of the usual family traditions, etc. Do we appreciate the emotional depths of these changes we are recommending? What can we do, with our expertise in homemaking skills, to better help such a client weather this huge wrench in her life patterns and identity within a family? (p. 634)*

As occupational therapists, we must do what is best for each individual aging adult in each individual situation. If a certain approach does not work for someone, it is our job to try something else, and to focus on what is most appropriate within the context of that person's life. We must continuously strive to create a client-centered environment in which the aging adult is able to function as independently as possible for as long as possible. The concluding section of this chapter offers a phenomenological perspective, to sensitize readers to the "emotional depths" to which Hasselkus refers.

## Meanings of Food and Meals

Food and meals are rich in occupational meaning, as they are filled with tradition, ritual, sensory engagement, memory, nostalgia, family, and community (Beagan & D'Sylva, 2011). Meals can mean different things at different times, depending on whether they occur in private or in public, in ordinary or extravagant contexts, with others or alone. The meanings attached to such occupations are personal and individual yet are always framed within a specific sociocultural context.

## Culture and Meaning

Culture plays a large role in the meaning of food and food preparation. Hocking et al. (2002) found that women in New Zealand and Thailand found meaning in foodwork related to tradition, gender roles, family and caring, extending hospitality, and protecting the health of their families. Similarly, cooking traditional foods for Christmas provided women in Eastern Kentucky a sense of tradition and ritual (Shordike and Pierce, 2005). The foods themselves, as well as the preparation methods and even the cooking utensils evoked sensory memories and nostalgia. In a comparison across all three studies, two major themes were noted across the cultures of Thailand, New Zealand, and Eastern Kentucky. By preserving the form, function, and meaning of the food preparation and sharing, participants in all three studies felt like they were protecting what matters in their cultural traditions. Furthermore, they felt a sense of ownership and responsibility in maintaining these food traditions during important holidays (Wright-St Clair et al., 2013).

Displacement (for a multitude of reasons, including migration) can create a situation in which food-related occupations become a way to transmit cultural traditions and identities. Preparing and eating traditional foods when away from home may confirm the familiar, reinforce belonging and strengthen ties to distant places or times (Beoku-Betts, 1995). Nostalgia can occur through smells, tastes, and textures, evoking memories of home, childhood, or particular people (Beagan & D'Sylva, 2011).

## Gender Differences

The importance of food preparation as an occupation that continues into later life seems to be greater for women than for men. This is based on the assertion that women are traditionally considered to be the gender that fills the role of meal preparer in the family unit. Although gender roles have shifted in recent decades, women generally continue to do the bulk of domestic labor, including meal preparation. In the United States, women spend twice as much time daily on "food preparation and cleanup" than their male counterparts, despite shrinking differences in time spent in paid employment (US Bureau of Labor Statistics, 2021). Statistics and qualitative studies of other countries tend to demonstrate at least the same, if not greater, skewing of domestic roles toward the female gender (Statistics Canada, 2005; Wright-St Clair et al., 2004; Hocking et al., 2002). Other studies have shown that even when men wanted to engage in meal-related occupations more equally, societal expectations (including masculinity and paid employment) hindered greater participation (Beagan & D'Sylva, 2011).

Oftentimes, traditions of food preparation are passed down through the generations, creating a situation in which women are trained from youth to fulfill these roles (Wright-St Clair et al., 2004). Interestingly, a woman's role in food-related occupations can simultaneously be considered an area of gender inequality and a means of exercising power. In a study of Armenian American women, it was acknowledged that food preparation was compulsory for women and could therefore be considered oppressive. However, it was also asserted that there was a sense of authority and control in the kitchen, as well as a place to bond with other women (Avakian, 2005).

For both men and women, eating is a biological need and is therefore a daily occupation that must be completed for survival. Outside of survival, both genders tend to prefer to eat food that aligns with their culture, traditions, and social contexts. For both genders, eating is related to what food is available to them, their personal physical and cognitive limitations, and their social surroundings.

## Long-Term Care

Earlier in this chapter, the importance of nutrition in several long-term care settings was discussed. For the occupational therapist, it is imperative to consider nutrition and feeding when treating patients in these settings. Aging adults who reside in long-term care facilities often are required to live in such a setting due to a lack of independence with basic and/or instrumental ADLs. Food preparation and feeding are both areas in which assistance might be needed. In a study of institutionalized aging adults in three skilled nursing facilities, only 29.4% of participants were able to feed themselves independently. Verbal cues were required for 7.8%, physical assistance was needed for 38.6%, and 24.2% of the participants were dependent for feeding. The study further found that although the vast majority of residents ingested adequate amounts of food, when inadequate intake was noted, it was more likely to be those who required physical assistance or were at the dependent level of feeding. Types of problems that increased the individual's risk of requiring physical assistance included improper positioning, dysphagia, upper extremity dysfunction, and visual deficits (Rogers and Snow, 1982).

It is essential that staff at long-term care facilities are educated in areas that could improve resident's intake and independence. Teaching nurses' aides, volunteers, and family members about proper positioning as well as methods of compensating for age-related visual and auditory changes could have a strong impact on how much and how well residents feed themselves. Simple changes like making sure that the resident is wearing prescribed glasses, that background noise is limited to allow for hearing and conversation, and that the dining area is well lit can make a difference in how a person functions during mealtime.

## Food at the End of Life

As discussed earlier in this chapter, nutrition is an important consideration for the person nearing the end of life, and how (or if) the feeding process occurs is best decided by the patient, relatives/caregivers, and medical team. As long as oral intake is possible, both palliative and hospice care programs will attempt meal services in various forms. However, as illnesses progress, issues such as dysphagia, weakness, and confusion can make oral intake more difficult, causing weight loss (Kang et al., 2018). According to the literature, approximately 50% of hospice patients are affected by malnutrition and weight loss, and infections increase due to malnutrition (Marley and Cunningham, 2015). Because of this, when difficulty with oral intake occurs, artificial nutrition and hydration (AN&H) can be considered. This can include options such as enteral nutrition (EN), parenteral nutrition (PN), or parenteral hydration (PH). There is discussion as to whether implementing AN&H goes against the ideals of palliative care or hospice care as an invasive procedure. However, many believe that AN&H interventions may be viewed as compassionate in order to avoid malnutrition and eventual starvation (Loofs and Haubrick, 2021). Attitudes surrounding AN&H usage may be influenced by culture and geographic identity. Within the United States, African American patients are significantly more likely than Caucasian patients to desire all measures of life support and are less likely to have a living will or power of attorney. Patterns of AN&H usage also seem to vary across rural/urban divides, with higher usage of tube feedings in urban areas compared to rural areas (Loofs and Haubrick, 2021).

Improved quality of life is one of the primary outcomes of all OT interventions, and evidence has been mounting that supports the profession's contribution to quality of life at the end of life (AOTA, 2020). Related to feeding and nutrition, the aim of OT can be to modify and adapt important aspects of the individual's feeding process while there is still oral intake. With both oral intake and AN&H, OT can be essential in educating caregivers on the importance of allowing their loved one to maintain as much self-control and be given choices whenever possible. There is an increased sense of self-worth when participating in familiar occupations, and OTs can be integral in helping maintain participation in these occupations for as long as possible (AOTA, 2016).

## The Role of Occupational Justice in Nutrition for Aging Adults

Occupational justice is defined as "the right of every individual to be able to meet basic needs and to have equal opportunities and life chances to reach toward her or his potential but specific to the individual's engagement in diverse and meaningful occupation" (Wilcock and Townsend, 2009, p. 193). Considered a basic need, nutrition and feeding are directly in the purview of the occupational therapist treating their clients through the lens of occupational justice. Many occupational therapists in traditional practice do not feel like they can promote occupational justice in a clinical setting. However, it has been argued that the basic aspects of OT practice, including being client-centered and empathetic, automatically begin to promote justice (Bailliard and Aldrich, 2017). By considering the aging adult holistically, including the culture, meaning, roles, and identities created through food, meals, and meal preparation as discussed above, the OT practitioner is enabling justice. Considering injustices, such as the deprivation that food insecurity can create, further promotes occupational justice for the aging adult.

## Food Insecurity

Risk factors for food insecurity are plentiful, especially for the aging adult. They may include sociodemographics, social isolation, inappropriate food intake, dependence, disability (including but not limited to acute or chronic disease, physical/cognitive/emotional impairment, oral health problems, and sensory impairment), and chronic medication use (Bickel et al., 2000; Bonnel, 2003). This can create issues with poor nutritional status, impaired health, inability to complete activities of daily living, and decreased quality of life (Bickel et al., 2000; Bonnel, 2003).

## Programs Available

Programs specific for the aging adult at a federal, state, and often local level are oftentimes accessible to combat food insecurity and all its effects. Federal programs are discussed early in this chapter. However, it is important that the occupational therapist working with people in the aging population are aware of what is available in their community to advocate for those with whom they work.

Through the Older Americans Act Nutrition Programs (OAANP), the Administration for Community Living's Administration on Aging (AoA) provides grants to individual states to support nutrition services for aging adults. The services vary by state but can include home delivered meals, meals in a group setting (such as senior centers or faith-based locations), as well as nutrition screenings, assessments, education, and counseling. Through these grants, some states also provide links to other in-home and community-based support groups, such as home health services, transportation options, home repair and modification programs, and fall prevention programs. Eligibility varies by state, however, federal criteria states that a person must be at least 60 years old or be a spouse (of any age) of someone at least 60 years old (Administration for Community Living, 2022).

Meals on Wheels, discussed earlier in this chapter, receives federal funding, but more than 70% of its budget is based on donations from individuals and businesses (Meals on Wheels America, 2022). Other agencies similar to Meals on Wheels exist throughout the country and world. Advocating for aging adult's access to nutritious meals is an important aspect of the OT provider's work, and therefore it is critical to be aware of what is available in the area in which services are provided.

## SUMMARY

As baby boomers age, and more adults move into the aging adult category, issues around nutrition and malnutrition will continue to grow. For those working with the aging adult, understanding the physiological changes that aging causes in terms of digestion, metabolism, and absorption will be essential to providing quality care. In addition to the changes that accompany aging, many adults also have one or more chronic diseases, which can require changes to eating behaviors and shift nutrient intake patterns. Incorporating personal and environmental adaptations/modifications along with educating the aging adult and/or their caregivers may be key to improving functional status for all aspects of food preparation and intake. However, it is also important to consider personal and cultural contexts and meaning in relation to food preparation and consumption in order to treat the aging adult in a holistic manner. Combining adequate and appropriate nutrition, while working with an aging adult who may not want to eat, requires that an interdisciplinary team works together to address all factors that can foster an enjoyable, well-balanced eating plan.

## Acknowledgment

The authors wish to thank Daphne Lo, Abhilash Desai, and Miriam Moss's contributions to the previous nutrition chapter in the first edition of *Occupational Therapy With Aging Adults*.

*The complete listing of the Bibliography and Chapter Questions and Answers are available in the accompanying enhanced eBook version included with the print purchase of this textbook. Visit Elsevier eBooks+ (eBooks.Health.Elsevier.com) to access this content.*

## CHAPTER 13

# Oral Health for Aging Adults

*Shirley A. Blanchard, PhD, BCPR, FAOTA and Jean J. Schensul, PhD*

## CHAPTER OUTLINE

## OBJECTIVES

- Define social determinants of oral health
- Discuss the relationship between prevention, general health, oral health, and quality of life in older adults
- Relate the interprofessional roles of dentistry, occupational therapy, and nursing for access to oral care for older adults
- Describe age-related changes in oral physiology
- Identify oral diseases that are prevalent among older adults; write a descriptive referral
- Explain how the *Occupational Therapy Practice Framework* guides interventions for oral care
- Discuss the significance of the long-term care environment for oral health
- Identify risk factors and preventive measures for aspiration pneumonia
- Provide recommendations for oral hygiene and denture care for those who need assistance or are unable to care for themselves
- Recommend assistive technology for oral care for elders with disabilities
- Identify strategies for addressing the challenges of providing oral care for patients with care-resistant behavior
- Describe patient and family education for oral care

For older adults, oral health (OH) both reflects and contributes to general health and quality of life. Eighty-five percent of older adults have at least one major chronic disease, and 50% have two or more chronic diseases (Centers for Disease Control and Prevention & Merck Institute of Aging and Health, 2004). Many studies have established associations between periodontal (gum) disease and chronic diseases such as cardiovascular disease, stroke, diabetes, and respiratory diseases. Systematic reviews have found that treating periodontal disease and improving oral hygiene has enhanced metabolic control for people with type 2 diabetes, prevented respiratory infections and death from pneumonia in clients in long-term care, and reduced cardiovascular disease (de Oliveira et al., 2010; Pace & McCullough, 2010; Simpson et al., 2010; Sjögren et al., 2008). Medications used to control chronic diseases often have oral side effects, including xerostomia (dry mouth), taste alteration, diminished bone health, tissue overgrowth, swelling, inflammation, and ulceration.

Good OH is required for three essential physiologic functions: mastication, speech, and protection. Tooth loss, precipitated by dental caries (tooth decay), periodontal disease, or injury, impairs both mastication and speech and may also lower self-esteem, restrict social contact, and inhibit intimacy (US Department of Health and Human Services, 2004). Diminished salivary flow, compromised by medications, irradiation, or disease, impedes both immunologic and mechanical protection. Oral and pharyngeal cancers result in significant disfigurement and have poor 5-year survival rates (Buchbinder et al., 1993). Oral pathogens can become bloodborne or aspirated, resulting in serious systemic disease. Poor OH increases the risk of upper respiratory infection, aspiration pneumonia, febrile episodes, rheumatic fever, bacterial endocarditis, glomerulonephritis, diabetes, cardiovascular disease, and cerebral and myocardial infarction (Shay & Ship, 1995; US Department of Health and Human Services, 2004). Pain from untreated oral diseases can hamper normal activities of daily living (ADLs) and disturb sleep (Table 13.1).

Mrs. Davidson's scenario is an example of the OH disparities often experienced by older adults, with dependence in ADLs and cognitive impairment as two important factors that contribute to these disparities (Jablonski et al., 2005).

## Health Disparities and Social Determinants of Oral Health

Health disparities are defined as "diminished health status of population subgroups defined by age, socioeconomic status, geography, disability status, and behavioral lifestyles" (National Institute of Dental and Craniofacial Research, 2002). Older adults experience OH disparities due to age and diseases (Table 13.2). However, in addition, racial/ethnic minority and low-income adults are affected by potentially lifelong exposure to structural and social factors that affect their access to dental treatment, their oral hygiene self-management, and their OH status. Structural/social determinants of health are defined by the World Health Organization (WHO, 2023) as:

*[T]he conditions in which people are born, grow, live, work, and age. These circumstances are shaped by the distribution of money, power, and resources at global, national, and local levels. The social determinants of health are mostly responsible for health inequities—the unfair and avoidable differences in health status seen within and between [social groups].*

Also included are commercial determinants of health, defined as the "strategies and approaches used by the private sector to promote products and choices that are detrimental to health" (Kickbusch et al., 2016), such as sweet and starchy foods and beverages that produce cavities and tobacco and alcohol products that cause or further oral disease.

**TABLE 13.1**  Medical Conditions With Oral Health Consequences (NIH/NIDCR, 2021)

| Medical Condition | Oral Health Consequence |
| --- | --- |
| Alzheimer disease and other progressive dementias | Poor oral hygiene, periodontal disease, dry mouth, dental caries risk |
| Anemias | Pale mucosa, atrophic glossitis, angular stomatitis, oral candidiasis, aphthous-like ulcers |
| Chronic kidney disease | Periodontitis |
| Diabetes | Periodontitis |
| Interpersonal violence, elder abuse | Oral and dental trauma (mandible facture, facial contusion and laceration, dental concussion) |
| Medications that impact the mouth (including antidepressants, antihistamines, herbal products) | Salivary gland dysfunction, gingival overgrowth, angioedema, oral pigmentation, lichenoid lesions, dysgeusia/taste changes, bleaching/petechiae, alveolar bon loss, mucositis/stomatitis, neuropathy, chemo-osteonecrosis |
| Neoplastic hematologic disease, including leukemia, multiple myeloma, lymphoma, and cancer chemotherapy | Mucositis, leukemic gingival infiltrates and inflammation, opportunistic infections, oral petechiae-ecchymosis, ulcers, tumor growth, periodontitis |
| Osteoarthritis | Poor oral hygiene, temporomandibular joint pain |
| Osteoporosis | Periodontitis, tooth loss |
| Radiation therapy for head and neck cancers | Oral mucositis, rampant caries, osteoradionecrosis, trismus of muscles of mastication, taste change |
| Sjögren syndrome (and other autoimmune diseases) | Dry mouth/mucosa, salivary gland enlargement, oral candidiasis, rampant caries, oral ulcerations, taste changes |
| Sleep disorders | Gingival inflammation, lower masticatory function |
| Stroke and acquired brain injury | Poor oral hygiene-neglect, dental caries, dysphagia, xerostomia, tooth loss, gingivitis/periodontitis |
| Systemic sclerosis | Microstomia, caries, dry mouth, periodontal disease, gingival recession, mandibular bone resorption |
| Thrombocytopenia and hemophilia | Petechiae and hemorrhagic bullae of mucosa, bleeding gingiva, spontaneous gingival bleeding |

**CASE EXAMPLE 13.1**    Mrs. Davidson

Mrs. Davidson is 88 years old and was admitted to a nursing care facility 2 months ago. Her medical history includes osteoarthritis, well-controlled hypertension, hyperlipidemia, and vascular dementia with subsequent memory loss. She has some teeth but has not had a dental check-up in many years. A dental screening revealed poor oral hygiene, inflamed and bleeding gums, only a few front teeth (no molars), and an area of irritation on the roof of her mouth.

Mrs. Davidson finished high school and worked intermittently as a cashier at a department store. She married and raised one son. She talks about missing her husband, son, and other friends who have passed away. She has few financial resources other than Medicare and Medicaid. Although she would have preferred to remain in her own home, she realized that she was unable to complete self-care and

access the community. Admission to a long-term care facility provided an opportunity for assistance in managing basic activities of daily living.

At the nursing home's monthly client care plan meeting, Mrs. Davidson's health status and needs are reviewed by an interprofessional team of care providers. Mrs. Davidson, along with her remaining family member, her daughter-in-law, agreed to the following goals:

a. improve her ability to care for her own oral hygiene;
b. reduce her resistant behavior when staff try to provide assistance with daily oral hygiene;
c. improve her nutritional intake; and
d. request a referral to a dentist regarding the missing teeth, possible difficulty chewing, and sores found in Mrs. Davidson's mouth.

**TABLE 13.2** Oral Health and Access to Care for Community-Dwelling Older Adults

| Oral Health Measure | 65+-Year-Olds | 65- to 74-Year-Olds | 75+-Year-Olds |
|---|---|---|---|
| Tooth loss[a,f] | 18.6% | 13.0% | 25.8% |
| Missing all teeth | 18.9% | 19.3% | 18.4% |
| Mean remaining teeth | | | |
| Untreated dental caries[a,f] | 18.9% | 18.5% | 19.4% |
| Coronal | | 12.4% | 16.6% |
| Root | | | |
| Periodontal disease[b] | 64.0% | | |
| Moderate or severe | | | |
| Xerostomia[c] | 10%–40% | | |
| Candidiasis infection[d] | Up to 65% | | |
| Wears dentures | | | |
| Orofacial pain[e] | 17.4% | | |
| TMJ (jaw joint) | 7.7% | | |
| Facial | 6.9% | | |
| Oral sores | 6.4% | | |
| Toothache | 12.0% | | |
| Burning mouth | 1.7% | | |
| Self-rated oral health[a] | 61.6% | 61.6% | 61.7% |
| Good–excellent | 38.4% | 38.4% | 38.3% |
| Fair–poor | | | |
| Dental visit past year[a] | 54.5% | 56.9% | 51.6% |

[a]Dye, B. A., Tan, S., Smith, V., Lewis, B. G., Barker, L. K., Thornton-Evans, G., Eke, P. I., Beltrán-Aguilar, E. D., Horowitz, A. M., & Li, C. H., & Li, C. H. (2007). Trends in oral health status: United States, 1988–1994 and 1999–2004. National Center for Health Statistics. *Vital Health Statistics, 11*(248), 1–92.
[b]Eke, P. I., Thornton-Evans, G. O., Wei, L., Borgnakke, W. S., Dye, B. A., & Genco, R. J. (2018). Periodontitis in US adults: National health and nutrition examination survey 2009–2014. *The Journal of the American Dental Association, 149*(7), 576–588.e576.
[c]Dental, Oral and Craniofacial Data Resource Center. (2002). *Oral health U.S., 2002.* NIDCR/NIH.
[d]Akpan, A., & Morgan, R. (2002). Oral candidiasis. *Postgraduate Medical Journal, 78*, 455–459.
[e]Riley, J. L., Gilbert, G. H., & Heft, M. W. (1998). Orofacial pain symptom prevalence: Selective sex differences in the elderly? *Pain, 76*, 97–104.
[f]Dye, B. A., Thornton-Evans, G., Li, X., & Iafolla, T. J. (2015). Dental caries and tooth loss in adults in the United States, 2011–2012. In *NCHS Data Brief*, No. 197. National Center for Health Statistics.

Healthy People (2030) (USD/HHS) identifies five general social determinants of health that include food insecurity, housing instability, lack of early childhood education, illiteracy, lack of engagement in civic participation, limited social cohesion, insufficient access to primary care, and negative environmental conditions. Lack of insurance to cover needed dental care is a major contributor to poor OH (Badr & Sabbah, 2020). Addressing these determinants has been shown to contribute to better oral and general health across the lifespan (Gomaa et al., 2019). These structural and social factors, which have contributed to historical inequities in accessing adequate dental services, underlie any encounters with vulnerable populations facing OH-related challenges and must be taken into consideration in relation to therapeutic approaches (Henshaw & Karpas, 2021; Smith et al., 2021).

OH disparities in older adults are manifested in dental caries (treated and untreated), periodontal disease, tooth loss and edentulism, and in access to quality dental treatment. Despite improvements in many of the measures for the OH of community-dwelling older adults during the past 40 years, disparities persist among racial and ethnic minorities and those with lower incomes and less education (Dye et al., 2007). While these problems appear at higher rates in all adults 65 and older, they are significantly higher in ethnic minority and low-income groups (Patel et al., 2020). The prevalence of dental caries in those 65 and over is twice as high for non-Hispanic blacks (29%) as compared to non-Hispanic whites (14%), and almost three times as high for Hispanics (36%) (NIH/NIDCR, 2021). Caries are three times as high for those classified as poor (33%) as those not poor (10%). For those 75 and older, untreated caries have declined significantly for all groups, despite continuing disparities (non-Hispanic whites 30% to 20%; non-Hispanic blacks 78% to 35%; and Mexican Americans 70% to 44% (NIH/NIDCR, 2021). Destructive periodontal disease affects 17% of adults aged 65 years or older, with higher prevalence and disease severity found among minorities, smokers, and those with lower incomes and less education. For periodontal disease, men fared worse than women (17% vs. 5%); Mexican Americans fared worse than non-Hispanic Blacks (24% vs. 17%), and both fared worse than whites (7%) (Dye et al., 2007; NIH/NIDCR, 2021). Periodontal disease can contribute to local and systemic infection and inflammation, bad breath, and tooth loss (Figure 13.1).

In terms of tooth loss, 19% of adults aged 65 years or older have no remaining teeth, and current smokers are more likely to have lost all their teeth (50%) (Dye et al., 2007, 2015). In general, older adults over age 65 years have an average of 19

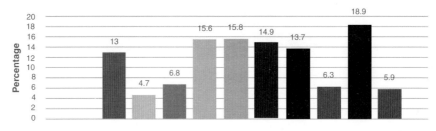

Percentage of adults 30+ with severe periodontitis by gender, poverty status, race/ethniciy and smoking status US 2009-2012 adapted from [67]

■ Men   ■ Women   ■ NHW   ■ NHB   ■ Hisp   ■ <FPL   ■ 1-2X FPL   ■ 2-4X FPL   ■ Smk   ■ NonSmk

**FIGURE 13.1**   Severe Periodontal Disease in Adults Age 30 and Older. (Adapted from Figure 3: Chapter 3B oral health across the life span – Older Adults, 3B-5 in Oral Health in America: Advances and Challenges. (2021). USDHHS, NIH, NIA, DCR, Bethesda, MD.)

remaining teeth, which is fewer than what is needed for an adequate functional dentition (Dye et al., 2007; Griffin et al., 2012). Older African Americans, however, have even fewer teeth, 15 on average (Dye et al., 2007). Tooth decay and periodontal disease continue to be the leading causes of tooth loss (Eke et al., 2018). Dental caries is as common a condition in older adults as it is in children, and it is more likely to remain untreated (Griffin et al., 2005). Nineteen percent of adults aged 65 years or older in the general population have untreated dental caries, whereas 27% of older Mexican Americans have untreated caries (Dye et al., 2015).

Two measures are commonly used to indicate perceptions of OH and well-being: perceived OH status and oral health quality of life (OHQOL). Thirty-eight percent of ALL community-dwelling older adults perceived their OH to be fair or poor (Griffin et al., 2012). These rates were higher for racial/ethnic minority older adults and for lower-income older adults of all racial/ethnic backgrounds. Over the past two decades, older adults have shown small increases in overall satisfaction with their OH (NIH/NIDCR, 2021). Although satisfaction has increased across all groups, including those 65 and above, for those rated as poor (below poverty level), disparities across ethnic/racial groups persist. Non-Hispanic whites reported highest level of satisfaction (81%), followed by non-Hispanic blacks (65%), leaving Mexican Americans far behind (45%). Then for those 75 years and above, only Mexican Americans improved, while the overall dissatisfaction rate for all others was 55%. A recent study (Li et al., 2018) using National Health and Nutrition Examination Survey (NHANES) survey data (2019) showed that perceived OH status was better in non-Hispanic whites, lower in English-speaking Hispanics, and lowest in Spanish-speaking Hispanics (Han, 2019). Income and education levels (lower) also made a significant difference.

OHQOL is also a potential indicator of OH disparities. African Americans report worse OH and quality of life than whites, and edentulous adults (those without teeth) express a worse quality of life than dentate individuals (those with teeth) (Dye et al., 2007; Hunt et al., 1995; Nuttall et al., 2001; Slade et al., 1996). These rates have generally persisted over time but vary across studies. For example, a study of OHQOL in low-income community-dwelling older adults showed no difference in OHQOL by racial/ethnic group,

age, gender, or income (Dye et al., 2007; Hunt et al., 1995; Nuttall et al., 2001; Slade et al., 1996). The study suggested that most residents had access to basic dental care, and the primary factor affecting OHQOL was the number of missing teeth (Reisine et al., 2021). In another recent study, however, race/ethnicity and education contributed to lower OHQOL (Proffitt, 2021).

The contributors to perceived OH and OHQOL are similar. Those who have lower perceived OH or OHQOL are more likely to have been affected by the limitations of inadequate income, poor access to quality foods, inadequate information about oral hygiene, and poor access to quality dental care or its long-term consequences (tooth loss and edentulism). Low perceived OH status and OHQOL are also associated with restricted food choices, reluctance to seek dental care because of fear of pain, and more limited communication with others, which constrains their social support system and promotes isolation and loneliness with associated health and mental health consequences.

In 2017, approximately 66% of older adults aged 65 years or older had a dental visit in the past 12 months, but as in the past, access to dental care in the past year among minority and low-income older adults has not increased proportionally (Dye et al., 2007; Katz et al., 1963), with non-Hispanic whites at 69%, leading all other groups by 12% to 15% (Kramarow, 2019). A major barrier to access to care is lack of dental insurance, which is typically not a retirement benefit. Neither Medicare nor the majority of state Medicaid programs cover preventive and/or restorative dental treatment for older adults; private insurance is often either unavailable or provides very limited coverage. As a result, older adults pay an increased portion of their dental expenses out-of-pocket, which may affect their treatment choices or ability to receive care (Griffin et al., 2012). Unmet dental needs remain high, especially among those with limited incomes and gaps in dental insurance (Bhoopathi et al., 2020). Recent efforts to include dental expenses in Medicare have failed to be approved by Congress, and the issue is not expected to be revisited in the near future.

Long-standing federal legislation, the Omnibus Budget Reconciliation Act of 1987, requires skilled nursing facilities to provide for both routine and emergency dental services to meet the needs of each resident, and many states require additional measures to ensure the OH of nursing home residents (Turnham, n.d.). Despite these laws, poor OH, inadequate mouth care, and limited access to dental care abound in long-term care settings (Smith et al., 2010; Wyatt et al., 2006). Currently, there are no federal laws governing OH in alternative long-term care facilities, such as group homes or assisted living centers, and state laws provide only general guidelines for personal care assistance (Smith et al., 2010). The NIH/NIDCR report (2021, 3B-46) (NIH/NIDCR, 2021) notes that guidelines for OH risk assessment and management are missing for nursing homes and should be established. A survey of alternative long-term care facilities in Michigan found that fewer than 20% of the facilities had a written plan for OH, provided a dental examination at admission, or had an agreement with a dentist to provide care (Smith et al., 2010).

Although Medicare and most state Medicaid programs do not reimburse for preventive or restorative dental treatments for older adults, chronic diseases that result in diminished function that interferes with self-care (such as feeding, oral care, chewing, or swallowing) may demonstrate a medical necessity for skilled intervention in a nursing home, home health, or outpatient setting. Occupational therapists may initiate referrals to dentists based on the results of an oral assessment, covered later in this chapter.

The health care reform proposed by the 2010 Federal Patient Protection and Affordable Care Act aims to provide health insurance coverage to those who are currently uninsured, slow the rise of health-care costs, reorganize the health delivery system, and improve the quality of care provided to all (Northridge et al., 2011). The broad goal is to create a more integrated and interprofessional public-health-oriented care-delivery system. Regrettably, dentistry and the importance of OH were not included in this model of client-centered medical homes (Northridge et al., 2011). Viewing the causal dynamics of the OH of older adults from a larger systems perspective illustrates the interplay of general health, nutrition, social engagement, quality of life, and policy on the development of effective OH promotion and interventions (Metcalf et al., 2011). Occupational therapists are important members of the interprofessional health-care team and are more likely than dentists to interact with frail and institutionalized older adults. A working knowledge of the OH issues associated with aging will greatly benefit interprofessional communication and referral for care.

## Age-Related Changes in Oral Health

Normal aging occurs for oral physiology as it does for the other body systems. Teeth will wear, gingiva (gums) will recede, oral tissue will atrophy, chewing efficiency will diminish, and although the sense of taste may change slowly, a decreased sense of smell results in a loss of flavor perception and food enjoyment (Ship & Mohammad, 1999). Normal aging may involve some tooth loss, dental caries (tooth decay), periodontal disease, xerostomia, infection, or pain, but these sequalae are more prevalent in older adults from racial/ethnic minority and low-income groups.

Currently, there are no nationally representative data on xerostomia, but prevalence estimates range from 10% to 40% of older adults (Dental, Oral and Craniofacial Data Resource Center, 2002). Xerostomia, or dry mouth, affects the ability to chew, taste, swallow, speak, and sleep. It can lead to increased plaque accumulation, dental caries, tooth loss, infections, inflammation, and uncomfortable dentures (Dental, Oral and Craniofacial Data Resource Center, 2002). Xerostomia can result from decreased salivary flow, changed salivary composition, systemic disease, or as a side effect of medications. There are more than 500 medications for which xerostomia is a potential side effect, including tricyclic antidepressants, antihistamines, antihypertensives, and diuretics, all drug classes commonly used by older adults (Fox, 1997).

Oral candidiasis (yeast infection) is the most common fungal infection in humans and is underdiagnosed among older adults—up to 65% of those who wear dentures experience candidiasis (Akpan & Morgan, 2002). Risk factors include decreased saliva, increasing age, antibiotic and steroid medications, dentures, high-carbohydrate diet, deficient vitamin $B_{12}$ and iron, smoking, diabetes, and immunosuppressive disorders. Candidiasis can present as acute white plaques that, when wiped away, expose a painful, red, ulcerated surface; as chronic white or red tissue; or at the corners of the mouth as painful, fissured, and encrusted cracks. Untreated candidiasis can result in altered taste, burning mouth symptoms, and difficulty swallowing and can disseminate throughout the body in immunocompromised clients, resulting in a mortality rate of 71% to 79% (Akpan & Morgan, 2002).

Pain is often regarded as a normal part of aging by both clients and their care providers. As a result, pain is underreported, underdiagnosed, and poorly managed in older adults (Institute of Medicine of the National Academies, 2011). Seventeen percent of older adults experience orofacial pain (often related to diabetes), including jaw joint pain, facial pain, oral sores, burning mouth, toothache pain, and reduced oral motility (Poole et al., 2010; Managing student behavior; Riley et al., 1998). Chronic pain is associated with increased frailty, social withdrawal, decreased performance in basic and/or instrumental activities of daily living (IADLs), and diminished quality of life (American Geriatrics Society, 2009; Rahim-Williams et al., 2009).

Prevention of OH deterioration occurs at the following three levels: primary, secondary, and tertiary. *Primary prevention* of dental caries and periodontal disease requires a focus on improving dietary habits, primarily avoidance of sugary and starchy foods, and regular and proper brushing and flossing, or cleaning between the teeth. Fluoride toothpaste and fluoride varnish applied by a dentist can help to prevent dental caries. Tobacco use and alcohol consumption should be discouraged because of their role in the development of oral lesions and cancers. *Secondary prevention* refers to early detection of disease, managed through regular dental care, medical provider screening for oral and pharyngeal cancers, and protective or prescribed anti-inflammatory antibacterial mouth rinses (e.g., chlorhexidine). Disease control and rehabilitation are the focus of *tertiary prevention*. The goal is to

---

**BOX 13.1**    Helpful Online Resources

**Smiles for Life: A National Oral Health Curriculum**
https://www.smilesforlifeoralhealth.org/teach-curriculum/
    Smiles for Life provides the nation's only comprehensive online oral health curriculum. Developed by the Society of Teachers of Family Medicine Group on Oral Health and now in its fourth edition, this curriculum is designed to enhance the role of primary care clinicians in the promotion of oral health for all age groups through the development and dissemination of high-quality educational resources. The following curriculum modules are especially relevant for the occupational therapy practitioner:
Module 1: The Relationship of Oral Health to Systemic Health
https://www.smilesforlifeoralhealth.org/teach-curriculum/
    course-1-relationship-to-oral-and-systemic-health/
Module 8: Geriatric Oral Health
https://www.smilesforlifeoralhealth.org/teach-curriculum/
    course-8-geriatric-oral-health/
    Teeth Wisdom
    https://teethwisdom.org/healthcare-resources/
oral-healthcare-resources-for-older-patients/
    Oral Health America's online portal provides education for older adults and their care advisors, connects vulnerable

populations to oral health-care resources in their own local communities, provides evidence-based resources for health professionals, and advocates for policy that provides for the oral health of older Americans.

**The State of Aging and Health in America Tooth Loss**
https://www.cdc.gov/aging/agingdata/data-portal/state-aging-health.html
    The *State of Aging and Health in America* is a report series that began as a joint effort of the Centers for Disease Control and Prevention's (CDC's) Healthy Aging Program and the Merck Company Foundation, and evolved into an interactive data website where professionals can get current data at the national, state, and selected local levels for 15 key indicators of older adult health, including complete tooth loss (edentulism).

**CDC Resources on Oral Health**
https://search.cdc.gov/search/?query=Oral%20Health&dpage=1
    Lists numerous sites on oral health.

---

preserve functioning that increases quality of life by reducing or preventing tooth loss, pain, and infection. This includes bridges and dentures, dental implants, scaling, and periodontal surgery. If caught early, oral cancers are generally treatable through the use of surgery, radiation, and/or chemotherapy, with the goal being quality of life and delayed mortality. All levels of prevention require the involvement of a dentist, dental surgeon, or dental hygienist. Primary prevention through OH and hygiene education can also be offered by trained caregivers and other professionals.

How can a non-dentist, specifically an occupational therapist, recognize these conditions and stages and know when to make a dental referral? The Academic Geriatric Resource Center of the University of California, San Francisco, has developed an online learning module for non-dental health professionals to conduct an OH assessment to screen for disease, dysfunction, and discomfort (Wiley Online Library, Academic Geriatric Resource Center) (see Box 13.1 for helpful online resources) (Wiley Online Library, Academic Geriatric Resource Center). The module outlines a systematic approach, beginning with an extraoral examination, followed by an intraoral examination, and concluding with an evaluation of the teeth and/or dentures. Both a geriatric oral health assessment screening tool and a demonstration video reinforce the learning material, and the module includes photos of the common oral conditions in older adults discussed earlier.

The geriatric oral health assessment screening tool was developed to aid in the evaluation and decision-making processes. The oral cavity can be prone to transient trauma, inflammation, and ulceration. These conditions often resolve themselves in 10 to 14 days. Therefore, if a soft tissue lesion is

observed during the intraoral examination, it can be re-evaluated in 2 weeks to determine whether it has healed. A lesion that is still present 2 weeks later requires a referral. When reporting your findings, note the lesion's general location, size, shape, and color; any pain or discomfort; whether there is blood or exudates; and whether the client knows how long it has been present. When writing a referral to a dentist, providing a description that includes these points greatly aids the dentist in focusing on the cause of concern.

Example of a referral note to a dentist on behalf of Mrs. Davidson: "Mrs. Davidson has only a few remaining teeth, her oral hygiene is poor, her gums bleed, and it has been many years since her last dental visit. Please evaluate the lesions on her upper left jaw, on the roof of the mouth, near the front teeth. There are two lesions, both of which are approximately 3 mm in diameter, irregular in shape, white, and not painful; no blood or pus is associated with the lesions; they cannot be removed by wiping with gauze; and the client was unaware of their presence."

Traditionally, in long-term care facilities, occupational therapists, speech pathologists, or nurses may assist the resident in the performance of oral hygiene and, as such, are ideally suited to perform periodic OH assessments.

## Occupational Therapy Practice Framework for Oral Health

Occupational therapy (OT) practice is guided by the *Occupational Therapy Practice Framework* (OTPF) (American Occupational Therapy Association, 2020). The therapeutic use of occupation includes persons, groups, or populations. The OTPF is based on the International Classification

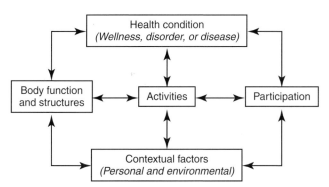

**FIGURE 13.2** International Classification of Functioning, Disability, and Health (ICF).

of Functioning, Disability, and Health (ICF) (World Health Organization, 2001). The ICF and the OTPF consider the effects of the health condition and disability on the whole person. For example, the health condition of osteoarthritis may cause neuromuscular and sensory changes in body structures that cause physical limitations in participation (performing oral hygiene). Access to the environment (such as the bathroom) secondary to using an assistive device or dependent mobility may also impede participation. This inaccessibility may result in a change in context. For example, Mrs. Davidson's health condition of vascular dementia impedes her memory. She is unable to participate in oral hygiene secondary to her inability to problem solve and initiate the task. Reduced sensation related to osteoarthritis interferes with her ability to perceive objects in her hand and perform grip and pinch. Although the bathroom is the typical location to brush one's teeth, because of a limitation in access to the environment, she may need to brush her teeth in the kitchen or dining room, or sit rather than stand at the sink. Context must also be considered; it may be more confusing for Mrs. Davidson to perform oral care in a different room in the middle of the day than following her typical early-morning routine. Fig. 13.2 summarizes the ICF model (how the health condition affects participation).

Occupational therapists use the occupational profile to ascertain the client's or person's previous level of occupational performance. The OTPF consists of occupations, contexts, performance patterns, performance skills, and client factors. ADLs are important occupations that include an older adult's ability to perform oral hygiene. Various performance skills and client factors are needed for oral care, including a stable head position in midline, upper extremity strength, gross and fine motor coordination, praxis (motor planning), visual perceptual skills, sensation, and cognition. Older adults may be limited in one or more of the aforementioned areas secondary to frailty, illness, injury, or disease sequelae. Table 13.3 depicts the OTPF matrix and the interaction of Mrs. Davidson's occupational profile and factors that affect her engagement in the occupation of oral hygiene.

According to Katz et al.'s classic study "Studies of Illness in the Aged" (Katz et al., 1963), older adults regain recovery in ADLs in a hierarchical or developmental fashion following an

episode of illness. Katz and his colleagues suggest that basic ADLs are regained in the following order: grooming (oral hygiene), feeding (eating and swallowing), continence, transferring, toileting, dressing (upper and lower extremities), and bathing. Intervention typically begins with oral hygiene and progresses to more challenging ADLs, such as dressing; bathing requires the highest level of performance skill (Katz et al., 1963).

Fig. 13.3 represents the Nagi model, which is a disablement model used in the *Physical Therapy Guide to Practice*. Again, Mrs. Davidson's medical condition is osteoarthritis, and her impairment limitations are strength and range of motion (ROM; difficulty reaching, placing, or manipulating oral care devices). The resulting activity limitations or barriers to function would manifest as a reduced plate-to-mouth pattern and an altered role for performing oral hygiene. An interprofessional collaboration between an occupational therapist, physical therapist, and dental hygienist may be warranted to reduce additional barriers to performance, in which case familiarity with the Nagi model would facilitate communication.

## Long-Term Care Settings

In 2016, 16% of the 49.2 million US adults aged 65 years and older, or approximately 8,327,100, required long-term care of some sort. Approximately 3% were in adult day care, 53.5% received home health care from an agency, 17.1% were in hospice care, 16% were in a nursing home facility, and the remainder, approximately 10% were in a residential care community (Harris-Kojetin et al., 2019; Poole et al., 2010). Older adults in long-term care settings may have comorbidities resulting in physical frailty, long-term cognitive or physical disabilities, and/or dementias, resulting in medical, cognitive, functional, and behavioral challenges. They require daily assistance with OH and hygiene and regular dental screening and care either on site, or readily accessible to prevent caries, pain, periodontal infection, and lesions. Their risk of caries and periodontal problems is exacerbated by xerostomia resulting from reduced saliva flow caused by the use of multiple medications and by dependence on soft foods, which may be difficult to remove from tooth surfaces or between teeth (Chávez et al., 2018). Oral hygiene education programs have had a positive impact on older adults in long-term care (Lago et al., 2017). Options for those with physical disabilities who are able to perform oral hygiene practices on their own are aids to brushing (e.g., toothbrushes with easy-to-hold handles) and easy-to-manage flossing tools. Those with long-term cognitive disabilities and dementias require administration of oral hygiene by caregivers, who may be family members or professional aides. A functional assessment that identifies and classifies the level of disability is useful in determining which behavioral interventions are most appropriate for a specific patient. Further, in the case of dementias, functional level changes over time, calling for repeated assessments and adjustments in accordance with need. Caregivers should be informed of the results of these assessments and how to respond appropriately

**TABLE 13-3** Occupational Therapy Practice Framework (OTPF) Matrix

| Domains | Occupations | Contexts | Performance Patterns | Performance Skills | Client Factors | Occupation and Activity Demand | Occupational Therapy Interventions | Approaches to Intervention | Outcomes Occupational Performance |
|---|---|---|---|---|---|---|---|---|---|
| Person Client Profile 88-year old female with Osteoarthritis, Impaired memory | ADL Oral hygiene IADL Health maintenance Decrease health risk behavior | Physical environment Accesses bathroom to perform oral care Expected to perform oral care by care-giver | Habits Performs oral care daily Routine Follows morning sequence of oral care | Motor skills Grips / manipulates Process skills Locates and organizes items for oral care Sequences task Social skills Requests assistance | Values independence Regulate response Strategies for memory | Utilizes toothbrush appropriately | Assistive technology for oral cares Large handle toothbrush Toothpaste dispenser | Restore daily oral care routine Educate staff and family | Improvement Perform oral care with set-up ↓ joint pain with Assistive Technology Increase self-efficacy Prevent gingivitis |

(Adapted from American Occupational Therapy Association. [2020]. Occupational therapy practice framework: Domain and process 4th ed.]. *American Journal of Occupational Therapy*, Vol. 74(Supplement_2), 7412410010p1– 7412410010p87. https://doi.org/10.5014/ajot.2020.74S2001

Guide to Physical Therapy Practice

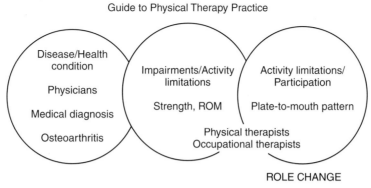

ROLE CHANGE

**FIGURE 13.3**   Interaction of Disablement Model and Health Professionals' Nagi Model. *ROM,* Range of motion. (Adapted from American Physical Therapy Association [APTA]. [2003]. *Guide to practice.* American Physical Therapy Association.)

to them. Research shows that caregivers need training and support to perform oral hygiene effectively with those with disabilities, including instruction in brushing, flossing, and denture cleaning techniques; use of motivational techniques and self-efficacy to promote maximum patient independence; and use of positive reinforcements to reduce stress and anxiety (Lago et al., 2017).

Those older adults with impaired cognitive functioning and associated anxiety, fear, paranoia, and emotional distress, who are less able or unable to cooperate in the context of dental hygiene practices and dental care may require sedation (oral to intravenous sedation and general anesthesia). Continued monitoring and screening are essential to avoid rapid deterioration of OH. Marchini and colleagues developed the Rapid Oral Health Deterioration Assessment (2019) (Marchini et al., 2019) to improve decision-making around OH care and caries treatment at different levels of need and believe it should be implemented regularly in long-term care settings (Craig et al., 2020).

OT practitioners provide a broad range of interventions in the long-term care setting. When providing interventions for older adults, who are often frail, it is important to consider barriers to performance. In addition to possible alterations in cognitive function, frailty among older adults is characterized by weight loss, fatigue, slowness, low activity level, and weakness. Collectively, impaired performance skills and frailty may result in the need for a higher level of care (Bailey, 2004).

The Federal Nursing Home Reform Act, or OBRA (the 1987 Omnibus Budget Reconciliation Act), created a national minimum set of standards of care and rights for persons living in certified nursing facilities (Turnham, n.d.). The Centers for Medicare and Medicaid Services (CMS) Minimum Data Set (MDS) for nursing home resident assessment and care screening full assessment form requires a reassessment of function every 30 days. Section G of the MDS includes performance of personal hygiene, which includes brushing teeth. The MDS uses a numerical rating scale from 0, which is independent, to 4, which is total assistance (Buchbinder et al., 1993; Centers for Medicare and Medicaid, 2022). Occupational therapists who consistently participate in the monthly recertification process have the advantage of identifying residents who

exhibit a change in function and who may benefit from skilled intervention.

Without intervention, older adults may experience altered roles and routines associated with good oral care and hygiene. For example, if there is a loss of memory and the older adult is accustomed to brushing his or her teeth at a set time of day and no one is aware of this routine, this seemingly simple ADL task is lost in translation. In Mrs. Davidson's case, this may also be related to her resistance to having others assist her with oral hygiene. By completing a thorough client and family interview or occupational profile and focusing on context and environment, routines can be restored that help motivate Mrs. Davidson to perform oral care or to expect and accept caregiver assistance in re-establishing a consistent routine for this basic ADL.

Age is also associated with a reduced sense of taste and smell (Imoscopi et al., 2012). For older adults like Mrs. Davidson, who have concomitant conditions, it is important to assess client factors that may contribute to loss of oral function. Lack of oral sensation and taste are examples of deficits in oral structures that may increase the necessity and preference for soft, sticky, and sweet foods, which results in dental caries. Combined with a decrease in healthy oral habits and difficulty in brushing and flossing, this leads to increased risks for periodontal disease and systemic inflammation.

Client factors include body functions such as oral motor muscle power, tone, sensation, and lingual control and coordination. Body structures, such as the cranial nerves, support the integration of facial, and oral mechanisms required for oral motor performance. Cranial nerves and oral structures must be evaluated along with the aforementioned performance skills. Evaluation of the sensory and motor components of the cranial nerves may reveal loss of oral sensation, motor weakness, or a risk for dysphagia. Table 13.4 presents the overlap in sensory and motor functions of the cranial nerves. Wolf et al. (1992) offer a diagram of the overlap between the sensory and motor functions of cranial nerves that contribute to oral motor performance (Fig. 13.4). Any loss of oral sensory or motor function may contribute to dysfunction in any of the four stages of swallowing and result in an unsafe self-performance of oral care.

**TABLE 13.4** Sensory and Motor Function of the Cranial Nerves

| Cranial Nerve | Purpose |
| --- | --- |
| Trigeminal V | Sensation: forehead, face, and jaw; biting, chewing, proprioception |
| Facial VII | Facial expression, elevate larynx, salivation |
| Glossopharyngeal IX | Taste (posterior one third of tongue), salivation |
| Vagus X | Initiates swallow, peristalsis in the esophagus, phonation, taste |
| Accessory XI | Swallowing, elevate larynx and pharynx (flexion of head, lateral rotation—sternocleido-mastoid) |
| Hypoglossal XII | Movement of tongue (position the tongue) |
| IX and X | Share gag reflex and phonation (speech production) |

Adapted from Bailey, P. (2004). *Neurological basis of swallowing.* https://www.coursehero.com/file/178261667/2004-HN-Neurologic-Representationpdf/.

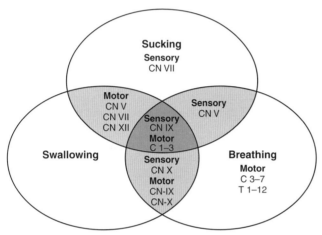

**FIGURE 13.4** Overlapping Function of the Cranial Nerves Involved in Sucking.

For example, upper motor neuron dysfunction may result in hypertonicity, a retracted tongue, and a positive bite reflex, whereas lower motor neuron dysfunction may result in oral and lingual hypotonicity, an imbalance of forces on the teeth, causing an open bite, altered facial expression, or problems with chewing, swallowing, drooling, and speaking (National Institute of Dental and Craniofacial Research, 2020). Table 13.5 summarizes the four stages of swallowing and their relation to oral structures and oral hygiene (Jones et al., 1994).

Aspiration pneumonia is the second most common nosocomial infection, accounting for 13% to 48% of infections in nursing homes, and it is the major reason for hospital admission, with a 20% to 50% mortality rate (Sjögren et al., 2008; Taylor et al., 2000). Although aspiration occurs in both healthy and frail individuals, it does not lead to pneumonia in the presence of an intact coughing reflex, good lung function, and a healthy immune system (Sjögren et al., 2008; Taylor et al., 2000). Risk factors for aspiration pneumonia include compromised general health (particularly chronic obstructive pulmonary disease [COPD] and diabetes), multiple medications, smoking, assistance required for feeding or oral care, tube feeding, missing teeth, dental caries, periodontal disease, poor oral hygiene, and denture use (Langmore et al., 1998; Taylor et al., 2000; Terpenning, 2005). The greatest risk factor for aspiration pneumonia is requiring feeding assistance.

Impaired head and body righting and positioning may result from decreased motor control, hypertonicity, hypotonicity, weakness, proprioception, and awareness of space or other perceptual dysfunction (Jenks & Smith, 2013). External supports, such as tumble forms or wheelchair seat inserts, may be used to improve base of support, posture, and midline head positioning (Northridge et al., 2011; Tumble Forms Image Dental Chair Positioning, 2012) (Fig. 13.5).

Studies have shown that receiving occupational, speech, and/or physical therapy to improve swallowing, positioning the client upright to maximize stability and support, feeding at a slower pace to allow longer chewing cycles before swallowing, and feeding smaller quantities per bite significantly reduced the incidence of aspiration pneumonia (Quagliarello et al., 2005; Sjögren et al., 2008; Terpenning et al., 2001). A systematic review of randomized clinical trials found that approximately one in 10 cases of death from pneumonia in long-term care residents may be prevented by improving daily oral hygiene (Sjögren et al., 2008). Additional prevention measures include referral to a dentist to receive treatment for dental caries and periodontal disease, use of various strategies to reduce xerostomia, limitation of tube feeding, increasing time spent out of bed, and smoking cessation (Langmore et al., 1998; Terpenning, 2005).

Oral motor performance in older adults and persons with disabilities who reside in nursing care facilities may also be limited secondary to impaired oral aperture (how far one can open the mouth). Limited oral aperture may be observed in clients who have a diagnosis of scleroderma, scar tissue associated with facial burns, Parkinson disease, and temporomandibular joint dysfunction. Preparatory methods, such as soft tissue mobilization, myofascial release (occipital release), electrical stimulation, or ultrasound, may be used to improve soft tissue extensibility. Mouth opening may be measured using assistive technology such as Therabite (Domsic & Medsger, 2011; New Jersey Education Association, 2010; Trail, 2004). Naylor (1982) reported that performing 18 weekly oral exercises using a stack of tongue blades may increase mouth opening for oral hygiene. When reduced oral aperture is chronic or

**TABLE 13.5**  Stages of Swallowing and Client Factors

| Stage of Swallowing | Client Factor | Barrier to Oral Hygiene |
|---|---|---|
| Stage I: Preparatory Stage | Impaired head and neck control<br>Upper extremity muscle weakness, loss of sensation, and gross and fine motor skills | Inability to perform plate-to-mouth pattern<br>Unable to hold and/or detect toothbrush in hand<br>Drooling and pocketing in the oral cavity<br>Reduced oral aperture |
| Stage II: Oral Phase | Inner and outer oral motor weakness, impaired oral sensation, lingual incoordination<br>Lip closure<br>Lack of control of saliva (thin liquids and toothpaste)<br>Reduced oral and lingual proprioception | Delayed swallow (oral pharyngeal weakness and pocketing)<br>May aspirate on toothpaste, thin liquids, and mouthwash<br>May be unable to detect toothbrush or food in the mouth<br>Consider temperature and texture of mouthwash and fluoride treatment |
| Stage III: Pharyngeal Phase | Contraction of pharynx and elevation of larynx, upper esophageal sphincter (UES) relaxes | Loss of motility and bolus control, toothpaste stuck in lower throat |
| Stage IV: Esophageal Phase | Cricopharyngeus contracts to prevent reflux | Must remain in upright position following oral hygiene to prevent reflux or aspiration |

Adapted from Jenks, K. L., & Smith, G. (2013). Eating and swallowing. In H. Pendleton & W. Schultz-Krohn (Eds.), *Pedretti's occupational therapy: Practice skills for physical dysfunction* (6th ed., pp. 617–621). Mosby.

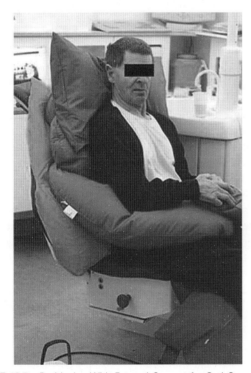

**FIGURE 13.5**  Positioning With External Support for Oral Care. (Picture adapted from Nunn, J., & Gorman, T. [2010]. Special care dentistry and the dental team. *Vital, 7,* 22–25.)

not reversible, thickened liquids or a pureed diet may be recommended. A child-size toothbrush may be needed to clean the teeth and oral cavity (Naylor, 1982).

Successful follow-through with the care plan will depend on the level of interprofessional assistance provided and the environment. The Ecology of Human Performance model of occupation suggests that the social and physical environment also influences behavior and occupational performance. The long-term care setting may have a positive or negative effect on self-care participation (Dunn et al., 1994). For example, having an accessible sink and a toothbrush is positive; inadequate assistance based on process skills or impaired memory would be negative. The first therapeutic intervention proposed in this model is to establish and restore occupational performance. The occupational therapist will identify barriers to performance and then design interventions that improve performance. Mrs. Davidson, for example, would benefit from contextual supports such as physical adaptations or environmental prompts.

Frail older adults often present with existing oral disease upon admission into long-term care due to their reduced ability to perform oral hygiene (Shay & Ship, 1995). Despite families and caregivers preferring that dental services be delivered within the facility, fewer than 20% of residents receive dental treatment, and daily mouth care is often inadequate (US Department of Health and Human Services, 2000; Wyatt et al., 2006). Barriers to receiving care within the facility include institutional-, client-, and provider-level impediments, such as complexity of the long-term care environment, lack of a dental operatory and equipment, challenging medical and behavior management, necessity of gaining informed consent, limited treatment options, time needed to provide service, unavailability of specialists, discomfort with providing treatment outside of a dental office setting, and low financial return (MacEntee et al., 2005; Wyatt et al., 2006).

Certified nursing assistants (CNAs) provide daily hygiene, including oral care. Jablonski et al. (2005) report that CNAs have the least education about diseases associated with inadequate oral care but make up 65% of the staff in long-term care facilities. Pyle et al. (1999) examined CNAs' knowledge of

OH, oral care-giving expectations, and oral care for 89 dependent residents. Results suggest that CNAs who had a history of tooth extraction were more likely to indicate that brushing teeth was important than those who had not experienced a tooth extraction (Pyle et al., 1999). Kaz and Schuchman (1988) hypothesized that oral care provided by CNAs in nursing homes would improve with education provided through a mobile dental clinic. Results showed that CNA delivery of oral hygiene to residents was inadequate and did not meet state reviewer and federal facility expectations and guidelines (Kaz & Schuchman, 1988).

Wardt et al. (1997) found that CNAs believed that oral care was more easily provided to residents who had dentures and that oral care in general was repulsive but would improve quality of life. Other research found that CNAs did not dislike performing oral hygiene but were unsure how to perform this self-care task, especially when the resident was resistant to care or combative. CNAs shared that oral care was omitted most often when assigned duties could not be completed (Chalmers et al., 1996). CNA knowledge and ability may improve with education by occupational therapists at the time of routine service delivery. Oral care performed in context and with demonstration by the occupational therapist may improve CNA self-efficacy (Chalmers et al., 1996; Wardt et al., 1997). Additional research is needed to support this premise.

## Occupational Therapy Assessments of Oral Health

Several OT assessments aid in determining taste perception and oral motor performance, as described in the following discussion.

Mrs. Davidson rates her health as good and has few complaints except that she does not much care for the food: "It tastes like cardboard." Initially, the occupational therapist may complete a sensory assessment of basic taste perceptions by applying a stimulus to the corresponding areas of the tongue: sweet (front and tip), salty (anterior and lateral), bitter (posterior), and sour (lateral and middle). If Mrs. Davidson is unable to identify basic taste perceptions, the practitioner will also assess basic olfactory sensation because smell (processed in the temporal lobe) is a component of taste. Similarly, the sense of smell may be assessed by having the client identify five common scents (such as coffee, garlic, cinnamon, vanilla, and lemon). Scents are presented one at a time with one nostril compressed (Laugerette et al., 2005; Palo Alto Medical Foundation, 2019; Pedretti, 1996; Imoscopi et al., 2012). With age, the number of taste buds and the sense of taste are diminished. Extreme heat and cold sensations, oral infections, dry mouth, smoking, spicy and sour foods, and medications (such as beta blockers and angiotensin-converting enzyme [ACE] inhibitors) alter taste. A referral to a primary care provider, dentist, pharmacist, and dietician would be beneficial to determine which factors may be contributing to her food tasting like cardboard. She needs some assistance

with self-feeding and has poor dentition. Thus, a thorough oral assessment, including motor and sensory function of cranial nerves, is indicated.

The outer oral motor assessment (Table 13.6) suggested by Logerman (1998) evaluates the resident's ability to perform facial expressions, lift eyebrows, and control lips (smile) (Everything Dysphagia, 2020; Logermann, 1998). The practitioner observes for bilateral facial symmetry. Asymmetry may indicate oral weakness or reduced tone. Working in the client's visual field helps to establish trust and facilitates understanding of assessment instructions.

The intraoral assessment (Table 13.7) examines oral structures, the tongue, and the swallowing mechanism. Like the outer oral assessment, it is important to note any weakness or deviation of the tongue to the stronger side or affected side. Manipulating the tongue forward and side to side from the oral cavity should result in a firm versus a mushy feel, which supports neuromuscular impairments.

A resident who has neurologic involvement may have a delayed swallow or deficits in any of the four stages of swallowing. Primitive reflexes, such as rooting, bite, and suck-swallow, may reappear in older adults who experience damage to upper motor neurons, the brainstem, or other cortical structures. An intact gag, palatal, and cough reflex protects the airway (Jenks & Smith, 2013). Collaborative assessment with speech pathology of oral structures and the swallowing mechanism will aid the practitioner in selecting safe and appropriate methods and assistive technology for oral hygiene.

Occupational therapists may also use standardized assessments to quantify the performance of oral hygiene. Common assessments include the Katz ADL index, the functional independence measure (FIM), the Barthel index, and the Rivermead ADL scale. Qualitative measures, such as the Canadian Occupational Performance Measure (COPM), may also be used.

The Katz index of ADLs (Katz et al., 1963) is a standardized assessment that evaluates level of independence or dependence in grooming, feeding, continence, transferring, toileting, dressing, and bathing. Although this assessment does not address oral care directly, similar motor and sensory

**TABLE 13.6** Examples of an outer oral Assessment

| Function | Instruction to Resident | Test Instruction |
|---|---|---|
| Facial expression | Lift your eyebrows Suck in your cheeks | Apply downward pressure to eyebrow Push air out in each cheek |
| Lip control | Smile Pucker your lips to make a kiss | Observe for symmetry |
| Jaw control | Open mouth as wide as possible | Observe head control; support under chin if needed |

Adapted from Jenks, K. L., & Smith, G. (2013). Eating and swallowing. In H. Pendleton & W. Schultz-Krohn (Eds.), *Pedretti's occupational therapy: Practice skills for physical dysfunction* (6th ed., pp. 617–621). Mosby.

**TABLE 13.7**  Examples of an Intraoral Assessment

| Function | Instruction to Resident | Test Instruction |
|---|---|---|
| Tongue protrusion | Stick out your tongue | Apply slight pressure to the tip of the tongue |
| Lateralization | Move your tongue side to side | Resist side to side with tongue blade |
| Tipping | Touch your tongue to the roof of your mouth, front and back | Apply downward pressure to tip of tongue |

Adapted from Jenks, K. L., & Smith, G. (2013). Eating and swallowing. In H. Pendleton & W. Schultz-Krohn (Eds.), *Pedretti's occupational therapy: Practice skills for physical dysfunction* (6th ed., pp. 617–621). Mosby.

**TABLE 13.8**  Adapted FIM Scores for Oral Hygiene

**Scoring**

7. Cleans teeth or dentures without assistance
6. Cleans teeth with assistive device (large handle toothbrush)
5. Standby assistance; remind to apply toothpaste to brush
4. Requires minimal assistance verbal cue; performs 75%
5. Requires moderate assistance, manual and verbal cues; performs 50%
6. Requires maximal assistance, hand over hand; performs 25%
7. Performs less than 25%; difficulty initiating

Adapted from Amundson, J., Brunner, A., & Ewers, M. (2012). *FIM scores as an indicator of length of stay and discharge destination in CVA patients: A retroactive outcomes study.* University of Wisconsin-La Crosse Journal of Undergraduate Research, III (pp. 263–270). https://www.uwlax.edu/urc/jur-online/2000/. *FIM*, Functional independence measure.

performance skills are required for grooming and feeding. A score of "A" on the index indicates complete independence in feeding, and a score of "G" indicates dependence in the aforementioned ADLs (Katz et al., 1963; Poole et al., 2010).

The FIM is similar to the Katz index of ADLs in that seven performance areas are scored, using a scale of 1 to 7 instead of A to G. Thirteen motor and five cognitive skills are evaluated. A score of 7 is total independence; 6 equals modified independence (uses an assistive device for oral hygiene or grooming); 5 requires supervision; 4 and 3 indicate minimal to moderate assistance; 2 indicates maximal assistance; and 1 indicates complete dependence (Table 13.8). An advantage of using the FIM is that it is quick to administer; a disadvantage is that it does not provide information about body structures or environmental barriers that may affect the performance of oral hygiene. The FIM also assesses process skills, such as social interaction, memory, comprehension, and problem solving, required to perform oral hygiene (Amundson et al., 2012).

The Barthel index is an assessment that scores improvements in rehabilitation of the chronically ill. Like the FIM, it is used to compare occupational performance upon admission and at the time of discharge. The assessment requires the client to perform 10 tasks while being observed. One of the tasks is performing oral hygiene. A score of 5 indicates independence in cleaning teeth; 0 indicates that the client requires assistance (Mahoney & Barthel, 1965).

The Rivermead ADL scale (Revised) was designed to assess basic and IADLs. IADLs are more complex activities than ADLs and are related to independent living (i.e., using the telephone, shopping, cooking, housekeeping, laundry, managing medications, managing finances, driving, or using public transportation). IADLs are very relevant to community-living older adults who can manage their own personal care but might require limited OT on an outpatient basis for these more complex tasks. An advantage of this scale is that the total score reflects level of disability and problem areas. Inpatient scores are compared with discharge scores to determine the level of progress. A score of 3 is independent, 2 requires verbal assistance, and 1 is dependent. The higher the score, the more independent is the resident. Oral hygiene is assessed under the "clean teeth section," which requires the resident to

manage the toothpaste, manipulate the toothbrush, and perform the task (Lincoln & Edmans, 1990).

The COPM uses an interview to help the client identify what he or she perceives to be problems with occupational performance. The client identifies the problems, prioritizes the problems in terms of importance, and then sets a goal for each problem. For example, Mrs. Davidson reports her problems and rates the problems in terms of importance on a scale of 1 to 5, with 5 being the least important (Table 13.9). Brushing her teeth is important to Mrs. Davidson; she rates her performance as poor and is not satisfied with her performance; she indicates that the size of the handle on the toothbrush is not important and that she may be able to initiate applying toothpaste.

Remember from earlier in the chapter that the following goals were set for Mrs. Davidson during the care plan meeting with her family members:
a. improve her ability to care for her own oral hygiene;
b. reduce her resistant behavior when staff try to provide assistance with daily oral hygiene;
c. improve her nutritional intake; and
d. request a referral to a dentist regarding the missing teeth, possible difficulty chewing, and sores found in Mrs. Davidson's mouth.

The occupational profile informs the practitioner about the client's prior level of function, what the client wants to achieve in therapy, and which occupations have meaning and improve quality of life. Therapists listen to the client and discuss realistic and obtainable goals; as Zirkel notes, "Your client is a real person who very well might have a real solution" (Zirkel, 2008).

Mrs. Davidson realizes that she needs assistance to perform oral care, but she may not be aware of how her physical and cognitive limitations affect her performance. Mrs. Davidson's role has changed; her independence is compromised by having a degenerative disease and dementia. Low self-esteem

**TABLE 13.9** Results of Mrs. Davidson's Canadian Occupational Performance Measure Interview

| Activity Problem | Importance | Rates Her Performance | Satisfaction With Current Performance |
| --- | --- | --- | --- |
| Brush her teeth | 1 | 5 | 5 |
| Hold regular-sized toothbrush | 5 | 5 | 5 |
| Apply toothpaste independently | 2 | 5 | 5 |

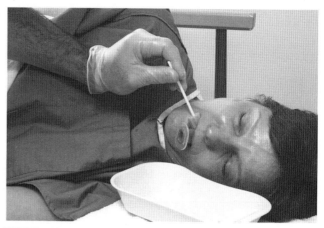

**FIGURE 13.6**    Toothette.

and self-efficacy may hinder motivation and the initiation of participation. Impaired memory may also compromise performance. Self-esteem may be restored by structuring participation in oral care so that she experiences success. Self-esteem may also be enhanced by fostering a sense of control over the task (Kaplan, 2002). For example, giving her a choice as to when she prefers to perform this task may make her feel like she has control over the task. Although memory may not be restored, consistent environmental prompts, such as establishing a morning routine, may be an effective first step to restoring participation (Kaplan, 2002).

## Oral Hygiene Promotion

Lifelong OH can be maintained with daily oral care. Health professionals who care for older adults have an important role in promoting oral hygiene practices, maintenance of dentures, and the need for referral to a dentist.

Oral sensory and motor performance may be improved through graded sensory input, oral exercise, or other methods of intervention. Persons with dementia or traumatic injury may exhibit oral hypersensitivity and benefit from graded tactile or sensory input to the oral cavity and gums. Rubbing the gums or using a moist Toothette (Fig. 13.6) to clean the oral cavity provides sensory stimulation, facilitates oral awareness, and desensitizes sensitive oral tissues. "Oral hygiene for the non-oral or oral client can be used as effective sensory stimulation of touch, texture, temperature, and taste" (Jenks & Smith, 2013).

Proprioceptive neuromuscular facilitation (PNF) head and neck patterns develop enhanced proprioceptive awareness, ROM, and the strength necessary to achieve midline stability. Occupational therapists should evaluate the client's specific needs to determine which type of PNF to apply, as well as its frequency and duration. When PNF is combined with shaker exercise (also called the head lift), the swallowing mechanism is strengthened. Graded sensory stimulation, such as alternating texture, taste, and temperature, may be performed by speech pathologists or occupational therapists who demonstrate competency in this area. Cold sensations, such as popsicles, may be used to improve oral muscle tone and facilitate the lingual praxis required for bolus control (manipulating toothpaste, managing saliva, and rinsing the mouth with approved consistency of liquids).

Oral and facial exercises, such as opening and closing the lips, puckering or pursing the lips as if to make a kiss, whistling, and moving the tongue side to side (lateralization), also support coordination and motor praxis. Oral and lingual exercise performed with graded resistance also facilitates inner and outer oral strengthening.

Occupational therapists prescribe strategies and low- and mid-technology devices for maintaining oral hygiene for a variety of health conditions. Low-technology devices include cylindrical foam to increase the size of the handle of the toothbrush; a mid-technology device would be a battery-operated or power toothbrush.

Osteoarthritis may result in joint pain; loss of ROM, pinch, and grip; and disuse atrophy. Because of disuse atrophy and reduced shoulder strength (such as external rotators), it may be difficult for Mrs. Davidson to reach against gravity. Devices such as an overhead suspension sling or mobile arm support (Fig. 13.7A and B) eliminate gravity for those whose muscle strength is less than grade 3 out of 5 (Table 13.10) (Killingsworth et al., 2013).

Toothbrushes are available in a variety of shapes and sizes based on consumer preferences; soft bristles are recommended to prevent damage to the gingiva and abrasion of tooth enamel. Toothbrushes can be modified for clients who have dexterity limitations. A common low-cost and effective low-technology solution is to slide cylindrical foam tubing over the handle of the toothbrush (US Department of Health and Human Services, 2004). The foam must be replaced often for infection control (due to the potential for bacterial growth). Scrap splinting material, such as Ezeform, may also be used to increase the handle circumference. Power toothbrushes facilitate brushing for both clients and caregivers and have been shown to decrease gingival bleeding and remove more plaque than manual toothbrushes (Davies, 2004). Power toothbrushes may be contraindicated for clients who have neurologic sequelae, such as seizures secondary to the autonomic nervous system's hypersensitivity to vibratory response.

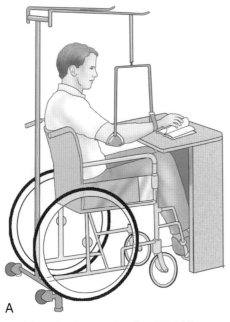

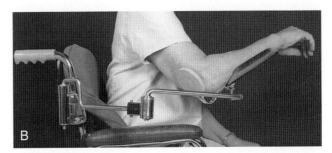

**FIGURE 13.7** (A) Overhead suspension sling. (B) Mobile arm support.

Superbrushes, such as the Collis-Curve toothbrush, have bristles positioned at multiple angles so that a simple back-and-forth motion cleans all sides of the teeth at the same time, which again is helpful both for clients with dexterity challenges and for caregivers (Box 13.2). Toothbrush alternatives that have very small heads, such as the single-tufted brush, proxy brush, and interdental brush, are ideal for cleaning between teeth with large gaps. Moistened soft sponge swabs, such as the Toothette shown in Fig. 13.6, can gently clean painful oral tissues and deliver glycerin or chlorhexidine (an antibacterial agent) to the tissues and teeth. For clients who require assistance in keeping their mouth open when receiving oral care, disposable mouth props are available (Fig. 13.8) (US Department of Health and Human Services, 2000). To reduce bacterial transmission, allow toothbrush bristles to dry between uses, label and keep separate from other people's brushes, store far away from toilets, periodically clean by soaking in chlorhexidine or hydrogen peroxide, and replace every 3 to 4 months or after an illness.

Mrs. Davidson is unable to grip her toothbrush secondary to pain. The occupational therapist may recommend joint protection by using a universal cuff (Fig. 13.9) to avoid the sustained finger flexion required to hold the toothbrush. A toothpaste dispenser that has a pump handle can be activated using the base of the hand or palm for additional joint protection (see Box 13.2).

Dental floss is available with pre-strung heads and extended handles to facilitate flossing for people or their caregivers with dexterity issues (Fig. 13.10). Those with active and/or recurrent dental caries benefit from fluoride varnish applications and high-fluoride-containing toothpaste, both available by prescription (Centers for Disease Control and Prevention, 2001). Rinsing with a prescription 0.12% chlorhexidine gluconate mouthwash is effective against the bacteria that cause periodontal disease (Ship & Mohammad, 1999). Frequent sips

**TABLE 13.10** Muscle Testing/Grading

| Grade | Strength | Movement |
|-------|----------|----------|
| 5 | 100% | AROM max resistance |
| 4 | Good 75% | Complete range of motion (ROM)<br>Mod Res |
| 3+ | Fair+ | Complete ROM<br>Min Res |
| 3 | Fair (50%) | ROM against gravity |
| 3− | Fair− | Some ROM against gravity |
| 2+ | Poor+ | Initiates motion against gravity |
| 2 | Poor (25%) | Complete ROM gravity eliminated |
| 2− | Poor− | Initiates motion if gravity eliminated |
| 1 | Trace | Slight contraction |
| 0 | None | No contraction palpated |

Adapted from Killingsworth, A., Pedretti, L. W., & Pendleton, H. (2013). Evaluation of muscle strength. In H. Pendleton & W. Krohn (Eds.), *Pedretti's occupational therapy practice skills for physical dysfunction* (pp. 529–574). Elsevier.

of water, stimulating saliva production with sugarless candy and gum, restricting caffeine intake, avoiding mouth rinses containing alcohol, using a vaporizer at bedtime, applying moisturizer to the lips, using commercial salivary substitutes, and prescribing casein phosphopeptide toothpaste alleviate the symptoms of xerostomia (Ship & Mohammad, 1999).

The occupational therapist must be aware of safety precautions when performing oral hygiene in clients who have dentures. Around-the-clock use of dentures causes inflammation of the underlying mucosal tissues and can lead to overgrowth of the soft tissues, bone resorption, and candidiasis infection (Zarb et al., 1997). Dentures should be

**BOX 13.2**    Assistive Technology for Oral Care

**Overhead Suspension Sling**

https://www.bing.com/images/search?view=detailV2&ccid=PTjfQ90E&id=7853230B5DA5583A5C659801D7FAB5335F8F7BB3&thid=OIP.PTjfQ90EssDdS4_6OdQAgAHaKW&mediaurl=https%3a%2f%2fth.bing.com%2fth%2fid%2fR.3d38df43dd04b2c0dd4b8ffa39d40080%-3frik%3ds3uPXzO1%252btcBmA%26riu%3dhttp%253a%252f%252fwww.ketteringsurgical.com%252fuploads%252fAiimed_FullImages%252f6678_d.jpg%26ehk%3dT6Y4TR2zZMxZo2rb8SkG1AnSILj6KMkSyn9bwU6dSY%253d%26pid%3dImgRaw%26r%3d0&exph=278&expw=199&q=overhead+suspension+sling&simid=608003563654166668&FORM=IRPRST&ck=5C00AD25C7E4B5743757C8EA5A9D5943&selectedIndex=0&idpp=overlayview&ajaxhist=0&ajaxserp=0

**Mobile Arm Support**

https://www.rehabmart.com/product/jaeco-multilink-mobile-arm-supports-8009.html

**Universal Cuff**

https://www.rehab-store.com/p-north-coast-medical-universal-quad-cuff.html?msclkid=a7d7558bbd921c93263f37d66b0d25a1&utm_source=bing&utm_medium=cpc&utm_campaign=ADL%20Shopping&utm_term=4585581970476530&utm_content=Norco%20ADL

**Cylindrical Foam**

https://www.amazon.com/6-Pack-Foam-Grip-Tubing-Latex-Free/dp/B06XTLQ95N/ref=asc_df_B06XTLQ95N/?tag=bingshoppinga-20&linkCode=df0&hvadid=80608056063458&hvnetw=o&hvqmt=e&hvbmt=be&hvdev=c&hvlocint=&hvlocphy=&hvtargid=pla-4584207588779451&psc=1

**Suctioned Denture Brush**

https://www.bing.com/search?q=suction+denture+brush&qs=n&form=QBRE&msbsrank=2_3__0&sp=-1&pq=suction+denture+brush&sc=3-21&sk=&cvid=2E593B-0BCD2A48B89D7CD0B61621E1FA

**Floss Holder**

https://www.bing.com/search?q=dental+floss+holder&qs=n&form=QBRE&msbsrank=6_7__0&sp=-1&pq=dental+floss+holder&sc=7-19&sk=&cvid=2E593B0BCD2A4-8B89D7CD0B61621E1FA

**Toothpaste Dispenser**

https://www.bing.com/search?q=toothpaste+dispenser&qs=LS&pq=toothpaste&sk=AS1LS2&sc=6-10&cvid=73757418099984FB2B77E271112E8640&FORM=QBRE&sp=4

**Weighted Universal Holder**

https://www.bing.com/search?q=weighted+toothbrush+for+tremors&FORM=R5FD2

**Collis Curve Toothbrush**

https://www.bing.com/search?q=collis+curved+toothbrush&qs=n&form=QBRE&msbsrank=6_7__0&qs=-1&pq=collis+curved+toothbrush&sc=7-24&sk=&cvid=4A2-BFD0CC532406A9B77EFBE63662C9E

**Mouth Prop**

https://www.bing.com/search?q=mouth+prop&qs=AS&pq=mouth+prop&sc=6-10&cvid=3B5A2D3E4BB943C5AADBEA0635959709&FORM=QBRE&sp=1&ghc=1

**Toothettes (Oral Foam Swabs)**

https://www.bing.com/search?q=toothettes&qs=n&form=QBRE&msbsrank=6_7__0&sp=-1&ghc=1&pq=toothettes&sc=7-10&sk=&cvid=0A48B614A80A4353BF47A6EA127762B3

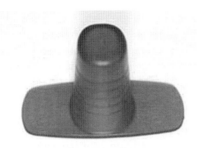

**FIGURE 13.8**  Mouth Prop.

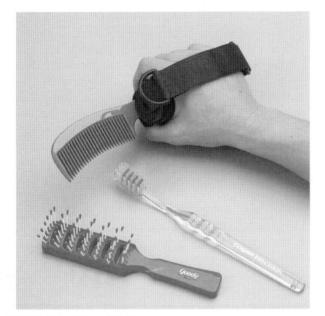

**FIGURE 13.9**  Universal Holder.

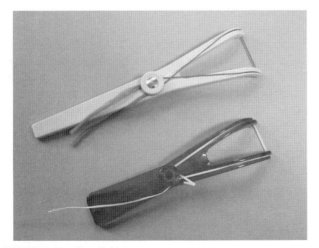

**FIGURE 13.10**  Floss Holder.

removed at night and placed in a container filled with water to prevent the acrylic from drying and possibly changing in dimension. Bacteria, stains, and calculus (tartar) collect on dentures and the oral tissues and, if not removed daily, can lead to odor, inflamed tissue, and candidiasis infection

(Zarb et al., 1997). Dentures should be thoroughly brushed daily and rinsed after meals when possible. Dentures should be cleaned with a soft toothbrush and mild liquid soap over a basin partially filled with water or lined with a wet wash-cloth to prevent breakage if dropped. Toothpaste contains abrasives that will wear away the denture acrylic and should be avoided. The oral tissues, tongue, and any remaining teeth should also be brushed daily with a soft toothbrush. Soaking dentures daily in water with a commercial denture cleanser tablet will remove most stains; however, avoid using bleach, as it will tarnish the metal framework of partial dentures and leach the color of acrylic dentures. Calculus depos-its can be removed by placing the denture in a plastic bag filled with cleanser and agitating it in an ultrasonic cleaner. Loose or unstable dentures require a referral to a dentist for relining or replacement. Denture adhesives and home reline kits should be avoided, as their use can adversely affect the position of the denture on the supporting tissues and make it difficult to keep the denture clean. Many states require the owner's name to be incorporated into the denture. The occupational therapist may also provide a suctioned denture brush to compensate for reduced dexterity or for the use of one-handed cleansing.

Upper extremity incoordination (ataxia) inhibits the dis-tal stability required for performing oral hygiene. Common clinical conditions associated with ataxia include multiple sclerosis, Parkinson disease, and cerebral palsy. Existing literature recommends weighted handheld assistive tech-nology. Weighted utensil holders (such as a toothbrush holder) provide some distal stability for clients who have intention tremor associated with multiple sclerosis. The lit-erature is inconsistent regarding the use of weights to reduce rest tremors, or the pill-rolling tremors associated with Parkinson disease. Trail (2004) recommends that the client reduce the degree of freedom of movement by holding the arms adducted and close to the body. Additional distal sta-bility may be achieved by using one hand to hold the other wrist; a prefabricated wrist cock-up splint may also be used to reduce the effects of pronation and supination associated with the pill-rolling tremors observed in Parkinson disease (Trail, 2004).

The use of fluoride is critical for preventing dental caries. Daily brushing with fluoride-containing toothpaste is recom-mended for all older adults, and adding a commercial 0.05% sodium fluoride mouth rinse provides additional benefits to those with a dry mouth or higher risk for decay (Centers for Disease Control and Prevention, 2001). Toothpastes are also commercially available with additional ingredients, depending on the needs of the consumer. Pastes designed to reduce plaque buildup contain triclosan or zinc citrate; those designed to reduce calculus contain zinc citrate or pyro-phosphate; those designed to reduce tooth sensitivity con-tain potassium nitrate, calcium carbonate, and arginine; and those designed to reduce dry mouth contain baking soda, lac-toperoxidase, glucose oxidase, lysozyme, and lactoferrin. To reduce gagging and accidental swallowing, use only a small, pea-sized amount of toothpaste.

## Care-Resistant Behaviors

Dementia is degenerative and progressive. Persons who have dementia need a consistent environment that provides structure and flexibility, and caregivers who realize that performance of oral hygiene is often slow and labored. Therapeutic interventions for ADLs focus on maximizing independence.

Clients with dementia may have decreased saliva, decreased denture use, and reduced dental access, as well as increased plaque, calculus, dental caries, mucosal lesions, and gingival bleeding and inflammation (Chalmers & Pearson, 2005). These clients may not be able to communicate their oral problems and instead manifest their discomfort or pain by not eating, pulling at the face or mouth, exhibiting aggression or restlessness, and chewing the lip, tongue, or hand (Chalmers & Pearson, 2005). Care-resistant behaviors, such as pushing away the caregiver, turning the face away from the care provider, or biting down on the toothbrush, are often invoked to oppose caregiving efforts. A successful pilot study of the Managing Oral Hygiene Using Threat Reduction (MOUTh) intervention found that using cues (polite one-step commands), bridging actions (older adult holds the same item as is being used in the mouth), and gestures (pantomimes of brushing) significantly reduced care-resistant behaviors and improved OH (Jablonski et al., 2011). Shanks (1996) also recommends the technique of triggering. For example, once the client starts the task, verbal encouragement such as "You do it; no one can brush your teeth as clean as you can," followed by praise, is an effective triggering technique (Shanks, 1996).

The occupational therapist may use the following strategies to increase participation in oral hygiene (Fraker, 2007; Gitlin & Corcoran, 2005; Jacobs & Jacobs, 2009; Shanks, 1996).

Occupational therapists may use the antecedent–behavior–consequences (ABC) model to understand the resistive behaviors associated with dementia. This model relies on the caregiver to identify the precipitating triggers of the resistant behavior (antecedent) and analyze the consequences. The caregiver determines and documents how long the behavior occurs (behavior), then plans an intervention (MacLin and Peterson, n.d.; Project IDEAL, Texas Council for Developmental Disabilities; National Institute of Dental and Craniofacial Research, 2004).

There are several strategies that caregivers may use for improving communication and reducing resistant behavior in a person who has dementia. First, gain eye contact, prepare the environment by minimizing distractions and clutter, identify yourself, and address the person by name. Avoid verbal expressions that may be taken literally. Do not speak in a childish manner. Speak to the person in a calm and moderately loud voice and state requests in a positive and supportive manner. Redirect or distract the person when he or she is agitated or distressed. Grade interactions from most to least complex (e.g., most complex: get ready to brush your teeth ["what do you need?"]; less complex: brush your teeth [use verbal cues, ask for specific information, e.g., "where is your toothbrush?"]; even less complex: help me brush your teeth [requires set up]; least complex: state the facts ["here is your toothbrush," perform with hand-over-hand guidance]. In mild and moderate stages of dementia, the occupational therapist may take step-by-step pictures of the client performing oral care. Picture instructions offer a non-threatening means of enhanced triggering (Piersol et al., 2012; Shanks, 1996).

Establishing an appropriate level of communication will reduce the possibility of resistant behavior. Use actual items with visual cues and hand-over-hand guidance. If there is resistance to hand-over-hand guidance, a mirror technique may be used; the caregiver performs oral care step by step using the same dental tools at the same time as the client.

The goal of behavior management is to respect the client's rights while delivering the necessary OH services. Although the client may have difficulty in appropriately expressing his or her feelings, take the time to first know the client's preferences and responses. The client may be more cooperative with a particular caregiver at a specific time of day, while listening to the television or radio, or when holding a comfort item. Additional suggestions include setting a routine time and place for oral care; identifying yourself and what you plan to do; using visual and verbal cues with short sentences and simple words; initiating tooth brushing but encouraging the client's participation by placing the brush in the client's hand and guiding it with your own; using positive reinforcement and maintaining a calm demeanor; and, above all, attempting to provide oral care every day (McNally et al., 2015).

Your recommendations to the interprofessional team regarding the care plan for Mrs. Davidson in Case Example 13.1 could include:

a. The diameter of the handle on her toothbrush could be increased with rubber tubing, making it easier for her to grip. If she can afford one, a power toothbrush would be easier for both her and a caregiver to use. If the facility can provide a superbrush, that would also be easier for her or a caregiver to use. Her missing teeth indicate that she may be at high risk for dental caries, so she should use a toothpaste containing fluoride and, if cooperative, rinse with a fluoride mouth rinse. Providing her with pre-strung dental floss on an extended handle would facilitate either her or a caregiver's ability to floss.

b. Some observational trial and error is necessary to optimize Mrs. Davidson's cooperation. What are her preferences for and responses to a particular caregiver, during a specific time of day, while listening to the television or radio, or when holding a comfort item? Additional suggestions include providing a routine time and place for oral care every day, using visual and verbal cues with short sentences and simple words for each step of what you are doing, allowing Mrs. Davidson to hold a toothbrush while you are performing her oral care, initiating tooth brushing but encouraging her participation by placing the brush in her hand and guiding it with your own, using positive reinforcement, and maintaining a calm demeanor.

c. Her complaint of bland-tasting food could indicate that a diminished sense of smell is affecting her enjoyment of food. Mrs. Davidson's missing teeth make it challenging for her to adequately chew her food, and her medications may be causing xerostomia, resulting in difficulty in swallowing food. She requires some feeding assistance due to her arthritis, putting her at risk for aspiration pneumonia. A combination of the following suggestions could be used:

- To stimulate her sense of smell and taste, add non-salt-containing spices to enliven the flavor, use more varied visual colors and textures of food, and add a daily multivitamin and mineral supplement.
- To address her xerostomia, actively encourage more water consumption during meals.
- To accommodate her compromised ability to chew, substitute fruit juices, or canned fruits for fresh fruit and vegetable juices or cooked and mashed vegetables for raw vegetables; offer ground meat or protein alternatives such as eggs, milk, cheese, and yogurt; and replace uncooked or partially cooked high-fiber whole grains with cooked grains (e.g., cooked cereals, rice, and bread pudding).
- To optimize her feeding assistance, slow the pace of eating and/or feeding and offer smaller-sized bites.
- To address her specific food interests, work with the dietitian to personalize her diet as much as possible.

## Patient and Family Education

Family caregivers and aides play a significant role in the care of older adults in long-term care institutions and community settings. Regardless of setting, caregivers may be called upon to deliver oral hygiene care, or to decide when it is required or performed inadequately. Training of caregivers should include (1) a description of OH and oral diseases in older adulthood and their causes and consequences; (2) disparities in OH; (3) OH problems in the context of disability or frailty; (4) oral hygiene challenges in dementia; (5) cognitive and behavioral management strategies; and (6) tools and practice in the administration of oral hygiene with trainer observation and feedback.

There is some evidence to suggest that training caregivers in the importance of oral hygiene and oral hygiene practices may improve the OH of older adults needing regular assistance including those with dementia (Lago et al., 2017; Zenthöfer et al., 2016). A 2020 review of four studies (Manchery et al., 2020) outlined interventions including lectures on the importance of OH and hygiene, demonstrations, monitored practice, and the use of games and instructional cards. The review showed mixed results, with several showing improvements in plaque score and denture cleaning, and only one showing improvement in gingivitis. The small amount of research on this topic suggests that trained caregivers can produce improved OH outcomes with dementia patients. The study notes that there is a clear need for further controlled intervention studies that might demonstrate consistent effects.

## Acknowledgment

The authors wish to thank Judith Barker and Susan Hyde's contributions to the previous oral health chapter in the first edition of *Occupational Therapy With Aging Adults*.

*The complete listing of the Bibliography and Chapter Questions and Answers are available in the accompanying enhanced eBook version included with the print purchase of this textbook. Visit Elsevier eBooks+ (eBooks.Health.Elsevier.com) to access this content.*

## CHAPTER 14

# Pharmacology, Pharmacy, and the Aging Adult: Implications for Occupational Therapy

*Hedva Barenholtz Levy, PharmD, BCPS, BCGP and Karen Frank Barney, PhD, MS, OTR, FAOTA*

## CHAPTER OUTLINE

## OBJECTIVES

- Recognize major environmental influences on medication use in older adults
- Define polypharmacy and explain its role in medication-related problems
- Identify common barriers to medication adherence among older adults
- Discuss the pharmacokinetic and pharmacodynamic changes that occur with age
- Define medication-related problems and recognize common examples experienced by older adults
- Describe how the occupational therapy process integrates with various pharmacology and medication-use issues

## Introduction

Medication use is pervasive among older adults. Forty-one percent of Medicare beneficiaries who are age 65 years or older have four or more chronic medical conditions, such as diabetes, heart disease, and hypertension (CMS Chronic Conditions, 2018). Treatment of these and other chronic conditions typically entails the use of multiple, long-term medications. However, medication use is not without consequences in this population.

Many newer medications have more potent effects, both therapeutic and adverse. Thus, the balance of benefit and risk for each medication prescribed and its impact on health outcomes for that individual must be considered. The benefit-risk balance is dependent on multiple factors that are affected by age and include pharmacologic, economic, and behavioral issues.

Increasingly, the impact of social determinants of health (SDOH) on the older client is being recognized. For clients age 65 and older, perceived poor mental and physical health; behavioral characteristics such as inactive lifestyle, poor diet, poor sleep, and alcohol use; and limited social associations are directly related to poor health status, increased emergency department visits, and hospitalizations (Krause, 2021). In addition, factors such as food insecurity, housing instability, and low social support can impact medication adherence (Wilder et al., 2021). Understanding these consequences and related implications of medication use in older clients will enable the occupational therapist to incorporate appropriate interventions and management strategies into daily practice.

## Setting the Stage for Medication Use

Private and public expenditures on health in the United States are the highest in the world. Health-care expenditures per capita in 2019 were $10,948, up from $8700 in 2013 (OECD, health spending, n.d.). Comparatively, per capita expenditures in Canada and Western European nations ranged from $5000 to $7000. Spending in Mexico, South America, and many Eastern European nations was less than $2000 per capita. Pharmaceutical spending for the same year showed a similar imbalance: per capita expenditures in the United States were $1376, compared with Canada and most European nations at $400 to $900, and with Mexico at $251. (OECD, pharma spending, n.d.). Clearly the United States leads global spending on medications. The 20 most commonly prescribed medications among Medicare beneficiaries are listed in Table 14.1, along with their category of use and drug class (CMS spending, 2020).

## Environmental Influences on Medication Use in Older Adults

Although greater prevalence of chronic conditions is the major reason for medication use among older adults, environmental and regulatory factors contribute to the widespread use of multiple medications in the United States. Familiarity with these factors lays the groundwork to understand the bigger picture of why older adults are exposed to more medications compared to other age groups, and subsequently are at increased risk for medication-related problems (MRPs).

## Medical and Pharmaceutical Advances

Adults are living longer as a result of advances in medical science and an improved understanding of and ability to prevent and treat many disease states. Similarly, more sophisticated developments in pharmaceutical research have led to new drug approvals. New pharmaceuticals are able to treat conditions that could not be treated in the past, such as cancer, stroke, and heart attack. Thus, adults not only are surviving previously devastating health conditions, but they are living longer and develop other medical conditions that require treatment, such as type 2 diabetes, heart failure, hypertension, neuropathy, and osteoporosis.

## Multiple Prescribers

Based on a sample from a Medicare population, beneficiaries on average have three physicians prescribing medications for them (Green et al., 2007). Thirty percent of Medicare beneficiaries see five or more specialists, a significant increase from just 17% in 2000 (Barnett et al., 2021). Fragmented care and lack of communication among physicians are potential factors that negatively affect client care. Physicians may not ask about or be willing to make changes to medications prescribed by other specialists, leading to increased risk of adverse drug reactions (ADRs) (Green et al., 2007), as well as greater potential for drug interactions and duplication of therapy. Until there is uniform access to a client's health record that enables improved communication between prescribing physicians, older adults and health-care providers need be diligent to create, maintain, and review a complete medication list for each client.

**TABLE 14.1** Twenty Most Commonly Prescribed Medications by Medicare Claims Data, 2020

| Drug Name (Brand Name) | Category of Use | Drug Class |
|---|---|---|
| Atorvastatin (Lipitor) | Cholesterol | HMG-CoA-reductase inhibitor (statin) |
| Amlodipine (Norvasc) | Cardiovascular | Calcium channel blocker |
| Levothyroxine (Synthroid, Others) | Thyroid | Thyroid product |
| Lisinopril (Prinivil, Zestril) | Cardiovascular | ACE inhibitor |
| Gabapentin (Neurontin) | Neurologic agent (seizures, atypical pain) | Gabapentinoid |
| Omeprazole (Prilosec) | Gastrointestinal | Proton pump inhibitor |
| Losartan (Cozaar) | Cardiovascular | Angiotensin receptor blocker (ARB) |
| Metoprolol succinate (Toprol-XL) | Cardiovascular | Beta blocker |
| Furosemide (Lasix) | Cardiovascular | Diuretic |
| Metformin (Glucophage) | Diabetes | Biguanide |
| Hydrocodone/acetaminophen (Vicodin, Norco) | Analgesic | Opioid combination |
| Simvastatin (Zocor) | Cholesterol | HMG-CoA-reductase inhibitor (statin) |
| Pantoprazole (Protonix) | Gastrointestinal | Proton pump inhibitor |
| Hydrochlorothiazide | Cardiovascular | Thiazide diuretic |
| Metoprolol tartrate (Lopressor) | Cardiovascular | Beta blocker |
| Tamsulosin (Flomax) | Urologic | Alpha-1 blocker |
| Rosuvastatin | Cholesterol | HMG-CoA-reductase inhibitor (statin) |
| Potassium chloride | Electrolyte | Electrolyte supplement |
| Carvedilol (Coreg) | Cardiovascular | Beta blocker |
| Apixaban (Eliquis) | Cardiovascular/direct-acting oral anticoagulant (DOAC) | Factor Xa inhibitor |

*ACE*, Angiotensin-converting enzyme; *CoA*, coenzyme A; *HMG*, hydroxyl-methylglutaryl.
From Centers for Medicare and Medicaid Services. *Medicare Part D Spending by Drug.* https://data.cms.gov/summary-statistics-on-use-and-payments/medicare-medicaid-spending-by-drug/medicare-part-d-spending-by-drug/data/2020. Accessed January 29, 2022.

## Availability of Nonprescription Products

In this chapter, the term nonprescription products refers to both over-the-counter (OTC) products and dietary supplements. Both are regulated by the Food and Drug Administration (FDA); however, OTC products are regulated as drugs, while dietary supplements are regulated as foods. Safety and efficacy implications of this distinction are described below. The nonprescription industry is large and continues to grow annually, with an estimated $40 billion market for OTC products and $43 billion market for dietary supplements (Sobotka & Kochanowski, 2020). Older adults commonly use these products in conjunction with prescribed medications, often without telling their physicians (Gardiner et al., 2006; Qato et al., 2016). Many do not consider these products as "medications" nor understand the fairly unregulated nature of the dietary supplement market (Sullivan et al., 2020). As such, clients may not include common and medically important medications such as aspirin, vitamins, or dietary supplements on their medication list. However, these nonprescription products indeed are drugs that can cause adverse drug effects and interact with drugs and disease states.

### Over-the-Counter Products

OTC options are vast, with over 300,000 products on the market (Drug Applications, 2020). Common OTC product categories used by older adults include analgesics, antacids, cough and cold products, and laxatives. Because OTC products are regulated as drugs by the FDA, manufacturers can only include ingredients that have been approved by the FDA and must abide by product labeling requirements (Rumore, 2020). An estimated 38% of older adults use OTC products on a regular basis, frequently alongside prescription medications (Qato et al., 2016). Since 1976, over 100 drugs have been reclassified from prescription to OTC status (Sobotka & Kochanowski, 2020). Notable recent switches include azelastine nasal spray, olopatadine allergy eye drops, topical diclofenac gel, and two intranasal steroid sprays, fluticasone and budesonide. Although available for use without physician supervision, OTC products still carry the risk of side effects and interactions; for example, acetaminophen can lead to liver toxicity; nonsteroidal antiinflammatory drugs (NSAIDs) ibuprofen, naproxen, and aspirin can cause significant bleeding. Indiscriminate use of OTC products can result in preventable adverse drug events, an area of great concern in older adults because they already are more vulnerable to medication-related harms.

Pharmaceutical companies add further to the maze of OTC options by inundating the market with new combinations of ingredients and brand-name extension products. Combination OTC products are a concern because a client might unknowingly ingest a single medication from multiple sources. A prime example for older clients is acetaminophen. This common analgesic and antipyretic is contained in many cough and cold products (e.g., Alka-Seltzer Plus), headache remedies (e.g., Excedrin), sleep products (e.g., Tylenol PM), and prescription pain medicines (e.g., Vicodin, Norco). If consumers are not aware of multiple sources of exposure, liver toxicity can result.

Brand-name extensions are another source of confusion (Clinical Resources, 2021; Sobotka & Kochanowski, 2020). Pharmaceutical manufacturers take advantage of trusted brand names to market OTC products that contain different ingredients. Unknowing consumers can be misled into choosing a product with a familiar name and end up consuming an ingredient different from what they or their physicians intended. Subsequently, adverse health outcomes can result. Common examples of brand-name extension products include Dulcolax® Chewy Fruit Bites that contain the laxative magnesium hydroxide rather than bisacodyl, which is found in the original product known as Dulcolax®; and Sudafed® PE that contains phenylephrine rather than pseudoephedrine, which is found in the original product Sudafed®. An example of brand-name confusion is illustrated by reports of clients who chose the wrong Dulcolax product for a colonoscopy preparation and subsequently needed to reschedule the procedure. Thus, clients always should be encouraged to consult with their community pharmacist when choosing an OTC product. Furthermore, it is important to view the actual OTC product packaging when conducting a medication review or creating a medication list, so as to document the correct OTC ingredients a client is taking.

### Dietary Supplements

As defined by the FDA, dietary supplements include herbal products, minerals, vitamins, and amino acids that are taken orally to supplement the diet (Tsourounis & Dennehy, 2020). Dietary supplement labeling may make structure-function claims, such as "calcium builds strong bones," but cannot link that effect to a disease state. The most common supplements among older adults are multivitamins, vitamin D, omega-3 fatty acids, calcium, and vitamin B12 (Mishra et al., 2021). Roughly two-thirds of older adults use one or more dietary supplements (Mishra et al., 2021; Qato et al., 2016), with 25% report using four or more in the past 30 days (Mishra et al., 2021). Dietary supplements are widely available, but unfortunately, "natural" does not always mean "safe," and presence on a store shelf does not guarantee effectiveness. The cost of many dietary supplements is significant, as well. In the author's (HBL) experience, older adults can be enticed by television advertisements for proprietary products that promise improved health or a cure-all. Too often, the claims are too good to be true, and the older adult has spent valuable money on a product with no proven health benefits.

The dietary supplement industry is underregulated compared with the prescription and OTC industry. Since passage of the Dietary Supplement Health and Education Act (DSHEA) in 1994, dietary supplements are regulated as foods. They do not require FDA approval and are not subjected to premarketing safety and effectiveness requirements mandated for drugs. The FDA can call for removal of a supplement from the market once it is found to be unsafe (Rumore, 2020). Quality issues with dietary supplements remain a safety concern, with contamination and mislabeling among the dangers (White, 2020). According to emergency department surveillance data, older adults accounted for 12% of visits related to dietary supplements and were more likely to be hospitalized compared to younger age groups. In addition, swallowing issues because of large tablet size—a result of lack of manufacturing regulations for dietary supplements—were the culprit in 38% of visits by older individuals (Geller et al., 2015).

Much still is unknown about safety and effectiveness of many dietary supplements. The mantra "buyer beware" is imperative. Clinical evidence is sparse, and too often based on small trials or case reports. Fortunately, more robust evidence is evolving. A recent meta-analysis identified atrial fibrillation as a potential adverse effect related to fish oil supplements, for example, adding to our understanding of risk-benefit with this product (Lombardi et al., 2021). As with OTC products, practitioners need to be aware of concerns regarding combining dietary supplements with prescription medications and educate their clients.

## Regulatory, Economic, and Cultural Influences

Regulatory, economic, and cultural changes impact medication use in direct and indirect ways. The presence of direct-to-consumer advertising (DTCA) of prescription drugs by pharmaceutical companies proliferated in 1997 following an easing of federal regulation. Only the United States and New Zealand allow DTCA for prescription drugs (Parekh & Shrank, 2018). Pharmaceutical companies spend roughly $6.5 billion annually in advertising, a tactic that serves them well. In a review of DTCA from 2016 to 2018, drugs that accounted for the highest Medicare expenditures also received the highest DTCA spending (US Government Accountability Office [US GAO], 2021).

The impact of DTCA remains controversial. On the benefit side, DTCA can lead to patients being more informed and empowered to talk with their physician about drug therapy options, side effects, and "delicate" health conditions, such as incontinence, erectile dysfunction, or depression. DTCA theoretically can address under-treatment of certain conditions and improve patient's medication adherence (Parekh & Shrank, 2018). On the negative side, critics argue that it encourages inappropriate use of medications, especially newer, higher-priced choices that may be unnecessary and ultimately increase medication costs and government spending via Medicare. Similarly effective options often are available at lesser cost for older adults, the majority of whom live on a fixed income. In addition, advertisements rarely present a balanced picture of the risks and benefits of therapy (Klara et al., 2018). Another concern is that the FDA is understaffed to adequately enforce DTCA regulations.

An increasing proportion of newly approved pharmaceuticals are so-called "specialty drugs," which refers to a range of high-cost outpatient drugs that treat complex health conditions such as hepatitis C, cancer, and autoimmune diseases. Often, special handling or storage requirements for these drugs are involved. Many specialty drugs are biologic agents, and are frequently marketed via DTCA: Enbrel, Keytruda,

Opdivo, and Xeljanz, for example. It is not uncommon for specialty drugs to cost tens or even hundreds of thousands of dollars. These medications must be accessed through specialty pharmacies that provide the needed expertise, including individualized patient education and monitoring that is necessary to ensure safe use and ongoing access to the therapy (Specialty Pharmacy, 2021). Many of the conditions treated with specialty drugs occur in older individuals.

Growth of the world wide web and internet access is another phenomenon that promotes medication use, both via advertisements and myriad websites offering health advice and information. An abundance of health information—albeit of questionable reliability and accuracy—is accessible to the general public. Clients often have greater awareness of diagnostic and treatment information and subsequently might be more willing to self-treat with nonprescription products or ask their physicians to prescribe medications for them. The reliability, accuracy, and recency of the material found on the internet remain a concern and a continual limitation of this source of health information. Undiscerning consumers are particularly vulnerable to the potential untoward effects of information gleaned from the internet.

## Polypharmacy

Polypharmacy can be defined simply as the use of multiple medications; however, the term is laden with negative connotations because of adverse consequences associated with injudicious prescribing. There is no standardized number of medications that defines polypharmacy. A threshold of five or more medications commonly is accepted. Using this definition, 36% of older adults experience polypharmacy, with 72% taking prescription and nonprescription medications concurrently (Qato et al., 2016). Community-dwelling older adults take an average of four prescription medications daily (Charlesworth et al., 2015). This number trends higher in populations with more comorbidities and greater frailty. Individuals in assisted living settings take seven medications on average, and nursing home residents typically take eight or more (Dwyer et al., 2010; Resnick et al., 2018).

The mere number of medicines a person takes is not always a measure of quality of prescribing, though. Older adults with multiple chronic conditions typically require polypharmacy to manage those conditions. For example, multiple medications commonly are needed to effectively manage heart failure, hypertension, or diabetes (Hoel et al., 2021). Indeed, multi-ingredient combination products have been developed to reduce pill burden to support appropriate polypharmacy.

In contrast, injudicious or overuse of medications can lead to negative health outcomes. Thus, polypharmacy can be defined qualitatively as the use of medications that are not clinically indicated or that are ineffective or harmful (Masnoon et al., 2017; Taghy et al., 2020). Consequences of inappropriate polypharmacy include decreased cognitive and physical function; decreased medication adherence; and increased ADRs, emergency department visits, and hospitalizations (Maher et al., 2014).

The burdens of polypharmacy on an older client can be overwhelming, especially for those who live independently. With more medications to take on a daily basis and potentially complex medication regimens, the greater the risk of an error, such as taking a wrong medication, taking it at the wrong time, or forgetting a dose. At the very least, clients should understand how and when to take their medications, as well as why drug therapy is prescribed. This basic information is central to the safe use of medications at home, yet many clients lack this level of health literacy.

Another implication of polypharmacy is high drug costs, which can present an undo economic and emotional burden for older clients on a fixed income. While Medicare Part D provides insurance coverage for medications, increases in drug costs have become a national concern (Hernandez et al., 2020). Many older adults continue to struggle to afford their medications. As a result, clients may choose not to fill a prescription, skip doses to extend the time before needing a refill, or exhibit other unsafe practices that can negatively impact health outcomes.

The prevalence and consequences of polypharmacy are well recognized. Efforts to improve the quality of prescribing for older clients are of paramount concern. Gerontology practitioners must focus on person-centered care when applying clinical practice guidelines to an older client, and resist pressure to prescribe before discussing risks and benefits with the client and/or caregiver. Strategies to optimize drug therapy are discussed below.

## Aging and Medication Adherence

Medication adherence, formerly termed compliance, is defined as the extent to which a person takes medications as prescribed. *Adherence* is the preferred term because it implies a collaborative approach between client and clinician regarding treatment decisions and medication-taking behavior (World Health Organization, 2003). Medication adherence has become an issue of national and global concern. Increased efforts have been made to promote awareness of nonadherence and rally a call to action across health-care disciplines to improve health outcomes (National Council on Patient Information and Education [NCPIE], 2007). It is estimated that 50% of patients are nonadherent to their drug therapy. Nonadherence is estimated to cost up to $300 billion annually in the United States (Nieman et al., 2017). Consequences in older adults include poor health outcomes and disease progression (Iuga & McGuire, 2014), which can negatively impact the ability to age in place.

Unfortunately, medication adherence problems are not always obvious, and nonadherence typically remains undetected until something unexpected or undesirable happens to a client. Box 14.1 provides examples of how nonadherence can be either purposeful or unintentional, overt or covert. Although the examples presented might seem straightforward, the reasons behind nonadherence rarely are. Importantly, most clients will not bring up adherence issues unless they are asked. Even then, they tend to be reluctant to admit nonadherence.

The World Health Organization (WHO) has developed five factors or dimensions of adherence to help define the myriad contributors to nonadherence (Table 14.2) (WHO, 2003): health system, social/economic, therapy-related, client-related, and condition-related. Among therapy-related barriers, the complexity of the medication regimen impacts the vast majority of older adults who have multiple chronic conditions and take multiple medications. In general, age alone does not impact the ability of a person to follow the instructions of how and when to take a medication. Rather, it is the multiplicity of instructions across several medications that leads to challenges. It is not uncommon that an older client might juggle medications that require administration at certain times of day (e.g., morning vs. bedtime) or with regard to meals (e.g., 1 hour before a meal vs. with food). Medicines that can be taken just once a day are associated with better adherence (Srivastava et al., 2013). Thus, even if the direct cost is higher for a once-daily formulation or therapeutic option, these choices typically are cost effective and preferred. In addition, the greater prevalence of multiple health conditions makes gerontological clients more susceptible to health problems that can arise from nonadherence.

Older adults typically experience multiple adherence barriers at once. Clients bring with them a unique set of physical, psychological, and emotional issues influenced by their SDOH and decades of life that ultimately impact the five

---

**BOX 14.1** Examples of Nonadherence

- Taking someone else's medication
- Taking more or less of a medication than prescribed
- Forgetting to take a dose or order a refill of a medication
- Skipping doses to make the supply last longer because of cost
- Skipping doses because of physical limitations (e.g., low vision, arthritis, tremors)
- Stopping a medication without physician's knowledge because of side effects or high cost

- Not ordering a refill of a medication because client does not know it needs to be continued
- Illiteracy that prevents the client from reading instructions correctly on the pharmacy label
- Not filling a new prescription because of cost or because the client refuses to take additional medications
- Choosing to skip the evening dose of a medication because the client has a social engagement away from home in the evening

**TABLE 14.2** World Health Organization Five Dimensions of Adherence

| Dimension | Examples |
| --- | --- |
| Health system–related factors | • Ease of scheduling appointments<br>• Drug formulary changes and restrictions<br>• Quality of communication with health-care providers |
| Condition-related factors | • Asymptomatic chronic diseases that lack physical cues (e.g., high blood pressure or cholesterol, osteoporosis)<br>• Mental health disorders (e.g., mood disorders, psychosis, dementia) |
| Patient-related factors | • Physical impairments (e.g., cognitive, vision, hearing, strength, and dexterity limitations)<br>• Psychological/behavioral (e.g., anger, stress, alcoholism) |
| Therapy-related factors | • Complexity of medication regimen<br>• Duration of therapy (usually life-long)<br>• Inconvenient therapies that interfere with lifestyle<br>• Medications with social stigma attached (e.g., for dementia)<br>• Medication side effects |
| Social- and economic-related factors | • Low literacy; limited English language proficiency<br>• Lack of health insurance<br>• Cost of medications<br>• Poor social support<br>• Cultural beliefs and attitudes |

From World Health Organization. (2003). *Adherence to long-term therapies: Evidence for action.* Retrieved from https://www.who.int/chp/knowledge/publications/adherence_full_report.pdf. Accessed January 29, 2022.

WHO adherence domains. Common overlapping barriers include having chronic conditions that impact functionality like arthritis or chronic obstructive pulmonary disease (COPD); asymptomatic conditions like high cholesterol or osteoporosis; poor vision; decreased memory; and distrust of the medical system. Indirect barriers such as lack of transportation or difficulty reaching one's health-care provider by phone also need to be considered. As a result, there is no one-size-fits-all approach to addressing adherence barriers in older adults. Success can be challenging. Approaches must be tailored to each client and ideally include ongoing support and reinforcement. Occupational therapists can play a critical role in addressing barriers as part of a multifactorial intervention plan for older adult clients.

Remembering to take medications is a common barrier. In addition to helping clients identify daily cues (e.g., mealtimes) for taking their medicines, there are a variety of memory supportive aids that can be utilized, depending on the specific barriers the client experiences. Reminder systems are some of the most common and accessible adherence tools. Calendars or medication charts posted on the refrigerator are simple and inexpensive. Pill organizers come in a variety of styles, ranging from a one-strip organizer with one compartment for each day of the week, to weekly organizers that have four daily compartments to accommodate medications that are dosed up to four times a day. Pill organizers should be checked to ensure the client can easily open the pill compartments, especially if arthritis or tremor is present. Other types of memory adherence aids include watches or "pagers" that can be programmed with alerts, or phone call reminder systems that record the voice of a family member or friend. Automated dispensing machines provide yet another option

when more controlled access to medications is warranted. Some pharmacies are able to dispense medications in special packaging that presorts medicines by time of day to facilitate adherence.

For clients with low vision, the pharmacy can be asked to provide large-print labels and written information in large font size, or a magnifier can be provided. Clients with arthritis can request prescriptions be filled with non-childproof tops. Eye-drop squeezers are available for clients with limited hand strength. Eye-drop guides can be used to facilitate administration of eye drops for clients who cannot keep their eyes open or have difficulty aiming the eye drop. Spacer devices that attach to metered dose inhalers (MDIs) can help clients who have difficulty coordinating drug actuation and breath inhalation. Note that spacer devices cannot be used with dry powder or soft mist inhalers.

Medication adherence is a complex topic with significant clinical, humanistic, and economic implications that are particularly notable in older adults. Solutions are rarely simple. Effective strategies to improve adherence tend to be multifactorial in nature and challenging to sustain (Kini & Ho, 2018). Understanding the nature and extent of medication nonadherence allows occupational therapists to be more aware of and ready to intervene to correct barriers their clients may face.

## AGE-RELATED CHANGES IN PHARMACOKINETICS AND PHARMACODYNAMICS

Changes in pharmacokinetics and pharmacodynamics are an important contributor to MRPs in older adults. To understand the impact of age on drug disposition in older patients and alterations in how older patients might respond to a medication, clinical research data are necessary. However, older adults commonly have complex medication and medical histories and frequently are excluded from drug trials. Subsequently, pharmacokinetic and pharmacodynamic data specific to the gerontological population for newly approved drugs often are insufficient to guide therapy because they are based on only a few hundred participants over the age of 65, and even fewer who are age 75 and older (Hinshaw et al., 2013; Lisi, 2021). Little is known about real-world safety for most new drugs until postmarketing data become available following widespread use in older patients. This section explains the nature of age-related pharmacokinetic and pharmacodynamic changes and provides examples of how these changes affect drug selection, monitoring, and, subsequently, safe use of medications in this population.

## Pharmacokinetics

Pharmacokinetics is the study of how the body handles a medication introduced into its system. Pharmacokinetics is comprised of four components: absorption, distribution, metabolism, and elimination. Age-related changes can occur in any of these components, often necessitating modification of dose or choice of drug. Table 14.3 lists common age-related changes in pharmacokinetics that affect medication use

(Donohoe et al., 2020; Drenth-van Maanen et al., 2020). Most commonly, drugs are taken orally and absorbed through the stomach, but drugs can be absorbed through the skin or mucosa, as with patches, rectal suppositories, or sublingual tablets. Decreased gastric motility seen with age can affect the reliability of absorption of certain medications; for example, variable effectiveness of furosemide in older adults is thought to be related to changes in gastric motility (Donohoe et al., 2020).

Drugs distribute in the body based on their chemical characteristics and can be characterized as distributing mostly into the water compartment (i.e., plasma), muscle tissue, or fat tissue. With age, the percentage of total body water and lean muscle mass declines and percentage of fat tissue increases. Thus, drugs that distribute primarily into lean muscle tissue or are hydrophilic are expected to be more "concentrated" in the aging body—that is, they have smaller volumes of distribution and thus smaller doses will be effective. Examples include digoxin, lithium, and angiotensin-converting-enzyme (ACE) inhibitors. In contrast, drugs that are lipophilic distribute into fat tissue, which is proportionately greater in older adults than in younger clients. The effect here is twofold: lipophilic drugs can take longer to reach equilibrium or constant levels in the body, and they can have a prolonged effect—therapeutic or adverse—because of increased accumulation in the fat

## TABLE 14.3 Effect of Aging on Pharmacokinetic Parameters

| Pharmacokinetic Parameter | Common Age-Related Changes | Comments |
|---|---|---|
| Absorption | Decreased motility, blood flow<br>Decreased acid production | Minimal clinical effects; extent of absorption typically not affected. Rate of absorption of drugs might be decreased. Certain drugs can further raise pH. |
| Distribution | Increased percentage of body fat<br>Decreased percentage of muscle mass, total body water<br>Changes in drug–protein binding (albumin and alpha$_1$-acid glycoprotein [AAG]) | Drugs that distribute in fat tissue (e.g., diazepam, trazodone, amiodarone) are cleared more slowly from body, leading to more severe consequences. Drugs that distribute in water or muscle tissue (e.g., digoxin, lithium, alcohol) typically require smaller dosages. Albumin levels can decrease with age; no change or slight increase in AAG with age. Clinical implications of changes in protein levels are limited, but important in select situations. |
| Metabolism | Decreased hepatic mass, hepatic blood flow<br>Decreased rate of certain metabolic pathways | Changes can lead to slower drug metabolism and prolonged exposure to certain drugs. Lower doses or avoidance might be warranted. Drugs that require metabolism to become activated might have reduced effect. Hepatic changes are variable across patients. |
| Elimination | Decreased renal blood flow, renal mass, and secretion of drugs into the kidneys<br>Decrease in kidney function estimated 1% per year after age 50, but variable across individuals | Approximately 30% of older adults have severe decrease in kidney function; 30% have moderate decrease; 30% have little change. Higher blood levels occur for drugs that rely on the kidney for elimination (e.g., atenolol, digoxin, lithium, allopurinol, famotidine) or whose metabolites are eliminated through the kidney (e.g., meperidine). |

From Drenth-van Maanen, A. C., Wilting I., & Jansen, P. A. (2020). Prescribing medicines to older people—how to consider the impact of ageing on human organ and body functions. *British Journal of Clinical Pharmacology, 86,* 1921–1930; and Donohoe, K. L., Price, E. T., Gendron, T. L., & Slattum, P. W. (2020). Geriatrics: The aging process in humans and its effects on physiology. In J. T. DiPiro, G. C. Yee, L. Posey, S. T. Haines, T. D. Nolin, & V. Ellingrod (Eds.), *Pharmacotherapy: A pathophysiologic approach* (11th ed.). McGraw Hill.

tissue, which serves as a drug reservoir. Thus, "start low, go slow" with drug dosing in older adults is an important mantra. Amiodarone and diazepam are examples of lipophilic drugs that should be used selectively and with extreme caution in older adults. Examples of drugs that are highly protein bound include amiodarone, warfarin, and phenytoin. Changes in protein binding are of importance in clients with poor nutritional status (Donohoe et al., 2020).

The liver is the main site of drug metabolism in the body. With age, there is reduced blood flow to the liver and reduced rate of drug metabolism. Many drugs rely on the liver to be transformed (i.e., metabolized) via enzymes into either inactive or hydrophilic molecules that are more readily eliminated from the body (Donohoe et al., 2020). Age-related changes that affect drug metabolism can lead to reduced clearance of the drug from the body and increased duration of action and side effect risks. Examples of drugs that have slowed metabolism in older adults and prolonged effects include several benzodiazepines (BZDs): diazepam, chlordiazepoxide, and alprazolam; propranolol, diltiazem, and theophylline. The effects of these drugs can be prolonged by hours or up to days compared to younger clients. Metabolism of warfarin can be slowed in older adults, prompting lower doses; however, its disposition in the body is complicated by additional pharmacokinetic and pharmacodynamic issues. Of, note, some drugs rely on metabolism to become active in the body, and thus might show reduced activity in older individuals (Donohoe et al., 2020; Drenth-van Maanen et al., 2020).

Finally, the kidneys are one of the major routes of drug elimination from the body. Renal function decline is an important source of age-related pharmacokinetic change. It is estimated that kidney function decreases 1% for each year after 50 years of age. The effect is variable, though, and up to 35% of older adults may have little or no change in kidney function (Donohoe et al., 2020; Drenth-van Maanen et al., 2020). Drugs that are primarily excreted via the kidneys can accumulate in the body, leading to prolonged therapeutic as well as adverse effects. Examples of drugs that require dosage adjustment secondary to reduced renal elimination are too numerous to list. Common examples used in older adults include allopurinol, digoxin, famotidine, gabapentin, lisinopril, lithium, and metformin. Many antibiotics are renally eliminated and require dose adjustments, too. Importantly, lack of dose adjustment based on age-related changes in kidney function is a significant cause of preventable adverse drug events (Chang et al., 2015).

In summary, age-related pharmacokinetic changes have a direct impact on drug dosing and selection and the potential for adverse effects and interactions. Changes in renal function and the liver's capacity to metabolize drugs are the most notable issues for older clients.

## Pharmacodynamics

The concept of pharmacodynamics addresses the physiologic response of the body to a drug—for example, the ability of a drug to slow the heart rate, dilate blood vessels, or cause sedation. The study of pharmacodynamics helps us understand the relationship between drug dose and response. Changes that occur with aging can alter the response of the body to a drug. Typically, older adults are more sensitive to both the desired and adverse effects of medications. Pharmacodynamic changes are more difficult to study because of inherent interplay with pharmacokinetic issues and difficulty in quantifying medication effects (e.g., sedation from BZDs). As a result, they are less well understood than pharmacokinetic changes. In addition, the effect of aging on pharmacodynamics is more variable among clients. Common examples of pharmacodynamic changes that affect medication use in older adults are summarized in Table 14.4 (Donohoe et al., 2020; Drenth-van Maanen et al., 2020; Schwartz & Abernethy, 2009).

**TABLE 14.4** Effects of Aging on Pharmacodynamic Parameters

| Examples of Changes With Aging | Examples of Clinical Effects |
|---|---|
| Decreased number of receptors | Decreased dopamine and muscarinic (cholinergic) receptors in CNS leads to increased risk of movement disorders or parkinsonism with antipsychotic agents and delirium or confusion with anticholinergic agents, respectively. |
| Decreased receptor sensitivity | Decreased response to beta-adrenergic stimuli and reduced cardiovascular response to beta-blockers (e.g., heart rate); possibly related to diminished number or density of beta-receptors. |
| Decreased baroreceptor function | Increased risk of orthostatic hypotension with diuretics, certain blood pressure medications (e.g., prazosin, doxazosin, nitrates), and tricyclic antidepressants (e.g., amitriptyline, doxepin). |
| Increased response (sensitivity) to medications | Increased sedation with benzodiazepines, antidepressants, opioid analgesics; increased sensitivity to central anticholinergic effects and antipsychotic agents; increased bleeding with warfarin. |

*CNS*, Central nervous system.
From Schwartz, J. B., & Abernethy, D. R. (2009). Aging and medications: past, present, future. *Clinical Pharmacology Therapy, 85*, 3–10; Drenth-van Maanen, A. C., Wilting, I., & Jansen, P. A. (2020). Prescribing medicines to older people—How to consider the impact of ageing on human organ and body functions. *British Journal of Clinical Pharmacology, 86*, 1921–1930; and Donohoe, K. L., Price, E. T., Gendron, T. L., & Slattum, P. W. (2020). Geriatrics: The aging process in humans and its effects on physiology. In J. T. DiPiro, G. C. Yee, L. Posey, S. T. Haines, T. D. Nolin, V. Ellingrod (Eds.), *Pharmacotherapy: A pathophysiologic approach* (11th ed.). McGraw Hill.

In general, older adults are more sensitive to the effects of medications compared with younger clients. Thus, lower starting doses and more gradual adjustments of drug therapy are warranted (i.e., "start low, go slow"). Decreased beta-receptor sensitivity has been documented with a corollary reduced response to beta-blocker drugs in older adults. However, changes in pharmacokinetics of beta-blocker drugs typically offset changes in receptor sensitivity, making dose adjustment unnecessary (Drenth-van Maanen et al., 2020; Schwartz & Abernethy, 2009). The influence of baroreceptor function is clinically important for medications that can induce orthostatic hypotension—namely, diuretics, antihypertensives, and tricyclic antidepressant drugs. Increased risk of orthostasis is directly linked to fall risk and potential fractures.

An exaggerated response to certain medications is fairly common. This is especially true for drugs that act in the central nervous system (CNS), such as sedatives and hypnotics, antidepressants, opioid pain medications, and alcohol. The starting dose for antidepressants and sleep medications typically is 50% of the dose used in individuals younger than 65, e.g. Side effects like drowsiness, dizziness, and confusion contribute to fall risk, thus, use of multiple CNS-active drugs should be minimized or avoided when possible.

Other examples of exaggerated response to medications in older adult clients include increased sensitivity to the anticoagulant effects of warfarin, hypoglycemia from insulin and sulfonylurea drugs (e.g., glyburide, glipizide), and movement disorders from antipsychotic medications. Older adults also are more sensitive to the anticholinergic side effects of medications. Anticholinergic side effects include peripheral effects like dry mouth, dry eyes, urinary retention, and constipation, and CNS effects like confusion and decreased memory. Issues regarding anticholinergic drugs are discussed in greater detail later in the chapter.

In summary, pharmacodynamic changes are extremely important in older adults, although more challenging to quantify. The aging body is more sensitive to drug effects, often necessitating lower initial doses and slow upward titration to allow the body to respond and reduce the risk of adverse drug events.

## Medication-Related Problems

An MRP is an event or circumstance involving drug therapy that interferes with an optimum outcome of therapy (Hepler & Strand, 1990). Medication use in older adults is associated with an increased risk of untoward events that stem from a range of contributing factors discussed above: environmental influences, polypharmacy, medication nonadherence, and age-related pharmacokinetic and pharmacodynamic changes. MRPs are estimated to cost $528.4 billion annually in the United States because of suboptimal prescribing (Watanabe et al., 2018). It is estimated that 28% to 72% of hospital admissions caused by an adverse drug event are preventable (Pirmohamed et al., 2004; Samoy et al., 2006; Sikdar et al., 2010), thus making MRP prevention an important topic when discussing safe and appropriate medication use in older clients.

MRPs can involve actual or potential problems. Examples of MRPs include:

- A client develops a duodenal ulcer while taking an NSAID (e.g., ibuprofen, naproxen) because she was not co-prescribed an acid-blocking drug along with the NSAID.
- A client is taking four CNS-active medications and experiences a fall.
- A patient does not use his inhaler because he does not understand its purpose and is seen in the emergency department with an exacerbation of COPD.
- A patient exhibits confusion and is found to have low vitamin $B_{12}$ levels resulting from long-term metformin therapy.

In these examples, the MRP could have been prevented with appropriate adjustment of therapy, monitoring, or patient education.

Eight categories of MRPs are described below (Hepler & Strand, 1990). These categories are useful as a framework to identify actual and potential sources of suboptimal medication use and more importantly, to pave the way for interventions to correct MRPs and improve health outcomes.

1. Untreated condition—The client has a medical problem that requires drug therapy but is not receiving a drug for that condition. Medical conditions can go untreated for several reasons. Clients might not tell their physicians about symptoms, such as incontinence, constipation, pain, or feeling depressed. Clients might improperly try to self-treat a symptom, when actual treatment requires medical attention. Physicians incorrectly might attribute symptoms to the aging process without further evaluation. Omission of therapy also is an example of an untreated indication. Examples include absence of a beta blocker following a heart attack or absence of an anticoagulant with atrial fibrillation. Explicit criteria for medication use have been developed to address omission of therapy in older adults and are discussed in a later section (O'Mahony et al., 2023).
2. Improper drug selection—The client has a valid clinical indication for taking the drug; however, a different drug is warranted because of safety or effectiveness concerns. Explicit criteria have been developed that identify potentially inappropriate medications (PIMs) in older adults and are discussed in a later section (American Geriatrics Society [AGS] Beers, 2023; O'Mahony et al., 2023).
3. Dose that is too low—The client has a medical condition that is being treated with too little of the correct drug. As discussed earlier, older adults typically are more sensitive to the effects of drugs and require lower initial doses. However, doses need to be titrated to reach effective or therapeutic doses. For example, a client is receiving pharmacotherapy to control blood pressure, but blood pressure remains elevated. Another example is a client who is initiated on the subtherapeutic starting dose of rivastigmine to treat Alzheimer disease, and the prescriber fails to titrate to reach an effective therapeutic dose.
4. Failure to receive a medication—The client has a medical problem that results from or progresses as a result of not receiving

a drug. Medications cannot be effective if clients do not have access to them or otherwise do not take them. Nonadherence falls within this category of MRPs and can result from myriad unique circumstances as discussed previously.

5. Dose that is too high—The client has a medical problem that is being treated with too much of the correct drug. Excessive dosing is one of the more common preventable MRPs in older adults. Age-related pharmacokinetic and pharmacodynamic changes often necessitate a lower dosage. Indeed, for many drugs, the initial gerontological dose is smaller than the usual adult dose, such as with warfarin and drugs used to treat insomnia, depression, or blood pressure. As discussed earlier, drugs that undergo renal elimination need to be dose adjusted.

6. ADR—The client has a medical problem that results from an ADR. ADR refers to any harmful or unintended response to a drug that occurs with normally used dosages (Edwards & Aronson, 2000). ADRs in older adults are the most common cause of emergency department visits (Budnitz et al., 2021). They may or may not be dose-related. Dose-related ADRs tend to be predictable, common, and an extension of a drug's known pharmacologic effects. Examples include tremor from excessive albuterol inhaler use, sedation from BZDs, and dry mouth from oxybutynin. A "hidden" cause of dose-related ADRs is drug interactions or reduced kidney function that lead to higher than expected drug concentrations in the body, even though the dose is within the usual range. In contrast, nondose-related reactions are unpredictable, less common, and unrelated to the pharmacologic effect of the drug. They are often more serious than dose-related reactions (Edwards & Aronson, 2000). Examples of these more serious reactions include hypersensitivity reactions, neutropenia, and platelet dysfunction. Careful drug selection, monitoring, and patient education can help reduce ADR occurrence. Unfortunately, ADRs in older adults are difficult to recognize. They might erroneously be attributed to aging or an existing medical condition and thus discounted as a drug-induced problem. Examples of nonspecific ADR symptoms include weakness, loss of appetite, depression, and decreased memory or confusion. Unidentified ADRs can lead to a prescribing cascade, in which additional medications are prescribed to treat an ADR.

7. Drug interaction—Drugs can interact with other drugs, as well as with disease states (e.g., NSAIDs can worsen heart failure or blood pressure control; prednisone can cause hyperglycemia and affect diabetes management) and foods or nutrients (e.g., grapefruit juice increases blood levels of diltiazem; metformin can decrease absorption of vitamin $B_{12}$ with long-term use). Drug interactions have a higher potential for serious clinical outcomes in older clients because of comorbidities and polypharmacy, as well as the presence of age-related physiologic changes discussed above. A drug interaction can be pharmacokinetic in nature, for example, if it affects the absorption, metabolism or elimination of a drug; or it can be pharmacodynamic in nature, for example, if it exacerbates or diminishes the

clinical effect of the drug. Examples of serious drug interactions in older adults include:

- ACE inhibitors or angiotensin receptor blockers when taken with diuretics that increase potassium levels (e.g., spironolactone, eplerenone) or potassium supplements can lead to hyperkalemia.
- Digoxin combined with amiodarone or verapamil can lead to digoxin toxicity.
- Increased bleeding with warfarin when combined with other drugs that increase bleeding risk, for example, NSAIDs, antiplatelet agents; or with drugs that inhibit warfarin metabolism.
- Lithium taken with ACE inhibitors or loop diuretics (e.g., furosemide, bumetanide) can lead to lithium toxicity.
- Opioid analgesics taken with BZDs, gabapentin, or pregabalin can lead to excessive sedation and respiratory depression.

Other examples of drug interactions noteworthy in older clients include hypotension from overly aggressive treatment of hypertension and fall risk associated with use of multiple CNS-active drugs. Identifying and preventing adverse events caused by a drug interaction is challenging, owing to significant interpatient variability. A combination that may not lead to clinical symptoms in one person could be detrimental in another. As pharmacogenomics testing becomes more commonplace, clinicians will have an additional tool through with to predict and avoid certain hepatic enzyme-based interactions.

8. Drug use without indication—The client is taking a drug without an evidence-based reason. Use of unnecessary medications increases a client's risk of drug interactions, ADRs, and other MRPs. Unfortunately, medications are more easily added to a client's regimen than discontinued. Drug use without an indication can occur in a variety of scenarios. Medications that were started during a hospitalization may no longer be appropriate upon discharge. For example, a proton pump inhibitor (PPI) might be started for ulcer prophylaxis in a critical care unit, continued throughout the hospitalization, and inadvertently written as a discharge medicine. Iron or vitamin $B_{12}$ replacement therapy might be continued once normal levels are restored or the underlying cause is addressed. Medications intended for short-term use, such as treatment for reflux symptoms or insomnia, might be continued despite resolution of symptoms. Finally, a medication might have been appropriately started concomitant with another medication (e.g., a PPI with an NSAID for ulcer prophylaxis or folic acid with methotrexate to prevent toxicity), but inappropriately continued once the other medication was stopped. These examples underscore the value of periodic medication reviews to detect this category of MRPs.

MRPs can negatively affect quality of life, clinical outcomes, and health-care costs. They can cause, aggravate, or contribute to a number of geriatric syndromes, such as confusion or delirium, dizziness, falls, and malnutrition. In turn, clients might experience reduced quality of life because of increased health problems, stress, or reduced cognitive or physical functioning. In addition, MRPs can cause or contribute to new medical conditions or worsen symptoms of an existing condition.

The importance of identifying, preventing, and/or correcting MRPs is paramount to the safe use of medications in older clients. Regular medication reviews by clinicians with geriatric pharmacy expertise are essential in this process. Clinicians should be quick to question the role of medications as a possible cause of new symptoms in older adults or when there is a lack of improvement despite drug therapy. In doing so, MRPs can be identified and corrected to maximize the positive outcomes of therapy while minimizing risks.

## Potentially Inappropriate and High-Risk Medications

Certain medications are considered to be high risk in older adults because of their propensity to cause or contribute to adverse drug events. For some medications, risk is deemed to outweigh benefit. For other medications, clinical benefit is high; however, these select medications also have the potential for serious adverse effects if certain safeguards are not in place. A better understanding of high-risk medications is essential to improving safe and appropriate use of pharmacotherapy among older clients.

## Potentially Inappropriate Medication Drug Listings

PIMs are defined as drugs whose risk is considered to outweigh clinical benefit in patients ≥65 years of age and for which safer alternatives are available. Specific drugs have been identified by geriatric experts that are considered to be PIMs. Two of the most well-known and best-studied PIM drug listings in older adults are the American Geriatrics Society (AGS) Beers Criteria (https://geriatricscareonline.org/ProductAbstract/american-geriatrics-society-updated-beers-criteria/CL001) and the Screening Tool of Older Person's Prescriptions/Screening Tool to Alert Doctors to Right Treatments (STOPP/START) criteria (https://link.springer.com/article/10.1007/s41999-023-00777-y) (AGS Beers, 2023; O'Mahony et al., 2023). These listings largely consist of explicit criteria, which by definition require minimal clinical interpretation when applying them to a given client. The tools should serve as guidelines and educational tools to improve prescribing, and in turn, health outcomes. They are not designed to be a litmus test for good or bad prescribing. Person-centered care remains essential.

The original Beers Criteria were created in 1991 by geriatrician Mark Beers, MD for use in frail nursing home residents. Following the untimely death of Dr. Beers, the AGS assumed responsibility for maintaining the criteria, with the goal of updating the listing every 3 years. The most recent version of AGS Beers Criteria was published in 2023 (AGS Beers, 2023). The current version consists of 37 drugs or drug classes that are recommended to be *avoided* or used only in certain clinical situations, plus a separate listing of 15 drugs or drug classes that are recommended to be used *with caution* in older adults. Drugs in this latter category generally are indicated for use in older clients; however, risk of adverse effects can be clinically significant. Examples of AGS Beers criteria are provided in Table 14.5 (AGS Beers, 2023).

**TABLE 14.5** Examples of the American Geriatrics Society Beers Criteria

| Drug/Drug Class | Rationale and Recommendation |
| --- | --- |
| First-generation antihistamines, e.g., chlorpheniramine, diphenhydramine, hydroxyzine | Highly anticholinergic; avoid |
| Alpha$_1$ blockers, peripheral, e.g., doxazosin, prazosin, terazosin | High risk of orthostatic hypotension; avoid use as an antihypertensive |
| Antidepressants: tricyclic agents (e.g., amitriptyline, nortriptyline, desipramine), paroxetine | Highly anticholinergic, sedating, orthostatic hypotension risk; avoid |
| Antipsychotics, first and second generation | Increased risk stroke, cognitive decline in persons with dementia; avoid for treating behavioral symptoms of dementia/delirium, unless other treatments have failed and older adult is threat to self or others |
| Benzodiazepines, e.g., alprazolam, lorazepam, triazolam, clonazepam, diazepam | Increased sensitivity; increased risk of cognitive impairment, falls, fractures, motor vehicle accidents; avoid (use may be appropriate for certain disorders such as seizures, severe generalized anxiety) |
| Sulfonylureas, glipizide, glimepiride, glyburide/glibenclamide | Risk of severe prolonged hypoglycemia; avoid |
| Proton pump inhibitors | Risk of *Clostridium difficile* infection, bone loss and fracture; avoid scheduled use for >8 wk unless high-risk patient for which maintenance use is justified |
| Nonsteroidal anti-inflammatory drugs (NSAIDs), non-selective | Increased risk of gastrointestinal bleeding or peptic ulcer disease in high-risk groups; avoid chronic use unless other alternatives not effective and patient can take proton pump inhibitor concomitantly |

From the 2023 American Geriatrics Society Beers Criteria Update Expert Panel. (2019). American Geriatrics Society 2019 updated AGS Beers Criteria for potentially inappropriate medication use in older adults. *Journal of the American Geriatrics Society, 67*(4), 674–694. https://doi.org/10.1111/jgs.15767.

In addition, the criteria include 9 disease states or syndromes for which specific drugs or drug classes should be avoided or used with caution, based on the potential to exacerbate the clinical condition. Examples of medications that are PIMs based on drug-disease or -syndrome interactions include the following (AGS Beers, 2023):

Heart failure: NSAIDs, diltiazem, verapamil

Syncope: cholinesterase inhibitors (agents for treating dementia), doxazosin, prazosin, terazosin (nonselective alpha blockers for treating hypertension)

Delirium: anticholinergic agents, BZDs, corticosteroids, $H_2$-receptor antagonists, non-BZD hypnotics (eszopiclone, zaleplon, zolpidem)

History of falls or fractures: antiepileptics, antipsychotics, BZDs, non-BZD hypnotics

Parkinson Disease: antiemetics (metoclopramide, prochlorperazine, promethazine), all antipsychotics (except clozapine, pimavanserin, and quetiapine)

The criteria also include separate tables that list clinically important drug-drug interactions, medications that are high-risk in the presence of kidney impairment, and a list of drugs with strong anticholinergic properties.

The STOPP and START criteria were developed in 2008 in Europe and revised most recently in 2023 (O'Mahony et al., 2023). STOPP version 3 consists of 133 criteria organized into 14 categories based on organ system or drug category—for example, cardiovascular, renal, respiratory, fall-risk drugs, analgesics. Examples are provided in Table 14.6 (O'Mahony et al., 2023). Its companion document, START is the first drug listing to address potential prescribing omission (PPO), that is, drugs that are indicated and thus recommended to be prescribed in older adults. START consists of 11 categories and 57 separate criteria identifying drug therapy that should be considered except for end-of-life or palliative care. Table 14.7 provides examples of criteria from START. PPOs are an important contributor to emergency department visits and hospitalizations (Wauters et al., 2016).

The AGS Beers Criteria and STOPP exhibit limited overlap, so it is noteworthy to consider drug classes that are common to both. These include anticholinergic drugs; antipsychotic agents when used to manage behavioral issues in patients with dementia; BZDs and non-BZD hypnotic drugs (such as zolpidem, eszoplicone, zaleplon); long-acting sulfonylureas (glyburide and chlorpropamide); and PPIs for longer than an 8-week duration unless an indication is present that justifies long-term use.

One of the biggest advantages to the AGS Beers Criteria is its frequent updates. START has the advantage of being the only tool to address PPOs that can lead to suboptimal outcomes. For any of the drugs included on AGS Beers and STOPP, risk is considered to be greater than clinical benefit, and alternative agents are preferred when possible.

## Anticholinergic Drugs

Drugs with anticholinergic effects are prominently included in both the AGS Beers and STOPP criteria, as mentioned above. A growing body of evidence supports an association between cumulative anticholinergic medication use and decreased cognitive and physical functioning, as well as irreversible dementia (Campbell et al., 2018; Landi et al., 2007; Richardson et al., 2018). Thus, it is important to limit exposure to anticholinergic drugs in older clients as much as possible.

The term *anticholinergic* refers to blockade or antagonism of receptors of the cholinergic system. The cholinergic nervous system relies on acetylcholine as its neurotransmitter. Fig. 14.1 illustrates the autonomic nervous system in a very simplistic manner, showing the role of acetylcholine versus norepinephrine transmission (Goldberg, 1988; Westfall et al., 2018). Acetylcholine plays a role both centrally and peripherally via the parasympathetic system. Namely, peripheral cholinergic transmission affects the eye, salivary and lacrimal glands, heart rate, gastric motility, and bladder contractions (Goldberg, 1988; Westfall et al., 2018). Central cholinergic transmission plays a major role in memory and learning (Schwartz & Abernethy, 2009). Consequently, blockade of acetylcholine activity by drugs with anticholinergic activity can result in an important constellation of side effects known as anticholinergic effects. Peripheral anticholinergic side effects include dry eyes, dry mouth, urinary retention, constipation, and blurred vision. Central anticholinergic side

**TABLE 14.6  Examples from Screening Tool of Older Person's Prescriptions (STOPP)**

| Category | Sample Criteria |
| --- | --- |
| Cardiovascular system | Verapamil or diltiazem with New York Heart Association (NYHA) Class III or IV heart failure |
| Coagulation system | NSAID and anticoagulant in combination |
| Central nervous system | Anticholinergics in patients with delirium or dementia |
| Musculoskeletal system | NSAID with severe hypertension |
| Urogenital system | Antimuscarinic drugs (e.g., oxybutynin, tolterodine, others) with dementia or chronic cognitive impairment |
| Drugs that predictably increase the risk of falls in older people | Benzodiazepines, antipsychotic drugs, hypnotic Z-drugs (e.g., zolpidem, zaleplon) |

*NSAID*, Nonsteroidal antiinflammatory drug; *PPI*, proton pump inhibitor.
From O'Mahony, D., O'Sullivan, D., Byrne, S., O'Connor, M. N., Ryan, C., & Gallagher, P. (2023). STOPP/START criteria for potentially inappropriate prescribing in older people: version 2. *Age and Ageing, 44*, 213–218.

**TABLE 14.7** Examples of Screening Tool to Alert Doctors to Right Treatments (START) Criteria: Therapy That Is Clinically Warranted

| Category | Sample Criteria |
| --- | --- |
| Cardiovascular system | Warfarin or newer direct oral anticoagulant drugs in the presence of atrial fibrillation |
| Coagulation system | Antiplatelet therapy with documented history of coronary, cerebral, or peripheral vascular disease |
| Central nervous system | Acetylcholinesterase inhibitor (donepezil, rivastigmine, galantamine) for mild to moderate Alzheimer dementia |
| Gastrointestinal system | Proton pump inhibitor with severe gastroesophageal reflux disease |
| Musculoskeletal system | Vitamin D in patient with known osteoporosis or previous fragility fracture |
| Musculoskeletal system | Vitamin D in older people with confirmed deficiency who are housebound, experiencing falls, or with osteopenia |
| Vaccines | Seasonal influenza vaccine annually |

From O'Mahony, D., O'Sullivan, D., Byrne, S., O'Connor, M. N., Ryan, C., & Gallagher, P. (2023). STOPP/START criteria for potentially inappropriate prescribing in older people: version 2. *Age and Ageing, 44,* 213–218.

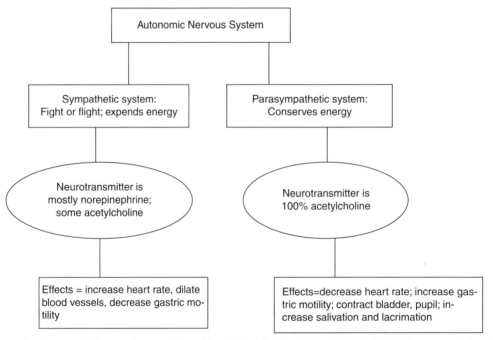

**FIGURE 14.1**    Schematic of Autonomic Nervous System. (Adapted from Westfall, T. C., & Westfall, D. P. [2018]. Neurotransmission: The autonomic and somatic nervous systems. In L. L. Brunton, J. S. Lazo, & K. L. Parker [Eds.], *Goodman & Gilman's the pharmacological basis of therapeutics* [11th ed.]. http://www.accesspharmacy.com/content.aspx?aID5956720. Accessed May 18, 2015; and Goldberg, S. [1988]. *Clinical neuroanatomy made ridiculously simple* [14th ed.]. MedMaster, Inc.)

effects include dizziness, weakness, sedation, decreased memory, and confusion. Drugs that block acetylcholine receptors, therefore, can have significant negative effects for older adults, yet look like common changes of aging. Importantly, anticholinergic medications should always be screened for as a cause of reversible confusion and memory impairment, with the goal of reducing anticholinergic load to limit the risk of irreversible damage. Table 14.8 lists medications that are considered to have strong anticholinergic activity (Aging Brain Care, 2012; AGS Beers, 2023).

## Anticoagulant and Antiplatelet Agents

Anticoagulant and antiplatelet agents consistently are associated with serious adverse events, namely bleeding complications. In a recent surveillance study, the anticoagulant warfarin was the number one drug associated with emergency department visits among adults ≥65 years of age (Budnitz et al., 2021). Close behind warfarin in this study were the newer direct oral anticoagulants (DOACs) apixaban (Eliquis) and rivaroxaban (Xarelto) along with antiplatelet agents clopidogrel and aspirin.

A safe rule of thumb is that any drug intended to "thin the blood" and prevent blood clots will increase the risk of bleeding and can be considered high-risk in older patients. Older clients are particularly sensitive to this adverse effect. Other DOACs include dabigatran (Pradaxa), betrixaban (Bevyxxa), and edoxaban (Savaysa). Other antiplatelet agents include prasugrel (Effient) and ticagrelor (Brilinta).

Note that these agents, including aspirin when used as primary prevention of cardiovascular disease, and selected DOACs, are included as PIMs because of bleeding concerns (AGS Beers, 2023; O'Mahony et al., 2023). Many older adults do not consider aspirin to be a "real" medication because of its OTC status and might omit it from their medication lists. Similarly, the NSAIDs ibuprofen and naproxen are available OTC and thus might not be reported to the health-care team. NSAIDs can exacerbate bleeding risk when used concomitantly with antiplatelet agents and anticoagulants. In clients age 65 and older who take an NSAID, PPI use is recommended to prevent gastrointestinal damage (AGS Beers, 2023; O'Mahony et al., 2023). Ultimately, careful monitoring and client education are mandatory for safe use of drugs that increase bleeding risk in older clients.

## Diabetes Medications

Insulin and some oral diabetes medications are considered high-risk because of the potential to cause hypoglycemia. Insulin, metformin, and glipizide consistently are among the most common medications leading to serious adverse events and emergency department visits in older clients (Budnitz

---

**TABLE 14.8** Commonly Used Medications With Strong Anticholinergic Effects[a]

| Generic Name | Brand Name | Use or Drug Category |
|---|---|---|
| Benztropine | Cogentin | Antiparkinson agent |
| Cyclobenzaprine | Flexeril | Skeletal muscle relaxant |
| Hydroxyzine | Vistaril | Antihistamine |
| Hyoscyamine | Levsin | Antispasmodic |
| Meclizine | Antivert | Antivertigo agent |
| Olanzapine | Zyprexa | Antipsychotic, second generation |
| Oxybutynin | Ditropan | Bladder antispasmodic (antimuscarinic) |
| Quetiapine | Seroquel | Antipsychotic, second generation |
| Solifenacin | VESIcare | Bladder antispasmodic (antimuscarinic) |
| Trospium | Sanctura | Bladder antispasmodic (antimuscarinic) |

[a]See also examples listed in Table 14.5.
From 2019 American Geriatrics Society Beers Criteria Update Expert Panel. (2019). American Geriatrics Society 2019 updated AGS Beers Criteria for potentially inappropriate medication use in older adults. *Journal of the American Geriatrics Society, 67*(4):674–694. https://doi.org/10.1111/jgs.15767; and Aging Brain Care. Anticholinergic cognitive burden scale, 2012 Update. https://corumpharmacy.com/wp-content/uploads/2020/08/Anticholinergic-cognitive-burden-scale.pdf. Accessed February 27, 2022.

---

et al., 2021). Insulin remains a reasonable option in selected clients with type 2 diabetes; however, its use in older adults can be complicated by poor vision, decreased dexterity, decreased cognitive function, and the need to coordinate timing with regard to meals. Any of these factors can affect an older client's ability to safely measure, administer, and use insulin over time. Of note, basal insulins such as glargine and detemir carry a low risk of hypoglycemia when used as monotherapy, but risk increases when combined with other hypoglycemic agents and insulin.

Among noninsulin diabetes drug therapy, oral hypoglycemic agents are of greatest concern. These agents primarily refer to the sulfonylurea drug class (e.g., glyburide, glipizide, and glimepiride). Hypoglycemic agents are so-called because they stimulate the release of insulin regardless of whether the individual has ingested a meal and can lead to severe hypoglycemia under conditions such as acute illness or reduced food intake. In contrast, metformin and other diabetes medications that do not directly stimulate insulin release carry a low risk of hypoglycemia when used as sole therapy. Clients who take medications to manage diabetes need to be educated carefully about the signs and symptoms of hypoglycemia. Older adults with diabetes who use beta blockers may experience unrecognized hypoglycemia because beta blockers mask common signs of hypoglycemia, such as increased heart rate and tremor, with the exception of sweating.

## Cardiovascular Agents

Among cardiovascular medications, diuretics, blood pressure medications, and digoxin commonly are related to adverse events leading to emergency department visits and hospitalizations. Diuretics have the propensity to cause electrolyte disturbances if not monitored properly—namely changes in potassium levels and cardiac conduction abnormalities—and to contribute to dehydration, hypotension, dizziness, and falls. Blood pressure medications can lead to serious adverse events because of the potential to exacerbate orthostatic hypotension and fall risk, and possibly increase fracture risk (Butt & Harvey, 2015). Hyperkalemia can result from the use of multiple cardiovascular agents that increase potassium levels, such as spironolactone with lisinopril or losartan (Abbas et al., 2015). Digoxin is a high-risk medication owing to its narrow window of safety, multiple drug interactions, and altered pharmacokinetics with age (Sikdar et al., 2010).

## Opioid Analgesics and Other Central Nervous System-Active Drugs

Opioid analgesics have emerged as high-risk medications in older adults because they are associated with sedation, falls, cognitive decline, and delirium (Naples et al., 2016). In addition, opioid analgesics can be involved in clinically important drug interactions when combined with BZDs due to an increased risk of overdose, or with gabapentin or pregabalin due to an increased risk of severe sedation, respiratory depression, and death (AGS Beers, 2023). Use of multiple CNS-active drugs are associated with increased risk of falls and fractures. The 2023 AGS Beers Criteria recommends avoiding the combined use of three or more of the following CNS-active drugs: opioid analgesics, antipsychotics, antiepileptics (including gabapentin and other agents to treat neuropathy), BZDs, non-BZD hypnotics, and the antidepressant drug classes of TCAs, selective serotonin reuptake inhibitors (SSRIs), and SNRIs.

## Fall-Risk Medications

Medications that consistently are identified with increased risk of falls in older adults include CNS-active drugs such as antidepressants, sedative/hypnotics, BZDs, and antipsychotic agents. Certain cardiovascular agents that are associated with fall risk include diuretics, nitrates, and digoxin. Other fall-risk drug classes are opioid analgesics, NSAIDs, and anticonvulsants. The mechanism by which drugs contribute to falls varies. CNS-active drugs contribute to side effects like sedation, dizziness, or confusion. Multiple blood pressure medicines can lead to orthostatic hypotension or low blood pressure, causing dizziness and fall risk. Both AGS Beers and STOPP include criteria that address fall-risk medication (AGS Beers, 2023; O'Mahony et al., 2023).

In summary, high-risk medications include consensus-based PIMs and additional high-risk drug categories. These medications need to be used judiciously and avoided when possible, in lieu of safer alternatives. Adequate monitoring and client education about side effects are needed. Identifying opportunities to discontinue or de-escalate high-risk medications is desirable.

## Strategies to Optimize Medication Use in Older Adults

Optimizing medication use in older adults most importantly should focus on limiting the number of medications prescribed and reducing inappropriate polypharmacy. When drug therapy is the treatment modality, medications should be selected and dosed carefully, giving appropriate consideration to age-related pharmacokinetic and pharmacodynamic issues for each drug. Every medication should have a valid clinical indication for ongoing use and monitoring parameters in place to document safety and effectiveness. PIMs should be avoided when possible and other high-risk medication used only when needed and with careful monitoring.

Deprescribing is defined as the clinically supervised process of stopping or reducing medications that might be causing harm or no longer are appropriate (Bloomfield et al., 2020). Ideally, health-care providers would be slow to prescribe because discontinuing drug therapy can be met with many challenges. Medication reviews for older clients can identify unnecessary or harmful medications for discontinuation on a case-by-case basis, but greater evidence to guide how and when to stop drug therapy is lacking. Barriers to deprescribing are common. In addition to the lack of training and evidence-based information to support clinicians, both patients and physicians worry about symptom recurrence or

disease worsening. Physicians typically are reluctant to alter another physician's prescribing. Reimbursement tends to incentivize prescribers to adhere to clinical practice guidelines, which focus on initiating therapy but not stopping it. As a means to counter the problem of polypharmacy, interest in deprescribing has escalated. The US Deprescribing Network (USDeN) was launched in 2019, joining similar international networks, and serves to foster and coordinate research in this area. Research is ongoing to guide best practices of how to stop or reduce medications and overcome barriers to deprescribe drug therapy.

Another component of optimizing medication use is to apply person-centered care. Ultimately, it is the client who must follow his daily regimen of medications and therapeutic lifestyle interventions. Making sure the client understands basic information about his medications that will help him take them correctly on a daily basis is paramount. Barriers to adherence need to be tailored to each client's unique situation.

Rising medication costs is a growing concern. For the majority of older clients who live on a fixed income, difficulty in affording medications can have a significant negative impact on health outcomes. There are several cost-saving strategies that can be encouraged. Ensure that clients proactively choose a Medicare Part D insurance plan that covers all or most of their prescription medications. This should be done annually during the enrollment period, as a plan's preferred drug list can change. Clients can ask their physician or pharmacist if there are less expensive therapeutic or generic alternatives for high-cost drugs. They also should speak with their physician when cost is an issue and check with their pharmacist about programs at the state level or assistance from pharmaceutical manufacturers. Trusted online resources include https://www.BenefitsCheckUp.org, https://www.ssa.gov/benefits/medicare/prescriptionhelp.html, and https://www.NeedyMeds.org.

Finally, a medication review by an expert in geriatric pharmacotherapy is of value for all older adults who take medications on a regular basis. A thorough medication review can identify and address the eight types of MRPs and high-risk medications. Occupational therapists can support clients in compiling a complete medication list that includes all OTC products and dietary supplements and encourage clients regarding the value of getting a regular medication review.

## The Role of Occupational Therapy in Promoting Safe Medication Use

While medication management is an interprofessional concern, utilizing expertise in activity analysis, occupational therapy staff have unique skills for implementing medication management as part of their activities of daily living evaluation and intervention with their clients (Schwartz & Smith, 2017). Thus, the *Occupational Therapy Practice Framework* (OTPF) (American Occupational Therapy Association [AOTA], 2020) includes Medication Management within the Instrumental Activities of Daily Living (IADL) Health Management section of

Table 2 (p. 32). For an individual to appropriately manage medications, the patients/client must successfully complete the following tasks: discuss their condition(s) with their physician, fill the prescription at a pharmacy, be able to interpret related health and prescription information, comply with the prescribed medication schedule, and refill the prescription, if indicated.

Generally, as part of the health-care team occupational therapists and occupational therapy assistants can promote safe medication use among aging adults by increasing awareness of both clients and caregivers about the risks and benefits of medication use, and interacting with physicians and pharmacists on behalf of the client regarding medication use, when indicated. High-risk medications described in this chapter illustrate how medications can cause serious adverse effects, such as bleeding and hypoglycemia, and contribute to drowsiness, dizziness, mental confusion or slowing, decreased memory, and fall risk. These potential drug side effects can hinder the occupational performance of activities of daily living (ADLs) and/or IADLs, thereby affecting overall quality of life. If the individual is referred for OT assessment and intervention, side effects may impede progress and have a negative effect on the ability of the older adult to reach their OT goals, as well as other positive short and long-term health outcomes. By being attuned to the possibility of MRPs, occupational therapy staff can support medication-related functional performance, as well as serve as advocates for their older adult clients.

Adherence is an important behavioral aspect to which occupational therapists can have a positive influence on health outcomes for the older client. Specifically, incorporating medication adherence into routine occupational goals that include establishing related habits and routines to support appropriate medication use can positively impact the client's health-related quality of life. Occupational therapy personnel can be advocates for clients if they appear not to be adherent to their medications by discussing with the physician and/or pharmacist their reasons, which may be physical, attitudinal, psychological, based upon affordability, or other reasons.

Observation of motor and cognitive skills and conversations with older patients/clients and their family members may reveal aging-related changes that impact medication management. These changes may include low vision, changes in grip and pinch strength, proprioception, tremors, lower cognitive or memory changes, and other conditions that impact the individual's ability to access and manage their medications. For example, mild cognitive impairment (MCI) has been shown to have a strong correlation with medication management errors Allen et al. (2022). Thus, OT intervention may positively impact medication use to avoid such errors.

When occupational performance limitations are identified, OT personnel can educate clients and their caregivers about adherence tools or adaptive devices that will support appropriate medication use. For example, occupational therapy

personnel can assist older adults in finding appropriate pill organizers and teach them proper scheduling and use, per their prescription. Features need to match the client's or caregiver's functional abilities and needs, including proper size, ease of filling, and ability to open the pill containers and organizers compartments. When pharmacists are aware of these needs, they typically assist in providing easier to open pill containers. OT practitioners may also recommend adaptive equipment to simplify opening pill containers. Other adherence tools can help clients handle eye drops, read prescription labels, or remind them to take medications on time, among other types of assistance. Thus, occupational therapy guidance can be invaluable in removing medication adherence barriers.

The information provided in this chapter can serve as a foundation to help occupational therapy personnel identify potential high-risk situations or signals of potential adverse drug events, and also feel empowered to communicate such concerns to the client's physician or pharmacist, as appropriate. Keep in mind that OT personnel working with aging adults may play an important role in their clients' successful medication management, especially when special needs or problems are identified. Changes in cognitive function or occupational performance, excessive or easy bruising, decreased stability, or falls, among other changes, all might indicate a MRP. By bringing concerns to the attention of the primary care provider or the client's pharmacist, what might be a preventable problem may be corrected. Using observation skills and developing rapport with the client will allow OT staff to determine whether any of the following medication management strategies are indicated:

- Reduce lack of adherence due to misinformation or misunderstandings about the need for medication use. Considerations include level of health literacy, cultural differences, role of family members, and/or caregivers, if any, and primary language (e.g., English as a second language).
- Bridge the information and understanding gaps between service providers and clients regarding medical terminology, medication names and uses, and potential or actual side effects.
- Facilitate removal of barriers to medication access, as described above.
- Collaborate with other disciplines and agencies to ensure advocacy and financial supports for affordable medication acquisition, when indicated.
- Ensure transportation for the client to their pharmacy, or facilitate delivery of medications.
- Develop strategies and routines to facilitate the client's independence in medication management whenever possible. Where total independence is not realistic, ensure that family or staff members support optimal medication use, allowing for the client's participation to the extent possible.
- Integrate medication use within the client's daily/weekly habits and routines. Table 14.9 provides common dosage

**TABLE 14.9** Medication Dosage Abbreviations

| Term | Directions |
|------|------------|
| QD[a] | Once a day |
| BID | Twice a day |
| TID | Three times a day |
| QID | Four times a day |
| QHS | Bedtime |
| ac | Before meals |
| pc | After meals |
| QOD[a] | Every other day |
| Q2H | Every 2 h |
| PO | By mouth |
| PRN | As needed |

[a]Because of the potential for QD and QOD to be confused, these are on the official "Do Not Use" list by Joint Commission.

abbreviations used for prescription drugs, to indicate the appropriate medication usage. Note also that labels (e.g., "Take with food," or those indicating potential side effects) may also appear on medication packaging, and should be reinforced with clients.

- Organize areas in the client's home for ease of medication use, considering both low- and high-technology options (Table 14.10) and cost.

Recall that the overall role of occupational therapy is to ensure that the client's medications are taken in a manner that supports the client's health and well-being in accordance with the physician's and pharmacist's counsel.

**TABLE 14.10** Occupational Therapy Strategies to Assist With Medication Use

| Individual Guidelines | **General** |
|---|---|
| | • When possible, client should use medical providers in one system that uses the same electronic record so that all doctors see the client's complete medication list. If this is not possible, extra care should be taken to prevent polypharmacy and other pharmaceutical complications. |
| | • Use one pharmacy. |
| | • Use medication calendar, either manual or cell phone daily planner, including a log for doctor visits and contact information. |
| | • If taking from the pill bottle, add rubber bands as reminders for doses to be taken, and remove when taken per day (or week). Other adaptations, such as turning the pill bottle upside down to represent having taken the pill afterwards, can also be used. |
| | • If medications are organized ahead of time with multiple pills in each organizer compartment, prior to having a medication refilled, add rubber bands to those compartments missing the medication, as reminders to add the medication to the organizer as soon as it is available. |
| | • Store pills in the same location, which may vary by time of day, and organize carefully. Use different color organizers for day and night. |
| | • Use note cards, cell phone, or other electronic apps for quick references. |
| | **Cognitive Simplification (for clients with limited health literacy, dementia, limited English proficiency, etc.)** |
| | • Use pictures, word signs, and simple language. |
| | • Encourage questions: |
| |   • What is each medication? |
| |   • Why is each medication used? |
| |   • When should the medication be taken? |
| |   • What does the label say? |
| |   • What happens if the pill is not taken? |
| |   • What are potential side effects? |
| |   • Where does the client get medicines and refills? |
| | **Upper Extremity Coordination and Strength** |
| | • Use alternate forms of pill containers (easy-open tops, blister packaging, pill opening devices). |
| | • Use assistive devices (syringe, weighted cups, pills in small paper cups). |
| | • Coordinate the time to take medication, based upon side effects. |
| | • Use automatic dispensers for eye drops or medications. |
| | **Swallowing Assistance** |
| | • Crush or split pills (with pharmacist approval), using a pill crusher or splitter. |
| | • Use foods such as applesauce, pudding, or ice cream to ease ingestion of pills. |
| | • Alternate forms of medications: gummies, liquid, chewable, patches, injections. |
| | • Use swallowing techniques (tip head back or forward, whichever works best for the client). |
| | • Use a pop or insulated bottle for water. |
| | • Use pill glide swallowing spray. |
| Request from Pharmacist | • Use blister packaging for pills if bottles are difficult to manage. |
| | • Remove child safety feature. |
| | • Provide information in Braille, native, or other languages. |
| | • Use different sizes or colors of bottles for pills that look similar. |
| | • Use generic equivalent medications. |
| | • Send reminders for refills, etc., via telephone, email, tablet/computer, or text messaging. |
| Family/Caregiver Assistance | Set up medications by week or more, as indicated. |
| | Provide reminder strategies, if indicated. |

*Continued*

**TABLE 14.10** Occupational Therapy Strategies to Assist With Medication Use—**cont'd**

| Low-Technology, Low-Cost Options | <ul><li>Add large print with colorful labels (colored tape or paint) to pill bottles.</li><li>Use color-coded, weekly/monthly, Braille, or large-print containers; use containers with removable days for travel.</li><li>Provide medication prompts, such as text messages, emails, telephone calls, and cell phone reminders.</li><li>Use pill storage containers in different colors and weekly or monthly organizers.</li><li>Use a separate small bag for pills when traveling; **always** store in carry-on bag so that medications would not be missed if luggage is lost.</li><li>Use a talking reminder clock.</li><li>Use a pill timer.</li><li>Use a pill splitter.</li><li>Use a pill dispenser or medication management wallet.</li></ul> |
|---|---|
| High-Technology, High-Cost Options | Glucose monitor and insulin pump<br>Automatic pill dispensers<br>Medicine cabinet with a light-emitting diode (LED) light and adjustable mirror<br>Electronic medicine cabinet with medication management features<br>Pill reminders:<br>    Pill container that sets off alarm<br>    Pager<br>    Key chain alarm<br>    Vibrating watch<br>    Email<br>    Text (Short Message Service [SMS])<br>    Alarm watch<br>    Glow cap<br>Cell phone, tablet, or computer apps:<br>    Remind client<br>    Provide refill reminders and tracking<br>    Record timing and dosing<br>    Track missed and taken doses<br>Ingestible sensor for measuring adherence (Hafezi et al., 2015)<br>Monthly medication system with reminder alarm<br>Unit dose systems<br>Home health services monitoring |

## CASE EXAMPLE 14.1    Medication Adherence, Fall Risk

**Subjective**

LW is a 68-year-old female who requested a medication review with a pharmacist because she is worried about taking lisinopril and simvastatin. Her brother had told her they were "not good for (her)."

**Past Medical History**

Transient ischemic attack (TIA) 5 years ago, hypertension (HTN), type 2 diabetes mellitus (T2DM), anxiety, sleep disorder, arthritis with back pain, osteoporosis; h/o fall in shower 2 years ago and broke ribs; status post (s/p) wrist fracture 4 months ago

**Medications**

*Prescription medications:* amitriptyline 10 mg once daily at bedtime, amlodipine 10 mg once daily at bedtime, clopidogrel 75 mg once daily in morning, lisinopril 20 mg once daily in morning, meloxicam 7.5 mg once daily (usually morning), metformin 500 mg twice daily

with meals, metoprolol tartrate 25 mg twice daily, simvastatin 20 mg once daily at bedtime, teriparatide (Forteo) 20 µg once daily (subcutaneous injection for osteoporosis), zolpidem 5 mg once daily at bedtime
*Nonprescription medications:* calcium 600 mg + vitamin D 100 units once daily

**Social History**

Client lives with spouse. Drinks 4 oz of wine "most" evenings. No history of tobacco use. Client does light housework during the day; no regular exercise program. Client uses pill organizer for medicines, but sometimes forgets to take her evening and bedtime medications.

**Objective:** height 5 ft. 2 in., weight 65 kg, blood pressure (BP) during visit today: 143/80 mm Hg

**Assessment**

**Adherence:** Client admits to skipping doses recently of lisinopril and simvastatin because she is concerned

*Continued*

| **CASE EXAMPLE 14.1**   Medication Adherence, Fall Risk—**cont'd** |

they are harmful. Refill record from her pharmacy shows refills are about 7 days late each month. Her current regimen requires administration times of breakfast, dinner, and bedtime, but she is consistent only in taking her morning doses. She shares that she has no set time to take her medications; she takes her morning doses because her husband reminds her when he takes his own, but later in the day, she is tired and does not remember. She also expresses frustration with difficulty opening her pill organizer ("my fingers just aren't so nimble"). Blood pressure is above goal of SBP <130 mm Hg for older adults despite being prescribed three antihypertensive drugs (amlodipine, lisinopril, metoprolol), likely impacted by poor adherence.

**Fall risk:** Fall-risk medications are amitriptyline and zolpidem. Multiple antihypertensives may exacerbate fall risk; need to ascertain if client experiences orthostatic hypotension. Alcohol in the evening can exacerbate fall risk.

**Insomnia:** Client says she has difficulty getting to sleep and she wakes up in the middle of the night and cannot get back to sleep. Amitriptyline and zolpidem (both for sleep) were prescribed by different physicians. These drugs are PIMs and can increase fall risk. They represent a duplication of therapy, as well.

**Drug interactions:** Meloxicam (an NSAID) added to clopidogrel increases bleeding risk. Meloxicam also can increase blood pressure.

**Osteoporosis:** Client is not getting enough calcium (600 mg through supplement plus about 200 mg/day through diet). Guidelines recommend 1200 mg calcium per day through diet (preferred) and supplements. Expert consensus recommends at least 800 units vitamin D per day. Need to ascertain dexterity to administer subcutaneous injection of teriparatide.

**Plan**

(Note: Occupational therapy personnel would especially reinforce the pharmacist's recommendations that are in italics.)

**Adherence:** Educate client about benefits exceeding risks of simvastatin and lisinopril for long-term cardiovascular benefit. *Client agreed to purchase a different type of pill organizer that is easier to open.* Evaluate eye-hand coordination, proprioception, pinch and hand strength, and provide related exercises, if needed. *Client agreed that dinner would be easier than bedtime to take her evening doses and her husband could help remind her; she also will keep pill organizer by the dining room table to cue her at dinner.* Pharmacist will recommend long-acting, once-daily formulations of metoprolol and metformin that client

could take in the morning to simplify regimen. Inform physician about poor adherence and potential impact on BP control.

**Fall risk:** *Educate client about fall-risk issues.* See "insomnia" re: amitriptyline and zolpidem (PIMs). *Educate client about interaction between CNS-active drugs and alcohol. Encourage client to rise slowly from sitting or other lower position to minimize orthostatic hypotension risk.* During their baseline assessment, occupational therapy (OT) personnel will develop an occupational profile to determine if certain activities place the client at greater risk for falls, and conduct a home/environmental safety assessment.

**Insomnia:** Recommend discontinue amitriptyline and zolpidem due to both drugs being PIMs and risk of adverse events (fall risk, confusion, decreased memory) outweighing possible benefit; patient already with h/o 2 falls. *Educate client about good sleep hygiene and optimal occupational performance in activities that may improve sleep pattern and minimize need for hypnotic medication. If OT personnel follow up intervention determines that these tips are insufficient, the OT personnel would recommend further consult with physician for other potential interventions.*

**Drug interaction/pharmacodynamic interaction:** Educate client about interaction between meloxicam and clopidogrel, if meloxicam cannot be stopped. Instruct her to monitor for signs of bleeding. Recommend addition of PPI as prophylaxis for gastrointestinal bleeding and ulcer risks as long as client is taking meloxicam. Pharmacist to recommend discontinuing meloxicam due to impact on BP and bleeding risk. *Alternatives to meloxicam for pain management include trial of acetaminophen 1000 mg TID and nondrug strategies (e.g., heat/cold, massage, mindfulness therapy, and meditation).*

**Osteoporosis:** Encourage increased dietary calcium intake; provide information on variety of dietary sources of calcium. Continue calcium carbonate, increasing to twice daily if needed, to achieve recommended amount of calcium per day. Continue teriparatide daily as instructed. *Ensure patient has dexterity to properly administer injections.* If not, need to discuss switching to alternative treatment option. *OT personnel would encourage the client to: (1) maintain strength through desired activities and exercise, in order to reduce fall risk, (2) limit alcohol consumption, (3) quit smoking, if indicated, and (4) use protective measures to reduce stress on the client's skeletal framework. The latter includes limiting heavy lifting, sliding or pushing objects when possible, and/or delegating if the task will present risk to the client.*

*CNS*, Central nervous system; *NSAIDs*, nonsteroidal antiinflammatory drugs; *PPI*, proton pump inhibitor.

**CASE EXAMPLE 14.2**   Over-the-Counter and Dietary Supplement Use

**Subjective**

MD is a 75-year-old male who requested a medication review to assess the several supplements he takes. "Are they all okay to take?" Client asks about adding St. John's wort to help his low mood.

**Past Medical History**

Type 2 diabetes, depression, hyperlipidemia, glaucoma, neuropathy, osteoarthritis in knees bilaterally; tremor in right hand

**Medications**

*Prescription medications:* atorvastatin 20 mg daily at bedtime, brimonidine 0.1% eye drops twice daily, citalopram 10 mg once daily

*OTC:* Ibuprofen 200 mg, three tablets before activity

*Vitamins and supplements:* alpha-lipoic acid (ALA) 100 mg once daily; vitamin B12 1000 µg daily; turmeric 600 mg per capsule, two capsules daily; glucosamine 1500 mg per two tablets, one tablet daily; Krill Oil (contains 1000 mg of omega-3 fatty acids) per capsule, 1 capsule daily

**Allergies:** NKDA

**Social history:** Client lives alone; attends senior center most days of the week for social activities and lunch. No longer drinks alcohol. Lost 27 kg over past several years as part of monitored weight loss program. No history of tobacco use. Client walks regularly "when his knees allow [him] to."

**Objective:** height 5 ft. 8 in.; weight 88 kg

**Assessment**

**Dietary supplements:** Client takes ALA and vitamin B12 for neuropathy symptoms in feet, states he is not sure if helping. He has been taking glucosamine for 3 months with no improvement in pain; just started turmeric and states no difference in pain yet. He also takes Krill Oil because he heard it is "good for you," but finds it very expensive. St. John's wort interacts with citalopram (and all selective serotonin reuptake inhibitor [SSRI] medications).

**Arthritis:** Client takes ibuprofen for bilateral knee pain about 5 days/week; however, has not informed his physician.

**Glaucoma:** Client has arthritis and noticeable tremor (untreated), which impacts ability to instill eye drops.

**Plan**

(Occupational therapy personnel would include in the client intervention a discussion of the individual's medication, supplements, and vitamin use; especially reinforce the pharmacist's recommendations that are in italics; and encourage the client to obtain clarifying information as indicated.)

**Supplements and vitamins:** ALA for peripheral neuropathy is *not harmful, but evidence for benefit is weak; client might wish to discontinue it.*

Client also takes vitamin B$_{12}$ for peripheral neuropathy; benefits are uncertain in presence of normal B$_{12}$ levels. Need to confirm B$_{12}$ levels, which will help guide benefit-risk assessment.

Client takes glucosamine for knee pain, but effective dose in clinical studies is 1500 mg/day, so client is taking subtherapeutic dose. Appropriate trial duration is 3 months, therefore, recommend that client increase dose and continue for 3 months at full dose to ascertain effectiveness. *Recommend to discontinue if no benefit seen.*

Client asked about St. John's wort. This supplement has same mechanism as SSRI antidepressants (including citalopram) and he should not initiate it. Remind client of importance of checking with his pharmacist before adding any supplement.

Client concerned about cost of Krill Oil. Krill Oil has no advantage over other fish oil products. However, fish oil is of questionable benefit for primary prevention of cardiovascular disease, according to most recent research. Thus, recommend stopping Krill Oil.

**Arthritis:** Ibuprofen offers some relief for patient to engage in physical occupations. Recommend to add acetaminophen if needed for additional pain control. *The individual may also be encouraged to bathe before engaging in activities that are primarily physical, as the warm water will increase blood flow and frequently reduce or prevent pain associated with these activities. Ensure good walking shoes; ask physician about use of knee brace or other recommendations.*

**Glaucoma:** Review and confirm proper eye-drop administration technique with client. *Obtain eye-drop guide for client due to hand tremor. Also, lying on his back on the bed to administer drops might be helpful. Occupational therapy can provide strategies for managing daily activities to mitigate effects of hand tremor and any related low vision.*

*OTC,* Over the counter.

*The complete listing of the Bibliography and Chapter Questions and Answers are available in the accompanying enhanced eBook version included with the print purchase of this textbook. Visit Elsevier eBooks+ (eBooks.Health.Elsevier.com) to access this content.*

CHAPTER 15

# Neurology and Cognition in Aging and Everyday Life

*Kristen Kehl-Floberg, MSOT, OTR/L, BCG and Dorothy Farrar Edwards, PhD*

## CHAPTER OUTLINE

## OBJECTIVES

- State the concepts, strengths, and limitations of theories of the aging brain
- Understand current evidence on aging, brain health, and occupational performance
- Connect the science of cognitive aging with occupational performance and participation
- Select reliable and valid assessment tools for evaluating the cognitive contributions to occupational performance of older adult clients
- Suggest best clinical practices for balancing agency, safety, and wellness in older adults with normal cognition

## Overview

Cognitive function is fundamental to daily life, yet it is one of the most complex phenomena of human existence. Occupational therapy practice with older adults exists at the intersection of aging, brain health, and occupational performance. "Normal" brain aging actually starts in early adulthood and accelerates into old age, the result of changes in the brain across the life course. The privilege and challenge of supporting older adults experiencing cognitive aging is to honor their years of experience, knowledge, and wisdom, while accurately characterizing cognitive contributions to occupational performance changes resulting from normal aging.

This chapter presents a review of scientific perspectives and evidence on the aging brain, a description of occupational therapy approaches for cognitive aging, inventories of cognitive assessment tools, and a short discussion of future directions of research and practice.

## Cognition: Definition and Epidemiology

*Cognition* is defined as the ability to think, learn, reason, and remember (Jankovic et al., 2022). Cognitive abilities provide us with the capacity to navigate the world in which we live, and are fundamental to occupational performance (Royall et al., 2007). *Cognitive loss* refers to a decrease from a previous baseline cognitive level that affects a person's ability to manage the roles and responsibilities of everyday life. *Cognitive aging* is the developmental change in cognition that occurs as the brain matures. Although cognitive aging has been thought of as only losses and occurring only in old age, it is now understood that cognitive aging includes a balance of gains as well as losses, and begins as early as the third decade (Salthouse, 2019).

Even subtle cognitive changes affect occupational performance because instrumental activities of daily living (IADLs) are characterized by cognitive complexity (Cornelis et al., 2017). Assessment and interventions to address late-life cognitive change are crucial areas of competence for occupational therapists working with older adults (Giles et al., 2020). According to the Centers for Disease Control and Prevention's Behavioral Risk Factor Surveillance System (BRFSS) survey (2015–2018), one in nine US adults over age 45 reported memory problems that have worsened over the past year, and about one-third of this group reported that this limited their ability to complete IADLs (Centers for Disease Control and Prevention, 2020); however, fewer than half of those reporting cognitively related IADL limitations discussed these issues with their primary health-care provider. Rigorous assessment of cognition is crucial when there is a question of whether a client's cognitive changes are normal or problematic (Box 15.1).

What's "Normal" and What's "Impaired"?

Whether, how, and in what way normal age-related cognitive changes transition to what may be considered pathological decline has been difficult to characterize. Although part of normal processes, cognitive changes are often felt as undesirable or limiting by those experiencing them (da Costa et al., 2016). Is this, then, "normal," or "pathological," or something else? Additional challenges arise in the actual definition and description of their experiences; mild impairments are often missed on clinical screening tools and clients are informed they don't meet any criteria for "significant" decline, despite the clients' experiences. The evolution of screening and diagnostic criteria (Lindbergh et al., 2016), the inherent challenges of studying longitudinal change in cognitive skills (Jankovic et al., 2022), and the limited number of studies of mild cognitive impairment and middle-age cognitive aging compared to studies of older adults and major neurocognitive disorder (NCD, previously "dementia") (Hughes et al., 2018) all create challenges to getting older adults with questions about their cognitive changes the help they may desire. OT practitioners can match functional cognition assessments with daily activities that the client finds challenging, thereby helping to bridge these gaps and support healthy cognitive aging.

## Theoretical Frameworks of the Aging Brain

The brain is the connective nexus between the person, environment, occupation, and performance. We engage our entire lifetime of experiences through the nervous system as the brain coordinates meaningful responses to, and participation in, these experiences through an exquisite network of perception, interpretation, purposeful action, and learning. Many scientific and clinical perspectives have been proposed to understand this phenomenal structure's aging process. Below we present several frameworks that are useful in occupational therapy practice with older adults.

### Biological Theories of the Aging Brain

Biological aging theories focus on the balance between cell death (senescence) and regeneration, with the goal of understanding why and how organisms age. Several biological theories of aging inform neurobiological theories and divide roughly into two camps: *damage* theories concerning oxidative stress, and *program* theories explaining genetic/epigenetic control of cellular and physiologic system processes (da Costa et al., 2016; Nakamura et al., 2017). Damage theory holds that protein damage from oxidative species is irreversible, which disrupts protein homeostasis (Nakamura et al., 2017). This may contribute to diseases involving protein damage in neurons, for instance, tauopathies such as Parkinson or Alzheimer diseases, which are characterized by excessive accumulation of protein and cellular waste (da Costa et al., 2016). In program theory, the metabolic signaling pathways are of interest, which may help explain cognitive decline comorbid with metabolic disease in many older adults (Lee et al., 2018; Nakamura et al., 2017). Program theory has

informed evidence that *epigenetic* factors (e.g., social and chemical environment, diet, and activity) moderate genetic expression (Akbarian et al., 2013). One clinically important insight from program theory is that the health trajectory of an aging brain can be supported and moderated by behavioral and external supports.

## Cognitive Aging and Development

In a shift from the biological assumptions of aging as an accumulation of losses, the *Cognitive Aging* perspective describes cognition in aging as a spectrum of normal, progressive changes that vary widely across individuals (Institute of Medicine, 2015). It constructs cognition as an interaction between *potential* and *limits*. Cognitive Aging classifies cognitive abilities into cognitive *mechanics* and *pragmatics* (or *crystallized* and *fluid* intelligence). One widely accepted model proposed by Baltes posits a mechanism for adapting to age-related cognitive changes. Age-related cognitive change is modeled as "selective optimization with compensation," a shifting balance between the two types of intelligence in service of function (Baltes, 1993). Crystallized intelligence facilitates automaticity, management of cognitive load, and over-learned skill; it includes procedural (or semantic) memory, and the fund of knowledge from accumulated experiences. Fluid intelligence facilitates planning, problem-solving, insight, and adaptation to novelty; it includes executive functions, attention, retrieval, and prospective memory (Harada et al., 2013). Crystallized abilities are supported by genetic, biological, and physiological structures, and demonstrate minor decline with age; fluid abilities appear to be more impacted by epigenetic factors, social determinants of health (SDOH), and between-person variation, and are more apparent in cognitive loss. Because cognition is a keystone to independence throughout adult life, a model that accounts for interactions between ability and decline is a powerful framework for occupational therapy practitioners (Royall et al., 2014).

## Psychological Theories of the Aging Brain
### Neuropsychology: Hierarchically Organized Structural Correlates of Behavior

Starting around the middle of the 19th century, scientists interested in the mind began attempting to understand human behavior and intelligence through experimental inquiry (Bloom, 2013). Early experimental psychologists believed they could answer questions about observable human behavior by identifying relationships between specific aspects of the human mind and specific anatomical parcels within the brain. The structural and functional picture of the brain that developed through these experiments was anatomically apportioned and hierarchical (ascending in complexity from brainstem to cerebellum to cerebrum) (Bloom, 2013). This perspective is still used today in the domain-focused assessment instruments based on these early localization studies. The multidisciplinary field of *neuroscience* which coalesced in the 1960s (Bloom, 2013; Dekkers, 2017) led to the discovery of interconnected neural networks reflected in the current multidisciplinary approach to cognitive health care for older adults, of which OT is a part.

## Everyday Cognition

Arising from applied psychology's interest in ecologically valid constructs of cognition, *Everyday Cognition* (EC) assesses memory and thinking skills using observation of decisions a client makes when presented with hypothetical contexts, settings, or tasks that represent those encountered by the individual in their life (Ayotte et al., 2012; Poon et al., 1993). Focusing on instrumental and social-emotional problem-solving, EC attempts to leverage the experiences, knowledge, and proficiency an adult brings to their completion of cognitively challenging daily tasks. This is its main divergence from neuropsychological assessments, which by contrast seek to isolate cognitive skill domains through novel and contextless challenges. EC assessment uses stimulus-response learning principles to structure paper-and-pencil questions measuring memory of a "stimulus" in hypothetical scenarios from daily life. It must be emphasized that, for the majority of these EC assessments, the client does not need to perform the actual task, only demonstrate reasoning on paper.

## Systems Theory Models

One of the most enduring impacts of the mid-twentieth-century shifts in scientific thought was the development of Systems Theory. Systems Theory describes complex systems consisting of *inputs*, *throughputs*, and *outputs* (Dekkers, 2017), and can be applied to cognition in several OT models. The Person-Environment-Occupation-Performance model (Law et al., 1996), one of the most widely used conceptual OT frameworks, is built on this framework. In PEOP, the output (cognitive performance) is supported by aspects from inputs (person, environment, and occupation) and shaped by through-put (transactions between P, E, and O).

The *Dynamic Interactional Model (DIM)* was built on the same foundation as PEOP but focuses more precisely on cognition (Toglia, 2018). DIM incorporated research on how people with normal cognition learn, process, and apply information. In DIM, cognitive performance is continuously shaped by the co-effects of person, occupation, and environment; DIM adds the unique contribution of a detailed delineation of several person factors of cognition. These are (1) person-level context, (2) several levels of self-awareness, and (3) *metacognition*, or the ability to use strategies and process skills to self-monitor and adapt during performance. DIM also recognizes contributions of the environment and the occupation's attributes in performance but emphasizes person-level skills and strategies. DIM is the foundational framework of several OT assessments and interventions including the Multicontext approach, the CO-OP approach, and the Weekly Calendar Planning Activity (see Table 15.4 for assessment tools).

Several other models of cognition have been developed for health-care interventions on a systems theory framework, including *Distributed Cognition* (Hollan et al., 2000; Hutchins,

1995) and the Systems Engineering Initiative for Patient Safety (SEIPS 2.0) (Holden et al., 2013). These models operationalize the environment's instrumentality to cognition and provide systems theory process modeling that is effective for evaluating health maintenance routines of older adults (Holden et al., 2015; Werner et al., 2021).

## Functional Cognition

The Functional Cognition framework is an OT approach that orients cognition unambiguously within occupational performance (Wesson & Giles, 2019). Functional cognition assessment and intervention approaches are performance-based, completed in context with the tools of daily life. Functional cognition interventions are structured to build on clients' priorities, assets, limitations, and the support required for success. The framework aims to describe the contribution of cognition to performance and to scale in-context performance for evaluation and scoring. It is inherently strengths-based, with intervention findings designed to inform treatment planning. FC shares common aspects of performance noted in the Systems Theory approaches. FC includes a range of OT evaluation approaches and instruments. See the Assessment section, and Table 15.4. Box 15.2 highlights cognitive frameworks for practice with older adults that come from the OT discipline.

## Population Health: Social Determinants of Health

Population health perspectives on cognition and aging are contextualized within communities and populations. To illustrate the relationships between cognition, aging, and the social and physical environments that affect whole populations, the US Department of Health and Human Services uses the SDOH model (DHHS Office of Disease Prevention and Health Promotion, 2020). This framework is based on population health evidence that exposure to different (often overlapping) conditions moderates brain health in aging. The Midlife in the United States Study (MIDUS) is a longitudinal study of adults from early midlife through old age (Hughes et al., 2018) exploring the role of psychological, social, and biological factors on age-related variations in health, including key aspects of cognition. Analyses of the MIDUS data have found that education and long-term stress accounted for differences in cognitive aging, and that ongoing engagement in meaningful activities promoted cognitive function in later life.

MIDUS and other longitudinal studies show that the effects of SDOH on cognitive abilities in late life are nested. For instance, the neighborhood of residence, a physical environment SDOH, predicts chronic health outcomes (Durfey

---

**BOX 15.2**  Cognition Frameworks by and for OT

- Dynamic Interaction Model (DIM)
- Functional Cognition
- Cognitive Functional Evaluation (CFP) Process

et al., 2019; Kind & Buckingham, 2018) and cognitive decline (Mayeda et al., 2016). The physical environment is in turn shaped by public policy, another SDOH. The remaining effects of "redlining" city planning policies (Mujahid et al., 2021), accessibility of the built environment for atypically abled individuals (Gell et al., 2015), and exposure to neurotoxins such as heavy metals from industrial pollution or lead-based paint (Paul et al., 2019), are all examples of these overlapping SDOH. SDOH also account for protective and supporting forces on aging and cognition. Education and sustained social engagement appear to positively moderate cognitive decline even in individuals who have imaging evidence of cortical atrophy (Perry et al., 2022; Wilson & Bennett, 2017).

## Evidence: The Science of Brain Aging and OT's Role

### Age-Related Physiologic Changes Impacting the Aging Brain

Normal aging includes physiologic, mental, and cognitive changes. This section lists changes that are typical of healthy aging, and ways OT can support brain health in aging adults.

### Structural Changes in the CNS and PNS

Structural changes in the brain are typical of normal aging and may be due to neuronal death, decrease in connectivity, or beta-amyloid protein accumulations at non-pathological levels (da Costa et al., 2016) (see also Chapter 9). Decreases in white matter mass and function, particularly in the orbito-frontal cortex, contribute most to these changes. Gray matter growth peaks around age 20, then declines steadily throughout life (Callaert et al., 2014); by late life, this is most notable in the prefrontal cortex, but it also affects temporal and hippocampal volume. This loss affects *neuroplasticity*, the adaptive re-routing of signal in response to demand through dendritic recruitment, growth, and pruning. Neuroadaptation occurs throughout the life course but becomes less efficient with advancing age. While adaptation still occurs in response to new challenges, decreased dendritic connectivity may cause learning to take more trials over a longer duration.

Changes to the peripheral nervous system's ability to efficiently conduct signals contribute to decreases in sensoriperceptual accuracy and reliability (see Chapter 9). This affects cognition by reducing the input to the central processing centers, which both provide less raw data for cognitive processes and reduce the baseline stimulation of the brain.

### Cardiovascular, Cardiopulmonary, and Metabolic Health

A healthy brain relies on a healthy heart, and this relationship's impact increases with age. Despite its small size (just 2% of lean body mass), the brain's metabolic activity requires 15% to 20% of the body's blood flow at rest (Kety, 1950). Normal cardiopulmonary changes can cause, or increase the risk of, decreased cognition. Lower blood volume is a factor in orthostatic hypotension which can lead to syncope and head trauma, and decreased lung function can limit available

intracerebral oxygen. Subcortical structures such as the hippocampus and limbic system have less circulatory redundancy than the cortex, so these regions tend to be vulnerable to disrupted oxygen transport (Markus, 2004). For example, persons with heart failure (HF) have been found to have about 2.6 times the incidence of cognitive decline (95% CI, 0.83 to 3.8) compared to the general population (Cannon et al., 2017). Metabolic disease, especially diabetes, is a single risk factor for cognitive decline, and an interactive risk factor with other CV disease risk factors.

### Sleep

Healthy sleep is crucial to all brain health and function, including cognition. Sleep disruption among otherwise-healthy older adults impacts cognitive aging, particularly higher-order cognition. Chronic sleep deprivation has been found to reduce the effectiveness of the glymphatic system, a waste-clearing cerebral metabolic process that appears important in managing accumulation of amyloid-beta (Bishir et al., 2020). Sleep disruption may contribute to or exacerbate age-related decreases in prospective memory (Fine et al., 2018). In a large cross-sectional study, Winer et al. (2021) found that hyper- or hyposomnolence, fractured sleep, and disrupted circadian cycles correlated with cognitive decline, greater amyloid-beta deposition, worse cardiovascular health, and depression. Thus, assessing and supporting sleep is a vital tool for supporting cognition.

### Cognition in Aging

A spectrum of cognitive change is consistently observed from middle through older age (Harada et al., 2013; Hughes et al., 2018; Salthouse, 2019). Although processing speed slows, global cognition is generally spared (Calso et al., 2016) potentially due to compensation or "cognitive reserve" (accumulated skills for cognitive flexibility and learning).

### Executive Functions

Frontal cortex functions are highly networked and complex, extending to the thalamus, the basal ganglia, sensory cortices, and back again; thus frontal functions may be affected by other cortical or subcortical structure changes. Some executive functions appear stable in aging, such as automatic inhibition, many aspects contributing to flexibility, and first-order theory of mind (an aspect of empathy and understanding others). Many executive functions rely on fluid intelligence, which tends to decline more than crystallized intelligence. Many people notice increased response time, decreased selective and divided attention, and increased time required to learn something new as they age. Hence, decision-making may become less efficient (Brown & Ridderinkhof, 2009). See Table 15.1 for a summary of normal executive function changes.

### Memory

Memory is complex and crucial to identity and the accumulation of experiences that create the wisdom treasured in older age. Typical normal aging involves both gains and losses in memory. Episodic memory declines very gradually from

**TABLE 15.1** Executive Function Changes and OT Supports

| Process | Change | OT Coaching/Education/Support |
|---|---|---|
| Processing speed | Decreases slightly each decade (age 30+) | Allow more time in conversation and new learning |
| **Executive Functions** | | |
| Attention | Stable for simple tasks, decreases for complex tasks requiring divided attention | Teach *chunking* (breaking a task into smaller parts with simpler cognitive demands in each part)<br>Reduce cognitive load by eliminating distraction |
| Insight/awareness | Stable to slight decrease | Coach on self-checking errors<br>Support using attention and planning strategies |
| Planning | May be affected by prospective memory | Establish reminders and scheduling devices embedded in routines |
| Visuospatial | Stable for simple tasks, decreases for complex tasks | Stepwise task aids such as checklists<br>Decrease environmental clutter |
| Learning | Requires more trials over longer period<br>Less efficient neuroadaptation | Grade novel skill development in small increments<br>Teach chunking and backwards-chaining (set the task up so that the client does just the last step, then progress "backward" through the steps one at a time).<br>Facilitate practice of new skills or strategies<br>Allow multiple trials and failures<br>Use teach-back |
| Reasoning | Slight decrease (age 50+)<br>Decision-making may become less efficient | Encourage allowing extra time for decisions, simplifying choices |
| Emotional regulation | Stable first-order theory of mind (*empathy and understanding of others*) | This skill is an asset contributing to caregiving skill and wisdom. |
| Inhibition | Stable | Use to compensate for decreased processes |

middle age, while semantic memory remains stable until late in old age. Non-declarative procedural (or semantic) memory remains stable and may increase throughout life. Memory changes may be underpinned by the separate change of decreased processing speed. Crystallized functions such as procedural memory relate to familiar and well-practiced knowledge and skills. However, decreased processing speed may partially explain decreased working memory, which can make it more difficult to retrieve and use knowledge, reason in novel situations, use metacognitive strategies and inhibit habitual responses. See Table 15.2 for OT strategies to support normal memory changes.

### History of Depression

Longitudinal and cross-sectional analyses have found associations between any history of depressive symptoms and decreased white matter and cognitive performance, but have not shown it to significantly affect long-term cognitive outcomes (Dotson et al., 2009). Depression can mimic symptoms of neurocognitive disorder (NCD), so screen for depression with clients reporting recent changes in their cognitive function (see also Chapter 17).

### Sensory Perceptual Processing

Coordinated and cross-linked associations between sensory inputs underlie cognition and functional cognitive performance. Older adults have been found to rely more than

younger adults on multiple inputs during social cognitive processing (Chaby et al., 2015), perhaps to adjust processing to age-related sensory loss. Presbycusis is positively correlated with age (see also Chapter 10) and has been found to strongly associate with cognitive decline (Griffiths et al., 2020; Johnson et al., 2021; Slade et al., 2020) suggesting that the brain relies on auditory input about the environment to maintain orientation and reserve (Uchida et al., 2021). Olfaction has also been found to diminish markedly in early cognitive decline (Tian et al., 2022). See Table 15.3 for how OT can support performance with normal perceptual changes.

### Implementing Evidence on the Neurology of Aging Through the OT Process

Normal cognitive aging is not a pathological process, and thus will not require intervention. However, clients with normal cognition are often referred for skilled OT related to other issues, and clients, caregivers/partners, or cross-disciplinary colleagues all may have reason to ask for an evaluation. In these cases, OT's role is to *delineate and support the contribution of cognition to occupational performance.* Cognition is not assessed by OT in the same way that a psychologist, speech/language pathologist, or gerontologist would assess it; inasmuch as cognition contributes to *performance*, it is its *contribution to performance* that is assessed.

**TABLE 15.2** Memory Process Changes and OT Supports

| Process | Change | OT Coaching/Education/Support |
|---|---|---|
| Prospective<br>*Planning for intended actions you will need to take in the future* | Decreases (age 70+)<br>Worsens with poor sleep | Embed health-promoting habits into routines (e.g., structuring spatiotemporal reminders, visual reminders, and checklists for complex routines).<br>Support sleep hygiene<br>Support attention (e.g., limit distractions) |
| Procedural/Semantic<br>*How to do something. Factual knowledge, motor learning, and procedures you've learned.* | Stable<br>Can be refreshed/cultivated | Encourage engagement with current events through reading, community outings, and participation in civic or faith groups |
| Working memory > Immediate recall<br>*Holding and retrieving 5–9 pieces of info for recall within 30 s* | Decreases slightly beginning in the 40s | Externalize info they will need in a moment, e.g., write down a phone number they must call as soon as they hang up, or use a placeholder while reading a recipe. |
| Working memory > Short-term/delayed recall<br>*Holding and recalling info after a few minutes to an hour* | Decreases slightly beginning in the 40s | Externalize info they will need in a few hours, e.g., plan a shopping outing by listing the places they need to travel in an efficient order, or writing down a new address they are going to and placing it in their wallet. |
| Retrieval<br>*Retrieving information from mid- to long-term memory without cues* | Decreased | Structure cueing through embedded reminders such as lists, electronic calendaring/reminder apps, or checklists for complex routines. |
| Temporal/Episodic<br>*Recalling an event, or the temporal order of sequential events, after a delay of weeks, months, or years* | Stable<br>Tends to be robust to age-related white matter changes | |

Note: Terminology sometimes differs between clinical and scientific vernaculars. Some terms may define multiple abilities depending on the audience/speaker.

**TABLE 15.3** Perceptual Process Changes and OT Supports

| Process | Change | OT Coaching/Education/Support |
|---|---|---|
| **\*Support Multi-Modal Inputs\*** | | |
| Tactile | Stable | Maximize the use of touch to supplement abilities that are diminishing. |
| Audition | Presbycusis is strongly associated with cognitive decline | Encourage hearing assessment and use of aids if prescribed.<br>Create a plan to sustain regular social engagement with adaptations for hearing loss.<br>Maximize sensory cross-linking and environmental stimuli through a rich environment, visual scanning, frequent social interaction. |
| Olfaction | Diminishes >75–80 years<br>May predict cognitive decline | Screen for mild cognitive impairment.<br>Screen for depression.<br>Assess client's favorite food characteristics other than flavor (e.g., texture, color, temperature) and help generate a list of nourishing foods they will still be able to enjoy (check food restrictions per medication list).<br>Create a checklist or chart for hydration and consistent meal/snack times.<br>Assess changes to food routines (e.g., spouse no longer in the home, decreased energy for cooking, moved further from grocery store).<br>Emphasize the social aspect of gatherings around food (e.g., continue a long-standing coffee outing with friends even if flavors are less enjoyable).<br>Design a system for labeling perishables with a "toss-by" date. |
| Vision | Vision-related falls and fall risk increase risk of head trauma and social isolation, both of which threaten cognition. | Use low-vision support strategies to decrease risk for falls and support safe community mobility options.<br>Encourage planning transportation options with family and community resources to prevent isolation. |

## Assessment: Discerning the Contribution of Cognition to Occupational Performance

Occupational therapists use a range of cognitive evaluation and intervention approaches. Instruments for functional cognitive evaluation are summarized in Table 15.4 (for an expanded review, see Wesson et al., 2016). We recommend a combination of observation of performance (non-standardized or standardized) and cognitive domain-specific skill assessment. Several frameworks provide guidance. Baseline Cognitive Screening (BCS) (Edwards et al., 2019) and the Cognitive Functional Evaluation-Extended (CFE-E) (Erez & Katz, 2019) are two well-developed approaches we cover in this text. Practitioners may choose elements from each approach that fit their time constraints, the relative position of their assessment in the continuum of care, and multidisciplinary team roles.

### Baseline Cognitive Screening

BCS uses standardized neuropsychological instruments in two stages; screening, and subsequent diagnostic testing as indicated, (Edwards et al., 2019). *Screening* tools are the most sensitive to change and are tuned to say whether a person may, potentially, have a cognitive impairment that impacts their function. Should a client's result on a screening test indicate potential impairment, a *diagnostic* tool is then used to confirm whether it exists, and its extent. This sequential approach progresses in specificity and predictive value, mirroring a biomedical assessment process prevalent in medical settings in which it may be most practical.

### Cognitive Functional Evaluation-Extended

The CFE-E consists of five stages: (1) interview/cognitive profile, (2) assessment of cognition within functional performance, (3) tests of single cognitive domains, (4) environments, and (5) quality of life and/or well-being (Erez & Katz, 2018; Erez & Katz, 2019). The CFE-E aims to assess the interactive complexity of cognitive contributions to performance, safety, and well-being; to this end, it is structured to include assessments of the personal, environmental, and occupational co-effects with cognition. These contexts interact with impairments, altering the degree of disability experienced. CFE-E is developed on the theoretical and taxonomical foundation of the *Occupational Therapy Practice Framework: Domain and Practice* (American Occupational Therapy Association, 2020), and (in its expansion to incorporate environment and quality of life) the PEOP model (Law et al., 1996). Because of this common language, it provides a model for occupational therapy interventions and OT's unique contribution in multidisciplinary collaboration.

Regardless of the approach chosen, assessment instruments must be checked for appropriateness to the population being served. Box 15.3 discusses the importance of this step for assessing cognitive health in older adults.

## TABLE 15.4  Cognitive Assessment Instruments Used in Functional Cognitive Assessment

| Instrument | Type | Training Required | ADL | Cues |
|---|---|---|---|---|
| **Screening Instruments** | | | | |
| Menu Task Assessment (MTA) | PB | No | IADL | Yes |
| Behavior Rating Inventory for Executive Function- Adult version (BRIEF-A) | IR, SR | No | IADL | N/A |
| Medi-Cog | NP/PB | No | None | No |
| Montreal Cognitive Assessment (MoCA) | NP | Yes | None | Some |
| Brief Inventory of Mental Status (BIMS) | NP | No | None | No |
| Saint Louis University Mental Status Examination (SLUMS) | NP | No | None | No |
| Trail Making Test (Parts A and B) | NP | No | None | Some |
| Short Blessed Test (SBT) | NP | No | None | No |
| Alzheimer's Disease Cooperative Study ADL scale (ADCS-ADL) | IR, SR | No | I/BADL | NA |
| Lawton IADL scale | IR, SR | No | IADL | NA |
| **Diagnostic Instruments** | | | | |
| Weekly Calendar Planning Activity (WCPA) | PB | No | IADL | Yes |
| Executive Function Performance Test (EFPT) | PB | No | IADL | Yes |
| Performance Assessment of Self-Care Skills (PASS) | PB | No | IADL | Yes |
| Assessment of Motor and Process Skills (AMPS) | PB | Yes | I/BADL | No |
| Performance Quality Rating Scale (PQRS) | PB | No | I/BADL | No |
| Kettle Test | PB | No | IADL | Some |

*D*, Diagnostic; *IADL*, instrumental activities of daily living; *IR*, informant report; *NP*, neuropsychological; *PB*, performance-based; *S*, screening; *SR*, self-report.
The MTA is from Edwards et al. (2019); the BRIEF-A is from Roth et al. (2005); the Medi-Cog is from Anderson et al. (2008); the MoCA is from Nasreddine et al. (2005); the BIMS is from Saliba et al. (2012); the SLUMS is from Tariq et al. (2006); the Trail Making Test is from Reitan (1932); the SBT comes from Blessed et al. (1968); the ADCS-ADL comes from Galasko et al. (1997); the Lawton IADL scale comes from Lawton and Brody (1969); the WCPA comes from Toglia (2015) ; the EFPT comes from Baum et al. (2008); the PASS comes from Rogers et al. (2016); the AMPS is from Fisher and Jones (2014); the PQRS is from Martini et al. (2015); the Kettle Test is from Hartman-Maeir et al. (2009).

**BOX 15.3**  Cognitive Testing in Diverse Populations

Many testing instruments contain bias due to over-representation of white participants in validation studies. New evidence exploring the phenomenon of higher incidence of neurocognitive disorder in Black versus white older adults suggests that many neuropsychological screening and diagnostic tests may contain racial bias, hence failing to accurately distinguish decline from preserved function in older Black adults. Weuve et al. (2018) followed participants in the Chicago Health and Aging Project for up to 18 years and found that older Black participants performed worse at baseline on four neuropsychological screening instruments than older white participants, but the rate of decline was similar across the two groups and was slower for Black participants' executive function (Weuve et al., 2018). This suggests that the test may underestimate cognitive ability across all cognitive levels in this group, potentiating over-diagnosis of decline. Additionally, sub-group analyses of normative samples have found different cut scores for different social groups on established tests. Milani et al. (2018) recommend Montreal Cognitive Assessment (MoCA) score thresholds that are lower for some racial and ethnic groups (Milani et al., 2018) compared to the initial normative sample in which racial demographics were not reported (Nasreddine et al., 2005). For whichever tool you use, obtain the latest psychometric evidence for your population to ensure you are interpreting the results fairly.

**BOX 15.4**  Client Self-Report of Functional Status

Self-report is the only modality we can use to assess experiences such as pain, quality of life, mood, and perspectives or attitudes. However, ***self-report alone should not be used to assess functional cognitive status***. It may be used to triangulate client's awareness of deficits and skills, but should not be relied on as the primary assessment modality because it requires the integration of cognitive skills such as memory, insight, safety and risk awareness, planning, and judgement, which can decrease in cognitive impairment (Okonkwo et al., 2009).

2014). Performance-based tests are also better at approximating the relationship between cognition and daily function, which is beneficial in an OT evaluation.

### Key Objectives: Awareness and Learning

Two cognitive domains are crucial for determining changes from normal cognitive aging and deciding on intervention approaches: *awareness* and *learning*. These two domains are nested; awareness is crucial to new learning, and learning from errors informs awareness. Awareness of deficits or skills is subdivided into three general levels: awareness of deficits/skills (or *intellectual* awareness), their real-time consequences (or *on-line* awareness), and their potential consequences (or *emergent* awareness). Subtle awareness deficits are a feature of amnestic mild cognitive impairment and early NCD, so are crucial to assess.

Tools for assessing awareness/insight and learning include:
- Triangulation, or identifying discrepancies between client report against observed performance in ADL and tests.
- Asking the client how they felt they did on a test or task.
- Cueing the client and observing their integration of the cue—do they correct course? (See Box 15.5.)
- Eliciting teach-back of any safety or other education provided.

### Considerations for Selecting an Approach (See Also Chapter 6)
#### Comprehensiveness

The CFE-E includes the greatest number of stages and assessment of concepts interrelated to cognition-related performance in daily life. BCS is comparatively narrow in focus, and as such its use should be predicated on a robust history and an understanding of the appropriateness of a test for the patient's diagnostic or population group.

#### Modality of Instruments

Tests may be cognitive domain-specific using a neuropsychologically based approach, performance-based (using structured or naturalistic task observation), or informant/self-report (to be used in addition, but not alone—see note in Box 15.4). Practice effects, or the achievement of a better score on a test through learning from repeated exposures, limits the use of neuropsychological tests for detecting subtle but functionally significant cognitive decline (Sanderson-Cimino et al., 2022). Review the chart thoroughly and inquire with family to assess testing history, use a test version that has not been used (if multiple forms are available) and do not re-use an instrument that is not designed for pre- and post-treatment testing with good test-retest reliability. Some performance-based tests avoid this issue through modifiable and dynamic test conditions so that practice is less likely to result in better performance (Puente et al.,

#### Observation of Occupational Performance

Structured observation through a standardized performance-based assessment is fundamental to cognitive assessment in OT. There are many excellent tools that provide structured observations of IADL performance (see Table 15.4). Unstructured IADL performance may be documented in terms of time to complete, errors and self-corrections made, cues required, safety risks noted, and client strategies for safe success. (A paper-and-pencil cognitive test is then compared to performance, and consistency/inconsistency between them is documented as support for intervention decisions.)

#### Observation of Environment

During task analysis, take note of the way the client sets up their surroundings, tools/materials, and medications or other health-management items. Observations may be enriched by posing open-ended questions concerning why the person has made these choices, and whether and how they help. Impacts of non-cognitive neurogenic impairments (e.g., hemiparesis,

BOX 15.5 Using Cues, or Not

Performance-based assessments have the benefit of being structured to permit the evaluator to test hypotheses about cognitive supports during the assessment. They integrate supports such as cueing and adaptations the client already employs in daily life (e.g., a medication list). In some instruments, cues may be scoring factors that contribute to both cut score values and intervention planning. The need for cues is then built into the intervention and goal planning, with a numeric score as support. For the purposes of assessing real-life performance, predicting service or caregiving needs, and creating effective intervention plans, offering cues to elicit best-possible performance is a practical divergence from singular reliance on decontextualized, domain-specific instruments in a neuropsychological "test-to-fail" approach, which generally forbid cueing. This is supported by the findings of Thomas and Marsiske (2014) who found that structured verbal cueing predicted change trajectories of cognitive performance on simulated ADL tests over time in older adults with and without MCI (Thomas & Marsiske, 2014). However, many tests forbid cueing. The standardized procedure of whichever test you choose must be followed faithfully to produce a useful finding.

**BOX 15.7** Resources for Planning and Self-Assessment

**Driving**
AARP Fitness to Drive Self-Assessment: http://fitness-todrive.phhp.ufl.edu/us/?intcmp=AE-ATO-ADS-ASSESS-ROW2-SPOT1
**Advance Directives** should be completed and notarized while cognition is still strong. https://www.nia.nih.gov/health/advance-care-planning-health-care-directives
Forms can vary from one state/county to another. State aging agencies, including legal guidance, may be found by searching for the client's area at https://eldercare.acl.gov/Public/Index.aspx

**Home Environment**
Home Safety Self-Assessment Tool (HSSAT): http://www2.erie.gov/seniorservices/sites/www2.erie.gov.seniorservices/files/uploads/Home%20Safety%20Self%20Assessment%20Booklet.pdf

**For Clients Who Are Caregivers**
Medline Plus: Caregiver Health: https://medlineplus.gov/caregiverhealth.html
Wisconsin Alzheimer's Institute Clinician and Caregiver training: https://wai.wisc.edu/dementia-capable-wisconsin/home-health-caregiver-education/

**BOX 15.6** Substitutions for Direct Observation of Activities of Daily Living

Because of their complexity and context-dependence, activities of daily living may not be practical to observe in some settings; in this case, use the occupational profile, observations of performance, and scores on standardized instruments to form recommendations on anticipated difficulties.

may not be able to effectively appraise their safety (da Costa et al., 2016).

IADL inquiry must include health management, driving and transportation, food and meal preparation, household management, financial management, caregiving, and leisure or social community participation; these are all keystones to safety and thriving.

### Intervention: Supporting Performance Throughout Age-Related Change

We have previously provided examples of OT support strategies for normal cognitive changes (see Tables 15.1–15.3). This section briefly describes decision tools and supports available to clients who demonstrate normal cognitive aging.

### Planning

Encourage clients to take advantage of their good cognitive health by planning for future needs. Creating advance directives, completing self-assessment of driving and home safety, engaging with caregiving supports if applicable, and creating a transition plan are time well spent. Caregivers are at higher risk for poor cognitive health outcomes secondary to activity restriction and social isolation; offer support resources and encourage them to check out their local Aging and Disabilities Resource Center. Tools available for free to consumers are listed in Box 15.7.

sensory deficits, or fatigue) may be distinguished through careful observation of this performance factor (Box 15.6).

### Impact on Occupational Performance: Activities of Daily Living

IADLs are crucial for OTs to assess and support. They are the most cognitively complex, layered, and interdependent responsibilities of adult life; this complexity makes them susceptible to errors, abandonment, or unsafe situations if cognitive changes occur, precipitating disability (Jekel et al., 2015). It is now well recognized and included in the diagnostic criteria for NCD that early decline can cause subtle but consequential decrements in IADL performance, particularly when the individual is under stress or in novel situations (Lindbergh et al., 2016; Rodakowski et al., 2014; Terhorst et al., 2017). Accurate self-appraisal of IADL performance is affected by age-related cognitive decline; for instance, older drivers with decreased insight

## CASE STUDY

Mr. E. is a 72 year-old man living in a medium sized city in a 2.5 story single-family home. He lives with and is the primary caregiver for his spouse, who has end-stage renal disease and moderate dementia. After retiring from his work as a high school math and science teacher, Mr. E. directed his neighborhood afterschool baseball program until his spouse began requiring 24/7 supervision three years ago. He drives and manages all household, financial, and medical routines. His medical history includes heart failure, atrial fibrillation, type 2 diabetes, and a car accident 40 years prior (restrained driver) resulting in concussion without loss of consciousness and left femoral neck fracture. You have received a referral for services for Mr. E. following a brief hospitalization for hyponatremia, dehydration, and decompensated heart failure. He is now back at home with new meds, has returned to driving, and is visited about daily by either his daughter who lives 30 minutes away or a neighbor. In the occupational profile, Mr. E. says he is most concerned about continuing to be able to take care of his spouse, but that this is getting more difficult because he can't leave her alone. When asked about what brought him to the hospital, he reports "I don't know what happened. My legs had gotten swollen and I just started feeling dizzy."

### Living for a Healthy Brain

Growing evidence suggests that choices such as controlling blood pressure, eating a plant-centered diet, and getting 150 minutes per week of moderate to vigorous physical activity (targeting aerobic, strength, and balance) has protective effects against cognitive decline and the onset of major NCD (Valenzuela et al., 2020; Zhao et al., 2018). The evidence on physical activity's preventative properties for cognitive decline is robust. Bauman et al. (2016) review found very strong evidence from clinical trials that both aerobic and strength training positively affected executive function, attention, and processing speed. This review also found evidence of a 28% reduction in the incidence of NCD, improved functional independence, larger hippocampal volumes, increased cerebral blood flow, and superior performance on cognitive tasks. Secondary prevention of cognitive impairment is also possible through physical activity's effect on cardiopulmonary function, metabolic health, hyperlipidemia, fall risk, and functional independence (see "Evidence: The Science of Brain Aging," this chapter). Evidence also suggests that social connectedness slows or reduces the impact of age-related cognitive changes including NCD (Wilson & Bennett, 2017). In addition to their singular effects, the three factors of sleep, nutrition, and physical activity may have interactive effects on cognition (Dominguez et al., 2021). While sleep disturbance has been found to independently contribute to short-term and chronic cognitive impairwment, more evidence is needed on interventions and best practices for sleep as primary prevention (Dominguez et al., 2021). Encourage clients to choose one or two areas they'd like to focus on and suggest ways to embed supports for these areas into existing meaningful routines.

### Emerging Areas

The Functional Cognitive approach has developed considerably in the past several decades. As such, many of these discoveries and developments have not reached the entire practicing body of OT. Thus we consider this to be an emerging practice area in the sense that practice uptake and feedback on this evidence is still evolving.

The use of machine learning and predictive modeling in health-care research is advancing rapidly and will likely result in new directions for practice and reimbursement. Because much of this research uses data from the electronic medical record (EMR), it is essential that OT practitioners document and/or advocate documentation of *functional performance*, not just assessment tool scores, in the medical records of OT clients. This will ensure that data on OT's impact on performance and cognitive disability is available for EMR-based analysis and that OT is hence included in future health-care models for aging adults.

## SUMMARY

Normal aging includes changes in functional cognition and the cognitively complex IADLs that rely on it. Many older adults naturally adjust and compensate for these changes with retained skills and new learning to continue to engage in occupations that are meaningful to them; however, health history, social history, and physiologic changes that increase in prevalence with advancing age all may complicate cognitive aging. OT can support older adults with normal age-related cognitive changes through rigorous assessment of functional cognition, and consultation and coaching to participate in activities that support cognitive health and planning for future cognitive changes.

*The complete listing of the Bibliography and Chapter Questions and Answers are available in the accompanying enhanced eBook version included with the print purchase of this textbook. Visit Elsevier eBooks+ (eBooks.Health.Elsevier.com) to access this content.*

## CHAPTER 16

# Cognitive Impairment, Dementia, and Occupational Therapy Intervention

*Ganesh M. Babulal, PhD, OTD, MSCI, MOT, OTR/L and Lili Liu, PhD, MSc (OT), BSc (OT), OT Reg. (Ont.)*

## CHAPTER OUTLINE

## OBJECTIVES

- Differentiate normal cognition from cognitive impairment and dementia
- Understand dementia as a global construct, various subtypes, and staging
- Identify screening measurements for ascertainment of cognitive impairment and dementia
- Describe the differential burden of dementia and how social determinants of health impact risk
- Examine the case studies and understand use of specific assessments, treatment options, and how client goals influence occupational therapy interventions

## Background and Operational Definitions

As the global population continues to grow (7.9 billion in 2021), there is a parallel increase among older adults (age 65 and older). The world population of older adults is projected to more than double from 700 million to 1.5 billion by mid-century. The corresponding growth is associated with an increase in life expectancy, where a 65-year-old can expect to live 17 years (2020)—this will increase to 19 years by 2050 (United Nations Department of Economic and Social Affairs Population Division, 2019). In a similar vein, the US population is aging rapidly, with over 10,000 adults turning 65 years daily. By 2050, more than 88 million Americans will be 65 years or older, representing more than a fifth of the population (see also Chapter 3). The accompanying longevity brings age-related changes in cognitive, motor, emotive, and sensory systems, which may confer a greater risk for chronic, non-communicable diseases. As a result, this will increase the global burden of disease, often impacting multiple systems and the growing prevalence of multimorbidity (two or more chronic conditions).

Cognition is abstractly defined as a global and dynamic set of mental processes involving perception, recall, reasoning, imagining, judgment, language, and problem-solving. Cognitive functioning can be parsed into specific substrates (e.g., executive function, working memory, divided attention) that may be studied, evaluated, and tested using questionnaires or tasks (see also Chapter 15). Conversely, emotions are a multidimensional process that innervates daily actions, goals, and behavior, often at a subconscious level. A simplistic dichotomy considers positive emotions are elicited when goals are met, control or satisfaction is gained, while negative emotions may arise during failure, pain, or discomfort (Ponzetti et al., 1999). There is a propensity to reduce and assess cognitive and emotive processes as independent constructs with little to no interaction. However, brain regions subserve both functions. For example, the amygdala supports attention and associative learning, while the dorsolateral prefrontal cortex is involved in emotional regulation and inhibition (Pessoa, 2008). Cognitive and emotive skills interact, support motivation, and afford completion of basic and instrumental activities of daily living (ADLs/IADLs), often in complex environmental settings.

While acute and acquired injuries may influence cognitive functioning in early to mid-life, chronic diseases like strokes and dementia may rise in prevalence in older adulthood to impact cognitive skills. An individual may experience a slow decline in cognitive abilities (e.g., processing speed, episodic recall); however, cognitive impairment and dementia are non-normative parts of aging. There is considerable variation in the cognitive functioning trajectory based on various individual risk factors, environmental affordances (or lack thereof), and daily activities. As a result, occupational therapy (OT) is optimally poised to intervene to support clients' independence in their daily activities based on their capabilities and environment.

## Dementia and Various Classifications

Dementia is an umbrella term that encompasses a group of symptoms that characterizes difficulty with memory, thinking, and communication, among others; in addition, it impacts an individual's ability to complete IADLs/ADLs. A decline in cognitive functioning typically begins with a gradual onset of mild symptoms (occasional memory loss, lapse in judgement) that advances to moderate impairment (IADL dependence, poor recall of recent events) and then progresses into a severe stage (ADL dependence, difficulty recognizing family or friends). In addition to changes in cognition, psychological changes in mood (depression, anxiety), personality, and neuropsychiatric symptoms (agitation, hallucination, delusions) can co-occur. There are multiple diseases and pathologies that impact the brain and influence the emergence of signs and symptoms of dementia. It is crucial to rule out potential reversible causes (e.g., diet, medication, hormonal imbalances) associated with conditions that may be classified or be termed "dementia" (see also Chapter 12). More importantly, dementia's progression is irreversible from *independence* to *assistance* and then complete *dependence*, which typifies the disease's time course irrespective of cause. Globally, approximately 55 million people are living with dementia. There is an average dementia prevalence of 8.8% in the United States among Americans aged 65 and older (Langa et al., 2017). In 2021, the estimated national cost of caring (acute, long-term care, hospice) for persons with dementia in the United States reached $355 billion USD, which did not include another $256.7 billion USD in unpaid caregiving provided by friends or family members (Alzheimer's Association, 2021). Typical forms of dementia include Alzheimer disease (AD), mixed (Vascular or Lewy body), Vascular, Lewy body, frontotemporal, and Parkinson disease dementia (PDD). Given the high cost of this debilitating and deadly set of diseases, it is essential to understand defining characteristics, including signs and symptoms, onset, progression, prognosis, and mortality.

## Alzheimer Disease

AD is the most common form of dementia (60% to 80% of cases), with an estimated 5.8 million US adults age 65 and older (Alzheimer's Association, 2021). By 2050, it is projected that number will increase to 12.7 million. Over the past 50 years, a venerable amount of research has examined the nosological complexities in diagnosing AD and analyzing the risk

factors. Age represents the single most significant risk factor, where the risk increases 2% to 5% for ages 65 to 74, 14% for ages 75 to 84, and 33% for age 85 and older. While several genes increase the risk for AD, the apolipoprotein E (APOE) e4 allele confers the greatest risk. An individual with a single copy of e4 has three times the risk, but two copies of e4 confers an 8- to 12-fold risk for developing AD (Loy et al., 2014). The lifetime risk for AD at age 65 or older is 21.1% for women and 11.6% for men, suggesting a higher risk for women (Chêne et al., 2015). The gold standard definition of AD is a pathological confirmation where the brain is preserved after death and examined for key proteins using stains that fluoresce under a microscope. However, given the limitations of that method, largely with access and cost, significant efforts were made over the past decade to find biomarkers in the body that may provide a glimpse or indicate that the disease has started. The progression of AD may be reimagined as a continuum. There is (1) a long preclinical stage (no symptoms), (2) an amnestic mild cognitive impairment (MCI) stage (mild symptoms), and (3) a dementia stage that encompasses a mild to severe progression.

## Preclinical Alzheimer Disease and Biomarkers

Preclinical AD is defined as a long asymptomatic period (15 to 20 years) when a person is cognitively normal, but the pathophysiological process of the disease has begun. This stage is operationalized as evidenced by abnormal levels measured by cerebrospinal fluid (CSF), imaging, and/or blood-based (plasma) biomarkers (Knopman et al., 2018; Sperling et al., 2011). Specifically, the hallmark of AD's pathophysiology is the abnormal accumulation of two key proteins: extracellular deposition of beta-amyloid (Aβ), more commonly known as plaques, and intracellular accumulation of tau or tangles. Abnormal levels of beta-amyloid or more colloquially termed as amyloid, and tau can be measured in CSF via lumbar puncture and via in vivo brain imaging using positron emission tomography (PET) and specific radioligands.

Before 2011, different diagnostic recommendations existed for defining the preclinical, amnestic, and symptomatic stages of AD. A conceptual model was proposed for the pathological-clinical continuum of AD with the caveat that not all individuals with biomarker evidence of AD will progress to the symptomatic stage (Sperling et al., 2011). The first stage concentrated solely on the degree of amyloid burden confirmed by either abnormal levels measured via PET or CSF biomarkers. The second stage added neurodegeneration as reflected by changes in several biomarkers, including CSF tau or ptau, hippocampal atrophy via magnetic resonance imaging (MRI), or network dysfunction via functional MRI. The third and final stage added cognitive decline as evidenced by subtle changes in daily activities, poor performance on cognitive tasks, or not meeting a clinical diagnosis for MCI. This tripartite staging, based on the emerging evidence at the time, excluded family history (e.g., autosomal dominant) or genetic risk (e.g., *APOE* gene) and was explicit in only being used for research (Sperling et al., 2011). However, since 2011, AD research has rapidly progressed with the development of new modalities and tracers (tau PET imaging) and biomarkers (plasma via blood-based).

## Mild Cognitive Impairment

Amnestic MCI is a transition phase due to AD characterized by continued brain changes from the preclinical stage coupled with very subtle impairment in a single cognitive domain, usually memory (Gauthier et al., 2006). Clients with MCI do not have significant impairment in their abilities to complete ADLs or IADLs. However, the client and their family and/or friends may notice these cognitive problems. The current prevalence of amnestic MCI is approximately 11.6 million Americans (Petersen et al., 2018). Among older adults with amnestic MCI, 15% will progress to AD within 2 years, and a third will progress within 5 years of diagnosis (Ward et al., 2013). Given the high rate of conversation for many clients, MCI represents the most salient manifestation of AD that is observable subjectively and objectively. Not all older adults with MCI will convert to AD. Those with amnestic MCI across multiple domains may have depression, or those with non-amnestic MCI (nonmemory-based) may convert to vascular or Lewy body dementia (Petersen, 2016). As a person ages, multimorbidity (two or more chronic conditions) increases and may reduce the sensitivity and specificity of a diagnosis. Additional laboratory, clinical, and neuropsychological testing can help to improve the accuracy of an amnestic MCI diagnosis.

## Mild Alzheimer Disease

As the pathological burden increases (entorhinal, frontal, and temporal cortices), there will be more difficulty remembering names or recent events. The memory loss will influence the successful completion of IADLs. A formal clinical diagnosis of AD is usually made during this stage. Most clients can function independently in daily life but require support (supervision to minimal assistance). There are emerging impairments in divided attention, reaction time, and juggling multiple tasks. Other symptoms include repetitive statements, a slower pace of activity, more difficulty with finances like paying bills, decreased judgment to complete some tasks safely like turning off a stove, and decreased spatial-temporal awareness with familiar places (e.g., getting lost). Physical abilities like range of motion, grip strength, and gait are intact and do not decline. While mood and personality may change, the client will continue to prefer their favorite activities, meals, and routines. A thorough interview with the client and a separate interview with a family member or friend can discern key symptoms distinctive to this stage and aid in a confident diagnosis. The mild AD stage can last for 2 to 10 years.

## Moderate Alzheimer Disease

In the moderate or longest stage of AD, the neuronal loss has spread into more significant portions of the frontal, occipital, temporal cortices, and hippocampus. Because these regions are directly impacted by the pathology, more observable impairments are observed with language, reasoning, and motor and sensory processing. Signs and symptoms most salient in this stage are increasing memory loss, reduced orientation to place and time, shortened attention span, and struggling to recognize distant relatives or friends/acquaintances. Overlearned behaviors like reading comprehension, verbal communication, and writing are impaired. A client in the moderate stage is often unable to follow a conversation or attend to a single person speaking in a room with others, and has difficulty organizing thoughts and adapting to new situations or unexpected changes. Motor planning is also impaired, like selecting the correct utensil to eat a meal or getting out of a chair. IADLs like driving, preparing a complex dinner, or managing finances are too difficult and will require maximum assistance. ADLs, including getting dressed, bathing, or brushing, require minimum to moderate assistance. There is a noted loss of impulse control characterized by making inappropriate comments or using vulgar language in front of others. There is an increasing prevalence of neuropsychiatric symptoms like delusions, hallucinations, mood swings, agitation, paranoia, and personality changes. These behaviors may become more noticeable during the late afternoon or transitioning into the night. Depression and anxiety symptoms will become more profound to be diagnosed as mood disorders in this stage of the disease. Additionally, falls are very common as the client transitions from one place to another or if they do not perceive or attend to common obstructions (e.g., rugs, cords). Greater supervision and care are often required at this stage, and many clients often transition from their home or assisted to long-term care.

## Severe Alzheimer Disease

In the last stage of AD, the pathology is diffuse throughout the cerebrum and cerebellum. The neuronal loss is most profound with cortical atrophy and whole-brain volume loss. Language ability is reduced to simple one-word commands (e.g., yes, no). The client may not recall important details about themselves like name or birthdate or recognize their families like a spouse or children. Many struggle with bowel and bladder control, often leading to incontinence or infections. Some clients will have difficulty with eating and drinking, which may lead to particles being deposited in the lungs leading to aspiration pneumonia. Ambulation is often challenging and may require a walker or wheelchair. Most ADLs may require maximum assistance to complete successfully.

## Late-Versus Early-Onset Alzheimer Disease

Most adults who develop AD at age 65 or older have what is termed late-onset AD (LOAD). Older age, having one or two copies of the APOE e4 allele, and a family history are all risk factors that contribute to the likelihood of developing LOAD. However, those diagnosed with AD before age 65 have early-onset AD (EOAD), sometimes in their 30s. Of all patients diagnosed with AD, approximately 5% to 10% have EOAD (Bateman et al., 2011). The only known risk factor for EOAD is an autosomal dominant inheritance pattern resulting from genetic mutations in one copy of the APP, PSEN1, or PSEN2 genes (Campion et al., 1999). Additionally, the heritability of EOAD is significantly higher, with estimates between 92% and

100% (Wingo et al., 2012). The clinical symptoms of EOAD are similar to LOAD with an early onset of anterograde episodic memory problems, followed by language, visuospatial, and motor impairments and then overall global cognitive decline (Reitz et al., 2020). One study found that depression, apathy, disinhibition, irritability, and changes in sleep were more common and severe in early EOAD compared to those with LOAD. Given the temporal course and onset of EOAD, the disease is more aggressive and survival time is shorter (Ringman et al., 2015).

## Vascular Dementia

Vascular dementia is the second most common cause of irreversible dementia and encompasses a range of disorders that contribute to cognitive impairment. The term vascular cognitive impairment is the preceding stage when vascular diseases are present or have an acute onset that precipitates in a rapid decline. Cerebrovascular disease encompasses several conditions that affect the blood flow and structures (blood vessels) of the brain (see also Chapter 9). Stroke (ischemic, hemorrhagic) is the most common cerebrovascular disease and a leading cause of disability, mobility limitation, and mortality. In addition to causing ~25% of all strokes worldwide, cerebral small vessel disease (CSVD) is the most common cause of vascular cognitive impairment and is a significant contributor to mixed dementias (i.e., presence of multiple neurodegenerative diseases, including AD (O'Brien et al., 2003; Pantoni, 2010). Deep cerebral microbleeds are the manifestation of severe hypertension leading to the risk of lacunar infracts and deep hemorrhages (Gao et al., 2018). In patients with AD, deep cerebral microbleeds were associated with an increased risk of cardiovascular events and mortality (Benedictus et al., 2015). White matter hyperintensities are lesions that signal axonal loss and demyelination—they are a risk factor associated with stroke, dementia, and impaired processing speed and cognitive decline (Prins & Scheltens, 2015). These "silent" symptoms of vascular risk, quantified through structural neuroimaging, are associated with impairments in processing speed and executive function, the high-level decision-making processes that older adults use to maintain activities vital to functional independence, such as driving. Clients affected by vascular cognitive impairment often struggle to live independently due to white and gray brain matter changes. Moderate or severe CSVD, as evidenced by the presence of white matter hyperintensities and neurodegeneration on MRI, can lead to impaired gait and balance, impairment in lower extremity performance, falls, strokes, depression, and ultimately dementia (Gorelick et al., 2011; Prins et al., 2005; Staals et al., 2014). Differentiating vascular dementia from AD is challenging given the level of integration with blood vessels within and surrounding the brain, in addition to risk factors for stroke (location, density, number, treatment) and AD dementia.

## Dementia With Lewy Body

Lewy body is an umbrella term that encapsulates a diagnosis of dementia with Lewy bodies (DLB) or PDD. A person has DLB if the dementia is classified as cognitive functioning that oscillates or changes (impaired vs. not), sleep behavior disturbances, visual hallucinations, and parkinsonism after the diagnosis. PDD is diagnosed starting 1 year or more after well-established Parkinson disease (Emre et al., 2007). Lewy body disease is a pathological disease made post-mortem of Lewy body pathology (abnormal aggregation of α-synuclein in the cortex) (Walker et al., 2015). Approximately 5% of older adults have pure DLB. Nearly 50% of AD cases have the co-occurrence of DLB, and the pathology is more frequent in the moderate to severe stages of AD (Cairns et al., 2015; Uchikado et al., 2006). Pathological studies of pure Lewy body support a stereotypic pattern of accumulation starting in the brainstem nuclei/olfactory regions and progressing to limbic areas and, in the most advanced stages, to the neocortex (McKeith et al., 2005). There are arguments to collapse both DLB and PDD into a simplified construct, but for the purposes of this chapter, we will keep them separate. In AD, the first loss of cognitive functioning occurs with memory; however, in DLB, the earliest loss appears to be with attention, visual perception, and executive functioning (McKeith et al., 2005). These symptoms are essential in distinguishing DLB from AD and PDD. As previously mentioned, cognitive function has more variance than AD, which has a more progressive decline. Yet, despite the oscillation in cognition, the client may appear more apathetic or may seem like they are daydreaming. REM sleep behavior disturbance (RBD) has also been found to be an early marker. One study of patients diagnosed with RBD found that upon a 10-year follow-up, over 75% of those with idiopathic RBD were then diagnosed with the neurodegenerative disorder (Iranzo et al., 2014). Caring for clients with DLB may address routines and patterns to support their sleep, redirect during episodes of visual hallucinations, address deficits in hand-eye coordination, and support visuospatial awareness as they complete their ADLs.

## Frontotemporal Dementia

Frontotemporal dementia (FTD), also called frontotemporal lobar degeneration (FTLD), is tied as the second most common cause of irreversible neurodegenerative dementia, ranking behind AD in adults younger than age 65. The age of onset occurs between ages 45 and 65, with an even distribution between sex, an average survival of 8 years, and it accounts for 5% to 10% of dementia cases (Neary et al., 2005). As its name suggests, this dementia is associated with degeneration of the prefrontal and anterior temporal lobes that become severely atrophied while the superior portions of the cortex become softer with additional aggregation of proteins like tau. There are three distinct clinical subgroups of FTD that have been described. The behavioral variant of FTD (bvFTD) is a syndrome distinguished by changes in behavior and personality and associated with cortical degeneration predominantly in the frontal lobes (Johnson et al., 2005). Clients present with a slow but progressive decline in social and emotional functions that reflects a degeneration of structures like the anterior cingulate, amygdala, striatum, and thalamus. The slow but insidious onset may be mistaken for a midlife crisis or mood disorder. The client may seem unmotivated or apathetic, insensitive, lack empathy, respond disrespectfully, fail to acknowledge behavior or insight into actions, and act impulsively.

The primary progressive aphasia (PPA) variant impacts the ability to communicate via speech, reading comprehension, or writing. There are three forms of PPA in FTD. Semantic PPA is the loss of words and ability to understand words, and possible loss of the ability to recognize faces and objects. Logopenic PPA is difficulty finding the correct words during communication; however, comprehension of words and use of grammar is intact. Nonfluent or Agrammatic PPA is the progressive loss of the ability to form words and articulate, specifically with the omission of short connecting words (to, from, the) and incorrect use of verb tenses. The normal flow of speech may appear restricted. The third class of variants is a movement disorder. Progressive supranuclear palsy occurs with ambulation and balance where there is an increased frequency of falls, increased rigidity in the upper extremity and body, and difficulty with ocular movement. Corticobasal syndrome is a movement disorder resulting from a progressive degeneration of nerve cells in specific brain regions. It may start unilaterally, but eventually, both sides will be affected, which can include rigidity, bradykinesia, dystonia, and apraxia (specifically limb despite strength being intact). Both progressive supranuclear palsy and corticobasal syndrome are tauopathies that impact neurons.

## Parkinson Disease Dementia

There are shared clinical, pathological, and symptoms between DLB and PDD. However, PDD is diagnosed following a formal diagnosis of PD based on established criteria and clinical assessment (Tolosa et al., 2006, 2021). Additionally, the aggregation of α-synuclein occurs deep in the substantia nigra and area of the brainstem, which results in a down-regulation and degeneration of neurons that produce dopamine. Like DLB, PDD has accompanying visual hallucinations but also has delusions. The hallmark phenotypic motor symptoms like rigidity, tremors (resting, intention, kinetic), gait problems (shuffling), masked facial expression, soft voice (hypophonia), and slower movements of PD become more profound in dementia. For those diagnosed with PD, the point prevalence of dementia is approximately 30%, with a mean onset time from onset of PD to PDD at 10 years (Aarsland & Kurz, 2010). For patients with PD that survived 20 years with the disease, the prevalence increased to 83%, with many showing dementia symptoms before they died (Hely et al., 2005). Caring for clients with PDD may focus on safety and environmental modification to remove any tripping hazards, provide physical support (e.g., grab bars), position belongings closer to them, structure ADLs with more time, and adaptive equipment.

## Mixed Dementia

Mixed dementia is defined as the co-occurrence of AD and vascular dementia or AD and Lewy body dementia, AD and PDD, or vascular dementia and Lewy body. The presence of vascular dementia, specifically infarcts, can lower the threshold and increase the likelihood of AD. In a modest study of a community sample of older adults, among those with dementia, 50% have at least one other dementia diagnosis (Schneider et al., 2007). In another pathology study of 120 brains, 30% were identified as having mixed dementia and were found to be significantly older patients (De Reuck et al., 2016). There may also be differences by race and ethnicity. Two studies found that African Americans and Hispanic older adults had more mixed dementia pathology and more significant atherosclerosis and cerebrovascular disease than non-Hispanic White older adults at autopsy (Barnes et al., 2015; Filshtein et al., 2019).

## Tools for Diagnosis Ascertainment

A primary care practitioner or neurologist will complete a thorough history and physical examination to assess whether a decline in cognitive abilities is present. They may refer the client to a neuropsychologist for a more in-depth examination using validated tests with norms to determine domain-specific impairment and severity. Clinical presentation, along with self- and family report, coupled with neuropsychological batteries, can provide robust diagnostics for the determination of dementia. There are numerous paper-and-pencil and electronic (via mobile applications) assessments of phenotypic symptoms screens that have strong reliability, validity, specificity, and sensitivity. The accompanying measures are not meant to serve as an exhaustive list but present some of the more widely used assessments of symptoms to provide an ascertainment of dementia.

### Dementia Screening and Testing for Generalists

The Assessing Dementia 8 (AD8) is a brief, simple, self-report screen of eight questions that probe memory, orientation, function, and judgment (Galvin et al., 2005). While it was initially developed for informants like a spouse, child, or friend who knows the client well, it has been found to be valid in persons with MCI or dementia. The client is asked to reflect and respond (Yes/No) as to whether they have experienced a change in the last several years on functions that might be impacted by cognitive (memory and thinking) problems. A score of two or higher suggests that cognitive impairment is likely to present, thus warranting further follow-up. Because it is self-report, it is prone to social desirability bias and stigma in providing honest answers. Since the symptoms are agnostic and only loosely connected to cognition, any mood disorder, neurodevelopmental, or chronic neurological disease may influence the response. The AD8 is free to use and requires minimal training beyond the instructions.

The Mini-Mental State Examination (MMSE) is one of the most prevalent cognitive screens to assess cognitive impairment and dementia in all of medicine and allied health (Folstein et al., 1975). The 30 items probe orientation to time and place, attention, recall, language, and visuospatial skills. A client's performance can be classified as normal, MCI, moderate, or severe, and the score can be adjusted based on the individual's age and education. The MMSE can help distinguish between dementia subtypes (e.g., AD, DLB, FTD) based on scores from specific cognitive domains. Limitations of the MMSE include poor discrimination between normal cognition and MCI, being dominantly visual dependent, having a ceiling effect for discriminating those in the preclinical stage (Spencer et al., 2013). The administration of the MMSE is straightforward based on the directions, but the measure incurs costs for the use of a single copy.

Similar to the MMSE, the Montreal Cognitive Assessment (MoCA) is a 30-item screen that assesses memory, visuospatial skills, attention, language, and orientation to determine if MCI is present irrespective of disease (Nasreddine et al., 2005). Since the MoCA is agnostic of etiology, it can be applicable to a range of neurological diseases and conditions beyond dementia (e.g., mood disorders, traumatic brain injury [TBI], sleep disorders, cancer). Unlike the MMSE, the MoCA has different versions to reduce practice effects, has an adapted version for visually impaired clients, and a basic version to account for low education or a lack of literacy. The MoCA is available in both paper (free) and a mobile app (purchase required) and requires certification.

The Rowland Universal Dementia Assessment Scale (RUDAS) is a brief, six-item screening for cognitive functioning that assesses memory, visuospatial abilities, body orientation, praxis, and language (Storey et al., 2004). The main purpose of the RUDAS is to assess cognition that minimizes cultural learning and language effects. A score of 22 or less out of 30 indicates potential cognitive impairment and suggests a more thorough examination. The RUDAS is free to use and has directions that allow anyone to administer it.

The Clinical Dementia Rating (CDR) is a standard stool used worldwide to stage dementia (Morris, 1993). Experienced clinicians integrate information from a neurological examination and separate interviews with the clients and a knowledgeable collateral source (family member or friend) to derive a CDR. Throughout the semi-structured interview, the clinician queries the client and the collateral source regarding whether there has been a change in memory, thinking, and behavior. The CDR is based on change across six domains: memory, orientation, judgment and problem-solving, community affairs, home and hobbies, and personal care. The CDR reflects whether an individual has dementia and, if so, the severity of dementia. Normal cognition is indicated by CDR 0, with CDRs of 0.5, 1, 2, and 3 representing very mild dementia, mild dementia, moderate dementia, and severe dementia, respectively. The CDR is free to use along with training and certification.

The Diagnostic and Statistical Manual of Mental Disorders-5 (DSM-5) is the current version published by the American Psychiatric Association and used to describe symptoms of all mental disorders (American Psychiatric Association, 2013). In the DSM-5, dementia is termed neurocognitive disorder (NCD), which has both a major and minor state (Blazer, 2013). Both forms include domains that may be affected and include social cognition, language, learning and memory, complex attention, executive ability, and perceptual—motor—visual

perception. Minor NCD is defined by having a modest decline in one or more cognitive domains based on self, a collateral source, or a clinician and poor performance on formal testing in the range of one to two standard deviations from established norms. However, the deficits do not interfere with IADLs, but more compensatory tools and strategies are required to maintain functional independence. Major NCD is present if there is a substantial decline from a prior level of functioning. Formal neuropsychological testing is two or more standard deviations from established norms, and the deficits interfere with IADLs. Minor or Major NCD stipulates that the deficiencies do not occur with delirium and are not attributable to a mood disorder like depression.

## Early Detection via Biomarkers

As discussed in the Preclinical AD stage subsection, biomarkers are extremely valuable given their clinical utility and confirmation of in vivo pathophysiology. While there are several biomarkers for different dementia subtypes, they are at various stages of development, validation, and clinical application. AD biomarkers are more established than others, given the prevalence of the disease and significant global research efforts to refine the sensitivity and specificity of the biomarkers. This section will focus on AD biomarkers.

Amyloid can be detected in both conventional CSF and PET imaging—levels of insoluble fibrillar amyloid are known to be present at lower concentrations in the brain and inversely in higher concentrations within the CSF among individuals in the preclinical stage of AD and as they progress to more advanced stages. The reduction of amyloid in the CSF is hypothesized to result from its aggregation in the brain, which inhibits diffusion into CSF (Blennow et al., 2010). Similarly, tau can now be detected via PET imaging and present in higher concentrations in the brain. In the CSF, the phosphorylation of tau or $ptau_{181}$ is another marker specific to the accumulation of the tangles of paired helical filament. Both $ptau_{181}$ (neurofibrillary tangles) and total tau (all different isoforms—neuronal and axonal) are present in higher concentrations in CSF. There have been significant gains in the past 5 years to identify and quantify these biomarkers in blood, specifically in plasma. Current research efforts are underway to validate parallel plasma biomarkers like amyloid ($A\beta_{1-42}$), tau, and $ptau_{181}$, and newer targets like neurofilament light (NFL) measuring axonal injury, and $ptau_{217}$, another marker of phosphorylation (Hampel et al., 2018; Janelidze et al., 2020). These biomarkers are associated with the derivation of the "preclinical AD" label and are an early indication that the disease process has started. Early detection of persons at risk of AD in the preclinical stage may help with clinical trials and structuring specific interventions that target modifiable risk factors associated with the decline due to AD.

## Global Perspectives and Differential Burden

Globally, dementia will increase from 55 million (2021) to 78 million by 2030 to 152 million by 2050. Six out of 10 persons with dementia worldwide currently live in low- and middle-income countries (LMICs) (Livingston et al., 2020). However, current estimates suggest that approximately 75% of persons with dementia are undiagnosed, and this number may be higher for LMICs (Gauthier et al., 2021). These countries already face major social, economic, and healthcare problems. Dementia is a critical issue in the national and regional agendas of LMICs, posing several challenges with regard to diagnosis, prognosis, care programs, and prevention (Mattap et al., 2021). Adaptations of international initiatives that have proven cost-effective to be used in these countries and the development of local solutions are strategies that can be put in place to respond to this scenario. However, this requires dedicated resources, established infrastructures, and trained clinicians that have the expertise to screen and diagnose dementia. As globalization, immigration, natural disasters, and conflicts have increased over the past few decades, a growing number of persons with dementia originally from LMICs are now seen in high-income countries.

With the growth of global diversity in ethnic and racial groups, the United States will also see an increase in African Americans, Hispanics, and Asians, while the non-Hispanic white population will decrease (Babulal, 2020). In the United States, African Americans are at twice the risk of dementia, and Hispanics are at one and a half times the risk of dementia compared to non-Hispanic whites. In addition to these disparities in dementia disease prevalence, minoritized groups have limited access to health care, including primary, emergency, and preventative maintenance, compared to non-Hispanic whites (Alzheimer's Association, 2021). These disparities accumulate as an increase in risk exposure, greater disease severity, and low access to health care intersect to reduce life expectancy across ethnoracial groups. The 2020 Lancet Commission on dementia identified 12 modifiable risk factors in a life-course model of dementia prevention, accounting for 40% of known risks, leaving 60% for unknown modifiable causes (Livingston et al., 2020). Risk factors include (1) low education in early life; (2) hearing loss, TBI, hypertension, alcohol abuse, and obesity in midlife; and (3) smoking, depression, physical inactivity, air pollution, and diabetes in later life. Occupational therapists are optimally positioned to support an inclusive and multidimensional framework in screening, assessing the client's needs, and understanding the impact of a dementia diagnosis on their IADLs, ADLs, and quality of life.

## Occupational Therapy Assessment and Intervention

OT intervention with older adults living with cognitive impairment begins with screening and assessment to understand a client's needs and determine ways to enhance the client's IADLs, ADLs, and quality of life. In this section, we present two programs of assessment and intervention that feature multidimensional frameworks. The first program uses *Cognitive Stimulation Therapy (CST)* as described by occupational therapists based in a rural region of the United States (See Box 16.1). Their screening and assessments of older adults encompass psychosocial, cognitive, and physical function. The second program, the *Geriatric Rehabilitation Program*, is presented by occupational therapists based in an urban setting in Canada (See Box 16.2). Similarly, their framework also includes mental health, cognitive, and physical function, as well as capacity assessment. These approaches aim to address outcomes of a client's goals related to IADLs, ADLs, and quality of life. Both programs use case examples to illustrate the approaches (See Case Examples of Ann, Mrs. B, Kay).

Later, in the section on caregiver considerations, we describe the *Care of Persons with Dementia in their Environments (COPE)* as an approach for engaging care partners.

---

**BOX 16.1**    Cognitive Stimulation Therapy for Persons Living With Dementia in a Rural Setting in the United States

Debbie Hayden, RN, BSN, OTR/L
    Director of Occupational Therapy, Perry County Health Care Systems
Janice Lundy, MHCA, MA, BSSW
    Director of Social Work and Geriatric Care Management, Perry County Health Care Systems
*Cognitive Stimulation Therapy (CST)* is a brief, evidence-based, psychological intervention for people with mild to moderate dementia. CST includes guidelines for structuring small, theme-based, group or individual sessions that provide stimulation and engagement, while providing an optimal learning environment and the social benefits of a group or one-on-one interaction. CST is easily adaptable to a variety of settings: home, outpatient clinics, care facilities, and community settings.
    Group CST is a 7-week, brief treatment program where, ideally, five to eight dementia patients meet twice weekly for 45 min or longer, for a total of 14 themed sessions (e.g., childhood, word association, categorizing objects) led by

two therapists. Group members should ideally be of similar stages of dementia, so activities can be delivered accordingly. The sessions are designed with a person-centered approach, incorporating key principles that optimize an individual's potential, while at the same time compensating for impairments.
    The design of CST supports a multidisciplinary approach to dementia intervention. Developed in the United Kingdom, CST group sessions were designed to be delivered by any professional with experience in dementia care, after participating in a brief training course. In the United States, the CST training focus is on clinical intervention for skilled health care professionals in clinical practice with persons living with dementia. Occupational, speech, and physical (if combined with an exercise component) therapists, clinical social workers, and psychologists are appropriate clinicians to deliver CST.

**Implementation of Cognitive Stimulation Therapy in Clinical Practice**
The key goal of CST is to improve cognitive function using techniques that exercise different cognitive skills. Key principles

*Continued*

## BOX 16.1 Cognitive Stimulation Therapy for Persons Living With Dementia in a Rural Setting in the United States—Cont'd

are strategically integrated into CST, with the aim of encouraging new ideas, thoughts, and associations. Some of these principles include focus on opinion versus fact; language, executive functioning, and mental stimulation; multi-sensory stimulation; reminiscence as an aid to orientation, and consistency and continuity between sessions.

CST is proven to benefit cognition and quality of life (Spector et al., 2003, 2010), and improve mood (Lobbia et al., 2018). Ongoing, weekly Maintenance CST (MCST) shows additional benefits in quality of life and improvements in ADLs at 3 months (Orrell et al., 2014). Feedback from participants finds CST to be a positive experience (Spector et al., 2011). CST is cost effective (D'Amico et al., 2015; Knapp et al., 2006) and as effective as the medications currently used to treat the symptoms of dementia (Livingston & Katona, 2000). CST is internationally adapted and currently used in over 34 countries.

An individual version (iCST), designed to be delivered by caregivers on a one-on-one basis, found improvements in care-dyad relationships and in quality of life of the caregiver. However, no change in cognition or quality of life was found in the person with dementia (Orrell et al., 2017). Recent evidence shows significant improvements in cognition with professional-led iCST (Gibbor et al., 2021).

### Cognitive Stimulation Therapy With Exercise

Physical movement was not a component of the original CST program but has been recently added as increasing evidence supports exercise as a key element in cognitive enhancement and reducing decline in people with dementia. CST programs now incorporate various forms of physical movement and exercise into their sessions.

### Assessment

Program effectiveness is evaluated using pre- and post-scores from quantitative measures along with qualitative feedback from both the participant and family or caregiver (see Table 16.1). In addition to standardized assessment tools, there are other considerations to determine if CST is an appropriate and effective intervention for a person with dementia, e.g., can the person have a meaningful conversation? Is the person's vision and hearing adequate to participate in activities and small group or one-on-one discussion? Can the person remain for the entire session?

### International Collaboration and Training

In 2015, University College London launched the International CST Center. The intention of the center is to create a network of CST experts who can share knowledge and collaborate on work to further develop CST. A list of countries and international training can be found at the CST International Center web page (University College London, 2022).

TABLE 16.1 Examples of Cognitive Stimulation Therapy Assessment Tools

| Assessments | Rational |
| --- | --- |
| Brief psychosocial history | General knowledge for session efficacy/patient cueing: |
| If possible, obtain collateral information from family/caregiver. | Name of parents/spouse; number/name of siblings/children; where they grew up/places they have lived; occupation/hobbies; possible areas of sensitivity (to avoid exposure to painful memories); brief mental health history? |
| QoL-AD (Logsdon et al., 2002) ADRQL (Kasper et al., 2009) DQoL (Brod et al., 1999) | Assess quality of life |
| CSDD (Alexopoulos et al., 1988) | Assess for depression as a possible reversible cause of dementia |
| Trail-Making A and B (Dawson et al., 2009) | Assess attention and visual skills. A-rote memory. B-executive function |
| Katz Index (Katz, 1983) | Assess activities of daily living |
| SBT (Katzman et al., 1983) | Assess orientation, memory, concentration, and registration |
| SLUMS (Tariq et al., 2006) MMSE (Folstein et al., 1975) MoCA (Nasreddine et al., 2005) | Assess global cognitive function |
| RGA (Morley, 2017) | Assess for geriatric syndromes and reversible causes of dementia |
| TUG (Podsiadlo & Richardson, 1991) | Assess functional mobility |
| FTSST (Csuka & McCarty, 1985) | Assess lower extremity strength and movement strategies |
| Hand Grip (Sousa-Santos & Amaral, 2017) | Assess upper body and general strength |
| Qualitative feedback post-intervention from patient and family/caregiver | Assess patient and family/caregiver perception of program effectiveness and level of enjoyment. |

*ADRQL,* Alzheimer disease–related quality of life; *CSDD,* Cornell scale for depression in dementia; *DqoL,* dementia quality of life; *FTSST,* five times sit-to-stand; *MMSE,* mini mental status exam; *MoCA,* Montreal cognitive assessment; *QOL-AD,* quality of life in Alzheimer's disease; *RGA,* rapid geriatric assessment; *SBT,* the short-blessed test; *SLUMS,* Saint Louis Mental Status Exam; *TUG,* timed up and go.

## BOX 16.2 Assessment and Intervention for Cognitive Decline in the Geriatric Rehabilitation Program in an Urban Setting in Canada

Betsey Williams, BScOT
  Occupational Therapist II
  Glenrose Rehabilitation Hospital in Edmonton, Alberta

Megan Kohls-Wiebe, MScRS (Rehab), BScOT, BSc
  Program Coordinator for START Psychiatry Hospital; OT Team Leader for Geriatric Psychiatry
  Glenrose Rehabilitation Hospital in Edmonton, Alberta

The Geriatric Rehabilitation Program (GRP) is located within a large freestanding rehabilitation facility in a major Canadian city. GRP provides comprehensive tertiary (higher level requiring specialized equipment and expertise during hospitalization) and quaternary (care with experimental medicine and procedures and specialized surgeries) rehabilitation services to older adults (age 65+ years) with high-level medical, physical, and mental health needs. GRP comprises a geriatric psychiatry day hospital and 4 inpatient geriatric rehabilitation units, with 65 beds for physical rehabilitation, 6 beds for post-stroke rehabilitation, 22 beds for psychiatric rehabilitation, and 11 beds for individuals with significant cognitive-behavioral issues. With its broad scope of practice, occupational therapy plays a central role in GRP in assessing and addressing cognitive, behavioral, social, emotional, and physical conditions impinging function and engagement in life activities. Our 12 occupational therapists and 6 occupational therapy assistants work within large close-knit, collaborative interdisciplinary teams.

### Assessment of Cognition
Cognition is multifaceted and its assessment may be complex. In order to fully and reliably understand cognitive functioning, particularly in the context of occupational performance, a thorough evaluation including impairment-based assessments, self- and proxy reports, and performance-based assessments is ideal (Dawson et al., 2009; Elliott, 2003; Godefroy, 2003; Goel et al., 1997; Hartman-Maeir et al., 2009; Katz & Hartman-Maeir, 2005; Kizony et al., 2011; Lezak, 1982; Poulin et al., 2013). For screening at admission we rely on self- and proxy reports. We tend to use impairment-based assessments for screening of global cognition and identification of impairment in specific cognitive domains (e.g., attention, orientation, visual construction, calculation). For assessment of higher-level executive functions (e.g., prioritizing, organizing, sequencing, self-monitoring, reasoning, judgment) required to engage in independent, purposeful, and self-directed behavior, we strive to use performance-based tools that are ecologically valid and congruent with occupational therapy philosophy and practice (Dawson et al., 2009; Elliott, 2003; Godefroy, 2003; Goel et al., 1997; Katz & Hartman-Maeir, 2005; Kizony et al., 2011; Lezak, 1982; Poulin et al., 2013).

### Screening at Admission
Within the first few days of admission, patients in both the inpatient and day-patient programs are screened by an occupational therapist. Screening is a three-pronged approach. First, we ask patients about their cognition (particularly memory issues), their functioning in ADL and IADL, and their community engagement. Where possible, we also get collateral information on cognition, function, and engagement from family or caregivers. Second, we administer a clock-drawing test (Agrell & Dehlin, 1998), where the patient must draw a circle, enter all the numbers on the clock, and set the time to 10 min past eleven. This provides quick information about spatial awareness, planning, executive function, memory, and following instructions. Third, we screen for depression and anxiety using standardized self-report tools including the Geriatric Depression Scale (GDS) (Douglas et al., 2007), Geriatric Anxiety Inventory (GAI) (Sheikh & Yesavage, 1986), Generalized Anxiety Disorder screener (GAD-7) (Pachana et al., 2007), or Patient Health Questionnaire (PHQ-9) (Spitzer et al., 2006). Although this may at first seem unrelated to cognition, it is well known that mood and anxiety issues impact significantly on cognitive functioning and engagement in daily life activities and quality of life. This process helps us differentiate whether a patient has true cognitive dysfunction or has a pseudo-impaired cognition (e.g., pseudo-dementia) resulting from depression or anxiety.

### Global Cognition Screening Tests
After basic screening for cognitive and functional issues at admission, occupational therapists typically move on to standardized cognitive screening to objectively look at global cognitive functioning, using one of the following: Montreal Cognitive Assessment (MoCA) (Spitzer et al., 1999), Saint Louis University Mental Status exam (SLUMS) (Nasreddine et al., 2005), Rowland University Dementia Assessment Scale (RUDAS) (Tariq et al., 2006), or Addenbrooke's Cognitive Examination-III (ACE-III) (Storey et al., 2004). We may also administer the Executive Interview (EXIT) (Hsieh et al., 2013) to look closer at executive functioning. If there are no issues identified with these cognitive screens, and patient and family have not identified issues, the patient is considered "generally cognitively intact" and no further testing is pursued.

### Functional Cognition Assessment
If screening suggests cognitive impairment or the patient and family or caregivers identify functional issues unrelated to physical impairments, assessment of functional cognition is initiated. Unlike cognitive screens, which look at basic cognitive domains in isolation, functional cognition tools assess a person's executive functions during actual performance of everyday occupations (see also Chapter 15). Executive functions are higher-level cognitive processes, which control the more basic cognitive functions (Dawson et al., 2009). They are integrative cognitive processes elicited in complex or novel situations, and are required for successful occupational engagement in real-world settings (Douglas et al., 2007; Goel et al., 1997; Katz & Hartman-Maeir, 2005; Kizony et al., 2011; Poulin et al., 2013). To assess functional cognition, we use a mix of standardized paper-and-pencil tests (Independent Living Skills [ILS] [Royall et al., 1992], Kohlman Evaluation of Living Skills-4th Edition [KELS-4] [Loeb, 1996], standardized performance-based tools (Executive Function Performance Test [EFPT] [Kohlman Thompson & Robnett, 2016], Executive

*Continued*

Function Route-Finding Task [EFRT] [Baum & Wolf, 2013], Kettle Test [Boyd & Sautter, 1993], and Multiple Errands Test) (Hartman-Maeir et al., 2005), as well as performance-based assessments for cooking, money management, and community transportation developed at our facility. We use a loose algorithm to direct which tools are chosen, based on: (1) the stage of cognitive decline, (2) the individual's tolerance for testing, (3) the activities the person will need to complete independently in their own life, and (4) the activities the patient will most likely struggle with based on the results of admission screening and global cognition screening assessments. For example, if a patient has known significant cognitive decline or very poor test tolerance, we would likely select the EFRT over the EFPT, because the latter is lengthy to administer and requires good test tolerance as well as high levels of attention, perseverance, and complex problem-solving. If a patient must use public transit to go to a day program, we would choose our facility-developed community transportation evaluation tool over the KELS-4, because the latter only assesses basic knowledge of community transportation, whereas the former evaluates actual performance out in the community.

### Driving Assessment

Driving is one of the most complex and potentially most dangerous occupations in which adults and older adults commonly engage. As such, if there are moderate or significant declines in basic cognitive domains or in executive functions, driving safety becomes a concern. In the Geriatric Rehabilitation Program, occupational therapists frequently identify a need to pursue driving assessments and will initiate the driving assessment process by completing two screening tools that predict possible failure of an on-road driver's test: Trail Making Test (Trails A & B) (Dawson et al., 2009) and the Motor-Free Visual Perception Test (MVPT) (Oosterman et al., 2010). If the results of these two tests predict poor on-road performance, the patient is counseled to cease driving. If the patient or family disagree with the test results or the findings are considered "borderline," we have an option to refer the individual for a full driver's assessment (including on-road evaluations) through the specialized driver evaluation clinic within our facility. (See also Chapter 21.)

### Capacity Assessment

Patients in the Geriatric Rehabilitation Program are often frail and cognitively impaired, with reduced decision-making abilities and increased vulnerability, which brings us to the topic of "capacity."

Capacity for decision-making is twofold: (1) an ability to understand information that is relevant to making a personal decision and (2) an ability to appreciate reasonable and foreseeable consequences of making a decision as well as not making a decision. We commonly address capacity domains related to health care, accommodations, and legal and financial matters.

Capacity in not an all-or-nothing concept. A person may retain capacity in one domain and not another. An older adult may maintain capacity for simple decisions in a specific domain but struggle or lack capacity for complex decisions within that same domain. For example, within the health-care domain, a patient with a cognitive impairment may not

experience difficulties making a decision about consenting to a vaccine but may struggle with a decision about having major surgery. In Canada (similar to the United States), there are legal measures in place to assign decision-making to another person or persons in the event the patient loses capacity in one or more domains (Colarusso & Hammill, 1972). Alternate decision-makers are typically family members and may be chosen by patients in advance. In the event the patient has not appointed someone to make decisions should the patient become incapacitated, court proceedings are required to identify and assign a suitable guardian or decision-maker (Colarusso & Hammill, 1972) (see also Chapter 2).

Although a patient may have a diagnosis of a cognitive impairment or mental illness, this does not necessarily mean they lack capacity. Older adults with intact insight and awareness are often able to make simple decisions with low risk, as their insight will help them to understand the risks involved in their decision. A person with cognitive impairment may be able to function well within their familiar environment with acceptable levels of risk.

In our program, capacity is assumed until proven otherwise; this is our first guiding principle. The onus is on the interdisciplinary team and assessor(s) to demonstrate lack of capacity versus the patient to demonstrating capacity. We do not assess most patients for capacity; we only proceed with investigating capacity when there is a robust reason identified for a capacity assessment. A "red flag" or trigger for assessment may come to light because a patient is struggling with or unable to make decisions, which puts patient or others at risk or harm. Sometimes a trigger is identified because there is conflict between what a patient wants and what the family wants. For example, the patient may insist on going home to live alone, but the family thinks it is too risky and wants the patient to move to a supportive living environment.

Another guiding principle is that taking away a person's capacity to decide, or right to liberty and freedom, is a serious step and should be a last resort, after all other options have been explored. Just because an older adult makes poor or bad decisions and takes risks, it does not mean the person lacks capacity. We act in a client-centered manner by involving patients in the capacity process and by considering the individual's general beliefs, cultural and religious beliefs and values, lifestyle, and past history of at-risk behavior. Older adults, like all adults, have the right to make questionable decisions and participate in risky behaviors. Many older adults are fiercely independent and have lived with risk for many years. To these individuals, living independently at risk is something they value above safety. In assessing capacity, our task is not to judge the behavior or decision, but to ascertain whether the person understands the foreseeable risks of their decisions and behaviors. Our aim is to minimize risk in areas of questionable decision-making while maximizing freedom. Sometimes this can be achieved without the need for a formal capacity assessment, so our first step is to gather data about the problematic decision-making domain and identify if there is a solution to the "trigger" or reason for questioning capacity. This process is guided by our onsite Capacity Assessment Process Worksheet (Parmar et al., 2015).

**BOX 16.2** Assessment and Intervention for Cognitive Decline in the Geriatric Rehabilitation Program in an Urban Setting in Canada—Cont'd

The Geriatric Rehabilitation Program comprises interdisciplinary teams and uses a team approach when assessing and determining a patient's capacity, such that the onus is not on one person or discipline to determine capacity. Occupational therapists play a central role in gathering details regarding the person's cognitive and executive functioning, strengths and limitations, functioning in daily living activities, living and community environments, and about the occupations the person needs to do as part of daily life and make recommendations to promote safety and independence in the least restrictive ways possible.

We are cognizant that decision-making capacity may change over time. A person may lack capacity in a specific domain on a temporary basis. For example, a client with an acute illness may lack capacity to make a domain-specific decision but may have their capacity reassessed and reinstated when they recover from their acute illness. As such, occupational therapists are typically involved in re-assessments of capacity as the patient's situation improves or deteriorates.

**Intervention for Cognitive Decline**

The experience of cognitive decline is unique to each individual. Which cognitive abilities are affected, which abilities remain intact, if and how cognitive decline progresses is multifactorial and is dependent on the interaction of a myriad of influences including genetics, education level, lifestyle, supports, environment, and others. As such, changes in cognition can be challenging to address, particularly within a rehabilitation setting with constant pressures associated with admission and discharge. Our approach in the program is to address any pressing cognitive issues affecting current safety and functioning, but always with an eye on the future, with the consideration that a patient's cognition may continue to decline over time. Below is a simplistic overview of our treatment approaches in the various stages of cognitive decline:

**Early Cognitive Changes (Mild Cognitive Impairment or Mild- Neurocognitive Disorder [NCD])**

In this stage, patients are often cognizant of their cognitive decline and still retain the capacity to learn some new skills and adapt to changes. In the Geriatric Rehabilitation Program, we provide opportunities for patients to learn and practice strategies to compensate for identified cognitive deficits (e.g., to use a daily schedule or calendar) and on simplifying or modifying activities and routines to reduce the cognitive demand of daily activities (e.g., use of blister-packed medication). In some of our program areas, we offer groups that focus on learning memory and attention strategies. Anxiety in response to recognized cognitive decline is common among our patients; to this end we offer stress management groups. Occupational therapists encourage regular engagement in a range of enjoyable activities that provide cognitive stimulation, social interaction, and physical exercise to help maintain function and quality of life. We refer or liaise patients to community programs and services that provide opportunities for such activities post discharge. Looking to the future, occupational therapists commonly recommend that patients begin exploring options for more supportive residences, meal-delivery services, private or public homecare services or companion services, and private or public transportation services.

**Middle-Stage Cognitive Changes (Early- to Mid-Dementia)**

In this stage, we concentrate on minimizing risks, while maintaining as much independence as possible. As dementia progresses, patients vary in their level of insight about the extent and nature of their cognitive decline and become less able to learn and generalize skills. Occupational therapists work with the interdisciplinary team to help patients and families put into place driving and transportation services, homecare services, and companion services as needed. Occupational therapists encourage patients and families to develop and practice scenarios to manage emergency situations such as a fire or a medical event so that the patient can "overlearn" what to do in such emergencies. They assist families in arranging emergency-response alert systems and medication-reminder, falls-detection and wandering-detection services. Occupational therapists commonly recommend relocation to a more supportive living environment (e.g., a retirement residence or senior's apartment building, see also Chapter 28) or environmental modifications such as disabling or removal of the stove or oven and the installation of shut-off faucets or stove shut-off timers. Occupational therapists may refer patients to seniors' or dementia-specific day programs in the community, progressing from least to most structured programs over time.

**Late-Stage Cognitive Decline (Mid- to Late-Dementia or Major-NCD)**

In this stage, the main focus is on protecting the individual. Patients at this point typically no longer show awareness of their cognitive issues and progressively become less aware of potential dangers in their environment, which increases the risk for unsafe situations and adverse events. In-hospital treatments concentrate on providing opportunities for physical, social, and cognitive stimulation. Occupational therapists also make recommendations to families or care homes for environmental modification to improve safety, ways to encourage engagement in self-care and social activities, and how to mitigate disruptive or unwanted behaviors, as well as recommending strategies for the family to get needed emotional supports and respite such as referral to the Alzheimer's Society programs. In addition, occupational therapists assist the interdisciplinary team and the family in relocation to a more secure living environment, such as a nursing home, with increased services and in late stages of cognitive decline assisting to set up 24-h care.

**Unique Populations**

Our rehabilitation facility is located in a multi-ethnic urban center, but also provides services to smaller communities within our province and within territories in northern Canada. As such, the facility serves a broad range of people from a wide variety of cultures and ethnicities, including Indigenous Canadians (First Nations, Inuit, and Métis). Fundamental to high-quality patient-centered care is cultural sensitivity and competency; this is particularly essential in dementia diagnosis, assessment, and treatment, where cultural and ethnic differences may become amplified because of cultural norms, beliefs, and expectations about aging and cognitive decline, as well as by the effects of existing marginalization of certain cultural groups within society.

## The Meaning of Autonomy and Independence in Inclusive Occupational Therapy

The United States and Canada are more ethnically diverse than ever. According to the United States Census Bureau, the US population was more diverse in 2020 than a decade ago. Although the White population continues to be the largest group, it has declined by 8.6% (Jensen et al., 2022). In contrast, the multiracial population has grown from 9 million to 33.8 million, an increase of 276%, and making up 10.3% of the US population. In Canada, over seven million identify with a visible minority group according to Canadian census (Statistics Canada, 2021), making up 22.3% of the Canadian population. The population of Indigenous peoples grew by 42.5% between 2006 and 2016, thus, are also the fastest growing population in Canada (Indigenous Services Canada, 2020). It is incumbent on occupational therapists to be *inclusive* in our assessments and interventions. As a profession, this means challenging the traditional concepts of autonomy and independence.

Although sometimes used interchangeably, autonomy and independence are separate constructs. Autonomy refers to liberty, self-rule or sovereignty, and freedom of will (Dworkin, 2015). Independence refers to the degree to which a person can perform a task or activity on one's own (Liu et al., 2022). One's "lack of independence shouldn't impact one's autonomy" (Liu et al., 2022, p. 2). In other words, one's ability to make decisions should be respected in the presence of disabilities. Even when living with progressive cognitive impairment and limited capacity, clients have rights to autonomy as outlined in the Canadian Charter of Rights for People Living with Dementia (Alzheimer Society of Canada, 2022; Liu et al., 2022, p. 49), AOTA 2020 Occupational Therapy Code of Ethics, and as described in the literature (Cohen-Mansfield, 2021). In particular, autonomy relates to respect, being oneself, and self-determination (Cohen-Mansfield, 2021) (see also Chapter 2, section on autonomy).

Autonomy and independence are Eurocentric concepts. Inclusive OT would consider autonomy and independence of clients at the intersections of gender, age, race, dis/ability, and culture. As such, occupational therapists could incorporate "relational autonomy" by reflecting on the impact of their interactions on clients' self-identities (Entwistle et al., 2010). For example, a client whose traditional culture values family roles may wish to include family members in decision making about interventions. With respect to independence, there is a tendency in Western culture to value independence as an end that can be achieved and maintained (Kirby, 2014). This is evident in the standardized outcome measures occupational therapists use, such as Functional Independence Measure, Independent Living Scale, and Barthel Index of Activities of Daily Living, measures that examine levels of independence in various abilities (Liu et al., 2022). Inclusive assessments would take into consideration factors beyond the client's function, such as social connections, physical environments, and access to community services and technology. These factors can be leveraged to allow a client to live with a desirable level of quality of life, while interdependent on social connections and assistive technologies.

## Role of Technology or AgeTech

"AgeTech" is a relatively new term that refers to the use of advanced technologies such as information and communication technologies (ICTs), robotics, mobile technologies, artificial intelligence (AI), ambient systems, and pervasive computing to drive technology-based innovation to benefit older adults (Pruchno, 2019). AgeTech overlaps with a similar but more broad term, "Gerontechnology," which is covered in Chapter 22, but the former refers to approaches to facilitate successful aging and assist older adults in meeting the domains of housing, communication, health, safety, comfort, mobility, leisure, and work (Ross et al., 2018).

AgeTech can support older adults living with dementia through cognitive health assessment, social connections, and mobility and transportation (Sixsmith et al., 2020). Digitized assessments automize documentation, some aspects of administration, such as timing, and allow therapists to use tools remotely. "Serious" (also called "therapeutic") mobile games, including games such as Bejewelled, Mahjong, Whack-a-Mole, and Word Search, have been used for assessment and intervention with older adults (Ríos Rincón et al., 2022). As assessments, they have been shown to distinguish between participants with and without dementia.

As interventions, engagement, positive affect, and MoCA scores have been shown to increase in older participants who used the above mobile games, and improvements were higher in participants with dementia (Ríos Rincón et al., 2022). However, changes are not always detected when using traditional outcome measures such as the MMSE, as illustrated in the following example. A study of dementia care residents using the Whack-a-Mole mobile game (Wallace et al., 2018) included one resident with an MMSE of 12/30, who was not oriented to person, place, or time at entry to the study. Her performance on the mobile game improved from level 1 to 7 over 5 weeks, and sustained this high level through weeks 6 to 10, despite a decline of MMSE score to 9/30 at study exit (Wallace et al., 2018). While needing additional studies with larger sample sizes, this finding suggests that traditional or standardized measures of cognitive function, while indicating decline, do not always capture improvements in abilities measured in other ways.

## AgeTech to Mitigate Risks of Critical Wandering

The concept of wandering has been subject to debate (Halek & Bartholomeyczik, 2012). The term wandering encompasses a range of behaviors (Kwak et al., 2015) and has been defined differently in publications (Algase et al., 2007; Lai et al., 2003), ranging from simple desirable locomotive behavior or purposeful walking with intention to escape, to mindless pacing with little awareness of surroundings (Algase et al., 2007; Lai et al., 2003). In some countries, such as the United Kingdom, the term wandering is avoided, as it is perceived to be stigmatizing. *Critical* wandering refers to wandering that results in persons with dementia going missing as a result of getting lost (Neubauer & Liu, 2021; Petonito et al., 2013).

The most common types of AgeTech to mitigate the risks of critical wandering are alarm products, monitors and locator technology, or devices with apps that help care partners track and locate a person with dementia. In a review of academic and gray literature, Neubauer et al. (2018) found 83 technologies, but only 19 (22%) were clinically tested. Of the 83 technologies, there were 26 types of devices with GPS, and alarms and sensors are the most common at 40% and 17%, respectively (Neubauer et al., 2018). As over 70% of the technologies were described in the grey literature, the authors recommended further research to strengthen the evidence for their use. OT practitioners who assist persons with dementia and their family care partners in selecting technologies to promote "safe wandering" are advised to consider factors that affect adoption and use of these technologies. Some of these factors are addressed in Chapter 22 as well as by Liu et al. (2022) and Neubauer & Liu (Neubauer & Liu, 2021) and include accessibility, affordability, perceived usefulness, privacy, and security. In one study on the acceptance of GPS wearable technologies with 45 dyads consisting of people with dementia and a family caregiver, GPS acceptance was high after participants used the devices for an average of 5.8 months (Liu et al., 2017). The participants thought that the technologies gave caregivers peace of mind and reduced anxiety in dyads when persons with dementia got lost.

AgeTech is only one strategy to mitigate risks associated with critical wandering. The Canadian Guideline for Safe Wandering (Neubauer & Liu, 2021) is a comprehensive guideline that provides proactive strategies ranging from no tech to high tech approaches. The guideline comes in three versions for use by the following populations: persons living with dementia, care partners such as family members, and facilities. Currently it is available in English and French for free online on Alzheimer Society websites in Canada.

## Caregiver Considerations

In this last section, we discuss family caregivers, or other members of a client's care circle, as partners in any OT framework that values *relational autonomy*. In other words, a client's wish to consult with their care circle during decision making should be normalized and not be viewed as a form of dependency. When a client is able to age in place with social and environmental support, this is a form of *interdependency* that facilitates and enables a client to meet personal goals. An example of engaging care partners in intervention is illustrated in the following description of the Care of Persons with Dementia in their Environments (COPE) program (See Box 16.3).

---

**BOX 16.3    Care of Persons With Dementia in Their Environments (COPE)**

Debbie Hayden, RN, BSN, OTR/L
    Director of Occupational Therapy, Perry County Health Care Systems
Janice Lundy, MHCA, MA, BSSW
    Director of Social Work and Geriatric Care Management, Perry County Health Care Systems
COPE is an evidenced-based approach to working with persons living with dementia with the goal of improving quality of life and well-being of the care dyad, along with improving the individual's functional level. COPE is a multidisciplinary, multicomponent program designed for persons with dementia who reside at home, have a care partner, and who are experiencing clinical symptoms of dementia such as decreasing

functional independence, behavioral and psychological symptoms, as well as care dyad distress (Gitlin & Piersol, 2015; Gitlin et al., 2009). Program effectiveness is evaluated through pre- and post-quantitative measures along with qualitative care partner feedback (See Tables 16.2 and 16.3).

COPE is delivered through 10–12 home sessions by occupational therapists trained in the program. The occupational therapist's role is in assessment, need identification, implementation of individualized intervention strategies, and education. The team may also include other medical or ancillary personnel trained in COPE (Gitlin & Piersol, 2015; Gitlin et al., 2009). For example, an advanced nurse practitioner may be involved to assess for reversible causes

---

**TABLE 16.2  Examples of Multidisciplinary Assessment Tools**

| | |
|---|---|
| Clinical Interview:<br>Caregiver profile<br>    Person with dementia profile<br>Interest Inventory<br>Caregiver approach to activity<br>Daily challenges | Assess daily routines, activities, functional level, and areas of concern; includes assessment of executive function. |
| Large Allen Cognitive Level Screen-5 (LACLS) (Allen et al., 2007)<br>Allen Diagnostic Module 2 (ADM-2)(Earhart, 2006) | Screen for cognitive level and capabilities |
| Timed Up and Go (TUG) (Podsiadlo & Richardson, 1991) | Assess physical mobility |
| Comportment Scale (Peavy et al., 1996) | Social behavior and appearance |
| Readiness to Change (Prochaska et al., 1997) | Assess care partner participation readiness |
| Observation of strategies (Gitlin & Piersol, 2015) | Assess interactions between care partner and person with dementia |
| Assessment of Physical Home Environment HEAP (Gitlin et al., 2002) | Safety |

*Continued*

**BOX 16.3**    Care of Persons With Dementia in their Environments (COPE)—Cont'd

of dementia. COPE consists of a three-phase protocol (Table 16.4) with the goal of aligning care partner expectations and environmental/task demands with the capabilities of the person living with dementia (Gitlin et al., 2010).

Research has shown caregivers receiving COPE reported greater perceived well-being. They also found that individuals living with dementia in the program experience less frequent and severe behavioral and psychological symptoms and greater engagement in meaningful activities (Fortinsky et al., 2020). In addition, persons with dementia who received COPE had less functional dependence and less dependence in IADL tasks (Gitlin et al., 2010).

**TABLE 16.3**  Additional Occupational Therapy Assessment Tools

| | |
|---|---|
| Bristol Activities of Daily Living (ADL) Assessment (Bucks et al., 1996) | Assess ADL function |
| Rapid Cognitive Screen (RCS) (Malmstrom et al., 2015) | Screen for dementia or presence of neurocognitive disorders |
| Functional Assessment Stage Test (FAST) (Sclan & Reisberg, 1992) | Functional assessment of cognitive level |
| Disability Assessment of Dementia (DAD) (Gélinas et al., 1999) | Assess ADL tasks with focus on initiation, planning, and effective performance |

**TABLE 16.4**  Three Phase COPE Protocol (Gitlin & Piersol, 2015)

| | |
|---|---|
| Phase I: Assessment phase (OT sessions 1–3) | Assess: COPE dyad, cognitive deficits/preserved capabilities of person with dementia, care partner communication style, identify problem areas, fall risk, and home safety. |
| Phase II: Implementation phase (OT sessions 4–8) | Provide care partner education on the capabilities of the person with dementia, develop individualized intervention strategies to address identified areas of concern, provide education and skills training for establishing a supportive environment, and education on strategies for care partner well-being. Introduce purposeful activity in this phase. |
| Phase III: Generalizability phase (OT sessions 9 & 10) | Reinforce education and skills training with goal for the care partner to be able to generalize skills learned to other problem areas or future concerns. |

*COPE,* Care of Persons with Dementia in their Environments; *OT,* occupational therapy.
**The tables are summaries of different assessments.**

## Caregivers as Proxies in Assessments of Older Adults With Dementia

The COPE program as described involves the care partner in each phase of the 10 OT sessions over three phases, thus, the client is actually the dyad. Even when older adults live in a residential care facility, apart from family members, there are important reasons to involve family members in the resident's care circle. Family members typically continue to provide care through visits or long-distance social interactions via technology.

This chapter has emphasized assessments and interventions that address ADLs in persons living with dementia. In a Danish study that interviewed 244 participants living with mild to severe dementia, and their caregivers, researchers determined that ability to perform ADLs, i.e., level of dependency, is the main factor affecting quality of life (Andersen et al., 2004). Other studies have also found an association between ADL performance and quality of life (Giebel et al., 2015). Progressive decline of cognitive capacity poses challenges in assessments of quality of life or life satisfaction and technology acceptance. In these circumstances, family caregivers who have known the client over their lifetime may offer valuable advice and direction in OT assessments and interventions. However, proxy ratings of quality-of-life measures do not always reflect accurately persons living with dementia, thus, it is recommended that self-rated *and* proxy-rated versions be used. Schölzel-Dorenbos et al. (2010) list 16 disease-specific quality-of-life measures for use with persons living with dementia. Of these, the authors recommend the Quality of Life-Alzheimer's Disease (QOL-AD) (Logsdon et al., 2002), as it is the most used questionnaire specific for dementia populations (Schölzel-Dorenbos et al., 2010). The 13-item scale has a self-report version for clients and a proxy-report version for caregivers, and can be used with clients who have low MMSE scores (Crespo et al., 2013; Schölzel-Dorenbos et al., 2010). The use of self-ratings demonstrates recognition and respect for a client's sense of autonomy and self-determination, regardless of the degree of cognitive impairment. In the early and moderate stages, inclusion of and correlation of self-ratings with proxy ratings can give occupational therapists an estimation of the accuracy of proxy ratings. This information provides a source of information in the later stage when the client is no longer able to complete self-ratings, and only proxy ratings are available. A third approach to assessment of quality of life is through observation of behaviors assumed to be related to quality of life (Crespo et al., 2013; Schölzel-Dorenbos et al., 2010).

Similar challenges apply to ratings of acceptance of technologies. With progression of one's dementia journey, a client may eventually be unable to respond to questions on their preferences for using AgeTech. In such cases, caregivers may serve as proxies. However, like quality-of-life measures, it is recommended that self-ratings, proxy ratings, and observations of behaviors be used by occupational therapists to obtain an accurate indication of a client's consent to use AgeTech. In the GPS study mentioned earlier, 45 client-caregiver dyads completed usability questionnaires before and after using one of three GPS wearable devices (Liu et al., 2018). Four of the six usability constructs were statistically significantly correlated between clients and caregivers: performance expectancy, social influence, behavioral intention to use, and actual use (Liu et al., 2018).

## SUMMARY

In this chapter we examined cognitive impairment, dementia, and occupational intervention. Cognitive impairment was described in the context of complex mental processes that affect ADLs. Dementia was examined with respect to types, prevalence rates, and clinical stages most often encountered by occupational therapists. Under OT intervention, we discussed screening, assessment, and types of OT programs. OT practitioners contributed descriptions and case examples from a rural site in the United States, and a geriatric rehabilitation program in an urban site in Canada. Both programs used multidimensional frameworks. In the latter part of the chapter, we examined the meaning of autonomy and independence and what this means in OT intervention. Inclusive assessments and interventions would consider the intersections of gender, age, race, dis/ability, and culture of our clients. Rather than autonomy and independence as the main driving constructs of our assessments, OT assessments and interventions would be more inclusive to underscore *relational autonomy* and *interdependence* in its frameworks. Relational autonomy is applied when caregivers are engaged in the assessment and intervention process, and clients' interdependence on caregivers and technology can enhance quality of life for clients living with dementia.

*The complete listing of the Bibliography and Chapter Questions and Answers are available in the accompanying enhanced eBook version included with the print purchase of this textbook. Visit Elsevier eBooks+ (eBooks.Health.Elsevier.com) to access this content.*

## CASE EXAMPLE  Ann

Ann is a 91-year-old female with a diagnosis of mild neurocognitive disorder. Ann was referred for CST assessment due to concerns with memory deficits impacting her ability to communicate (word-find deficits) and interact with her family. Standardized assessments performed included: SLUMS, KATZ Index, Trail-Making A and B, QOL-AD, CSDD, TUG, FTSST (see Table 16.1).

Ann's performance on SLUMS indicated mild neurocognitive disorder with a score of 21/30. KATZ Index indicated general independence with ADLs. Family reports Ann is independent in most IADL tasks with exception of family-assist for financial management. Trail-Making Test A and B showed some visual and executive function deficits. The CSDD and QOL-AD, performed by the social worker, were negative for depression and showed moderate quality of life, which corresponded with family's report. Physical measures using TUG/FTSS were in low normal range. Ann was able to have meaningful conversations, and exhibited no visual or auditory deficits. She was found to be a good candidate for group CST with exercise and participated in 14 sessions delivered by an occupational therapy and social worker.

Goals included independent or self-cueing (use of name tags) for recall of group members' names, engagement in reciprocal language without prompts, improved cognition evidenced by improvement in SLUMS performance by 3–4 points, and improved communication with reduction of word-find deficits.

Ann's post-assessment indicated the following goals were met: recalling group members' names, engagement in reciprocal language without prompts, improved cognition evidenced by a 5-point increase in SLUMS score (26/30). Improvements in word-find deficits, and global communication were reported by family. Ann's QOL-AD score improved by 4 points, and she reported enjoyment in participating in CST. She stated feeling stronger, which correlated with marked improvements in TUG/FTSST. It was recommended that Ann continue weekly MCST.

## CASE EXAMPLE  Mrs. B

Mrs. B is a 73-year-old woman of Canadian Indigenous descent. She grew up in Northern Canada and was sent to residential schools as a child. She completed Grade 7 at age 13 before running away from school. At 17, she trained as a nurse's aide and worked at a small hospital until her retirement at age 65. She lives alone in a small two-bedroom house in the city. Her adult children brought her to the emergency room at a local hospital after she experienced a fall in the community. She was found to have a fractured pelvis and left femur. After being stabilized in the acute care hospital, she was transferred to our facility for physical rehabilitation in the Geriatric Rehabilitation Program. The inter-hospital transfer papers listed "advanced cognitive impairment, probable dementia" among her diagnoses. Additional comments about the patient included: "Slow to respond, doesn't follow directions, forgetful. SLUMS score–20/30."

*Continued*

**CASE EXAMPLE   Mrs. B —Cont'd**

When the Geriatric Rehabilitation Program occupational therapist asked the patient admission screening questions about cognition and functioning in ADL and IADL, the patient did not identify any concerns. This was supported by collateral information obtained from the patient's family. The patient declined to do the clock drawing test and the mood or anxiety screening questionnaires. However, the patient was friendly, forthcoming, chatty, and engaged during the admission screening. The occupational therapist noted in the chart "Patient's cognition appears generally intact."

When the occupational therapist administered global cognitive screening tests a week later, the MoCA score was 18/30 (indicating dementia) and Mrs. B seemed reluctant to respond at times and did not answer some questions. The patient often replied to questions with comments like "I don't know" or "I can't do that." The EXIT score was 20/50, suggesting executive impairment. While these tests scores were consistent with the previous SLUMS score, the occupational therapist charted that these scores did not seem to match the patient's presentation on the unit, nor the patient's and family's report of patient functioning.

The occupational therapist met with the patient and family to discuss the results of the SLUMS, MoCA, and EXIT. The patient was clearly upset over the findings. The assessments brought back memories of Indigenous residential school where, as a child, she was shamed by the teachers for not performing up to their standards. Since then, exams had instilled a fear in her. She said the "beep" sounds made by the timer triggered anxiety in her and paralyzed her from answering questions. She also complained that so many questions were "fired" at her in such a short time, and she was not given enough time to answer them. The family confirmed that, in their culture, it is respectful to wait for answers to a question before asking another, to allow time for silence and reflection. When the family inquired about the content of the tests, they said the test items were not culturally sensitive and that they did not reflect the experiences and education of the patient. Mrs. B echoed the family's concerns and said, "What do these tests have to do with my life anyway?"

The patient and family made it clear that they felt the occupational therapy and treatment team had not shown the patient the respect she was due. Mrs. B was concerned about the poor scores on the cognitive screening tests being on her "permanent record" in the hospital chart, and she worried about being "hauled off" to a care home against her will, just as she had been with the residential schools. After much discussion about what was important to Mrs. B and her family, the occupational therapist offered an alternate approach for further testing, if the patient was interested. The patient and family agreed to the new plan, in which the therapist would use testing scenarios that were more relevant to the patient.

The occupational therapist proceeded with functional-cognitive testing using performance-based items framed as tasks the patient may do with her family or friends. Mrs. B said this approach made sense to her. For example, the Kettle Test was framed as the patient having a friend over for coffee and a chat. With the EFPT, the cooking item was framed as making a new recipe of oats for her grandchild; for the Telephone item, she decided to look up the number for a grocery store in her neighborhood and phoned there to inquire about grocery delivery, and so on. The results of the functional cognitive testing suggested no issues with executive function, activity performance, or safety. Despite being asked to do novel tasks in a novel environment as part of the testing, the patient said, "It didn't feel like testing, I was just doing things anyone would do."

While standardized cognitive screening tests like the MoCA and SLUMS are quick and easy to administer and score, and they have clear advantages for mitigating biases and inconsistencies of non-standardized assessments, these tests (and the standardized way in which they are administered) come with cultural and education biases which can negatively impact performance and hence diagnosis of patients. This highlights the importance of basing clinical opinions about a patient's cognition on different sources, of getting to know the patient, of understanding the cultural and educational background before testing, and of using a variety of approaches in cognitive testing in order to obtain a valid picture of cognitive functioning within the context of a patient's life.

**CASE EXAMPLE   Kay**

Kay is a 72-year-old female with a diagnosis of vascular dementia and depression. Identified areas of concern included lack of interaction with family, memory deficits, decreasing functional independence, excessive sleep/inactivity, and orientation deficits. COPE was initiated with the goal of identifying her current cognitive level and capabilities in order to provide recommendations for communication, task simplification, purposeful activities, and environmental modifications at a level consistent with her capability and cognitive level. Assessments showed moderate to severe dementia. Deficits were noted in initiation, planning/organization, and proficiency and completion of ADL/IADL tasks, along with moderate dependency for ADL/IADL tasks. The assessments included: LACLS, ADM-2, DAD, Bristol, RCS, and FAST (see Tables 16.2 and 16.3). Interest inventory indicated interest in John Wayne movies, cats, baseball and football games, music, watching musicals, and flowers. A Timed Up and Go test score of 35.5 s indicated fall risk and mobility deficits.

Examples of Intervention Strategies:
- Care Partner Education—on use of therapeutic lying (telling "white lies" in order to temporarily placate the person with dementia), name and framing strategies, the person with dementia's current capabilities, use of redirection, use of simple one- to two-word commands, and stress reduction.
- Purposeful Activity Prescription—included listening to music, watching favorite ball games, movies, musicals, simple floral arrangements, and simple exercise.
- Environmental Modifications—recommendations for a shower bench and handheld shower.
- Task Modification—placing items in line of sight (water bottle to increase fluid intake). Simplifying task directions and use of prompts.

Outcomes: Improved engagement in activities, less sleeping, increased participation in IADL/ADL tasks with less resistance, and care partner generalization of learned information.

## CHAPTER 17

# Aging Adults and Mental Health: Engaging in Meaningful Occupations

*Lauren Angela Selingo, MSOT, OTR, Michelle Perryman-Fox, PhD, MSc, BA (Hons), Vimita Patel, MD, George Grossberg, MD, and Virginia C. Stoffel, PhD, OT, FAOTA*

## CHAPTER OUTLINE

## OBJECTIVES

- Understand how occupations might be disrupted for older persons living with psychiatric and substance use disorders as well as common symptoms, presentations, and the relationship between disorders and aging processes
- Consider the psychosocial implications of social expectations of older persons, the effects upon their mental health, and engagement in occupation
- Identify with the roles, attributes, and distinct values of the interprofessional mental health team to facilitate older persons' purposeful engagement in occupation
- Identify occupational therapy approaches, interventions, and evaluations to support older persons' engagement in occupation when psychiatric or substance use disorders impact their lives

## Introduction

### Older Adults' Current Mental Health

Whether you are an occupational therapy (OT) student, practicing occupational therapist (OT), occupational therapy assistant (OTA), or mental health professional who has come to this text with the desire to explore OT's role in mental health intervention, welcome!

OT is a profession whose origins are rooted in the treatment of mental health disorders (Stoffel & Moyers, 2004); our skill sets in this area are critical, as globally, older adult populations (60 years of age and over) are projected to experience an increase in mental health challenges between now and 2050, and 20% of older adults have been estimated to have a mental health or neurological condition as of 2017 (World Health Organization [WHO], 2017). OT practitioners who work with older adults across settings (for example, inpatient, long-term care facilities, outpatient clinics, or community senior centers) are likely interacting with individuals who present with mental health needs.

### Chapter Approach

The purpose of the chapter is to provide introductory knowledge regarding older adult mental health factors, diagnoses, barriers, and facilitators to older adults' engagement in desired occupations, and the role of OT practitioners and interprofessional care team members across therapy processes.

This chapter is authored by three occupational therapists with varying international experience—two from the United States and one from the United Kingdom, along with two physicians with psychiatric and medical backgrounds. International perspectives on older adults' mental health care are incorporated across the chapter.

The authors recognize that their perspectives regarding older adults, mental health, and the OT process within mental health care are shaped by personal characteristics and experiences in practicing as medical professionals in differing settings and institutions. It is in the spirit of critical reflexivity or "beliefs, values, and social and systemic structures" and "how such dimensions influence our daily professional practice" (Kinsella et al., 2012, p. 214) that the authors invite you to approach this work. Beyond this chapter, it is encouraged that the reader seek additional resources from alternative voices and perspectives to enhance learning. The experiences of two older adults from different health-care systems within the United States (Robert) and the United Kingdom (Anne) will be presented. The OT process (screening, evaluation, intervention, and discharge) will be used to enable the reader to bridge the gap between theory, evidence, and practice. When engaging with the case studies, it is important to remember that the US model of health care works on a privatized system and the United Kingdom is a social model of health care.

Evidence-informed reasoning questions are included in each section to promote critical reflection. The aim is to expand the reader's reflective practice skills, meaning "... a way for professionals to learn through reflection on their experience, as a way to generate knowledge in and from practice, as a means to acknowledge practitioner experience knowledge as significant, and as an approach to negotiating the challenging complexities of professional practice" (Kinsella et al., 2012, p. 211). The reader is encouraged to engage with the questions in the boxes to pause, reflect, and examine the case studies. As you read the chapter, engage in the creative process of writing your thoughts down, and remember there are no "right" and "wrong" answers, as incorporating new knowledge into practice takes time and experience (Harries & Duncan, 2011) and all reasoning is contextual.

To initiate the personal reflective process across the chapter, think about the following questions in the Reflection Break 1 box:

## REFLECTION BREAK 1

**Exploring Personal Assumptions and Implicit Biases**

Before you read on, consider these questions:
1. When you think of older persons, what do you picture?
2. What are the factors you initially assume about older persons' mental health and well-being?
3. What questions are you hoping will be raised regarding older adults and mental health as you move into this chapter?

## Community Participation, Personal Engagement, and Access to Health Care for Older Adults

Our understanding, perspectives, and assumptions of old age influence our therapeutic approach to practice and service provision. It is essential to understand that everyone experiences the aging process no matter how old we are, yet we

understand that the "end cycle of life," "...is socially constructed either by cultural assumptions or, more than often, policy and legislation" (McIntyre, 2013, p. 17). With the proportion of older people living with a mental health diagnosis on the rise, such diagnoses have a significant impact on older adults' autonomy, rights, quality of life, functionality, and occupational choices meaning, "the process that leads to engagement as a result of intrinsic and extrinsic factors" (Brennan & Gallagher, 2017).

Older people are not a homogeneous group. We all have varying skills, needs, resources, and interests. Despite this, assumptions regarding older people as a population and their choices of occupation remain. Ageism is defined as the denial of basic human rights of older persons and is considered one of the most pervasive prejudices across human society (Brownell, 2010). Ageist attitudes result in categorizing people solely on the basis of their age and assumptions regarding "shared" occupations (e.g., the belief that older adults avoid using technologies) (Reynolds & Lim, 2013). This indicates discriminatory attitudes and actions within general society as well as the health and social care factors. Prevalent beliefs equate old age with being depressed, lonely, or confused. However, it is essential to be cautious when speculating about the psychology of aging adults because of the significant danger in believing that as we become old, we must fall into these categories (Birren et al., 2018). Such assumptions can limit both older adults' and OT practitioners perceptions of older adults' realities and capabilities (Birren et al., 2018).

Older adults are underserved in the area of mental health due to the stereotypes and the previous experiences of their access to care and health services (Bodner et al., 2018). This gap in care is concerning, given that the world population is aging, and increasing numbers of older adults (age 65 and older) are projected to be living with a mental health condition by 2050 (about 20%) (WHO, 2017). Due to the stigma surrounding older adults' mental health, such conditions are under-identified by health-care professionals (Bodner et al., 2018). Wuthrich and Frei's (2015) study used questionnaires before and after treatment to ascertain 60 older persons' (aged 60 to 79 years) barriers to engaging in health care. Findings indicated that lacking access to resources such as transportation, holding beliefs that it is typical to be anxious and depressed at older ages, assuming that psychological therapy is less likely to be effective for older persons, and a lack of unhelpful therapy due to therapists' lacking of understanding of older persons' unique challenges, served as barriers to participation in care services, amongst other variables (Wuthrich & Frei, 2015). Consequently, with the restriction of engagement in health care services, the risk of a person experiencing significant occupational deprivation, meaning, "a prolonged restriction in participating in necessary or meaningful activities due to circumstances outside of the individual's control" is enhanced (Whiteford, 2010, p. 201). For older persons, continued ageist perspectives, lack of education, and subsequent access to health-care services can impact engagement in purposeful occupation, long-term health, and well-being.

## Redefining Occupations

Bearing in mind the impact of ageism and that people are shaped by their personal contextual factors, we can examine the potential changes that older adults can experience. First, it is important to understand the concept of occupational engagement, or "the involvement in an occupation with current positive personal value attached to it," and "a fluctuating state influenced by complex and multiple internal and external factors" (Morris & Cox, 2017). Activities of daily living (ADLs) (e.g., dressing, bathing) (Holstein et al., 2007) and instrumental activities of daily living (IADLs) (e.g., medication management, shopping) can require additional levels of physical or cognitive assistance for older adults (Gontijo Guerra et al., 2021). Engagement in valued occupations such as work, community and social participation, physical activity, and leisure pursuits all support health outcomes for older adults and one's quality of life

(Stav et al., 2012). In considering the importance of continued participation in desired occupations (Stav et al., 2012), changes in older adults' physical skills may challenge their understanding of themselves within the context of their occupations (Mulholland & Jackson, 2018).

When collaborating with older adults to promote re-immersion in one's desired occupations and address barriers and facilitators to occupational engagement, it is important to be aware of potential mental health diagnoses and symptoms older adults may be experiencing for the first time, or across their lives. Box 17.1 includes brief descriptions of common mental health diagnoses that older adults can experience as adapted from the American Psychiatric Association (APA) Diagnostic and Statistical Manual of Mental Disorders (5th edition) (DSM-5) (2013).

Older adults with mental health challenges should not be and are not defined by their diagnosis; there are complex personal factors and facets that make up who they are as occupational beings, as illustrated in Robert's and Anne's case studies.

### BOX 17.1 DSM-5 Criteria for Common Mental Health Diagnoses That Can Present in Older Adults

| | |
|---|---|
| Major Depressive Disorder | Five or more symptoms during a 2-week period, representing a change of functioning, and at least one of the symptoms should be either (1) depressed mood or (2) loss of interest or pleasure.<br>1. Depressed mood most of the day, nearly every day.<br>2. Markedly diminished interest or pleasure in activities most of the day, nearly every day.<br>3. Change in appetite nearly every day, resulting in body weight change of 5% in a month.<br>4. Psychomotor agitation or retardation (observable by others).<br>5. Fatigue almost every day.<br>6. Feelings of worthlessness or guilt almost every day.<br>7. Reduced ability to concentrate nearly every day.<br>8. Persistent thoughts of death, suicidal ideation without a specific plan, or a suicide attempt or a specific plan for committing suicide.<br>These symptoms must cause the person significant distress or functional impairment. Substance abuse or another medical condition must be ruled out. |
| Generalized Anxiety Disorder | Excessive anxiety and worry, occurring most days for at least 6 months, about many topics or activities. Individuals find it extremely difficult to control this anxiety.<br>The following symptoms are associated (at least three needed for diagnosis):<br>1. Restlessness<br>2. Feeling easily tired<br>3. Impaired concentration<br>4. Irritability<br>5. Muscle tension<br>6. Restless sleep, difficulty falling or staying asleep |
| Bipolar I Disorder Manic Episode | At least 1 week of elevated, expansive, or irritable mood. Additionally, three or more of the following symptoms are seen:<br>1. Grandiosity<br>2. Decreased need for sleep<br>3. Pressured speech (rapid talking)<br>4. Flight of ideas<br>5. Distractibility<br>6. Increase in goal-directed activity or psychomotor agitation<br>7. Excessively indulging in pleasurable activities without regard for consequences |

*(Continued)*

| BOX 17.1 | DSM-5 Criteria for Common Mental Health Diagnoses That Can Present in Older Adults—Cont'd |
|---|---|
| Post-traumatic Stress Disorder | Exposure to actual or threatened death, serious injury, or sexual violence in at least one of the following ways:<br>1. Directly experiencing trauma<br>2. Witnessing trauma occurring to others<br>3. Learning about trauma occurring to a close family member or friend<br>4. Indirect aversive exposure to details of the traumatic event<br><br>Presence of one (or more) of the following intrusion symptoms associated with the traumatic event:<br>1. Distressing memories of the traumatic event<br>2. Recurrent distressing dreams<br>3. Flashbacks of the trauma<br>4. Psychological distress at reminders of the trauma<br>5. Physical reactions to reminders of the trauma<br>Persistent avoidance of stimuli associated with the traumatic event:<br>1. Avoidance of distressing memories, thoughts, or feelings<br>2. Avoidance of external reminders of trauma<br><br>Negative change in cognition and mood associated with the traumatic event:<br>1. Impairment of memory of trauma due to dissociative amnesia<br>2. Negative beliefs or expectations about oneself or the world<br>3. Cognitions related to trauma that lead the individual to blame self or others<br>4. Persistently negative emotional states<br>5. Reduced interest or participation in activities<br>6. Feelings of detachment from others<br>7. Persistent inability to experience positive emotion<br><br>Marked alteration in arousal and reactivity:<br>1. Irritability and anger<br>2. Recklessness<br>3. Hypervigilance<br>4. Exaggerated startle response<br>5. Problems with concentration<br>6. Sleep disturbances |
| Delirium | 1. Disturbances in attention and awareness (reduced orientation to the environment).<br>2. This disturbance develops over a short period of time (usually hours to a few days) and represents a change from baseline attention and awareness. It tends to fluctuate in severity during the course of a day.<br>3. A disturbance in cognition (e.g., memory deficit, disorientation, language, visuospatial ability, or perception).<br>4. The disturbances are not better explained by another preexisting neurocognitive disorder.<br>5. There is evidence that the disturbance is a direct physiological consequence of an underlying medical condition, substance intoxication or withdrawal, or toxin. |
| Major Neurocognitive Disorder (formerly Dementia) | Significant cognitive decline from a previous baseline level in one or more cognitive domains:<br>1. Learning and memory<br>2. Language<br>3. Executive function<br>4. Complex attention<br>5. Perceptual motor<br>6. Social cognition<br>The cognitive deficits interfere with performance of activities of daily living such as managing finances and medications. Cognition is not altered due to delirium or another psychiatric disorder. |

Adapted from the American Psychiatric Association. (2013). *Diagnostic and statistical manual of mental health disorders* (5th ed.). Arlington, VA.

## Learning About the Person: Interviews, Observations, Screening, and Assessments

Older adults can experience ageist assumptions regarding their needs and well-being, and continued therapy may be unhelpful due to therapists' lack of understanding of persons' unique challenges, which may inhibit older adults' access to skilled mental health care (Wuthrich & Frei, 2015). With this in mind, the OT practitioner working with older adults needs to intentionally use a person-centered approach (Tonga et al., 2015) through a combination of collaborative methods to provide a picture of what the person's occupational performance motivations,

## Case Studies: Introduction to Robert and Anne

### Robert

Robert is a 75-year-old Latino man who is living alone in his multi-level suburban home after the recent death of his wife in a small US city. He loves to socialize with his neighbors and attends his local church twice a week. Robert has been fairly healthy throughout his life, with a brief episode of depression in his late 20s. Robert chose to be alcohol-free as he found it exacerbated his depression. He has three children in their 40s and 50s, with his closest child (his son) living 3 hours away. Robert has worked as an accountant throughout his adulthood and enjoys completing large puzzles with his wife in his free time. Prior to his wife's passing, the couple was taking care of their three grandchildren over a weekend once every 2 months while his son and his wife travel. After his wife's passing, Robert tells his children he can continue to do the daily chores he and his wife would share (his wife would cook meals, do the laundry, and clean the home, while Robert would wash the dishes, complete larger home management projects, manage finances, and complete yard work). Robert's son comes to the house once a month to assist with yard work and larger home management tasks, and the family has set up a meal delivery service to provide dinners for Robert 4 days a week to ease the level of kitchen clean-up he must do. Robert is very close with his neighbors who live on either side of his home; they frequently drop off meals, manage his yard care on the weekends, take him to church, and spend time talking with Robert whenever he sits outside on his porch. During the months following his wife's death, Robert's children note that he appears to be struggling with his grief, and intermittently reaches out to them multiple times a week over the phone. His neighbors also begin to worry about Robert, as he frequently does not answer the door, and often forgets to bring in meals that his neighbors leave on his porch or those delivered by the delivery service, which is highly unusual for him. He does not come outside to sit on his porch as often, and when he does, he is not his usual, animated self.

Six months after the death of his wife, Robert's children notice that he is increasingly acting unusually; he does not answer their calls, and when his children are able to get a hold of him, his speech is frequently slurred, his conversations are difficult to follow, and he is confused about the time of day and who he is speaking to at times. His neighbors do not see Robert sitting on his porch anymore, and one neighbor becomes so concerned when Robert does not answer the door after multiple visits from neighbors that she calls his son, who is finally able to get a hold of Robert by calling him. When his son comes to visit earlier than usual, he finds that Robert has not been keeping up with the household chores; he appears unkempt and confused at times. Robert's son tells him that he and his wife will be postponing their travel plans, that Robert will not have to take care of his grandchildren, and that his son will be visiting the following month.

Consider…

- What health issues and diagnosis(es) might you consider that Robert might have based on his current functioning?

### Anne

Anne is a 95-year-old white female who lives alone in a one-bedroom flat on the third floor or a housing building in the United Kingdom in a large, urban city. Anne is known for her strong will and independence; she is not receiving support for her daily needs, activities of daily living, or instrumental activities of daily living. She lightly cleans her flat once a week, and enjoys taking on cooking challenges when preparing meals for herself. She receives assistance from her niece and nephew who visit biweekly to support with management of her finances and heavier cleaning tasks. Anne does the majority of her shopping by herself, and will walk to and from shops that are near her building to shop for food and personal care items. Anne's husband passed away over a decade ago, and she has no living children, as her son died when he was 15 years old. She is known to be the athlete and the dancer of the family and loves to spend time with people around her. She will attend local concerts with friends or family members around once a month, she often hosts bridge games at her flat. Anne has not had any significant medical needs throughout her life, and regularly attends check-ins with her general practitioner, who recently recommended that Anne use a four-point rolling walker for support when ambulating for long distances. Anne has been hesitant to implement this recommendation, as she is concerned that using the walker will significantly impair her ability to engage in her home care tasks and social activities. She has not been taking the walker with her when running errands about the local community. Her niece is particularly concerned about Anne going out into the community without her walker, as she has been noticing that Anne has recently been having difficulties with safe mobility in the home and has been struggling with safely entering and exiting her shower, which has a slight step. Anne has also been reporting that she is skipping meals due to a lack of appetite. When Anne's niece has brought up her concerns with Anne, Anne tends to change the subject of conversation, and does not appear to wish to discuss her current functioning in and outside of the home.

Consider…

- Given Anne's personal factors, mental and physical factors, what occupational issues (Trentham & Dunal, 2009) might she be at risk for?

supports and barriers are, and tapping into the goals defined by the person in order to fully participate in their important and meaningful occupations. Starting with the occupational profile (American Occupational Therapy Association [AOTA], 2020), a picture of the older adult's everyday life emerges. Using an interview process, daily activities related to what the person wants and needs to do are explored, strengths are identified, and environmental resources are apprised. In the course of exploring habits and routines, the occupational therapist collaborates with the older adult to note occupations that contribute to one's mental health and well-being (such as social connectedness and restful sleep), and those that may put the person's wellness at risk (such as the use of tobacco, negative thinking, or lack of engagement in personally meaningful occupations). The occupational profile highlights the person's strengths and guides the collaborative process from which the older adult and OT practitioner develop the intervention planning process. The Activity Card Sort, second edition (Baum & Edwards, 2019), including 89 cards with photos of instrumental, leisure, and social activities, might be a useful resource.

In building your own occupational profile for Anne and Robert, you can consider the following questions in the Reflection Break 2 box:

---

### REFLECTION BREAK 2

**Learning About Anne and Robert**

1. What do you identify as their valued occupations?
2. Who are the people in their lives who play a critical role in carrying out their daily and weekly routines?
3. What changes do you see in their occupational performance that might reflect mental distress?
4. What information might you need to more fully understand Robert and Anne's situations?
5. Who might also play a key role in finding the optimal solutions to their health and wellness (family, medical, community, and peer supports)?
6. What social determinants of health are considered to impact on Robert and Anne's situation (barriers and facilitators)?

---

Should additional information be needed to further explore potential facilitators and barriers to everyday life, and document the intervention effectiveness, several OT assessments might be selected to complete a comprehensive assessment.

The Canadian Model of Occupational Participation (CanMOP) (Egan & Restall, 2022), which was formerly known as the Canadian Model of Occupational Performance (COPM) and the Canadian Model of Occupational Performance and Engagement (CMOP-E) guides the Canadian Measure of Occupational Performance assessment tool (Law et al., 2019), and provides provide insight into the person's concerns related to their occupational engagement in the areas of self-care, leisure, and productivity. The model and assessment highlight the importance of individuals' ability to choose to engage in occupations that are meaningful to them, as well

as their satisfaction with their performance, and their personal environment (Egan & Restall, 2022; Law et al., 2019). The Role Checklist Version 3 (Scott et al., 2017) engages in a reflection of past, current, and future occupational roles, with a focus on building future roles with an understanding of past and current roles. The Canadian Personal Recovery Outcome Measure (Barbic, 2018) provides a snapshot of personal well-being in the past week based on agreement with 30 descriptors of statements reflecting outcomes of mental health recovery that takes into consideration the item difficulty as well as the person's ability. Items considered to be associated with early recovery include:

- "I am motivated to keep myself well."
- "I sleep well."
- "I have a purpose in life."
- "I have new interests."
- "I can be an advocate for myself."
- "I am respected by others."
- "I contribute to my community."
- "I have peace of mind."

Each of these tools offers insights into the mental health and other life challenges the person faces and provides a means of tracking progress and change over time when used as a baseline with re-evaluations.

Several screening tools will offer insights into the severity of depression, anxiety, and substance use (Hospital Anxiety and Depression Scale, Bjelland, et al., 2002; Geriatric Depression Scale, Parmelee & Katz, 1990), as well as the Screening and Brief Intervention for Referral and Treatment (SBIRT) for alcohol and substance use disorders (https://www.samhsa.gov/sbirt) may be indicated. Depending on the severity of depression, anxiety, and harmful substance use, referral with other members of the treatment team might be indicated, with the OT practitioner carefully monitoring for suicidal thinking and actively facilitating the older adult and caregivers' engagement in strategies for coping and harm reduction.

Measures associated with assessing/evaluating functional cognition might help to shape realistic expectations around safety, autonomy, and caregiver engagement. The Cognitive Performance Test (Burns, 2018) generates a profile of cognitive function around ADLs, IADLs, and independent living care. Chapter 15 (Neurology and Cognition) and Chapter 16 (Cognitive Impairment and Occupational Therapy Interventions) provide additional measures used as OT cognitive and performance assessments.

All of the information generated in the evaluation process will help shape where and how the older adult might receive OT services (e.g., primary care, specialized inpatient, outpatient, day care, community, in-home and telehealth care). Providing assistance with accessing programs and services to meet the identified needs and support the person's goals are important contributions of the OT practitioner, who also observes as an advocate and ally, should barriers such as racism, classism, ageism, ableism, or sexism interfere with the older adult's ability to engage in everyday occupations.

Turning to Robert and Anne, apply your clinical reasoning to the changes presented in their functional status and consider answering the questions posed in their case studies that follow.

## Case Studies: Clarifying and Meeting Robert and Anne's Health Needs

### Robert

Robert's son observes during his visit the following month, that the home appears to be in a worse state, with Robert appearing disoriented and speaking to people who are not present, including his mother and wife, both of whom are deceased. Concerned, Robert's son takes him to the emergency room, as he is worried that Robert may have had a stroke. Once at the emergency department, Robert is eventually diagnosed by a psychiatrist as having schizophrenia. Robert's son, the primary decision-maker of the family, agrees with the psychiatrist's recommendation that Robert be admitted to the hospital's inpatient behavioral health unit for treatment.

Consider...

- Think back to your previous assumptions regarding Robert's potential diagnosis and health condition. What might be the pitfalls of assuming a diagnosis based on age and gender?

To assess Robert, the occupational therapist on the unit chooses to use the Canadian Measure of Occupational Performance (CMOP), as the assessment will allow Robert to review his ability to engage in and his satisfaction across numerous occupations and allows for personal re-assessment across the treatment process (Law et al., 2019). When completing the COPM, Robert scores a 2 for satisfaction and performance in multiple self-care activities, including personal care and community management, a 1 for performance and 2 for satisfaction in productivity activities including household management, and a 4 for performance and 3 for satisfaction in quiet leisure and socialization activities (Law et al., 2019).

Consider...

- In recalling Robert's occupational history and personal roles, what occupations and skills might you want to target during therapy, given Robert's COPM results?
- How might Robert's cultural background influence your assessments, interventions, interactions with, and recommendations for Robert?

### Anne

About 3 months after Anne's niece begins to notice changes in Anne's eating and mobility patterns, Anne experiences numerous falls in the home and in the community in quick succession, with the most recent and severe fall occurring within her local store whilst attempting to buy biscuits. Anne's niece takes her to the hospital, whereupon admission, Anne presents with acute confusion and a suspected infection. During the admissions process, she becomes agitated and frightened, and chooses not to answer questions that the medical team presents to her. Anne's niece shares information regarding Anne's most recent functioning and falls to the accident and emergency room care team. Anne is then transferred to a medical ward. While there, Anne also demonstrates difficulties in engaging in activities of daily living, such as dressing and toileting, as she struggles with staying focused and recalling the steps of each task. She is referred to the occupational therapy team to understand how her current cognition and physical abilities are impacting her functioning. Due to Anne's confusion, she was unable to engage in purposeful conversation regarding her occupational history. Therefore, with her best interest in mind, the multidisciplinary frailty team contacted Anne's niece to establish her social history to understand her level of previous function compared to her current presentation.

Anne's niece reports when visiting Anne, she has been known to experience bouts of paranoia and suspected short-term memory challenges, such as leaving doors and windows open, and voicing concerns that she has been robbed. It was reported that Anne has recently demonstrated a significant reduction in her oral intake, with snacks serving as her primary source of nutrition throughout the day. Consequently, she has lost weight.

As a result of Anne's disoriented presentation, when evaluating her, the occupational therapist inquired as to the length of time she has demonstrated hyperactive confusion (disorientation to day and time, pacing, hyperactive speech), and how long her reduced water and food intake has been occurring. Anne's niece reported these symptoms as worsening over a 2-week period.

Consider...

- In applying your knowledge of delirium, what do you think the occupational therapist should do in this incidence where there was a dramatic reduction of function following hyper delirium?
- Who would you need to discuss this with on the medical team?

In assessing Anne's current functioning, the occupational therapist observes her engaging in multiple ADLs and IADLs, including toileting, dressing, using the phone, and completing a light meal preparation task (which involved Anne making a cup of tea). During the observations, the occupational therapist notices that Anne struggles with staying on task and the sequencing of many of the task steps. The occupational therapist communicates the results of the assessment observations, family reports, and Anne's redacted fluid intake to her medical team, which includes the nurse, care coordinator, and a social worker. It is suspected by the team that Anne has experienced a urinary tract infection, which has exacerbated Anne's suspected onset of memory loss through hyper delirium, causing significant bouts of confusion and aggression. Anne is placed on a 2-week round of antibiotics and intravenous fluids as a medical intervention.

Consider the following questions in the Reflection Break 3 box:

---

**REFLECTION BREAK 3**

**Evaluating Anne and Robert**

1. Do you feel that Robert meets the diagnostic criteria for schizophrenia and that Anne presents with hyper delirium?
2. What might you do if you as Anne's or Roberts' therapist notice changes in the symptoms they are displaying during your initial interactions and their evaluations?
3. In addition to conducting standardized tests or observing participation in daily activities within Robert's and Anne's evaluations, what types of additional topics might be important for Robert and Anne to talk about in exploring their current functioning and personal contexts?
4. If Anne or Robert are unable to provide you with some of the information you need in creating an occupational profile, who might they direct you to talk with?

---

## Designing Persons' Goals and Interventions

### Goals, Interventions, and Outcomes

Occupational therapy is a person-centered, occupation-driven profession (Mee & Sumsion, 2001), meaning persons actively engage in collaboration with the OT practitioner regarding their personal goals, desired occupations, interventions, and progress evaluation. Within mental health settings, person-centered goal setting is linked to better long- term independence and self-support outcomes (DeAngelis et al., 2019), and personal occupations can serve an important role in developing personal satisfaction and empowerment within (Hultqvist et al., 2015).

Evidence-informed interventions (interventions and practice that are driven by research evidence with additional focus on the personal contexts of the person who is receiving treatment) (Miles & Loughlin, 2011) that address the person's desired occupations and personal needs should be implemented. One guiding method to structuring therapy includes a strengths-based approach (Tse et al., 2016), which focuses on the person's goals, and "assets" (Tse et al., 2016). Personal self-determination is emphasized, with the therapist serving as a facilitator throughout treatment (Tse et al., 2016). Within Robert's and Anne's case studies, a strengths-based approach may include the OT practitioner incorporating Robert's and Anne's preferred leisure occupations, needed activities of daily living and instrumental activities of daily living tasks, and families into treatment interventions and education (Tse et al., 2016).

Occupational Therapy services can address a wide variety of preparatory and occupation-based skills (American Occupational Therapy Association (AOTA), 2020). Services can be delivered individually, within groups, or through consultative services (Burson et al., 2017). A brief exploration into potential topics and occupations that occupational therapy practitioners can address in their collaboration with older adults follows.

### Prevention, Health, and Wellness Promotion

Interventions targeting prevention, health, and wellness are aimed at reestablishing and maintaining holistic well-being (including physical, mental, and social functioning) (Burson et al., 2017). Treatment can focus on interventions that promote physical and mental well-being and preventative measures; these can include creating personal schedules that promote optimal sleep, exercise, and leisure engagement, and self-care plans that address the following aspects of self-care (physical, emotional, psychological, spiritual) (AOTA, 2020; Burson et al., 2017). Orientation and cognitive adaptation activities such as journaling, calendar planning, seasonal activities, task-chunking, and the use of descriptive sensory exploration can all serve as tools for orienting to person, time, and place (Brown, 2011).

Individuals can learn about and practice self-management skills for health promotion surrounding symptom and condition management, both within treatment and personal daily contexts (e.g., interactions with others, during desired occupations) through coping and adaptive skills, including meditation, psychoeducation, interpersonal skill training (Rotheram-Borus, 1988 as cited in Haertl & Christiansen, 2011), and creative expressions (Haertl & Christiansen, 2011).

### Medication Management

Medication management can serve as an important area of self-management, as older adults with mental health diagnoses may be given multiple medications to address symptoms and promote daily functioning (Siebert et al., 2017). Occupational therapy practitioners can promote the use of medications for symptom management through education regarding the medications a person is taking or is recommended to take through group and/or individual therapy (Siebert et al., 2017). Therapists can work with the people they serve to ensure that they are taking medications in the correct dosages and at the recommended times (Siebert et al., 2017). Occupational therapy practitioners can explore their habits regarding medication use or nonuse and incorporate their goals into medication management using motivational interviewing techniques (Siebert et al., 2017). Collaborating with people to identify compensatory and adaptive strategies, such as pillboxes or alarms, and establishing routines can be useful for those who may need cognitive adaptations to promote engagement in daily occupations (Sanders & Van Oss, 2013; Siebert et al., 2017). Ensuring that people have access to printed medication directions and using "teach back" methods also serve a role in collaborating with other health-care professionals (e.g., pharmacists, psychiatrists) (Siebert et al., 2017) to establish a medication plan that is manageable for the person, given their personal contexts and capabilities (Sanders & Van Oss, 2013; Siebert et al., 2017).

## Cognitive and Emotional Regulation

Cognitive and emotional regulation strategies are a key facet of treatment for older adults with mental health diagnoses. Descriptions and applications of two approaches will be illustrated next.

Cognitive behavioral therapy (CBT) is an intervention approach composed of numerous models (Buttler et al., 2006, as cited in McCraith, 2011). While occupational therapy practitioners are not CBT therapists, they *can* use CBT approaches to guide their therapy (McCraith, 2011). From an OT perspective, a CBT approach addresses personal cognitions and beliefs that prevent one's engagement in desired occupations (McCraith, 2011). The intervention focus is placed on personal growth in gaining new perspectives, cognitive processes, and behaviors that promote occupational engagement and that can be used in addressing challenges that arise within one's daily life (McCraith, 2011). Given our profession's emphasis on occupational performance, OT practitioners' use of CBT approaches should be tied to collaborating with the person to promote changes in "surface-level automatic thoughts, intermediate assumptions, and "rules for living"" that impact engagement in one's desired occupations (McCraith, 2011).

Robert's occupational therapist could use a CBT approach when Robert comments, "I don't see the point in sitting on the porch anymore; I have nothing to say and the neighbors are always nosey." The occupational therapist could use Socratic questioning, or open-ended questions that promote collaborative discovery of solutions that benefit the person, given a specific problem. This would involve discussing the potential outcomes of Robert choosing to sit on his porch and engage with neighbors, with attention paid to considering the likelihood of each outcome (e.g., "what was the last interaction you had with a neighbor, did you share anything with them?") (McCraith, 2011). The occupational therapist must take care in avoiding over-interpretation of Robert's responses and must promote Robert's engagement in personal discovery surrounding his social occupational engagement (McCraith, 2011).

Emotional regulation or "efforts to control emotional states" is a key factor in promoting participation in one's desired occupations (Scheinhoz, 2011). Emotions play a role in how we cognitively process the world around us, and allow us to assess and understand experiences before, as, and after they occur (Scheinhoz, 2011). Regarding mental health, we can experience emotional dysregulation at times, which can include difficulties with responding to situations with emotions that are not "adaptive," given the particular situation (Schore, 2003, as cited in Scheinhoz, 2011). Dysregulation can present as difficulties with "moving on" from a strong emotion after an extended period of time (Scheinhoz, 2011). Occupational therapy practitioners can work with people on establishing emotional regulatory skills using a wide variety of approaches, including cognitive therapy, dialectical behavioral therapy, and skills training (e.g., mindfulness, distress tolerance) (Scheinhoz, 2011). Given Anne's recent agitation, her occupational therapist might work on emotional regulation skill-building with her by collaborating to find calming tools, such as music, that can be used when Anne is feeling angry or agitated during her admission (Scheinhoz, 2011). The therapist can provide education to care staff about what music Anne prefers when she is feeling agitated, and can collaborate with Anne to identify ways in which Anne can sense when she is feeling angry and verbally communicate to staff when she would like music to be played in her room (Scheinhoz, 2011).

## Activities of Daily Living, Instrumental Activities of Daily Living, and Home and Community Adaptations

Engagement in ADLs (e.g., sleeping, bathing, dressing, eating) and IADLs (e.g., food preparation, money management, home maintenance) are critical aspects of participation in daily life and completion of necessary occupations (AOTA, 2020). Symptoms that derive from depression, bipolar disorder, and other diagnoses can pose challenges to engaging in the spectrum of daily activities (Spangler, 2011), which makes an occupational therapist's skill sets in examining the whole person, their contexts, environments, and potential adaptations critical for re-engaging older adults in their desired occupations (AOTA, 2012). Considering and addressing social occupations with older adults is also highly important, as those who are living in rural settings may be impacted by loneliness or depression that contribute to difficulties in completing daily care activities and social engagement (Garabrant & Liu, 2021).

An important person-centered intervention OT practitioners can use targeting ADLs and IADLs includes occupational reflection, "a structured reflective process during which a person carefully analyzes the impact of their daily occupational patterns and routines on their health and well-being" (Bailliard et al., 2021). When engaging in occupational reflection, older adults can explore creating "activity patterns" and what beneficial changes they might implement within their habits and routines to promote healthy functioning following discharge (Bailliard et al., 2021). Personal reflection can more closely examine how one's engagement in various occupations impacts one's mental health, and the positive and negative factors one might experience when engaging in such occupations (Bailliard et al., 2021). Occupational reflection can promote personal connections to one's social environment and recognition of the positive implications of participating in social occupations (Bailliard et al., 2021). Overall, occupational reflection can serve as an important tool in growing personal insight into the effect of one's desired occupations on one's health, and it has been demonstrated to be an effective tool when used with adults with mental health diagnoses (Bailliard et al., 2021).

Collaborating with the person and their family and caregivers to identify potential home and community adaptations to increase safety and increase occupational performance in desired tasks may be needed (AOTA, 2012; Castaneda et al., 2013). Therapists may work with individuals to identify potential modifications to commonly accessed environments (e.g., sensory-based adaptations, medication location, in-home assistance) to promote full engagement (AOTA, 2016). For Robert, treatment targeting ADLs and IADLs may include collaborative family planning to establish additional in-home supports and adaptations (e.g., visual reminders for where items are stored in the kitchen, removing non-commonly used items from the counters and other spaces in the home, and establishing regular times when Robert's children meet with him to review occupational needs). For Anne, developing visual aids for orientation (e.g., a daily schedule that includes meals, and when she receives therapy) and food and water intake within her commonly accessed environments could be included within treatment to promote engagement in feeding and eating tasks.

### Social Participation and Community Integration

In addressing social participation and community engagement, attention should be paid to older adults' physical mobility skills and needs to prevent barriers to social occupations (Charles & Carstensen, 2010). Older adults may re-examine personal priorities, with increased focus placed on critical relationships (Charles & Carstensen, 2010). Emotional regulation skills can improve, and older adults may experience a decrease in the occurrence of negatively valenced feelings as they participate in social occupations (Charles & Carstensen, 2010). Social engagements serve as support in older adults' quality of life, including engagement in spiritual practices and maintaining one's social roles through participation in activities (Levasseur et al., 2009). From a community participation perspective, there are many factors that can promote or hinder older adult participation in their communities, including social and policy-based systems (Theis & Furner, 2011). Consideration regarding older adults' physical environment should also play a significant role, with older adults benefiting from increased seating availability within community spaces, and community support systems that meet mobility needs (Vaughan et al., 2016).

Participation in social occupations (including the desire or ability to participate) may be affected by mental health symptoms; therefore, older adults may benefit from targeted social skill-building interventions (Mann et al., 2017). Engagement in peer support, whether through virtual or in-person formats, intends to promote social relationships and role development and personal decision-making, which may be implemented in facilitating participation in social occupations (Davidson et al., 1999). Family participation in therapy and psychoeducation to address creating positive relationships, ways of supporting the person engaging in treatment, and social interaction skills also serve as important interventions in increasing re-engagement in desired social pursuits (Davidson et al., 1999).

### Grief, Bereavement, and Harm Reduction Related to Pain and Substance Use

Box 17.2 provides brief descriptions of bereavement and harm reduction factors to be aware of.

### Sensory Regulation

For older adults with sensory regulation difficulties, there are numerous sensory models that can be considered for intervention approaches (e.g., Jane Ayres' Sensory Integration Theory, 1972; Dunn's Model of Sensory Processing, 1997; Brown & Nicholson, 2011). Sensory modulation program activities have been beneficial in exploring and building skills

---

**BOX 17.2**    Grief and Bereavement and Harm Reduction Factors

| Grief and Bereavement | Harm Reduction Related to Pain and Substance Use |
|---|---|
| Older adults may experience numerous losses (independence, spouses, family, friends) as they continue to age (Pickens, 2011, p. 766). For individuals with mental health diagnoses, grief and bereavement surrounding the loss of a loved one can manifest uniquely (Pickens, 2011, pp. 767–768). Emphasis on participation in IADLs, with a focus on autonomous decision-making, particularly if an individual has lost a spouse or partner who assisted with tasks can serve in reconnecting individuals to their preferred occupations (Pickens, 2011, pp. 767–768). Encouraging individuals' exploration of grief expression and memorializing the deceased (e.g., engaging in activities and with physical spaces and individuals that the deceased person loved) can also serve as the focus of interventions (Pickens, 2011, p. 767). Recognizing that families may create shared rituals surrounding grief can allow for opportunities for collaborative occupational engagement between individuals and their loved ones (Pickens, 2011, p. 767). | Older adults may use substances such as alcohol and prescription medications at harmful levels to manage chronic pain or injuries. In approaching harmful substance use, a harm reduction approach may be implemented (Rao, 2014, p. 344). Such models emphasize decreasing the negative side effects and risks of substance use (Rao, 2014, p. 344). Interventions can include collaborating with the individual to identify strategies for limiting substance use and using motivational interviewing to explore change behaviors surrounding use (Rao, 2014, p. 344). This approach includes symptom tracking related to physical health/functioning to mitigate personal harm and relapse prevention that focuses on social engagement (e.g., Alcoholics Anonymous) (Rao, 2014, p. 344). |

around modulation of sensory stimuli (Champagne, 2008). Sensorimotor activities such as exercise, mindfulness activities that implement sensory feedback, and hand-based creative tasks may address these skills (Champagne, 2008). Sensory modalities can include weighted blankets, sound therapy, brushing techniques, and aromatherapy (Champagne, 2008). Therapists may facilitate exploration into what sensory input individuals prefer for stimulation and modulation through sensory carts and enhancements to the therapy environment (Champagne, 2008). Individuals can create sensory "kits," or boxes that contain sensory items that enable them to achieve a specific, personalized purpose, such as sobriety or relaxation (Champagne, 2008). The kit and other modalities can be used to create a tailored sensory "diet" that may be used for sensory regulation within and outside of therapy (Champagne, 2008). The role of sensory regulation in adult mental health care is an area of intervention that deserves continued attention and research to develop effective, person-driven interventions (Brown & Nicholson, 2011).

## Leisure Skills

Leisure should not be overlooked as an important occupation in older adults' lives (Chen & Chippendale, 2018). Engagement

and re-engagement in leisure activities may serve as valuable coping skills for diagnoses such as depression (Nimrod et al., 2012). In their study on the meaning of leisure for those who have mental health diagnoses, Craik and Pieris (2006) note that there have been numerous definitions of leisure across the OT profession, including that leisure is, "a complex phenomenon with three principal elements: time, occupation and experience." What one older adult might consider a leisure activity may differ from another, but leisure occupations that are personally identified can be implemented into therapy; for some, this may include cooking and baking, while for others, desired leisure pursuits may include expressive arts (Craik & Pieris, 2006). In turning to the case studies regarding leisure-based interventions, for example, Anne's love of playing bridge could be translated into treatment through the use of card games within orientation and sequencing tasks, while Robert could use puzzles as a coping strategy for when he is feeling overwhelmed or experiencing grief.

In further considering the relationship between collaborative goal setting and potential interventions, we can further explore Robert and Anne's experiences when receiving OT services.

## Case Studies: Providing Person-Centered Care

### Robert

After conducting the COPM, the occupational therapist, in collaboration with Robert, sets the following goals:

Short-Term Goal (7 Days):

1. Robert will be able to self-initiate three self-orientation strategies when he is experiencing disorientation, and use at least one technique with no verbal cues in three out of four trials for increased orientation to self, time, date, and location for optimal engagement in desired daily occupations.
2. Robert will be able to self-initiate three self-modulation techniques when he is experiencing negative symptoms, and use at least one technique with no verbal cues in three out of four trials for optimal engagement in desired daily occupations.
3. Robert will be able to use a medication management device (pill box) with no more than minimal verbal cues for taking the correct medication at the correct time for optimal symptom management and engagement in desired daily occupations.

Long-Term Goal (14 Days):

1. Robert will consistently independently use personally identified self-orientation and self-modulation techniques when experiencing disorientation and/or diagnosis symptoms for optimal engagement in desired daily occupations.
2. Robert will consistently independently self-administer needed medications using a medication management device for optimal symptom management and engagement in desired daily occupations.

### Anne

During her admission, Anne's occupational therapist, in addition to physical rehabilitation interventions, focuses on cognitive interventions that promote sensory regulation and mood stabilization, given Anne's difficulties with attending to tasks and sequencing. Anne's occupational therapy goals center around feeding and eating, gaining safety and independence with self-dressing, and orientation for the purposes of engaging in her preferred occupations.

The occupational therapist uses Anne's favorite soothing music to promote her engagement in self-dressing and eating tasks. At times Anne will become agitated during treatment and state, "I don't want to be here and you can't make me stay." She is usually receptive to therapeutic listening on behalf of the therapist. The occupational therapist blends multiple sensory stimuli with cognitive interventions to promote orientation and attention with Anne, including which of these allows Anne to describe the sounds, smells, and visual input she is experiencing in her room. Finally, the therapist works with Anne on creating a verbal story narrative surrounding mealtimes to support Anne's oral intake and participation in feeding and eating activities. Anne continues to decline in her physical functioning and is then further moved to two different wards, where she has multiple falls and behavioral challenges (continued fluctuating mood, aggression, and disorientation). The occupational therapist provides verbal and written hand-offs to new members of Anne's care team regarding her sensory and orientation preferences and needs, with the therapist describing Anne's treatment course and needs in verbal communication with Anne's care team and in her documentation. As a result of Anne's prolonged stay in the hospital setting with ongoing cognition support, Anne developed hospital-acquired pneumonia; she was then retransferred to the short-stay ward within the hospital, where the occupational therapist inquired about Anne. It was advised that Anne was now to be receiving end-of-life care.

*Continued*

## Case Studies:     Providing Person-Centered Care—Cont'd

### Robert

While admitted, Robert is prescribed Risperdal for his symptoms (Keepers et al., 2020). Robert actively participates in the provided group therapy sessions, which include a focus on medication and symptom management, sensory modulation, and emotional processing, all of which are structured around a dialectical behavioral therapy lens. Robert's symptoms are improving; however, he is affected by depression, and struggles with these symptoms both in and outside of group therapy sessions. The OTA on the unit also notices that Robert is not ambulating safely and appears to be at risk for falls. The care team refers Robert to a physical therapist from the hospital's inpatient rehabilitation department, who assesses Robert and provides him with a four-wheeled walker. Prior to discharging, the occupational therapist also conducts the Cognitive Performance Test and determines that Robert is unsafe to be living at home alone.

Consider...

- Are these goals occupation-based? Might they be meaningful to Robert based on what you know about him?
- What recommendations might you give the family surrounding Robert's discharge destination, personal adaptations to promote occupational independence, and safety plan based on his score(s)?

Robert is understandably upset about the assessment's findings, the rapid changes in his health and mobility, and being away from home. The occupational therapist provides supportive listening and problem-solving methods in collaboration with Robert; some days are tougher than others, and there are times when Robert likes to reflect with the occupational therapist on the life he had: "I was so happy, I had my wife, my kids, my grandkids...things were good, even when the kids moved out and got their own lives, we had each other...now everything seems so different; I feel like a different person, each day is harder than the last one..."

Consider...

- What are some ways in which you could respond to Robert when he talks to you about how he is feeling?
- How could you incorporate his positive feelings and memories surrounding his family into treatment?

### Anne

Consider...

- Are the targeted skills within Anne's therapy goals occupation-based? Might they be meaningful to Anne based on what you know about her?
- What are some ways an occupational therapy practitioner could support Anne in transitioning to end-of-life care?
- What are some ways the occupational therapist could support Anne's family in Anne's transition to end-of-life care?

---

The people we serve, including persons such as Anne and Robert, may receive medical interventions to assist with their mental health symptoms and increase their ability to participate in their preferred occupations. Box 17.3 provides information on some of the medical and procedural interventions that are available for addressing mental health symptoms.

### The Care Team

There are many health-care professionals who contribute to older adults' care in mental health settings. Care providers collaborate with one another and the person to assess their needs, create a person-centered treatment plan, and provide updates on the person's functioning and response to treatment. The interdisciplinary team also works to ensure that the person has the appropriate support as they are discharged, whether that be in-home services, outpatient services, support groups, and/or personalized adaptations. Box 17.4 provides brief descriptions of the various care team members who may serve older adults.

Professionals across the care team are invaluable in ensuring that individuals' goals are met, progress is monitored, and people have a discharge plan in place to best meet their needs. Across settings and teams, OT practitioners serve as valuable voices in promoting the use of strengths (Tse et al., 2016) and occupation-based approaches to older adults' care (Mee & Sumsion, 2001). Compassion, empathy, humility, reflexivity, and a collaborative spirit should underpin the process of intervention planning and personal interactions.

Anne and Robert may have different or similar care team members given their needs; in thinking about the role of interprofessional care team members in their care, consider the following in Reflection Break 4 box.

| BOX 17.3 | Medical and Procedural Interventions for Older Adults' Mental Health Symptoms |

| Medical/Procedural Intervention | Indication(s) in Older Adults |
| --- | --- |
| Selective serotonin reuptake inhibitors (Zoloft, Celexa, Lexapro) | Major depressive disorder (MDD) (Karasu et al., 2000), generalized anxiety disorder (GAD), and other anxiety disorders (APA, 1998), posttraumatic stress disorder (PTSD) (Benedek et al., 2009). |
| Buspirone | GAD (Laakmann et al., 1998) |
| Mood stabilizers (lithium, anticonvulsants such as Depakote and Lamictal) | Bipolar disorder (APA, 2002) |
| Atypical antipsychotics (Risperdal, Zyprexa, Seroquel, Abilify) | Late-life schizophrenia (Keepers et al., 2020), bipolar disorder (APA, 2002) |
| Cholinesterase inhibitors (Aricept, Razadyne, Exelon), Namenda | Cognitive symptoms of dementia (Rabins et al., 2017) |
| Aducanumab | People with Alzheimer's disease with mild cognitive impairment (Dhillon, 2021) |
| Electroconvulsive therapy (ECT) | Severe major depression, suicide risk, mania, intolerance or poor response to medications, catatonia, good response to previous ECT (Mankad et al., 2010) |
| Psychotherapy (including cognitive-behavioral therapy, family therapy, group therapy) (Makover, 2017) | MDD, GAD, bipolar disorder, PTSD, and multiple other psychiatric disorders |

### REFLECTION BREAK 4

**The Role of the Interprofessional Care Team**

1. What health-care professionals might be on Anne and Robert's care teams, and what role might the occupational therapist have in interacting with those care team members?
2. Were the occupational therapist to be the care coordinator for Anne or Robert, what are some tools and skills you might need in communicating their needs and current functioning to other care team members?
3. What aspects of Anne and Robert's care and functioning would be critical to discuss at each care team meeting?

## The Road Forward

As members of the health and human service team, OT practitioners provide important input to monitoring the ongoing and unfolding needs of those they serve, requiring updates and reassessing and interacting with the older adult and their family/caregivers. This can involve "systematic observation and informal, but dynamic, interactive reevaluation to constantly assess the person's ability" (Donoso et al., 2019), thereby building on the occupational profile and data from the initial evaluation with an eye towards progress and goal attainment.

### Evaluation Purpose for Outcomes, Transition, or Discontinuation of Services

It is wise to consider that evaluation is a complex process in which the information and evidence we use is interpreted in relation to the people we serve. For practice, these purposes include: (1) the opportunity to establish whether people are benefiting from the therapeutic input or service and identify the changes in their participation, (2) ensuring that the therapeutic process is prioritizing people's needs (while delivering services), (3) facilitating transition to a different provider, program, service, or level of care, and (4) providing documentation that goals have been met or the person no longer chooses to be involved in the program, requiring attention to a discharge plan that attends to the person's needs around their occupational performance (AOTA, 2020). Preparing for transitions such as discharge from formal services to community support, from health providers to self-care or care provided by family, friends, or peers with similar lived experiences is initiated by the OT practitioners as a final stage in the OT process.

### Discharge and Recovery

Preparing for discharge and transition involves an intentional interpersonal focus initiated by the OT practitioner, called "therapeutic use of self" (AOTA, 2020). One way moving forward might be facilitated by summarizing the journey of working together, eliciting reflections from the older adult as to how they feel about what they accomplished, what they are looking forward to, any fears or concerns they have, and who they plan to connect with in support of their social, emotional and physical health needs. Helping the person and their family caregivers to identify what they see as triggers that might signal a need to reactivate their status with the intervention team, and finding supportive environments meeting the values, preferences, and pragmatics of the person's life are important to address.

**BOX 17.4**    Older Adults' Mental Health-Care Team Member Roles in Collaboration with the Person

| Title | Role |
|---|---|
| Occupational Therapist | • Evaluates the person's previous and current mental health, functional, and occupational performance<br>• Collaborates with the person to develop person-centered goals<br>• Engages the person in evidence-informed interventions targeting personal goals<br>• Provides the person and their caregivers/family members with recommendations for successful home and community engagement<br>• Communicates change in function to care team, including the occupational therapy assistant<br>• Collaborates with the person, their family and caregivers, and the team to optimize the discharge process and re-engagement in the community |
| Occupational Therapy Assistant | • Collaborates with the person to develop person-centered goals<br>• Engages the person in evidence-informed interventions targeting personal goals<br>• Provides the person and their caregivers/family members with recommendations for successful home and community engagement<br>• Communicates change in function to care team, including occupational therapist<br>• Collaborates with the person, their family and caregivers, and the team to optimize the discharge process and re-engagement in the community |
| Psychiatrist | • Evaluates, diagnoses, and monitors a person's past and current mental functioning, including diagnosis symptoms, cognition, and functional abilities.<br>• Prescribes medication for managing diagnosis symptoms and educates individuals on medication and potential side effects<br>• Collaborates with the person and significant others to determine appropriate length of stay for the individual<br>• Makes recommendations/orders for additional services during admission and at discharge<br>• Communicates changes in the person's needs or status to other care team members |
| Nurse | • Evaluates the person's functioning on a daily basis and monitors vitals<br>• Administers medications and provides education on medication purpose and side effects<br>• Promotes the person's participation in daily programming and services<br>• Communicates changes in the person's needs or status to other care team members<br>• May provide recommendations to psychiatrist to re-evaluate the person's medications based on their reports of side effects/changes in functioning |
| Certified Nursing Assistant | • Assists the person with activities of daily living as needed<br>• Assists the person with mobility needs to/from programming<br>• Assists with maintaining safety precautions across care environment<br>• Communicates changes in the person's needs or status to other care team members |
| Social Worker | • Evaluates the person's personal and residency factors<br>• Communicates changes in the person's needs or status to other care team members<br>• Conducts interventions with the person, which can include education on self-esteem, self-care practices, and engaging in healthy relationships |
| Care Team Coordinator | • Can be one of the other health professionals listed (e.g., the occupational therapist serves as the person's care team coordinator)<br>• Oversees and organizes care team huddle meetings, progress meetings, and evaluation and discharge meetings<br>• Communicates changes in the person's needs or status to other care team members |
| Chaplain | • Provides spiritual programming through group and individual methods<br>• Collaborates with the person to identify the role of spirituality in recovery and health-care maintenance<br>• Provides psychosocial support. |
| Peer Support Specialist | • Collaborates with the person on psychosocial and skill-building support that is guided by peer support specialist's experiences and expertise<br>• Provides emotional support<br>• Uses their personal experiences with change to encourage change talk |
| Significant Others | • Provides emotional support<br>• Engages collaborates with the care team and loved ones<br>• Provides history regarding the person's health, prior functioning levels, and personal factor history to care team as needed<br>• Engages in education on interventions, home adaptations, and the person's needs with care team members<br>• Engages in discharge planning with care team and the person<br>• Provides support when transitioning between facilities and discharge destinations |

One concept associated with mental health is the journey of recovery– that is, living a life of meaning and purpose, experiencing health, having a place one calls home and being connected to one another in the community and a sense of belonging (Barbic, 2018). For those who view their engagement with mental health services as the start of their recovery journey, the practitioner works with the person to engage with accessible assistance services that will support, expand and sustain their sense of recovery, finding acceptance with living with mental health challenges that may ebb and flow.

Table 17.1 identifies a number of informal and formal supports that could be valuable resources for the older adult and their family/caregivers. A study of the Wellness Recovery Action Program for Healthy Aging (WRAP-HA) (available at https://www.ahpnet.com/Products-Services# Wellness-Recovery-Action-Plan) based on a peer-to-peer model, has demonstrated growing evidence of enhancing well-being and recovery, decreasing loneliness and isolation, reducing psychiatric symptoms, enhancing hopefulness, increasing empowerment, improving quality of life, and increasing self-advocacy with treatment providers (Cook et al., 2012). OT practitioners who work collaboratively with peer support specialists are in a strong position to impact sustainable health and well-being for this population of older adults.

In returning to Robert and Anne as they near the end of their engagement in OT services, the occupational therapist serves an important role in ensuring that Robert and Anne have a smooth discharge process and have the care and community supports they need. As you finish reading about Robert and Anne, consider the following in the Reflection 5 box.

**TABLE 17.1** Recovery Supports

| Recovery Support | Role |
|---|---|
| Family, friends, neighbors, and caregivers | • Provide psychosocial and emotional support<br>• Assist with occupations requiring physical and cognitive supports<br>• Assist with implementing education provided in treatment into the older adult's daily contexts and environments |
| United States: National Alliance on Mental Illness (NAMI) https://www.nami.org/Home | • Helplines<br>• Education and resources on mental health supports for family members and caregivers<br>• Advocacy efforts surrounding mental health awareness<br>• National and state-based organization access |
| United Kingdom: Mental Health Foundation https://www.mentalhealth.org.uk/ | • Advocacy efforts surrounding mental health awareness<br>• Education, podcasts, and publications on mental health<br>• Personal resources for mental health support |
| United States: Mental Health America https://mhanational.org/ | • Nonprofit organization focusing on programs and initiatives that promote mental health and prevent mental health challenges<br>• Educational resources on recovery and support<br>• Access to professional help and resources<br>• Provide education on managing one's mental health and diagnoses for family and friends, providers, and oneself |
| United Kingdom: National Health Service Long-Term Plan https://www.england.nhs.uk/mental-health/adults/older-people/ | • Guiding plan for UK health care through 2023/2024 that includes focus on the mental health of older adults<br>• Looks to increase access to mental health-care supports<br>• Designed to remove barriers to care<br>• Focuses on improving mental health through one-to-one and community mental health supports |
| Community Programming | • Accessible to all<br>• Can provide education and programming on mental health and mental health diagnoses<br>• Supports social engagement and community building |
| Senior Centers | • Available to all<br>• Can provide light meals, activities and programming throughout the day, and caregiver support<br>• Can provide programming on mental health<br>• Support social engagement and community building |

## Case Studies: Robert's and Anne's Road Ahead

### Robert

In conducting discharge planning with Robert's care team and family (led by his son), the occupational therapist finds that Robert's family is unable to provide him with the level of support he would need to safely remain living in his home, and they do not have the finances to fully cover Robert's living expenses in an assisted living facility. Robert strongly desires to stay in the home he and his family shared, and struggles with conversing about alternative living options with the occupational therapist, social worker, and other care team members. He often says to the team, "You just don't understand, I have so many memories in that house, it's my home...I need to be there" The occupational therapist and care team continue to meet with Robert and his family (when possible) to discuss potential discharge destinations and solutions. Despite the care team's belief that Robert would be best supported in assisted living, Robert's son, in agreement with his other family members, decides that Robert will remain living in his home.

Consider....

- How might you navigate discussing the differences between the care team's recommendations regarding Robert's safety and discharge destination and Robert's son's preferences?
- What recommendations might you need to make given that Robert will be discharging to his home? What support services and adaptations might Robert need to be successful?

The care team facilitates a plan to provide Robert with home care multiple times a week, with a plan to reassess his needs in three months. After Robert discharges, the occupational therapist calls Robert to see how he is feeling, reviews his medication management, personal safety, and walker safety plans, and provides psychosocial support to Robert as he continues to manage his symptoms and adjust to his new home care routine.

Consider...

- What supportive services might Robert benefit from long term if he continues to remain in his home (such as outpatient services, in-home health, community and family supports)?
- What might next steps look like for Robert if upon reassessment at the 3-month mark, he is experiencing difficulties with living safely in his home?

### Anne

Anne's care team, including her occupational therapist, meet with Anne's niece and additional family members to discuss Anne's wishes and review her end-of-life care plan. Anne has provisions in her advance decision document that outline her desire to enter palliative care as she enters the end of her life. The care team discusses Anne's desire to enter palliative care with her family present, and ultimately Anne and her family choose to transfer Anne to a nearby palliative care ward. In discharging to the ward, Anne's occupational therapist provides the family and palliative care team with sensory and orientation preferences and needs, as well as additional recommendations for comforting sensory input, orientation activities, ways to engage Anne in end-of-life reminiscence activities. After Anne's transition to palliative care, the occupational therapist reaches out to Anne's family to ensure that she is comfortable and has her needs addressed; Anne's niece confirms this.

Consider...

- What are some topics/areas that Anne's care team could explore with Anne during end-of-life reminiscence activities?

## REFLECTION BREAK 5

### The Discharge Process

1. When might Robert and Anne feel prepared for discharge given their goals for therapy and discharge destinations?
2. What personal skill sets and characteristics do you possess that might be important to use when having difficult decisions with Anne and Robert or their families regarding their current functioning and discharge destinations?
3. How do you see yourself supporting older adults after they discharge from occupational therapy services?

## Conclusion

Older adults may experience new and exacerbating mental health challenges that affect their ability to engage in the occupations that matter to them. Personal factors such as ageism, assumptions on the realities of older adulthood, social engagement, and community access all serve as critical barriers and or facilitators that OT practitioners must consider when collaborating with people across treatment. Personal reflection and critical reflexivity, evidence-informed reasoning, and compassion should ground interactions with older adults to ensure that OT practitioners are providing optimal, person-driven care.

Evaluations for older adults receiving mental health treatment may include focus on cognition, orientation, or occupational performance. Interventions for older adults can occur across settings, and address both preparatory skills and occupation-based activities. The OT practitioner can approach treatment by incorporating older adults' preferred activities through an occupation-based approach, and individuals' skill sets, interpersonal relationships, strengths, and preexisting community support. There are many varying health professionals who serve as part of an individuals' care team.

It is critical that we are aware of the impact of who we are as individuals and OT practitioners on our interactions with those we serve and view each person we treat as someone who is worthy of dignity and compassion. We must promote personal autonomy and decision-making wherever possible across the course of therapy. Intervention for older adults may include a variety of approaches and skills addressed, all with the goal of empowering people and returning them to the occupations in which they need and want to participate. Ensuring that we are taking care of our personal mental health and well-being as practitioners is also important in providing individuals with the best treatment possible (Scanlan & Still, 2013).

You were encouraged to read about and reflect on Robert and Anne's experiences with mental health services, with both having different personal, mental health, and occupational contexts. For Robert, health management and psychosocial support were all critical aspects of the care process. Flexibility with discharge planning on behalf of the care team was an important factor in ensuring that Robert was returning to his home with the best occupational support for him and his family. For Anne, the occupational therapist's support and personalized sensory modulation and orientation interventions, and their continued involvement across Anne's admissions, demonstrate the important role of OT both during and after direct care. At the heart of both Anne's and Robert's care was a focus on promoting occupational engagement; Anne and Robert's case studies represent people we may serve in OT, as well as potential interventions and discharge paths in which people may engage.

OT practitioners are invaluable members of older adults' mental health- care teams. We can use our unique skill sets in addressing occupational engagement with older adults who are experiencing changes in their mental health function and promote a return to the desired activities that make life meaningful. As you conclude the chapter, consider this Reflection Break 6 box.

---

### REFLECTION BREAK 6

1. Were any of your assumptions about older adults and mental health factors challenged throughout the chapter?
2. What can you do in the future to continue to practice critical reflexivity regarding older adults with mental health diagnoses?
3. What questions that you came to the chapter with did you feel were answered by the content?
4. What questions were not answered, or what topics do you feel you need to conduct further research on?
5. What material from the chapter do you see yourself applying to your practice?

---

*The complete listing of the Bibliography and Chapter Questions and Answers are available in the accompanying enhanced eBook version included with the print purchase of this textbook. Visit Elsevier eBooks+ (eBooks.Health.Elsevier.com) to access this content.*

## CHAPTER 18

# Spirituality, Resilience, and Aging

*Lydia Manning, MGS, PhD, Thuli Mthembu, PhD, MPH, BSc OT, Lauren Bouchard, MS, PhD, and Julia Buschbacher, BS*

## CHAPTER OUTLINE

## OBJECTIVES

- Define the basics of spirituality and resilience in tandem with adaptation
- Discuss the connections between aging and spiritual resilience in older adults
- Clarify appropriate use of spirituality and/or religion in everyday practice
- Assist practitioners in incorporating spirituality into Occupational Therapy interventions
- Discuss the importance of *Ubuntu* in the well-being of older adults as part of intergenerational solidarity and relations

The changes and related life events and health shocks associated with aging invite people to engage in the process of meaningful adaptation and response to adversity. How individuals respond to troubles and traumas in the form of adaptation is internal and external. The end goal is often to have mastery of one's environment and energetic position. The essence of occupational therapy (OT) is to create settings and support abilities where practitioners promote the successful performance of meaningful occupations by individuals in a holistic way in their quest to navigate their environment and energy. What roles do spirituality and resilience play in the practice of OT? What factors determine how people adapt to the changes, life events, and health shocks associated with aging?

This chapter reviews the commonly agreed-upon understandings of resilience and spirituality relating to aging. We consider the connections between spirituality, resilience, and OT. The sections are organized to address the critical domains of the respective constructs, experiences, and practices. We summarize the connections between spirituality, resilience, adaption, and aging and offer suggestions for interventions related to OT. We also explore factors that promote integration and optimal adaptation over the life course.

## Defining Resilience

Resilience is an adaptation to adversity wherein a person rebounds or "bounces back" from stressful life experiences (Lavretsky, 2014). Resilience can be operationalized as a trait (e.g., psychological resilience; Gulbrandsen, 2016; Taylor & Carr, 2021), process (Zautra et al., 2010), outcome (Fullen & Gorby, 2016; Joyce et al., 2018; Koni et al., 2019), or identity and way of being (Manning & Bouchard, 2020). Resilience can also be viewed as physiological (e.g., heightened reactivity; Obradović, 2012), psychological/emotional (O'Rourke et al., 2010; Takahashi et al., 2016; Taylor & Carr, 2021), relational (i.e., familial; Walsh, 2020; communal; Bartholomaeus et al., 2019), and spiritual (Manning, 2014; Manning et al., 2019).

Given the prevalence of lifetime adversity, resilience is vital to aging well, as older adults who exhibit resilience can thrive with proper support (Domajnko & Pahor, 2015; Manning & Bouchard, 2020; Taylor & Carr, 2021). In addition to cumulative lifetime adversity, older adults also face new challenges in old age, such as disability, health limitations, ageism, inaccessibility, and social isolation (Hayman et al., 2017). Researchers have shown that resilience is key to well-being throughout these challenges and successful aging in general; however various pathways of resilience are key to an understanding of the construct itself (Lavretsky, 2014).

## Psychological

First, psychological resilience is a popular way of understanding resilience as a reserve of coping resources, which allows for successful adaptation to stressful events (Taylor & Carr, 2021). This means that a person may cope amid ongoing stressors (e.g., advanced age; Browne-Yung, 2017; Hayman et al., 2017) without facing debilitation in their daily lives. From a strengths-based perspective, many older adults have a wealth of psychological resources, including life perspective, wisdom, and meaning-making, even amid dire circumstances such as the COVID-19 pandemic (e.g., Fuller & Huseth-Zosel, 2021).

Others have found that psychological resilience is crucial to coping with stigmatized health conditions (Takahashi et al., 2016). Taylor and Carr (2021) found that psychological resilience ultimately predicted positive health outcomes for older people. Finally, others have noted that resilient coping is a significant predictor of psychological well-being (Tomás et al., 2012) and community well-being affects older adults' positive aging at an individual level (Bartholomaeus et al., 2019).

## Physiological

The physiological aspects of resilience are key to occupational therapists and others due to the nature of rebounding from illness, disability, or other physical limitations. Whitson et al. (2018, p. 493) asserted that physical resilience concerns "an individual's ability to resist functional decline or recover physical health following a stressor." According to Obradović (2012), lifetime adversity (especially beginning in childhood) may increase physiological reactivity to stress and adversity. Children who have experienced early trauma and parental abuse are especially susceptible to physiological changes, which impact nervous system homeostasis (Obradović, 2012). This is especially true when the amount of risk surpasses general levels of support and resources. Chronic adversity (e.g., poverty, social marginalization, ongoing trauma) may impact the ability to rebound from stress across the life course due to the physiological changes in the nervous system (Obradović, 2012).

Similarly, Whitson et al. (2018) describe "physiological reserves" as key to older adults rebounding and maintaining physical resilience. Physical resilience is especially crucial in older adults who face increased levels of health limitations due to chronic disease and/or disability (Whitson et al., 2018). While physical resilience may be especially important to occupational therapists and health providers, it is also vital to note how the functional decline of older adults may be related to other types of resilience (Manning et al., 2016).

## Relational

Next, relational aspects of resilience include familial and communal resilience. Often, resilience is discussed as an individual affair without regard to the social contexts of the individual; however, human beings live in groups and are fundamentally interconnected socially. This social interconnection within families and larger community groups can be advantageous in bouncing back from adversity. Western cultures tend to value resilience as a solo effort; however, resilience cannot be fully understood without knowledge of the social resources, capital, and infrastructure of communities (Aldrich & Meyer, 2015; Cohen et al., 2016).

Community resilience is often mentioned in disaster literature, especially among older adults who may be vulnerable due to physical and cognitive limitations (Nicosia et al., 2022; Timalsina et al., 2021). For example, interventions including movement, group interaction, and emotional processing for older adults with cognitive impairments may be associated with a renewed sense of continuity even during devastating natural disasters such as wildfires (Nicosia et al., 2022). Timalsina et al. (2021) reported that community integration and preparedness are key for older adults in Nepal amid frequent earthquakes. The older adults who reported lower resilience scores faced greater challenges at a communal level due to lack of resources, displacement, and socioeconomic barriers to adaptation.

Community resilience has also been noted regarding the environmental and ecological connections to physical and mental health. Community resilience can be defined as "how people overcome stress, trauma, and other life challenges by drawing from social networks and cultural resources embedded in communities" (Kirmayer et al., 2009).

Older adults are in a unique position in terms of community resilience depending on the cultural nuances of old age in variable societies. For example, older adults may be considered leaders, elders, or mentors in positions of high esteem, or they may be overlooked, isolated, and undervalued depending on the values of the community. Similarly, older adults may have variable experiences in older age as social connectedness and familial support also play a role (Hayman et al., 2017). Thus, social support—from both familial and communal sources—enhances older adults' relationships and health outcomes during times of transition or crisis (Martin et al., 2015).

## Spiritual

Many older adults express the importance of spirituality and/or religion as integral to their worldview, and spiritual resilience may play a salient role as well (Manning, 2013; Manning et al., 2019). For many older adults, religious beliefs, rituals, and communities play a continual role in navigating the hardships of life (Bouchard et al., 2021). For some, religiosity is directly linked to spirituality (e.g., Jewish faith as connected to a daily sense of the divine in ritual); however, spiritual resilience is not always based upon formal religious practice and may, in fact, be completely divorced from formal religious dogma.

Spiritual resilience is an important factor to consider in OT when focusing on the well-being of older adults. It has been indicated that older adults aim to achieve the meaning and purpose of life by engaging in diverse and preferred occupations to sustain their internal resources as part of spiritual resilience (Ormel et al., 1999). While a variety of definitions of the term *spiritual resilience* have been suggested, it can be defined as the ability to draw from one's "spiritual beliefs or religious practices as the most important means for coping" with hardships related to problematic and traumatic situations that influence people's health, quality of and well-being (Duke, 2017, p. 3). However, according to Manning et al.

(2019), spiritual resilience refers to "the ability to sustain one's sense of self and purpose through a set of beliefs, principles, or values while encountering adversity, stress, and trauma by using internal and external spiritual resources" (p. 172).

## Defining Spirituality

For the purposes of this chapter, spirituality must be separately defined from spiritual resilience. The definition of spirituality itself varies due to differences in conceptualization (Atchley, 2009; Johnson, 2016; Manning, 2012; McFadden, 2005; Wink & Dillon, 2003; Zinnbauer & Pargament, 2005). Zinnbauer and Pargament (2005) defined spirituality as the search for the sacred—that is special, set apart from the ordinary, and deserving of reverence. Atchley (2009) defined spirituality as a realm of human experience encapsulating an intense awareness of the present, transcendence of the personal self, and a feeling of connection with all of life. Spirituality is a way of being in the world that affords individuals opportunities for connection and meaning. These connections and processes of meaning-making require adaptation and actions that allow one to navigate their environment better.

Researchers have established that spirituality and spiritual practices positively correlate with health and well-being outcomes for older adults. According to Koenig (2012), participation in religious/spiritual practices helps older adults to cope with illnesses and stressful situations, including chronic pain, cardiovascular disease, cancer, diabetes, natural disasters, bereavement, and acts of terrorism. Researchers have found that frequent spiritual experiences are linked to decreased anxiety and depression, as well as increased happiness and self-esteem (Ellison & Fan, 2008; Koenig, 2012; Lee, 2011).

Spirituality, adaptation, and aging are also positively linked. The concept of positive aging, which "embraces the idea of making the most of opportunities, innovations, and research which promote a person's sense of independence, dignity, well-being, good health and enable their participation in society," connects to spiritual adaptation strategies during the COVID-19 pandemic (Stock et al., 2017, p. 5). Several qualitative studies conducted amid the pandemic address older adults' coping strategies, noting that spirituality provides a sense of strength, comfort, hope, and peace of mind during the challenges of social isolation (Lucchetti et al., 2021; Sadang et al., 2021). According to Malone and Dadswell (2018), spirituality is a source of strength, comfort, and hope in difficult times and brings about a sense of community and belonging. These factors suggest that spirituality can play a role in positive aging.

Underpinning much of the discourse on spirituality and aging are the theoretical and empirical offerings from key contributors in this subfield. For example, when addressing the body of literature on spirituality and aging, it is vital to explore the developmental theory of gerotranscendence, an approach used in understanding aging as development proposed by Tornstam in 2005. This theory attempts to understand the aging process not from a pathological perspective, as many first and second-wave gerontological theories do

(i.e., disengagement and activity theories), but from a perspective that celebrates a developmental process involving the highest level of supremely positive human development (Tornstam, 2005). Gerotranscendence comprises three major dimensions: the cosmic, the self, and social and personal relationships.

Within each of these dimensions, there are complex sub-dimensions involving interaction with time and previous experiences, the confrontation of the self and ego-integrity, and the interactions with social and personal spheres or the material and mundane. This theory assumes there to be a development (both natural and implicit) that happens as individuals age. For some older adults, this positive development is accentuated or blocked as they move throughout their life course. This theory suggests that all humans have the potential to reach gerotranscendence.

Atchley (1997) claimed that, while spirituality is quite popular in mainstream culture and the academy, its "soft" nature from a scientific viewpoint causes "spirituality to be stereotyped by scientific gerontology as a suspect enterprise" (p. 327). This stereotyping occurs because spirituality deals with aspects of human life not easily measured by conventional scientific methods (Atchley, 1997). Regardless of such spiritual experiences and spirituality being challenging to measure, there are increasing numbers of people willing to discuss their spirituality with researchers (Atchley, 2000, 2008). Attempting to examine and explore how spirituality operates in people's lives is crucial. It needs to be incorporated into the methods and modalities we employ as we aim to support and bolster the ability of people to navigate hardship and adapt to accommodate adversities and transitions over the life course.

## Connections Between Spirituality, Resilience, and Aging

As noted above, resilience is universally understood as a form of adaptation or flourishing in the face of adversity (Hildon, 2008; Masten, 2001; Van Kessel, 2013). Resilience is achieved through utilizing various internal and external resources (Van Kessel, 2013). Spirituality and resilience as constructs and experiences are intimately linked to people as they age. Manning et al. (2019) argued that spirituality plays an essential role in how people demonstrate resilience in later life and found that as individuals in their study aged, spirituality became a more significant source of strength.

Efforts to bolster resilience for older adults have focused on individual efforts such as cognitive behavioral therapy, mindfulness (Joyce et al., 2018), and self-compassion (Delaney, 2018). Other interventions include group dynamics or a combination of reframing and group dynamics (Fullen & Gorby, 2016; Fullen et al., 2018). It is plausible that contemplative practices such as mindfulness hold promise in helping older adults to learn and practice resilience as part of their spirituality. Practitioners can create resilience-based interventions for older adults by designing programs or interventions that include mindfulness or meditation training to reduce stress and improve mood. Virtual social support programs or other opportunities for meaningful interaction may also improve interpersonal resilience.

Benefits of spirituality and resilience often include positive health outcomes, having meaning and purpose, the use of positive coping strategies, and the ability to positively adapt in the face of adversity. It is commonly understood that while aging presents many positive experiences and changes, it also invites the possibility of loss and decline. In other words, with aging, there are often negative losses such as the decline of body and mind, loss of friends and family, and a higher prevalence of chronic conditions and related impairments (Hayman et al., 2017). These realities invite people to rely on enhanced strategies, including spiritual coping, support, or resources, to manage the unique context of advanced age.

## The Vital Role of Adaptation in Growing Older

While aging is a process of continually negotiating gains and losses across various life domains, Nikitin and Freund (2019) argued that most older adults successfully adapt to these shifting balances of resource gains and losses. Growing older involves continual and dynamic adaptations in peoples' internal capabilities and external environments, which comprise the person-environment (P-E) fit theory. Adaptations within P-E fit have been widely conceptualized (Baltes, 1997; Chaudhury & Oswald, 2019; Golant, 2011; Lawton & Nahemow, 1973). Lawton and Nahemow (1973) propose that when a person's level of competence—whether it be cognitive, emotional, physical, or social—decreases, their behaviors are more strongly influenced by the environment (see Chapters 4 and 20). Chaudhury and Oswald (2019) acknowledge that older adults' sense of agency and belonging are intertwined, specifically as "social-physical agency, in the long run, decreases over time, social-physical belonging increases over time" (p. 4). Older adults' functioning and means of adaptation vary depending on their health status, functional activities, built environment, and social environment (Webb et al., 2010).

Baltes' (1997) Selection, Optimization, and Compensation (SOC) theory addresses the vital role of adaptations during aging. SOC states that older adults can select desirable goals and purposefully act to optimize them; however, if the desired goals cannot be achieved, older adults will use strategies to compensate for declines (Baltes, 1997). In other words, aging embodies an inherent dynamic between gains and losses. According to Zhang and Radhakrishnan (2018), studies have found that older adults living with multiple chronic conditions greatly benefit from SOC adaptations, including improved balance, activities of daily living, self-rated health, and subjective well-being, in addition to decreased pain and depression (see also Chapter 4).

Aging invites important questions, such as "how do people maximize gains and minimize losses in a manner that reflects optimal adaptation to the changes in the availability of resources throughout their lives?" It is plausible that the practice of OT is crucial to helping people positively adapt

to the myriad of changes and adversities that occur in life according to their wants, needs, and expectations. For many older adults, these opportunities for adaptation will involve spirituality and resilience as elements on their pathways to optimal aging.

Understanding resilience, spiritual resilience, and spirituality is vital to OT because the internal spiritual resources are congruent with the client factors (i.e., values, beliefs, and spirituality) and performance patterns related to habits, routines, roles, and rituals (AOTA, 2020). Similar to Manning et al. (2019) conceptualization of external spiritual resources, OT focuses on the contexts, which include the environmental and personal factors, as part of the geographical life-space for older adults that enable or hinder engagement and participation in occupations (AOTA, 2020). This corroborates with Douma et al. (2021) explanation of geographical life-space as "the spatial area in which a person lives, gets out and about, interacts, participates, conducts his or her societal roles, and engages in activities in the course of everyday life" (p. 1). Optimal aging requires older adults to be able to masterfully navigate these geographical life spaces; this requires the need for one to engage in adaptation.

## Occupational Justice and Older Adults

In the OT profession, occupational justice has been used to "support individuals and communities to participate in valued occupations as part of a just and empowering society" (Hadden et al., 2020, p. 118) (see also Chapter 31). In this chapter, the term occupational justice will be used in its broadest sense to refer to all "equitable or fair opportunities and resources to do, be, belong and become what people have the potential to be and the absence of avoidable harm" (Hocking, 2017, p. 32). It promotes strengthening community actions directed at creating supportive environments that enable vulnerable groups like older adults to participate in occupations that are contextually driven through advocating and mediating for occupational opportunities. However, Wolf et al. (2010) indicate that occupational justice can be violated when people are deprived of the physical, social, economic, or cultural resources or opportunities to engage in valued and satisfying occupations. This can result in outcomes of occupational injustices related to occupational deprivation, alienation, marginalization, and imbalance (du Toit et al., 2019; Wolf et al., 2010).

Occupational therapists should seek to ameliorate the occupational injustices experienced by older adults in diverse communities. The OT endeavors should align with the meliorism perspective that accentuates active "experimentation and transformative change" in everyday life with the involvement of all stakeholders (Baranek et al., 2020). Consequently, occupational therapists would be able to promote older adults' capacities to make decisions as they navigate their daily lives, routines, and habits (Baranek et al., 2020). According to the WFOT (2021) Position Statement on Occupational Therapy and Ageing Across the Life Course, occupational therapists have the responsibility to: "…adopt a rights-based approach for combating occupational injustice and marginalization to promote opportunity for all people to freely engage in necessary and chosen occupations."

Much has been published on occupational injustices. These studies indicated that discrimination, injustice, health inequalities, disparities, and structural and contextual factors could enable or prevent older adults' participation and engagement in everyday occupations (Cox, 2020; Lewis & Lemieux, 2021; Orellano-Colón et al., 2015; Wamara & Carvalho, 2019). Adversities originating from these injustices include the serious and widespread disturbances resulting from the recent COVID-19 pandemic and its related lockdown regulations and rules to control the transmission of the virus (Cox, 2020; Sinn & Kuepfer, 2021; United Nations, 2021a). Along with the occupational injustices that influence older adults' participation and engagement in everyday occupations, chronic and comorbid conditions such as rheumatoid arthritis, diabetes mellitus, cardiac conditions, and musculoskeletal pains may present additional challenges (De Coninck et al., 2021; Karttunen et al., 2014; Urtamo et al., 2019).

These conditions are common among older adults, resulting in functional decline, restrictions, and limitations of activity and participation (Urtamo et al., 2019; Karttunen et al., 2014). Nevertheless, evidence from a qualitative study that investigated the perspectives of older adults on their functioning, social participation, and health and the factors influencing these elements suggest that traditions and religious activities motivate older adults to remain active as part of social participation and social connectedness (De Coninck et al., 2021). In OT, spirituality is considered an aspect of client performance that enables people to cope with occupational challenges, disruptions, and adversities (AOTA, 2020; Mthembu et al., 2017a). As occupational therapists, we should work with older adults to identify and access spiritual resources at both the individual- and community levels to foster adaptation and resilience.

## Spiritual Resilience and Occupational Therapy

Older adults have accumulated various life experiences, dealing with chronic health problems, finances, death, and losses of close friends and relatives (Ramsey & Blieszner, 1999). Many have learned to navigate internal and external spiritual resources to achieve mental hardiness. Successful survivors of multiple life crises may become resilient as a result, leading to eventual wisdom and resilience of a spiritual nature.

However, as OT embraces older adults' spiritual resilience, we should strive to understand the common factors relative to social support, spiritual connections, efficacy, locus of control, and their life experiences (Duke, 2017; Mthembu et al., 2015; Manning, 2013). Concerning social support, occupational therapists should enable older adults as capable citizens to shape their communities and be involved in community projects, church, and family gatherings (Duke, 2017; Mthembu et al., 2015, 2017a).

Regarding spiritual connections, OT needs to enable older adults to engage in eudaimonic occupations that would sustain

their "reliance on spirituality to overcome hardship over the life course" to strengthen their spiritual and occupational resilience (Brown, 2021; Manning, 2013, p. 568; Thibeault, 2011; Zafran, 2020). It is necessary here to clarify exactly what is meant by occupational resilience from an OT perspective. Brown (2021) describes occupational resilience as "a person's ability to successfully and creatively navigate and negotiate life stressors, challenging environments and difficult events, whereby changes and modifications to daily occupations and occupational participation are required" (p. 104). Following spiritual connections, the eudaimonic occupations are crucial in older adults because they foster optimism, spirituality, resilience, and belonging during demanding and adverse events in life (Thibeault, 2011; Zafran, 2020).

Five occupations of a eudaimonic nature give older adults meaning and purpose in life: (1) *connecting occupations*, activities that provide opportunities to connect with family, friends, and community, to experience social support and a sense of belongingness (Hammell, 2014; Thibeault, 2011; Zafran, 2020); (2) *centering occupations*, that enable older adults to experience awareness, calmness, and inner strength; (3) *creative occupations*, in which older adults play, have fun, create, discover, explore, and experience happiness (Brown, 2021); (4) *contemplative occupations*, such as journaling, prayer, long walks in nature, which provides opportunities to see the full picture from present, past, and future; and (5) *contributing occupations* that allow older adults to give back to the younger generations, communities, groups, and organizations that hold us up. This resonates with the notion of occupational legacy, whereby older adults pass on their legacy beliefs to their communities as part of intergenerational solidarity (Meuser et al., 2019; Mthembu, 2021).

Older adults who engage in contributing occupations tend to experience positive mental and physical health, longevity, and a sense of belongingness because they add to others' well-being as part of a collective effort (Hammell, 2014). These eudaimonic occupations are essential in strengthening the spiritual and occupational resilience of older adults (Mthembu et al., 2015; Manning, 2013). In focusing on older adults' spiritual and occupational resilience, occupational therapists would contribute to achieving Good Health and Well-being as goal three of the 17 Sustainable Developmental Goals (United Nations, 2021b). This is vital in the profession of OT because it strengthens the promotion of health by enabling older adults to take control over and improve their health while developing personal skills and resilience capabilities (Ziglio, 2017).

In strengthening the spiritual and occupational resilience of older adults, OT would need to provide effective primary health-care services related to prevention, rehabilitation, promotion, palliative, and healing processes and address occupational disruptions (Ziglio, 2017). Whiteford (2000) refers to occupational disruptions as restrictions that hinder participation in valued occupations, which are beyond the older adults' control and undermine their health and well-being. Therefore, occupational therapists need to collaborate with older adults to mitigate occupational disruptions by adopting the strategies of occupational capital, which include "internal capacities and external support" (Cameron et al., 2016). Internal capacities, such as older adults' motivation, energy, positive self-image, optimism, and confidence, should be considered, as they form part of resilience. Enabling and underlying such internal capacities are internal physiological pathways that include optimal allostasis, immune competence, and cerebral activation asymmetry helps occupational therapist fosters resilience so that older adults could thrive and flourish during challenging difficulties (Ryff et al., 1998).

In addition to internal capacities, occupational therapists may enhance external support by incorporating the seven pathways to resilience found to be relevant across cultures, consisting of access to material, relationships, identity, cohesion, power and control, social justice, and cultural adherence (Ungar et al., 2007). Both internal capacities and external resources are key in promoting the resilience of older adults when they need to address a range of adversities affecting their occupational performance. This is significant in understanding how spirituality and resilience can be integrated into OT practice.

## Current Models Integrating Spirituality and Resilience Into Occupational Therapy Practice

One may argue that understanding both spirituality and resilience should be integrated into occupational practice as part of assessments and interventions used in existing programs (Mthembu et al., 2017a; Sadri Damirchi et al., 2018; Soomar et al., 2018; Richards et al., 2007). Occupational therapists need to ensure that assessments and interventions that are aimed at promoting successful and healthy aging should integrate spirituality as part of individuals, groups, and communities (Mthembu et al., 2017a, 2017b; Soomar et al., 2018). This could be possibly implemented by adopting current models of integration.

From an OT perspective, spiritual resilience can be integrated using existing models, such as the Kawa (River) Model (Blieszner & Ramsey, 2002) and the Canadian Model of Occupational Performance and Engagement (CMOP-E) (Fijal & Beagan, 2019; Polatajko et al., 2007). These models can be used to describe behavior or motivation and interventions with older adults.

## The Kawa Model and Moody's Five Stages of the Soul

The Kawa Model is originally a Japanese OT framework developed to foster a socially and culturally compatible worldview of occupation and well-being. It was developed to enable Japanese occupational therapists to gain insight into the cultural differences that shape clients' views of their reality in life (Lim & Iwama, 2006). This framework is significant in OT practice because it assists occupational therapists from an Asian background in strongly focusing on collective actions and efforts that enable the relationship between the clients and the environment. In strengthening the collective perspective, Lim and Iwama (2006) highlight that an individual

should be perceived as part of the community, the environment, and the family. This further indicates that occupational therapists should consider the clients' culture, beliefs, and rituals. In the Kawa Model, a river metaphor is used to reflect the life flow and the journey of life, which can be useful in guiding OT assessment and intervention for older adults (Gregg et al., 2015).

The Kawa model is made up of five elements, which are: water signifying life flow; river sidewalls and bottom, demonstrating the physical and social environment; rocks representing life circumstances; driftwood representing a person's assets and liabilities; and spaces representing the areas and opportunities in which occupational therapists can support the older adults. In support of spiritual resilience, the river banks, rocks, and driftwood can be utilized to "represent support, barriers, challenges, and opportunities" (Lape et al., 2019, p. 1).

These components are significant to the understanding of the role of spiritual resilience in older adults, as represented by the driftwood that epitomizes the assets and liabilities. The Kawa Model is important in OT because it can be used as part of narrative interactions through communication and productive relationships with older adults and knowledge exchange (Lape et al., 2019; Nelson & Allison, 2007; Newbury & Lape, 2021). Using pictorial images and pictures to initiate life narratives are effective strategies that occupational therapists may use as part of the Kawa Model. This will facilitate the trusting relationship between the older adults and occupational therapists. Occupational therapists may use the Kawa Model to structure healthy aging interventions to enhance older adults' understanding of their own difficulties relative to the potential for adaptation.

In critiquing the Kawa Model, Wada (2011, p. 230) identified gaps connected to the absence of inner self, active belonging, and "challenges of addressing issues related to occupations, and introduced the concept of *seken* (day-to-day community)." According to Kurihara (2007), *seken* refers to the appearance of the total network of social relations that surround an individual. It conveys the corresponding cultural norms and values regulating social behavior and hints at how such relations and behavior are maintained. Therefore, it is important for occupational therapists to have a better understanding of the person and environment so that they may be able to facilitate the "notion of inner self and *seken*," which promotes belonging (Wada, 2011). This will further assist in raising "occupational therapists' awareness of the challenges that individuals face in the process of belonging," which can influence their spiritual resilience (Wada, 2011, p. 235).

Occupational therapists might facilitate the integration of inner self and *seken* by adopting Moody's five stages of the soul, namely the call, the search, the struggle, the breakthrough, and the return (Moody & Carrol, 1997). These stages are important in OT because they provide solutions for the flow of life of older adults. Occupational therapists can use the stories generated from the Kawa Model to encourage older adults to engage in reflections on their lives as they relate to the five stages. It has been reported that the stages of soul assist older adults in "achieving a set of skills that promote personal, social, and spiritual well-being" (Fogle & Holley, 2019, p. 430). The stages of the soul are presented in the following case study.

## The Case Study

Leah was an 87-year-old black female who was a domestic worker during the apartheid era. She raised her six children as a single parent and tried to meet their needs. For all of her life, she was a full member of St. John's Faith Apostolic Church. She was a dedicated member, practicing all the expected activities. During her last stage of late adulthood, she was longing for more engagement in religious observation activities. Her children assisted her in attending the services and supported her throughout the last stage of her life. She was diagnosed with hypertension and diabetes mellitus, and later on, she had a neurocognitive disorder that resulted in her not recalling some of the short-term memory activities. However, in 2014, she had an amputation because of poor blood supply in her lower extremities, and she passed away in April 2014.

## Application of Moody's Five Stages of Soul to Case Study

*The call* is a first stage where a new level of spirituality is explored through the major life changes. The 87-year-old black female, Leah, experienced difficulties related to the health conditions that influenced her participation in religious activities. However, she was assisted by her family to engage in religious activities such as prayer, connecting with the familiar environments that facilitated reflections about life. *The search* is the second stage that involves responding to the call by exposing the self to new spiritual ideas. This was evident for Leah because she had an opportunity to visit a church that helped her to engage in other religious activities that assisted her to gain insight into herself.

The third stage, *the struggle*, is the most difficult stage, because older adults may experience depression and anger. Leah experienced the most difficulties because of her diabetes mellitus and neurocognitive decline. It was a difficult time for the 87-year-old black female and her family because she required an amputation. However, the *stage of breakthrough* was not achieved because she did not establish a new sense of love for others and a connection with life and purpose. The *stage of return* involves coming back to everyday life after the breakthrough, which is something that did not happen with the 87-year-old black female because she passed away 3 days after the amputation.

## The Canadian Model of Occupational Performance and Engagement

In supporting the harmony and life flow depicted in the Kawa Model, Polatajko et al. (2007) present the CMOP-E, which encourages the dynamic interdependent relationship between the person, occupation, and environment. The person is the center of the CMOP-E model, encompassing cognitive,

affective, and physical performance components/skills. In the CMOP-E, spirituality is considered the person's core that influences human occupation. According to Polatajko et al. (2007), people's spirituality is believed to be molded and articulated through engagement in occupations. Occupational therapists use client-centered approaches, which enable older adults to select activities such as religious observation to tap their spirituality.

The CMOP-E model presents the environmental component as one that influences the person, the occupation, and spirituality. The environment comprises physical, cultural, institutional, and social aspects. These aspects of the environment play a significant role in availing the person of occupational opportunities. Within the CMOP-E, occupation consists of self-care, productivity, and leisure.

Both the Kawa Model and CMOP-E support the harmonious interdependent relationship between the person, occupation, and environment; however, there are moments where disruptions occur among the components, which results in occupational dysfunction. In times when older adults are experiencing occupational dysfunction, spiritual resilience may assist the older adults to create or recreate accepting the conditions, finding solutions, and striving for balance among daily occupations (Santoso et al., 2015). This could be possible when occupational therapists collaborate with older adults to facilitate the process of spiritual resilience, drawing from the inner self, belongingness, and social environments (Cameron, 2021; Santoso et al., 2015; Wada, 2011). The occupational therapists might use the elements of the Kawa Model and Stages of Soul to facilitate the process of spiritual resilience.

However, to facilitate older adults' spiritual resilience, occupational therapists should adopt an anti-colonial lens that views health care as a social relationship between people (Hunter & Pride, 2021). This is significant for the profession because these models would "endorse social change and actively address colonial power inequities" (Hunter & Pride, 2021, p. 329). Occupational therapists may deal with the rocks in the Kawa Model, which form part of the social inequalities that influence older adults' social participation in their community, family, and peers. Furthermore, occupational therapists may deal with the social environments in CMOP-E that enable connectedness and interdependent relationships. Therefore, occupational therapists would need to consider the spiritual resilience of older adults who "experience health inequities linked to part of access to culturally-relevant health care" (White & Beagan, 2020, p. 200).

In OT practice, ethical places are significant because occupational therapists should treat older adults with respect, apply justice, provide intervention that would benefit the older adults without causing any harm, and allow them to make informed decisions. Thus, the ethical spaces may strengthen the older adults' spiritual resilience because they may engage in "cross-cultural conversation in pursuit of ethically engaging diversity and disperses claims to the human order" (Ermine, 2007, p. 202). It is pertinent that occupational therapists should adopt Kawa and CMOP-E models to facilitate spiritual resilience by providing the older adults with opportunities to share strategies that they have used to "address complex social, historical, and political factors" (Hunter & Pride, 2021, p. 333). Through the visual images and stories, older adults may share their skills on how they have conquered life's challenges.

In OT practice, spiritual resilience can be considered as part of older adults experiencing psychological happiness and resilience (Mthembu et al., 2017a, b; Richards et al., 2007; Sadri Damirchi et al., 2018).

In a semi-experimental pretest-posttest design with a control group conducted with elders in Rasht, Sadri Damirchi et al. (2018) found that group therapy provides a unique opportunity for integrating spirituality. This resonates with the belief that spirituality is a protective factor that underpins older adults' spiritual resilience (Manning et al., 2019; Duke, 2017; Manning, 2013). Therefore, these models will assist occupational therapists to accompany and support older adults in their life journeys as they deal with many challenges. The accompaniment will be strengthened by the philosophy of *Ubuntu*, which includes compassion, reciprocity, dignity, humanity, and mutuality in the interests of communality in light of justice and mutual caring (Chigangaidze, 2021, p. 276).

## Importance of *Ubuntu* in the Well-being of Older Adults

*Ubuntu* is the most significant construct that is explained through an African Ethno-philosophy, which is grounded in a communal way of humanness, interdependence, social connectedness, and interpersonal relationships (Cornell & van Marle, 2005; Hammell, 2014; Mthembu & Duncan, 2021; Ngubane-Mokiwa, 2018). The construct of *Ubuntu* is congruent with Sisulu's (2003, p. 6) assertion that an individual's identity is determined by the difference that they "have made to the lives of others" as part of communal well-being. Similar to the contribution to others, Nolte and Downing's (2019, p. 12–13) concept analysis study highlights a variety of attributes related to *Ubuntu*, which comprise "respect and dignity, solidarity, spirituality, reciprocity, harmony, mutuality, affinity, and kinship." These attributes are resonant with the OT profession, and they are important in the promotion of the well-being of older adults. Consequently, the evidence reviewed here suggests a pertinent role for OT "to promote concern for humankind and address broader occupational needs in society" as part of the decolonial turn (Mahoney & Kiraly-Alvarez, 2019, p. 4). Thus, Hammell (2017) advocates that OT should "advance the right of all people to engage in occupations that contribute positively to their own well-being and the well-being of their communities" (p. 209).

Older adults are perceived as custodians of indigenous knowledge that is passed on to generations through the process of caregiving, which fosters *Ubuntu* as part of legacy beliefs (Chisale, 2018; Meuser et al., 2019). *Ubuntu* acknowledges that older adults are open, engaging, and vulnerable

organisms within the world, which indicates OT should challenge societal issues that affect older adults' occupational lives and well-being (Mthembu & Duncan, 2021; Mahoney & Kiraly-Alvarez, 2019) (see also Chapter 31, OTs as change-agents). It becomes clear that occupational therapists should collaborate with individuals, families, communities, and other stakeholders to form partnerships enabling population-based wellness (WHO, 2017). This is consistent with du Toit et al.'s (2019) invitation that the OT profession needs "to develop practice addressing occupational injustice within collectives," which will promote "citizenship, agency and self-determination" among older adults (p. 578).

It is important to consider *Ubuntu* in the OT profession when embarking on projects that promote collaborative engagement of older adults in everyday occupations. Collaborative engagement in everyday occupations could provide older adults with opportunities to share their life experiences with younger generations in communities as part of the occupational legacy in passing on traditions, beliefs, cultural activities, and rituals (Mthembu, 2021). Occupational therapists may enhance the process of spiritual resilience by enabling older adults to engage in occupations that will allow older adults to meet the "human needs to belong, connect, and contribute" (Hammell, 2014, p. 46). Creating a supportive environment for older adults to engage in connecting and contributing occupations will enable them to meet the "axiological human needs subsistence, protection, affection, understanding, participation, idleness, and creation, identity, and freedom." These needs are enunciated in "cultural and socio-economic contexts through the existential categories of *being, having, doing,* and *interacting*" (Guillen-Royo, 2020): *Being* is concerned with individual or collective characteristics; *having* is focused on institutional arrangements, technologies, societal values, and habits; *doing* is associated with personal or collective actions, and *interacting* refers to the characteristics of physical and natural environments (p. 116).

OT professionals should enable older adults to flourish through their human capabilities that promote developing personal skills needed for the good life in a truly human way (Nussbaum, 2000, 2003). Nussbaum's (2000) human capabilities that are central to human life consist of: (1) ability to live a normal lengthy life; (2) ability to have good bodily health; (3) ability to have bodily integrity, freedom of movement, freedom from violence and abuse; (4) ability to use the senses, imagination, and thought; (5) ability to experience emotional development through attachments with others; (6) ability to practical reason through engagement in critical reflection; (7) ability to experience affiliation and live with others in a respective and dignified way and not discriminate others; (8) ability to have the gratitude of living with other species; (9) ability to play and enjoy a variety of valued occupations; and (10) ability to have one's control over environment both political and material. These human capabilities are crucial in sustaining spiritual resilience because older adults use their potential so that they can be able to promote wellness and social justice. Thus, the importance of *Ubuntu* resonates with a sense of belongingness, the psychological need for relatedness, interdependent relationships, contribution to others, and connecting occupations.

WHO (2017) states that older adults who experience occupational challenges due to adversities originating from different health conditions should be assisted to attain their intrinsic capacity and compensate for the loss of capacity. This has implications for OT practice to provide care, support, and environmental actions that will maintain functional abilities and promote the well-being of older adults by protecting their occupational rights and autonomy. Nevertheless, Hammell (2017) warns that OT should not only focus on the abilities of individuals whose lives are already impacted by illness, injury, or impairment but also on creating opportunities for achieving well-being through the occupational engagement of all those whose capabilities are inhibited by injustices.

Although *Ubuntu* has been identified as an important part of well-being among older adults, Chisale (2018) raises concern that the caregiving part of *Ubuntu* appears to be a double-edged sword that promotes women's equality and dignity but also perpetuates the hegemony of masculinity and patriarchal values that dehumanizes and preserves the gendered stereotypes of caregiving. This is important to note, as Morris (2021) argues that some occupations tend to have dark sides, which indicates that the gender inclusiveness in caregiving as part of *Ubuntu* might conceal the negative aspect (Chisale, 2018).

The African Ethno-philosophy emphasizes that *Ubuntu* involves morality, which is passed on to the younger generations as part of the occupational legacy in families and communities. In anchoring *Ubuntu* morality, Letseka (2013) espouses that older adults in society have ethical responsibilities to initiate and individuate young generations into *Ubuntu* morality so that they "become citizens that are inclined to treat others with justice and fairness at all times" (p. 351). Consequently, Letseka (2013) propounds that "moral norms and virtues such as kindness, generosity, compassion, benevolence, and respect and concern for others" can be adopted as part of humanness. These virtues resonate with the ethos of OT and can be considered as part of intergenerational solidarity enabling social cohesion between generations. *Ubuntu* is related to spirituality because these concepts promote interdependence and connectedness among people.

## Conclusion

The central theme of this chapter was to consider how spirituality and resilience are involved in the adaptation process necessary to optimally age. The connections between spirituality, resilience, and OT were explained, and it was concluded that OT, when aligning with spirituality, can be congruent with the unique characteristics of older adults (i.e., values, beliefs, and spirituality) and performance patterns related to habits, routines, roles, and rituals. The critical domains of the respective constructs, experiences, and practices were considered, and the connections between spirituality, resilience, adaptation, and aging were summarized. Overall, the chapter provides perspectives on how older adults can maximize gains and minimize losses in a manner reflecting optimal adaptation and aging while relying on practices of OT that incorporate elements of spirituality and resilience. Additionally, we engaged global and intergenerational perspectives to explore how people benefit from models and practices of OT that embody a humanistic and just approach.

*The complete listing of the Bibliography and Chapter Questions and Answers are available in the accompanying enhanced eBook version included with the print purchase of this textbook. Visit Elsevier eBooks+ (eBooks.Health.Elsevier.com) to access this content.*

## CHAPTER 19

# Diverse Understandings of 'Successful Aging'

*Debbie Laliberte Rudman, PhD, OT Reg. (Ont.), Sarah Lamb, PhD, and Selena E. Washington, PhD*

## CHAPTER OUTLINE

## OBJECTIVES

- Provide an overview of the origins and development of the contemporary paradigm of 'successful aging,' inclusive of various inter-related terms (e.g., active aging, healthy aging, productive aging)
- Critically consider the assumptions and limits of contemporary aging models aligned with the successful aging paradigm
- Address why diversity matters when considering meanings of 'successful aging' and possibilities for 'aging well'
- Explore evidence addressing occupation as a contributor to 'aging well'
- Gain exposure to programs and approaches that address occupation to support 'aging well'

What does it mean to age successfully? If you reflect on people in your life or people in the media whom you view as aging successfully, what characteristics seem to define success? How do those characteristics reflect the society in which you exist? How might these characteristics be differentially achievable, or valued, depending on an individual's social location, for example, in terms of gender, race, class, culture, or disability status? These questions are important to address—as individuals and as a profession—given that how 'successful aging' is thought, talked, and written about—that is, how it is discursively constructed—shapes what come to be taken for granted as the ways individuals and societies, including health care systems and professionals, should manage aging (Laliberte Rudman, 2017; Lamb, 2014). As well, discourses of successful aging shape occupational possibilities for older adults, marking out particular occupations and ways of doing occupations as appropriate, ideal, and possible and as worthy of supporting through social and health care systems and policies. At the same time, such discourses exclude and fail to support other types of occupations and ways of doing occupations, shaping occupational injustices for those older adults who do not have the capacities and resources that align with dominant ideals of successful aging or who hold alternative understandings of what it means to age well (Canadian Association of Occupational Therapists [CAOT], 2011; Laliberte Rudman, 2006, 2017; Trentham, 2019).

Within the broader context of population aging (see Chapter 3), along with other social transformations such as heightened global mobility, increasing economic globalization, and changing family structures, questions of how to define and achieve successful aging at individual to societal levels have been increasingly prioritized in gerontology, health care, and social policy (Calasanti & King, 2021; de Medeiros et al., 2016). Within the North American context and increasingly on a global scale, a particular paradigm of successful aging has become dominant over the past few decades, one that emphasizes continued health, independence, productivity, individual responsibility, and youthfulness (Lamb, 2014; Laliberte Rudman, 2017; Neilson, 2009). Although this paradigm of successful aging seems well aligned with occupational therapy's focus on enabling health and well-being through occupation and has enhanced knowledge regarding factors that can support older adults in maintaining health and well-being, it is also crucial to be aware of how uncritical promotion of discourses and practices aligned with this paradigm may deepen inequities, contribute to ageism, limit occupational possibilities, and promote viewing particular older adults as having "failed" at aging. Essentially, a one-size-fits-all model for addressing successful aging is an inadequate approach given that older adults are not a homogenous group (Calasanti & King, 2021; Lamb et al., 2017; Laliberte Rudman, 2006).

In this chapter, we encourage occupational therapists to understand and support diverse understandings of aging well. In agreement with Calasanti and King (2021), we propose moving away from "any universal model of an ideal old age, just as we would reject models for ideal womanhood or being healthy people of color in a racist society" (p. 1824).

In turn, we encourage occupational therapists to celebrate and support many ways of aging. We begin by providing an overview of the dominant successful aging paradigm, starting with addressing one of the most prominent models influencing research, health care practice, and social policy in many Western societies, specifically Rowe and Kahn's model of successful aging (Calasanti & King, 2021; Rowe & Kahn, 2015). We then summarize key characteristics of the dominant successful aging paradigm as it has developed over time, including how various versions, such as positive aging, active aging and healthy aging, have been incorporated into social policies within North America and globally (Asquith, 2009; Laliberte Rudman, 2017). Although acknowledging the contributions of this paradigm in turning attention to continued possibilities for well-being, occupation, and social contributions in later phases of life, we also point to key concerns regarding determinantal social, occupational, and political effects arising from how this idealized vision of aging has been developed and promoted. In the second section of the chapter, we share examples of other ways of thinking about what it means to age well and illustrate why it is vital to attend to diversity in OT practice with older adults. In the final section, we turn to specific examples of social programs and OT practice and research approaches addressing aging well.

## Dominant Paradigm of Successful Aging: Origin, Development, and Critiques

Since the 1960s, many gerontological researchers have focused on developing models that delineate the components and predictors of aging well (de Medeiros et al., 2016). Although various terms have been used to denote a vision of aging well, such as productive, optimal, positive, active, or healthy aging (Asquith, 2009; de Medeiros et al., 2016), many of these terms and models are aligned with a broader successful aging movement originating in the United States in the mid-1960s, when the term successful aging was coined by gerontologist Robert Havighurst (Katz & Calasanti, 2015; Lamb, 2014). This successful aging movement has grown into a paradigm (Lamb et al., 2017), that is, a particular constellation of ideas, values, and beliefs dominant within a field (Kuhn, 1996). The influence of the successful aging paradigm has extended beyond gerontological research into health care, popular media, social policy, consumer markets, and other social arenas, shaping how many people, academics, health care professionals, and governments in North America have come to understand aging and how aging should be managed by individuals and societies (Lamb et al., 2017; Laliberte Rudman, 2017; Pack et al., 2019).

### Origins—Rowe and Kahn's Model of Successful Aging

Key characteristics of the paradigm of successful aging can be traced back to the seminal work of physician John Rowe and psychologist Robert Kahn, completed as part of the MacArthur Foundation Study of Aging in the United States

(Calasanti & King, 2021; de Medeiros et al., 2016; Rowe & Kahn, 1997, 1998, 2015). This multistate longitudinal study, conducted from 1988 to 1996, sought to deepen understanding of factors that differentiated older adults who experienced "normal" age-related declines in physical and cognitive function from those who maintained high function (Rowe & Kahn, 1997, 1998). This work resulted in a three-component definition of successful aging, specifically, "low probability of disease and disease-related disability, high cognitive and physical functional capacity, and active engagement with life" (Rowe & Kahn, 1997, p. 433). This model focuses on involvement in productive and social activities, as well as the responsibility of individuals to modify their lifestyles to reduce risks for disease, disability, and dependency (Rowe & Kahn, 2015). Overall, this model emphasizes individual agency and everyone's ability to shape their own aging process, an emphasis that has become a key defining feature of the contemporary successful aging paradigm. This emphasis is exemplified in the following quote from Rowe and Kahn's *Successful Aging* book published in 1998: "In short, successful aging is dependent on individual choices and behaviors. It can be attained through individual choice and effort" (p. 37).

On one hand, Rowe and Kahn's model is often viewed as making positive contributions by promoting an optimistic approach and counteracting longstanding negative conceptualizations of aging which framed decline, disengagement, and dependency as inevitable (Katz & Calasanti, 2015). In addition, it has served as the basis for a substantial body of research addressing factors that predict and enhance health and functioning amongst older adults, and has informed medical, health care, and social practices and programs that aim to support older adults' functioning and societal contributions (Calasanti & King, 2021; Stowe & Cooney, 2015). Of specific relevance to OT this model has facilitated the generation of research evidence regarding the contributions of social and productive occupations to health and well-being for older adults. For example, several longitudinal studies have connected participation in social and productive activities to longevity, self-reported happiness, physical function, cognitive function, and other measures of health and well-being (Evans et al., 2019; Fratigilioni et al., 2004; Glass et al., 1999; Menec, 2003; Russell et al., 2019). Such studies provide evidence supporting OT interventions aimed at enabling older adults to engage in a range of social and productive occupations (de Medeiros et al., 2016; Stav et al., 2012; Stevens-Ratchford & Diaz, 2003).

However, as will be further discussed in the following sections, this model of successful aging and the broader paradigm of successful aging that has developed since the 1980s have also been extensively critiqued. In order to support the occupational rights, health, and well-being of diverse older adults, it is crucial that occupational therapists are critically aware of the limitations and boundaries of this dominant paradigm, given that particular emphases and omissions obscure inequalities, perpetuate ageism, narrowly define appropriate occupations for older adults, and promote a narrow Western-centric view of aging well (Asquith, 2009; Calasanti & King,

2021; Laliberte Rudman, 2006, 2017; Lamb, 2014). Prior to addressing these critiques, key characteristics of the contemporary successful aging paradigm are summarized.

## On-Going Development of the 'Successful Aging' Paradigm

Since the late 1980s, an idealized vision of successful aging, with its foundation in the markers established in Rowe and Kahn's model, has pervaded North American society and extended out globally (Katz & Calasanti, 2015; Dillaway & Brynes, 2009; Lamb et al., 2017). Despite many critiques, successful aging remains a dominant conceptual framework in gerontology (Dillaway & Brynes, 2009; Lamb, 2014). Hundreds of models of successful aging, which have adapted and extended Rowe and Kahn's model, have been proposed and studied, and research institutes focused on successful aging have thrived (Katz & Calasanti, 2015; Rowe & Kahn, 2015). Various models consistent with successful aging, such as productive aging and active aging, have also been incorporated into position statements of OT professional associations (American Occupational Therapy Association [AOTA], 2016; World Federation of Occupational Therapists [WFOT], 2021), and have guided OT research (Smallfield & Elliott, 2020).

In addition, often underpinned by concerns regarding an aging "crisis," national and international policies have promoted ideal visions of aging consistent with the successful aging paradigm to manage potential economic, health and other sociopolitical implications of population aging (Asquith, 2009; Laliberte Rudman, 2016; Neilson, 2009). For example, in 2002, the World Health Organization (WHO) published and promoted a policy framework for Active Aging, with active aging defined as "a process of optimizing opportunities for health, participation, and security" (p. 12). Within this highly influential document, the WHO urged its member states to enact policies aimed at maintaining independence and autonomy, optimizing quality of life, and delaying disability (Raymond & Grenier, 2013). In 2006, with the publication of a document titled *Work Longer, Live Longer,* the Organization for Economic Cooperation and Development (OECD) spawned a focus on productive aging, which has increasingly been narrowly defined as on-going involvement in the labor force. Since that time, policy shifts aimed at both extending work lives and decreasing the economic costs of aging populations have been instituted in many national contexts. For example, several nations have integrated policies banning mandatory retirement, increasing the age of eligibility for public pensions, and restricting access to disability-related income systems (Laliberte Rudman, 2016; Laliberte Rudman & Aldrich, 2021; OECD, 2019).

In addition, ideas consistent with the successful aging paradigm have pervaded various types of public media, self-help books, and consumer markets, including an ever-expanding anti-aging industry (Lamb, 2014; Lamb et al., 2017; Petersen, 2018). A quick search on Google for self-help books addressing aging published in recent years reveals titles such as *Successful Aging: A Neuroscientist Explores the Power and Potential of Our Lives, Boundless: Upgrade Your Brain, Optimize Your Body, and Defy Aging* (Greenfield, 2020), and *The Longevity Paradox: How to Die Young at a Ripe Old Age* (Grundy, 2019). Fueled by the promise of achieving successful aging, particularly achieving agelessness, the value of the global anti-aging industry was predicted to expand from approximately US$140 billion to US$216 billion between 2015 and 2021 (Petersen, 2018).

Across these various academic, political, professional, consumer, and other social arenas, key aspects of the contemporary successful paradigm are often evident. These aspects include an emphasis on individual responsibility for achieving security and well-being in later life; maintaining independence and avoiding dependence; being productive and socially engaged; and maintaining a youthful mind, body, and lifestyle (Laliberte Rudman, 2016, 2017; Lamb, 2014; Lamb et al., 2017; Stowe & Cooney, 2015). This paradigm has established a "gold standard" (Dillaway & Brynes, 2009, p. 706), normative model of aging that has a significant influence, particularly in North America, on how health care professionals, researchers, politicians, and others have come to think about and act in relation to aging (Laliberte Rudman, 2017; Lamb, 2014). Indeed, perhaps not surprisingly given the ways in which this paradigm centers outcomes aligned with values and beliefs upheld in many Western societies (Lamb et al., 2017; Trentham, 2019), research has revealed that this paradigm is appealing to many aging and older North Americans, particularly among those with the financial, health, and other resources to participate in the productive, consumer, body management, and other types of occupations held out as contributing to successful aging (Laliberte Rudman, 2015; Lamb, 2014, 2018; Pack et al., 2019). Moreover, as the successful aging paradigm has evolved and spread into many aspects of North American and other Western contexts, it has increasingly been framed as a "duty to age well," one that older adults are expected to work towards not only to maintain personal well-being but also to avoid becoming a societal burden or social embarrassment (Asquith, 2009; Laliberte Rudman, 2016; Lamb, 2018).

As occupational therapists, we can welcome optimistic views of aging that support continued occupational engagement at the same time as being critical of specific ways the successful aging paradigm has been taken up within contemporary society. As detailed in the next section, it is crucial to be aware of the exclusionary effects of this paradigm as well as its potential to reinforce ageism and support state retreat from funding for services for older adults. To support the occupational rights of all older adults, such as those with disabilities, those who are living in poverty, those who are racialized, and those with varied cultural and religious backgrounds, occupational therapists need to advocate for and use understandings of aging well that are more inclusive of diverse older adults and diverse types and ways of doing occupations in later life (CAOT, 2011; Laliberte Rudman, 2017; Trentham, 2019).

## Critiques of the Successful Aging Paradigm— Implications for Occupation and Occupational Therapy

As noted above, a key defining feature of the successful aging paradigm is an individualistic emphasis on the ability, and responsibility, to proactively manage one's lifestyle and engage in a never-ending project aimed at achieving prolonged health and independence (Laliberte Rudman, 2017; Lamb et al., 2017). As stated by Dillaway and Brynes (2009), successful aging discourses convey "that individuals should be able to overcome personal barriers and work toward successful aging at all times; indeed, this is their responsibility" (p. 705). This emphasis on individual responsibility and personal control over the aging process and its outcomes has been critiqued by many authors, given that it neglects historical, social, and structural forces that shape social inequalities and health conditions, such as those tied to race, gender, and social class (Calasanti & King, 2021; Lamb, 2014, 2018; Simons et al., 2016; Stowe & Cooney, 2015). Such social inequalities, which result from group-based disadvantages and inequitable social conditions and resources, cannot be overcome through individual choices alone and create differential possibilities for aging well across the life course (Calasanti & King, 2021; Laliberte Rudman, 2017; Stowe & Cooney, 2015). For example, within the United States, intersecting socioeconomic inequalities tied to factors such as race, class, gender, and ability mean that individuals experience income disparities and differential access to health care that profoundly impact health and wellbeing in later life. In turn, "given these financial realities, it follows that many people aged 65 and older—and women more than men, as well as minority group members and poor or working-class people—are constrained in their health and lifestyle choices" (Katz & Calasanti, 2015, p. 30). In neglecting these social inequalities, the dominant paradigm of successful aging excludes older adults who face financial, health, and other types of barriers to making what have come to be constructed as the ideal and correct lifestyle "choices," as well as those whose cultural and social locations mean that they may hold alternative understandings of success (Lamb, 2017; Liang & Luo 2012; Raymond & Grenier, 2013). Moreover, given the focus on personal responsibility, the successful aging paradigm has been politically taken up in ways that frame those who are viewed as failing to age successfully, such as those who experience dependence and disability, as irresponsible and undeserving of support (Laliberte Rudman, 2017; Stowe & Cooney, 2015). It is vital for occupational therapists to work against such framings, instead committing to advocating for services and programs that address social inequalities and their implications for the aging process (CAOT, 2011; Laliberte Rudman, 2017). Indeed, critical gerontologists have pointed to how the successful aging paradigm has been taken up within many nations since the 1980s within neoliberal measures that have restricted and dismantled various protective measures for older adults, such as public pensions and publicly funded health services (Calasanti & King, 2021; Raymond & Grenier, 2013).

Another key critique of the successful aging paradigm is that it has failed to overcome ageism because it promotes "a vision of the ideal person as not really aging at all in later life" (Lamb et al., 2017, p. 11) and promotes fear of bodily, cognitive, and other signs of oldness (Calasanti & King, 2021; Lamb, 2018). Oldness continues to be framed as something that must be continually defied, and those who are deemed to be old are devalued and may be excluded from possibilities for meaningful participation (Lamb, 2014, 2018; Raymond & Grenier, 2013). For example, several qualitative studies addressing how older adults in North America understand and negotiate successful aging have revealed ways that such older adults seek to distance themselves from oldness; for example, by socially distancing themselves from people whom they perceive as old and resisting the use of assistive devices that could be seen as markers of being old (Laliberte Rudman, 2015; Lamb, 2018; Lamb et al., 2017; Pack et al., 2019). Moreover, the promise of avoiding oldness offered through the successful aging paradigm is likely to set up tensions, contradictions, and self-blame even for aging adults who can participate in the practices it promotes, given that many are likely to eventually experience signs and symptoms they associate with oldness despite their attempts to defy aging (Laliberte Rudman, 2015; Lamb, 2014, 2018; Pack et al., 2019). As such, the dominant successful aging paradigm fails to create positive possibilities for older adults who experience disability, decline, and dependency, and can promote self-blame and social blaming of those deemed to be "old." Thus, given that occupational therapists often work with older adults who do experience health challenges and disabilities, it is important to avoid unreflexively perpetuating ageist attitudes and practices embedded in this dominant paradigm and to integrate approaches that support the personhood, dignity, and desired occupational engagement of older adult clients. For example, Trentham (2019) advocates shifting away from a Western ethnocentric preoccupation with independence in OT with older adults, framing it as an "unattainable goal and a mirage, particularly for the diversity of seniors served by occupational therapists" (p. 199). In turn, Trentham proposes that occupational therapists shift towards supporting interdependence and focus on occupations older adult clients "really value and how they want to engage in them, whether on their own or with the support and engagement of those in relation to them" (p. 200).

A final critique of the successful aging paradigm important for occupational therapists is that this paradigm promotes a very narrow view of what occupations are ideal possible, and health-promoting for older adults while also ignoring inequalities in the financial, health, social, and other resources required to participate in the occupations promoted (Laliberte Rudman, 2006). Overall, occupations tied to contributing to society, through production or consumption, and to self-maintenance are prioritized (Laliberte Rudman, 2006, 2017; Lamb, 2014). Productive occupations have been increasingly narrowly defined as involvement in the paid labor market, such that other ways that older adults make productive contributions to society, such as through caregiving, volunteering, or political advocacy, may become progressively neglected (Laliberte Rudman, 2016; Moulaert & Biggs, 2013). Moreover, the ways in which ageism functions as a barrier to sustained engagement in the paid labor force for many older adults is also neglected, further intensifying financial, social, and occupational inequities for older adults who face intersectional barriers tied to age, race, gender, educational status, and other social identity markers (Laliberte Rudman, 2016; Laliberte Rudman & Aldrich, 2021). Consumer-based occupations often focus on services and products designed to enable the maintenance of youthful bodies, minds, and lifestyles, such as studying Italian in Florence, jetting off to a trek in Nepal, or even skydiving, as President George H.W. Bush did on his 80th birthday (Fountain, 2005). Many of these idealized occupations required substantial financial and health resources to participate, further excluding older adults who experience social inequalities (Laliberte, 2006).

Given the broad conceptualization of occupation in OT, the expanding body of knowledge regarding the multiple interconnections between diverse occupations and well-being, and the growing awareness of the sociopolitical production of occupational injustices, occupational therapists and scientists have a key role to play in broadening discourses of aging and expanding occupational possibilities (Laliberte Rudman, 2017). Moving forward, important directions include working with diverse older adults, as individuals and collectively, to generate knowledge and awareness of the various ways that older adults engage in occupations that contribute to the well-being of themselves, their families, and communities, as well as engaging in interdisciplinary scholarship that has attended to other ways of understanding and enacting aging (Calasanti & King, 2021; Raymond & Grenier, 2013; Trentham, 2019).

## Attending to Diversity in Conceptualizing and Addressing 'Aging Well'

Anthropologists, sociologists, and critical gerontologists have examined the extraordinarily popular paradigm of successful aging—and its corollaries, healthy and active aging—probing both the paradigm's underlying cultural assumptions as well as alternative ways of conceptualizing aging well. We can see from studies on cultural values surrounding aging that, first, many groups do not emphasize independence to the same degree as emphasized in prevailing North American successful aging models. Second, many individuals and cultural groups are much more accepting of aging and its changes than successful aging models imply.

It is not surprising that diverse models of what it can mean to age well exist cross-culturally (e.g., Lamb, 2015, 2017; Sokolovsky, 2020). The literature is too vast to summarize here, but common cross-cultural understandings of aging well center on ideals of appropriate interdependence over the life course and the provisioning of elder care within multigenerational families. Rowe and Kahn present as a straightforward fact: "Older people, like younger ones, want to be independent. This is the principal goal of many elders, and

few issues strike greater fear than the prospect of depending on others" (1998, p. 42). Yet it is important to consider that throughout Asia and most of the developing world—and among many non-white racial-ethnic groups within the United States—living intimately with others in a condition of appropriate inter/dependence is generally regarded as much more normal and valued than is living fully independently in older age (e.g., Brijnath, 2012; Calvo, 2018; Cliggett, 2005, pp. 13–15; Ikels, 2004, p. 9; Lamb, 2009; Lewis, 2011). While full dependency is not wished for by most people in any cultural context, beyond white middle- to upper-class North America, it is very common for elders and their communities to find it entirely appropriate to reside with, depend on, and receive care from kin—even intimate bodily care as necessary—just as most people find it entirely appropriate and valued for minor children to be dependent on their parents. As one example, Rocío Calvo finds that greater reported satisfaction in later life for Latinos may be tied to cultural emphases within Latinx communities on family support instead of individual self-reliance. Calvo (2018) reports: "Hispanic immigrants in our study co-resided with their adult children more often than any other group. Interestingly, while living with their children made older Hispanics happy, it had the opposite effect among older Whites."

Further, many individuals and groups cross-culturally do not emphasize agelessness and striving not to be "old" to the extent promoted by prevailing North American successful aging discourses. An alternative Indian Hindu perspective, for instance, is that life fundamentally entails change, decline, and transience—not only in old age but as an essential feature of the human material condition. Coming to realize this transience can be a positive and enlightening move, potentially making both aging and dying meaningful (Lamb, 2014). Some in India are even puzzled by the successful aging discourse now circulating around the world, including in their nation. They enjoy trying to be healthy and active, such as by taking morning walks and eating well, but one of Lamb's research participants asked of 'successful aging': "What's the point? Are the Americans trying to avoid being old? Or, is it because people want to live more and more and don't want to die?"

Even within North America, we see vibrant alternatives to the successful aging paradigm's emphasis on individual control over the aging process, agelessness, and fending off "oldness." For instance, popular Christian media and fieldwork with US Catholic nuns suggest that successful aging may clash with Christian values in its rejection of old age. Life stages are considered part of God's plan, not to be altered by human intervention or criticized by human actors (Corwin, 2021; Thacker, 2019). Many older Americans who have actually reached a stage they identify as "old" also convey perspectives that are much more accepting of change in old age than successful aging discourse. Sociologist Meika Loe (2017) finds that many North Americans age 85 and beyond emphasize "comfortable" rather than "ageless" aging, for instance, and reporter John Leland (2022) of the *New York Times* explores how many among the oldest old strive for "pleasures within reach" rather than aspirations of younger times. In a collection of essays written in her eighties, author Ursula Le Guin (2017) pushes back against the "fairy tale" language prevailing in US society: "You're not old! Nobody's old. We're all living happily ever after" (p. 17), arguing: "To tell me my old age doesn't exist is to tell me that I don't exist. Erase my age, you erase my life—me" (p. 14).

In addition, lower-income older Americans commonly convey a sense of powerlessness to achieve ideals of healthy aging—due to external obstacles beyond their control, ranging from lack of access to healthy foods and good medical care, to having worked in toxic environments, to living in bedbug-infested buildings, which hinder one's ability to socialize and go out and do things (Lamb, 2018, 2020). The notion that willpower and lifestyle choices can be harnessed to achieve health in aging can feel alienating to those who have contended with structural inequalities throughout life.

In closing this section reflecting on diverse conceptualizations of aging well, it is important to point out that the prevailing successful aging paradigm—emphasizing values of independence, productivity, individual control, and agelessness—is not simply an academic, gerontological, and medical model. It is also a cultural one, emerging from and reinforcing widespread cultural values and assumptions held by many laypeople, not only professionals, in North America (Lamb, 2014; Lamb et al., 2017). So, many clients of occupational therapists will themselves believe in and espouse 'successful-aging' ideals, such as that being "old" or needing help with activities of daily living is bad and embarrassing. Pushing back against her medical team's recommendation that she use a cane, one older white American in her eighties refused, "I don't want a cane." "Why?" anthropologist Sarah Lamb asked. She replied straightforwardly, "Because it makes me old." Understanding the pervasiveness of successful aging discourses is thus important to inform how occupational therapists approach interventions, pointing to the need to explore how such discourses may influence what clients view as acceptable and unacceptable approaches to supporting their occupational participation.

## Evidence-Based Community Health Promotion and Wellness Programs

The previous section makes it clear that the definition of successful aging must be considered in regard to cultural relevance, in addition to social conditions and resources. Rosal and Bodenlos (2009) define culture as "what is learned, shared, transmitted intergenerationally, and reflected in a group's values, beliefs, norms, behaviors, communication, and social roles" (p. 39). In this section, we will focus on programs that consider how aging individuals are positioned to age well with the aforementioned factors taken into consideration. Through an intersectional lens, we provide three examples of programmatic implementation in the United States that address the facilitation of occupational engagement and demonstrate how 'aging well,' in diverse expressions, can be supported through evidence-based program initiatives.

The **Community Aging in Place, Advancing Better Living for Elders (CAPABLE)** program model created by the John Hopkins School of Nursing (Szanton et al., 2021) is an evidence-based, client-directed, 5-month program. The program combines services from an occupational therapist, registered nurse, and a maintenance/home contractor to provide home safety modifications, install assistive devices, and provide basic home repairs. Connecting this to aging well, the program improves the conditions and resources that older clients have to move forward in occupational engagement. This evidence-based program demonstrated significant improvement in activities of daily living (ADLs) and instrumental activities of daily living (IADLs), as well as health outcomes, such as pain and depression. The program realized these positive outcomes while reducing health care costs, finding up to $22,000 in medical savings for dual eligible beneficiaries (private insurance and Medicare) over a period of two years. In a study with low-income older adults on Medicaid and Medicare who participated, this program resulted in 75% of participants improving their self-care functioning over the course of five months (Szanton et al., 2021).

The **Falls Free Coalition** is a national effort led by United States National Council on Aging (NCOA) to address the growing public health issue of fall-related injuries and deaths in older adults. The effort focuses on advocacy, awareness, and educational initiatives, including building community infrastructure to reduce falls among older adults. Three national organizations, the National Council on Aging, the Archstone Foundation, and the Home Safety Council, collaborated to create the national FallsFree Coalition (NCOA, 2022). The Coalition's collaborative leadership now includes state departments of aging, public health departments, and health-care providers. In 2021, a year impacted by the COVID-19 pandemic, 370 million older adults learned about the importance of fall prevention through traditional media, new media, and community outreach (NCOA, 2022). NCOA also launched the Falls Free Checkup, a digital screening tool modeled after the 12-question screener included in the Centers for Disease Control and Prevention's Stopping Elderly Accidents, Deaths, and Injuries (STEADI; Stevens & Phelan, 2013).

The **Well Elderly Studies 1 and 2** were landmark studies examining the role of occupational therapy in promoting aging well. Based on research examining the complex, interlocking physical, psychosocial, economic, and social factors influences the occupational performance, health, and well-being of older adults, Florence Clark and colleagues (1997) designed and evaluated the effectiveness of an OT primary prevention program that targeted urban, multi-ethnic, community-dwelling seniors. They conducted a 9-month randomized control study with 361 well older adults, aged 60 and older, living in Los Angeles. urban dwelling. A key underlying hypothesis was that an OT intervention, based on principles of fostering meaningful and productive activities, could enhance function, maximize health, and promote health. Research participants were randomly assigned to one of the three groups: a social control group that participated in general group social activities ($n = 122$); a non-treatment control group ($n$ = 119); and the OT treatment group ($n$ = 122). Participants in the treatment group participated in a specifically designed program, Lifestyle Redesign, carried out by trained occupational therapists. The researchers hypothesized that participation in a social activity group would be less effective in promoting daily function, physical well-being, and psychosocial well-being than participation in the primary prevention Lifestyle Redesign program.

The Well Elderly Study 1 found significant benefits from the Lifestyle Redesign program delivered by occupational therapists across various health, function, and quality-of-life (QoL) domains (Clark et al., 1997). This study provided the most comprehensive evidence to date of the effectiveness of occupational therapy primary prevention interventions with older adults. The participants in the Lifestyle Redesign treatment group demonstrated significant improvements in functioning or a relative reduction in the extent of functional decline, as compared with those in the social skills and no-treatment control groups. Overall, participants in the Lifestyle Redesign treatment group demonstrated significant gains in 10 of the 15 outcome measures studied, as compared with the control groups, providing solid evidence of the comprehensive effectiveness of this primary preventive OT intervention with well older adults. Clark et al. (2012) conducted a follow-up randomized control trial, Well Elderly 2, to replicate previous findings regarding the impact and cost-effectiveness of the Lifestyle Redesign intervention, and to understand the mechanisms underlying those effects. In this second study, relative to the control groups, the intervention group showed more favorable change scores regarding pain, vitality, social functioning, mental health, composite mental functioning, symptoms of depression, as well as life satisfaction, and a significant greater increase in quality-adjusted life years (Clark et al., 2012).

Many subsequent studies have investigated the Lifestyle Redesign program, with some occurring in countries other than the United States. For example, the program was used with a group of French-speaking Canadian older adults and was found to result in improved knowledge about health, social participation, leisure, and mobility (Levasseur et al., 2019). As another example, recognizing the importance of addressing cultural relevance, the Lifestyle Redesign intervention protocol was adapted for use in Israel. The Israeli

Lifestyle Program (ILP) aimed to enhance health and functioning of older adults, with results suggesting this program had potential to improve occupational performance, quality of life, and depressive symptoms (Maeir et al., 2021). Lifestyle Redesign has also adapted when applied with older adults with different socioeconomic, health, and cultural backgrounds, such as with Latino (Schepens Niemiec et al., 2019) and Swedish older adults (Johansson & Björklund, 2016). These examples demonstrate that evidence-based knowledge needs to be translated into practice to ensure fit with sociocultural contexts; aspects such as appropriateness, acceptability, fidelity, and timeliness of the intervention should be assessed prior to implementing a program within a specific context (Glasdam et al., 2021).

## SUMMARY

Occupational therapists need to be critically reflexive regarding how they, and the broader society in which they are embedded, think about what it means to age successfully. As outlined in this chapter, the dominant paradigm of successful aging, while supporting the continued importance of on-going, meaningful occupational participation in later life, presents a narrow view of what it means to age well. This narrow view, with its emphases on individual responsibility, continued youthfulness, and the avoidance of disease and disability, has been critiqued for being ageist, Western-centric, and exclusionary. From an occupational perspective, there is a need to be cautious regarding how the dominant successful aging paradigm can limit occupational possibilities for older adults and shape occupational injustices. As such, it is important to be aware of the diverse ways older adults understand what it means to age well, and to work with older adults to support occupational participation in later life in ways that support diverse ways of being and doing in later life.

*The complete listing of the Bibliography and Chapter Questions and Answers are available in the accompanying enhanced eBook version included with the print purchase of this textbook. Visit Elsevier eBooks+ (eBooks.Health.Elsevier.com) to access this content.*

CHAPTER 20

# The Physical Environment and Aging

*Graham D. Rowles, PhD, FGSA, FAGHE, Malcolm P. Cutchin, PhD, FGSA, Margaret A. Perkinson, PhD, FGSA, FAGHE, FSfAA, and Karen Frank Barney, PhD, MS, OTR, FAOTA*

## CHAPTER OUTLINE

## OBJECTIVES

- Review alternative historical and contemporary theoretical approaches to understanding the relationship between a person and their physical environment.
- Understand older adults' use of and attribution of meaning to their physical environment.
- Recognize the need for and alternative approaches toward environmental modification and adaptation associated with both aging in place and relocation.
- Provide approaches to effective occupational therapy practice that acknowledge the role of the physical environment in affecting well-being.
- Understand the approaches to conducting occupational therapy assessments of physical environments and interventions that support the occupational performance of older adults.
- Recognize diversity and social exclusion with respect to participation in the physical environment.

It has long been recognized that behavior, physical and mental health, quality of life, and well-being are influenced, indeed, shaped by the physical environment, and especially so in old age (Evans, 2003; Shipp & Branch, 1999; Wahl et al., 2012). In this chapter, we consider the way characteristics of physical settings (both the natural and built environment) interact with the changing capabilities of the aging adult to create patterns of behavior, lifestyles, and the experience of "being in place"

that are more or less adaptive for older adults (Rowles, 1991, 2018). Being in place is the sense of well-being that results from identifying with and being "at one" with one's environment. At any point in time, a person's experience of "being in place" or its opposite, feeling "out of place," expresses a state of being along a multidimensional continuum that evolves during accommodation to changing personal capabilities and environmental challenges. In old age, the dynamic homeostasis between the opportunities and constraints exerted by the environment and the person's changing (generally reduced) capabilities evolves in an ongoing process of adaptation. At first, such adaptation may occur through both subconscious and deliberate accommodation (for example, environmental modification or lowered occupational performance motivations and expectations). Eventually, it may become necessary for the individual to relocate to a more supportive environment. Indeed, we may envisage an array of possible trajectories of relocation where an individual might move along a continuum of supportive living options, perhaps from an independent residence to a congregate or assisted living facility and then to a nursing home as their circumstances change, although not necessarily in an invariant linear progression.

This general perspective on the changing relationship between the older individual and their physical environment has been expressed in a number of theories. We describe how these ecological theories evolved over the past three-quarters of a century, beginning with Kurt Lewin's (1951) seminal articulation of field theory and the basic $B = f(P, E)$ equation (where $B$ = Behavior, $P$ = Person, and $E$ = Environment) and progressing through the classic ecological theory of Lawton and Nahemow (1973), to a series of contemporary perspectives (Chaudhury & Oswald, 2019). Comparable perspectives have emerged in occupational therapy (OT) and occupational science. Such perspectives, including Person-Environment-Occupational Performance (Baum et al., 2014), Person-Environment-Occupation (Law et al., 1996), and the Model of Human Occupation (Kielhofner, 1995), led to the expanded $B = f(P, E, A)$ conceptualization of Iwarsson (2004) (where $A$ = Activity), and to more recent post ecological transactional representations such as the Deweyan pragmatist perspective developed by Cutchin and colleagues (Cutchin, 2004; Cutchin & Dickie, 2013; Rhodus & Rowles, 2022). These models provide a foundation for OT with aging adults, allowing for diverse behavioral and socioemotional interventions with individuals, as well as environmental modifications to enhance adjustment and well-being.

Against this theoretical background, we provide a contemporary account of the way older people use their physical environment and develop implicit mental awareness and engagement with the settings of their life. Over time, the blending of habitual patterns of use and awareness imbue the environments of a person's life with meanings that directly influence their sense of well-being. In the contemporary world, few lives are lived in their entirety in a single location. For most people, life involves multiple relocations to new settings over the life course—a process over which, depending on age and circumstance, the person exerts a greater or lesser degree of personal control. This process involves a constant making and remaking of place that in old age becomes increasingly problematic as personal capability and resources decline (Oswald & Rowles, 2006; Rowles & Watkins, 2003). We present a model of the way in which, with respect to the recreation of one especially important place in most people's life, their home, relocation involves continuously attempting to make or remake a place of meaning and identity. Making and remaking home is more difficult for some people than for others; in old age, it may become especially hard. This is where gerontologists, planners, architects, interior designers, physical therapists, occupational scientists, and especially occupational therapists have a critical role to play.

The final portion of the chapter shifts to intervention. First, we consider contemporary approaches to creating optimal physical environments for older adults—from the microscale of the individual dwelling to the macro level of neighborhoods and communities—that support and maximize health and well-being, not only for older adults but all people. Second, we explore the role of OT environments and the interventions of occupational therapists as ways to proactively enhance quality of life by facilitating optimal adaptations to changing circumstances through maximizing the role of the physical environment in supporting a preferred lifestyle.

## Aging and Environmental Press

The notion of "environmental press" is first credited to the psychologist Henry Murray, who coined the phrase to refer to any external environmental characteristic that influences behavior (Murray, 1938). As we grow older, the configuration of our residence increasingly shapes and limits our behavior and use of space. On a microscale, getting in and out of the bathtub or the shower becomes more problematic. Even if there are convenient handrails, our aging bodies no longer have the strength to pull ourselves out of the tub or the slipperiness of the shower floor becomes increasingly hazardous to an unsteady body. High shelves in the cupboards where we store occasionally used items become less safely accessible. We no longer use upstairs rooms because our stairs become a physical barrier. Indeed, the physical constraints of our residence lead to increasing "environmental centralization" as we confine ourselves to a more limited portion of our residence (Rubinstein, 1989), or "set up" within a single room (Rowles, 1981). Outside our dwelling,

the physical environment of the immediate surroundings can be similarly constraining. The once easily traversed slope of a lengthy driveway may make it difficult to access a roadside mailbox, especially in inclement weather. The snow that we frolicked in as a child, in old age becomes a daunting physical barrier that may put us at risk for falls and related injuries. And in the neighborhood beyond our residence, we may find that the physical environment becomes increasingly hostile with cracked sidewalks, poor lighting, dangerous slopes, lack of places to sit and rest, excessive noise, heavy traffic, crime-ridden neighborhoods, and other barriers that increasingly limit our activity space (Balfour & Kaplan, 2002). There is evidence that the physical setting of many neighborhoods discourages walking by older adults (Bonaccorsi et al., 2020; Michael et al., 2006). Growing concern with nurturing age-friendly neighborhoods and communities is a reflection of increasing recognition of the degree to which many current neighborhood environments are incompatible with the needs of older residents, lead to lifestyle constraints on environmental participation, limit options for maintaining a high quality of life, and constitute significant threats to well-being (Yen et al., 2009). Such concerns have been amplified by both voluntary and involuntary COVID-19-related lockdowns.

## Aging and Environmental Competence

Effects of the physical environment are mediated by changes in individual capabilities that generally accompany the experience of growing old. Normative changes limit environmental participation. Reduced lung capacity (caused by the tendency to lean forward as a result of the compression of our spinal column, weakening of the diaphragm, and reduced elasticity of lung tissue), calcification of ligaments, muscular atrophy and loss of strength, balance impairment (only partially compensated for by a widened gait), lowered "reserve capacity" of our physiological systems, and slowed reaction times often act in combination to limit mobility and make environmental participation and occupational performance more difficult. (See also Chapters 8 and 9.) Such changes are accentuated by sensory changes (Paraskevoudi et al., 2018). With respect to sight, increasingly impaired depth perception, reduced peripheral vision, increased difficulties in distinguishing among colors (particularly in the blue-green end of the spectrum), increased susceptibility to glare, and the increasing opacity of the lens all make the physical environment seem more daunting and environmental negotiation more difficult. Such changes are often accentuated by hearing loss including presbycusis, associated with growing difficulty in locating and distinguishing among sounds and filtering out background noise. (See Chapter 10 for additional discussion of low vision and hearing impairment.)

Normative physiological and sensory changes are made more problematic by an array of primarily chronic health conditions ranging from arthritis to heart disease that often accompany old age. The combined effect of normative changes and health impairment is to reduce environmental participation and occupational performance by making older adults increasingly reluctant to venture forth from their homes, particularly at night and during busy times of the day (Rudman et al., 2006). As a result of the well-documented consequence of this—the tendency to spend an increasing proportion of each day at home—the design and configuration of interior physical environments become increasingly important in sustaining well-being (Rowles et al., 2003). This is particularly so in the context of the COVID-19 pandemic (Wiles, 2022).

## Reconciling Environmental Press and Environmental Competence: Theoretical Foundations

Over the past century, the tension between the increased impact of environmental press and the limitations imposed by declining individual competence has been reflected in theoretical perspectives that provide an important framework for interpreting the environmental participation potential of older adults. Lewin's (1951) field theory and ecological equation (discussed earlier) has been elaborated through increasingly sophisticated conceptualizations of his B = f (P, E) formulation. The most influential of these was the ecological model developed by Lawton and Nahemow (1973). The ecological model focuses on the individual's adaptation level, the point at which personal competence and environmental press are in a state of equilibrium. As indicated in Fig. 20.1, at point A, there is perfect balance between the press exerted by the environment and the competence of the individual to handle that level of press. But person/environment adaptation is not a static equilibrium—the fragile balance between individual competence (capability) and environmental constraint (press)—is constantly evolving as either

the individual's competence or the press of the environment changes (Fig. 20.1) (See also Chapter 4.)

It is useful to explain this dynamic equilibrium through an illustration. Imagine a 78-year-old person, Mr. Fellows, living alone in a suburban residence where he and his wife successfully raised their family. The children left home decades before, and his wife died 2 years ago. As he moves into his eighties, reduced physical strength, increasingly debilitating arthritis, a chronic heart condition, and impaired vision make mowing the lawn, climbing the stairs to the bedroom, and handling daily chores increasingly difficult. As his condition worsens, Mr. Fellows' competence level drops from point A to point B where, as you will note, he is at the margin of maximum performance potential and close to moving into the zone of negative affect and maladaptive behavior. At this point, the level of environmental press is too strong for Mr. Fellows to function effectively. He has two options. The first is to attempt to effectively increase his level of competence through options that might include an exercise program to improve his strength or environmental or behavioral modifications (for example moving his bedroom downstairs or hiring a neighbor's son to mow his lawn).

There is generally a limit to such in situ modifications. For many people, the eventual outcome is the need to move to a more supportive environment (with less environmental press). So, Mr. Fellows moves to an assisted living facility, point C in Fig. 20.1, a location where he can establish a new adaptation level reflecting his level of competence. And the process continues in an ongoing process of constant adjustment of his adaptation level to changing individual competence and environmental press.

Lawton and Nahemow's model occupied center stage for several decades. However, it is being increasingly transcended by more sophisticated perspectives generated in environmental gerontology and occupational science. A key contribution in this regard has been the work of Iwarsson and her colleagues in adding the notion of activity and presenting a transactional perspective (Iwarsson, 2004; Iwarsson & Stahl, 2003). This body of work indicated that the relationship between person and environment could be better understood by adding activity (A) as a mediating variable. Thus, the equation now becomes B = f(P, E, A). Expanding on Lawton's notion of environmental proactivity (Lawton, 1989), in this perspective, the individual is regarded as having greater agency than in previous models and is explicitly viewed as able to influence the nature of the person/environment interaction through his or her behavior or activity repertoire. With respect to the physical environment, the person is no longer viewed as passive, merely responding to environmental stimuli. Mr. Fellows might manifest his agency by purchasing a riding lawnmower, installing a stair elevator, or increasing his environmental competence by beginning an exercise program.

A second contemporary perspective builds on this idea of agency and adds greater emphasis on the lived experience of the environment by adding the idea of belonging. Chaudhury and Oswald (2019), building on previous work (Wahl et al., 2012), propose an integrative model of person-environment

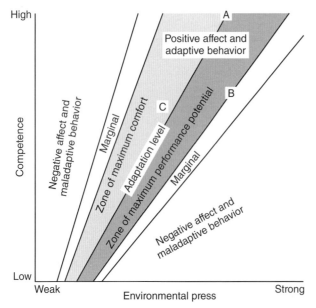

**FIGURE 20.1**   The Ecological Model. (Reproduced with modification from Lawton, M. P., & Nahemow, L. [1973]. Ecology and the aging process. In C. Eisdorfer & M. P. Lawton [Eds.], *The psychology of adult development and aging* [pp. 619–674]. Washington, DC: American Psychological Association.)

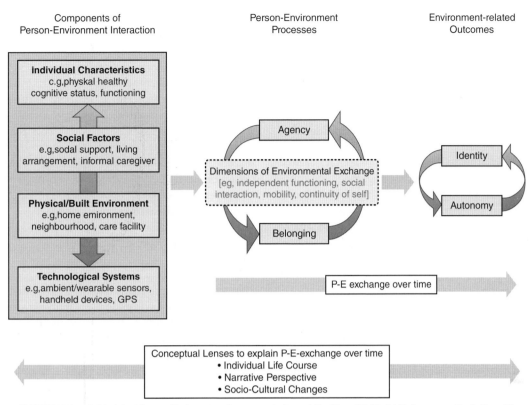

Components of
Person-Environment Interaction

Person-Environment
Processes

Environment-related
Outcomes

**FIGURE 20.2**   A Model of Person-Environment Processes in Later Life. (From Wahl, H-W., Iwarsson, S., & Oswald, F. [2012]. Aging well and the environment: Toward an integrative model and research agenda for the future. *The Gerontologist, 52*[3], 306–316.)

exchange over time (Fig. 20.2). This model comprises three interrelated components: person-environment interaction (involving *individual characteristics*, *social factors*, the *physical/built environment*, and *technological systems*); person-environment processes (expressed in the mutually reciprocal fusion of *agency* and *belonging*); and environment-related outcomes (manifest in the interwoven relationship between *identity* and *autonomy* and ultimately well-being). In addition to adding a temporal component by acknowledging the evolution of the person-environment relationship with advancing age, this model moves us toward a more fully transactional perspective in which person and environment cease to be separate entities but rather become coconstitutive and blurred.

While a transactional perspective is an element of both the PEA model and Chaudhury and Oswald's integrative model, it is the fulcrum of Cutchin's conceptualization of the human-environment relationship. Building on the pragmatism of John Dewey, Cutchin and colleagues developed a more fully transactional understanding of the dynamic person-environment relationship that focuses on situational dynamics as a whole and on how person and place are continually evolving through inquiry and action (Cutchin & Dickie, 2013). As part of this perspective, *place integration* was developed as a concept for framing the dynamics of people and their concrete, problematic situations, where both habits and creative solutions are used to recoordinate transactional relationships of the older person and place and enhance well-being (Cutchin, 2004; Johansson et al., 2013). As a result, place integration is a continual process of actively creating, maintaining, and recreating person-place relationships through

time and emergent and evolving situations. This represents a complete shift from a sequential stimulus-response model, where the individual is influenced by the environment and the environment is modified by the individual, to a model whereby person and place are simultaneously coevolving through action in an ongoing situation that is constantly in process. Importantly, this perspective was developed with significant attention to occupation as a key form of the inquiry and action that drives transactional adjustment of person-environment relationships (Cutchin, 2013).

## Aging and Use of the Physical Environment

Theoretical perspectives provide important alternative ways of understanding the person-environment relationship and the manner in which this relationship might relate to experienced dimensions of identity, well-being, and autonomy and to aging well. At a more pragmatic level, it is useful to provide an informational backdrop with respect to the fundamental dimensions through which individuals experience their physical environment.

At the most basic level, people of all ages experience their environment through its **use**, what many occupational scientists would term *occupational performance*. The infant rolls around in the limited space of her crib. The grade school child frequents the garden and the neighborhood (at least that component of the neighborhood that is sanctioned by the watchful parent). The teenager, particularly when they have received the geographical liberation of a driving license, travels more broadly and frequents an array of settings where typically he or she meets with age peer group friends. During their working life, most people in Western cultures typically frequent a series of residential spaces as they move from an apartment to a first home to the dwelling where they raise their family and perhaps eventually to the place where they elect to retire. In each space and at each time of life, individuals trace an activity space that tends to become remarkably routine and repetitive. Activity spaces can be considered at a series of different scales (Webber et al., 2010). There is a daily rhythm and routine to the manner in which residential space is utilized—the bedroom for sleeping, the living room or den for television watching in the evening, the kitchen at certain times of day for family gatherings or eating, and the dining room for special occasions. Use of this environment may become so routinized that we find ourselves on "automatic pilot" as we traverse familiar space without thinking, using the proprioceptive abilities that David Seamon termed *body awareness of the environment* (Seamon, 1979).

Similarly, a regular temporal periodicity often evolves as we trace a daily route through physical space to and from home (first places) to work (second places), and to special places like cafes, churches, and other primarily social locations (third places) we frequent (Finlay et al., 2019; Markiewicz, 2019; Oldenburg, 1999). Such patterns provide regularity in our use of the environment: often, they are framed in relation to either moving away from or returning to our dwelling. As we use that limited portion of the physical environment that defines our pattern of daily activity, we gain a familiarity with its characteristics. For each person, use of the physical setting is reflected in a unique imprint. And the reciprocity between person and environment in its use becomes habitual, generating a sense of comfort that in most cases evolves into a preference as we become more and more attuned to the familiar. Indeed, for most people, this process of habituation, on scales ranging from the residence through the neighborhood, to the community and beyond, results in a unique manifestation of relationship with the physical environment (Kastenbaum, 1980/1981; Rowles, 2000). Inasmuch as our patterns of regular environmental use intersect with those of others whose lives are shaped by comparable space/time routines, we become part of a place ballet of intricately intertwined life worlds (Seamon & Nordin, 1980). Over time, use of the physical environment becomes taken for granted. We do not think about specific paths and physical locations (either within or beyond our residence). They become the places of life experience within which we are fully oriented. Occupational scientists have illustrated how such taken-for-granted relationships with the environment do not last forever. Change in the person or environment can disrupt habits that previously enabled occupational performance and well-being in particular environments (Cutchin, 2007; Fritz, 2014). Yet the science on habit suggests that people, including older adults, can develop new habits to create positive relationships with environments after change or problems occur (Fritz & Cutchin, 2016).

Although habits can be redeveloped in environments after disruption, as people grow older, everyday physical activity spaces tend to become progressively more restricted both spatially and temporally (Hendrickson & Mann, 2005). Declining physical capabilities and the increased effort of maintaining a geographically extensive activity space, as well as loss of significant social roles (e.g., retirement, empty nest) and subsequent loss of economic wherewithal, mean that we tend to spend more time at home (Cohen-Mansfield et al., 2012; Marottoli et al., 2000). We become increasingly reluctant to drive at night and limit excursions beyond the dwelling to those daytime hours when traffic on the roads is limited (Webber et al., 2010). And as we become frail, our patterns of taken-for-granted use of the space within the residence may reflect an increasing medicalization of our home as we gradually reconfigure the furniture and patterns of use and activity to accommodate disability and increasing medical need (Fange & Ivanoff, 2009).

## Aging and the Meaning of the Physical Environment

Use of the physical environment is grounded in **cognitive awareness** of the environment on multiple scales (from the configuration of furniture and rooms, through the layout of our neighborhood, to the street patterns of the larger community in which we reside). Cognitive differentiation of the spaces we inhabit provides "mental maps" of the myriad spaces of our life. These mental maps are images of known spaces that we call to mind when we think of particular locations; they provide a cognitive atlas that we use for orientation in moving from place to place, whether it is crossing our living room without bumping into furniture or successfully traversing the city to visit a friend or shop for groceries (Catney et al., 2018; Vitman-Schorr & Ayalon, 2020). Over our lifetime, we develop countless mental maps that form a latent reservoir of environmental knowledge that can be resurrected at will. Over time, mental maps of the physical environment are built and modified as the spaces we inhabit change and as experience with the environment changes, either becoming more detailed with repeated use or increasingly vague and inchoate as a result of reduced use (Phillips, 2013). Our mental map of a specific neighborhood may evolve over time as buildings are demolished and replaced by others or the configuration of roads is altered during neighborhood transition. As we grow older, reduced participation in environments beyond our home and neighborhood may lead to growing inaccuracy of our mental map as our image of a particular space becomes increasingly based on recall. Indeed, we are often surprised and a little disoriented when, visiting a location we have not visited for some time, we discover how different it has become. One emerging perspective is to view this process as neuro-geographical embodiment, where body-mind-environment assemblages are contingent and ever shifting through the life course (Naughton, 2022). In this context, it is interesting to note that cognitive mapping/spatial navigation ability is a stronger predictor of preclinical dementia than traditional psychometric assessments.

Both use and cognitive awareness are implicated in a third level of environmental experience, the **meanings** with which places are imbued. Over time, we develop emotional affiliation (both positive and negative) with environments as they become increasingly a part of our persona. Locations where important life events transpired may come to hold a special place in consciousness and heart as they become a part of the intricate tapestry of our relationship with the environments of our life: the location of a tragic motor accident, the park where we walked with the person who eventually became our spouse, the café where we were sitting when we learned we were to become a parent, or the gravesite of a close relative with the headstone inscription that sustains them in our consciousness even beyond their death. The mechanisms through which this transpires are beginning to be understood (Gatersleben et al., 2020; Levy, 2011). Over time, our environment becomes increasingly differentiated through repeated use, through selective incorporation within our mental map of our world and meanings relating to our personal history of occupation.

For many people, the residence is the ultimate seat of meaning, a location that assumes increasing significance as it evolves from being merely a "house" or dwelling—the locus of activities—to a "home," a place that becomes the repository of identity and an expression of our persona. There is a voluminous literature on the concept of home that identifies the plethora of interwoven meanings embraced in this construct. Whether our home is an arrangement of cardboard boxes under a freeway overpass, a tent in a refugee camp, a rude hut or cabin, a spacious apartment, or a suburban residence, the place that is home has been shown to embrace diverse dimensions of affinity (Board & McCormack, 2018; Chaudhury, 2008; Rowles & Chaudhury, 2005). These include the territoriality of a point of origin and centering (Mallett, 2004; Rubinstein, 1989)—the place from which we depart and to which we return (Case, 1996; Hagerstrand, 1970). But home becomes imbued with an array of meanings beyond this: it becomes a source of identity (Marcus, 1995; Rubinstein & de Medeiros, 2005), self-expression (Smith, 1994), security/safety (Dahlin-Ivanoff et al., 2007), privacy (Smith, 1994), refuge (Roush & Cox, 2000), continuity (Sixsmith, 1986), ownership (Bate, 2018), social relationship (Sixsmith, 1986), belonging (Rubinstein, 2005), familiarity (Rubinstein, 1989), and freedom (Dahlin-Ivanoff et al., 2007). Each of these dimensions should be considered as dynamic; their expression changes with evolving circumstances. For example, the increasing level of home confinement occasioned by the COVID-19 pandemic has transformed the meaning of home for many people (Cutchin & Rowles, 2022; Gezici Yalçın & Düzen, 2021). For some, this included transition to virtual exercise programs and the modification of rooms to include related exercise equipment, transforming the meaning of the home environment.

In the process of creating home, we transform a space into a place (Rowles & Watkins, 2003). An important feature of creating and maintaining a sense of home is the role possessions play in shaping and reinforcing the meaning of the self in place (Coleman & Wiles, 2020). Many people surround themselves with personal objects and mementoes that reflect and project their identity and reinforce a sense of being at home. The Teddy Bear and security blanket of infancy and childhood may give way to the posters that adorn a dormitory room at college. As people move through life, there is a pattern of accumulation of artifacts that reflect the story of their life (Rowles & Watkins, 2003). The growth of a family becomes expressed in an array of framed photographs on the sideboard. Statuettes and vases accumulated on holiday trips or received as gifts remind us of important experiences. Rugs, furniture, and items gradually accumulated over time increasingly come to reflect the personality of a home and its residents. Indeed, some homes become museums of life. The importance of personal artifacts is clearly apparent in the angst that many people experience when they age and find themselves having to divest themselves of some of these possessions as they move to progressively smaller living quarters (Ekerdt et al., 2012; Magnusson, 2018).

## Aging, Relocation, and Making and Remaking Place

A temporal perspective on the acquisition and divestiture of artifacts provides a useful segue to explicit consideration of the role of time in shaping the meaning of the physical environment as this evolves over a lifetime. For most people, and certainly for U.S. residents who relocate to a different residence on average more than 11 times over their life course (US Bureau of Census, 2015), life involves processes of constant adaptation to a changing physical environment, either through in situ adjustments such as the need to close off an upstairs room, or the need to relocate to an entirely new setting as a result of failing health and environmental competence. This process is represented in Fig. 20.3. Moves may be ephemeral (for example, the overnight stay at a motel where we are forced to recreate a very temporary semblance of home) or permanent (the move to a new dwelling); however, the process is essentially the same, involving having to give up a familiar setting and create a new sense of being in place, or at home, in a different and initially unfamiliar physical space. Here, we focus on the process of permanent relocation.

While processes involved are complex and multidimensional, relocation essentially involves three interwoven components that are expressed differently and over which we have different levels of control at different points during our life (Rowles & Bernard, 2013). First, each relocation necessitates *abandonment* of a familiar mode of being in place: it requires giving up familiar patterns in the use of space, the redundancy of well-established mental maps of the places we inhabit, and threat to the emotional affiliation of places of meaning in our life as we may no longer be able to frequent and experience these spaces and as they fade into memory. Second, relocation to a new physical setting necessitates *creation* of a new mode of being in place as we establish new patterns in our use of the environment, as we create new mental images to provide us with an orientation to the new setting, and as we develop new senses of emotional affiliation related to the events that transpire in the new setting. Each new setting provides constraints on establishing a familiar mode of being in place; our new residence may not have the fireplace that provided both physical and psychological warmth as we stared into the flickering flames. There may be no windowsills for our plants. But there may be new opportunities: central heating means that we no longer have the chore of stepping out into the cold to gather logs from the stack on the back porch; a sun lounge may provide an even better setting for our African Violets.

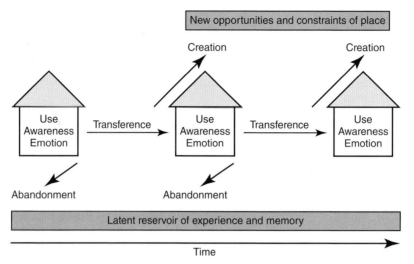

**FIGURE 20.3**    The Experience of Relocation: Remaking Home. (Reproduced from Rowles, G. D., & Bernard, M. [2013]. The meaning and significance of place in old age. In G. D. Rowles & M. Bernard [Eds.], *Environmental gerontology: Making meaningful places in old age* [pp. 3–24]. New York, NY: Springer Publishing Company.)

Both abandonment and creation are eased by a third process, environmental *transference*, our ability to transport elements of our old and familiar environment into a new and unfamiliar setting as we engage in the process of making the unknown familiar. Such transference may involve relocating furniture and possessions. Indeed, we may "set up" by arranging furniture and positioning treasured artifacts in our new abode in a way that mimics their placement in the home we left behind. Subject to the constraints of the new setting, we may also evolve a rhythm and routine in the pattern of daily life that reflects a continuation of our former lifestyle. We may rise at the same time, watch the same television programs, and attempt to establish a relationship with our new neighbors comparable to the one we had before. It is also possible to facilitate transference by retaining our links with former settings through return visits, ongoing contact with former neighbors, or retaining a vicarious affiliation as we monitor events in our former neighborhood or community through the media. And, of course, unless we are cognitively impaired, our memories never leave us. We can always return to the places of our past by tapping a vast reservoir of experiences and memories.

Over time, we constantly make and remake place as we move from environment to environment. Indeed, life entails an ongoing and never-ending quest for achieving a sense of being in place—being at one with our physical environment. Perhaps the most important factor in this process is the degree to which we have control. During early life, our autonomy and control are limited. Our being in place and whether or not we relocate are shaped by our parents. As adults, control and ability to shape our environment are generally much greater. We can decide where we want to live and the types of environment we wish to frequent according to individual or family preference. Some people favor the vibrancy and excitement of a gentrifying inner city neighborhood with a local deli, lots of bars and restaurants, local festivals, and ready access to art galleries and concerts. For others, the more tranquil milieu of a rural setting with a slower pace of life

focused on the pleasures of gardening and companionship of a few neighbors is preferred. But as the limitations of old age begin to have effect, generally not until our seventh and eighth decades, we may become frail and find ourselves with progressively less decisional autonomy and control over our physical environment as family members, physicians, and social services professionals have increasing input into determining our environmental circumstances.

Changing environmental potential and what M. Powell Lawton, a founder of environmental gerontology, termed *environmental vulnerability* make the physical environments we create—on scales from the entire neighborhood and community down to the design of an individual nursing home room—critical. Does society create environments conducive to the changing environmental experience of older adults and others who are environmentally vulnerable? And to what extent does the practice of OT facilitate and maximize environmental engagement and occupational performance? In the final sections of this chapter, we turn to these issues.

## Creating Physical Environments for Aging: Barriers and Opportunities

More than four decades ago, Joseph A. Koncelik (1979, p. 110) wrote, "Thoughtless environmental design 'speaks' to people with sensory losses, telling them that they are incapacitated, senile, slow, weak, and perhaps too stupid to survive." Unfortunately, despite the passage of the Americans with Disabilities Act in 1990, many community environments continue to speak the same way and provide significant challenges to those who are environmentally vulnerable. In too many cities, traffic lights remain timed too rapidly to facilitate safe pedestrian crossing (Lachapelle & Cloutier, 2017). Supplemental auditory prompts for walk lights are rare. There are still too few places to sit and rest. Sidewalks remain uneven, in poor repair, or absent, and public spaces are poorly designed, precluding occupational participation and social interaction (Peace, 2013). Even medical facilities, including physician offices, urgent care centers, and hospitals, frequently don't provide environmental supports to enable easy navigation for aging adults with mobility, visual, auditory, and/or other sensory or functional limitations.

There are some grounds for optimism. Initially facilitated by the World Health Organization's *Healthy Cities Project* of the 1980s and reinforced by the *Global Age-Friendly Cities Project*, another World Health Organization initiative launched in 2005 in 33 cities around the world (including New York, NY, and Portland, OR), there has been a movement toward a more comprehensive approach to creating "livable" cities and communities. Increasingly, such highly publicized initiatives are being complemented by smaller-scale projects and programs in cities and communities throughout the world. In the United States, livable and age-friendly city initiatives are present in a plethora of locations at different scales. By 2012, Andrew Sharlach identified 292 age-friendly initiatives representing four approaches: community planning, system coordination and program development, colocation of services, and the development of consumer associations (Sharlach, 2012). Many of these initiatives focus on enhancing the physical characteristics and accessibility of neighborhood environments. We are beginning to embrace the idea of "'…complete streets,' that enable multiple types of mobility, including walking, self-propelled and electric wheelchairs, golf-carts, bicycles, public transit, as well as automobiles" (Sharlach, 2012, p. 29). There is also growing evidence of innovation in the emergence of new housing and service models enabling older adults to age-in-place (Hou & Cao, 2021). These trends are reinforced by measures to assess the physical characteristics of neighborhoods, including accessibility, amount of greenery, density, diversity, location, street pattern, block size, setback of dwellings from the street, and street topography, with respect to ability to support the mobility and well-being of older residents (Burton et al., 2011; Kan et al., 2020). We are rapidly developing an array of tools to assess older adults' needs and preferences with respect to their community environment. While these are positive developments, it is important to temper optimism with caution. Currently, few "age-friendly" or "livable" community initiatives have significant governmental support or command sufficient recurring resources from the private sector to instill confidence in their long-term sustainability or transformative effectiveness in nurturing supportive neighborhood physical environments for environmentally vulnerable older adults. (See also Chapter 32 on creating age-inclusive communities.)

Moving from the community to the individual residence, there has been parallel development of initiatives to facilitate the optimal physical design of residential environments. Three trends provide promise for enhancing occupational performance. First is **increasing ability to measure the fit between an individual and their physical setting** and to use such measurement instruments as a basis for assessing need and promoting effective design intervention. One important example here is the Housing Enabler Instrument developed by occupational therapist Suzanne Iwarsson and her colleagues

(Iwarsson, 2004; Iwarsson et al., 2009). The Housing Enabler integrates an assessment of functional limitations and identification of physical barriers in the residence to create an accessibility score reflecting the unique outcome of the relationship between environmental needs and environmental press for a single individual. A second and often related tool, a "usability in my home" measure (Fange & Iwarsson, 1999; Fänge & Iwarsson, 2003), provides an approach to measuring the degree to which the physical environment is perceived by the individual to be supportive of activities of daily living (ADLs) (including personal hygiene, getting dressed, grooming, and using toilet facilities) and instrumental activities of daily living (IADLs) (including but not limited to cooking, laundry, washing dishes, and cleaning). With the development of abbreviated versions of such instruments, we can anticipate continuing improvement in the ability to objectively measure the residential environmental needs and preferences of older adults (Carlsson et al., 2009).

A second major development over the past several decades has been the emergence of **smart homes and smart home technologies** (Pal et al., 2018). Efforts to improve housing accessibility and use through more sensitive design such as the installation of ramps, lever door handles, lowering counter surfaces, installing pull-out and other types of adaptive kitchen shelving, and elder-friendly bathroom design with grab bars and the introduction of surfaces to minimize slipping and the risk of falls are now being supplemented by innovations that involve sophisticated technologies. Body-worn sensors monitor activities (Atallah et al., 2009). Motion-sensitive lighting is becoming common. Monitoring from a distance is also an increasingly recognized option. It is now possible to use wireless sensors to monitor use of electrical devices, cabinet sensors, bed use patterns, flow of water (indicating the use of facilities), and motion sensors to chart the use of individual rooms (Gaddam et al., 2011; Kaye et al., 2011). The basic idea is that the older individual is enabled to maintain independence at home because the occurrence of unusual patterns can trigger supportive intervention. Camera-based surveillance systems for home monitoring have also emerged as an option for facilitating older adults' continuing ability to live alone. The frontier of technology in smart home design of the future lies in robot technologies currently being developed in laboratories throughout the world. (See also Chapter 22 for additional technological advances.)

The potential impact of smart technology is not limited to home environments. Future residential care facilities may offer "assisted cognitive systems" that are embedded in physical environments and are sensitive and responsive to residents' actions and needs (Cook et al., 2009). A prototype dementia residential care facility, Oatfield Estates in Oregon, employs the concept of "layered architecture" to monitor all activities, doors, lights, and appliances within the building. Notable among its supports to residents are the "Activity Compass," which helps to direct residents to indoor destinations, and the "Adaptive Prompter" that uses information from embedded sensor networks to guide a resident through selected activities, such as grooming or dressing (Kautz et al., 2002).

A major issue in the introduction of smart home, camera surveillance, and ambient intelligence alternatives is their acceptability by older adults. Research indicates reluctance of some older adults to be monitored in their home by cameras, but there appears to be a surprisingly high level of acceptance by older adults provided that appropriate levels of privacy are maintained (Courtney, 2008; Zwijsen et al., 2011). The tension between the need for surveillance invasiveness and the preservation of appropriate levels of privacy remains an ongoing challenge in the evolution of technologies that facilitate aging in place (Ehrari et al., 2018; Rubeis, 2020).

Placing the changing environmental needs of older adults in the broader context of the life course leads to a third major development in creating physical environments conducive to the needs of older adults. One can make a strong argument that we should not be seeking to create environments for older adults but rather environments for all people at all stages of life. This is the fundamental premise of **universal design**, which focuses on basic principles to facilitate the optimal design of environments for all users. There are seven broadly accepted principles of universal design (Carr et al., 2013; Story, 1998) (Table 20.1). Each principle provides a template for design decisions that optimize the potential for older adults to age in place.

A particular need in the evolution of universal design is for community-level change to accommodate intergenerational needs (Thang & Kaplan, 2013). Recent estimates indicate a significant increase in multigenerational housing—young adults returning home and grandparents living with their children (Duncan & Levner, 2013). In addition, central cities in North America have grown faster in terms of both younger and older populations in comparison with surrounding suburbs, due to the attraction of walking to shopping, restaurants, and other centrally located destinations. These factors may provide added impetus for the increased use of universal design principles in residential and other building construction (Duncan & Levner, 2013). Application of universal design principles enhances occupational performance for all generations; its implementation is intuitively attractive in community planning, new construction, and retrofitting housing.

An important issue with respect to smart homes and universal design is the availability of such options. There is a danger of developing many theoretical options but few pragmatic choices for the majority of older adults. Sophisticated smart home technologies are currently primarily to be found in the model homes developed in research universities and experimental laboratories such as the Georgia Institute of Technology "Aware Home," the "Gator Tech Smart House" at the University of Florida, or the "Place Lab" at MIT. The costs of translating such innovative models into commercially viable housing options are likely to be considerable and it may be many years before older adults are able to fully harness such technologies.

## The Role of the Physical Environment in Occupational Therapy with Older Adults

While the use of sophisticated technologies offers significant supportive prospects for the future, most occupational therapists live in a world of the present as they confront the day-to-day challenges of older adults trying to adapt to changing physical capabilities in their home and community environments. No technology can replace an informed and caring practitioner. However, as environmental design and technology provide us with a widening array of alternatives, occupational therapists can enhance their contribution to the patient/client's health and well-being by being especially sensitive to the role of the physical environment in supporting

**TABLE 20.1**  Principles of Universal Design

| Universal Design Principle | Description | Example |
|---|---|---|
| (1) Equitable use | Useful and marketable to people with diverse abilities | Doors that automatically open |
| (2) Flexibility of use | Accommodates a wide range of individual preferences and abilities | Automated teller machines' buttons far enough apart to be pressed accurately |
| (3) Simple and intuitive use | Easy to understand, regardless of user's experience, knowledge, language skills, or current concentration level | Providing furniture assembly instructions in a series of clear illustrations instead of text |
| (4) Perceptible information | Communicates necessary information effectively to the user, regardless of ambient conditions or the user's sensory abilities | Computer software that relays information visually through text and pictures, and audibly through speakers |
| (5) Tolerance for error | Minimizes hazards and the adverse consequences of accidental or unintended actions | Hallways that return to common areas rather than stop in dead ends, a failsafe feature |
| (6) Low physical effort | Can be used efficiently and comfortably with a minimum of fatigue | Bottle caps that are easy to grip and require only a small range of motion to open |
| (7) Size/space for approach/use | Appropriate size and space are provided for approach, reach, manipulation, and use regardless of the user's body size, posture, or mobility | Wall-mounted components (e.g., toilet paper) that are visible, easy to reach, and easy for all arm and hand sizes to use |

Reproduced from Carr, K., Weir, P. L., Azar, D., & Azar, N. R. (2013). *Journal of Aging Research* (as adapted from Story, 1998).

| **BOX 20.1** | Fundamental OT Principles for Environmentally Sensitive Interventions With Aging Adults |

1. When interacting with a new older client, whether in the community, office, clinic, or an institution, anticipate their physical environmental needs, so that if assessment processes are undertaken, the individual is not placed at a disadvantage:
   a. Ensure adequate lighting within the intervention space.
   b. Minimize or eliminate background noises.
   c. Provide the client with a chair with arms, if indicated.
   d. Ensure that any materials that the client may need or be asked to manipulate be within a distance of "easy reach." This includes seated tasks or those in bed.
   e. Facilitate cognition, time, and space orientation through use of clocks, signage, or additional visual cues.
   f. If the older client is away from home or other familiar environments when the OT intervention is conducted, include questions about the ease of use of their home and community environment, and arrange for a home visit, whenever indicated, to observe the client's occupational performance.

2. Conduct an environmental assessment in every intervention setting, whether community based (agency or home) or institutional.
   a. Whenever possible, conduct a thorough review of the environment, noting strengths as well as areas in need of improvement or total change to ensure good occupational performance person-environment fit.
   b. If a thorough review isn't possible, note the most obvious conditions in need of change, and follow up to ensure that changes that fit occupational performance abilities have been made.
   c. Make short- and long-term recommendations for additions and/or changes, based upon the needs of the aging clients served and the ability of the setting to comply. Wherever possible, advocate for aging-sensitive design of the environment, using the most current evidence to support recommendations for additions or changes.

effective therapy. Occupational therapists are known for their creative, holistic approaches that support adaptation, despite typical and sometimes debilitating aging related changes (see Box 20.1).

Assessment of occupational performance outside the older client's home and other familiar environments is likely to be a less accurate reflection of abilities in all areas of performance. Consider the physical environmental tenets introduced earlier: Typically, the older adult will find performance of activities more meaningful within a familiar space, such as their home, reflecting their "place integration." Therefore, motivation to perform is likely to be greater than in unfamiliar spaces. In the client's home, their demonstration of performance skills is likely to be optimal, and reflect more routine and taken-for-granted patterns of movement within an "automatic pilot" mode that would be likely absent in a hospital room, clinic, or other physical spaces. The OT will ideally be able to observe the client's implementation of their normal routines and habits and build upon well-established mental maps and patterns of physical functioning. If the client is unable to demonstrate fully, family members or others who are familiar with the individual's preferred routines may be sources of information critical to optimizing future occupational performance at home.

## Physical Environment as Context and Target of Occupational Therapy Interventions

At all levels of care, occupational therapists (OTs) and OT assistants (OTAs) are well positioned to facilitate the older adult's interactive relationship with the physical environment, to the extent that the individual's physical and psychosocial abilities allow. The *Occupational Therapy Practice Framework* (OTPF-4) describes aspects of the OT domain, which serves as the foundation for OT practice in the United States. It includes Context: Environmental Factors and Personal Factors as one of five domains within which interventions are conducted, described in the OTPF as the broad construct that encompasses environmental factors and personal factors. Environmental factors are aspects of the physical, social, and attitudinal surroundings in which people live and conduct their lives (American Occupational Therapy Association [AOTA], 2020, Table 4, p. 36.) Thus, the physical environment is viewed as a contextual component that interfaces with the client's personal factors, and also mediates daily life occupations.

Older adults encounter the need for environmental OT interventions for a variety of reasons, due to pressing physical and psychosocial problems, as well as needs or problems that they have determined or of which they may be unaware. On behalf of aging adults, OT services are provided at three different levels: (1) directly with individuals and/or family/caregiver(s); (2) through consultation and administration with community organizations, designers, and architects; and (3) through consultation and/or administration with governmental, nongovernmental, and/or international agencies (Barney, 2012, p. 1879). Thus, OTs may be direct providers of services, administrators, and/or consultants, depending upon the nature of the identified needs and setting. Historically, OTs have conducted environmental assessments that consider the occupational competence of older clients living at home. Individually tailored recommendations for short- and long-term goals and interventions are established collaboratively with the client, and the OT assists the individual in remediating aspects of the physical environment that hinder occupational performance. For example, some of the most common physical environmental adaptations are grab bars, higher toilet seats, bath benches, and handheld shower heads that are recommended and installed in bathrooms to promote safety and compensate for diminished strength, coordination, or

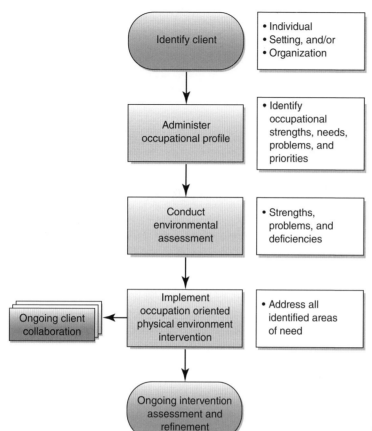

**FIGURE 20.4** Universal occupational therapy physical environmental intervention process.

range of motion. Nevertheless, recommendations can cover all aspects of occupational performance within the physical environment, including performance in the dwelling, doorways, yard, grounds, neighborhood, and/or community.

OTs may intervene as well on behalf of optimizing the physical environment in planning new building structures and land use applications with architects and urban planners, and across a range of settings within the medical continuum of care. Health-care-related interventions may include consultations regarding the environmental design and retrofitting of facilities, including primary care clinics and physician offices, acute and subacute care settings, home health-care environments, and long-term care settings such as residential and skilled care settings, and palliative and hospice care environments.

Additionally, at the community level, OTs conduct community-based wellness and injury prevention programs to facilitate the older individual's accommodation to the physical design of their current residential settings and neighborhoods. OTs are also involved in advocating and planning for livable communities and aging in place initiatives at the community, state and national level, to promote programs and developments that support a goodness of fit with typical aging changes that older adults experience. Since older adult sleep performance and quality of sleep may be affected by aspects of the built environment, including noise, safety, light, and neighborhood characteristics (Teslow & Molitor, 2021), OT interventions may involve collaboration in developing

problem-solving approaches with neighborhood and government officials. Additional environmental quality concerns regarding air, water, soil, lead, and/or other exposures that place neighborhoods at risk should be reported, audited, and remediated by the relevant government agency, typically in communication with the US Environmental Protection Agency (EPA).

The nature of interactions and the extent to which the OT may facilitate the older adults' environmental competence vary according to the amount of contact and the relationship that the OT has with the individual and service-related administrative personnel. Occupational therapists need to be proactive in advocating for supportive environments that correspond with the service delivery patterns in the settings and influence-related administrative policies and procedures.

Beyond the macro-level contributions of informed advocacy, implementation of physical environment-sensitive OT interventions follows a similar process, whether the client is an individual, a setting within the established health-care system, a community-based organization, or neighborhood (Fig. 20.4). Once the client is identified, an occupational profile, either a standardized version for individuals or one tailored to the setting, should be conducted to identify the occupational strengths, needs, problems, and priorities in completing occupational performance that is appropriate and meaningful to the client. Once such a profile is established, then an environmental assessment can be performed to determine the current level of environmental press on the client, and what, if any, appropriate measures might be taken to address revealed problems, deficiencies, and needs. A summary of both short- and long-term goals for remediation can then be completed, taking into consideration the feasibility and cost, if any, for recommendations made. Next, an occupation-oriented physical environmental intervention that addresses identified problems, needs, and deficiencies is designed, with ongoing consultation with the client, and significant others, including coresidents and/or family members, as indicated, to ensure that the client's needs are met. Finally, an assessment process for determining the ongoing and potentially changing needs of the client should be operationalized, including integrated plans for continuous assessment and refinement, as needed, as shown later.

Physical environment–related OT interventions focus on supporting the client's age-related changes and/or comorbidities that affect ability to age in place and participate in desired activities/occupations. To be most effective, such interventions must address the aspects of being in place (use, cognitive awareness, emotional significance, and meanings) identified earlier in this chapter. It is important to acknowledge and respect each individual's occupational performance abilities together with their preferred habits and routines, and sense of being in place. Awareness of the rhythms and routines of daily life, processes of habituation, the place ballets that form the choreography of everyday life, the complex mental maps that constitute each person's orientation within their life space, and the emotional capital that is invested in the places of a person's life are essential elements of environmentally sensitive and meaningful interventions. Within this wider understanding of experiential and environmental context, interventions may often include not only adaptive accommodations but also employ appropriate assistive devices that compensate for occupational performance deficits (Barney, 2012, p. 1887). Within this rubric, the aims of intervention become to (1) continually collaborate with the older adult/group/neighborhood or community to plan and implement truly client-centered care, (2) tailor the approaches to meet the elderly patient's/client's activity needs and potential, and (3) facilitate maximization of the older adult's autonomy and continued participation in society. Interventions must be appropriate and meaningful within the framework of the client's lived experience in order to ensure that the individual or group is enabled to maximize overall well-being and achieve the best possible quality of life.

Fundamental concerns of OT practitioners include supporting the older adult's, group's, or population's autonomy in setting priorities and making decisions regarding their participation, and maintaining a level of mastery and control over their environment and lifestyle. OT personnel therefore foster an enabling therapeutic relationship with older adults of all ability levels throughout the continuum of medical care or in community settings, together with their families and/or other support systems. The emphasis of OT intervention on the older adult's ability to participate in meaningful occupations promotes cost-effective care, individual competence, and optimal quality of life (AOTA OTPF, 2020; Clark, 2012; Clark

et al., 1997; Jackson et al., 1998). Acknowledging the role of the physical environment in this process is a critical component of this endeavor that is too often neglected. Frequently, the constraints of therapists' workload expectations in many health-care settings foster a limited approach to OT interventions, resulting in processes that emphasize improvement in components of older adults' physical function, without due consideration to environmental press or supports and related psychological well-being. Evidence-based OT interventions holistically include all components of well-being and quality of life, including the physical environment's meaning and level of support for older adults. Often in health-care settings, OTs have the opportunity to recommend supportive environmental features and interventions that can benefit all participants, as well as collaborate with older adults individually in maximizing their function and overall quality of life. Thus, the occupational therapist needs to view each setting and individual served as an occasion to evaluate and recommend physical environmental adaptations, wherever indicated.

## Assessing the Effectiveness of Occupational Therapy–Based Environmental Interventions with Older Adults

Recent literature reviews (Carnemolla & Bridge, 2020; Garin et al., 2014; Ransolin et al., 2022; Rijnaard et al., 2016; Sánchez-González et al., 2020; Valipoor et al., 2020; Wahl et al., 2009) have identified a growing body of research on the impact of environmental interventions on the function and well-being of older adults in various settings, including hospitals (Taylor & Hignett, 2016; van den Berg et al., 2021), assisted living facilities (Cutler, 2007), nursing homes (Cutler et al., 2006; van der Velde-van Buuringen et al., 2021; van Hoof et al., 2015), dementia care facilities (Jones & van der Eerden, 2008; van Hoof et al., 2010) and home environments (Canham et al., 2018; Clarke, 2014; Clemson et al., 2019; Gitlin et al., 2006, 2009; Horvath et al., 2013). Iwarsson et al. (2009) and Wahl et al. (2009) both concluded that, compared to simple counts of total numbers of environmental hazards in a home, indicators of person-environment fit in home environments were stronger predictors of older adult function (e.g., frequency of falls), thus reinforcing our earlier discussion of the utility of the P-E conceptual model. A close examination of one "gold standard" OT-based environmental intervention for older adults, the Environmental Skill-Building Program (ESP) (later renamed the Skills$_2$Care$^R$) (Gitlin et al., 2003, 2005, 2010), underscores the power of the person-environment fit model to effectively guide research and inform practice related to older clients' physical environments. The ESP was a randomized clinical trial of a home-based OT intervention that focused on the role of the physical environment in supporting dementia family caregiving and care receiver function. It was one of six longitudinal NIH-supported interventions in the Resources for Enhancing Alzheimer's Caregiver Health (REACH) initiative, a multisite program designed to conduct social and behavioral research on interventions to enhance dementia family caregiving (Schulz et al., 2003). The goal of the ESP intervention was to "help family caregivers reduce the disparity between environmental press and personal competence by providing skills to effectively manipulate dimensions of the home environment to manage daily problems associated with dementia care" (Gitlin et al., 2003, p. 536). After baseline assessments, caregivers were randomly assigned to either the experimental or control group. Members of the experimental group received the environmental intervention, i.e., six OT sessions, which entailed (1) caregiver training on Alzheimer's disease (AD) and on the impact (both supportive and detrimental) of the physical environment on their relatives' ADL functions and troublesome behaviors, (2) instruction on problem-solving strategies (including identification of triggers of problematic behaviors) that involved manipulating or modifying the physical and social environment, (3) implementation of individualized environmental strategies, and (4) the generalization of these strategies to emerging problems or issues (p. 536). Strategies that modified the physical environment included installation of equipment (e.g., grab bars); removing, rearranging, or labeling objects; purposeful placement of objects (e.g., laying out clothing or hygiene products to facilitate dressing and grooming); and use of color contrasts. Other strategies addressed alteration of tasks (e.g., simplification techniques, cueing, planning routines, providing graded activities) and alteration of the social environment (e.g., communicating with formal care providers, coordinating care tasks among family and friends). The interventions were individualized and client based, based on OT needs assessments and assessments of the home to identify which of 11 caregiving domains the caregiver wanted to address. OTs continued training and reinforcement of strategies in subsequent sessions and continued to define attainable, concrete goals, assist in problem solving, and provide constructive feedback. Appropriate equipment and assistive devices were ordered and installed, and OTs trained caregivers in their use. Three follow-up assessments were conducted at 6-month intervals.

At the 6-month follow-up, caregivers in the intervention group demonstrated significantly improved skills (i.e., greater use of effective strategies) and had significantly less need for help in providing daily care, indicating enhancement of the personal competence factor as defined in the P-E model. They also reported significantly fewer negative behavioral occurrences by their relative with dementia compared to the caregiver controls, thus diminishing the demands of environmental press on the caregiver. At the 12-month follow-up assessment, compared to the controls, caregivers in the intervention group reported improved affect and a trend for maintenance of skills and reduced negative behavioral occurrences (Gitlin et al., 2009). The researchers concluded that the sustained positive impact of the intervention had a clinically significant effect, given the ongoing decline of the care receiver that is typical of the AD trajectory.

While evidence-based interventions are proven to work, unfortunately, they are not generally incorporated into practice settings (Kwan et al., 2022; Sox et al., 2008). It is essential to study the implementation as well as efficacy of randomized

trials, to facilitate incorporation of proven interventions into general use. Gitlin and colleagues (2010) proceeded to evaluate the implementation of ESP, regarding whether it could be integrated into a large OT home care practice and reimbursed by Medicare B. A 2-year study with 21 OTs and 41 caregivers indicated that although there was some degree of inconsistency in problem-solving training by the OTs, caregiver enactment of ESP strategies was highly successful. They concluded that optimal implementation would require additional OT training and coaching.

## Widening Horizons

It is appropriate to conclude by envisaging a future agenda for a physical environment-sensitive occupational science that moves beyond the ideas presented in this chapter. Such an agenda would expand the field and enhance the effectiveness of OT. Critical to this agenda will be building on more sophisticated theoretical perspectives that recognize the transactional nature of older people's being in place and focus on situational aspects of place integration and care as they evolve over time (Rhodus & Rowles, 2023). The agenda would include greater consideration of the need to facilitate ongoing connections with nature (through home garden use, the design of sunrooms, modification of windows to maximize potentials for "setting up," and visual surveillance of the world beyond the threshold for those who are home or institution bound) (Corley et al., 2021; Reynolds, 2011; Rowles, 1981). The agenda also would examine how environmental quality and lifelong exposures to harmful agents might affect occupational performance, with implications for all ages across a variety of physical environmental exposures, both urban and rural.

The agenda would include more sophisticated understanding of design features such as the role of stairs; the paradox of steps as both an environmental barrier and beneficial to health (Shipp & Branch, 1999). It would include developing ever more sophisticated personal and equipment-related technologies to facilitate continuing environmental participation (Verbrugge et al., 1997). It would include recognition and more refined understanding of the importance of abandonment, creation, and transference as elements of the making and remaking of home (Fig. 20.3) and the development of intervention strategies to facilitate minimally stressful relocation (Hertz et al., 2005). It would include exploration of "place therapy" (Chaudhury, 2003; Scheidt & Norris-Baker, 1999), the manner in which physical environments and the places of people's lives may be therapeutic and used proactively as a focus of OT (Pálsdóttir et al., 2018; Whalley Hammell, 2021a). Finally, increased recognition of the role of the physical environment may even extend to exploration of the role that the settings in which OT is conducted play in influencing the effectiveness of such therapy (Skubik-Peplaski et al., 2012).

Moving forward, two interwoven concerns are of paramount importance in assessing the role of the physical environment in relation to well-being and the role that occupational therapists must play in ensuring the best possible outcomes. First, it is essential to recognize the great diversity not only of physical environments but also of modes of being in place of different populations. In this chapter we have viewed aging primarily through a white, middle class, Western lens. But variations in ethnicity, race, socioeconomic status, culture, access to resources, and social history make for the creation of a kaleidoscope of physical settings and how they are experienced. Growing old in Chinatown is very different from the experience of aging in a Chicago suburb. Rural Iowa provides an entirely different setting from Manhattan or the Bronx in New York City. Furthermore, North American aging lived experiences are different from European, Central or South American, African, Australian, New Zealand, and Asian aging experiences. There is also increasing recognition of the diversity of populations and the role that social exclusion plays in the way people are enabled or precluded from establishing an optimal sense of being in place in the neighborhoods and communities where they reside (Walsh et al., 2020). Moving forward, OT, to be truly effective, must seek to understand diversity and occupational deprivation as this relates to the opportunities and constraints of the physical environment with the goal of furthering occupational justice and inclusivity (Malfitano et al., 2019; Whiteford et al., 2020).

Second, in seeking advances both in understanding and practice, it is important to critically assess the transformative effects of the COVID-19 pandemic and the potential for emerging diseases to change the daily lives of older adults and expose inequity and injustice (Hoffman et al., 2020). In this chapter, we have tangentially noted this issue in a number of places. But more is needed. As occupational therapists grapple with a "new normal," there is a need to

reframe entire domains of practice with respect to aging and the physical environment to take into account major societal changes such as increased focus on working from home, transformations of home and community spaces, increased spatial distancing, growing reliance on mobile technologies and virtual communication, and changes in patterns of service delivery and lifestyles that may become more or less permanent. While some may view this as a daunting challenge, we see it as an opportunity for advancing OT in exciting new socially and environmentally responsible directions (Whalley Hammell, 2021b).

We end this chapter with words from Richard J. Jackson's important 2003 editorial (Jackson, 2003, p. 1383):

*"Whereas our generation may reap some benefits from the new field of the built environment and health, with a little vision and a lot of good science and hard work, our children and grandchildren will be able to walk or bicycle home from their workplaces through attractive communities designed to promote the physical and mental health of all people."*

To add to Jackson's words, our hope is that this sentiment can be extended to especially embrace those who are the most environmentally vulnerable—older adults and both older and younger persons with disabling conditions. Occupational science and OT have the capacity to make this so.

*The complete listing of the Bibliography and Chapter Questions and Answers are available in the accompanying enhanced eBook version included with the print purchase of this textbook. Visit Elsevier eBooks+ (eBooks.Health.Elsevier.com) to access this content.*

## CHAPTER 21

# Driving and Transportation: Aging Drivers

*Ganesh M. Babulal, PhD, OTD, MSCI, MOT, OTR/L and Anne E. Dickerson, PhD, OTR/L, SCDCM, FAOTA, FGSA*

## CHAPTER OUTLINE

## OBJECTIVES

- Explain the importance and complexity of driving and community mobility as instrumental activities of daily living (IADLs)
- Understand the relationship between aging, disease, and disorder on driving outcomes
- Analyze the uses and limitations of different types of driving assessment tools and evaluation processes
- Demonstrate the ability to plan and implement interventions for remediation of driving disability with aging adults
- Review the role of technology in supporting driving behavior and remediating driving impairment
- Identify solutions and strategies in planning for a non-driving future

## Overview of an Aging Population of Drivers

Life expectancy in the United States (US) has steadily increased over the past three decades due to a reduction in communicable diseases and expanded access to health care. At age 65, a female can expect to live 20.5 additional years, while a male can expect to live 18.1 more years in the US (Payne, 2018). By 2060, approximately 95 million Americans (20%) will be ≥65 years of age, representing nearly a quarter of the US population. Along with this subsequent growth, there will be an increase in older drivers, where 25% of all drivers will be in this age band by mid-century (National Highway Traffic Safety, 2020). In 2019, among the 42 million licensed drivers age 65 and older, there were 8000 deaths and more than 250,000 injuries resulting from motor vehicle crashes (MVCs) (Federal Highway Administration, 2020). Drivers aged 80 and older consistently have a higher crash-related mortality rate than middle-aged adults due to a higher risk of injuries resulting from an MVC (Cox & Cicchino, 2021). Older adults are aging in place in their independent residences, engaging in the workforce longer—many finding a second career, and are well integrated within their communities, often living in them across multiple decades. Self-driving (referred to henceforth as driving) provides a means for transportation/mobility, access, and participation and confers a sense of autonomy, independence, and agency.

Driving is one of the most complex instrumental activities of daily living (IADLs) that individuals engage in spanning decades across their lives. The demands of this dynamic activity require the rapid, sustained, and coordinated deployment of several conscious and subconscious functional systems (cognitive, motor, sensory, and affective). The management and coordination of resources across systems typically occur in response to a continually changing natural (e.g., weather, light) and built environment (e.g., road conditions, other drivers, construction). Additionally, the driver must cope with internal factors like physical and psychological stress, sleepiness, and exhaustion. Despite driving being an overlearned task, age-related decline may moderately impact one or more abilities (e.g., reaction time, strength, range-of-motion, sensation) that support the driver-vehicle task interface. While these modest and gradual changes may limit driving performance, they often do not impact driving safety. However, chronic conditions like arthritis, cerebrovascular disease, neuropathy, cataracts, and dementia impair function and increase the risk of crashes, resulting in increased related injury and mortality among older drivers. Thus, the goal of this chapter will be to provide the tools, evidence, and guidance to make the most appropriate screening, evaluation, and/or intervention decisions about driving fitness for all clients seen by occupational therapy.

## Driving and Community Mobility as an Instrumental Activity of Daily Living

"I might as well be dead." Every occupational therapy practitioner who has needed to tell an older adult that they need to cease driving has heard a variation of that statement. While driving is the primary mode of transportation for older adults in the United States (Coughlin & D'Ambrosio, 2012) and for those in rural areas, often the only means of transportation, it is not the primary reason for this heartfelt statement. Baby Boomers grew up with the automobile industry and were the first generation where they owned their vehicles as teens and parents. For the generation that grew up in the 1950s and 1960s, driving was their method of *social networking* (Dickerson, 2016). It was the most important means of seeing friends, attending social events, and embracing their freedom. As such, the actual act of driving was and continues to be an essential occupation. Regardless of whether the individual can return to driving or not after a medical condition or with advanced aging, the practitioner must address the therapeutic intervention of community mobility *and* the emotionality associated with this most important IADL among older adults.

According to the *Occupational Therapy Practice Framework* (American Occupational Therapy Association [AOTA], 2016), occupational therapy practitioners provide evaluation and intervention services in all areas of occupation (e.g., sleep and rest, work, leisure, and social participation). However, ADLs and IADLs are the backbone of our profession (Doucet, 2014). The Centers for Medicare and Medicaid Services (CMS) understand that services need to be based on a person's ability to return to purposeful activity (Doucet, 2014). As demonstrated in the outcome study on readmissions (Rogers et al., 2017), occupational therapy was the only service that reduced hospital readmissions. The authors posited that since occupational therapy focused on meeting patients' functional and social needs, only occupational therapy made a difference. These results also reinforce that occupational therapy needs to focus on clients' daily tasks and social participation needs. In other words, a therapist should address functional deficits so the client can return to everyday tasks they need and want to do, including driving since driving is one of the most essential IADLs for clients (Dickerson et al., 2013). Driving for most adults underlies all the other occupations including work, education, play, leisure, and social participation, as well as most of the other IADLs (e.g., shopping, health management, money management, caregiving). Accordingly, practitioners appreciate that although driving a personal vehicle is a licensed privilege, community mobility is a right of all people (WFOT, 2019). Thus, occupational therapy practitioners have an ethical obligation to address driving and community mobility.

While there are many reasons driving and community mobility are not addressed, including brief rehabilitation stays, there may be a lack of confidence and competence among occupational therapy practitioners (Dickerson et al., 2011). Practitioners may be hesitant to speak about driving due to the lack of clear roles guiding the occupational therapy process for the IADL of driving and community mobility and the specialization of driving rehabilitation. However, consider that therapists are not experts in cooking, money management, or medication management. Yet, when observing clients unable to prepare a simple meal, manage a budget, or take their medication appropriately, practitioners feel confident in addressing these deficits as indicators that the client may not have the capacity to live independently. As experts in *activity analysis*, this reasoning also applies to the complex task of driving. If a client cannot appropriately make a sandwich for lunch or manage their medication, it is appropriate to put a "***stop***" on driving. Accordingly, it is also important to understand this "hold" on driving is not the final determination, only the licensing agencies have that responsibility. Nevertheless, the practitioner needs to use their professional clinical reasoning to make a justifiable recommendation considering the risk level of the IADL of driving and community mobility. Occupational therapy practitioners need to appreciate that they have the essential knowledge, skills, and abilities to screen, evaluate, and plan interventions based on a client's capacities in driving and community mobility for the client to maintain or expand their participation in their community supporting quality of life (AOTA, 2016).

## Understanding Driving Behaviors

A difference between driving and other complex IADLs is that driving is done within a highly dynamic environment. While shopping is a complex IADL, if a person with dementia becomes confused in a store, they may impede the flow of other shoppers or cause difficulty for a cashier, but they are unlikely to cause harm to anyone else. When a person with dementia gets confused while driving a vehicle, the potential risk of injury or worse increases beyond that individual. The question is, why don't individuals with dementia, family members, or health practitioners recognize this risk? While there may be multiple reasons, the one reason pertinent to this discussion is that the person with dementia can drive. Michon's hierarchy of driving behaviors explains this phenomenon.

Michon's framework has three levels, operational, tactical, and strategic. The ***operational*** level is the lowest level consisting of the overlearned human-machine interactions necessary to control the vehicle, such as using the brake, turning the steering wheel, and pressing the accelerator. These are the intuitive skills of the driver such that a driver on a familiar route they use daily will often arrive without any real memory of getting there. Persons with dementia retain these overlearned skills because of motor memory—it is indeed "like riding a bike." It is also why it is impossible to tell someone with dementia, they cannot drive because they can. What needs to be said instead is that they are not *fit to drive* because of the disease process.

The *tactical* level includes behaviors related to immediate decisions during driving maneuvers such as slowing down for weather and road changes, stopping for a yellow light, making a turn, and other routine maneuvers. Tactical decisions are governed by traffic rules and are also overlearned and practiced habits. Additionally, increased roadway designs to improve safety (e.g., protected left turns, arrows painted on lanes, channeling of lanes) has made it easier for an impaired driver, since fewer critical decisions are necessary with such embedded protections.

The *strategic* level involves decisions about the mode of transportation (e.g., vehicle, walking, biking), the goal of the trip, and how to get to the destination. The strategic level is also manifested during the driving process. For example, when an emergency vehicle blocks the usual route home, the driver must recognize the situation and negotiate another route. These unexpected route changes are often the cause of older adults with cognitive impairment getting lost in familiar areas. While they can physically drive and respond to basic road rules, their capacity to problem-solve in reaction to a new, dynamic situation is significantly impaired. Table 21.1 expands on the three levels with areas of function and the person factors to be assessed for each of the levels.

## Driving Fitness

*Fitness to drive* is defined as "a description of a driver's skills and abilities that indicates the individual is capable of fully controlling their vehicle, responding to the dynamic driving environment, and obeying the rules of the road and traffic laws" (Transportation Research Board [TRB], 2016a). Older adults are generally safe drivers overall, having the lowest risk of collisions compared with other age groups. This is partly due to lower exposure to the risk factors of being on the road during rush hour, night driving, and avoidance of high-speed interstates. Additionally, research has demonstrated that it is

not "age" that leads to declines in driving but instead the functional impairments associated with medical conditions that put **older drivers** at risk (Dickerson et al., 2019b). Thus, *medical fitness to drive* is defined as "when fitness to drive is due to a change or progression in a medical condition that requires consideration or assessment of driving risk" (TRB, 2016a).

With normal aging, a person may have slower information processing speeds and motor responses. Older adults compensate by driving more slowly and conservatively, as with most activities. It is not until drivers are over the age of 80 years that crash risk increases significantly when, for example, intersections require quick information processing and immediate decisions (e.g., yield signs, flashing signals) (Cox & Cicchino, 2021). Moreover, the frailty and fragility of some older adults put them more at risk to die of a crash than younger or middle-aged adults, which is why driver safety is so essential (Pomidor, 2019). Additionally, as one ages, there is a higher likelihood that the number and implications of medical conditions increase as one ages (Kent, 2010). Thus, the older adults at risk are typically clients who have medical conditions with functional impairments that will affect driving skills. However, it is important to also understand that drivers of any age who have a disability may benefit from the skilled services of occupational therapy practitioners who will address an individual's unique needs, thus promoting engagement in the occupation of driving and community mobility.

## Client Factors

Evaluation of driving fitness is generally based on an assessment of sensation (primarily vision), motor, and cognition, including visuo-perceptual skills. Since the infamous 2003 Santa Monica crash in which 86-year-old George Weller crashed through barricades and killed 10 people, researchers have sought to find the "one" assessment that will predict when someone is unfit to drive. In more recent years, research has clearly shown that there is not, nor will likely be, one definitive tool to determine fitness to drive (Aksan et al., 2015; Anderson et al., 2012; Bédard et al., 2013; Dickerson et al., 2014). In fact, fitness to drive depends on many factors beyond a score on a test, specifically, diagnosis (in terms of prognosis), age, context/environment (e.g., rural, urban, farm), and driving experience (e.g., novice, experienced driver, professional driver).

### Vision

While most licensing agencies have strict guidelines and tests for visual acuity, there is scant evidence that visual acuity is significant for driving fitness. However, cataracts are a major concern associated with driving, since they develop gradually over time, and the older adult may not recognize the gradual changes. Fortunately, identification and removal of cataracts effectively improve driving safety, and if done early, MVCs can be reduced by 21% (Mennemeyer et al., 2013). Visual fields may also decline over time with ptosis or drooping of the eyelid found commonly in the older population. However, most field cuts are consequences of medical conditions (Pomidor, 2019). While significant field cuts or visual neglect precludes driving, with field cuts, there are large individual differences, with some evidence indicating

**TABLE 21.1** Hierarchy of Driving Behaviors With Associated Areas of Function and Person Factors to Assess

| Levels | Driving Skills | Area of Function | Person Factors to be Assessed (Examples, Not All Inclusive) |
|---|---|---|---|
| Operational | Vehicle operation | Motor skills Visual skills | ROM, coordination, endurance, proprioception, sensation, strength, |
| Tactical | Rules of the road | *Discrete* cognitive skills | Attention (divided, sustained), memory, processing speed, multi-tasking |
| Strategic | Wayfinding, navigation | Executive functioning | Insight, judgment, problem solving |

Created by author (A. Dickerson).

that good drivers can compensate for field cuts (Wood, 2019). Finally, contrast sensitivity is associated with more driving errors (Carr et al., 2016; Dickerson et al., 2014); however, it is a normal aging process and should be a topic of education about how to avoid driving at dusk or dawn rather than a criterion for cessation. (For more information on vision, see Chapter 10.)

## Motor

While driving requires motor abilities, driving has become much less physically demanding with the improvements in technology. Even physically frail older adults may have the capacity to continue to drive (Pomidor, 2019), although safe and unsafe drivers have been classified using physical factors such as balance (Lacherez et al., 2014). Additionally, range of motion issues can be easily compensated with backup cameras, fisheye/panoramic mirrors, or blind-side warnings. On the other hand, proprioception in the lower extremities is essential for modulating the brake and accelerator and avoiding the "pedal confusion" paradigm which is found as the common reason for crashes through store fronts or garage walls. Though not a normal process of aging, common conditions such as diabetes should be a red flag to test sensation and proprioception of the legs and feet. Other conditions with motor deficits (e.g., stroke, spinal cord, traumatic brain injury [TBI]) often allow the individual to drive with vehicle modifications as long as there are minimal cognitive deficits. Cognition is the most critical factor for determining fitness to drive.

## Cognition

Driving requires visual and cognitive processing that occurs quickly in a dynamic environment. Research evidence describing the relationship between each of the critical cognitive processes for driving, such as attention (selective and divided), visual perception and processing, memory, executive functioning, and insight, is beyond the scope of this chapter. (See Chapter 15 for more information on cognition.) However, research has clearly shown that different cognitive assessments are necessary to determine fitness to drive (Aksan et al., 2015). More specifically, three key domains are identified: processing speed, visuospatial abilities, and memory (Anderson et al., 2012) or processing speed, executive function, and higher-level cognition (Anstey et al., 2012). As skilled evaluators of complex IADLs, occupational therapists need to promote occupation-based assessments in assisting with determining fitness to drive. One example is the *Assessment of Motor and Process Skills* (Fisher & Bray Jones, 2014), which has been demonstrated to differentiate between medical-at-risk drivers and medically fit drivers (Dickerson et al., 2011).

## Common Conditions Impacting Driving and Community Mobility

### Stroke

A cerebrovascular accident, more colloquially known as stroke, is perhaps one of the most studied and critically examined conditions that directly impact driving (Fisk et al., 1997). In the United States, stroke is the fifth leading cause of death and a leading cause of disability, with an annual incidence of 795,000 (Virani et al., 2021). Stroke can be classified as either ischemic (or infarct) or hemorrhagic (rupture/bleeding), which share common risk factors and can result in different severity and outcomes. While the incidence of stroke increases with age, several established medical risk factors increase the likelihood (e.g., heart disease, hyperlipidemia, hypertension, obesity, diabetes mellitus II, history of smoking, and prior history of strokes) (Feigin et al., 2016). Social determinants of health, such as access to healthy foods/diets, physical and psychological stress, coping mechanisms, climate, personal crime, and poverty, increase the likelihood by indirectly acting upon risk factors.

The consequences of stroke or post-stroke sequelae are heterogeneous and can include: (1) cognitive impairment, like memory recall, executive function (planning, decision making), or attention, (2) language deficits, like aphasia or communication and comprehension of written and verbal information, (3) visual impairments, like field cuts, (4) mood disorders, like depression, anxiety, apathy, or anger, (5) affective-cognitive disorders, like anosognosia or prosopagnosia, and (6) partial to complete loss of muscle function nerve disruption (Babulal & Connor, 2014). Some post-stroke conditions may be detected immediately, while others may arise months during recovery, and others may spontaneously improve with time or via medical intervention. Given the multidimensional impact a stroke can have on the body, the resulting sequelae can impair one or more systems that support driving safely. Post-stroke physical and visual impairments, like hemiplegia and field cuts, are more salient and often aggressively targeted during rehabilitation to improve recovery back to baseline or as close as possible (Legh-Smith et al., 1986; Richards et al., 2008). A comprehensive driving evaluation conducted by a driving rehabilitation specialist/occupational therapist may assess overall performance, identify domain-specific deficits, synthesize medical history with task activity to provide safety recommendations and limitations while also offering strategies and compensatory approaches to avoid driving risks (Devos et al., 2011; Unsworth et al., 2019). Driving simulators and on-road assessments can evaluate specific processing and functioning domains required to ensure driving capabilities and appropriate performance. Cognitive assessments have been used as off-road predictors to forecast a return to driving after short- and long-term recovery. Paper and pencil measures, such as the Trail Making tasks, the Rey–Osterreith Complex Figure Design, and the Useful Field of View Test (UFOV), reasonably correlate with the predictive outcome on a road-test (Marshall et al., 2007). The intersectionality across clinical assessments of multiple systems (motor, sensory, cognition, mood), medical history, medication, comorbidities, and demographic factors influence fitness-to-drive factors and a return to driving.

### Dementia

The term dementia refers to an umbrella or a family of disorders that broadly describe a set of symptoms that an individual may have difficulty with, including memory, thinking, and language. As dementia progresses into more severe stages, the loss of function will directly impair a client's ability to complete IADLs and subsequent ADLs. There are approximately 55 million persons with dementia, and this number is expected to reach over 150 million by 2050. In the United States, the annual prevalence of dementia among Americans age 65 and older is 8.8%, and this number is expected to double by 2050, especially in the absence of disease-modifying treatments (Langa et al., 2017; Nichols et al., 2019). More common etiologies of dementia include Alzheimer disease, mixed (vascular or Lewy body), and vascular dementia, which ranks in order of disease prevalence. Other less common forms include Lewy body, frontotemporal, and Parkinson disease dementia (PDD). The overall characteristics of dementia and global decline are rooted in cognitive abilities, so assessing cognitive function and neural substrates that support function has been a focus of practitioners. Dementia is a slow progression over many years, transitioning from cognitively normal health to impairments and then dementia. Stereotypic changes in cognitive functioning begin with a gradual onset of (1) *mild symptoms* (occasional memory loss, lapse in judgment), which then evolves into (2) *moderate impairment* (IADL dependence, poor recall of recent events, unable to recognize friends, acquaintances), and then coalesce into (3) *severe impairment* (ADL dependence, inability to encode/store memory, unable to recognizing family or friends). There are also comorbid conditions like depression, apathy, anxiety, and neuropsychiatric symptoms that can co-occur with dementia.

There have been well-established studies using driving simulators, and on-the-road assessments that demonstrate clients with moderate to severe dementia are not fit to drive and are more likely to fail a driving test or are at a higher risk for crashes regardless of dementia etiology (Adler et al., 2005; Brown & Ott, 2004). A recent systematic review found that individuals with vascular, Lewy body, frontotemporal, and PDD had a parallel stepwise higher risk of driving safety as their dementia progressed (Toepper & Falkenstein, 2019). However, Alzheimer disease seemed more variable, with minimal risk in the early stages but higher risk at the moderate and severe stages. The clinical dementia rating (CDR) is a scale that stages a person with dementia. A rating of 0 indicates normality; 0.5, very mild; 1, mild; 2, moderate; and 3, severe. One study found that older drivers with CDR 0 were the least likely to fail a road test, followed by CDR 0.5, and then CDR 1—difficulty with lane changes, use of signals, and controlling speed were specific behaviors that indicate decline (Duchek et al., 2003). Since symptoms of dementia can emerge 15 to 20 years before a client becomes symptomatic, the development of molecular biomarkers provides an early indication that the pathophysiological process has started. Recent research studies have shifted to examining biomarkers of disease pathology in older adults who are cognitively normal (e.g., CDR 0). Older drivers without dementia or decline but with positive biomarkers made 2.5 more errors on a road test and were faster to receive a rating of marginal/fail on that road test compared to those with normal biomarker levels (Roe et al., 2017a, 2017b). Advancement of

driving assessments using in-vehicle global positioning system (GPS) dataloggers allows for evaluating driving behavior in the actual environments that older adults navigate daily (Babulal et al., 2016; Eby et al., 2012). Studies using GPS dataloggers among cognitively normal older drivers have found a decline in daily driving occurring behaviors faster among those with abnormal biomarkers (Babulal et al., 2021; Roe et al., 2019). This suggests that changes in driving occur well before an older adult becomes cognitively impaired or symptomatic (Bayat et al., 2021). (For more information on dementia, see Chapter 16.)

## Other Progressive Neurological Conditions

The variation of dementia subtypes resulting from different etiologies can influence disease onset, phenotype, and resulting functional impairments that directly impact ADLs/IADLs. For example, dementia with Lewy body (DLB) and PDD share pathology (aggregation of the protein α-synuclein) and clinical symptoms, typically the manifestation of overt motor impairments. However, DLB is characterized by rapid changes in cognitive function accompanied by hallucinations, while PDD is established, generally 1 year or later following a diagnosis of PD based on clinical assessment and uniform criteria (Walker et al., 2019). Unlike DLB, the stereotypic motor phenotypes like rigidity, tremors, and slower movements of PD become more severe as the disease progresses. There is a rich body of literature on PD on driving (Heikkilä et al., 1998). A systematic review found that drivers with PD are more likely to fail a road test compared to age-matched controls, with operational and tactical skill being noted as predictive of overall driving and a combination of visual, cognitive, and motor deficits influencing performance (Devos et al., 2015). A naturalistic study using an instrumented vehicle found that drivers with PD took more time to complete a route, maintained slower speeds, longer brake times, and had lower brake pressure compared to controls (Phokaewvarangkul et al., 2019). Since DLB tends to co-occur with AD, limited studies examine pure DLB and driving outcomes (Gorrie et al., 2007).

Multiple sclerosis (MS) impacts the central nervous system because of the immune system attacking myelin sheathing (a fatty layer surrounding nerve fiber) in the nerve cells of the brain and spinal cord. The neuroinflammation disrupts cellular communication and can result in cognitive impairment, fatigue, numbness and tingling, unstable mood, muscle weakness, pain, and unstable gait. The multisystemic impact of MS influences driving performance and driving risk. Fatigue is a significant issue that impacts drivers with MS compared to healthy controls, influencing their endurance and ability to control the vehicle (Chipchase et al., 2003). Several studies show adjustment-to-stimuli (slow or impaired reaction to roadway information) on the road, and gap acceptance errors (poor judgment on time-to-distance to cross safely in response to others on the road) predicted which drivers with MS would pass or fail a road test (Krasniuk et al., 2017). Another study examined persons with MS and found they had more challenges with attention, information processing, working memory, and visuomotor coordination tasks compared to controls, and drivers with MS and cognitively impaired performed more poorly on a road test compared to those MS drivers without impairment (Badenes et al., 2014). Current protocols on driving simulators are being developed to probe specific facets of driving, like the environment (e.g., urban, suburban), cognitive processing, and street complexities, to determine strategies that may help with remediation and potential inventions to preserve driving skills (Krasniuk et al., 2022).

## Sleep and Sleep Apnea

Sleep is crucial for driving, and drowsy driving (absence of alcohol, medication, or illicit drugs) was found to be responsible for 91,000 crashes, 50,000 injuries, and nearly 800 deaths in 2017 (National Highway Traffic Safety Administration, 2021). Being awake for approximately 18 hours was comparable to having a blood alcohol content of 0.05% (Williamson & Feyer, 2000). The deleterious effect of sleep on driving can be seen with increased blinking, difficulty focusing (missing signs/exits), lane drifting, tailgating, poor short-term memory, and increased aggression (Higgins et al., 2017; Maia et al., 2013; Sunwoo et al., 2017). In addition to the risk sleep deprivation has on driving, numerous neurological diseases also impact the circadian rhythm and sleep. For example, rapid eye moment (REM) sleep disturbances are one of the earlier indicators of DLB, and sudden onset of sleep was associated with a risk of crashes among drivers with PD (Iranzo et al., 2014; Meindorfner et al., 2005).

Obstructive sleep apnea (OSA) is a common and often underdiagnosed sleep disorder that affects an estimated 54 million Americans and causes daytime sleepiness, snoring, headaches, feeling fatigued, and forgetfulness (Benjafield et al., 2019; Lévy et al., 2015; Young et al., 1993). OSA occurs because of a partial or complete obstruction of the upper airway, which requires the diaphragm, heart, and other chest musculature to work harder to open the airway for respiration. The cessation of a regular breathing pattern is marked by apneic episodes that may include pausing, snorting, and gasping for air to resupply the oxygen-deprived central nervous system (CNS). Apneic episodes may occur hundreds of times in severe cases. As a result, OSA has an immediate impact on the quality and quantity of sleep, interrupts transition into sleep stages, and directly reduces sleep quality (Lee et al., 2016). The risk factors for OSA include narrow airway, weight (heavier), age (older), large tonsils, hypertension, diabetes, smoking, and alcohol use (Franklin & Lindberg, 2015). The health-related consequences of OSA can range from fatigue during the waking hours to an increased risk for a heart attack, stroke, heart failure, and even cognitive impairment (Yaffe et al., 2011). Individuals with OSA are at risk for impaired driving and increased risks of crashes. The confluence of being drowsy, fatigued, and having impairment in multiple cognitive processes reduces performance and increases driving risk. OSA is a condition that can be remedied by conservative approaches like weight loss and lifestyle changes or machines using continuous positive airway pressure. Additionally, surgical intervention like rhinoplasty to fix a deviated septum or uvulopalatopharyngoplasty to increase the upper airway and support increases the volume of air.

## Evaluation of Driving and Community Mobility

When considering the IADL of driving, identifying potential safety risks is not significantly different from identifying safety issues of other complex IADLs. When the client is at risk for falls or safety doing their ADL/IADLs, the therapist informs the client and family/caregivers of the implications of risk and the strategies that might be used to mitigate any unwanted outcomes. With driving, that process is not any more complex, but it is more ***complicated***. This is because the potential risk involves the client and potentially affects **the public**. The risk of a crash significantly increases with medical conditions, particularly with cognitive impairment (Pomidor, 2019; Society & Pomidor, 2016). Since driving and community mobility are well within the scope of occupational therapy practice, it is the ethical obligation of the occupational therapy practitioner to identify risk (Slater, 2014). Additionally, occupational therapy has been recognized as the "go-to" profession for driver evaluation and rehabilitation (Dickerson et al., 2018; Society & Pomidor, 2016). Moreover, occupational therapy practitioners need to address this IADL with all clients, or it will be a practice area lost to other less qualified service providers who are already designing certificate programs that purport to evaluate older adults effectively (Dickerson, 2012). Understanding driving rehabilitation's process and specialty area are important to understand how occupational therapy practitioners can appropriately address driving.

## Driving Rehabilitation and Driver Rehabilitation Specialist

A **driver rehabilitation specialist** (DRS) is a general term for a diverse group of providers without specific licensing or educational requirements. Those who use the initials DRS have diverse backgrounds (e.g., engineers, driving instructors, health care professionals), and there is no consistency between states. The reason is mainly based on the history of driving rehabilitation.

Driving rehabilitation developed after the proliferation of the automobile when adaptations to vehicles were created to allow individuals to return to driving despite physical impairments (Hyde, 2006). Occupational therapists, driver educators, and engineers collaborated to provide driver rehabilitation based on medical and vocational rehabilitation service models (Pellerito, 2006) with a focus on *compensatory* rehabilitation. This was done through vehicle modification and adaptive equipment for individuals with specific *physical* impairments (e.g., spinal cord injuries, amputations, spina bifida, dwarfism). Over time, driving rehabilitation programs expanded to include clients with acquired brain injury and/or older adults with physical and cognitive disorders. With the advancement of medical practice and technology (e.g., driving simulators), driving rehabilitation has become restorative, not just compensatory. Thus, it is essential for driver rehabilitation specialists to have a medically based education to evaluate fitness-to-drive from a cognitive perspective and adjust the vehicle to physical deficits. With these more complex services, there is a clear need for more differentiation of services. Occupational therapy is the ideal profession to fulfill the requirement of appropriate professionals with general skills to meet the screening, evaluation, and intervention services and those who become DRS to provide the very specialized services of driving rehabilitation.

## Diversity in Driving Programs

To bring clarity to the increasing diversity of driver services and complexity of driving rehabilitation as a service, the *Spectrum of Driver Services* was created to illustrate the diverse types of services related to driving. The *Spectrum* document explains the range of available services (Fig. 21.1). The significant features include:

1. The differentiation of driver services is between community-based education (e.g., driver safety programs, driving schools); medically based assessment, education, and referral (e.g., driver screening, IADL evaluations); and driving rehabilitation programs.

2. For the type of program, common credentials, providers' knowledge, and specific services, the chart illustrates the differences between educational programs from the medically based services, including differentiation between screening for driving risk, an IADL assessment completed by a generalist occupational therapist, and the specialized services provided by the DRS.

3. Most important is the outcome of each program type. Driver safety programs provide education and awareness, and driving schools may enhance skills for healthy older drivers. However, these two programs should not be the intervention resource for individuals with medical conditions. Medically at-risk drivers should be referred to the programs that provide medically based assessment, evaluation, and/or the specialized programs.

The *Spectrum* also differentiates the "levels" of driving rehabilitation programs (Fig. 21.2). If an older adult needs adaptive equipment to compensate for a physical impairment, they should be referred to a *Low Tech* program that has modified vehicles. Those who need a "high tech" modification, such as driving from a wheelchair, should be referred to the services of a *High Tech* program. Finally, the *Basic* program is appropriate for older adults with cognitive impairment. It is critical to understand that the word ***basic*** does not imply simplistic; it refers to the fact only a "basic" vehicle is needed for the evaluation. In fact, evaluations and interventions for clients with cognitive impairment are often more complex than adapting a vehicle for an amputee (low tech).

While the *Spectrum of Driver Services* offers an overall conceptualization of driving services and driving rehabilitation based on vehicle modification, it does not differentiate the ***diversity of clients*** with an array of diagnoses in combination with complex environmental and contextual factors. Thus, the next section is a new model of conceptualizing driving evaluations.

## Driving Evaluations Based on Diagnosis

An occupational therapist who specializes in driving rehabilitation performs a ***comprehensive driving evaluation*** to determine an individual's fitness to drive. The comprehensive driving evaluation is a complete assessment of an individual's driving knowledge, skills, and abilities that typically includes: (1) a medical and driving history review; (2) an assessment of sensory-perceptual, cognitive, and functional psychomotor abilities (usually called a clinical driving evaluation or clinical assessment); (3) an on-road assessment in a vehicle, as appropriate; (4) an adaptive equipment evaluation, as appropriate; and (5) a report of the results with recommendations including transportation options (TRB, 2016b). The outcome of this evaluation typically results in one of the following: (1) the driver is fit to drive and needs no further intervention, (2) rehabilitation is required of underlying human factors (e.g., cognition, physical, sensory), (3) compensation through training (e.g., driving simulator, using GPS), (4) compensation through adaptation of the vehicle (e.g., hand controls, steering knob for one-handed turning), or (5) cessation of driving counseling and planning.

As with any occupational therapy process, an evaluation should be tailored to the individual client's needs and goals. However, medical systems tend to favor standardized protocols for evaluation, including specialized driving evaluations. Many driving rehabilitation specialists, especially at the novice levels of practice, use extensive testing following the same pattern using the same assessment tools for every client (Dickerson et al., 2014). Only recently have there been clear distinctions between the types of comprehensive driving evaluation (Dickerson & Schold Davis, 2020) with important distinctions of skill levels for completing the assessments. Essentially, as an occupational therapy practitioner, it is more important to understand driving rehabilitation in terms of these categories of clients to refer them to the right service/ professional at the right time. The four categories include Physical, Developmental, Neuro-Cognitive, and Complex Medical.

### Physical

The ***Physical*** category consists of diagnoses solely based on physical impairment (no cognitive impairment). This may include persons with amputations, spinal cord injuries, and other disabilities that will require vehicle modification for adult clients. The evaluation will focus on the client's **physical** strengths and limitations and a plan for modifying a vehicle for independent driving. The DRS should be a low- or high-tech provider using the *Spectrum* document, depending on the need. As this category does not include cognitive or neurological processes, the evaluation shifts from a medical provider to needing the skills of a rehabilitation engineer or certified driver rehabilitation specialist with sufficient training in vehicle modification and equipment.

### Developmental

The ***Developmental*** is a distinctive category for a new driver. Evaluation and intervention for a client with a disability who has no experience behind the wheel is a unique challenge that takes an experienced driving rehabilitation specialist who also needs to evaluate the driver's readiness to drive. This category is

## Spectrum of Driver Services: Right Services for the Right People at the Right Time

A description consumers and health care providers can use to
distinguish the type of services needed for an older adult.

 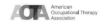

| | COMMUNITY-BASED EDUCATION | | MEDICALLY-BASED ASSESSMENT, EDUCATION AND REFERRAL | | SPECIALIZED EVALUATION AND TRAINING |
|---|---|---|---|---|---|
| **Program Type** | Driver Safety Programs | Driving School | Driver Screen | Clinical IADL Evaluation | Driver Rehabilitation Programs (Includes Driver Evaluation) |
| **Typical Providers and Credentials** | Program specific credentials (e.g. AARP and AAA Driver Improvement Program). | Licensed Driving Instructor (LDI) certified by state licensing agency or Dept. of Education. | Health care professional (e.g., physician, social worker, neuropsychologist). | Occupational Therapy Practitioner (Generalist or Driver Rehabilitation Specialist#). Other health professional degree with expertise in Instrumental Activities of Daily Living (IADL). | Driver Rehabilitation Specialist#, Certified Driver Rehabilitation Specialist*, Occupational Therapist with Specialty Certification in Driving and Community Mobility+. |
| **Required Provider's Knowledge** | Program specific knowledge. Trained in course content and delivery. | Instructs novice or relocated drivers, excluding medical or aging conditions that might interfere with driving, for purposes of teaching / training / refreshing / updating driving skills. | Knowledge of relevant medical conditions, assessment, referral, and / or intervention processes. Understand the limits and value of assessment tools, including simulation, as a measurement of fitness to drive. | Knowledge of medical conditions and the implication for community mobility including driving. Assess the cognitive, visual, perceptual, behavioral and physical limitations that may impact driving performance. Knowledge of available services. Understands the limits and value of assessment tools, including simulation, as a measurement of fitness to drive. | Applies knowledge of medical conditions with implications to driving. Assesses the cognitive, visual, perceptual, behavioral and physical limitations that may impact driving performance. Integrates the clinical findings with assessment of on-road performance. Synthesizes client and caregiver needs, assists in decisions about equipment and vehicle modification options available. Coordinates multidisciplinary providers and resources, including driver education, health care team, vehicle choice and modifications, community services, funding / payers, driver licensing agencies, training and education, and caregiver support. |
| **Typical Services Provided** | 1) Classroom or computer based refresher for licensed drivers: review of rules of the road, driving techniques, driving strategies, state laws, etc. 2) Enhanced self-awareness, choices, and capability to self-limit. | 1) Enhance driving performance. 2) Acquire driver permit or license. 3) Counsel with family members for student driver skill development. 4) Recommend continued training and / or undergoing licensing test. 5) Remedial Programs (e.g., license reinstatement course for teens / adults, license point reduction courses). | 1) Counsel on risks associated with specific conditions (e.g., medications, fractures, post-surgery). 2) Investigate driving risk associated with changes in vision, cognition, and sensory-motor function. 3) Determine actions for the at-risk driver: • Refer to IADL evaluation, driver rehabilitation program, and / or other services. • Discuss driving cessation; provide access to counseling and education for alternative transportation options. 4) Follow reporting / referral structure for licensing recommendations. | 1) Evaluate and interpret risks associated with changes in vision, cognition, and sensory-motor functions due to acute or chronic conditions. 2) Facilitate remediation of deficits to advance client readiness for driver rehabilitation services. 3) Develop an individualized transportation plan considering client diagnosis and risks, family, caregiver, environmental and community options and limitations: • Discuss resources for vehicle adaptations (e.g., scooter lift). • Facilitate client training on community transportation options (e.g., mobility managers, dementia-friendly transportation). • Discuss driving cessation. For clients with poor self-awareness, collaborate with caregivers on cessation strategies. • Refer to driver rehabilitation program. 4) Document driver safety risk and recommended intervention plan to guide further action. 5) Follow professional ethics on referrals to the driver licensing authority. | Programs are distinguished by complexity of evaluations, types of equipment, vehicles, and expertise of provider. 1) Navigate driver license compliance and basic eligibility through intake of driving and medical history. 2) Evaluate and interpret risks associated with changes in vision, cognition, and sensory-motor functions in the driving context by the medically trained provider. 3) Perform a comprehensive driving evaluation (clinical and on-road). 4) Advise client and caregivers about evaluation results, and provide resources, counseling, education, and / or intervention plan. 5) Intervention may include training with compensatory strategies, skills, and vehicle adaptations or modifications for drivers and passengers. 6) Advocate for clients in access to funding resources and / or reimbursement. 7) Provide documentation about fitness to drive to the physician and / or driver-licensing agency in compliance with regulations. 8) Prescribe equipment in compliance with state regulations and collaborate with Mobility Equipment Dealer^ for fitting and training. 9) Present resources and options for continued community mobility if recommending driving cessation or transition from driving. Recommendations may include (but not restricted to): 1) drive unrestricted; 2) drive with restrictions; 3) cessation of driving pending rehabilitation or training; 4) planned re-evaluation for progressive disorders; 5) driving cessation; 6) referral to another program. |
| **Outcome** | Provides education and awareness. | Enhances skills for healthy drivers. | Indicates risk or need for follow-up for medically at-risk drivers. | | Determines fitness to drive and provides rehabilitative services. |

#DRS – Health professional degree with specialty training in driver evaluation and rehabilitation.   *CDRS – Certified Driver Rehabilitation Specialist-Credentialed by ADED (Association for Driver Rehabilitation Specialists).   +SCDCM – Specialty Certified in Driving and Community Mobility by AOTA (American Occupational Therapy Association). ^Quality Approved Provider by NMEDA (National Mobility Equipment Dealers Association).

*Driver Rehabilitation Programs: Defining Program Models, Services, and Expertise.*
Occupational Therapy In Health Care, 28(2):177–187, 2014

**FIG. 21.1**   Spectrum of Driver Services: Right Services for the Right People at the Right Time. (Funded by the National Highway Safety Administration.)

## Spectrum of Driver Rehabilitation Program Services

A description consumers and health care providers can use to distinguish the services provided by driver rehabilitation programs which best fits a client's need.

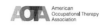

| Program Type | DRIVER REHABILITATION PROGRAMS<br>Determine fitness to drive and / or provide rehabilitative services. | | |
|---|---|---|---|
| Levels of Program and Typical Provider Credentials | BASIC<br><br>Provider is a Driver Rehabilitation Specialist (DRS)# with professional background in occupational therapy, other allied health field, driver education or a professional team of CDRS or SCDCM with LDI**. | LOW TECH<br><br>Driver Rehabilitation Specialist#, Certified Driver Rehabilitation Specialist*, Occupational Therapist with Specialty Certification in Driving and Community Mobility+, or in combination with LDI.<br><br>Certification in Driver Rehabilitation is recommended as the provider for comprehensive driving evaluation and training. | HIGH TECH<br><br>Driver Rehabilitation Specialist#, Certified Driver Rehabilitation Specialist*, Occupational Therapist with Specialty Certification in Driving and Community Mobility+.<br><br>Certification in Driver Rehabilitation is recommended as the provider for comprehensive driving evaluation and training with advanced skills and expertise to complete complex client and vehicle evaluation and training. |
| Program Service | Offers driver evaluation, training and education.<br><br>May include use of adaptive driving aids that do not affect operation of primary or secondary controls (e.g., seat cushions or additional mirrors).<br><br>May include transportation planning (transition and options), cessation planning, and recommendations for clients as passengers. | Offers comprehensive driving evaluation, training and education, with or without adaptive driving aids that affect the operation of primary or secondary controls, vehicle ingress / egress, and mobility device storage / securement. May include use of adaptive driving aids such as seat cushions or additional mirrors.<br><br>At the Low Tech level, adaptive equipment for primary control is typically mechanical. Secondary controls may include wireless or remote access.<br><br>May include transportation planning (transition and options), cessation planning, and recommendations for clients who plan to ride as passengers only. | Offers a wide variety of adaptive equipment and vehicle options for comprehensive driving evaluation, training and education, including all services available in Low Tech and Basic programs. At this level, providers have the ability to alter positioning of primary and secondary controls based on client's need or ability level.<br><br>High Tech adaptive equipment for primary and secondary controls includes devices that meet the following conditions:<br><br>1) capable of controlling vehicle functions or driving controls, and<br><br>2) consists of a programmable computerized system that interfaces / integrates with an electronic system in the vehicle. |
| Access to Driver's Position | Requires independent transfer into OEM^ driver's seat in vehicle. | Addresses transfers, seating and position into OEM^ driver's seat. May make recommendations for assistive devices to access driver's seat, improved positioning, wheelchair securement systems, and / or mechanical wheelchair loading devices. | Access to the vehicle typically requires ramp or lift and may require adaptation to OEM^ driver's seat. Access to driver position may be dependent on use of a transfer seat base, or clients may drive from their wheelchair. Provider evaluates and recommends vehicle structural modifications to accommodate products such as ramps, lifts, wheelchair and scooter hoists, transfer seat bases, wheelchairs suitable to utilize as a driver seat, and / or wheelchair securement systems. |
| Typical Vehicle Modification: Primary Controls: Gas, Brake, Steering | Uses OEM^ controls. | Primary driving control examples:<br><br>A) mechanical gas / brake hand control;<br><br>B) left foot accelerator pedal;<br><br>C) pedal extensions;<br><br>D) park brake lever or electronic park brake;<br><br>E) steering device (spinner knob, tri-pin, C-cuff). | Primary driving control examples (in addition to Low Tech options):<br><br>A) powered gas / brake systems;<br><br>B) power park brake integrated with a powered gas / brake system;<br><br>C) variable effort steering systems;<br><br>D) reduced diameter steering wheel, horizontal steering, steering wheel extension, joystick controls;<br><br>E) reduced effort brake systems. |
| Typical Vehicle Modification: Secondary Controls | Uses OEM^ controls. | Secondary driving control examples:<br><br>A) remote horn button;<br><br>B) turn signal modification (remote, crossover lever);<br><br>C) remote wiper controls;<br><br>D) gear selector modification;<br><br>E) key / ignition adaptions. | Electronic systems to access secondary and accessory controls.<br><br>Secondary driving control examples (in addition to Low Tech options):<br><br>A) remote panels, touch pads or switch arrays that interface with OEM^ electronics;<br><br>B) wiring extension for OEM^ electronics;<br><br>C) powered transmission shifter. |

#DRS - Health professional degree with specialty training in driver evaluation and rehabilitation.    *CDRS – Certified Driver Rehabilitation Specialist – Credentialed by ADED (Association for Driver Rehabilitation Specialists).    +SCDCM – Specialty Certified in Driving and Community Mobility by AOTA (American Occupational Therapy Association)    ^OEM – Original Equipment installed by Manufacturer. **LDI-licensed driving instructor.

*Driver Rehabilitation Programs: Defining Program Models, Services, and Expertise.*
Occupational Therapy In Health Care, 28(2):177–187, 2014

**FIG. 21.2**    Spectrum of Driver Services: Right Services for the Right People at the Right Time. (Funded by the National Highway Safety Administration.)

typically reserved for young adults with diagnoses such as cerebral palsy, autism spectrum disorder, attention-deficit/hyperactivity disorder (ADHD), spina bifida, dwarfism, and others.

### Neuro-Cognitive

The ***Neuro-Cognitive*** category is probably the most common type of comprehensive driving evaluation done by the occupational therapist/driving rehabilitation specialists and is for individuals with any type of neurological or cognitive impairment. For those with primarily cognitive impairment, such as dementia, the focus is on determining the degree of risk with the ongoing loss of executive function and speed of processing.

For disorders with both physical and cognitive components (e.g., stroke, Parkinson disease [PD]), the client's cognitive ability must be sufficient to be able to understand how to compensate for the physical impairments. This type of evaluation requires a deep understanding of neurology, activity analysis, and functional performance, and it is essential for the driving rehabilitation specialist to also be an occupational therapist.

### Complex-Medical

Finally, the ***Complex-Medical*** category is the driving evaluation of those with complicated diagnoses or a combination of diagnostic categories. When an older adult has uncontrolled diabetes, it is common to have a lower extremity amputation and sleep apnea, requiring a comprehensive driving evaluation uniquely designed to address multiple issues. TBIs may also have various issues that increase the complexity of addressing driving and/or community mobility. In many cases, the occupational therapist may be working with family members to work out transportation issues instead of independent driving.

While these four categories are not inclusive of all driving evaluation candidates, they do offer a way to communicate knowledge and skill level with the anticipation that practitioners using these categories explain their services will also improve service delivery.

## Framework for Determining Driving Risk by Generalists

To assist occupational therapy practitioners in meeting the ethical obligation of addressing the highly valued occupation of driving, the OT-DRIVE framework was created. This framework is based on a traffic light analogy: green, red, and yellow. The older adult, who has been driving, is seen by an occupational therapist for evaluation and intervention due to a hip replacement. With no cognitive deficits, this client would be seen as "green," not needing any specialized evaluation for driving fitness except for the standard guidelines for hip replacement. The client who is medically compromised by their medical condition (e.g., dementia, stroke, advanced age) and unfit to drive is "red." Finally, the client who is "yellow" shows a mixed evaluation picture. Specifically, the medical condition impacts driving, but the degree of risk is not precise. Thus, a referral to a specialized evaluation is necessary (Fig. 21.3).

To use OT-DRIVE, start with the "OT" as the occupational therapist using their expertise to evaluate sensorimotor, visual-perceptual, and cognitive factors. This process should also include the occupational therapy profile (interview) to determine if driving is one of the occupations valued by the client. Thus, the "D" is for **Develop**. Determine the client's readiness for driving and other forms of transportation, and address where they currently are situated and the expected potential for the future. The "R" is for **Readiness**. Using the colors "green," "yellow," and "red" assist in illustrating the occupational therapist's judgment about the client's status and/or their potential based on their diagnosis and evaluation results. Justification for either the decision of "cessation" (red) or "specialized evaluation" (yellow) should be based on results of a performance evaluation(s) with clear recommendations for the client and/or family. If a referral for a driving evaluation for driving competency needs to be deferred for some reason (e.g., not recovered), it should not be forgotten. Even a therapist in acute care should be able to give guidelines of what "to do" when function is restored and the client would like to pursue driving.

"I" is for **Intervention**. For healthy older adults with an acute issue, this is a unique opportunity to offer cautionary guidance for restrictions based on their diagnoses (e.g., use of hand splint driving, hip precautions) and health promotion strategies. For those clients in the red zone, the focus should be on the development of a transportation plan to ensure

continuous community mobility. Transportation planning is crucial for individuals with progressive conditions, as driving cessation is inevitable. Planning will assist the client and family members, as driving cessation should never be a crisis—the worse outcome being a crash. Families need clear and concrete education, such as the *Occupational Therapy Checklist of Community Mobility Skills* (Dickerson & Schold Davis, 2020), which matches the physical and cognitive skills to which type of transportation is needed. Finally, intervention for the yellow level is focused on restoring or optimizing the critical abilities for safe driving in the domains of vision, cognition, and physical, as well as helping the client understand that their efforts to address these areas are critical for returning to driving.

The "V" is for **Verification** of the treatment plan with the client, family, physician, and team. As education has always been part of the occupational therapy process, the "E" is for **Education**. For green, occupational therapy practitioners can offer valuable information on maintaining fitness to drive, improved safety with vehicle technologies, and future transportation planning. For the red or yellow, while driving is not an option at this point in their recovery, the expertise of the occupational therapist is crucial in determining the *potential* for recovery, or for those who have to cease permanently, the need to plan for alternatives to maintain social participation.

For clients who may need the expertise of a specialized driving evaluation, it is critical to understand the timing of referral is significantly different depending on the type of and degree of impairment. In cases with primarily motor impairments (e.g., amputation, spinal cord), the best practice strategy is to converse early with a specialist so possibilities (i.e., purchase of a specialized vehicle) can be explored to support success in their future transportation.

## The Generalist's Resource to Integrate Driving

Based on the OT-DRIVE framework, the *Generalist's Resource to Integrate Driving (GRID)* was developed to assist generalists in determining the next steps in integrating driving into everyday practice. Using the structure of red, green, and yellow as functional markers for driving performance risk, the GRID provides specific guidelines for generalists to evaluate, create, and implement intervention plans to develop or restore the client's valued IADL of driving and community mobility.

The GRID consists of a table (Table 21.2). The first column lists *client factors* that include the major factors to consider when screening or assessing driver fitness. These are not all the possible client factors, but factors that are most relevant (e.g., seizures, crashes), most related to driver fitness (e.g., visual skills, cognitive), and/or commonly understood by generalist occupational therapists. The second column is the critical contextual factors that offer relevant and specific information that must be considered when determining the driving risk levels. Finally, the last three columns indicate the scores to assess the client in terms of red (indicator of cessation), green (indicator of no risk), or yellow (needs further evaluation). Some boxes do not have a color or score because there are no specific screening tools to gain a score, or it is a

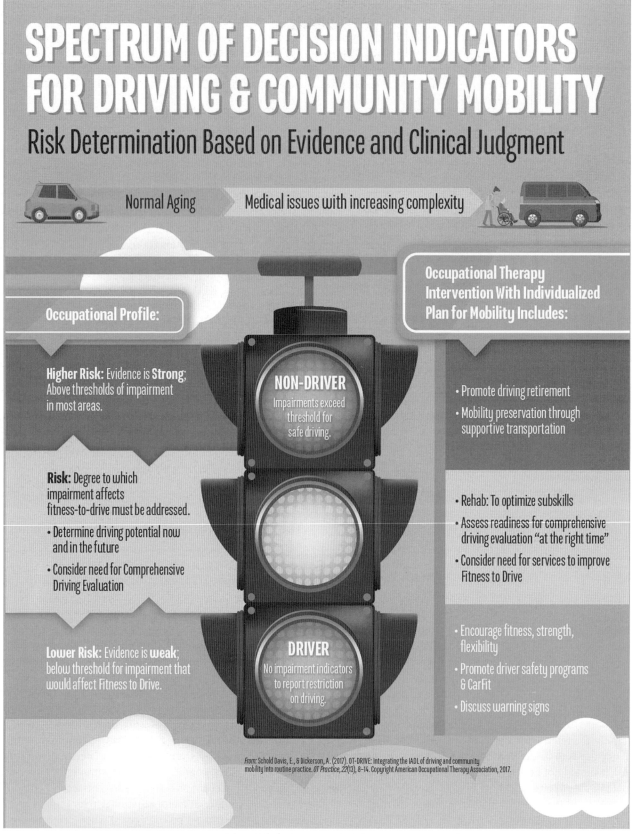

**FIG. 21.3**    Spectrum of decision indicators for driving based on the OT-DRIVE Model. (Courtesy: American Occupational Therapy Association.)

**TABLE 21.2** Generalist's Resource to Integrate Driving (GRID)

### Generalist's Resource to Integrate Driving (GRID)

| Client Factors | Contextual Factors | GREEN | YELLOW: Refer | RED |
|---|---|---|---|---|
| **Medical** | | | | |
| Seizures | Most states have strict criteria for seizures. | ☐ Controlled | ☐ Other medical concerns | ☐ Uncontrolled or recent. |
| Diabetes Control | Some states have criteria. | Decision to refer based on outcomes from screening on physical, vision, sensation and cognition | | ☐ Uncontrolled &/or poor insight or compliance |
| Neurological Status | Consider whether condition is progressive, nonprogressive, stable, remediable. | | | |
| **Falls** | Flag: Multiple falls. | | | |
| **Crashes** | Flag: At-fault crash; multiple minor crashes. | | | |
| **Insight** | Recognition of deficits and how they affect their driving risk. | | If refer to DRS, share information about level of insight. | |
| **Physical Skills** | | | | |
| Strength | Impaired physical capabilities alone should not prevent anyone from being referred. | ☐ Within functional limits | ☐ Impairment that may impact driving. | |
| ROM | | | | |
| Sensation | Individuals who have difficulty understanding the instructions for completing these physical screens should be evaluated primarily on cognition for driving risk. | ☐ No problems | ☐ Impaired sensation either foot | ☐ Unable to follow directions |
| Rapid Pace Walk | | ☐ 5.0 - 7.9 seconds | ☐ 8 or more seconds | |
| Brake Reaction | | ☐ 0.35 - 0.65 seconds | ☐ 0.66 - 1.0 seconds | |
| **Visual Skills** | State Vision Requirements dictate RED | | | |
| Distance Acuity | Acuity is a criterion for driving at all state licensing agencies, but the measure varies between states. If outside of state legal limits, send to a vision specialist for evaluation. | ☐ 20/10 to 20/40 acuity. | ☐ 20/50 to 20/70 | ☐ Vision clearly impacting any ADL/IADL safety issues |
| Visual fields | Some states have visual field criteria, if outside legal limits, send for a vision specialist evaluation **before** a driving evaluation. | ☐ Full visual fields | ☐ Questionable visual fields. | ☐ Obvious neglect or field cut |
| **Cognitive / Perceptual Skills** | | | | |
| AMPS | Occupational performance measure, weigh motor and process scores based on diagnosis. Must be certified rater. | ☐ Motor 2.0 - 4.0 Process 1.3 - 4.0 | ☐ Motor -2.0 to 1.9 and Process 1.0 and up OR Motor 2.0+ and Process is 0.9 - 1.2 | ☐ Process 0.8 or below |
| Trail Making A | Always do the Trails A example first. Time includes cueing for mistakes. | ☐ 0-39 seconds without errors. | ☐ Completed and taking over 40 seconds with or with mistakes. | ☐ Unable to complete |
| Trail Making B | Trails A and Trails B example should be completed. Time includes cueing for mistakes. Stop after 5 minutes. | ☐ 0-90 seconds (with or without corrections) | ☐ Between 1.5 - 3.5 min (with or without corrections) | Any time over 3.5 minutes ☐ with/out corrections; or cannot complete |
| Clock drawing | This clock drawing should follow the directions and scoring from the CADrES from *AGS Clinician's Guide* (Version 3 or 4). | ☐ 0-1 errors | ☐ 2-5 errors | ☐ Obvious distortion with missing elements |
| BCAT* | Brief Cognitive Assessment; Total = 50; should be certified. | ☐ At least 44 out of 50 | ☐ Between 25 to 43 | ☐ Score of 0 to 24 |
| MOCA | Full MOCA; Total = 30 points; should be certified. | ☐ At least a score of 27 | ☐ Between 16 - 26 pts. | ☐ Score of 0 to 15 pts. |
| Snellgrove Maze | This screening tool was designed for dementia; thus, scoring may not be valid for individuals with other types of conditions. | ☐ 0 to 60 seconds & 0 errors | ☐ 0 - 60 seconds with 1-2 errors; 61-90 seconds with 0-2 errors. | ☐ More than 90 seconds, or multiple errors, Cannot do. |

Use with permission:  Anne Dickerson (dickersona@ecu.edu); Susan Touchinsky (susie@adaptivemobility.com) or Terri Cassidy (terri@healthpromotionpartners.com)

Created by Dickerson, A., Touchinsky, S., and Cassidy, T.; Used with permission.

factor that the occupational therapist needs to use their clinical judgment to determine.

The screening scores used for differentiating green, yellow, and red are based on the three pillars of evidence-based medicine (Sackett et al., 1996): (1) research evidence for each screening tool listed, (2) expertise of occupational therapists with significant driving rehabilitation experience, and (3) the clear understanding that driving is a highly valued activity of clients and there are different degrees of risk in diverse contexts. Specifically, the most substantial evidence for using an assessment is used with diverse sample populations. The analysis includes sensitivity and specificity, offering a full range of cut-off scores with their rate of true positives and true negatives. Unfortunately, many research studies that develop cut-off scores are based on a particular population (e.g., dementia) and, therefore, may not be valid for other populations (e.g., stroke, TBI). Cut-off scores are typically based on the concept that a particular score indicates whether the individual is "likely" to pass or fail a driving outcome. The score ranges used in the GRID are designed to indicate that the individual "likely" needs further or specialized evaluation, not for making a licensing decision. However, for those with client factors

clearly in the red, the best practice is to provide occupational therapy interventions to meet the client's community mobility needs by means other than driving to ensure continued social participation. Finally, while there is a list of multiple assessment tools, not all need to be completed. However, it is important to address all the client factors (e.g., medical, falls, crashes, insight, physical skills, visual skills, cognitive/perceptual skills), most of which are likely already in the medical history (e.g., seizures, diabetes control, neurological status). All that needs to be added would be driving history, specifically asking if there are any recent crashes. The following bullets offer other important points to consider when using the GRID.

- Most states require a driver to be seizure free for at least six months; a therapist should check in their state.
- Some states also have requirements about the clients' control of their diabetes. If the diabetes is not under control, the client should not be driving (red). Whether they are green or yellow will depend on the other assessment tools.
- Insight is a therapist's judgement about a client's ability to understand their impairments and take appropriate action. Certainly, this is an important observation to communicate with any referral to an OT-DRS.

Accordingly, if there is no insight, driving should be prohibited with a family member needing to be involved.

- Visual distance acuity is a state-mandated requirement. If the client does not meet the visual requirement for the state, a referral to a visual specialist is the starting point.
- While visual acuity is not associated with crashes (Desapriya et al., 2014), it is important to check for field cuts in individuals with TBI, stroke, or other brain impairments. Instead of determining the exact visual acuity (e.g., 20/20, 20/30, 20/50), if the individual does not have *functional vision* to do everyday tasks, they should not drive.
- Impaired physical capabilities alone should not prevent anyone from being referred, as the OT-DRS can typically find compensatory strategies or equipment. However, if an individual has difficulty understanding the instructions for completing any physical screens, this deficit should be considered in terms of the **cognition risk** rather than a physical risk.
- In the opinion of the GRID's developers and others (Doucet & Gutman, 2013; Gillen, 2013), the *Assessment of Motor and Process Skills* (Fisher & Bray Jones, 2014) is the best occupational therapy evaluation for assessing the IADL of driving. The cutoff scores are based on analysis of over 230 rated drivers. However, occupational therapists are skilled in activity analysis and can use their own judgement in observing other complex IADLs.
- While the other assessments tools listed (e.g., Trail Making Test A & B, Clock- Drawing Test, Brief Cognitive Assessment Tool (BCAT), Montreal Cognitive Assessment [MoCA], Snellgrove Maze) are screening tools, used in the hands of an experienced occupational therapist, they can be used for evaluation. Moreover, you do **not** use all of them. For example, you use the BCAT **or** the MoCA; the Snellgrove Maze was researched on persons with dementia (Snellgrove, 2009), so with a different diagnosis, you need to interpret the results cautiously.
- The Clock-Drawing Test is one of the few that is free of bias from diverse cultural backgrounds and educational levels but has some controversy with how it is scored. Several studies in the literature (Mendez et al., 1992; Shulman et al., 1986; Sunderland et al., 1989) have indicated that the scales by Shulman et al., Mendez et al., and Sunderland et al. showed greater diagnostic accuracy and similar results compared with neuropsychiatric exams.

In summary, the GRID is a clinical reasoning tool. It is not designed to fill in all the boxes using one test, and there is no right or wrong. It can be used as a referral guideline, an actual referral document to send to an OT-DRS or plan interventions, *"We have to work on these areas before we say that you can drive or before we refer you to a DRS/OT."* Regardless, the emphasis should be on occupation-based assessments. While the AMPS is the only performance-based assessment on the GRID, there are others. Use them along with your clinical expertise and astute observation skills to determine the degree of "risk" in the highly complex task of driving.

## Driving Performance

The evaluation of on-road performance is considered distinctive to the practice of the driving rehabilitation and requires an occupational therapist with specialized skills (Dickerson et al., 2012). While additional education is necessary, essentially, the process of observing the on-road performance is the same as other occupational therapy performance assessments since the evaluation is done in the *natural context of the driving environment*. For example, to determine if a client is safe to cook independently, it is best to observe that client in the kitchen making a meal. Thus, it would be best to have the client drive in their natural driving environment to get the best picture of driving competence. The on-road assessment is described as a valid method for determining fitness to drive (Justiss et al., 2006). The challenge is providing a "real enough" driving opportunity to determine driving competence while ensuring the driver's safety and that of the DRS (observers) and other road users. Along with cost, it is the primary justification for developing strategies for general occupational therapists to screen for driving fitness and only sending those who require an on-road assessment (the "yellows") rather than sending *all* clients for the on-road performance assessment (reds and greens!).

## Road Test Versus a Driving Evaluation

What is a driving evaluation? To a licensing agency, it is a 15- to 20-minute test of competency to attain a license. To an occupational therapist with driving rehabilitation expertise, it is a specialized assessment to determine medical fitness to drive. It is important to consider Michon's hierarchy of driving behaviors to understand the differences.

Fig. 21.4 illustrates the three levels of driving behaviors. Driving schools teach novice drivers how to operate and handle the vehicle (operational) and the rules of the road (tactical) and appropriately test at these two levels. Driving instructors direct their students by ordering them to "turn right here, get in this lane"—no self-navigation. The driving instructor's focus is on the new driver by ensuring they stay in their lane, use appropriate pressure on the brake, and leave enough distance between their personal vehicle and other vehicles. After the basic skills are internalized in the driving school, navigation and wayfinding skills are assumed to be reviewed later with parents or mastered with ongoing practice. As stated earlier, state licensing agencies' 10- to 15-minute driving test or evaluation is only concerned with operational and tactical—it is for the novice driver. Therefore, individuals with cognitive impairment often "pass" a driving test by the state—there is no higher cognitive functioning (i.e., strategic) is required. In fact, some states have curtailed "different" tests for older adults because it is considered ageist, and rightly so. Fitness to drive is not based on age but on functional ability. Thus, only when an individual is getting a comprehensive driving evaluation for medical fitness to drive are all three levels examined. Accordingly, occupational therapy practitioners must address driving fitness with all medically-at-risk clients who intend to return to driving.

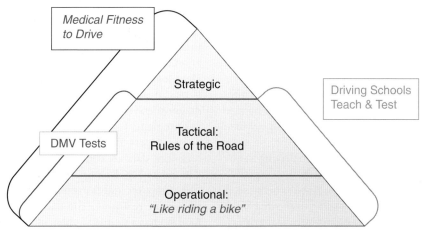

**FIG. 21.4**  Levels of driving behaviors. Michon model redefined (Transportation Research Board, 2016a,b). (Created by A. Dickerson.)

## Driving Simulators

Like the "driving evaluation," a driving simulator is a term that covers a wide range of possibilities, from a simple steering wheel connected to a game console to a fully immersed vehicle in surround sound and video. However, the type of simulator that best represents an effective tool for occupational therapy is the ***interactive driving simulator*** offered by three or four companies that have specifically designed systems for occupational therapy practitioners and/or driving rehabilitation specialists. An interactive driving simulator is defined as a computer-controlled environment that represents selected aspects of the driving experience considered to be representational of real-world driving (TRB, 2016a). The word "interactive" implies that the client responds to the stimuli on the screens with their actions incorporated into the system and continues using those responses. These functional models offer an array of "scenarios" or snippets of driving tasks that are classified by difficulty (e.g., easy, medium difficulty, hard), environments (e.g., urban, rural, foggy, night), hazards (e.g., traffic, pedestrians crossing the road, deer, sudden stops), and an array of traffic maneuvers (e.g., traffic signals, different types of intersections, hills). Some models have additional scenarios of preparatory tasks (i.e., building the skills for using the accelerator or brake pedals, steering accuracy) or multitasking activities (i.e., counting activities, remembering directions, attending to objects appearing on the screens or in mirrors). Simulators allow objective measurements of clients' responses to designated driving tasks and scenarios and how the responses influence subsequent events within the limits of the parameters of the simulation program through the accelerator, brake, and steering components.

There is now clear evidence for the efficacy of using driving simulators for both assessment and intervention in driver rehabilitation (Bedard et al., 2010; Classen & Brooks, 2014). For example, Mazer and colleagues demonstrated in a randomized controlled study with individuals with non-progressive neurological conditions (including stroke) with moderate deficits were more likely to pass an on-road assessment after 16 hours of training on a high-fidelity simulator when compared to those enrolled in a traditional intervention (Mazer et al., 2015). These results are representative of many other studies that suggest driving simulator skills can be generalized to real-world driving, including older adults (Dickerson et al., 2017; Stinchcombe et al., 2017).

The growing research evidence has two significant implications for occupational therapy practice. First, the studies support the concept that performing occupation-based activities provide greater rehabilitation potential. That is not to say that component-based therapy is not useful, but the integration and use of functional tasks at the right level of challenge will improve function over component-based exercise. The second implication is the recognition of recovery of function often occurs over time. Therefore, it is important to make sure clients have adequate resources and information for pursuing driving rehabilitation beyond the short time they are in rehabilitation services.

One of the advantages of the driving simulator is that it can be programmed to present drivers with challenging situations that would be unethical or dangerous in the real world. Similarly, if an unfit driver commits a critical error in the driver simulator, there are no safety consequences for the driver, the therapist, or other road users. Simulated driving evaluations can present drivers with the same situations, allowing some standardization of performance needed to determine driving fitness, which is in contrast to the open road where the driving environment is dependent upon weather and other road users.

On the other hand, one untapped use of the driving simulator is occupational therapy intervention. For clients for whom driving is a valued occupation, using the driving simulator to improve multitasking, motor coordination, attention, scanning, and many other discrete skills is a powerful motivator for working to meet therapy goals. As occupational therapists, we use cooking activities to improve process and motor skills, not teaching them to be chefs. Similarly, using a driving simulator to improve functional capacities should not be coded as "driving" but therapeutic activity. Moreover, the manufacturers of these specialized interactive driving simulators are keen to work with occupational therapy practitioners to meet their needs and typically willing to improve and upgrade scenarios needed by their users.

Driving simulators do have barriers to use in practice. The first is a higher cost, however, their price is relatively similar to other major pieces of equipment, and if used consistently with all types of clients, the cost is recovered. Another barrier to using driver simulators is *simulator adaptation syndrome* or simulator sickness. Simulator sickness is like motion sickness—a physical discomfort experienced when driving a simulated vehicle. It likely occurs because of the incompatible sensations of visual, auditory, and motion systems being seen on the screen. Yet, there is no bodily feeling of moving since you are seated in the simulator. Symptoms include dizziness, headache, cold sweats, nausea, and vomiting. Clients are more susceptible if they are over 70 years of age and female. The contextual design of the scenarios (e.g., curves, turns, stops), duration of the scenario, simulator configuration, and calibration of the brake and accelerator also contribute. However, mitigation strategies can be effective and include diet (not an empty stomach), a cool room temperature and airflow, and keeping turns to a minimum (Stern & Akinwuntan, 2012). Moreover, many of the more straightforward or shorter scenarios of simulators are designed for the lowest risk of simulator sickness, and building a tolerance for using simulators is possible with a skilled practitioner (Stern & Akinwuntan, 2012).

Another barrier to driving simulators is training. Driving simulators may seem deceptively easy to use. However, a driving simulator is a very complex tool, and the occupational therapist wanting to use it "needs to seek and obtain the appropriate education and training to use this tool effectively, appropriately, and with the knowledge to minimize simulator sickness" (Classen & Brooks, 2014). Fortunately, a textbook is available for occupational therapy practitioners that includes descriptions of types of simulators, information on how to use simulators, evaluation and intervention for a wide variety of populations, and practical knowledge for using driving simulators for clients (Classen & American Occupational Therapy, 2017).

## Naturalistic Driving

Since driving is an overlearned task, controlled conditions like a road test or driving simulator may not reflect driving as it occurs daily or expose errors made by experienced or cognitively normal drivers outside of these controlled conditions. Some critical considerations include vehicle preference (e.g., truck, van, car), specific local or regional laws governing driving, and behavior/customs of driving (e.g., more honking in larger cities). These are not necessarily accounted for within the road test assessment. Some limitations of all road tests include the use of an unfamiliar car, driving on unfamiliar roads, performance anxiety (poor performance) or the Hawthorne effect (better performance due to being watched), and reliability of the evaluator and the scoring system (Eby et al., 2012). One alternative method is to record, store, and assess naturalistic driving behaviors using GPS methods.

These are in-vehicle data loggers, which provide precise data on distance traveled per trip, number of trips per day, time and location, speeding, hard braking, sudden acceleration, ability to detect minor and major vehicle impacts. Data loggers have several novel key advantages. The device is placed under the dashboard and plugs into the onboard diagnostic systems (OBD II) port with minimal installation requirements (~1 minute). It is not readily visible to drivers or passengers and has a minimal impact on driving behaviors. Raw data are collected and transformed into analyzable data related to driving. All data are extracted from the vehicle's computer and transmitted via mobile towers to secured servers in real-time. The data extraction and transmission method has a significant benefit; if a vehicle is driven in areas where the signal is lost, data are collected and then re-transmitted when a strong signal is established. As a result, one can capture the individual's driving behavior in their vehicle as an environment over substantial periods of time in order to examine changes in driving behaviors (Babulal et al., 2016; Babulal et al., 2017; Roe et al., 2019).

## Report (Self/Collateral Source)

Personal accounts of driving activity and behavior provide invaluable information that may not be discernable from laboratory-controlled or naturalistic methodologies. If the driver is aware of changes in their behavior or changes are observed by a family member or friend, this information can support a more comprehensive assessment in the absence of objective data. The Driving Habits Questionnaire (DHQ) is a self-reported form that captures information about driving behavior and preferences (e.g., avoiding rush hour, inclement weather, night driving), driving area, space, number of miles and trips, crashes, and traffic citations experienced over the past year (Owsley et al., 1999). We know that the process of aging is associated with increased self-regulation and more restricted driving space (Langford & Koppel, 2006). The DHQ is the conventional measure of driving self-regulation (Wong et al., 2015), has good test-retest reliability (Song et al., 2015), and is acceptable to older adults (Molnar et al., 2007). This can inform an occupational therapist's evaluation of the driving performance and behavior.

## Transportation Planning

### Aging in Place

Older adults want to remain in their homes and communities. As occupational therapists, it is our duty to work with clients towards their valued goals, including remaining in their homes and connected to their communities. However, the reality is that for many older adults, there will be a time when driving retirement is necessary. We know that men outlive their driving ability by 6 years and women by 10 years (Foley et al., 2002). This is often very difficult to accept (Patomella et al., 2009) and in fact, many individuals continue to drive regardless of the medical recommendation (Coughlin & D'Ambrosio, 2012).

Typically, if driving is not possible due to medical impairments, public transportation is not an option for the same functional reasons (Silverstein et al., 2016). This will further eliminate many social activities that are important to maintain contact with others. Although transportation network companies or E-hail (e.g., taxis, Uber, Lyft) may be seen as expensive, one strategy is to work out a budget with the client to show that these services may be cheaper than owning a car and paying for maintenance, gas, parking, and insurance.

## Maintaining Community Mobility

With clients who must retire from driving, the occupational therapy practitioner needs to address their community mobility needs through transportation planning, beyond just offering the client and family information and a list of resources. Analyzing the actual transportation needs of the client—that is, where they need and want to go with family and friends, not only assists with planning but helps the therapist address the client's anxiety of not knowing what to do. A new tool has been developed to assist in this process called the *Checklist of Community Mobility* (Dickerson & Schold Davis, 2020). Based on the same concept as the OT-DRIVE, the Checklist was designed to use the occupational therapist's expert knowledge of functional capacities to describe the supports needed for the client's successful negotiation of the environmental complexities of community mobility. Using the listed functional areas, the therapist determines if the client can perform the required tasks independently, with assistance, or with difficulty. Then using the guidance statements on the Checklist, the therapist can assist the client, family member, or social worker with the appropriate type of transportation needed for the client. For example, if a person with dementia can walk and climb stairs but cannot communicate with a driver or problem-solve, that individual would need a specialized service that provides door-through-door assistance. While this Checklist cannot specify services in geographic areas, the tool can educate family members and transportation providers. Fig. 21.5 is a copy of the Checklist.

Finally, since IADL driving and community mobility have an essential role for older adults, we, as occupational therapists, can play an important role in health promotion. We must promote **Transportation Planning**. Just as people plan for financial and work retirement, they must plan when they will no longer be able to drive. As therapists, we understand the need to stay connected to our community and participate socially with family and friends. Thus, we must provide information and strategies for this process. As part of a funded demonstration project from the National Highway Traffic Safety Administration, a website was developed by an occupational therapist called *Plan for the Road Ahead*. It is a website dedicated to older adults planning for their future transportation and is free of advertisements. It includes many interactive tools for therapists to use with their clients and/or for older adults on their own.

## Role of Technology in Improving Safety

With technology growing exponentially, self-driving cars' concept may be the answer in the future. However, the idea that fully automated motor vehicles are ready to roll out and take away our transportation problems is simply inaccurate. While some functioning "driverless" vehicles exist, at this point, their range, speed, and abilities are limited. Moreover, what is often overlooked is that the infrastructure (e.g., roads, buildings, traffic signals) also needs the technology to communicate with a vehicle, and at this point, perfect weather conditions are required. Driving in snow, rain, or rural areas would not be possible. Other issues yet to be resolved include the legal ramifications of crashes, situational awareness if and when a driver needs to take control immediately, and determining the criteria for a "license" to use an automated vehicle. Finally, it is crucial to understand that it will take years to make the transition when a driverless vehicle becomes available. Presently, it takes at least two decades for new technology to be on most registered vehicles. For example, as of 2014, rearview cameras and video displays are required on new vehicles. However, the Highway Loss Data Institute (HLDI) predicts that it will not be until 2039 that 95% of registered vehicles will have rear cameras (Bulletin, 2012; Cicchino, 2018).

However, amazing strides have been made in automating aspects of driving to improve driver safety and comfort. They are captured across two general categories: crash avoidance systems (CAS) and Advanced Driver Assistance Systems (ADAS). CAS provides warnings to prevent potential crashes, such as lane departure warnings, forward collision warnings, and blind-spot warnings. Current research has found that forward collision warning systems have decreased front-to-rear crashes by 27%, front-to-rear crashes with injuries by 20%, and large truck-to-rear crashes by 44% (Cicchino, 2018). In another study, rates from lane change crashes with blind side monitoring systems were 14% lower than crashes of vehicles without blind spot warnings (Cicchino, 2018). Also, the combination of rear-vision cameras and parking assistance reduced backing crash involvement by 42% (Cicchino, 2019). For older adults, rear cameras cut crashes by 40% for drivers 70 and older, compared to 15% for younger drivers (Cicchino, 2017).

ADAS provides timely information to assist drivers by providing night vision enhancement, navigational assistance, adaptive cruise control, and adaptive headlights. While these systems may be helpful for older adults, they only work if they are used. Research from manufacturers on the status of systems being on and off reported that lane maintenance systems are more frequently considered annoying and are turned "off" in 25% to 79% of the vehicles, depending on the vehicle type (Cicchino, 2017).

## Barriers to Technology

There are barriers to adopting the ADAS technology by older adults (Trubswetter & Bengler, 2013). First, older adults do not necessarily perceive the systems as useful and demonstrate a lack of trust. This is likely because older drivers do not fully understand the operations of the technology and actually may incorrectly use the assistance (Dickerson et al., 2019a). For example, they may mistakenly attribute collision prevention features to adaptive cruise control. In addition, a study found when

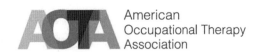

aota.org

**Occupational Therapy Checklist of Community Mobility Skills (CCMS)**

**Objective:** This tool merges individual functional mobility with demands required by transportation type to assist in indentifying transportation options that support and/or increase safe and effective community mobility.

**Directions:** Indicate the level of independence/assistance needed for each functional area. Identify the types of transportation options available in the community (indicate the support offered if possible). Then, highlight transportation options most feasible to support the individual's mobility. Consider also that each destination may require a different transporation option.

| Functional Areas: Is the individual able to: | Perform Independently | Perform with assistance | Perform with difficulty/unable | Comments |
|---|---|---|---|---|
| 1. Walk one block | | | | |
| 2. Walk briskly to cross street with pace of "Walk" signal | | | | |
| 3. Climb two steps | | | | |
| 4. Climb two sets of stairs | | | | |
| 5. Physically maneuver in a new environment | | | | |
| 6. Get in and out of a car | | | | |
| 7. Ready and independently wait near entrance/exit | | | | |
| 8. Secure own seatbelt | | | | |
| 9. Manage personal mobility devices (e.g., cane, walker, wheelchair) | | | | |
| 10. Read and decipher a schedule | | | | |
| 11. Read and decipher a map | | | | |
| 12. Manage money/money card | | | | |
| 13. Recognize the need and have the ability to call 911 | | | | |
| 14. Consistently use a cellphone | | | | |
| 15. Communicate all needs with driver | | | | |
| 16. Problem solve when a problem occurs with transportation | | | | |
| 17. Know, recognize, and communicate location (pickup and destination) | | | | |
| 18. Communicate identification information and/or phone number | | | | |
| 19. Communicate date and time of trip | | | | |
| 20. Use voice-based travel technology | | | | |

**Public Transportation (e.g., bus, subway, train)**
*Requires individual to be able to:*
A. Walk various lengths to the designated stops for pickup and destinations
B. Handle one to four steps to board/get off
C. Have good mobility, including balance
D. Appropriately handle a crowded social environment or the need to wait
E. Manage money and/or money card**
F. Communicate needs of when they need to stop**
G. Have higher cognitive skills for complex environments**
H. Read a schedule and/or route**
I. Cognitively adjust if service is running behind or ahead of schedule**

**Guidance Statements for Public Transport:**
● If the individual can perform abilities 1 through 20, they will likely be successful in using public transportation.
● If the individual can perform abilities 1 through 9 independently, but needs assistance with abilities 10 through 20, a companion is recommended.
● If the individual can perform abilities 1 through 9 independently, with potential to learn abilities 12, 13, 14, and 15 for a specific routine route, consider mobility manangement.

Transportation while seated in wheelchair: consult accessible transit, paratransit, or Driving Rehabilitation

***indicates could be completed by a companion escort/caregiver***

**Transportation Network Services (TNS)**
**(e.g., taxi, Uber, Lyft, Go-Go Grandparent):**
*Requires individual to be able to:*
A. Walk at least short distances to locate car
B. Enter and exit a car independently
C. Fasten own seatbelt with no assistance
D. Manage all mobility equipment with minimal assistance
E. Communicate needs to driver including destination and location**
F. Navigate unfamiliar environments**
G. Manage money/money card/electronic account**
H. Able to recognize the need and have the ability to call 911**
I. Consistently use a cell phone
J. Problem solve unexpected events

**Guidance Statements for TNS:**
● If the individual can perform abilities 1 through 20, they will likely be successful in using TNS.
● If the individual can perform abilities 1 through 9 independently, but need assistance with abilities 10 through 20, a companion is recommended.
● If the individual can perform abilities 1 through 9 independently, identifies specific destination needs and can use a phone, programs with added support may be successful (such as Go-Go Grandparent)

**Supplemental/Assisted Ride Programs offer:**
I. Door through door—The driver will assist individual to and from their home as well as at destination; may provide limited assistance with a new environment.
II. Door to door—The driver will assist individual in/out of car and to door, however, rider has to navigate to and from destination independently.
III. Curb to curb—The driver will pick up and drop off individual at curb.
*Required skills vary depending on type of transportation; Individuals should be able to:*
A. Transfer in/out of a car with limited assistance from driver
B. Buckle their seat belt with limited assistance from driver
C. Identify self and contact information
D. Call and schedule a ride**
E. Appropriately handle money/money card/ticket system**
F. Communicate needs during the trip with the driver**
G. Report location to driver**
H. Use a cell phone**
I. Handle medical/mobility equipment such as a cane, walker or wheelchair with limited assistance from driver
J. Able to recognize the need and have the ability to call 911**
**Guidance Statements for Ride Programs:**
Program services and supports vary greatly. Typically a needs assessment is conducted to set up an individualized program. The rider may then consistently access the services.

**FIG. 21.5**    Occupational therapy checklist of community mobility skills (CCMS). (Courtesy: American Occupational Therapy Association.)

training older adults on the use of the in-vehicle information systems (e.g., hands-free commands), the workload of the driver was increased, and practice did not eliminate interference with driving. Therefore, more research is needed to understand older adults' use of the technology, including the older adults' unique needs and learning styles. Work also needs to consider behavioral adaptations (e.g., less use of turn signals with blind-spot detection), real-world safety benefits, and most importantly, the effect on situational awareness or the ability to take over when using automation (e.g., adaptive cruise control) (Dickerson et al., 2019a).

There is no question that these technologies can increase the safety of older adults and have real-world benefits. However, occupational therapists need to work with their clients and family members to determine if the client has the capacity to learn and understand the new systems. Of course, the most significant barrier is cost. Most of these systems are on the top models of manufacturers and, even then, are considered options. Nevertheless, for the older drivers who can afford them with the cognitive ability to learn and understand their use, the new systems may prolong the driving life of these drivers. A knowledgeable therapist can offer meaningful information.

## Global Positioning System Use for Wayfinding

An excellent low-cost option to improve safety is an electronic navigational system using GPS. A study examined if GPS use improved older drivers' safety on unfamiliar routes by comparing performance between drivers familiar and unfamiliar with GPS (Thomas et al., 2020). It also explored whether training with GPS impacted performance for those who were unfamiliar. Results demonstrated that all drivers made fewer driving errors when using GPS than using paper directions when driving in unknown areas, and those familiar with the GPS did better. The study also found that drivers in their 60s made fewer mistakes than those in their 70s. When asked to program a GPS, naturally, those participants who previously used the GPS did better than those who had not used one.

In the second study (Thomas et al., 2020), three types of training were used to learn how to use the GPS: video training only, video and hands-on training, and a control group. Not surprisingly, the hands-on group did significantly better than the control group and the video-only group. There was also a significant difference between the control and video-only groups. The results of these studies have important implications for occupational therapy practitioners. First, therapists should encourage their clients to use a GPS, especially for unfamiliar areas. If they are unfamiliar, providing information on using them is helpful. Unlike vehicle technology, a GPS device is relatively inexpensive and is easily installed in any age or type vehicle. However, as with recommendations, occupational therapy practitioners must use their clinical judgment. Using a GPS may not be appropriate with cognitively impaired drivers, as GPS technology is sometimes wrong or cannot predict a closed roadway or street under construction. Cognitively impaired drivers may blindly follow the GPS instead of making a judgment that technology has made an error. Therefore, a GPS should not be recommended when driving cessation should be the outcome.

## Autonomous Vehicles

Technological advances over several decades have propelled the development and testing of driverless, self-driving, or autonomous vehicles (AVs) at an unprecedented pace. These vehicles rely upon an exceptionally sophisticated system of cameras, lasers, sensors, GPS, robotic mapping algorithm, and computer vision, all continuously working in real-time to navigate a vehicle. Adoption of AVs is anticipated to significantly reduce crashes and resulting injuries and fatalities, while also saving billions annually (Fagnant & Kockelman, 2015). The popularity of AVs in the media has only increased since companies like Google, Tesla, and Lyft have invested money and time into AV technology to test their AV fleets on public roads.

In 2014, the Society for Automotive Engineers (SAE) published the Taxonomy for Automated Driving System, which has since become the industry standard for outlining specific parameters that define automation levels (0 to 5), ranging from none to full automation of all driving modes. The AV industry is currently transitioning from partial automation (level 2) to conditional automation (level 3). At SAE level 3, automation is only available to some driving modes, and the driver is still responsible for resuming manual control following a warning signal. Currently, no automotive manufacturer offers a level 3 AV. It is unclear how long it will take to get to level 5; some estimates project into 2050 with sustained progress and funding (Jeon et al., 2016; Milakis et al., 2017). Current estimates of consumer cost of a level 3 AV are difficult to find; however, a self-driving sensor alone costs $75,000. Technology costs will need to be radically reduced to improve affordability while retaining reliable AV sensors. Research into how AVs impact travel demands, traffic flow, decision-making processes, emissions, and energy consumption is slowly emerging. There are no federal or state guidelines on licensing and testing for AVs. Similarly, legislation concerning liability, blame, and burden of proof in collisions and AV misuse (e.g., drunk driving, recklessness) are unwritten (Fagnant & Kockelman, 2015). Finally, the acceptability of AVs and managing expectations of the general public need to be addressed. A survey of 5000 drivers across the world showed that drivers were very concerned with software hacking, how to handle legal issues with crashes, the safety of AVs, data transmission from AVs (Kyriakidis et al., 2015). Greater automation increases driver dependency and reduces the ability to intervene in the event of a cyber-attack resulting in compromised AV security and privacy (Milakis et al., 2017). Motion sickness is also very common in travel via AVs and needs to be remedied (Diels & Bos, 2016). Adoption and use of AVs in the aging population will require technological training and driver education programs to update driving skills (Yang & Coughlin, 2014).

*The complete listing of the Bibliography and Chapter Questions and Answers are available in the accompanying enhanced eBook version included with the print purchase of this textbook. Visit Elsevier eBooks+ (eBooks.Health.Elsevier.com) to access this content.*

# CHAPTER 22

# Assistive Technology: Supports for Aging Adults

*Kimberly A. Furphy, DHSc, OTR and David C. Burdick, PhD, FGSA, FAGHE*

## CHAPTER OUTLINE

## OBJECTIVES

- Appreciate how population aging increases the need for occupational therapy services, and how the application of various assistive technologies can enhance those services
- Understand and apply some conceptual models linking humans to their environmental contexts when adding multiple technologies
- Understand and appreciate other fields' conceptual models to improve one's interprofessional competencies
- Become more aware of various low- and high- technology devices and technologies that can aid in the provision of occupational therapy services to the aged and disabled
- Understand that despite the push for the latest gadgets and gizmos, several low-technology devices continue to best serve older clients
- Understand and practice in a care environment that will increasingly utilize automation, home and behavior monitoring, telehealth, and other smart technologies
- Apply general concepts learned about the strengths and weaknesses of current and emerging AgeTech technologies

covered in this chapter to opportunities and threats posed by future technological developments
- Demonstrate increased ability to find additional information and resources on the topics addressed in this chapter

## Introduction

Readers of other chapters now understand the "megatrend" of population aging, and important recent paradigm shifts (e.g., successful aging, interdisciplinary collaboration/competencies, aging in place, and perhaps Institute for Health Care Improvement [2020] 4Ms: What Matters, Mentation, Medication, and Mobility) that provide context to their work. These developments will increasingly affect service provision by occupational therapy (OT) and other health professions to older adults in coming years. This chapter builds upon this knowledge and presents technological innovation as another dramatic megatrend and potential "game-changer" for OT service provision in diverse settings. When properly designed, deployed, maintained, available, and used, technological tools can allow older adults to maintain independence longer, reduce costs, and contribute to a sense of empowerment, life satisfaction, and well-being. Technological tools that do not possess these characteristics can result in frustration, unnecessary expense, abandonment, and harm through risks of higher morbidity and mortality. So, "buyer beware" is an appropriate caution in this discussion. Several factors impact one's decision to utilize assistive devices, including affordability, accessibility and knowledge of the availability of the device, prior experience with the device, ease of learning and the user-friendliness of the device (Lee & Coughlin, 2015). A daunting and growing array of hardware, software, and online products makes it difficult for consumers and providers to choose what is best. For example, AssistiveTechnology.us provides information on equipment vendors, funding resources, and resources for obtaining AT devices. Such resources assist the consumer and practitioner find, select, and acquire appropriate technological tools (Table 22.1).

**Acknowledgements:** The authors wish to thank our co-author from the original 2016 version of this chapter, Dr. Debra Lindstrom-Hazel, for her substantial contributions, and Kerstin Maguire, Health Sciences major, Gerontology minor, and pre-Physical Therapy student at Stockton University, for her assistance in updating references and citations, updating review questions, and in drafting an abstract.

**TABLE 22.1** Listing of Assistive Devices by Intended Function or Special Feature: Function, Description, and Major Categories

| Device Function Type and Description | Major Categories |
|---|---|
| Aids for Daily Living: Products to aid in activities of daily living | Bathing, carrying, childcare, clothing, dispenser aids, dressing, drinking, feeding, grooming/hygiene, handle padding, health care, holding, reaching, time, smoking, toileting, transfer |
| Blind and Low Vision: Products for people with visual disabilities | Computers, educational aids, health care, information storage, kitchen aids, labeling, magnification, office equipment, orientation and mobility, reading, recreation, sensors, telephones, time, tools, travel, typing, writing (braille) |
| Communication: Products to help people with disabilities related to speech, writing, and other methods of communication | Alternative and augmentative communication, head wands, mouth sticks, signal systems, telephones, typing, writing |
| Computers: Products to allow people with disabilities to use desktop and laptop computers and other kinds of information technology | Software, hardware, computer accessories |
| Controls: Products that provide people with disabilities with the ability to start, stop, or adjust electric or electronic devices | Environmental controls, control switches |
| Deaf and Hard of Hearing: Products for people with hearing disabilities | Amplification, driving, hearing aids, recreational electronics, sign language, signal switches, speech training, telephones, time |
| Education: Products to provide people with disabilities with access to educational materials and instruction in school and in other learning environments | Classroom, instructional materials |
| Environmental Adaptations: Products that make the built environment more accessible | Indoor environment, furniture, outdoor environment, vertical accessibility, houses, polling place accessibility, lighting, signs |
| Housekeeping: Products that assist in cooking, cleaning, and other household activities; adapted appliances | Food preparation, housekeeping, general cleaning, ironing, laundry, shopping |
| Orthotics: Braces and other products to support or supplement joints or limbs | Head and neck, lower extremity, torso, upper extremity |
| Prosthetics: Products for amputees | Lower extremity, upper extremity |
| Recreation: Products to assist people with disabilities with their leisure and athletic activities | Crafts, electronics, gardening, music, photography, sewing, sports, toys |
| Safety and Security: Products to protect health and home | Alarm and security systems, childproof devices, electric cords, lights, locks |
| Seating: Products that assist people to sit comfortably and safely | Seating systems, cushions, therapeutic seats |
| Therapeutic Aids: Products that assist in treatment for health problems and therapy and training for certain disabilities | Ambulation training, biofeedback, evaluation, exercise, fine and gross motor skills, perceptual motor, positioning, pressure/massage modality equipment, respiratory aids, rolls, sensory integration, stimulators, therapy furnishings, thermal/water modality equipment, traction |
| Transportation: Products to enable people with disabilities to drive or ride in cars, vans, trucks, and buses | Mass-transit vehicles and facilities, vehicles, vehicle accessories |
| Walking: Products to aid people with disabilities who are able to walk or stand with assistance | Canes, crutches, standing walkers |
| Wheeled Mobility: Products and accessories that enable people with mobility disabilities to move freely indoors and outdoors | Wheelchairs (manual, sport, and powered), wheelchair alternatives (scooters), wheelchair accessories, carts, transporters, stretchers |
| Workplace: Products to aid people with disabilities at work | Agricultural equipment, office equipment, tools, vocational assessment, vocational training, workstations |

Adapted from AssistiveTechnology.us.

In this chapter, we first provide a brief introduction to the concepts of technology, gerontechnology, and AgeTech as a conceptual framework and roadmap for what follows. Next, we address effective low-technology devices that support activities of daily living (ADLs) and instrumental activities of daily living (IADLs). The current authors (Furphy & Burdick) have made several revisions to this section from the first edition (Furphy et al. 2016) but wish to acknowledge the significant contributions made in the first edition by our co-author Debra Lindstrom-Hazel. We then turn to higher-tech devices, often electronic, involving computer and/or telecommunications technology, frequently called intelligent assistive technologies (IATs) or more recently "AgeTech" (Fang, 2022, Woods, 2019), that support the work of occupational therapists and enhance the well-being of their older adult clients. These areas include telehealth, telemedicine, robotics, smart houses, and other computer assistive technologies. In this section of the chapter, we have made the most significant alterations and updates due to dramatic developments and new technologies such as smartphone apps, artificial intelligence (AI), and virtual reality (VR).

There have been dramatic developments in the field of gerontechnology (defined below), in the past 20 years. Joseph Coughlin, director of the MIT AgeLab, suggests that we have entered the "Fourth Wave" of technology and aging, which focuses on the wants of older adults and not just their needs, and where the fruits of significant research and market forces related to the "silver economy" and aging of the baby boomers have made technology use more ubiquitous ("Technology has become the new toilet paper" during the COVID-19 epidemic). In this "Fourth Wave," he argues that policy innovations must encourage equity and inclusion, build on previous waves, and briefly describes how we should make broadband like water, provide smart buyers and advisors, provide trusted training, ensure affordability, and establish safeguards (Coughlin, 2020).

## Technology, Tools, and Gerontechnology

We first provide definitions, intended to guide the OT provider in understanding and applying information subsequently addressed in the chapter. *Technology* generally refers to the practical application of basic knowledge. It usually extends capacities or capabilities over space and time and increases efficiency in carrying out various tasks. Earlier we used the term *technological tool*. A tool is either "a handheld device—including smartphone apps—that aids in the accomplishment of a task," "something used in performing an operation or necessary task in the practice of a vocation or profession," or simply "a means to an end" (Tool, 2015). Although the term *technological tool* seems redundant, we use it to promote an important concept—our gadgets and gizmos do not just appear out of nowhere, and do not operate (effectively, at least) in a vacuum. Instead, they must be understood and used as part of a broader multidimensional and dialectic context. *Multidimensional* because they involve individuals and groups (clients, caregivers, designers, manufacturers, distributors, salespersons, providers) within organizational,

economic, and environmental contexts. *Dialectic* because these relationships are multi-directional, reciprocal, and ever-changing (Kutzik & Burdick, 2014).

*Gerontechnology* studies the complex relationship of biopsychosocial aspects of human aging and multiple forms of technology, primarily information/communication technology (computers and mobile devices), assistive devices, medical devices, and home modifications. *Gerontechnology* refers to the application of this study to the development and deployment of technological tools that help to meet the needs and fulfill the wishes of older adults, and that provide enhanced quality of life and life satisfaction, through support for aging in place, community/family engagement, and participation in ADLs. Gerontechnology involves scholars and researchers from a wide variety of basic and applied sciences and from the arts and humanities who, for example, consider ethical issues.

## Themes and Issues Concerning Gerontechnology and Occupational Therapy Practice

As you read the chapter, it will be helpful to keep in mind the following themes and issues that have bearing on the effective utilization of technological devices:

**Cost and Payment Options:** What does it cost to *purchase* and *maintain* a device, app, or online service? Do supplies need continual replenishment? Are "loan closets" available/accessible that provide free use of recycled medical equipment? Do third parties pay for purchase, training, maintenance, and supplies?

**Barriers to Use**: Besides cost, are there other barriers to device or service use? Barriers include emotional concerns (e.g., perceived stigmatization) and cognitive barriers such as lack of awareness that a product/solution exists. Other barriers include difficulty in use or lack of adequate instructions; ethical considerations, such as privacy and monitoring technologies; and access barriers such as limited vendors and limited, inefficient, or ineffective repair services. Inordinate fears about online consumer fraud can be mitigated with adequate training and safeguards, allowing elders to safely and comfortably conduct online financial transactions. We elaborate on some of these issues later in the chapter.

**Durability and Adaptability:** These two characteristics relate to cost and efficacy. Regardless of the type (high-technology or low-technology), is it durable if the device is intended for long-term use? Is it still useful if the person's condition worsens (or improves)? Can it adapt if user needs change?

**Evidence-Based and Best Practice:** Which devices are evidence-based interventions and "best practice" for specific conditions? Do they result from translational research (basic research that directly benefits humans)? Unfortunately, many businesses market and sell products of dubious quality and value. It is crucial, yet often difficult, to differentiate between appropriate/effective products and modern variants of "snake oil" using "technobabble" to confuse and deceive unsuspecting older adults and care partners. Between the two extremes are devices and technologies that vary by cost and effectiveness. Clearly, high-technology is not necessary or appropriate when low-technology or human assistance/intervention are available, affordable, and appropriate.

**Enabling Versus Disabling:** The provision of technological devices to an older person can have an array of outcomes based upon the specific interaction of that person's needs and abilities and the demand characteristics of their environment. Lawton and Nahemow's Ecological Model (Lawton, 1980; see also Chapter 20) helps predict these results by comparing an individual competence in functional domain with the demand (or press) characteristics of one's environment. When competence is slightly above press, the individual can complete a task with minimal effort. The model describes this as being in a *state of maximum comfort*. If the press is slightly above competence, the individual is in *the maximum performance potential zone*, likened to setting the bar just slightly above the person's capabilities. In this case, there is a rehabilitative opportunity that OTs should consider. To be avoided are situations where press and competence are widely mismatched, because the result is commonly negative emotions (ranging from frustration to boredom) and/or maladaptive behaviors (declining capacities, harmful or risky activities). Occupational therapists are accustomed to providing appropriate technologies to reduce the press, creating better balance between press and competence, and yielding desirable and therapeutic outcomes. Yet, client overdependence on assistive devices can, for example, precipitate further declines in clients' abilities, make them more likely to fall when ambulating, or limit their ability to access multiple environments if the assistive devices are tied to the environments in which they are housed.

## Other General Considerations: Demographics, Secular Trends, and Conceptual Models

The demographic imperative presented by population aging in the United States, Europe, Asia, and elsewhere requires new care models and approaches. In 2019, the number of persons in the United States over 65 years of age had grown to 54.1 million, comprising 16% of the total population (Administration for Community Living, 2021). The older population is projected to continue to grow, reaching 80 million by 2050, at which time there will also be an estimated 19 million people over 85 years of age (Ortman et al., 2014). Burgeoning numbers of people who are old and old-old and suffering from chronic conditions and impairments in ADLs and IADLs, coupled with a shortage of family caregivers, growing ethnic and cultural diversity, issues of health-care reform and the push for cost containment, and other social changes, have all enhanced the role of occupational therapists and the importance of assistive technologies.

Population aging and other secular trends (such as increasing obesity and type 2 diabetes) have a clear influence on the prevalence and effects of ADL and IADL limitations. Although during the 1990s there were consistent findings of a slow but consistent decline in disability rates among older persons in the United States (particularly in IADLs), more recent research may indicate that this trend has reversed. Growing evidence suggests that the first year or two of COVID-19 lockdown and social distancing may have led to declines in physical, psychological, and social function among older adults, which would also lead to declining capacity in ADLs and IADLs that could be mitigated by or rehabilitated with appropriate technological devices (Flanagan et al., 2020; Hoffman et al., 2021; Kirwan et al., 2020).

The growing movement in North America, Europe, and Asia toward the development of interprofessional competencies in gerontological care is also a significant paradigm shift that is effectively addressed and intertwined throughout this book, and that has enhanced importance in this chapter (Choi & Park, 2021; Goldberg et al., 2012; Politynska et al., 2012). Whereas a social worker's comfort zone for interdisciplinarity includes teammates from nursing, medicine, psychology, and perhaps OT or physical therapy, the modern occupational therapist involved in technological applications may need to work with those specialists in addition to those from human factors/ergonomics, neuroscience, telecommunications, computer and industrial design, and others. (See also Chapter 30 regarding interdisciplinary processes.)

In considering the influence of technologies in the care of older adults and people with disabilities, it is useful to consider conceptual models and rubrics, such as Lawton and Nahemow's. Helpful review of conceptual models for assistive technologies are provided by Lenker & Paquet (2003) and Burdick (2016, 2018). Birkland's (2019) Information and Communication Technology (ICT) User Typology, discussed below in our "High Technology" section, is also valuable.

Chapter 4 also considers other models for the general provision of OT. The Rehabilitation Engineering and Assistive Technology Society of North America (RESNA) includes the Human, Activity, Assistive Technology (HAAT) Model in training for the RESNA Assistive Technology Practitioner Certification Exam. HAAT encourages assistive technology practitioners, human factors engineers, and psychologists to consider the complex interactions of three variables: (1) a person, (2) acting or behaving, in (3) a context, especially when the use of assistive technology is part of that context (Cook et al., 2020).

Fozard (2005), a major contributor to the study of gerontechnology, designed a useful classification matrix to elucidate the array of domains where technologies have potential influence and the nature of their influence. The technologies discussed in this chapter can be recommended by occupational therapists and used by older adults to have multiple and spreading effects on physical, psychological/emotional, social, spiritual, and economic well-being. Fozard (2005) classifies human activity into five areas or domains (Health & Self-Esteem, Housing & Daily Living, Mobility & Transport, Communication & Governance, and Work & Leisure) and four effects (Prevention or Delay of Decline, Compensation for Age-Related Loss, Care Support & Organization, and Enhanced Satisfaction with Quality of Life). It is essential for the occupational therapist always to be mindful of the nature of the technology/device recommended or utilized, the potential domain(s) of its effects, and the scope or range of potential influence on the older adult's life and well-being. This taxonomy relates to both our earlier discussion of press/competence and the technology categories described next.

Although occupational therapists have their own taxonomies and professional jargon, it is important to develop comfort with the models/methods of other professions that work with older adults.

## Contextual Complexities for Application of Technology in Occupational Therapy Practice

A recent review of the literature on smartphone and tablet use by older adults demonstrates the complexities of the issues involved. Focusing on articles studying everyday smartphone or tablet use for cognition, memory, or ADLs, the authors found that these devices are "seen by users as acceptable, enjoyable, and non-stigmatizing alternatives to conventional assistive technology devices," but barriers include limited digital literacy, less than optimal accommodation for sensory/motor capacities of elders, and limited input from or collaboration with researchers and clinicians (Wilson et al., 2022, p. 1). While over 70% of older adults used the Internet in 2021 (up from 12% in 2000) and 90% of older adults now own cell phones, only 60% have smartphones. Looking more closely at the data, the authors noted that socioeconomic barriers must also be addressed: those with a high school education or less, with income less than $30,000, from rural settings, and Black/African American elders were least likely to use technology. Persistent gaps are also reported between those with and without disabilities. So, we (collectively) have our work cut out for us, and issues of diversity, equity, and inclusion and intersectionality must be considered as trends are evaluated.

Each year, MIT Technology Review magazine publishes a list of 10 breakthrough technologies. The reader might google this phrase "MIT 10 breakthrough technologies" and add the year for a point-in-time update of recent developments. The number one development in 2022 was listed as "The End of Passwords" (Editors, 2022). This may end an annoyance for many users and be particularly useful in helping elders to accomplish IADLs via online services and smartphone apps.

The COVID-19 pandemic seems to have dramatically accelerated older adults' usage of technology. As the next cohort (50- to 64-year-olds) age, digital technology use will become more universal and occupational therapists can expect to more easily utilize a wide array of digital/electronic technologies with their older clients.

## Low-Technology Devices

### Activities of Daily Living and Instrumental Activities of Daily Living

As people age, their physical capabilities change which can impact their desire to participate in favored activities, but taking care of themselves and their homes often remain important occupational tasks for them to complete. Individuals can use assistive technology to improve their functional independence and safety when completing necessary and favored tasks, but the use of adaptive devices is very individualized (Haggblom-Kronlof & Sonn, 2007). Occupational therapists must help the older adult and family members/caregivers determine which occupational tasks the person wants/needs to complete and then assist them in choosing best method/device to complete that task safely and satisfactorily.

What people need and want to do depend on their interests; their physical, perceptual/sensory, psychosocial, and cognitive abilities; their living environment; and the type of assistance available to them. For instance, ADLs (e.g., dressing, grooming, and bathing among others) that many people need and want to complete are often very similar. However, the IADLs (e.g., meal preparation, laundry, home management among others) people choose to engage in are more individualized. In addition, the level of assistance a person may need to perform ADLs versus IADLs often varies because IADLs often require more complex physical and cognitive functions. To determine the appropriate low-technology assistive devices needed, occupational therapists and consumers can compare device features and pricing by searching for potential devices in a search engine such as Google. Most manufacturers and distributors now provide extensive web pages and print catalogs that older adults and their families can browse to see available equipment or to get ideas for making their own devices (e.g., via 3D printing) to help them do the tasks they want to do.

People's perceptions of and their satisfaction with how well they can complete the task when using the device impacts their interest in using adaptive devices. Lee and Coughlin (2015) reported on multiple studies that found failure to use assistive technologies effectively results from poor design, unclear/overly complicated instructions, or a combination of both.

### Basic Activities of Daily Living

People with mobility limitations often find bathrooms the most challenging place in the home to navigate. People who use a wheelchair or scooter sometimes have trouble getting through narrow bathroom doors necessitating door removal or remodeling to widen the doorway to allow wheelchair access to use the commode and shower/tub safely with assistance. Getting onto and off the commode can also cause difficulty, and a raised toilet seat, strategically placed grab bars, and toilet safety frames around the toilet can improve safety without high cost or inconvenience.

Getting in and out of the bathtub can be very difficult for individuals with poor balance and/or the inability to lift their legs. Appropriately placed grab bars help individuals getting into and out of the tub. Some bathroom contractors can cut out a piece of the bathtub so that the person can step into the tub to sit on a bath bench and use a handheld shower while sitting in the tub. Or the contractor can remove the tub/shower combination to place a prefabricated no-step/low-step shower stall in the footprint of the original tub. Tub seats/benches allow individuals to enter a tub without stepping over the tub ledge, but rather by sitting and rotating their legs into the tub. Simple solutions like replacing shower doors with a tension rod and shower curtain allow for ease of transfer when using a tub seat or bench (Case Example 22.1).

A variety of low-technology assistive devices can enable individuals with different disabilities to perform other basic self-care tasks. Individuals with arthritis who have difficulty grasping feeding utensils can use utensils with built-up handles to compensate for the lack of range of motion in the fingers when grasping utensils (see Case Example 22.1). Other individuals who may have difficulty reaching their feet for lower body dressing may benefit from using a sock donner, dressing stick, long-handled shoehorn, and/or reacher to don their clothing. Still others might use long-handled bath sponges or wash mitts to complete bathing tasks safely and effectively. The variety of low-technology devices is great and are addressed further in Chapters 12 and 13.

### Instrumental Activities of Daily Living
#### Cooking/Meal Preparation

Although some people choose to have others do much of their meal preparation for them (e.g., microwaving frozen meals, having prepared meals delivered to their home, or choosing to eat in restaurants or congregate meal sites), meal preparation is an essential occupational task for some older adults. A growing variety of meal kits and delivery options

has grown in recent years and may be a nutritious and therapeutic option for elders who enjoy and may benefit from meal preparation. These include Blue Apron, Freshly, Hello Fresh, Purple Carrot, and others reviewed in Bon Appetit (Hopkins, 2022).

Osteoarthritis in the hands is prevalent among older adults and often impairs their ability to accomplish functional tasks. Adaptive devices can often allow people with arthritis to complete tasks more efficiently and safely. Many universally designed kitchen gadgets (e.g., electric jar openers, large-handled peelers) are available in department and kitchen stores to ease food preparation for everyone.

Having devices readily available for "touching/testing" in home goods stores simplifies the task of determining whether the device meets one's needs, and often increases acceptance as it allows the user to experience the features of the device and its potential benefits. Additionally, manufacturers, distributors, websites, and stores selling these devices would do well to provide clear instructions on various device characteristics and guidance on how to choose the right product in sales displays and not just in the instructions available after the product is retrieved from its packaging. Hammel (2004) reported that "word of mouth" among older friends regarding useful assistive devices is often the most common catalyst for the decision of adoption by older adults. One might have expected a modern evolution of the "Tupperware Parties"

---

### CASE EXAMPLE 22.1   Low-Technology Devices for Activities of Daily Living and Instrumental Activities of Daily Living

Mary and Ed have been married for 68 years and live in the home Ed built shortly after they wed. Mary, who was a stay-at-home mother, is 86 years old and has advanced rheumatoid arthritis. She uses a rolling walker outside but has not used a device in her home, as she prefers to "counter surf." However, she recently fell twice at home. Ed, 88 years old, is a retired union carpenter. He has lower body orthopedic issues resulting from a fall at work when he was 54. He ambulates with a straight cane but seems to be getting progressively weaker and needs a more supportive device. Mary and Ed are Catholics who attend church regularly. They have two daughters and one son, and eight grandchildren. Their children and grandchildren assist them as able.

Their home is a 1200-square-foot ranch-style home with a detached garage. There are four 6-inch steps that lead to small landings at the house's front living room and rear kitchen entrances. Both entrances have railings on both sides. The kitchen is a galley-style kitchen with a table that seats four people. The door to the basement staircase is also in the kitchen. There is a railing on one side of the basement stairs. The laundry is in the basement. There are two small bedrooms, a small family room, and a larger living room. The bathroom is very small, with the tub/shower combination with sliding doors straight ahead as you enter and the sink and toilet on the right.

Mary had expressed concern that she was having trouble doing her housework and meal preparation due to her lack of balance and strength. Ed was concerned about accessing

the basement, toilet, and tub more safely due to his lack of lower extremity range of motion and strength.

After evaluation, their occupational therapist recommended railings on both sides of the basement steps for safety. She also suggested that Mary and Ed avoid the basement and that family or a laundry service do the laundry for them. She did not recommend a higher toilet because Mary is 4'11" and Ed is 5'4", so their son placed Versa-frame armrests on their toilet to assist with sitting and standing to reduce effort. The occupational therapist suggested the family remove the shower door and replace it with a curtain. In doing so, Mary and Ed could then safely transfer to and use a shower chair and handheld shower. The family purchased a walker tray for Mary to use with her walker while preparing meals to prevent further falls. They also purchased a narrow-based quad cane for Ed to use instead of the straight cane to provide him with more support.

For meal preparation, the occupational therapist recommended several large-handled utensils and devices for cutting and preparation of food. In addition, she recommended a cutting board with food stabilizers built into the board to stabilize food while cutting, a mini food processor, and showed her how to move heavy pots from the stove to the sink without having to lift them for draining.

The family implemented these low-cost modifications, allowing Mary and Ed to stay in their home for two more years before moving to an assistive living center due to further physical decline.

begun in the 1950s to demonstrate new plastic storage containers, to demonstrate various gadgets and gizmos to assist elders in aging in place. Some of this occurs on social media; Bonvissuto (2022) reports on one tech design showcase for aging in place and senior living recently opened in Columbus, Ohio.

A person's safety is an important component of meal preparation. The ability to safely use the stove, oven, microwave, and cutting utensils must be determined before making meal preparation recommendations (see Case Example 22.1). Some examples of kitchen devices that can minimize the stress on the hand joints include tools with larger and softer handles, cutting utensils that use the whole hand instead of several fingers, electric choppers or food processors to minimize hand-chopping, and electric mixers that stabilize and rotate the mixing bowl.

People can also make other adaptations for food preparation and cleanup, including accessible locations for the microwave or other frequently used appliances. Locating a microwave above the stove may have seemed like a great idea when someone was able to reach up and remove the hot dish easily, but as hand and shoulder strength diminish, and wrists become arthritic, the microwave may be safer at a waist-high level (on the counter or table) to make it safer to take hot dishes out and set them on a hot pad on the counter instead of lifting them down from a microwave at shoulder height.

A person's kitchen habits and routines can help determine the best location for appliances and storage locations for frequently used utensils/tools and foods for easy access. Many appliance options are available in kitchen departments to help users optimize their food preparation abilities if they have the financial resources to make changes, such as having a dishwasher drawer or small oven right under the counter. Homebuilders/renovators and kitchen designers are slowly addressing these issues. The National Association of Home Builders (NAHB) provides training and credentialing for Certified Aging in Place Specialists (CAPS), who consider appropriate design in the kitchen, bathroom, garage, and other areas of the home. The occupational therapist can help make such recommendations to older clients and provide referrals to home modification contractors.

Forgetfulness in the kitchen can lead to spoiled food, or worse, to fire hazards. Door-open beepers on refrigerator/freezers that sound an alarm after 30 seconds and easily used timers and auto-shutoff or alarms on ranges and ovens dramatically reduce risks and have become more common in newer appliance models.

### Cleaning and Laundry

As people age, their interest and ability in cleaning and laundry vary significantly. Consideration of the older adult's physical, sensory/perceptual, and cognitive abilities is essential for the safe completion of these activities. With all appliances, it is crucial to evaluate the older adult's ability to safely reach and use the controls before recommending independent completion of a task. If someone considers cleaning an important occupational task, and the person is determined to be safe

in that task completion, the occupational therapist may assist with finding devices that will allow for safe and efficient completion of desired tasks. Devices available for making home management easier are also commercially available at many stores or online.

A significant barrier to an older adult independently doing their own laundry is the location of the washer and dryer. It may be a safe task if they are on the main floor and the controls are understandable and within reach. If the washer and dryer are in a basement, which is common in older houses, the safety in going up and down stairs while carrying a basket of clothing must be determined when making recommendations for independently completing laundry. Stacked washers/dryers, particularly near the master bedroom, may be a convenient space saver, but may create specific impediments for those with various handicaps. Moreover, front- versus top-loading designs present different opportunities and hardships, based on the functional capabilities of each user. Height-modifiable laundry baskets on wheels allow users to scoop laundry from a separate front-loading washing machine and dryer into the basket rather than lifting and transferring the laundry.

When proper product placement and design cannot overcome impediments to successful and safe use, exploration of options for having someone else complete these home management tasks may be necessary. Also, when attempting to effectively fit a person to their environmental situation, appliances, assistive devices, fixtures, and so forth, it is important to project forward in time and accommodate further declines in the individual's capacity. Selecting a device that becomes obsolete within months due to a decline in the user's capacity can be expensive, frustrating, and dangerous.

### Avocation

The location of vocational and avocational equipment and materials is critical to safe and efficient use as a person plans how to best stay actively engaged in meaningful activities and to age in place. This may mean, for example, moving a basement workshop to one stall of a two-stall garage, raising garden beds, moving a sewing machine to the ground floor, or changing the location and setup of the computer. Someone is more likely to stay engaged in a hobby if they can easily and safely get to the location of the equipment and materials.

Gardening can be extremely rewarding and therapeutic for older adults and encourages physical activity and stretching. A wide and growing variety of adaptive devices can make things easier for garden and outdoor work for people with osteoarthritis and limited strength, endurance, and balance. Perennials are generally preferable to annuals where capacity is limited. Raised beds and container gardening are also preferable (Fig. 22.1), and there are various ways to simplify watering. A variety of adapted tools is available to assist in playing cards, board games, and other recreational activities. These tools assist with problems related to decreased fine motor skill, decreased strength, and low vision among other issues that the older adult experiences (Box 22.1).

The occupational therapist must understand each person's individualized interests, needs, and abilities to make

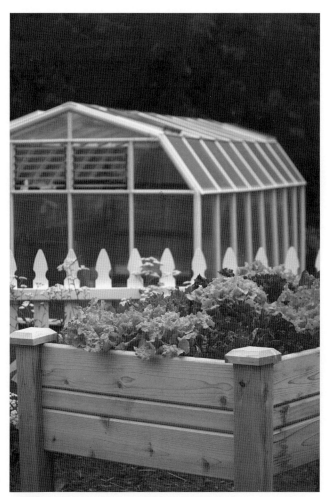

**FIG. 22.1**    Raised garden bed. (Photo © istock.com)

recommendations for meaningful engagement and participation in avocational activities of clients' choosing that will enhance their life satisfaction and personal well-being.

## Functional Mobility

Mobility aids are assistive devices commonly used by older adults and, excluding wheelchairs, are often obtained without medical consultation or fitting (Sehgal et al., 2021). Walkers and canes are much easier for people to use in homes, but without proper fitting may actually increase the risk of falls (West et al., 2015). Salespersons may help fit a mobility device to the person if purchased online or from local medical supply companies, but it is always best if the individual seeks the expertise of a licensed occupational or physical therapist to ensure correct fit.

Individuals often obtain wheelchairs through medical consultation and proper fitting or without a fitting for general mobility needs. Wheelchairs improve mobility, cognitive functioning, socialization, independence, a sense of freedom, flexibility and joint mobility, muscle strength, endurance, and balance (Woloszyn et al., 2020). However, it is often challenging to get the wheelchair and the person into and out of homes and move through narrow hallways within homes. In addition, wheelchairs are more difficult to transport in private cars and vans than are walkers and canes.

Many wheelchairs are manual, but powered mobility devices, such as power wheelchairs and scooters, are also available for use by older adults. Individuals often use powered wheelchairs and scooters when they are unable to walk distances on their own and unable to use their upper extremities to propel themselves in a wheelchair. Scooters are a popular choice for many older adults, as they are reportedly easier to manage in homes (once they are in the home and if there is enough space) but are very difficult to transport in private cars or vans without specialty lifts (Edwards & McCluskey, 2010). Powered mobility devices can be beneficial for moving around inside the home and in the community, but the process to transport them requires a mechanical lift on a vehicle because of their size and weight.

### Getting Into and out of Cars/Driving

Several new technologies assist with various aspects of driving, for example, crash avoidance, driving assistive systems, wayfinding (see Chapter 21). Even if driving is no longer an option for some clients, the car is the most common and preferred method of transportation for more than 90% of older adults (Binette & Vasold, 2018). There are a variety of assistive devices available that can assist individuals to use their car more easily and safely. A rotation disc on the car seat can help the seated client swing their legs into and out of the car. A temporary grab handle placed into the latching mechanism on the door can help people get safely into and out of the vehicle. Additionally, a limited number of car makes and models provide front driver and passenger seats that swivel toward the doorway to allow easier entry and egress. The occupational therapist must provide recommendations for safe transfers for different types of vehicles because getting into a standard sedan is very different from getting into a sports car, pick-up truck, mini-van, or sport utility vehicle.

The CarFit program (Fig. 22.2), offered jointly by the American Occupational Therapy Association (AOTA), AARP, and the American Automobile Association (AAA), is an educational program for older adults designed to maximize their safety, comfort, and mobility through making adjustments in their cars that facilitate optimal fit (e.g., seat position and mirror settings).

### Community Mobility

A person's ability to get around the community is critical for staying actively engaged in meaningful activities (Qin & Taylor, 2020). This may involve walking, bicycling for some, driving, or getting rides through privately arranged transportation, rideshare (e.g., Uber, Lyft), taxi services, community-provided passenger services, or public transportation.

The majority of persons in the United States, including older adults, who do not live in cities with adequate mass transit systems prefer to drive their own car for its convenience and sense of independence. We will discuss a few high-technology developments in a later section. Even if public transit services are available/accessible, older adults who have never used public transit may be unwilling or unable to learn how to use it when they can no longer drive.

---

**BOX 22.1**    Technology Websites and Related Resources Topically Organized

**General/Contextual Issues:**

Reframing Aging Initiative: www.reframingaging.org

Age and Ability Inclusive Toolkit: https://ageismtoolkit.vcu.edu/

Online Financial Health/Literacy: https://fintech.aarpfoundation.org/

**Aging and Climate Change:**

Aging & the Climate Crisis. (2022, Summer). *Generations*. Complete Issue. https://generations.asaging.org/summer-2022

Climate Change in an Aging Society E-Newsletter, sponsored by Climate Change and Consciousness (https://www.cccearth.org). E-mail HRMoody@yahoo.com to subscribe.
    www.grayisgreen.org

**Websites with a variety of assistive technology devices:**

https://enablingdevices.com/shop/

http://www.infogrip.com/

https://www.lighthousetoolsforliving.com/Assistive-Technology.html

http://www.maxiaids.com/

https://www.rehabmart.com/all-categories.asp

https://shop.maddak.com/index.php

**Equipment for assistance with activities of daily living (ADLs):**

https://www.discountmedicalsupplies.com/aids-to-daily-living/accessories.html

https://www.discountmedicalsupplies.com/aids-to-daily-living/dressing-aids.html

http://www.tubcut.com/

https://www.bathfitter.com/us-en/

https://www.ncmedical.com/categories/Assistive-Devices-ADL_12839533.html

https://www.performancehealth.com/products/home-care-daily-living

http://www.wrightstuff.biz/getting-ready.html

https://www.rehabmart.com/bathing-toileting.html

https://www.rehabmart.com/independent-living.html

http://www.harriscomm.com/equipment/alarm-clocks.html

**Equipment for assistance with cooking/meal preparation:**

https://www.ncmedical.com/categories/Food-Prep_12863001.html

https://www.ncmedical.com/categories/Kitchen_12839995.html

https://www.rehabmart.com/post/aging-in-place-heres-8-kitchen-tools-to-make-cooking-easy

**Equipment related to avocations:**

https://www.thewrightstuff.com/adaptive-garden-tools.html

https://www.rehabmart.com/category/card_games.html

https://www.enasco.com/c/Senior-Activities-Nasco

https://www.oldagesolutions.org/assistive-devices/leisure-activities/

http://www.allaboutvision.com/lowvision/reading.html

**Equipment related to transportation and driving:**

https://www.arthritissupplies.com/car-mobility-aids.html

https://www.aarp.org/auto/trends-lifestyle/info-2019/car-accessories-for-disabled-adults.html

http://www.programsforelderly.com/safety-independent-transportation-network.php

https://www.flickr.com/photos/completestreets/sets/72157617261981677/

https://www.arthritissupplies.com/car-mobility-aids.html

https://www.medicare.org/articles/auto-mobility-aids-for-assisting-senior-drivers/

**Equipment related to communication:**

http://www.sc.edu/scatp/aacsymbols.html

http://www.harriscomm.com/equipment/alarm-clocks.html

**Equipment related to environmental control:**

http://www.smarthome.com/_/index.aspx

http://www.x10.com/homepage.html

http://www.innotechsystems.com/accenda/index.html

https://home.google.com/welcome/

https://itouchless.com/products/sensor-ez-faucet-ezf003c

**Equipment related to computer access:**

http://www.logitech.com/en-us/mice-pointers/trackballs

http://www.evoluent.com/

https://www.zoomtext.com/

https://www.infogrip.com/products/

https://www.maxiaids.com/computers

**Useful Organization Websites**

**AOTA Communities of Practice:** https://www.aota.org/community/communities-of-practice

**National Digital Inclusion Alliance:** https://www.digitalinclusion.org/digital-navigator-model/

**Human Factors and Ergonomic Society:** https://www.hfes.org/

**American Society on Aging Connected Communities:** https://asaging.connectedcommunity.org/home

**LeadingAge: CAST (Center for Aging Services Technologies):** http://www.leadingage.org/cast.aspx

**Gerontological Society of America: GSA-TAG (Formal Interest Group on Technology & Aging):** https://www.geron.org/membership/interest-groups#technology

https://www.geron.org/membership/interest-groups#technology

**RESNA Special Interest Groups:** https://www.resna.org/Membership/Special-Interest-Groups-SIGs

**LinkedIn (e.g., Gerontechnology) and Facebook discussion groups**

---

Distance to the bus stop, perceived cost, fear of crime, feelings of lost privacy, confusing bus schedules, and the need for transfers are all potential disincentives for older adults to use public transit. Only 15% of older adults reported using mass transit in 2018, and 82% indicated that driving their own vehicle is their primary way of getting around (AASHTO, 2018). Public transit's real and perceived shortcomings must be addressed, but it may still not be available or an acceptable option for some older adults, particularly in rural and suburban areas.

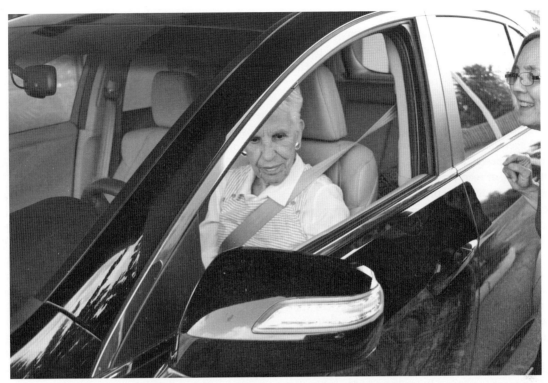

**FIG. 22.2**    CarFit program assessment. (Photo © istock.com)

Some communities have reasonable transportation options for older adults through paratransit systems, local taxi services, faith-based organizational transportation services, and community services such as a transportation network that allows people to join the network and receive car rides at a reasonable rate. One innovative network in 10 states is the Independent Transportation Network America ("About ITN", n.d.), where older adults can receive ride vouchers in exchange for donating their cars to the network's fleet of vehicles. This type of system allows more safety, autonomy, and dignity because the participating older adults have bought into this network that provides enhanced flexibility and convenience. The National Aging and Disability Transportation Center (NADTC.org) and others are also helping to improve accessible transportation for older adults and people who are disabled.

One option for older adults who live in communities where friends, stores, restaurants, community centers, and other places of destination are within walking distance is to get to desired locations by walking or by using their current ambulation devices. This walking/rolling is only appropriate if there are safe sidewalks and bike lanes that are barrier-free and safe crossings for streets that they need to cross. Complete Streets (2020) is an innovative program throughout the United States that helps communities focus on safety on the roads for drivers, cyclists, parents pushing strollers, and pedestrians/rollers. Complete Streets focuses on safe access for all users and factors that allow buses to operate on time. Modifications include auditory and visual alerts and countdown indicators for street crossing, the provision of enough time to get across during the walk sequence, and the implementation of curb cuts for motorized scooters, wheelchairs, and strollers.

Federal policy developments and initiatives will continue to improve sustainable and livable communities for residents of all ages. For example, the US Department of Housing and Urban Development (HUD) has partnered with the Environmental Protection Agency (EPA) and the Department of Transportation (DOT) to enhance the livability of communities. The guiding principles in this partnership include: (1) enhancing integration of multimodal transportation infrastructure and facilities, (2) providing safe and adequate accommodations for all users, (3) increasing community connectivity and cohesion, (4) integrating mobility services and automation to help improve overall quality of life, and (5) decreasing overall cost of moving people, goods, and services (US Department of Transportation, 2022).

### Service Animals

Trained service animals assist people with disabilities in performing various tasks to help them compensate for hearing, visual, sensory, motor, or cognitive deficits. Because these areas decline with age, it is appropriate to consider service animals as a viable alternative to human assistance at one end of a continuum and technological devices at the other. People are most familiar with guide dogs that assist the visually impaired with mobility in different environments. Other types of animals, such as trained monkeys and miniature horses, assist in accomplishing various tasks. Some animals pull wheelchairs for those who cannot push one independently or fatigue easily. Some animals help retrieve items from the refrigerator or pick up items from the floor for those who cannot reach those areas. Service dogs can be specifically trained to alert an individual to blood sugar changes or to alert and protect individuals affected by seizure disorders. Still, others act as therapeutic companion animals. Research has shown that individuals with physical or hearing impairments who have a service animal show increased independence, social participation, participation in recreation, and quality of life (Hall et al., 2017).

## Communication

Older adults can have difficulties with communicating clearly due to various age-related changes or diseases that affect their ability to produce speech, hear speech, see someone communicating with them, or read written words.

When people have difficulty producing words due to aphasia or motor apraxia, or difficulty producing clear speech due to dysarthria or hearing difficulties, this can significantly affect their quality of life. No-tech, low-technology, and high-technology assistive devices can help individuals communicate by supplementing their current speech ability, replacing their difficulty in communicating verbally, or compensating for their vision and/or hearing sensory loss. Devices that compensate for speech are called augmentative and alternative communication (AAC) devices. These will be addressed later in the chapter in the high-technology section.

Unaided speech options (no-tech) include the use of gestures, body language, and sign language, which enable the individual to get their meaning across without the use of devices. Low-technology options include writing on a tablet, pointing to items on a picture, phrase, letter, or word board, or choosing a word or phrase from a booklet that contains words and phrases the individual most commonly uses. If the older adult has difficulty communicating, the occupational therapist must consult with a speech and language pathologist to include the most appropriate communication words and symbols for that person's current capabilities. The speech and language pathologist would determine the words/pictures used for a low-technology communication board, and the occupational therapist would determine the access means to the device. There are various ways that a person can access a communication device. The person conveying the message can use their finger or an alternative pointing device (e.g., a head pointer or laser pointer) to point to choices on the board. The individual could also use eye gaze to indicate their choice as the partner in the conversation watches where the individual's eyes are looking to determine the individual's choice.

Functional communication can also become difficult for older adults if they experience a loss of hearing or vision that is not corrected through traditional compensation devices such as glasses/contacts and hearing aids. Referrals to appropriate professionals (e.g., optometrists, ophthalmologists, or audiologists) are needed to find the best device or adaptation possible to maximize a person's functional communication in light of any sensory impairment. Hearing aids are expensive and unaffordable for many older adults, because they are not currently a covered benefit for Medicare recipients. Not hearing what is going on around you is always frustrating. Older adults and their families can become extremely frustrated when they purchase hearing aids out of pocket, and they do not totally compensate for a hearing loss. In this case,

the older adult often ends up not using them. In 2022, there is some indication price reductions may occur due to advanced technology and market forces.

Other devices to compensate for a hearing impairment include adaptive alerting mechanisms such as alarm clocks that shake a bed, light-activated doorbells and warning systems, and telephone systems with extra-loud volume control. Most newer television sets have settings to activate closed captions on television programs to allow someone with a hearing limitation to understand the content of programs by reading the closed captioning on the screen.

When communicating with people who have visual or auditory sensory impairments, it is essential to communicate in quiet environments with sufficient ambient lighting while also reducing glare on the eyes of the older adult. Seating the client where the glare is behind their back, rather than in their eyes, can dramatically improve their ability to pick up nonverbal cues and to use limited lip-reading. (See Chapter 10 for additional suggestions on dealing with low vision and hearing impairments.)

Compensations for problems with communication due to vision loss include enlarged print, colored overlays, brighter light, magnification (handheld magnifying glasses or increased magnification on a computer screen), and text-to-speech programs (simple programs are a part of most computer operating systems, but much more sophisticated programs are also available commercially). The following section of this chapter discusses high-technology compensations. Refer to the websites in Box 22.1 for examples of available programs.

## Cost and Payment Options for Durable Medical Equipment

Many of the assistive devices discussed so far—canes, walkers, wheelchairs, commodes, and so forth—are generally classified as *durable medical equipment* (DME). Such equipment is available for purchase from a wide variety of sources and vendors. Medicare Part B covers DME if it is prescribed by a physician, is used for a specific medical reason (i.e., medically necessary), can be used repeatedly, and is expected to last 3 years ("Durable medical equipment", n.d.). Medicare pays for different equipment in different ways (i.e., rent, buy, or choice of rent or buy) and individuals need to meet their Part B deductible before being covered. Once the deductible is met, the individual is responsible for 20% of the Medicare approved amount (i.e., amount the supplier agrees to receive) for the device. It is important to note that not all DME is covered via Medicare. For instance, tub seats and benches are not covered by Medicare, nor are adapted feeding or dressing devices, among others. In this instance, an individual may have a secondary insurance carrier who would pay for the non-Medicare covered device or the individual would have to pay out-of-pocket. The insurance coverage guidelines for DME can be daunting for the patient and their caregivers to understand and navigate. Health-care professionals should have a basic understanding of the guidelines, but equipment retail store employees can assist with navigating the process.

## High-Technology Devices, Apps, and Services

Now that we have surveyed the many low-technology devices that occupational therapists and other professionals can use to assist older adults in maintaining their independence, we will now review some high-technology alternatives in the areas of health and self-esteem, housing and daily living, communication, and governance (including compensation for cognitive decline), work, and leisure (following Fozard's matrix). Remember, when a low-technology and low-cost alternative does a comparable or better job than the latest and greatest, we suggest that, particularly for the current older cohort, it is best to "keep it simple."

### General Considerations: Cost, Access, Bandwidth, Digital Divide

Before jumping into a discussion of the potential benefits of specific high-technology devices and services, we need to briefly refer to macro level issues, concerns, and developments regarding the context in which one may wish to use various technological tools. The "digital divide" by age, race, class, income, and education has been a key concern for many scholars and practitioners in recent years. For example, the International Association of Gerontology and Geriatrics convened an expert panel from the continents in October 2021 to discuss opportunities and risks regarding the application of technology to the lives of older adults. The goal of most elders in most regions is to "age in place." Thankfully, many elders are eager and willing to use technology, but many others are unable or unwilling. Kamber (2022) provides an excellent overview and argument as to why we must close the gap between the groups.

As learned during the COVID-19 pandemic, a less than optimal communications infrastructure (particularly in rural areas) and prohibitively high costs for low-income individuals were barriers to online teaching and learning at the K-12 and post-secondary levels (Hoffman et al., 2021). Various efforts were mounted due to the COVID-19 pandemic to reduce the digital divide, providing training and support to elders and others who lacked digital access, knowledge, or proficiency. In early 2022, the US Congress passed the Bipartisan Infrastructure Law (Infrastructure Investment and Jobs Act) that promises that all Americans will have access to reliable high-speed broadband Internet. The White House notes that by some estimates, 30 million Americans lack such access and that $65 billion would be spent to increase access and that affordability would be considered to reduce the digital divide. CNBC reported that the administration had received commitment from 20 Internet service providers to provide free Internet to low-income households (Feiner, 2022), and Gleckman (2022) predicts that this plan will be a "huge help to older adults" in enhancing access to telehealth, remote monitoring, virtual services, and programming.

Several recent studies have noted that a significant majority of elders have positive attitudes about the current and potential benefits of technology in their lives. Despite other

barriers and risks, this is a strength to build on, countering prevalent ageist myths in society that elders lack interest in or capacity for technology use. An optimistic belief by practitioners regarding their older clients' ability to adapt, change, and grow may be one of the best predictors of that practitioner's effectiveness with their clients (Burdick, 1983). Tice and Perkins (1996) suggest that practitioners focus on identifying and building upon clients' strengths, rather than dwelling on their weaknesses and disabilities.

As with low-technology devices, your interventions should be tailored to each client's wishes, needs, and capacities. Birkland's (2019) typology of elders' likelihood of adapting new technologies may be helpful in best matching each client to appropriate technological tools. The model describes five ICT user types (Enthusiasts, Practicalists, Socializers, Traditionalists, and Guardians), each with its own likely relationship to technology. The important takeaway is that an understanding of each client's type and preferences may assist the occupational therapist in encouraging their client to adopt various technological tools to improve their objective well-being, subjective life-satisfaction, and ability to age in place.

### Activities of Daily Living

Many high-technology devices can help caregivers in the home to provide care for older adults particularly with mobility within the home during ADL and IADL task performance. Ceiling-supported transfer systems, bathtub lifts to get a person into and out of the tub (Fig. 22.3), stair glides, elevators within the home, and outdoor lifts into a home are options that one may consider if the funding for those high-technology devices is available. (See Box 22.2 for listing of apps that can assist with ADL performance.)

### Instrumental Activities of Daily Living

For many older adults, the loss of the ability to do higher level IADL tasks, such as shopping and banking, often occurs before the loss of basic ADLs (Coventry et al., 2020). The inability to prepare one's own meal or shop for the food necessary for meal prep impacts an individual's functional independence significantly. Although, as previously discussed, tasks such as

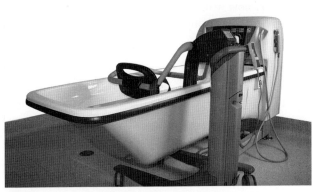

**FIG.22.3** Bathtub lift. (Courtesy of Geraldine B. Ellenberger.)

| **Box 22.2** | Apps for Various Functional Skills and Occupations |

**Apps for Cognitive Compensation and Remediation:**
*Constant Therapy:* https://thelearningcorp.com/constant-therapy/
*Lumosity:* https://www.lumosity.com/en/
*Rehab Coach:* https://play.google.com/store/apps/details?id=com.blackfrogweb.rehabcoach&hl=en_US
*Mind Mate:* https://www.mindmate-app.com/
*Alz Calls:* https://alzcalls.com/

**Apps for Communication Compensation and Remediation:**
*Dragon Anywhere:* https://www.nuance.com/dragon/dragon-anywhere.html
*Tactus Therapy Apps:* https://tactustherapy.com/apps/
*AmuseIT:* http://www.amuseit.nz/?fbclid=IwAR2EE9Gz0U_yiHgFompLtaVwvljj1I4lcm0llSj_GKaVF55NwNuq11Z91A4

**Apps for Recreation and Fitness:**
*Audible:* https://www.audible.com/howtolisten
*Old Time Radio Shows:* https://oldtimeradioshows.co/
*Old Time Radio 24:* https://apps.apple.com/us/app/old-time-radio-24-yesterday-usa-radiotimes-shows/id1071613208
*Tai Chi for Seniors Pro:* https://apps.apple.com/us/app/tai-chi-for-seniors-pro/id577042546
*Pocket Yoga:* https://www.pocketyoga.com/apps/pocket-yoga/?rewrite-strtolower-url=Apps/PocketYoga
*Librivox:* https://play.google.com/store/apps/details?id=com.scdgroup.app.audio_book_librivox&hl=en_US&gl=US

**Apps for Activities of Daily Living and Instrumental Activities of Daily Living:**
*Medisafe:* https://www.medisafeapp.com/
*Good Rx:* https://www.goodrx.com/mobile
*ShopWell:* https://apps.apple.com/us/app/shopwell-better-food-choices/id393422300
*iBP Blood Pressure:* https://apps.apple.com/us/app/ibp-blood-pressure/id306526794
*Pillboxie:* https://apps.apple.com/us/app/pillboxie/id417367089
*Sciddy:* https://appadvice.com/app/sciddy/493269707

**Apps for Vision Compensation and Remediation:**
*Magnifying Glass with Light Pro:* https://apps.apple.com/us/app/magnifying-glass-w-light-pro/id477968382
*Brighter and Bigger:* https://asada.website/brighterandbigger/e/

**Apps for Community Mobility:**
*Life 360:* https://www.life360.com/
*Park-N-Find:* https://apps.apple.com/us/app/park-n-find/id1068711953
*Lyft:* https://apps.apple.com/us/app/lyft/id529379082
*Uber:* https://apps.apple.com/us/app/uber-request-a-ride/id368677368

meal preparation can be compensated for using meal delivery services, there are some ways to compensate for IADL deficits through a variety of apps or online services.

Individuals can complete banking online using their bank's website or app. Being able to take a picture of a check to deposit it into an account means those who are no longer driving or who have mobility deficits can remain independent in banking tasks. Grocery stores offer online shopping, ordering and delivery service or partner with other providers, like Instacart, that limit the individuals' need to rely on others for transportation and assistance. Online shopping options through Amazon and Walmart allow individuals to purchase household items that are delivered to their front door. (See Box 22.2 for listing of apps that can assist with IADL performance.)

### Driving

Modern vehicles provide more standard wayfinding (e.g., global positioning system [GPS]), collision avoidance, lane departure warnings or corrections, rear facing cameras, and other devices that can make driving safer for the older or impaired driver (see Chapter 21). Some vehicles have automatic parallel parking capacity (e.g., intelligent parking assist system [IPAS] and advanced parking guidance system [APGS]). While fully self-driving cars have taken longer to

develop than some car companies and futurists had predicted (particularly for suburban and rural areas), recent developments in the application of reinforcement learning to AI may accelerate the timeline where self-driving cars become an everyday reality (Heaven, 2022). A study from Juniper Research (2015) forecasts that by 2025 there will be almost 20 million fully autonomous (FAV) or self-driving vehicles on the road. This technology could be a "game changer," as it will provide a myriad of opportunities for the older adult to interact with others, decrease their social isolation, improve their functioning in community tasks, and will remove a major trigger for concern and disagreement for families with older relatives.

### Augmentative and Alternative Communication and Smartphones

High-technology options for communication include electronic devices that produce speech as the individual points to pictures or types words on a speech-generating device (SGD). Software for various tablet devices is becoming much more prevalent and useful. These devices are called augmentative and alternative communication devices.

Many high-technology devices come with a touchscreen that the individual can touch to choose words or phrases to convey. Other devices come equipped with a camera that detects where the person is looking to use eye gaze to select words or phrases they want to convey. Still, others offer the individual the option of using switch scanning to choose letters, words, or phrases. The development of tablets such as the Apple iPad and the proliferation of smartphone use has made access to AAC for many individuals a cost-effective reality, because there are numerous apps available to download that aid in speech production for those with speech problems (Case Example 22.2).

There has been some criticism of the use of AAC devices because of fears that the individual will become too dependent on the devices and consequently never develop or regain the ability to speak after suffering a disabling condition affecting speech, such as a cerebrovascular accident (CVA). However, studies have shown positive results regarding using AAC devices for individuals with Alzheimer disease (Fried-Oken et al., 2012), strokes (Dietz et al., 2020), and Parkinson disease (Beukelman et al., 2007).

## Home Automation and Electronic Aids to Daily Living

Individuals are living longer, yet options for supported living environments for older individuals have not kept pace with this growth. The support available from and provided by family members has diminished in recent decades due to the need for family members to work, the migration of family members away from their aging parents, and a lower fertility rate (National Academies of Science, Engineering, and Medicine, 2016). Family support will continue to decline because of fewer adult offspring born to baby boomers than among previous cohorts. In addition, many older adults choose to remain in their own homes due to the familiarity of the environment, the control afforded by living in their own homes, and their desire to remain independent for as long as possible (Kasper et al., 2019; see also Chapters 20 and 32). Consequently, there is a growing need for supportive approaches, programs, and devices that encourage individuals to remain living independently in their own homes and to "age in place."

Aging is associated with a variety of health disorders, conditions, and declines that jeopardize successful aging-in-place. For example, mobility issues, declines in sensory function, and falls can inhibit an individual's ability to remain safe and independent in their own home. In recent years, technological advances in home automation have enabled individuals to age in place more safely and independently. Home automation options can range from standalone remotely operated lighting to smart homes in which functions can be accessed within a home's WiFi network or via the Internet to run lights and appliances in the home, monitor the residents' activity level, provide reminders for those with cognitive impairments, or assist with tracking residents' health through blood pressure or blood sugar monitoring (Demiris & Hensel, 2008; van Hoof et al., 2011).

The availability of high-speed broadband Internet service is moving toward a new level of download and upload speeds through traditional wired cable connections. Likewise, cellphone speeds and bandwidth that support mobile smartphone usage is being dramatically improved, thanks to the deployment of 5 G Internet by most of the main providers. Both developments have hastened the development of "the internet of things" (IoT), which mostly involves communication among various devices within one's home WiFi Network. So, home monitoring, control of lighting, security cameras, heating/cooling, and other devices are contributing to further development of "Smart Homes", which until this time has been more aspirational than reality. In coming years, occupational therapists will have a wider variety of IoT applications available to use with or recommend to older clients. It is important to note the various barriers to use described above, and the need to carefully monitor developments in the industry with respect to privacy, maintenance of critical functions in times of service disruption caused by electrical outages, denial of service hacking, or other factors.

Home automation technology has significantly advanced in recent years, although home automation was available as far back as the 1934 World's Fair in Chicago. Since then, availability in personal homes has been most possible since 1975 with the development of X-10 technology that transmits and interprets signals sent from a remote control into functions such as "on" and "off" to control various devices in a person's home ("A brief history," 2019). While X-10 technology remains a popular means of communication with electronic devices for home automation despite issues with signal reliability, wireless alternatives with higher bandwidths have become more popular (e.g., Zigbee, Z-Wave). Faster home Wi-Fi networks with additional signal strength

---

## CASE EXAMPLE 22.2   Augmentative Communication

Jean is a 72-year-old woman diagnosed with a cerebrovascular accident 1 year ago, resulting in severe expressive aphasia. In the past year, she has not seen many improvements in her ability to speak so that others can understand her.

Jean is getting increasingly frustrated when trying to communicate her needs to others. Her husband has asked for assistance in providing his wife with a means to communicate. After evaluation, Jean's speech-language pathologist and occupational therapist determined that she could type and spell and was cognitively intact. Because of these characteristics, she was deemed a good candidate for a speech-generating augmentative and alternative communication (ACS) device. With a device that she can use to either spell out her needs or point to words to create sentences to indicate her needs, Jean will be able to communicate effectively with her family and friends. After evaluation with several ACS options, her therapists determined that a speech-generating app on her phone provided her with the best function and convenience with communicating her needs.

and range along with the projected rapid development and adoption of 5 G and the IoT is expected to be a major catalyst for greater use of technology to assist older adults in aging in place (Carnemolla, 2018).

Home automation devices have significant implications for keeping older adults safe and independent in their own homes. Research demonstrates that home automation devices have reduced the prevalence of falls, have improved the quality of life of older adult users, and decreased the number of caregiving hours provided to those who require assistance with ADLs and IADLs (Ma et al., 2021).

Steele and colleagues (2017) note that while assistive technology was once a specialized practice field of OT, now the wide range and availability of mainstream products mean that generalists in OT have many new tools at their disposal. Virtually anything in a home can run via automation. Devices with only two functions, like "on/off" or "open/close," are most easily automated and found in single, standalone controllers. Devices that require configuration of functions, such as temperature or volume control (e.g., Google Nest via Google Home; Amazon's Alexa SmartHome) sometimes involve a combination of technologies found in electronic aids to daily living (EADLs) (once known as environmental control units [ECUs]) (Case Example 22.3).

Single, standalone controllers, such as "The Clapper," operate a single device. They can be operated via touch, sound, voice, or proximity. Individuals often use these simple control devices to operate appliances with two functions and are the easiest for older adults to set up and use. Similar standalone devices for control of the home allow older adults the ability to turn the water on and off without having to turn faucets due to a weak grasp, but rather by proximity to the receiver. Some overhead lights and fans come standard with a remote control to allow users to operate them without walking to a wall switch or reaching for a pull string. These simple modifications may reduce the number of falls in an individual with mobility and balance problems. Motion detectors for light operation and hallways and bathrooms can reduce the number of falls that older adults have during nighttime toileting activities.

Philips Hue Smart LED lighting and similar systems provide a wide array of lighting options and routines for lighting through the home controlled by a smartphone app, computer, or voice commands via virtual assistants that may provide ease for a physically impaired elder to adjust multiple lights without the need to reach to wall switches and hard to reach lamp switches. Routines can be set to mimic the brightness of sunrise and sunset, which may help in maintaining appropriate sleep cycles. These lights have also been studied for their benefits among individuals with Alzheimer disease and other neurocognitive disorders to reduce agitation, for example, and to reduce "sundowner syndrome" (Clay, 2019). Alternative television (TV) remote controls come with larger buttons for the visually impaired or are operated by voice commands for those with limited fine motor skill and strength that inhibits their ability to operate the buttons on standard remote-control devices. Several cable TV operators now provide apps for iPads and other tablets that allow convenient viewing of program schedules and remote control.

## Smart Homes

Smart home automation initially occurred to allow individual control heating/ventilation, security systems, and lighting from a centralized in-home console. Today, with the advent of mobile devices, the notion of smart home has evolved, with broader implications for older adults' safety, security, general well-being, and enjoyment, as they are increasingly allowed and encouraged to age in place. Smart home technology can monitor the resident's activities, specifically regarding falls, medication schedule management, and tracking of what a resident had to eat. Family members and providers can monitor them on several behavioral parameters from remote settings.

### Barriers and Facilitators of Smart Home Technology

Harris et al. (2021) provide a very useful review of the facilitators and barriers to older adults' use of many of the smart

---

## CASE EXAMPLE 22.3 Environmental Control

Anne Marie is a 62-year-old woman diagnosed with multiple sclerosis when she was 45 years old. She has progressively lost function in all her extremities and can only control the movements in her neck. Anne Marie is quite verbal, has no difficulty with projecting her voice, and is cognitively intact. She spends most of her day in her hospital bed because her personal care assistant finds it challenging to get her up and into her wheelchair, and when up, Anne Marie fatigues after an hour or so.

Recently, Anne Marie has had more difficulty accepting her dependence upon her personal care assistant for simple tasks such as changing the channels on the television. She has asked for assistance in determining the best electronic aid to daily living (EADL) to allow her to control television functions, to turn her bedside lamp on and off, and make and receive phone calls independently.

After evaluation, her occupational therapist determined that the most appropriate device would be controlled through voice-recognition technology. With a voice-controlled system, Anne Marie would effectively control her identified devices. The recommended EADL device should have television control, light control, and telephone access since those are the functions Anne-Marie identified as goals. With such a system in place, Anne Marie can operate her television, make and receive telephone calls, and operate her bedside lamp independently. Virtual assistants such as Alexa (with the Amazon Echo Show device) and Google Home (perhaps with the Google Nest Hub device) would be appropriate to recommend to Anne Marie.

technologies (e.g., smartphones, smart security technologies, digital home assistants, and others) that have appeared in recent years. They note that, despite older adults' rapid increases in the use of technology (most are catching up quickly) there are still areas of concern. Their review is particularly appropriate for occupational therapists as they discuss impediments and catalysts for the use of technology in assisting with ADLs and IADLs. The main facilitator of smartphone use was user's perceived usefulness in daily life. The main barriers for smartphone use were found to be ignorance of features and cost. Barriers for use of Smart Security Technology (such as smart doorbells and entrance monitors, smart door locks, and smart cameras) were ignorance on how to use or access. Digital Home Assistants (e.g., Amazon Echo and Google Home) were reported as used at least some of the time by 30 of the 80 study participants, yet over half had never used one. Kadylak and colleagues (2021) used a longitudinal approach to assess the varied use of Amazon Alexa by a small group of elders. They noted that the digital assistant could assist with ADLs (calling caregivers to assist with transfer), IADLs (medication reminders, creating shopping lists), and enhanced ADLs (such as music listening, checking on the weather, playing games, and contacting others), particularly for individuals with mobility limitations. They found that participants often because attached to their device, gave their device a name (anthropomorphized), and that they helped to reduce loneliness and boredom. "I don't want everybody to know I don't know something, but I don't mind asking Alexa. She seems like my friend." While Alexa can speak with various accents and languages, as this chapter was finalized came news (Palmer, 2022) that Amazon has demonstrated a new feature under development that could allow Alexa to mimic anyone's voice, "including a dead relative." Imagine having one's favorite grandma, born in 1899, reminding the elder, "Don't forget to wash behind your ears" as she did when you were a toddler. The cassette recording from 1972 she first heard a recording of her own voice would provide Alexa the necessary voice clip.

Major new research initiatives have emerged in late 2021 and early 2022 that will increasingly apply the power of "big data" and AI to assisting elders to age in place. For example, in 2021, Johns Hopkins University received a $20 million grant to increase the rapid development and deployment of AI devices to encourage healthy and independent living (Blount, 2021). The initiative involves researchers and practitioners from several schools and disciplines at the university. Two such devices cited were gait monitoring to predict and prevent falls by elders, and another that monitors facial expressions and speech patterns that might indicate early stages of dementia. The MIT AgeLab has recently added an Artificial Intelligence and Longevity initiative to other priorities, including Caregiving and Well-Being, Home Logistics and Services, Retirement and Longevity Planning, Transportation and Livable Communities, and COVID and Life Tomorrow. See: https://agelab.mit.edu/artificial-intelligence-and-longevity/overview/

## Robotics

Robotics is the newest technology that can assist older adults with control over items in their environment and completion of ADLs and IADLs. Although still in relative infancy, home robotic technology worldwide has been gaining interest as a form of assistance in keeping older adults in their homes longer. Research areas have included service robots that can help older adults with medication management, robotic garments that monitor activity level, breathing, and heart rate, and robotic devices that assist the older adult with transfers to and from various surfaces. Results indicate that these devices positively influence older adults' physical and psychosocial functioning (Lin et al., 2018). In addition, robotic companion pets have been demonstrated to have high acceptance rates and positive outcomes for emotional and physical well-being (Rebola & Malle, 2021). Researchers have recently found that older adults are likely to accept robotic care instead of human assistance for tasks such as housekeeping/cleaning, removing trash, and doing laundry, but prefer humans when they need assistance with bathing/toileting, dressing, and other more personal tasks. They are more likely to accept robotic assistance for these other tasks if it helps avoid institutional care (Georgia Institute of Technology, 2012).

Amazon premiered their Astro Robot with Alexa in late 2021 for $999, but it currently is not much more than a fun mobile home monitor, that can respond with assistance like the stationary Alexa stations. (Basu, 2021). South Korea leads the way internationally in the development of robotics; Japan, with the oldest average age on earth, is leading the way in development of robotics for long-term care. Freakonomics Radio (Kanfer, 2021) suggests that while robots will take many jobs from humans, newer collaborative robots ("cobots") will dramatically change how work gets done in several fields.

Although sophisticated multifunction robotic devices are currently cost-prohibitive and of limited availability for most older adults to obtain, we believe that they will become much more common in the next decade and that volume sales will reduce costs, much as has occurred in personal computing.

Currently, some simpler robotic technologies are available on the mainstream market that can assist older adults with completing some home management tasks. A handful of commercially available robotic vacuums (e.g., Roomba) can help older individuals maintain carpets and floors, despite balance, strength, and mobility issues. In addition, physically impaired older adults wishing to maintain their lawns can use a robotic lawnmower. Robotic pool and rain-gutter cleaners are other examples of automated robotic technologies that allow older adults to age in place and maintain independence.

## Virtual Reality

Therapeutic use of immersive VR technologies in health care has also grown measurably in recent years and is projected to continue to grow rapidly as federal grant funding and technology sector investments grow. "The V.R. segment in health care alone, which according to some estimates is already valued at billions of dollars, is expected to grow by multiples of that in the next few years, with researchers seeing potential for it to help with everything from anxiety and depression to rehabilitation after strokes to surgeons strategizing where to cut and stitch" (Ouyang, 2022, np). Immersive VR for general recreational use is expected to experience dramatic growth in the coming years, as witnessed by Facebook's rebranding as "Meta" and Mark Zuckerberg's description of "The Metaverse" at Connect 2021 (Meta, 2021).

Occupational therapists use VR systems to provide intervention for various functional problems including cognitive, hand and upper extremity, mobility, balance, postural control, and psychosocial deficits. VR allows patients to safely participate in simulated occupations when the patient does not have the ability to participate in the actual activities due to sensory, motor, cognitive, or psychosocial deficits. VR systems employ several theories of neuroscience and motor learning focusing on repetitive, intensive, modifiable task-oriented practice especially when an individual has motor planning difficulties. In other cases, VR assists individuals with cognitive or psychosocial deficits to safely practice occupations with real-time feedback to ensure success in performance of occupations. Some VR systems are also combined with robotic devices to allow individuals the ability to practice problematic movements using robotic limbs to play a game or participate in an activity.

There are three types of VR systems that therapists use with patients. Some VR systems produce the image of a simulated activity on a screen while the individual manipulates a controller to complete a task. Many of these nonimmersive VR systems utilize gaming technology to allow the individual to practice specific movements to improve the individual's ability to use that movement functionally. The Nintendo Wii was perhaps the first "VR" gaming system older adults used in rehabilitation settings to improve upper extremity function, balance, and various other skills using gaming technology. Since then, therapists use devices like the MusicGlove to improve hand function in individuals with orthopedic and neurologic conditions. There are various other nonimmersive VR systems available, and many are not as cost prohibitive as the other types of VR systems to be discussed next. Nonimmersive VR systems are best used to improve a specific skill like range of motion or standing balance rather than improve function in a specific occupation.

The second type of VR system is semi-immersive and utilizes a larger screen and control devices to simulate activities that individuals want to perform better. An example of a semi-immersive VR system is a driving training simulator such as the STISTIM Drive or the EF-CAR REHAB driving simulators. This type of VR system has the advantage of reduced cybersickness, which is increased in a fully immersive VR system (An & Park, 2018).

Others immerse the individual in virtual environments and require the individual to function in the virtual environment while wearing a head-mounted monitor. These systems often employ apps that individuals use to practice tasks in the virtual environment that might be difficult or unsafe to perform in a nonvirtual environment. An example of an immersive rehabilitation VR system is the REAL System. One major disadvantage of the immersive VR system is cybersickness that some individuals experience while participating in the virtual environment.

Studies have shown that older adults find VR enjoyable and useful in improving function in various occupations (Lina et al., 2020). Others have shown the VR interventions improved the physical functioning of older adults reducing their risk for falls and improving their function in daily life tasks (Molina et al., 2014). Regular exposure to and immersion in natural settings has long been demonstrated to have positive benefits to individuals of all ages. A recent mixed-method feasibility study (Kalantari et al., 2022) provides promising evidence that VR provides low-cost therapeutic benefits for elders in clinical and recreational settings, especially for those who lack direct access to nature.

Occupational therapists sometimes utilize reminiscence therapy to trigger improvements in procedural memory among individuals suffering from mild cognitive impairment or dementia. (Baillon et al., 2005.) Preliminary findings indicate that VR-supported reminiscence provides several benefits for individuals with dementia in long-term care settings (Fuchs, 2022), and in connecting cognitively impaired residents with family living at a distance (Afifi et al., 2021). Among the benefits reported by Fuchs is a 70% reduction in the use of antipsychotic medications among VR using residents. There are some negative side effects that should be considered, including dizziness and headaches and overuse is discouraged to keep users connected with real surroundings. According to the article, there are currently six companies providing VR reminiscence therapy for older adults in hundreds of long-term care communities worldwide.

## Computer Assistive Technology

People use computers to accomplish many things in their daily lives. They use computers to communicate and socialize with family, friends, co-workers, and clients. People use computers to manage their homes, pay their bills, and shop online. They use computers to pursue recreational interests, create videos and music, and research items of interest. Unlike younger generations, many older adults never used computers in the classroom or their work environments. They may not attempt to learn the technology out of fear of doing something wrong or not being successful, privacy concerns, stigma, and fear of dependence, among others (Yusif et al., 2016). However, as computers have become more prevalent in work environments, more people, including the baby boomers, have been exposed to computers and are comfortable using them. Boot and Ortiz (2021, November 14) in summarizing demographic trends from the Pew Research Center noted that the gap between age groups in Internet use has continued to narrow over the past 20 years. During COVID-19's early years, the biggest shift was among those 50 to 64, whose Internet use rate approached 100%, equivalent to younger groups. In 2021, 75% of those aged 65+ reported using the Internet.

Operating a computer may present particular challenges for novice and experienced older adult computer users. Aging causes visual problems that may make seeing the computer screen difficult or hinder an individual's ability to see the letters on the computer keyboard. Range-of-motion or strength limitations might make it difficult for an individual to reach all the keys on a keyboard, move the computer mouse effectively, or click on icons to open files, folders, and Internet sites. Fine motor coordination problems may make operating a computer mouse difficult or may make hitting the correct keys on the keyboard impossible.

Fortunately, as computer technology has improved, so has the development of assistive technology devices and software and operating system modifications that make using the computer easier for older adults despite any deficits or disorders (Fig. 22.4). The following are some examples of hardware and software devices that can enable an older adult to operate a computer more easily.

## Computer Input Compensations: Mouse Modifications

A person must accomplish several standard tasks to operate a computer. An individual needs to use the computer mouse effectively to maneuver the pointer/cursor in all directions on the computer monitor to open icons, files, and folders. Some older adults have difficulty accomplishing this because of decreased strength and range of motion that occur due to various orthopedic and neurological conditions. Several devices are available that the older adult can use.

For those with limited upper extremity function, trackballs are perhaps the most common alternative to the standard mouse. They allow the individual to move the cursor on the screen by moving a ball that sits on top of a base. Essentially, the individual can accomplish cursor movements by the trackball close to the body or in their hand and move the ball with minimal finger and wrist movement. Some trackballs have a larger base and ball, others can be held in the hand and operated with thumb movement over the ball.

MouseKeys, a built-in accessibility feature in both Mac and Windows operating systems, allows an individual to move the mouse cursor and perform all mouse functions via the number pad on the keyboard. This option is suitable for people who cannot move the standard mouse due to range-of-motion or strength issues but who have sufficient fine motor control to operate the keyboard keys.

Individuals with range-of-motion and strength issues can use various alternative joysticks to operate the cursor. People generally use computer joysticks for computer gaming but can also use them to replace the standard mouse. These are also good alternative mouse options for people who are familiar with joystick operation on power wheelchairs, because they are comfortable with the control required to use these devices.

The trackpad, commonly seen on laptop computers, is a final alternative to the mouse for individuals with compromised upper extremity function. Trackpads also can be added to desktop computers to enable individuals with poor proximal upper extremity range of motion and strength to reposition the trackpad closer to compensate for their deficits and utilize their fingers to move the cursor by dragging them along the trackpad.

For individuals with little to no upper extremity function, electronic head-pointing devices enable them to operate the computer mouse. These devices require the individual to wear a reflective dot or device on the head that transmits an infrared or ultrasound signal to a camera placed on the computer monitor. The camera detects the position of the individual's head and moves the cursor on the screen accordingly. Of course, to operate this device effectively, the individual needs sufficient head and neck range of motion and strength.

A second skill an individual needs to operate a computer mouse is the ability to click the buttons on the mouse to open files, folders, and Internet sites. Single- or double-clicking on the right or left buttons on the standard mouse usually accomplishes these tasks. Sometimes individuals have difficulty performing mouse clicks due to poor fine motor strength or coordination. There are numerous software and hardware solutions and devices and operating system configurations that will help individuals compensate for deficits in mouse-click operation. Changing mouse tracking sensitivity and required double-click speed can help, as can alternatives to double-clicking. Some software programs enable the individual to perform mouse-click, double-click, click-and-drag, and various other functions simply by holding the cursor over the item that needs to be opened or moved. That is, the individual must be able to activate a function such as double-click by dwelling over the double-click icon on the program menu on the screen. Once the individual activates double-click, they move the cursor to the program's icon to open it. Once there, the individual allows the cursor to dwell over the icon for a preset period, for instance, 3 seconds, which opens the program. The individual can use any pointing device described previously to move the cursor. People who operate the mouse with an electronic head-pointing device or cannot isolate a finger to press the buttons on the standard mouse, trackball, or joystick often use this type of program.

Easy reconfiguration of Windows and Mac operating systems facilitates computer use by individuals who cannot perform the double-click or click-and-drag functions. By

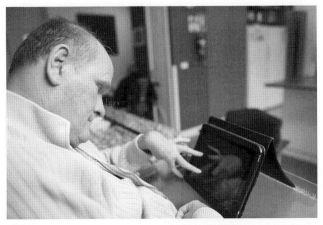

**FIG.22.4**   Using the computer. (Photo © istock.com)

reconfiguring the settings, an individual can use a single click instead of the double click to open programs and can perform click-and-drag options without holding down the button while dragging and moving items. Instructions for doing this reconfiguration can be found on the help menu for the operating system, videos on YouTube, and Internet sites using a search engine.

A final way to perform mouse clicks is via use of a software program that enables users to operate a switch to click on-screen objects. In most cases, a horizontal bar that starts at the top of the screen and moves slowly downward accomplishes this. When the bar reaches the desired object on the screen, the user hits the switch, thereby freezing the line. The user then presses the switch again to activate a pointer that moves horizontally along the line. Once the pointer reaches the desired item, the user then hits the switch again, opening the item.

Older adults suffering from carpal tunnel syndrome and other repetitive stress disorders may have difficulty operating the computer mouse due to pain and discomfort. There are numerous types of ergonomic pointing devices available. These ergonomic pointing devices place the forearm and hand in a better position to reduce the strain placed on the upper extremity structures typically affected by overuse with mouse function.

### Computer Input Compensations: Keyboard Modifications

Sometimes older adults have difficulty hitting one key at a time, releasing the keys quickly enough, reaching all the keys on the keyboard, or isolating their fingers to hit keys due to upper extremity strength, range-of-motion, and coordination issues (Case Example 22.4).

Low-technology items such as typing sticks, mouth sticks, and head pointers allow individuals who cannot isolate their fingers due to coordination issues to hit individual keys. These devices offer individuals single-digit access to typing, which is a very slow means of typing. However, for individuals with little or no funding for devices, these are affordable options for many who want computer access at a low cost.

Due to orthopedic or neurological conditions, individuals with range-of-motion issues often require the use of an alternatively sized keyboard to operate the keyboard most effectively. Smaller keyboards limit the individual's need to reach far from one side of the keyboard to the other to reach all the keys. However, with the smaller keyboard size, the size of the keys is usually decreased. Therefore, good fine motor skill is generally necessary to use these keyboards.

An alternative to the smaller keyboard is an alternatively configured keyboard in which the layout of the keys is different from the standard QWERTY. These layouts place the most frequently used letters in the center of the keyboard and letters that are frequently used in combination, such as *t* and *h*, near each other. This layout reduces the amount of movement a person needs to make to type common words. This option for keyboarding is effective for one-handed keyboard users and for those who fatigue easily with standard keyboard use due to range-of-motion issues, but who cannot use a smaller keyboard due to fine motor issues.

A larger keyboard with larger keys is an option for individuals with poor fine motor control but good proximal range of motion and strength. This modification will eliminate the number of undesired characters appearing on the screen due to coordination deficits.

Older adults suffering from carpal tunnel syndrome and other repetitive stress disorders can also benefit from the numerous types of ergonomic keyboards available. These keyboards place the keys in a more ergonomic position to reduce the stress placed on the upper extremity structures typically affected by overuse of computer operation.

Morse code is another alternative means of letter and number input. Individuals using Morse code for letter input can use either a single or double switch to perform the series of dots and dashes used to produce letters. This option is excellent for computer input for individuals familiar with Morse code and those who have little to no functioning in most of the body and cannot afford the eye-gaze systems discussed later in this section.

---

**CASE EXAMPLE 22.4**   Computer Access

Andrew is a 68-year-old man with diabetes diagnosed with a cerebrovascular accident 2 years ago. He cannot use his left arm functionally but has intact function in his right, dominant extremity. He has a history of diabetic retinopathy, which has caused his vision to decline enough that he has difficulty reading his pill bottles and the newspaper.

Andrew has used a computer over the last 10 years to communicate with family members and friends across the country via email and a videoconferencing software program he had used at work. He has noticed a decline in his ability to see items he has typed on the computer monitor, and he has indicated a desire to be able to type more efficiently using his right hand. He has asked for assistance in finding software and hardware that might allow him better access to his computer.

After evaluation, his occupational therapist determined that Andrew would benefit from adaptations to his computer for input, processing, and output. For input, a keyboard with better one-hand access would be optimal. Often, these keyboards are smaller in size to allow the one-handed computer user to access all the keys more easily. Another recommendation would be for Andrew to use a word-prediction program to improve his typing speed by limiting the number of keystrokes he would need to produce text, making his typing more efficient. The final recommendation would be for Andrew to use a screen-reader and magnifier software program to compensate for his declining visual function. With these adaptations, Andrew should be able to use the computer and continue to communicate with his family and friends more effectively.

Computer keyboarding can also be accomplished via the use of an on-screen keyboard. Both Mac and Windows operating systems have on-screen keyboards in their standard accessibility features. Projections of images of keyboards onto the computer screen allow the user to click on individual letters, dwell over individual letters for a predetermined time, or via switch scanning, to make letter choices as each row on the keyboard is scanned. With click-and-dwell options, users can point to the letters using any pointing device discussed previously. Scanning is an extremely slow means of letter input but may be the only option for some individuals with minimal physical function.

Speech-recognition programs allow the user to perform both mouse and keyboard functions via the use of the voice. The individual first needs to program the voice so that the computer recognizes what the user says. Once programmed, the user can dictate text and perform keyboard and mouse functions via voice. Both Mac and Windows operating systems offer speech-recognition features in their newer operating systems. However, these programs do not allow the degree of functionality afforded by other commercial speech-recognition programs, such as Dragon Naturally Speaking. These speech-recognition programs are appropriate for individuals familiar with the standard keyboard functions because everything that was accomplished via the keyboard needs translation into voice command. Therefore, a fair degree of cognitive skill is required to learn how to use and operate these programs. Speech-recognition programs (and add-ons to standard programs) are an excellent alternative means of computer access for those with poor upper extremity functioning coupled with poor head control but who have good respiratory function.

Eye-gaze systems are perhaps the newest option in computer input for those with no other options due to minimal functioning of other body parts typically used for computer operation. With these systems, the individual simply needs to look at items on the screen to open them or look at letters on an on-screen keyboard to input words and data. The user accomplishes letter input via a camera placed on the monitor that detects the position of the individual's eyes via reflection of light off the retina. These systems are often cost-prohibitive for many people because medical insurance does not cover computer input, but they do cover them for electronic AAC device access.

Some computer users have difficulty with fine motor skills, which causes them to hit two keys at a time, placing unwanted characters in the document. Keyguards are low-tech items placed on the keyboard to reduce the number of unwanted characters typed by hitting two keys at a time. Windows and Mac operating systems both have a feature called filter keys that ignore the unwanted keystrokes by requiring the individual to hold down a key for a predetermined amount of time before recognizing it as a keystroke. The individual can configure filter keys so that they must release a key and push it again before a repeat character can appear on the screen. Filter keys can also be configured to ignore repeat keystrokes for those who have difficulty releasing keys quickly enough such that numerous repeated characters appear on the screen.

## Computer Productivity/Processing Compensations

The computer access assistive technology described thus far can provide individuals with enhanced ability to operate the computer mouse and keyboard. In some cases, such as with character input via switch scanning, the ability to efficiently produce documents is compromised. Speed and productivity are important in today's workforce and in other activities, such as shopping online, because some sites limit the amount of time allowed for text entry into order forms.

### Word Prediction

One way to speed up letter input is software programs that predict the words an individual is trying to type based on the first few letters typed. These word-prediction settings allow the individual to use fewer keystrokes to type a word or phrase. That is, when the person types the letters *t* and *h*, for example, a menu of words that commonly begin with those letters is presented. If the desired word or phrase is in the list, the person chooses the word(s) without having to type everything. Word prediction is especially effective in reducing the time a person spends in typing longer words.

### Abbreviation Expansion

Abbreviation expansion programs are another way to improve efficiency and productivity with computer input. With abbreviation expansion, the user simply needs to type in an abbreviation, such as *OT*, and once that combination of letters is recognized, the entire phrase *occupational therapy* will replace the *OT* originally typed. As you can see, the number of keystrokes required to type *occupational therapy* would dramatically decrease, which would, in turn, speed up productivity.

### Macros

A final way to speed up letter and number input is through keyboard and mouse macros. Macros allow the individual to record common phrases or mouse actions and transform them from longer keystrokes or mouse movements into shorter sequences of keystrokes. For example, if an individual needed to type their name and address repetitively on multiple documents, they could record the name and address through the Macro Recorder, then apply a sequence of keystrokes, such as Alt-A, to represent the name and address. The next time the person needs to type the name and address, they simply hit the Alt and A key in Microsoft or Shift plus A keys in MacIntosh and the name and address will appear.

All these productivity options can dramatically improve the efficiency of the computer user. In a world where speed and productivity are paramount, they are necessary accommodations for computer access for older adults with functional limitations due to age-related changes or various diseases. For older adults with repetitive stress disorders and arthritis, decreasing the number of times they need to press a keyboard key might allow them to complete keyboarding tasks with less pain and discomfort. For older people with progressive disorders, reducing the number of keystrokes can assist in keeping fatigue at bay.

### Computer Output Compensations

Numerous low- and high-technology compensations and devices allow individuals with visual deficits to "see" what is present on the computer monitor. Perhaps the easiest compensations that an older adult with mild visual impairments can use are to enlarge the text size and increase the space between individual letters in web-browsing, word processing, and email programs while the individual is viewing materials or inputting text. These changes enable better visualization of the typed text without paying for any other computer modifications because these options come standard in most software programs.

To compensate for more severe visual deficits, images on the monitor can be enlarged by other means. Low-technology screen magnifiers can be placed over the existing monitor to enlarge what is present on the screen. These are easy to obtain but do not offer as much functionality as some of the other high-tech screen-magnification options. Both Mac and Windows operating systems provide an electronic screen-magnification accessibility feature. There are also numerous commercially available screen-magnification software programs for purchase and several free programs available via Internet searches. These electronic magnification programs magnify either the whole screen or parts of the screen to enable those with visual impairments to see the screen better.

Two other options that allow individuals to "see" what is on the screen are screen readers and text-to-speech programs. These programs will read aloud icons and menus on the desktop and in programs and read what is typed in a document via individual letters, whole words, complete sentences, or any combination of these. Of course, to use these programs the individual must hear effectively, which may be a problem with some older adults. Also, consideration of environmental factors that might affect the use of these programs is necessary. For example, older adults could not use programs in a classroom situation or libraries unless headphones are attached to the computer. Several commercially available screen readers/text-to-speech programs and a few freeware programs are available for download. Mac and Windows operating systems offer a screen-reader option as a standard part of their accessibility features, and they are part of Microsoft and Google program suites.

### Computer Use: Psychosocial Effects

Computers offer individuals the ability to manage their households, participate in leisure and recreational activities, create, communicate, and research information. Computer use may also have added benefits for older adults. Research has shown that computer use for the older adult can have positive psychosocial value. Several studies have shown that computer use can positively influence the quality of life of the older adult (Erickson & Johnson, 2011; Werner et al., 2011). Opalinski

(2001) and Hendrix (2000) found that computer use allowed older individuals to acquire new skills and gain knowledge, thereby increasing their feelings of control, self-esteem, and self-efficacy. Other researchers found that by increasing the older person's interaction with others via the Internet, loneliness decreased, rates of suicide declined, independence in ADLs improved, and medication needs for ailments such as arthritis decreased (Czaja & Lee, 2007; White et al., 2002). Lyden and colleagues (2021) provide a useful tool to guide OT and other providers in interventions to increase or maintain social engagement among clients with mild cognitive impairment.

Options for compensating for functional deficits that affect the older individual's ability to use a computer are numerous, as shown in this discussion. These options, coupled with the fact that computers have proven benefits for the older user, make it clear that professionals working with the older adult population should not disregard the use of computers with their older clients in trying to bring about functional gains. Unfortunately, most medical insurance plans will not pay for computer modifications that are not medically necessary, and many older individuals are on fixed incomes and unable to purchase some of the technology discussed previously. It is important for the professional working with the older adult population to think "out of the box" for creative options for obtaining these devices. For example, grants are available that might finance a computer center in a senior housing complex. OT professionals might also search various online "freecycle" sites that provide gently used devices free of charge or for a nominal fee.

### Mobile Devices and Apps

Mobile devices have become more mainstream, and they have taken on a more significant role in the lives of older adults. Many options provide older adults with mobile means for communication, health monitoring, environmental control, and cognitive stimulation.

Mobile phones can be very simple, such as a specially designed flip phone that opens to answer and closes to hang up, or that has just one button to push for a live operator who connects the caller with predetermined contacts. The Jitterbug flip phone was consistently rated high in usability for older adults due to its larger buttons, brighter displays, and simplified operations compared with many other phones on the market. But cell phones that are not smartphones (which is still the case for almost half of the current older cell phone users) miss the opportunity provided by a wide array of apps in both the iPhone and Android domains. Jitterbug's Smart3 and others attempt simplify smartphone use for older adults.

For more tech-savvy users, smartphones allow for voice calls, text messages, browsing the Internet, reading e-mail, social networking, taking photos and videos, and utilizing apps. They can serve as global positioning and AAC devices, and some apps can detect falls and alert family and responders. Even the very simple cell phones also have "reminder" features to allow someone to receive alarms and reminders to compensate for minor cognitive limitations.

Many older adults use mobile device technologies to communicate with family, friends, and community resources. Text messaging has become a popular way for older adults to communicate with their younger family members because this is often the preferred method of communication for pre-teens and teens. Text messaging has its inherent difficulties for the older adult. For example, "text speak" or text jargon is often difficult for the older adult to understand. In addition, for older adults with arthritic hands, typing on the small keypads available on most mobile devices often inhibits the effective use of text messaging. Finally, the small screen and available text fonts often inhibit those with visual problems from using this feature effectively. Luckily, as mobile carriers have recognized the growing number of older adult mobile technology consumers, more features are being built into new devices to accommodate these problems. In addition, individuals can download numerous apps for free or for a nominal fee. These apps can enlarge the keypad available on touchscreen devices, make the fonts larger, or read aloud what they type onto the screen. There are also devices, such as Jitterbug, that are explicitly designed with the older adult user in mind.

People can also communicate with friends and family through apps like WhatsApp and Zoom, using smartphones, smartwatches, and tablets. According to an AARP survey conducted during the COVID-19 pandemic, roughly a third of Americans 45 and older reported feeling lonely. This loneliness affects the health of older adults putting them at a "higher risk of dementia, greater rates of depression and nearly four times the risk of death among heart patients" (Davis, 2020). Videoconferencing apps or video/voice communication apps have become popular with older adults to combat the effects of loneliness by giving the older adult a means to communicate face to face with friends and family who may not live close geographically. There are also intergenerational programs available that connect older adults with younger strangers to combat isolation. Programs such as "Big and Mini" and "Eldera," among others, match elders with younger individuals to end social isolation and bridge generations (Halpert, 2022).

Another benefit to using WhatsApp and similar apps to communicate is its use of Voice Over Internet Protocol (VOIP). Standard cell phone technology sacrifices audio quality to carry more conversations on a given cell tower; however the deployment of 5G promises to improve signal quality. Because of normal age-related declines in hearing high-pitched sounds (referred to as presbycusis) and the consequential difficulties in differentiating among similar consonants, "regular" cell phone calls are difficult for older adults to hear, particularly in noisy environments. Since WhatsApp uses VOIP voice calling and communication is clearer for the older adult to hear, making similar VOIP apps a better option for them.

With the emphasis today on reducing health-care expenditures, mobile monitoring devices that give physicians daily updates on client health can be at the forefront of the cost-saving measures necessary in lowering health-care costs. It is possible to monitor sleep, ambulation, medication reminders/adherence, blood pressure, glucose levels, and other health measures through mobile technologies and apps and other peripherals that are both easy to use and often inexpensive.

Mobile technologies have also provided older adults with alternatives to the traditional medical alert systems if a fall or other medical emergency occurs. Smart watches can detect serious falls and respond by asking the individual whether help is needed. Mobile technologies have enabled active older adults to leave their homes where they may have previously been tethered to a medical alarm base station, such as that available from Lifecall. Services such as those offered by Great Call's 5 Star Urgent Response allow the older adult to leave home yet still access help at any location with wireless coverage.

Control of electronic devices in one's home is also possible through mobile technologies and apps. Apps enable the smartphone to be used as a remote control and offer access to devices in the environment connected to peripherals that interface with the app. The older adult with mobility problems would not need to get up from bed to turn the lights on for those nighttime bathroom trips or would be able to adjust the temperature settings in the home or remotely lock doors should the individual forget to do so before a long trip. Both Apple and Android operating systems offer numerous apps for environmental control. In addition, television and Internet service providers provide environmental control through their services and most often allow for access to controls through a mobile app.

Age-related cognitive declines affect the older adult's ability to age successfully but can be slowed, mitigated, or compensated for through mental stimulation and cognitive strategies. Cognitive psychologists have long documented different types of memory (i.e., long-term, short-term, episodic, iconic, echoic, procedural, and prospective—see Chapter 15). Time- and event-based prospective memory—remembering to do something—often show declines with advanced age, and reminder devices can be of assistance. A recent study (Charness et al., 2021) notes that current reminder devices have some shortcomings, particularly as they are not effectively matched to specific user needs. They are developing and testing a prototype D.R.E.A.M. System (Digital Reminder for Everyday Activity Memory) that proposes to address current shortcomings in reminder systems, helping to remind user about a wide variety of needed tasks (e.g., medication use, time to leave for a doctor's appointment, need to defrost food for dinner, reminder to call a friend to wish a happy birthday, etc.). The program has implications for normal aging but is currently focusing on assisting individuals with mild cognitive impairment (MCI), traumatic brain injury (TBI) and post-stroke cognitive impairment (PSCI) to remember tasks categorized on a Tablet App in categories of Health, Home, and Social. An estimated 40% of individuals aged 80 to 84, and 60% for those 85 and over, suffer from MCI (Gillis et al., 2019).

Mobile technologies and apps provide cognitive stimulation to the older adult, thereby reducing the effects of diseases such as dementia and providing for leisure outlets and social interaction. Research has shown that mobile technologies have improved the functioning of adults with dementia through apps that target specific areas of cognitive functioning such as memory and problem solving (but recall that mobile technologies have inherent access problems for the older adult, as previously discussed) (Coppola et al., 2013). Lumosity's Human Cognition Project conducted research into the effectiveness of the brain games it offers and found that individuals who are undergoing chemotherapy or who are recovering from strokes demonstrated improved mental awareness and information processing as benefits of daily participation in the brain games. In addition, apps such as "Words with Friends" provide the older adult with mental stimulation and the ability to engage in a leisure activity with family and friends or even complete strangers.

Mobile technologies offer the older adult more cost-effective, user-friendly communication, health monitoring, environmental control, and cognitive stimulation options. It is best to match the technology with the needs of individuals based on their skills and desire to incorporate technology into their everyday lives. It is also important to note that as mobile technology becomes more prevalent in society, the incidence of "technophobia" will continue to decline.

### Telehealth/Telemedicine Devices and Services

*Telehealth* and *telemedicine* are two terms that have been used interchangeably to describe the exchange of health information between individuals in their homes and remote health-care professionals through video and audio technologies (Colucci et al., 2019). The term *telemedicine* is more correctly used to describe the clinical services provided through electronic means to improve a client's health status. *Telehealth* involves clinical services and medical education, administration, and research. Using technology to remotely monitor an individual's health and safety has shown great promise in helping people to avoid diseases and injuries and to maintain good health. The use of telehealth and telemedicine increased dramatically as a result of COVID-19. States, such as South Carolina, provided tablets, instruction on digital literacy, and free or reduced-price Internet access to rural elders (Wicklund, 2021). As described earlier in this chapter, a growing network of digital navigators is helping to reduce the digital divide and to assist elders before their first telehealth visit (Goforth, 2021, July).

Various types of telehealth devices are now used in monitoring residents' health in their homes (Cimperman et al., 2016). Devices can monitor cardiac functions, blood sugar levels, weight, general activity, sleep patterns, and other health-related parameters. Some telehealth devices measure only one item, such as blood pressure, whereas others are bundled to provide remote health-care providers with an overall picture of a client's daily health. Daily tracking and monitoring health measures has significant implications for keeping older adults healthy. For instance, information on weight gain in a client with congestive heart failure can provide the physician with information about the individual's

heart function, enabling the physician to provide immediate intervention without the client waiting for the next available appointment. Systems that gather and analyze data show the greatest promise for cost-effective care provision.

A variety of options for mobile health (mHealth) monitoring through smartphones, wearable sensors (e.g., fitness trackers), and other mobile devices can collect health-related data, communicate with health-care providers, and provide real-time feedback for interventions to users (Cajamarca et al., 2019).

## SUMMARY

This chapter provides fundamental and reasonably up-to-date information on how to understand and effectively utilize assistive technologies to support the wants and needs of older adults. These include the ability to age in place and to enhance or maintain a high quality of life, as well as objective and subjective measures of well-being despite a variety of conditions and disabilities that become more common in the later years. However, there is a catch. Some materials that are up to date as we complete this chapter may become obsolete by the time you read it because the application of technology in OT practice is rapidly changing.

Constantly during preparation of this manuscript, we noted new developments, products, services, research, and resources to consider for inclusion. So, it becomes crucial to ask, "How did we address this challenge, and how should the reader?"

First, we began with some fundamental guiding principles, paradigms, and models—from OT and allied disciplines, gerontology, psychology, and others. Your commitment to understanding these principles will enhance your ability to apply them to your practice, increase your ability to independently assess the value of new technologies as they appear over time, and enhance your interprofessional competencies. Connecting, communicating, and collaborating with specialists from other disciplines is particularly important when considering or using technological tools to enhance your client's well-being.

Next, we turned to a discussion of low-technology devices. These are less likely to change as rapidly as the high-technology, electronic, mobile devices, and *continue to be the most useful in many situations*, despite the never-ending push to use the latest, greatest gadgets and gizmos. The long-handled shoehorn sometimes works better than Velcro closures, the trip to the store continues to provide a whole host of biopsychosocial benefits compared to home delivery services, and the "high-touch" intervention of a human therapist will be difficult to replace with the most sophisticated robot. The lesson here is to pay close attention to the tried-and-true technologies presented in the low-technology section of this chapter.

We definitely need our "early adopters" to continually push the envelope. Just as National Aeronautics and Space Administration (NASA), Neil Armstrong, and the *Apollo* astronauts helped us develop the technologies necessary to get to the moon, we need explorers in health-care delivery.

Whether or not you are comfortable and effective as an early adopter has a lot to do with your personality, your training, your organization's leadership and risk-tolerance attitude, and your organization's financial resources. However, regardless of your preferences, it is imperative to keep your client's wants, needs, and best interests at the forefront as you help them decide what is best for them. Remember, "What Matters" to the client is the first of 4Ms in an Age Friendly Healthcare System (Institute for Health Care Improvement, 2020, June).

Our discussion next turned to high-technology options. We focused primarily on IAT, including environmental control devices for in-home care and daily living support. We also covered the swiftly changing fields of telehealth, telemedicine, tele-homecare, personal care robots, VR, and AI. Somehow, we snuck in service animals, and you may have asked, "What's this doing here" before you realized that the training of these animals and the array of services they provide are truly remarkable. Our high-technology section next discussed computer assistive technologies before concluding with mobile devices. We focused on input, output, and productivity/processing compensation issues for computers.

As you think about the section on computer assistive technology, you may believe that computers are obsolete—the name of the game is mobile devices. This may be somewhat true, but the difficulties in computer use by older adults, and the technological adjustments made to overcome these difficulties, are perhaps even more pronounced and poorly addressed when it comes to supporting the successful use of mobile devices by older adults. Small screen displays, glare on screens in bright/outdoor environments, limited bandwidth barriers to high-speed uploads/downloads, and other issues make mobile-enabled health deployment for older adults a work in progress.

How else should you prepare for continual change in your work with older adult clients, in collaboration with other occupational therapists and specialists from other fields? Get accustomed to knowing what organizations provide the best objective trustworthy information about new devices. The AOTA, the Human Factors and Ergonomic Society, the American Society on Aging, the Center for Aging Services Technologies (CAST) of LeadingAge, and the Gerontological Society of America are all helpful sources. There are also useful discussion groups on LinkedIn (e.g., gerontechnology) and Facebook that can help you stay ahead of the curve.

*The complete listing of the Bibliography and Chapter Questions and Answers are available in the accompanying enhanced eBook version included with the print purchase of this textbook. Visit Elsevier eBooks+ (eBooks.Health.Elsevier.com) to access this content.*

## CHAPTER 23

# Family, Friends, and Social Contexts in Later Life

*Margaret A. Perkinson, PhD, FGSA, FAGHE, FSfAA and Karen Frank Barney, PhD, MS, OTR, FAOTA*

## CHAPTER OUTLINE

## OBJECTIVES

- Understand changing family dynamics in the United States over time and different generations.
- Describe the changing roles of aging adults as their children reach adulthood.
- Explain how occupational therapy personnel can encourage positive relationships among two or more generations and extended family members.
- Understand the role of occupational therapy in facilitating functional familial habits, routines, and occupations.
- Discuss the roles and meaningfulness of friends among older adults.

The social contexts of older adults, including families, vary widely throughout the world, depending upon customs and norms of the country, region, religious or nonreligious practices, and specific family circumstances, such as deaths of spouses or children, never-married with children, individuals or couples without children, adoptions, disabling conditions, employment or retirement status, incarceration, or acceptance or rejection of members for various reasons. It is likely that most occupational therapy (OT) personnel have experienced life within a family unit for all or part of their lives, yet within their practice will need to relate to a variety of family structures and living circumstances of the patients/clients they serve that differ from their own life experience. Occupational therapists (OTs) and OT assistants (OTAs) are expected to promote functional familial participation within their interactions with family members as they provide OT interventions within whatever circumstances they encounter (Reitz & Scaffa, 2020). Should dysfunctional interactions be observed or detected within the family, friend, or coworker relationships, OT staff should enlist additional interprofessional or other qualified providers to assist with problem solving, always using a client-centered approach.

## Changing Family Structures and Dynamics in the 21st Century

As discussed in Chapters 1 and 3, the impact of the demographic transition on the experience of later life can hardly be overstated. The increase in general length of life and decline in fertility rates have resulted in radical changes in family structure and relationships (Smock & Schwartz, 2020). Families in the relatively recent past consisted of two, at most three, generations, with multiple siblings in each generation, resulting in a pyramid-shaped family structure. Current demographic changes have had a direct effect on average family size and composition: compared with families of past eras, contemporary families are more likely to include multiple generations (due to increased length of life), with fewer members in each succeeding generation (due to decline in fertility rates), resulting in a "beanpole" family structure (Bengston, 2004). This transformation of family structure has major implications for family relationships and dynamics, for example, the nature of spousal relationships in longer-lasting postchildrearing or nonchildrearing marriages, the nature of relationships between parents and their older and fewer adult children and grandchildren, and the changing availability of informal kin-based support for care of older adults (National Institute on Aging [NIA], 2007). Intergenerational relationships assume greater importance within families with fewer members within generations and with longer years of shared lives between generations (Bengston, 2004).

Current changes in the ways families are formed, maintained, and dissolved result in new and varied family structures and relationships. Types of living arrangements currently experienced by older adults are far more varied than in the past. In 2021, 60% of older adults who lived in the community lived with their spouse or partner. About 27% of all older adults lived alone—21% of older men and 33%

of older women (US Census Bureau, 2021). Of older adults (aged 57 to 85 years) in a partner relationship, 62% were in a first marriage, 28% were remarried, 3% were in unmarried cohabitation, and 7% were in a LAT (living apart together) relationship (Lewin, 2017).

## Childless Older Adults

The age at first marriage is increasing globally, contributing to the general decline in fertility. An estimated 16.5% of older adults were childless in 2021 (US Census Bureau, 2021), and the number of childless younger women is rising, especially in East Asia (Cheng, 2020). In the United States, the percentage of women without any children by the end of their reproductive years doubled between the mid-1970s and the mid-2000s, from about 10% to 20%. However, since then, the portion of women who remain childless has been declining to around 15% (Frejka, 2017).

## Never-Marrieds

The total number of Americans who have never been married is historically high. Compared with 1960, when 9% had never married, 1 in 5 adults ages 25 or older (42 million) were not married within the last decade (Wang & Parker, 2014). A variety of factors contribute to this phenomenon: later life marriages, cohabitation and raising children outside of marriage, hard economic times, changing demographics and cultural norms.

In 2021, approximately 6% of persons aged 65 years and older in the United States had never married (US Census Bureau, 2022). That number is projected to increase to 11% by 2060 (US Census Bureau, 2017). Approximately 25% of older Black women have never married. Older never-married persons are 5 times as likely to live below the US federal poverty line (Lin et al., 2017).

## Cohabitation and Living Apart Together

Social norms regarding premarital relationships are becoming less restrictive among both older and younger adults (Cherlin, 2010). Growing numbers of older adults live outside traditional family structures. Two that are gaining in popularity are "cohabitation," a coresidential intimate partnership, in which partners are not married/remarried, and "living apart together (LAT)," a noncoresidential intimate partnership in which partners maintain separate households and share living quarters on a temporary or intermittent basis (De Jong Gierveld, 2004; Levin, 2004). In 2000, an estimated 950,000 adults over age 50 lived with an unmarried partner. By 2016, that number had increased to over four million (Brown, Lin et al., 2019). For many older adults, cohabitation represents an alternative to marriage and is replacing remarriage following widowhood or divorce (Brown et al., 2017). Financial benefits of cohabitation are significant. Unmarried couples can continue to receive pension benefits and Social Security that may terminate upon remarriage.

For younger adults, transient LAT generally represents a temporary period prior to cohabitation (Turcotte, 2013). Long-term, stable LAT relationships are more common among older adults (Connidis et al., 2017; Lewin, 2017). With cohabitation and LAT on the rise, older adult couplings are assuming a more companionate form of relationship (Carr & Utz, 2020). Cohabitation among older adults can function as a long-term alternative to marriage (King & Scott, 2005), tending to be quite stable, with an average duration of almost 10 years (Brown et al., 2012). Only a minority of older cohabiting couples wed or break up.

### Needs of Childless and Unmarried Older Adults

Unpaired older adults may need more support as they age, if they encounter health-related and occupational challenges. For example, an individual living alone and experiencing usual and customary age-related changes may find that reaching objects high or low, managing basic activities of daily living (BADLs) (fundamental self-care activities) and instrumental activities of daily living (IADLs) (cooking, cleaning, pet care, mobilizing, maintaining finances, transporting oneself, shopping, and any other requisite occupations to support living in a community), and participating in leisure occupations have become more difficult over time. When one lacks a partner whose abilities can support and supplement one's own needs related to these changes, challenging occupations become even more demanding, and outside support may be required.

Some, but not all, never-married individuals have family support, which enables them to continue to be functional if the support relates directly to their declining abilities. Those whose families are not present or who limit support may have increasing challenges, physically and mentally, over time. Thus, it is important for OT staff to discern what, if any, support is available and to what extent, in order to provide fully relevant interventions with these individuals.

### Later Life Marriages: Courtship in Later Life

Men and women find themselves seeking relationships in later life for a variety of reasons, including never having been married, divorce, or death of a spouse. Familial, cultural, ethnic, and/or religious norms and expectations may play a role in how the individual finds a mate in later years, if they are so inspired. Older individuals find potential mates in various ways. These include participation in a wide variety of work and social groups, including recreational, religious, neighborhood-based and congregate housing, musical, political, travel, theater, and sports. Although they are less likely than younger adults to use online sites or apps for dating, they may utilize sites that focus on specific interests of older adults (Brown, 2020). Aging adults may also reflect upon earlier friendships that may have romantic potential, such as high school or college friends, workforce colleagues, and neighbors, any of which could potentially result in a romantic relationship (see Fig. 23.1).

### Gender Differences in Late Life Marriage and Divorce

Men and women experience marriage in later life in quite different ways (Carr & Utz, 2020). In 2021, 69% of men and only 47% of women aged 65 and over in the United States were married (US Census Bureau, 2022). The differences were even starker for the oldest old. For those aged 85 years and over in the United States, 60% of men and only 17% of women were married, due in large part to the fact that women live generally longer than men and tend to marry older men, and men are more likely to remarry after widowhood or divorce. Until relatively recently, most marriages in later life ended with widowhood, and divorce in mid- and later-life was uncommon (Brown, Lin et al., 2019). The rise in "gray divorce" now accounts for approximately one-third of the dissolutions of late-life marriages (Brown & Wright, 2017). From 1990 to 2010, gray divorce among persons aged 50+ years more than doubled (Lin et al., 2016). In 2015, 18.1% of older women and 14.3% of older men were divorced. In 1990, 1 in 10 divorced individuals were over age 50, in 2010, that number climbed to over 25% (Brown & Lin, 2012).

The experience of postdivorce differs by gender: women generally encounter drastic declines in income and economic well-being, while men generally suffer the "social penalty," i.e., loss of friends and support from adult children, due to weaker social ties prior to divorce (Lin, 2008). Repartnering after divorce further weakens fathers' relationships with their adult children (Kalmijn, 2013a; Noël-Miller, 2011). Although similar in level of education, unmarried older adults are four times more likely to live in poverty and twice as likely to experience disability compared to their married counterparts (Lin & Brown, 2012).

Approximately 37% of men and 22% of women repartnered within 10 years of gray divorce, more frequently through cohabitation rather than remarriage, especially for men (Brown, Lin

et al., 2019). Repartnering following widowhood is less common than repartnering following divorce, especially for women (Brown et al., 2018; Vespa, 2012).

Negative and distressed communication leading to conflict and distancing is a major cause for divorce (Frye, 2018; Mark & Jozkowski, 2013; Wilde & Dozois, 2019). Growing apart also is a commonly cited reason for divorce (Bair, 2007). Divorce rates vary widely by country. More developed nations have higher incidences of divorce than lesser developed nations. Other reasons for lesser divorce rates may be religious practices and societal norms.

## The Impact of COVID-19 on Marriage in Later Life

Compared to younger people, older adults reported less pandemic-related stress, less life change, less social isolation, and less negative impact on the quality of their relationships (Birditt et al., 2021). Data drawn from the 2020 National Social Life, Health, and Aging Project COVID-19 Study indicated that during the pandemic, the quality of relationships of couples aged 50 years and older stayed the same for 67%, improved for 23%, and declined for 10% of the couples in the sample (Wong et al., 2023). Deepened marital relationships may be one response to the COVID-19 pandemic. Most individuals altered their occupations, with couples spending more time together at home, even though individual tasks might be different. Habits and routines have typically been adapted or discarded to maintain a safe home environment. Staying as safe as possible has been a larger challenge for older adults, who are more susceptible to COVID-19, requiring relative isolation from the outside world, wearing masks

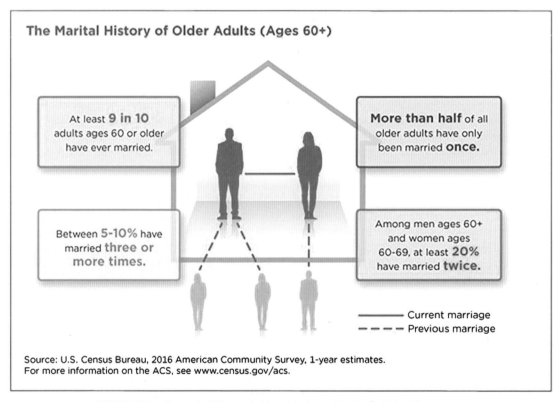

FIGURE 23.1   The marital history of older adults (ages 60+) in the United States.

routinely, and also ordering groceries, clothing, and household goods online, or having someone younger who is less at risk for infection shop for them. During the enforced isolation of the COVID-19 lockdowns, the intensity and nature of older adults' shared occupations, such as meal preparation, fitness, reading, pet care, or types of entertainment, may have deepened—this is clearly a prime research topic that should be explored.

## Long-Lasting Marriages

The long-term marriage literature indicates that five "C's" are highly relevant to long-term marital satisfaction: (1) commitment, (2) caring, (3) communication, (4) conflict and compromise, and (5) contract—marital partners' expectations of each other and their marriages (Sharlin et al., 2018). Marital longevity for some relates to having lived through the global Great Depression in the 1930s, as well as World War II or other major stressors. Many have practiced a religious faith that reinforced marital values.

Marital satisfaction appears to be more related to the quality of interactions than to income and duration of the marriage (Dhaliwal, 2021). Numerous sources state that marriages that last 50 or more years reflect the following traits: willingness to compromise, being willing to show emotion and be vulnerable, trusting fully in their spouse, showing physical affection, respecting one another, appreciating all time spent together, being best friends, having good problem-solving strategies and communication skills, and making the marriage a priority in their lives (Ben-Ze'ev, 2019; Dhaliwal, 2021; Kaslow & Sharlin, 2022; Norgren et al., 2004).

Gender differences may soften with age, with men becoming more nurturing, and women more assertive (Bachand & Caron, 2001). Setting and pursuing goals in older adulthood may increasingly involve a spouse as a support for engaging in and/or completing a wide variety of activities (Zambrano et al., 2022). These occupations may include BADLs and IADLs when physical and/or mental functional performance has declined, managing household tasks, traveling to medical appointments that often increase in number with age, maintaining participation and productivity in organizations and social groups, continuing familial or other roles, traveling for recreational purposes, and participating in new occupations.

These concepts also apply to couples in the lesbian, gay, bisexual, transgender, queer, or questioning (LGBTQ+) community, whether married or not, who tend to maintain long-term relationships until one partner's death (Michelson & Harrison, 2021). However, not all long-lasting marriages are totally fulfilling; they may be maintained for economic, social, cultural, religious, or other reasons (Batista da Costa & Pereira Mosmann, 2021). Thus, OT personnel must develop discerning relationships with older couples, as individuals, to determine how to best develop rapport with each spouse to support their individual and collective aspirations and goal attainment, as well as identify interprofessional resources to alleviate spousal abuse, if it is reported or suspected.

## Widowhood

Approximately 30% of women aged 65 and older were widowed in 2021, as opposed to 11% of older men (US Census Bureau, Annual Social and Economic Supplement, 2022). Both widows and widowers have a 66% higher risk of dying within the first 90 days of losing their spouse due to self-neglect, lack of a support network, and lifestyle changes that follow the death of a spouse (Moon et al., 2014).

Widowed persons have higher levels of informal social participation than nonwidowed persons, but comparable levels of formal social participation (Utz et al., 2002). Social participation levels tend to decrease before the death of a spouse, primarily because of poor spousal health and heightened caregiving demands, and increase following the loss, because of increased support from friends and relatives. Marital status can be a strong determinant of friendship patterns in later life, with married older adults aligning with other married adults, and single/unmarried older adults (especially women) also gravitating toward each other (Perkinson & Rockemann, 1996). A newly widowed woman may find a new (and possibly larger) set of women now open to potential friendships because of her change to singlehood.

A majority of widowed persons use social participation as an active coping strategy to deal with the negative effects of widowhood (Utz et al., 2002). Social participation in informal activities such as visiting friends and telephone contact assumes great importance in daily life in late-life bereavement. Formal social participation (e.g., membership in clubs or social organizations) may not provide the emotional and instrumental support that informal social participation does, thus explaining why formal social participation levels remain constant after widowhood.

Older adults, particularly those experiencing devastating or stressful losses and transitions such as widowhood, tend to rely on their convoy of lifelong social relations and support, i.e., cohort members who share similar life experiences and historical contexts and with whom they derive support, self-definition, and a sense of stability and continuity (Antonucci & Jackson, 1987; Kahn & Antonucci, 1980).

A longitudinal analysis of secondary data from the 1996–2012 University of Michigan Health and Retirement Study found that widowhood status of participants aged 50 years and older was related to cognitive decline (Shin et al., 2018). Protective factors against this decline included higher education status and having at least one living sibling. Utilizing the same dataset and its accompanying Consumption and Activities Mail Survey, Lee et al. (2019) investigated the effects of leisure engagement on cognition among the 2,827 participants. Their results showed that engagement in mental activities mitigated the effect of widowhood on cognition. Findings did not include the effects of intergenerational support. These findings reinforce the need for OT intervention to support mental activity engagement for this population.

The Chinese Longitudinal Healthy Longevity Survey 2002–2014 examined the impact of widowhood over time. Understandably, loneliness accompanies widowhood acutely and is long-lasting; however, remarriage may mitigate the effects of the initial loneliness. Even though the loneliness slightly decreased over time, it may still be significant after 40 years of bereavement (Yang & Gu, 2021).

In general, loneliness is associated with many physical and psychological health risks, including depression (Luanaigh & Lawlor, 2008), cognitive impairment (Zhou et al., 2018), mortality (Luo & Waite, 2014), and poor self-rated health (Tsur et al., 2019). Therefore, OT personnel should be discerning about detecting loneliness in older men and women who have been widowed or never married, so that relevant support and meaningful occupational engagement can be integrated into OT interventions and recommendations.

OT personnel need to be objective about intervening in marital relationships, since each couple has their own history, but can benefit from interventions that encourage developing mutual occupational interests or accepting and respecting different occupational choices, if that supports the marriage best. More or less mutual occupational engagement may be desirable, depending upon the couple's interests and abilities.

## Parent-Adult Child Relationships

The nature of the lifecourse is not static but is influenced by opportunities for employment and social and cultural trends of a given historic period, as has been illustrated throughout this text. This flux is not confined to the period of later life; it also is reflected in the radical changes that the period of young adulthood has undergone since the 1950s (Fingerman, 2017). Classified as adults in the past, persons aged 18 to 30 years are now seen as striding an "interim period" of prolonged youth (Fingerman, 2017). This shift in young adulthood has significant implications for the experience of midlife parenthood and the nature and quality of parent-adult child relationships.

Changes in parent-adult child ties are reflected in increased contact between the generations, increased support from parents to grown children, and increased affection between generations (Fingerman, 2017). Whereas frequency of contact with adult children averaged about once a week in the past, now over 50% of older adults report daily contact with a grown child (Fingerman, 2016). From 1970 to 1990, parents spent the most money on their teen-aged children. Since 2000, most money designated to offspring has gone to children under age 6 and young adults aged 18+ years (Kornich & Furstenberg, 2013).

By 2015, intergenerational residence became the modal resident pattern for 18 to 34 year olds, replacing coresidence with romantic partners (Fry, 2015, 2016). For 25 to 34 year olds, 9.5% of males and 6.6% of females lived with their parents in 1970, expanding to 20.4% of males and 13.1% of females in 2019. These percentages increased further in 2020 to 22% of males and 13.4% of females due to COVID-19 lockdowns (US Census Bureau, 2022). Major reasons for adult children living with parents include poor job prospects, the high cost of housing, and delay in age of marriage (Fingerman, 2017). Almost one-third (32%) of young adults living with parents were neither working nor going to school (Fry, 2016; Vespa, 2017), due to disability, raising their own children, addiction, and/or life problems (Fingerman, 2017).

Most adult children eventually "leave the nest," and establish a work life and home of their own. Relationships with their parents have been described as "collective ambivalence," since quality and contact within relationships vary (Kalmijn, 2013b; Ward, 2008). More than half (58%) of younger adults (18 to 24 years old) in the United States are living with their parents (US Census Bureau, 2022).

Many "boomerang kids," adult children who returned to live at home (Bly, 2006; Farris, 2020), are partially or fully college-educated and gainfully employed and contribute to a "crowded nest." Besides occurring within the United States, this phenomenon also occurs in Spain (Holdsworth, 2005; 2006) and other European societies, for example, Italy and Germany (Luetzelberger, 2014). The long-term implications of this phenomenon are unknown; however, OT practitioners must consider these dynamics within intervention processes, should the adult children remain in their parent's homes.

If the intergenerational relationships are good, aging adults have a ready and able support system that truly cares about their well-being. Related evidence regarding extended coresidence is positive, as it promotes intergenerational solidarity throughout time (Leopold, 2012). However, if relationships are strained or negative, and especially if abuse is inferred or observed, then protective measures should be taken collaboratively within one's interprofessional team, police, and/or other legal authorities, if indicated.

## Grandparenthood/Step-Grandparenthood

Shifting patterns of 21st century family formation are reflected in the evolving role of grandparents as providers of care (Doley et al., 2015). Approximately 10% of US grandparents live with at least one grandchild (Casper et al., 2016). Of the 7 million households with coresident grandparents, 60% of these grandparents functioned as head of household. One-third of these households lacked the parent "skipped generation," that is, a household with only the grandparent and grandchild generations.

In 2016 to 2020, 1.1 million grandparents aged 60 and older were responsible for most of the basic care of coresident grandchildren under age 18. Of these grandparents, 407,000 were employed; 33% were unmarried (i.e., never married, widowed, or divorced); 31% had a disability; 16% lived below the poverty level; and 23% spoke a language other than English.

Grandparents have increased opportunities for having an important influence on their grandchildren due to increased life expectancy, decreases in family size, the rise of single parent families, and increases in maternal employment in the United States (Dunifon & Bajracharya, 2012). Grandparent roles vary, due to cultural and economic differences, as well as circumstances in which the grandparent is raising the grandchild. A practice example in Chapter 31, OTs as Change Agents, highlights the critical OT role of organized grandmothers who are raising their children's children, due to a devastating HIV/AIDS epidemic that resulted in the deaths of thousands of parents (Iwelunmor et al., 2006).

In rural Thailand, grandparents frequently care for grandchildren, due to the migration of parents seeking work elsewhere. Role confusion has resulted regarding that of the parents vs grandparents (Tangchonlatip et al., 2016). In other locations, grandparents have primary responsibility for their grandchildren on an interim basis, due to many different circumstances related to parental employment or dysfunction (Dunifon, 2013).

## Family Caregiving

Family caregivers represent the major proportion of the community-based long-term care workforce in the United States and provide an estimated 70% to 90% of community healthcare (Adelman et al., 2014; James et al., 2016; McGhan & McCaugherty, 2017). They represent the foundation of the US health-care system. In addition to assisting with BADLs and IADLs, family caregivers often serve as gatekeepers to health and social service systems for those unable to negotiate such systems on their own. Family caregivers often interpret and evaluate symptoms of an illness or condition, help to decide how symptoms should be managed, and eventually decide when and how professional health-care providers should become involved (Perkinson et al., 2020). In providing family-centered care, OT practitioners should approach the process of family caregiving as a cooccupation (Reid et al., 2022; Warren & Sakellariou, 2019) and focus on supporting the family system, rather than the care recipient alone. The family carer knows the care recipient in ways that the professional health-care providers do not, and should be regarded as a pivotal member of the care team.

In 2017 to 2018, 40.4 million family caregivers provided unpaid care to a family or nonfamily member aged 65 and older; 60% provided assistance with BADLs and 99% provided assistance with IADLs, amounting to approximately 24 hours of care per week (AARP & National Alliance for Caregiving, 2020). The estimated value of family caregiving services in 2017 was approximately $470 billion annually (Reinhard et al., 2019).

Most caregivers of adults care for a relative (89%), typically a parent or parent-in-law (50%), spouse or partner (12%), grandparent or grandparent-in-law (8%), or adult child (6%). Ten percent provide care to a friend or neighbor. Many caregivers live together with their care recipient (40%), up from 2015 (34%).

### Caregiver Stress

Care provided by a family member or friends can be stressful, since it entails physical and psychological strain over an extended period (Lovell & Wetherell, 2011; Pearlin et al., 1990). As mentioned before, families often provide home care that saves billions of dollars annually if services were provided by purchased sources (Langa et al., 2001), often at a significant cost to themselves if wages are lost in the process (Earle & Heymann, 2012). Other personal costs can involve decreased health status, including mental and physical health consequences (Lovell & Wetherell, 2011; Schulz & Sherwood, 2017), as well as decreased opportunities for meaningful occupations. The latter has been especially true for women

during the COVID-19 pandemic, as overlapping responsibilities during typical work days have grown exponentially. Still unknown is the full pandemic impact on faculty and student caregivers (Parrish et al., 2021).

### Medicalization of Caregiving

Revised US Medicare reimbursement policies have resulted in older patients being discharged to the community at earlier stages of recovery, often requiring family caregivers to perform medical tasks typically performed by advanced health professionals, for example, injections, tube feedings, wound care, catheter and colostomy care, and other complex procedures (Feinberg et al., 2011; Perkinson et al., 2020; Reinhard et al., 2012). Fifty-seven percent of caregivers for older adults assist with medical and nursing tasks (Reinhard & Feinberg, 2015). Many caregivers receive insufficient guidance in such tasks (Ward & Marshall, 2003), adding to caregiver stress. If OT staff providing home health-care services note such family caregiver concerns or stressors, they should facilitate additional supportive communication with the medical and/or nursing staff, as well as intervening with strategies that may simplify caregiver workload and support their engagement in meaningful occupations.

### Work Demands

Over 50% of adult caregivers of parents are employed (Johnson & Weiner, 2006). Of those, 60% report that demands of caregiving negatively affect work performance (Fortinsky, 2011), resulting in tardiness, absenteeism, declining work performance, lost career opportunities, and dropping out of the workforce altogether (Calvano, 2013; Griggs et al., 2019; Peng et al., 2019).

### Care Recipient Needs and Behaviors

Incontinence, wandering, and disruptive behaviors are significant sources of caregiver stress (Beach et al., 2005). The progression of the care recipient's condition presents constantly new care demands, requiring adjusting to and learning new caregiving tasks (Perkinson et al., 2011). OT staff should utilize interview and observation skills to facilitate interventions for mitigation of these challenges, wherever possible.

### Family Conflict

Disagreements among family members regarding various aspects of caregiving (e.g., interpretation and management of symptoms, choice of treatments, costs of care, decisions regarding relocation to a more intensive care setting) are not unusual (Flynn & Mulcahy, 2013; Perkinson et al., 2020). Perceptions of unequal contributions by family members to caregiving may be especially divisive (Barca et al., 2014; Perkinson et al., 2020). While working to maintain rapport with family members, staff may assist in clarifying concerns within the OT scope of practice and refer family members to relevant sources for further resolution regarding disagreements.

### Negative Impact on Existing Social Support and Ties

Caregiving demands may eventually become all encompassing, leaving little time or energy for outside activities

(Leggett et al., 2011). Spousal caregivers often find themselves socially isolated as a result of attenuated social networks (Greenwood & Smith, 2015). The inability of the care receiver to maintain previous levels of shared experience, companionship, and intimacy may represent an even greater loss (Monin & Schulz, 2009). Thus, OT personnel should use supportive, empathic approaches and provide relevant resources, whenever indicated.

Despite the significant demands of family caregiving, there is growing recognition of the positive aspects of this role (Brown & Brown, 2014; Kim et al., 2019) and its benefits to positive physical and psychological health for the caregiver (Fredman et al., 2010; O'Reilly et al., 2015; Roth et al., 2015).

### Caregiving Assessments

OT personnel need to use astute interview and observation skills, as well as develop and maintain strong rapport with caregivers and clients, to discern unmet needs and design occupational profiles and interventions that will ease stress, support functional occupational performance, and promote optimal meaning for all involved in the caregiving/receiving process. In addition to observational and interview methodologies, excellent inventories of caregiving assessments identify a large number and wide variety of practice-oriented tools (Cameron et al., 2009; Family Caregiver Alliance, 2012). The National Academy of Sciences set of basic principles and guidelines for caregiving assessments offers helpful guidance for choosing among the many options (Schulz & Eden, 2016). Additional OT-related criteria are available to identify aspects of caregiving most relevant to specific family situations and to evaluate the rigor and appropriateness of specific caregiving measures (Bear-Lehman et al., 2016). (See also Chapter 6, Screening and Assessment.)

### Caregiving Interventions

More than 200 interventions for family caregivers of older adults have been developed and tested in randomized control trials (Gitlin et al., 2015; Maslow, 2012). Excellent inventories of family caregiving evidence-based interventions, model programs, and emerging practices are available, including the Family Caregiver Alliance (nd) and the Rosalynn Carter Institute for Caregivers. Furthermore, the World Health Organization (WHO) developed a comprehensive approach for caring for older adults and included caregiver approaches (Peña-Rosas, 2019). However, they did not specify OT or a focus on what is meaningful for the older individual. Therefore, our profession needs to be proactive with the WHO regarding understanding our profession and the potential for improving the overall health-related quality of life of older adults.

### Siblings

Aging siblings may experience varied relationships. In one study, older female siblings separated by geographic distance neither expected nor received support from each other. Nevertheless, these older siblings considered their relationship to be very important and wanted either the same or greater amount of contact. Thus, family ties appear to remain strong (Langer & Love, 2019). If distance is a factor and more contact is desired, OT personnel can facilitate that process via virtual means, if all siblings have access to and use cell phones, tablets, and/or computers.

### Sexuality and Intimacy

The WHO (2006) defines sexuality as "…a central aspect of being human throughout life [that] encompasses sex, gender identities and roles, sexual orientation, eroticism, pleasure, intimacy and reproduction. Sexuality is experienced and expressed in thoughts, fantasies, desires, beliefs, attitudes, values, behaviors, practices, roles and relationships. Sexuality is influenced by the interaction of biological, psychological, social, economic, political, cultural, legal, historical, religious and spiritual factors." Intimacy entails feelings of closeness and connectedness with or without physical touch.

Compared to their experience of sexuality in youth, older couples may enjoy greater sexual satisfaction due to fewer distractions, more time and privacy, elimination of the threat of pregnancy, and enhanced ability to express their needs and wants. Emotional maturity in later life increases a sense of confidence, enhances communication skills, and decreases inhibitions, contributing to more satisfying sexual experiences. However, age-related physical changes may impede sexual expression for some, and protection from venereal disease may be indicated as well. Various health conditions, such as declining energy, chronic pain from arthritis and other conditions, and self-consciousness stemming from a negative body image associated with aging, may adversely impact later life sexuality. Furthermore, declining hormone levels and changes in neurological and circulatory functioning may cause sexual problems, such as erectile dysfunction and vaginal pain or discomfort.

Erectile dysfunction or impotence becomes more common among men after age 40, when testosterone levels begin to drop. Vaginal changes for women include thinner and stiffer vaginal walls and decreased lubrication. Menopause may be accompanied by hot flashes, mood changes, and/or sleep disorders. Declining levels of estrogen may result in diminished sex drive. Other causes of decreased sexual functioning include overuse of alcohol, joint pain that accompanies arthritis, dementia, depression, diabetes, heart disease, incontinence, medications (especially for pain, hypertension, Parkinson's disease, antihistamines, antidepressants, and sedatives), obesity, and stroke. Lack of a suitable partner also may be an issue, especially for older women (Schwartz et al., 2014). (See also Chapter 9, Physiological and Neurological System Changes with Aging, and Chapter 14, Pharmacology, Pharmacy and the Aging Adult.)

Recent research reflects increasingly permissive attitudes toward sexual activity among aging adults (Graf et al., 2021). Nevertheless, many adults find a discussion of sexual occupations and aging uncomfortable (de Vries, 2009). This discomfort is real, yet potentially ageist. Consider that this dissonance implies inequality among adults (Scherer, 2009), and is contraindicated for OT practice, whether the individual engages individually, or with same or opposite sex partners. Aging adults may still have strong sexual drive, albeit different from earlier decades in their lives, and aging-related changes may have altered their sexual health status and ability to engage as they did in younger years (Graf et al., 2021). OT staff should include sexuality in their queries with aging adults about performance of activities of daily living and, when indicated, include findings in the client's occupational profile, providing guidance and support for this aspect of individual or social participation (AOTA, 2020).

### Sexual and Gender Minorities: Lesbian, Gay, Bisexual, Transgender, Queer, or Questioning

Older adults who identify as a member of a sexual and/or gender minority include lesbians and gays, as well as persons who are bisexual or transgender. Data from the first national federally funded study on LGBTQ+ aging and health (Fredriksen-Goldsen & Kim, 2017; Fredriksen-Goldsen et al., 2011) reveal the following:

#### *Resilience*

Ninety-one percent of LGBTQ+ older adults engage regularly in wellness activities; 82% engage in moderate physical activities; 89% feel positive about belonging to their LGBTQ+ communities; and 38% attend spiritual or religious activities at least once a month.

#### *Risks*

Sixty-eight percent experienced verbal harassment; 43% were threatened with violence; 82% have been victimized at least once; 64% have been victimized at least three times; 53% report loneliness; and 31% experience depression.

#### *Access to Care*

Twenty-one percent do not disclose their sexual or gender identity to their doctor; 15% fear accessing health care outside the LGBTQ+ community; and 13% have been denied health care or provided with inferior health care.

#### *Caregiving and LGBTQ+*

Rates of caregiving by men (26%) and women (30%) are high. Fifteen percent of caregivers provide care to a partner or spouse, 32% to a friend, 16% to a parent, 2% to an adult child, and 7% to other relatives. Caregivers are more likely than noncaregivers to report a disability, depression, victimization, and verbal and physical abuse (Anderson & Flatt, 2018).

OT personnel should interact with all older patients/clients with sensitivity to their needs and whatever relationships in which they engage, regardless of one's own personal values. If OTs or OTAs aren't comfortable providing care to individuals with differing sexual preferences, they should discuss with their supervisor to identify someone else to provide optimal OT services.

### Elder Abuse

The NIA (2020) identified six major types of abuse of older adults:

(1) Physical abuse: Entails use of physical force to inflict bodily harm. This includes the use of restraints against the older person's will.

(2) Emotional/psychological abuse: Entails the infliction of anguish or pain through verbal and/or nonverbal actions. This includes hurtful words, threatening, ignoring, and isolating the older adult—keeping them from seeing friends and relatives.

(3) Neglect: Ignoring the needs of the older adult, including withholding food, medications, and/or access to health care.

(4) Abandonment: Deserting the older adult who needs help, leaving them alone with no plan for care.

(5) Sexual abuse: Involves nonconsensual sexual contact, forcing the older adult to be part of sexual acts.

(6) Financial abuse: Entails stealing, changing names on legal documents such as wills, forging checks, illegal or improper use of the older adult's funds, property, and/or assets.

A systematic review of the prevalence of elder abuse and neglect in the United States (Cooper et al., 2008) reported that 6% of older adults experienced significant abuse within the prior month, and 5.6% of older couples recounted physical violence in their relationship within the last year. Nearly 25% reported significant psychological abuse; within the past year, 5% of family caregivers admitted to physical abuse to those with dementia. Reports of abuse to adult protective services were limited (1%–2%).

Should OT staff suspect or witness abuse or neglect, if possible, they should judiciously intervene, attempting to deescalate the situation, while working to ensure the safety of all parties involved, report the incident(s) to the appropriate local authorities, and assist in connecting those affected to appropriate support services (Pathak et al., 2019).

### Impact of Migration on Families

"Transnational families" are familial groups whose members live separated from each other some or most of the time, while continuing to feel "a sense of collective welfare, unity, and familyhood across national borders" (Bryceson & Vuorela, 2002). The UN estimated the number of international migrants to be 281 million in 2020 (IOM World Migration Report, 2022), or 3.6% of the global population. Persons 64+ years old represented approximately 12.2% of international migrants, and that percentage has remained steady over time (IOM World Migration Report, 2022). If families served by OT staff aren't connected with local resources to support international familyhood, OT personnel should be aware of their concerns and needs as well as connect them with agencies, social workers, or others who can facilitate this process.

### Demographics

Immigration tends to proceed along "migration corridors" (e.g., from Syria to Turkey, Central America to the United States), originating in low- and mid-income countries. The majority (approximately two-thirds) of those participating in international migration do so voluntarily for work, family, and study, and regard their moves as stepping stones to opportunity. Labeled "economic migrants," they seek better economic prospects from more politically stable countries (Bryceson, 2019). The remittances that they send back home represent significant sources of income for their families and wealth for their homelands (approximately $702 billion in 2020) (IOM World Migration Report, 2022).

The situation differs radically for involuntary migrants, i.e., those displaced by conflict and persecution, severe economic and political insecurity, and/or natural disasters (e.g., earthquakes, typhoons). Internationally displaced refugees and asylum seekers numbered approximately 26.4 million in 2022; the numbers of the internally displaced persons (those forced to leave their homes to move to other parts of the country) were even greater—55 million in 2022. Depression has been associated with forced migration, which has been historically considered as a major stressful event and is common in parts of the world, such as China (Zheng et al., 2021), and more recently in other areas, including Afghanistan, parts of eastern Europe, and south and central America (Shultz & Rechkemmer, 2018).

Despite preferences to remain in their homes for most, relocation takes place for older adults for a variety of reasons, impacting aspects of their health status (Reed et al., 2016). These relocations may negatively affect mental and physical health, as well as the individual's rating of their health status (Reed et al., 2016; Thapa et al., 2018). It is thus an imperative that OT personnel include interventions that are relevant and meaningful for these families that include older adults who are trying to establish new relationships, habits, routines, roles, and relationships within environments that are unfamiliar to them (Barney, 1991). Interprofessional support may be indicated, according to their needs and interests.

### Historic Trends in Migration

Changing patterns of immigration to the United States have resulted in shifts in numbers and composition of migrant elders. Before 1970, over 50% of non–US-born older adults migrated from Europe and Canada. More recent immigrants now come to the United States from Latin America, Asia, and Africa (Abdul-Malak & Wang, 2016).

COVID-19 has had a significant impact on global mobility in general. During the peak of the pandemic, 108,000 COVID-19-related international travel restrictions were imposed globally (IOM World Migration Report, 2022), resulting in trapped and stranded migrant populations on a massive scale (McAuliffe, 2021).

### The Impact of Technology on the Experience of Migration

Global digitalization has greatly altered the everyday lives of migrants. Digital technology has become a lifeline that enables adaptations and safe, meaningful lives in unfamiliar locations, while remaining connected to home (Dekker et al., 2018; McAuliffe & Blower, 2021). Various apps are available to support better integration into destination countries and enhanced ability to maintain social ties and monetary support to families and home countries (Bhabha et al., 2021). Online chatbots support social integration to new environments, using

machine-learning technologies to provide individualized psychological support and guidance in negotiating complex migration policies and visa requirements and supporting way-finding in unfamiliar cities. The Mobile Money app has been a critically important resource for unbanked migrants, enabling cheap, safe, and fast transfers of remittances; facilitating digital cash transfers and digital identities; and enabling migrants' access to credit (Kitimbo, 2021).

Information and communication technology (ICT) has transformed the social dynamics of migrant families. Mass migrations in the 19th century (e.g., from Europe to the United States) entailed permanent moves, with little opportunity to maintain contact with families and countries of origin (Moberg, 1951). In contrast, 21st century innovations in technology, transportation, and global banking offer multiple ways to maintain communication and support with those who remained behind (Bryceson, 2019; Wang & Lim, 2021).

ICTs represent the "social glue of transnationalism," enabling constant connectivity and a continued sense of family. Migrants and family members who remained behind can maintain continued involvement in each others' everyday lives and occupations and perform familial duties from afar (Wang & Lim, 2021). This may include virtual attendance and participation in family and local gatherings, events, and rituals (Nyamnjoh, 2019, 2021). Even supervision and caregiving within a process that has been termed *digital kinning* of older adults across continents are possible via the use of this technology (Baldassar & Wilding, 2020). The second author's neighbor uses this approach in addition to trips to Africa to ensure that her father, a retired professor, receives good care.

### Adjustment to Migration by Older Adults and Their Families

The act of migration represents a major disruption to one's "being in place," that is, the sense of well-being that results from identification and being "at one" with one's environment. Such a move entails abandonment of familiar settings and modes of being to create a new sense of place in a different, unfamiliar physical and sociocultural space. (See Chapter 20, Physical Environment, for a detailed explanation of processes entailed in transforming unfamiliar "spaces" into "places" of meaning and identity and attaining "place integration.") Recent migrants must develop new mental maps to orient to their physical environment, negotiate new routines and patterns of use of that environment through adaptations of previous occupations, and optimally develop emotional attachments to their new settings as a result of events or occupations that transpire there (Zemke, 2004).

There are two main categories of older adults who are affected by migration: those who relocate with their families to a foreign country and those who remain behind. The two groups encounter different challenges in their attempts to recalibrate daily lives.

### Late-Life Immigrants

Late-life immigrants, foreign-born adults who have relocated to a nonnative country at age 65 years or older, are faced with the dilemma of "aging-out-of-place." They are mostly "invited elders" (Choi, 2012), who relinquish long-established bonds to their homeland to assist their immigrant adult children in a foreign land. Such a move requires an array of major adjustments to a different culture, language, physical space, and socioeconomic environment, disrupting personal and familial roles, routines, sense of place, and identity. The loss of habitual behaviors, routines, relationships, occupations, and shared understandings represents major disruptions that require continued renegotiations of everyday life within the destination setting (Huot & Laliberte, 2010; Laliberte, 2002).

### Challenges of Migration

Wijekoon et al.'s (2021) study of Sinhalese late-life immigration to Canada illustrates the challenges that older migrants are likely to face and possible strategies to meet them. The fact that older adults typically follow their adult children in migration often results in a heightened dependency on those children to navigate unfamiliar situations, with major implications for the balance of power within the familial household. With less authority and input into family decision making, the older parents must either adjust or surrender altogether familiar family roles that previously gave structure, meaning, and purpose to daily life and personal identity (Wijekoon et al., 2021). As the adult children acculturate to the ways of their new home, normative expectations within the household may shift, impacting significant aspects of daily life. For example, the once familiar role of grandparent may need to be renegotiated to conform to new norms regarding child discipline, calling for a less authoritarian approach to modeling child behavior. OT staff should approach each older migrant's needs to address the strategies that are best suited for that individual, taking into consideration the family unit's needs.

Diminished sense of influence and authority within the household, coupled with a strong sense of dependency, may lead the older adult to lower expectations of what might be asked of other family members. They may selectively prioritize needs to focus on the most essential occupations, e.g., going to medical appointments, as opposed to more "trivial" occupations, e.g., socializing with ethnic peers (Wijekoon et al., 2021).

Older migrants often admit to feeling like an outsider, disoriented and alienated from a new environment so different from their homeland. Lack of fluency is a major issue, making it almost impossible to go out alone. Unfamiliarity with local culture presents barriers to even the simplest conversations, e.g., discussions of national sports or local politics. An unfamiliar health-care system presents daunting obstacles to needed services and medications. Possible changes of weather may call for major adjustments of daily routines and even clothing.

### Strategies for Meeting Migration Challenges

Wijekoon et al. (2021) documented strategies that older migrants have used to deal with the previously mentioned challenges. A wide variety of occupations help to maintain a sense of continuity with life left behind. Many make conscious efforts to recreate a sense of home by engaging in ethnic peer networks, retaining their mother language, wearing ethnic clothing, cooking ethnic dishes, and participating in native traditions and services of worship. By performing basic household chores, such as cooking, laundry, and yard work, that do not require fluency in the new language, older migrants can make significant contributions to their families, thus restoring, at least in part, a sense of worth, identity, and continuity with the past. Providing childcare to grandchildren allows opportunities to pass down family values and traditions from their native culture. Older migrants also may provide valued cultural services, such as sewing traditional garments, building lanterns for Buddhist celebrations, and sharing cultural knowledge.

Participation in religious occupations, such as meditation, chanting, attending services, and reading sacred texts in the temple, provides access to ethnic peer networks and fosters a sense of solidarity with newly established compatible friends. Such relationships and occupations provide opportunities to reflect on challenges of migration with their peers and share strategies for coping and adapting.

Successful adaptation to migration required striking a balance between attempts to maintain continuity with the past and modification of a variety of occupations to achieve a better fit with their new home (Wijekoon et al., 2021). To achieve that fit, older migrants need to reevaluate past roles and norms and renegotiate them to be compatible with those of their new home. For example, later life is no longer viewed as a time of rest and relaxation, as was the case in the homeland; postretirement capacities and participation are framed as more vigorous, allowing full-time occupation in domestic tasks and possible employment. With incorporation of Western/Canadian values, in this study, expectations of filial piety were reduced or dropped altogether. Even the most simple habits were modified to "blend in." For example, the appropriate way to greet someone morphed from a deep bow to a hearty handshake. Relinquishing certain norms and expectations confers a degree of freedom, i.e., the requirement to dress a certain way in public. However, in many ways, the late-life migrant needs to "start over" and relearn "how things work."

### Left-Behind Communities and the Elders Who Remain

Support provided by those who migrate out to their older adults who remain behind represents a significant flow of resources. For example, data from the large-scale Cambodian Rural Urban Migration Project (Zimmer et al., 2022) indicate that 77% of both international and rural to urban migrants provided financial support to stay-behind families. Rural to urban migrants were most likely to provide instrumental as well as monetary support, and both types of support were more likely to be provided by women migrants to female-headed households.

Distance prevents international migrants from providing adequate instrumental support to their relatives who remain behind. Schröder-Butterfill's (2022) research on a German-speaking minority group residing in Romania illustrates how left-behind communities and their older adults transformed and recreated networks of care in the face of significant out-migration. Older adults renegotiated household roles, stepping in when they could to perform essential duties, such as childcare, cooking, cleaning, and other household tasks. They also renegotiated practices of care, what types of care were acceptable and permitted, and who stepped in to provide it (Lawreniuk & Parsons, 2017). While existing local support ties intensified, those ties also expanded and were renegotiated. It was necessary to enlist new informal care providers who previously were not involved in providing support, i.e., those with neighborly ties that extended across ethnic boundaries. Religious networks that had previously focused on spiritual care readjusted to become quasi-welfare institutions, providing meals-on-wheels and in-home visits and developing a church-based care home. The "left-behind" sending communities were transformed in their adjustment to out-migration, just as surely as the migrants themselves and the family members who remained behind (Schröder-Butterfill, 2022).

## Reinforcing Familial Relationships and Shared Values

As indicated earlier, there are numerous ways that families may remain connected, whether living in the same community or at a distance. Older family members living in the same community may serve as caregivers for their grandchildren when parents are employed or away from home or for other reasons (Fingerman et al., 2012). When invited, grandparents who live at a distance from younger generations may care for grandchildren while parents are away for business or other purposes.

When older and younger generations live at a distance and thus do not often connect in person, the development of computer and cell phone technology offers additional ways of connecting, either of which can be mutually beneficial. From following each other on social media, to direct communication via email, or texting pictures with commentary, these modes can promote intergenerational rapport even between continents.

### Family Rituals and Routines

Many family traditions revolve around births, birthdays, and holiday celebrations and involve meaningful rituals that are passed from one generation to another (Nelson-Becker & Stangster, 2019). Some are based upon religious practices, such as in the Christian, Jewish, or Muslim faiths. Celebration of holidays is typically meaningful for older family members, who enjoy sharing time with their younger generations, siblings, and/or cousins and friends and cooking holiday meals or treats using recipes passed down from earlier generations (Wright-St Clair et al., 2013).

From an occupational science perspective, these ritualized routines and daily habits comprise meaningful occupational performance from early ages and provide structure and expectations of the occupations that comprise daily life and celebratory occasions, for all individuals, and are especially important for members with disabling conditions (Boyd et al., 2014; Segal, 2004). Older family members having opportunities to share past experiences and ongoing routines, family

recipes, crafts, or other skills with younger generations or friends can serve as meaningful occupations for all participants (Carlson et al., 1998; Denham, 2003, Fiese & Parks, 2002).

### Shared Occupations

Some grandparents have daily or regularly scheduled time with their grandchildren in their homes and have opportunities to pass on intergenerational traditions such as cooking and hobbies or various skills including sewing, knitting, crocheting, wood-working and other crafts, athletic, or musical avocations. These are meaningful occupations typically for both generations, and typically need to be scheduled around both generations' abilities and needs. Grandparents living in the same region as the next generation have more opportunities for shared occupations, which usually are planned according to the different generations' needs and interests. However, when grandchildren live at a distance, more effort needs to be made to experience mutually gratifying occupations. The second author's grandchildren are in this category; thus, extra days before holidays for preparing traditional family recipes have been incorporated into schedules, as well as trips or special activities with individual grandchildren to further bond with them and enjoy time together.

Many of the second author's teenage sewing projects were facilitated by a cousin's wife, both of whom were the age of grandparents, and since most of ours were deceased, they served as wonderful substitutes. Additionally, since we lived in the same city, we enjoyed many meals, holidays, and special events together. These were all very meaningful to us as children.

### Reminiscing with Family Members

Reflections of memories from the past are a common practice among older adults (Butler, 1963), for whom time "seems to fly" as one ages. Reminiscing and life review foster the creation of bonds between people and help older adults to cope with important life events and find meaning to life (Westerhof & Bohlmeijer, 2014). Most reminiscing reflects positive feelings and reactions; however, occasionally sadness accompanies reflection, associated with nostalgia (Cappeliez et al., 2008). Commonly, reminiscing occurs within families, often with older members sharing information about their childhood, young adulthood, work life, and pets, whether at home or away. Reminiscing may occur between siblings, cousins, and other relatives, many of whom enjoy telling stories about their past (Salmon & Reese, 2016).

### Ethical Wills

Similar to a legal will that ensures that material goods are passed on to the persons and/or causes of choice, an ethical will ensures that one's values and beliefs, parting thoughts, and wishes are documented and passed on to persons most dear (Perkinson, 2018). Sometimes called *legacy letters*, ethical wills provide a way to transmit one's life lessons, feelings, and final thoughts to future generations. There is no format or right way to write one. It might contain family history and stories; expressions of blessings and love or perhaps forgiveness;

articulation of cultural and spiritual values, traditions, and beliefs; validation of pride in children and grandchildren and hopes for their future well-being; expressions of gratitude and requests for ways one would like to be remembered—all the cherished intangibles, the knowledge and wisdom accumulated over a lifetime, to be preserved and shared with those most dear. An ethical will might be of far greater value to descendants than the legal will.

How does one write an ethical will? Again, there is no one right way to do it. The older adult might start by thinking of the most important events in their life and experiences or persons of greatest significance. Why did the events or people hold such importance? When did the older adult feel most happy, content, worthy, or seek forgiveness from the next generation? Can they see common elements or patterns in these memories? What are the life lessons that they want to share and underscore to those they love?

The process of writing an ethical will or legacy letter is similar to writing a life review. The act of identifying, documenting, and reflecting on the most important elements of a lifetime helps to put things in perspective and find meaning in one's existence. Both have the potential to foster and promote personal growth. The ethical will differs from a life review in that it goes beyond reflection and review; its primary purpose is to share the outcome of that review with those who matter.

An excellent example of an ethical will was presented as a lecture by Randy Pausch, a professor at Carnegie Mellon University who died of pancreatic cancer at the age of 47. He shared his life lessons with his students in the moving, witty, and profound "The Last Lecture: Really Achieving Your Childhood Dreams," which is available on YouTube: www.bit.ly/LectureVideo.

One need not be at the end of life to write an ethical will. It is just as relevant to review and evaluate one's life at times of major transitions and share those reflections with those closely impacted by that transition. An excellent example of such a legacy letter was written by Barack Obama, *A Letter to My Daughters*, penned at the start of his presidency, January 18, 2009, available online: www.bit.ly/LifeLegacies.

## Friends and Social Networks

### Social Networks and Convoys of Social Support

The **Convoy Model of Social Support** (Antonucci & Akiyama, 1987; Antonucci et al., 2014) suggests that the social connections and networks that people develop and accumulate throughout their lives differ in levels of closeness and are maintained over time by exchanges of social support. This model envisions each person as moving through life surrounded by a convoy, or personal network of individuals from whom they give and receive social support.

Convoys are dynamic and lifelong, changing in some ways but remaining stable in others. They may be pictured as a set of three concentric circles of support network members (Kahn & Antonucci, 1980), each representing different levels of closeness to the focal person. The inner circle represents "people to whom you feel so close that it is hard to imagine life without them." The middle circle represents "people to whom you may not feel quite that close but who are still important to you." Their connections suggest a degree of closeness and relationships that are more than the simple fulfillment of role requirements. The outer circle represents "people whom you have not already mentioned but who are close enough and important enough in your life that they should be placed in your personal network" (Antonucci, 1986). Members of the third circle are considered to be close to the focal person but usually in a very role-prescribed manner. For example, one might have a close and important relationship with a coworker, but this relationship does not transcend the work environment or continue after retirement.

As the global context is rapidly aging and becoming more mobile, the number of older adults facing challenges maintaining social networks as they continue to work, retire, move to a new residence, or lose a loved one is changing (Menkin et al., 2017). Ongoing social support continues to be important for personal development, health, and well-being into old age, and friendships with former coworkers are frequently an important dimension of meaningfulness for aging adults (Djundeva et al., 2018).

During the COVID-19 pandemic lockdown period, when many older adults practiced self-isolation, they were motivated to experience positive emotions because they perceive their length of life as more limited, compared with younger adults. To maintain this positivity, older people organize their social environments and invest more in closer and satisfying relationships (e.g., with family, friends, neighbors, and coworkers), since they provide emotionally meaningful interactions (Cavallini et al., 2021). Evidence for older adults regulating their emotions by focusing on positive emotional states derived from the perception of closeness to family, friends, and coworkers may thus have prevailed during the pandemic (Antonucci, 1986; Djundeva et al., 2018). Summed together, the three circles represent the overall social convoy of the individual. When examined separately, they represent distinct levels of closeness within the overall convoy.

The convoy model suggests that structural and functional characteristics among convoy members vary in a meaningful and predictable manner by life-cycle stage (age) and feelings of closeness (circle placement) (Fuller et al., 2020; Zhang et al., 2011). Relationships with people in the innermost circle of the convoy, such as one's spouse, parents, children, and other close family members, remain relatively stable throughout life and involve the exchange of many different types of support. In contrast, relationships with coworkers, neighbors, and acquaintances, that is, people in the periphery of the convoy, tend to be less stable. These peripheral relationships are more vulnerable to changing situations than family relationships are and may end due to changes in jobs, social roles, location, or other life events. Thus, the frequency, type, and reciprocity of social exchanges with peripheral relationships tend to decrease with age.

While the Social Convoy model focuses on the composition of later life networks, identifying members and their characteristics, the **Socioemotional Selectivity Theory** focuses on age-related changes in social goals and patterns of interaction with those network members (Carstensen, 1993; Carstensen et al., 1999). With increasing age and end-of-life realizations, motivational goals change. Rather than seeking to acquire information from many diverse social relationships, as seen with adolescents and young adults, older adults shift to focus on emotional aspects of relationships. By selectively restricting their social life, they prioritize time spent with members of the innermost circle of their social convoy, their emotionally close significant others.

## Neighborhoods and the Impact of Residential Context on Social Networks

Early research indicated that characteristics of neighborhoods may impact the quality of life of older residents. *Social Integration of the Aged* (Rosow, 1967), examined the relationships between life in age-dense and age-integrated environments and various aspects of social life of older adults (e.g., size and composition of social networks, frequency of social interaction, life satisfaction, and quality of life). Neighborhood age-density contributed to formation of friendships, especially among those within their same age group, gender, and marital and social status, depending upon the proximity of neighbors. He found this to be especially true of those within the working class, compared with middle class residents. Multiple changes in the older person's life roles, including retirement or death of a partner, nearly doubled their socialization if they lived in an age-dense neighborhood.

## Impact of Relocation

Residential moves by older adults ages 60 and older increased by 1.4 million from 2010 to 2019 in the United States. The 2017 American Housing Survey and the American Community Survey 2014–2018 from the US Census Bureau were used to determine patterns of moves within older age groups. Findings indicated that the motivations of baby boomers younger than 70 are more diverse than older cohorts (Li et al., 2022).

When geographical change of a household occurs, whether due to aging preferences, as in Americans moving from colder regions to the sunbelt, or for economic, health, oppression, loss of spouse, desire to be nearer to their families, or other reasons, OT personnel need to be cognizant of the individual's need and motivation for moving and observant regarding their psychological status as they adapt to new environments, since relocation effects vary significantly (Bradley & Van Willigen, 2010). OT staff should consider how to promote the continuation of past occupations, if they continue to be relevant, and/or involvement in new occupations that are commensurate with the older individual's interests and abilities. Especially if the individual is living alone, enjoys assisting others, and is physically and mentally able to do so, volunteering should be considered, since volunteer work after relocation has been shown to have a significantly positive impact on the adjustment and physical health of older persons who relocate (Gonzales et al., 2019).

## Negative Aspects of Neighborhoods

The health and well-being of older adults are affected by many factors in their neighborhood, and those over the age of 50 may be more affected than younger age groups (Population Reference Bureau, 2022). Especially if the older adult has spent many years in their communities, they have experienced higher levels of exposure to neighborhood conditions than younger residents. These exposures may include pollution, crime, poorer governmental and legal infrastructures, limited access to grocery stores, deteriorated streets and sidewalks, and fewer health-care resources, factors that may make it difficult to determine the neighborhood feature(s) that are responsible for specific health conditions that may occur concurrently or over time. Living in disadvantaged, high-poverty neighborhoods is associated with many negative outcomes, including weak social ties, limitations in accessing health care and other supportive services, limited physical activity options leading to mobility limitations, health problems, and high stress (Population Reference Bureau, 2022). (For more information on the social dynamics of older adults' neighborhoods and their impact on the development of personal networks and quality of life, see Chapter 20, The Physical Environment and Aging.)

## Leisure Activities

Participation in leisure activities has been associated with life satisfaction, personal well-being, and quality of life (Fernández-Mayoralas et al., 2015). Older adults' interests in leisure activities typically don't change over time; however, individual differences are apparent and varied. When diminished physical function or depressive symptoms are present, these impact participation (Chang et al., 2014; Janke et al., 2006). Physical function symptoms can involve a variety of challenges, including vision, hearing, musculoskeletal, neurologic, and energy levels that limit the amount, frequency, or extent of participation. If depression or dementia is present, these symptoms may also limit the client's abilities.

Initially through developing an occupational profile that typically includes utilizing standardized assessments, OT staff work with clients to identify short- and long-term goals that relate to the patient's/client's current status and incorporate meaningful occupations that the individual would like to initiate or continue, either by themselves or with family members or others. Note that Chapters 6 and 7 provide extensive explanations of this process. Some relevant occupations may relate to a diagnosis and prior participation, whether long-term or may present new interests. A determination needs to be made regarding whether these occupations are realistic in a customary format, including the ability to adapt these activities for maximum client gratification. When an occupation in its typical format seems unrealistic, yet the client continues their interest in the activity, by applying creativity to occupational analysis, OT staff can convert active occupations, such as golfing, to modified versions including board games or other versions of the occupation. Gardening adaptations may include areas immediately adjacent to sidewalks, to enable easy accessibility, or wheelchair gardens—elevated boxes in which individuals may plant and nurture seedlings—or other versions that enable walker or wheelchair use. Adapted versions of meaningful occupations are primarily limited to OT staff creativity, which is one of our profession's strengths.

Sports are occupational categories that include individual and group participation, either active or spectator versions. Although engaging in competitive sports is usually associated with young adults, increasingly, older persons participate in competitive events, even including triathlons (Brown, Cotter et al., 2019). In 2009, 28,000 older athletes ages 56–90 years from 95 countries competed in Sydney, Australia, in 28 sports included in the World Masters Games. Forty-four participants identified themes that motivated them to participate, as follows: (1) they like a challenge to test their abilities, (2) they discovered that they could win in their age group, (3) they are motivated to work harder, (4) they are able to compare themselves with others in their age group, and (5) the competitions encourage them to travel and establish ongoing friendships (Dionigi et al., 2011).

Reducing sedentary behavior and risk management are fundamental to participation in sports activities, due to aging-related changes. The promotion of physical activity in older adults should emphasize moderate-intensity aerobic and muscle-strengthening activity, coordination, flexibility, and balance, as well as physical self-concept (Conde-Pipó et al., 2021; Nelson et al., 2007; Pedersen et al., 2013; Pedersen et al., 2017).

Most older adults who engage in active sports are motivated by the physical, psychological, and social benefits. Walking, swimming, yoga, pickleball, tennis, racquetball, Tai Chi, croquet, and golf are all occupations that reduce the risk of injury, especially as our bodies and fitness levels change (Dionigi et al., 2013; Nelson et al., 2007). Additionally, spectator sports have demonstrated positive effects among older adults, including their overall sense of belonging and subjective well-being. This occurs through attending sporting events, identifying with the team, and collective psychological support (Inoue et al., 2020). Subjective well-being is associated with the team's performance. Interestingly, the social well-being benefits of team identification are greater for middle-age and older fans of poorly performing teams (Inoue et al., 2022).

Living in a downtown condo community that is situated close enough to walk to professional baseball, football, ice hockey, and soccer games, for over 20 years, the chapter's second author has observed extensive camaraderie and team spirit among our residents. Many of these neighbors have season tickets and related sports apparel and truly enjoy these experiences as couples or in groups. Her observations are in sync with the Inoue et al. (2022) studies.

Family reunions, especially for African Americans, are a highly meaningful experience and an opportunity to share intergenerational family histories and are used for bridging intergenerational gaps and surviving many social challenges. Family reunions have served as rituals of historical and cultural appreciation, resistance in the face of oppression, and transitions into the future (McCoy, 2011). Additionally,

Choi et al. (2016) found that among Korean older adults, participation in religious activities, friendship organizations, and both family and school reunions may help preserve cognitive function in individuals aged 45 years or older. High school reunions offer opportunities for older adults to reflect and reengage with individuals in meaningful ways, yet have mixed meanings for many individuals (Capps, 2011). For those who experienced positive high school experiences, academically and/or socially, these are opportunities to gather together again in meaningful ways. However, if older adults use social media and have experienced less than their perceived optimal life, they may be reminded daily of differences in lifestyles, accomplishments, and opportunities that their classmates have had (Midgley et al., 2021). If OT personnel sense that this occupation contributes to feelings of being lesser than classmates and promotes depressive symptoms, an instrumental approach would be to identify an alternative or another occupation that is currently more fulfilling.

## Cultural Differences

Culture is a system of learned behavioral patterns, values, beliefs, customs, expectations, and ways of life that are shared and passed down through members of a group. One's cultural context represents an essential dimension of the environment encountered by older adults, as represented in the Person-Environment-Occupation-Participation Model. Culture may be considered as the lens through which one interprets and assigns value to a vast array of phenomena including experiences, relationships, sensations, etc. (Perkinson & Solimeo, 2014). For example, shared expectations regarding caregiving identify the nature and frequency of care, location in which it transpires, persons involved and division of labor, standards defining "good" care and appropriate care-providing/care-receiving behaviors, and acceptable limits on caregiving (Perkinson, 1995). While the expectations are shared by members of a given social/cultural group (e.g., spousal residents of a US retirement community, Chinese elder parents and adult children), the socialization to and implementation of the group's caregiving norms may vary among group members, depending on the ability and motivation of those involved, as well as the "moral force" or strength of particular caregiving values and beliefs.

A number of studies have compared the influence of different cultural orientations on socioemotional aging processes. These comparisons typically involve Western (i.e., Euro-Americans) with East Asians influenced by Confucian thought (Fung, 2013; Fung et al., 2001; Markus & Kitayama, 1991). Independent Western cultural values tend to emphasize individual autonomy from birth; value persons as individuals; maintain physical space between children and parents; support individual expression of self via language, feelings, and actions; and, separately, maintain a certain amount of distance to support their children's development as unique individuals (Keller, 2003, Keller et al., 2004). In contrast, socialization to interdependent Eastern cultural values encourages children to think of themselves as members of social groups, whose needs are viewed as more important than those of individuals

(Keller et al., 2004). Recent research has questioned prevailing theorizing around individualism-collectivism and models of selfhood, calling for evidence from locations other than Western and Confucian East Asian societies (Krys et al., 2022) to support these claims.

It is important to incorporate culturally specific approaches and cross-cultural interprofessional work in therapeutic and related supportive interventions (Morrow-Howell & Yang, 2013; Perkinson, 2019). With current and projected increased migration patterns and integration of different cultures, OT personnel need to be highly adaptable and adept in finding relevant resources, agencies, and individuals who can assist in ensuring successful, culturally appropriate interventions.

## Social Isolation and the Impact of the Pandemic

Social isolation and loneliness may be toxic to health, especially for older adults (Lubben, 2017; Valtorta et al., 2016), representing strong risk factors for chronic disease and death (Cacioppo & Cacioppo, 2014; Holt-Lunstad et al., 2015). Family caregivers often find themselves socially isolated and lonely due to attenuated social networks and social supports (Greenwood & Smith, 2015; Leggett et al., 2011). However, it is important to remember that being alone does not always equate with loneliness. For some, it affords peaceful solitude, enabling personal growth and self-awareness, increased focus on self-care, comfort from being alone, and freedom to pursue one's interests without distraction (Brehm et al., 2002).

Social isolation/loneliness places specific subgroups, such as immigrants and LGBTQ+ persons, at heightened risk for a variety of medical conditions, including a 50% increased risk of dementia. Additional deleterious effects include premature death and the following increased risks: 29% for heart disease and heart failure with a related 4 times increased risk of death, +68% for hospitalization, +57% for emergency department admissions, and +32% for stroke (CDC, 2022).

During the COVID-19 pandemic, social isolation and loneliness were seen as behavioral epidemics among aging adults throughout the United States, Europe, and China, adding to an already significant problem (Gerst-Emerson & Jayawardhana, 2015; Luo et al., 2012; Wang et al., 2011). The

protective guidance of lockdowns for vulnerable older adults, with or without health conditions, exacerbated an already precarious situation. COVID-related lockdowns were particularly stringent in the United Kingdom, where individuals were told to "shield" themselves for at least 3 months and to limit admissions to health systems. Thus, many older adults had few outside contacts, and long-term care facilities halted visitors—this occurred in the United States as well, in consideration of the heightened risk of autoimmune, cardiovascular, mental health, and neurocognitive problems in the older population (Vrach & Tomar, 2020).

The second author of this chapter and her husband, now in their late 70s, limited contacts to their condo community, but seldom interacted, and always wore masks during the pre-immunization period. While awaiting immunization availability, younger neighbors volunteered to purchase groceries weekly for a year, other purchases were made online, workouts were with a geriatric trainer in our condo, using our cell phones, and regular scheduled family gatherings were done virtually. The couple's dog was instrumental in getting them sanely through the pandemic lockdown period; not everyone wants a pet, but she is a sweet companion who kept both of them laughing, moving via walks outside, and engaged in her care around daily routines.

### Ways to Promote Social Interaction and Relationships

OT personnel should use their observation and interpersonal skills to determine the socialization levels and needs of aging adults, while respecting individual gender, class, education level, and cultural differences and occupational preferences, unless those activities seem inappropriate (e.g., negatively affect the individual or reinforce unhealthy or illegal patterns of behavior). If the older adult client needs and desires more socialization, occupations recommended should be aligned with their interests. Many organizations or activities may be considered, including volunteer work, during the therapeutic intervention process. Additionally, many communities have organizations designed specifically to meet aging adults' social needs.

Shared housing is an option that ensures a level of socialization with mutual benefits and has gained in popularity

## CASE STUDY 23.1

When grandparents live a distance from grandchildren, mutual experiences and related opportunities for bonding and sharing family histories, everyday and other life events, and development of close relationships may be much more limited than if grandparents live in the same household or community. If technological supports are accessible, and parents allow connections between grandparents and grandchildren to utilize these media, such adaptive approaches can assist in developing and maintaining the relationships and mitigate some of the effects of the geographical distance between the generations. Creative approaches need to be employed to maintain the intergenerational engagement. For example,

this chapter's second author's family planned a year ahead several years in a row, to ensure that all grandchildren (cousins) ages 7–12 who lived at a distance could attend "camp" with them in a cabin on a lake for 1 week together in the summers. The advance planning was necessary due to other activities to which the grandchildren were typically committed. Once together, they were able to get to know and "catch up" with each other each year and enjoy a wide variety of "camp" occupations. Time will tell regarding whether these events assisted in grandparent/grandchild and cousin bonding, but to date, among these grandchildren who are now young adults and teenagers, that seems to be so.

## CASE STUDY 23.2

This chapter's second author organized a virtual monthly visit with her three sisters during the pandemic across different time zones. It has been successful to date in keeping these sisters connected and informed about each other's lives, and periodically first cousins are also included in these visits. In addition, she has helped to organize similar weekly virtual gatherings with her husband's siblings. These reunions are especially meaningful because until quite recently, they were unaware of each other's existence. Her husband discovered his biological siblings for the first time at age 75 through DNA testing; he was adopted as an infant during the World War II era; for decades until recently in the United States, identities of birth parents were not disclosed. Imagine learning that one has a brother and sister they have never known before! With willing parties, there is much catching up and learning about family history and current occupational pursuits, all of which is very meaningful to participants.

## CASE STUDY 23.3

In 1998, in their late 50s after their children were away from home, the second author of this chapter and her husband learned of an innovative opportunity—a plan to transform a historic landmark building in downtown St. Louis, Missouri, into a multiuse site, including a hotel, restaurants, and condominiums. They had considered condominium living for years, as part of their transition from a single-family home in the suburbs, once their children were "out of the nest," to an environment that could support aging in place. Regarding this concept, this site offered enormous advantages and amenities:

- Reduced maintenance of exterior and interior physical spaces, with support provided by hotel staff and condominium association infrastructures
- As many extra bedrooms as needed (beyond our guest bedroom and bath), an appealing feature to accommodate out-of-town family and friends; residents benefit from hotel discounts
- Resident neighbors as a unique "community" representing diverse ages, cultures, races, religions, work and retirement roles, and other backgrounds
- Fitness room and swimming pool shared with the hotel
- Room service availability
- Secure parking in the building
- Patio at the top of the building with gas grills for condo residents
- Mass transit (bus, metro transit, and railroad) directly across the street
- Grocery stores, pharmacies, restaurants, library, houses of worship, parks, theaters, aquarium, three major sports venues, auditoriums, concerts, museums, courts, major parades, and other attractions within easy walking or short driving distance. Major medical centers are less than 10 minutes away; these include physicians and hospitals.

Standard designs were offered to convert the building for condominium residents, but the couple was allowed to alter those plans. Thus, they requested that their unit be fully accessible—at or above the federal standards, to support their aging-related needs. The second author of this chapter also advocated for accessibility and "aging-friendly" design and services throughout the building, resulting in modifications to the original plan, to accommodate neighbors with mobility limitations. Thus, an elevator to the 13th floor pool and a lift for the pool provide adaptations for neighbors regardless of ability levels.

This couple has lived in this neighborhood for 22 years and are very appreciative of not only the fundamental support it provides but also the residential environment. Neighbors are of diverse ages, races, cultures, religions, professions, vocations, and lifestyles, with frequent planned and spontaneous social gatherings. Annual events, such as holiday decorating and a holiday dinner, bring neighbors together, as well as regular book club meetings, exercise, and other activities that include athletes and graduate students, as well as those with established professions or vocations and retirees, all who all thrive together.

over the past decades in the United States. Options include the following (Lambert, 2022):

- Home sharing—two or more decide to share a house; there are several versions of this option.
- Board and care—persons may share a bedroom or have their own room; meals are served together in a dining room.
- Cohousing—this option includes sharing chores and meal preparation and is typically intergenerational
- College life—this includes university-based retirement communities located on university campuses. Amenities include non- or for-credit college classes, and access to all activities on the campus, including medical centers. The intergenerational atmosphere is very appealing for some aging adults.
- Living with adult children—this may be precipitated by a variety of reasons stemming from two or more generations, and may be within the parents' or adult child's home or on the same grounds in a separate home.

Thus, it behooves the OT practitioner to become aware of resources that can facilitate optimal socialization for aging adults, and develop networks of contacts for facilitating these types of shared housing if relevant to the OT service provided.

*The complete listing of the Bibliography and Chapter Questions and Answers are available in the accompanying enhanced eBook version included with the print purchase of this textbook. Visit Elsevier eBooks+ (eBooks.Health.Elsevier.com) to access this content.*

## CHAPTER 24

# Arts, Humanities, and Occupational Therapy with Older People: An Aesthetic Lens on Practice

*Susan Coppola, OTD, OT/L, FAOTA and Desmond O'Neill, MD, FRCPI, FGSA, AGSF*

## CHAPTER OUTLINE

## OBJECTIVES

- Describe the development and application of arts and humanities in professional practice.
- Understand better the key importance of arts and humanities in the daily occupations of older adults and the challenges posed by aesthetic deprivation.
- Recognize the partners from arts and health and humanities disciplines as collaborators to develop programs in arts and health.
- Gain awareness of exemplars, resources, and knowledge frameworks that underpin successful arts and health programs for older adults.
- Consider how best to incorporate arts and humanities into education, professional development, and research in occupational therapy practice.

## Introduction to Arts and Humanities Informing Health-Care Practice

It is increasingly apparent that the knowledge base that health-care professionals require for effective and insightful practice across the lifespan needs to draw on a broad range of sources. This should not come as a surprise given the complex interaction between the many elements of the biopsychosocial approach to well-being and illness. A major development in this regard has been a growing recognition that the scholarship and techniques of arts and humanities can assist us in a number of ways. This includes understanding the processes of aging in a more authentic fashion and the journeys of older clients through illness and disability in developing more effective ways of engaging and supporting the transitions between well-being and illness. Known under the descriptor of medical and/or health humanities, these approaches can also augment professional well-being and reflective practice. This has been complemented by a parallel development in gerontology, termed *Cultural Gerontology* (Europe) and *Humanities and Aging* (North America) (O'Neill, 2015).

The humanities and arts represent a range of disciplines, including (but not confined to) literature, music, visual art, dance, history, philosophy, theology, anthropology, law, and cinema. There is increasing interest and evidence for introducing arts and humanities into professional education and continuing professional development of health-care professionals, including occupational therapists (Coppola et al., 2017; Kinsella & Bidinosti, 2016). However, given the broad spread of arts and humanities, this is not as straightforward as developing a course in more tightly defined areas such as anatomy and physiology. The challenge arises in part from the very different methodological approaches of the arts and humanities compared to the empirical sciences. The humanities and arts focus on techniques such as close reading, critical analysis, comparative, and historical frameworks. For occupational therapy (OT), as with other disciplines, these challenges are also encountered when incorporating related aspects of professional practice, such as ethics and spirituality. With humanities minimized or even absent from professional education, as a group, we have limited understanding of their importance in reasoning and in older adults' lives.

## Arts, Humanities, Leisure, and Well-Being

The arts, humanities, and leisure activities are critically important to well-being and resilience for all of us, a domain that has been relatively neglected until recently (Moss & O'Neill, 2014). This is typified by a ground-breaking study, which indicated that patients recovering from stroke who did not have access to their favored music CDs recovered less well than those who had such access (Sarkamo et al., 2008). There is also clear evidence of better health and well-being among those who engage with receptive arts activities, such as music, theater, cinema, dance, etc. (Fancourt & Finn, 2019). Increasingly, studies are showing qualitative benefits of active arts engagement (Cohn et al., 2017; Groot et al., 2021; Ho et al., 2019; Keisari et al., 2021). Music interventions tailored to older individuals have been shown to improve pain, depression, and agitation (Dunphy et al., 2019; Huber et al., 2021; Schroeder et al., 2018). These findings are reflective of the key place of aesthetics in Maslow's (1970) revision of the hierarchy of needs, ranking at a high-level feeding into self-actualization. Additionally, the power of humanities to express oneself and form deep connections to others responds to Maslow's theory of the human need for love and belonging. Unfortunately, Maslow's hierarchy has been misinterpreted in health-related settings to prioritize resources toward older adult's physical survival and safety, while neglecting the essential need for meaning, belonging, pleasant experience, and purpose to life.

*Aesthetics* is a term that we tend not to use frequently in everyday language, but is deeply embedded in our everyday lives. Therefore, it calls for the profession's increased interest in the aesthetics of everyday as a matter of importance. For the philosopher Dewey, aesthetics was not just high art but extended to a broad range of cultural activity and represented the highest level of our interactions with our environment, and was also embedded in many everyday activities—"an extension of the power of rites and ceremonies to unite men, through a shared celebration, to all incidents and scenes of life" (Dewey, 1934, p. 275). The potency of arts, leisure, and humanities arises from many aspects, including their engendering a sense of belonging to a wider sharing of emotions and experiences with friends, family, and society, supporting searches for meaning, enjoyment, relaxation, and reflection. These activities touch in a complex manner many interlinked domains, including psychological, biological, social, behavioral, and spiritual, which in turn relate to health behaviors, health, and well-being (Fancourt et al., 2021). Recognizing and meeting the challenges of aesthetic deprivation are important in general and critical in addressing the barriers to access to aesthetic supports that older adults often encounter in illness, disability, and social deprivation (Moss et al., 2015).

It is important to note that the concept of culture here is not so-called "high culture," but the way that culture is present, expressed, and perpetuated in—music, clothing, household objects, dance, stories, and more—with juxtaposition of colors, designs, objects, movement, and sounds. The body of literature on benefits of cultural activity in aging is centered on English-speaking places (Bernardo & Carvalho, 2020).

## Arts as a Lens for Understanding the Longevity Dividend

One of the major barriers to effective care for older people is widespread ageism across society, professions, and health-care systems. This discrimination on the basis of old age often feeds off what has been termed the *failure model of aging*. The emphasis on age-related disease and disability can deflect attention from the huge gains to us all of increased longevity, and not just in terms of increased lifespan. Attention to late life creativity can provide a useful focus for influencing students, professionals, and the public on the gains of later life. It is remarkable how the late works of most great artists represent the pinnacle of their achievements, a distillation of life experience and wisdom, and a search for meaning at its most intense. This can be seen in the late movies of Clint Eastwood, late song albums of Leonard Cohen, paintings of Matisse, and sculpture of Louise Bourgeois in their ninth decades, and a host of other great artists in every sphere of achievement (O'Neill, 2011). In a broader sense, this focus can also lead to a reflection on the everyday creativity we see among older people in adapting to changes (O'Neill, 2019), which in turn can also explain theories of optimal aging such as Selection, Optimization and Compensation (Baltes & Baltes, 1990) and the Socio-Emotional Selectivity theories (Carstensen, 1992).

## Developing a Platform for Engaging With Arts, Humanities, and Aging

OT arises from a tradition that is rooted in activity, engagement, and creativity. This is a receptive terrain within which to develop frameworks for practice that include arts and humanities into the fabric of care and support for older people. Important resources for creating a therapeutic approach enriched with arts and humanities are the three interrelated key foci of engagement between arts, humanities, and health, namely, arts therapies, arts and health practitioners, and medical/health humanities. Although each key focus has its own academic direction and development, there are also considerable areas of overlap and indeed potential artificial barriers between the activities, particularly between arts therapists and arts and health practitioners. Some mistrust may arise regarding role boundaries, often because of concerns over resources and funding streams. Patterns of working together may vary from location to location, and it is a professional obligation to pursue harmonious collaboration. Occupational therapists who wish to further integrate arts and humanities into their practice with older people should seek out connections with practitioners in each of these disciplines. A helpful model for thinking about teamwork has been proposed by Moss (2016). This allows for a range of coordinated activities and also liberates arts and humanities practice from institutional settings (see Fig. 24.1).

The arts therapists are likely to be the professionals most familiar to occupational therapists. Both emphasize a diagnostic and personalized therapeutic approach to engagement with the individual patient/client, as is common in other forms of therapist frameworks. Shared perspectives may lead to group-based work with a given art form. Arts therapists have formal professional training with clinical placements. Arts and health practitioners tend to have a broader reach,

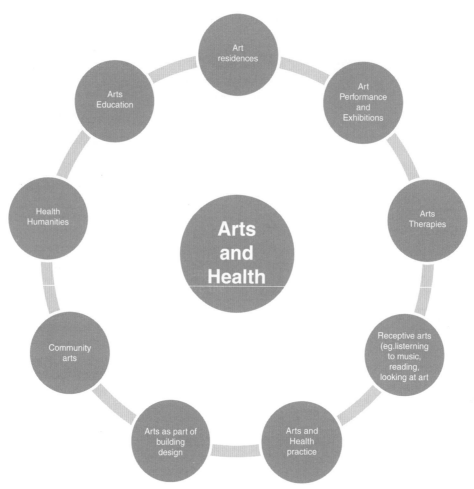

**FIGURE 24.1**     A new paradigm for arts and health. (From Moss, H. [2016]. Arts and Health: A New Paradigm. *Voices: A World Forum for Music Therapy, 16*, 1–16, with permission.)

arising from many aspects of arts practice, such as community arts, and in certain health-care settings have formal roles such as directors of arts and health promotion. In the United States, these are often recreation therapists. A helpful focus for working with arts and humanities practitioners is through the emergence of training programs for artists in health-care (Moss & O'Neill, 2009), which have similarities with elements of arts therapies programs. Medical and health humanities scholars and faculty may arise in diverse faculty settings, sometimes health-care, sometimes arts and humanities, and increasingly in more formalized joint working. Weaving through these activities and discourses are activities such as artists in residence from all aspects of the arts, and linkages with community arts programs. The spectrum of arts and humanities informed practice runs across the spectrum of care from prevention to palliation. Depending on the location of practice, there may be further collaboration possible, from community arts programs for those living at home to activities coordinators in nursing homes (Buettner & Voelkl, 2006). In general, the focus of the art therapist is expressive and OT is skill developing, and yet overlap is evident (Davidow, 2018).

## Programs in the Community for Older Adults

Community programs that target arts-based engagement of older adults are growing rapidly. Some are designed to engage older adults' particular access for visual and hearing impairments in museums, whereas others target performing arts venues. Many programs have been placed online, due to the COVID pandemic, and others can be found locally.

Programs focused on aging and arts are growing as our population ages; here, we name a few national programs:

The National Endowment for the Arts: Accessibility: Creative Aging Program—offers facts, recommendations, and research supporting aging and the arts (https://www.arts.gov/impact/accessibility/creativity-and-aging).

Museums and Creative Aging—is an initiative of the American Alliance of Museums (https://www.aam-us.org/programs/museums-creative-aging/).

Lifetime Arts https://www.lifetimearts.org/.

National Center for Creative Aging—https://creativeagingresource.org/organization/national-center-for-creative-aging-ncca/.

An example of local programs is Compas Artful Aging (https://www.compas.org/artful-aging) in Minnesota.

Many programs promote access to the visual and performance arts for people across the lifespan with impairments. This includes audio description and object handling for people with visual impairments, and for those with hearing impairments—signing, closed caption, and hearing systems. Arts Access focuses on audio description (https://artsaccessinc.org/). Art Beyond Sight is a multimodality arts and culture accessibility organization (http://www.artbeyondsight.org/mei/). The roles that occupational therapists can play in art museums are emerging around the world (see, for example, Salasar et al., 2016). These are typically consultation and collaborations, such as the second author's work with UNC Ackland Art Museum to develop a program for people with dementia that involved tours led by a docent and occupational therapist or student. In this program, the docent was the content expert, and the occupational therapist provided adaptations for engagement.

## Community Programs for People With Dementia

The work of Ann Basting has been influential in reimagining community and creativity in the lives of older adults with dementia (Basting, 2020). Her strengths-based approach, called "Timeslips," includes creative activities, such as dance, art, and theater, that form the basis for engagement. In nursing homes, Timeslips has shown to have a positive impact on residents' engagement and alertness, staff-resident interactions, and staff views of residents (Fritsch et al., 2009; Swinnen & de Medeiros, 2018).

Music and Memory (https://musicandmemory.org/) is a nonprofit organization that trains people to provide personalized music to people with cognitive and physical impairments. There are certified trainers throughout the United States and in many other countries. A well-known program is a tailored program called "Music on my Mind." Singing opportunities through religious or other coral groups is a potent occupation for many people with dementia.

Many museums are developing programs for people with dementia. One well-developed example based on engagement of participants is Meet me at MoMA: The MoMA Alzheimer's Project: Making Art Accessible to People with Dementia (https://www.moma.org/visit/accessibility/meetme/). With these resources and possibilities in mind, practitioners are encouraged to seek local resources for arts engagement and work with community partners to advance programs as part of our role in occupational possibilities and participation for older adults with varying abilities (Isaac & Hamilton, 2020).

## Applying Arts and Humanities in Occupational Therapy Practice

*"Art is not the possession of the few who are recognized writers, painters, musicians; it is the authentic expression of any and all individuality…" (John Dewey)*

OT's ultimate goal is participation in personally meaningful and health-promoting occupations. This outcome is well supported in gerontology research showing such participation as consequential to health and well-being (Menec, 2003). Bentz et al. (2021) found that for older adults with advanced cancer, 89% of occupations that brought joy were leisure, and many of those were arts and humanities based. Often dismissed as distractors or fillers of time, creative occupations have healing powers (Livingston, 2019). Benefits of arts and humanities are noted in social and biomedical literature, from narrative accounts to neurosciences, further validating increased use of these occupations with older adults (Carr et al., 2009; Chang & Chou, 2015; Fraser et al., 2015; Teater & Baldwin, 2014). There has been strong interest in intergenerational arts practice since the 1980s, although there is a generally weak evidence base for the effectiveness of intergenerational practice regardless of the domain. An encouraging study from the United Kingdom suggests that this is worth pursuing (Douse et al., 2020). In addition, intergenerational practice resonates with the emerging impetus of the Age-Friendly University enterprise (Vrkljan et al., 2019) and trends in intergenerational practice in OT.

Occupations used in OT's origins consisted of making beautiful and useful objects, often arts and crafts, using textiles and other raw materials. Fabrication of an aesthetic product served as therapeutic medium for meaning, well-being, and recovery. Today, those particular arts and crafts are dated, and rarely used. Yet, recent research supports the value of craft hobbies as creative activities that support life satisfaction for older adults through their impact on identity, spirituality, calming, and recognition (Adams-Price et al., 2018). There are areas of distinction and overlap between art and craft. Art is considered a creative expression of emotions and ideas that enlist technique and materials. Crafts involve technique and materials that may enlist creativity. Here, we consider both as related occupations.

In many settings, OT's scope with older adults has narrowed to survival, chiefly basic self-care skills and prevention of medically adverse events, and interventions that will reduce costs and burden of care. This practice is centered on the body, not the life nor the experience of the person (Dancewicz & Bissett, 2020). In this context, many therapists suffer from moral distress about meaninglessness for themselves and older clients (Hasselkus & Dickie, 1997). Ageist, fragmented, and strained systems constrain humanistic instincts about the quality of life during clients' waking hours, to instead focus on the brief therapy session. In institutional settings, it takes commitment and respect to turn role boundaries into teamwork with arts, recreation, and leisure therapies. Collaboration focused on clients can discern how art activities, art therapy, and art in therapy each benefit clients. Moreover, pervasive disparities for marginalized older adults (Fluharty et al., 2021) are a pressing call for teamwork with nurses, physicians, social workers, physical therapists, and others to create these occupational possibilities for older adults (Lewis & Lemieux, 2021; Rudman, 2006). Indeed, infusing creativity into care can lead us to more humanistic and meaningful practice (Basting, 2020).

A therapeutic repertoire that includes arts and humanities requires overcoming misperceptions. Some presume that art is fine art appreciated by privileged people, or that practice with arts or crafts is outdated and unscientific, or that art is separate from everyday life and occupations. Young therapists can reflect on arts and humanities in their own lives—customized playlists, spoken word poetry, tattoos, singing, dance, fashion, religious art—to find parallels for understanding arts and humanities in the lives of older adults. Such aesthetics are integral to expressions of belonging within a cultural group and statements of one's unique and evolving personal identity. Such preferences are telling of important dimensions of life stories that can inform all aspects of intervention. Arts and humanities occupations are embedded in cultures and therefore central to client-centered practice of learning and intervening meaningfully and respectfully with older persons.

Occupational therapists can bring the richness of arts and humanities into practice in varied ways. Most obviously, they can be important *occupations* directly addressed, such as playing the piano or photography. Arts and humanities can also contribute to the sensory *environment*, creating a favorable context for occupations. Additionally, everyday occupations are infused with *meaning through aesthetic choices*. This section will discuss arts and humanities in these three ways, as occupations, within contexts, and infused in occupation.

## Arts and Humanities as Occupations

Wilcock's (1998) framework for quality of life as consisting of *doing, being, belonging, and becoming* is useful to interpret meanings of arts and humanities occupations. Participation means acts of *doing*, which can range from witnessing a performance, going to museums, to making arts. *Being* is about how the occupation is experienced as well as how it is incorporated into identity in the form of interests, abilities, or preferences. *Becoming* is about learning and changing through experiences. *Belonging* is about connection in identifying with others who share an interest. Occupations are often chosen to associate with particular people (Rudman et al., 1997). Having choices to do, be, become, and belong is integral to quality of life and identity, of being a particular person, a vital element of client-centered practice.

A major part of arts and aesthetic engagement of most of the population, including older people, is receptive rather than participative in nature, and one of the key priorities of arts-informed practice is to the greatest extent possible align the activities to the personal preferences of those we support. This is a practice best understood as curatorship (Moss & O'Neill, 2019), and it is an evolving skill and practice, using insights from the arts and humanities and health to balance the older person's individual preferences with available resources and opportunities. It is not that older people cannot be introduced to new arts forms and participatory arts, but our practices in arts and humanities should mirror the wider concept of person-centered care. Sounding out what are the arts and leisure activities of older people should be an integral component of assessment and can be aided by a range of screening measures, such as the Pleasant Events Schedule (MacPhillamy & Lewinsohn, 1982). OT literature has exemplars of facilitating participation in community arts programs (Edwards & Owen-Booth, 2021).

In OT, arts engagement can be potent and diverse. Arts activities, like painting and piano playing, are often utilized pragmatically, as interventions to improve impairments in fine motor skills or attention span. Evidence supports use of meaningful occupations over exercises (Nagayama et al., 2017; Nielsen et al., 2017) and the value of creative activities as intervention (Hansen et al., 2021). Our bodies self-organize to do purposeful tasks, with precision, recruiting more than just the isolated muscles that are activated with rote tasks. Creative arts in OT can benefit a person's feelings of control, sense of self, purpose, expression, illness experience, social support, and identity (Perruzza & Kinsella, 2010). In late life and palliative care, they can support coping with decline in ability alongside existential concerns (La Cour et al., 2007). Creative activities offer myriad ways to be adapted, individualized for successful experiences and for personal expression. In long-term care, art activities can benefit mood, communication, reminiscence, and social relationships (Durocher et al., 2021). Arts and humanities products—like a poem, photo album, or recording—can become gifts that express feelings for others and serve as legacies. Arts can serve to process life stories and experiences, such as the theater project of older lesbian, gay, bisexual, transgender, queer, or questioning (LGBTQ+) men (Morgan & Rubio III, 2019). And indeed arts can fill time in ways that are satisfying.

## Considerations for Interventions With Arts and Humanities

It is not necessary for an older person to identify as an artist to have an interest, talent, or goal relating to arts and humanities. Preserving that identity or interest may be consequential to important aspects of recovery and well-being. A client may have a long-standing interest in quilt design, gospel music, poetry, dance, or other culturally important expressions. They may enjoy other creative occupations such as gardening, cooking, and collecting. Indeed, there are many parallels to interest in sports, in the artistry of performance of any occupation.

It is helpful to support intensity of involvement in particular areas of interest. Arts and humanities have been shown to influence well-being if there is repeated or sustained involvement, but not for short-term experiences (Tymoszuk et al., 2020). Consider how joining a regular singing group can generate opportunity for personal growth, contribute to routines and social connections, and offer a reason to get out of bed and dressed for the day.

Choice and control in activities are key to older adults finding them beneficial (Everard, 1999; Rudman et al., 1997). Client-centered practice is based on this premise. Yet, in many settings, success of an art making or music program is measured by gathering older adults in proximity to be an audience or to do the same activity. Materials are distributed in an orderly fashion. Staff make pragmatic decisions to maintain control, based on beliefs about what is "good for" participants. For some older adults, the high level of staff control provides helpful structure. For others, more freedom and choices within activities are needed to make the activity beneficial. Customizing experiences is key, as for example it is personalized music that shows the most benefits (Leggieri et al., 2019).

Interests change. People may not want to participate in things they no longer do well or in the same way (Bentz et al., 2021). An activity may be culturally inappropriate or humiliating, or may kindle feelings of loss, as noted in Robert Murphy's (2001) autobiography that described the craft of making a doormat in OT as an indignity.

Being pressured to participate in an activity that is disliked—such as coloring, dancing, or listening to a type of music—can be harmful to identity (Rudman et al., 1997). Older persons may participate to be kind to caregivers, to support an identity as a cooperative person. They may participate in an unpleasant activity simply to be with others.

It is essential to learn and critically consider what constitutes meaningful and "culturally safe" occupations for a person, from the lens of diversity. The need for learning about the person is amplified when working with an older adult of another culture, race, religion, gender identity, ideology, age, or other distinction. Practitioners must humbly examine and question their own assumptions and stereotypes that a person would like a particular type of dance, music, or art based on any of these distinctions. An invitation to participate in an activity without pressure is key. A person may want to try something new.

Close observation can uncover genuine and evolving preferences. When an older adult has limited verbal communication, practitioners notice signs of involvement or flow experiences in activities (Csikszentmihalyi & Csikzentmihaly, 1990; King, 1978). Signs of engagement include eye gaze, posture, communication, and body language. Reading these signs requires knowing enough about the person to, for example, interpret whether a frown means disapproval, fatigue, or concentration, or whether a smile implies anxiousness or happiness. Simple moments of pleasure, engagement, and interpersonal connection are significant outcomes for some. For others, a longer duration in an activity may be needed for a good outcome. Such engagement can offer benefits of rest for care partners, and also potential shared experiences. Arts offer opportunity to create things together, like a video, art work, or story.

Occupational therapists have distinct skills and creativity to analyze, grade, modify, adapt, and scaffold occupations and environments to enable occupations. It is a complex problem-solving process to, for example, help an older adult with cognitive, mobility, and vision impairments go to a concert. In addition to the pragmatics of planning, getting ready, getting there, being there, and getting home, there are the nuances of how these processes are experienced by the person and care partners who put effort into making these events happen. Drawing upon the expertise of care partners and ensuring their satisfaction with the experience are integral to the work of occupational therapists.

Temporal aspects of participation are complex. A misunderstanding about the occupations of older adults is that if there is something they like to do they should do it all the time and persist for a long time. However, satisfaction is associated not with the amount of time spent but with congruence between desired amount of time in an activity and how much time is spent in it (Ray & Heppe, 1986). Timing of when and how long a person knits, paints, or plays guitar may vary. Once a week might feel like enough to the person. In some situations, encouraging a person to participate or persist can be helpful. It takes skill to anticipate when encouragement seems like nagging that diminishes the joy of an occupation. An older adult may fatigue easily from the physical, cognitive, and emotional effort of even pleasurable occupations. Creating an unrushed, relaxed atmosphere can help. Time itself can be experienced differently as we age, as passing more quickly with age and with being limited.

When use of arts in traditional practice is challenged by others, practitioners should keep in mind that emerging research is supporting arts and humanities practices in physical rehabilitation and recovery. Case stories tell of creative "making", like knitting, as vital to recovery (Fortuna, 2022). Art programs during stroke rehabilitation show promise for mental well-being for self-selected patients (Morris et al., 2016, 2019). Meaningful occupations have been found to be more effective than impairment-focused exercises in rehabilitation for various conditions (Collis et.al., 2020; Lin et al., 1997). An art program for stroke survivors contributed to improved mental well-being, confidence, connections, and quality of life, yet more research is needed (Baumann et al., 2013; Beesley et al., 2011; Pang et al., 2021). A qualitative study by Symons and colleagues (2011) revealed that art contributed to clients' enjoyment, confidence, future planning, and recovery during rehabilitation for neurologic conditions. It is well established that dance can improve physical function and have psychosocial benefits as well (Hwang & Brawn, 2015; Morris et al., 2019). Although evidence based, these practices are difficult to adopt where team members and older clients have expectations for what OT interventions should look like. Rote exercise is the predominant intervention by OTs in skilled nursing facilities (Jewell et al., 2019), offering time efficiency for staff. Clinical spaces are often filled with rote exercise equipment and decontextualized cognitive activities, despite the "Choosing Wisely" national campaign with the American Board of Internal Medicine and American Occupational Therapy Association that deems nonoccupationally embedded interventions as "questionable" and producing "suboptimal outcomes" (American Board of Internal Medicine Foundation, 2018; Gillen et al., 2019). From the client perspective, a meaningful arts-based project that carries across therapy sessions may optimize their recovery.

## Aesthetics in the Environment

Aesthetics are often a part of everyday living—music, colors, scents—that can bring pleasure. Boldness, loudness, complexity, and meanings of visual art or music can create an emotional climate that may range from boring to agitating. Clinical spaces may feel stark or cluttered with odd juxtapositions of medical and personal objects, jarring announcements from a loudspeaker, or noxious smells, all especially disquieting if sensory processing or discrimination is a challenge. It comes as no surprise that music-based interventions in acute care have benefits for people with dementia (Sousa et al., 2020). Cognitive changes produce vulnerability to stressors and call for attention to aesthetically pleasing environments to promote well-being. Further, with sensory loss, other senses may become more prominent and draw attention to the benefits of, for example, a person with low vision experiencing pleasant music.

Medical environments prevail in the experienced world of many older adults. Consider instead the aesthetics of walking in nature, seeing a sunset, of being on a boat. Safety concerns may keep people confined to indoor places and disrupt aesthetic and emotional ties to nature, the desire to move, and embodied experiences of happiness or freedom. Aesthetics that promote movement, creativity, and social connections are absent in the sounds of clinical environments. In the story of dancer Ronald K. Brown's stroke rehabilitation, it was music that brought back movement ability (Kourlas, 2022). Adaptations to the visual environment in aging can go beyond illumination, contrast, and size to incorporate the aesthetics color, design, sound, and texture. Occupational therapists can influence aesthetic experiences of older adults, with attention to small things, like arranging photographs and eliminating noise, to broader collaborations to enhance lived environments.

## Aesthetics in Everyday Occupations

A humanities perspective helps therapists practice aesthetically by thinking not just about tasks and skills but also about occupations as they are infused with experiences of beauty, connection, and meaning. To varying degrees, there is a personal aesthetic associated with our identities that we infuse into everyday occupations—when selecting clothes, applying make-up, shaving, or wearing a necklace or baseball cap. A person may feel humiliated if seen without these key aspects of their personal identity. The hospital gown and "workout clothes" are convenient for donning/doffing; they save staff time. Personally significant accessories like a purse, hat, watch, ring, or belt are problematic in this context. This standardization/homogenization can strip away aesthetics of cultural and gender identities, and the symbols that make a person a particular person. In a study of Iranian elders, Izadi-Avanji et al. (2021) found aesthetics to contribute to feelings of inner peace, connectedness to family and significant others, and to a sense of independence and well-being. Occupations are practical, and they are also about quality of life brought about by harmonious aesthetically pleasing experience (Cutchin, 2013).

Arts and humanities remind practitioners to think about what is beautiful to each person that reflects their identity. As one older adult said, "I will use a walker only if it is red." Asking about personal aesthetics might seem to be a frivolous question for an older adult who is recovering from a stroke. Yet setting goals for restoring identity and joy and moving toward beauty may be the most fruitful way forward.

## Experiences of Using Arts and Humanities With Older Adults

### Case Study 24-1 by Allison Calhoun, MS, OTR/L The Collage

W had recently moved into the assisted living facility where I worked. Her move was prompted by several falls with injuries and worsening cognitive impairment. She had never married and had no children. W was a well-known member of the local artist community. She had built a house with an artist studio that looked out into the woods through a wall of glass. As I got to know her, I learned she created woodcuts, often with themes of the moon or intricate depictions of letters of the alphabet, using a specific multistep process. W was mobile with a walker and standby assist for short distances when I began working with her. Our goals were related to improving safety and function and to help her transition to living as meaningfully and purposefully in a small new assisted living room. W was kind and well-loved and was used to being independent and to living alone. This transition was a change for her. She was showing some signs of depression and was feeling that she no longer had full control over her life.

As I talked with W about her interests, she told me about her woodcuts and began explaining the process of making them to me. She had drawers full of materials and artist proof prints of woodcuts that I found stunning. Meanwhile, she pointed out small imperfections in each one of them, and indicated that they were not of adequate quality to be sold or displayed in a show. I also realized as I worked with her that her process of making woodcuts could not be replicated adequately in the assisted living room, nor could she accurately remember all of the steps or their sequence. While recognizing how being an artist had been vital to her identity, her livelihood, and her overall persona, I knew that she probably could no longer create her art in exactly the same way as she had before. She and I continued to talk, and we came up with the idea together to make a collage out of her old artist proofs. I was apprehensive at first to be an accomplice to her cutting up her artwork. I shared the idea with her nieces, who were overjoyed to have her do anything that brought her joy. We agreed to see where the project took us. From that day forward, I was able to weave in her therapy goals of initiating, sequencing, imagining, standing safety, and stamina while working on the collage projects, which all translated to improved safety and engagement in daily routines and enhanced mood. The other wonderful outcome was that friends in her artist community would come visit her and help her work on the collage project as well. One friend brought a card table to use. Another friend brought special glue. Over the course of our therapy sessions and beyond, she created five original collages. She named each one of them by seeking "votes" from her friends when they came to visit. Ultimately, her family and friends facilitated an opportunity for W to have a show highlighting her artwork over the years. The collages she made were part of the show, and several of them sold! Use of her art as a therapeutic medium added meaningful life to her years.

## Case Study 24-2 by Allison Calhoun, MS, OTR/L
## The Dance

I met a participant at a local adult day center while introducing and orienting some OT students to the site. G had recently started to attend the center each day. She had been diagnosed with dementia, and her family was seeking opportunities for socialization and for respite for her husband and daughter who lived with her. I soon learned through talking with G and gathering some details from the facility staff that she had been a ballet dancer. Her performance in a dance production was what had attracted the eye of her husband many years previously. G was clearly frustrated with her difficulty in communicating and participating at the center. I spoke with her daughter when she picked her up later that day, and she tearfully said that so much of her mom seemed to be fading away. I mentioned that we had talked about dancing, and that her eyes lit up when I mentioned ballet. Her mom had also eagerly shown me dance moves. I told G's daughter that one of the OT students was a dancer and that I would like to pair up to talk about dance with her mom. I asked her daughter to send in her ballet shoes. What resulted were some beautiful encounters between the OT student and G. They talked and danced, and G became more articulate, smiled more, and seemed more confident. Her daughter also mentioned that her mom was happier and calmer at home, too.

## Education and Research

As the profile of arts and humanities in OT continues to expand, it will be important to integrate key elements into education and continuing professional development. A very useful toolkit for curricular development in the medical and health humanities has been developed by the Health Humanities Consortium (https://healthhumanitiesconsortium.com/; Albright & Carytsas, 2021). A similar development in arts and health has been developed by the National Organization for Arts in Health (https://thenoah.net/), which can help to inform those aspects relevant to occupational therapists in practice.

Research and scholarship is a core element of professional practice, and our knowledge base for arts and humanities in clinical practice remains in a relatively underdeveloped state. It is important to retain a broad perspective on the nature of such research, and to avoid an undue emphasis on a quasi-pharmacological approach to "prescribing" arts and humanities in practice, as eloquently phrased by two leading scholars in a

paper titled "Shall I Compare Thee to a Dose of Donepezil?" (De Medeiros & Basting, 2014). Much of the research base is still of variable quality, and this represents a significant opportunity for research in OT. A useful handbook has been developed on research in health humanities that can provide guidance on techniques and likely sources of interdisciplinary support (Klugman & Lamb, 2019). Interdisciplinary research presents unique challenges and opportunities, and a complementary book on how to navigate such relationships provides helpful advice on developing these key relationships (Callard & Fitzgerald, 2015). (See also Chapter 30 for more on interdisciplinary processes.)

## SUMMARY

This chapter offers rationale and principles for therapists to consider arts and humanities as consequential to social participation and quality of life. In it, we call for a turn toward what is beautiful and profound, from the dominant discourse in aging of preventing decline, falls, and disease. Meaningful practice with older adults calls upon therapists to consider a wide range of occupations and expressions to align with clients' diverse interests, identities, and cultures. Infusing arts and humanities requires overcoming misperceptions about aging and about what constitutes arts and humanities, and to consider participation as ranging from active doing/making to receptive experiences. Arts and humanities can infuse personal expression, interpersonal connections, and aesthetic experiences into daily life, which are matters of particular importance in the deprived life situations of many older adults. OT is uniquely positioned to uncover and make possible these forms of occupations, to infuse pleasant aesthetic experiences in the ambient environment, and to see aesthetics as *part of* everyday occupations. Arts and humanities occupations are integral to culture and identity and are therefore consequential to client-centered practice for intervening meaningfully and respectfully with older persons and their families. Practitioners are called upon to use creativity, teamwork, and outreach to community programs and resources to build these opportunities of meaning and pleasure for older clients and practitioners themselves.

*The complete listing of the Bibliography and Chapter Questions and Answers are available in the accompanying enhanced eBook version included with the print purchase of this textbook. Visit Elsevier eBooks+ (eBooks.Health.Elsevier.com) to access this content.*

CHAPTER **25**

# Health-Care Systems and Services Overview

*Beth Fields, PhD, OTR/L, BCG, Miriam Rodin, MD, PhD, and Karen Frank Barney, PhD, MS, OTR, FAOTA*

## CHAPTER OUTLINE

## OBJECTIVES

- Understand the importance of health and health care
- Compare and contrast health system models of high-income countries
- Define and distinguish between types of health-care services along the continuum of care
- Articulate core components of health-care quality
- Discuss the role of occupational therapy within interprofessional systems of care for aging adults

## Health and Health Care

### Health

Health is defined in numerous ways by various sources. For nearly eight decades the World Health Organization (WHO) has maintained the following definition: "Health is a state of complete physical, mental, and social well-being, and not merely the absence of disease or infirmity" (WHO, 2022). However, the WHO definition has been recently challenged by various sources who indicate that managing disease, not solely its absence, reflects a healthy life, especially when considering aging adults. Otherwise, a large portion of the life course is ignored. Global inequities regarding the experience of health and well-being exist, partially due to a lack of awareness or policies that enable people to participate in doing, being, or aiming to become, that enable people to participate according to their needs, capacities, and potential (Wilcock, 2006). This is true throughout the lifespan, although historically these tenets have been applied primarily to younger age groups.

Since populations in most nations in both the developed and developing world are aging, a definition of health that informs national systems that serve aging adults is indicated (Fallon & Karlawish, 2019; Rudnicka et al., 2020). Thus, health can be defined narrowly as the absence of illness or disease or more broadly as "a state of physical and mental well-being that facilitates the achievements of individual and societal goals" (Gettel et al., 2021). The latter definition reflects the growing body of research showing that every aspect of a person's life affects health status. Physical well-being may be thought of as an objective process, while mental well-being can be considered as a subjective process (Neves, 2021). Thus, health is increasingly seen as a multidimensional concept incorporating physical, mental, social, and spiritual well-being. This broader definition is consistent with the occupational therapy profession's focus on meaningful engagement in occupations to support health-related quality of life throughout the life course (Hubbard & Huang, 2020).

Health-related quality of life (HRQoL) and wellbeing are constructs promoted by the US Center for Disease Control and Prevention (CDC) (Office of Disease Prevention and Health Promotion, 2022), Center for Health Statistics (CHS), and Office of Disease Prevention and Health Promotion for all individuals. Based on status indicators from Healthy People 2020 final results, they established their objectives for Healthy People 2030 (Giroir, 2021), emphasizing improving the quality of life for older adults in the following example categories:

1. *General:* Increase the amount of physical activity and decrease hospital admissions for diabetes and pressure ulcer- related hospital admissions.
2. *Dementias:* Increase the number of older adults or their caregivers who are aware of their diagnosis, reduce the proportion of preventable dementia hospitalizations, and increase the number of individuals who discuss their subjective cognitive decline with their health-care provider.
3. *Infectious Disease*: Reduce the rate of hospital admissions among older adults with urinary tract infections and reduce health care–associated infections.
4. *Injury Prevention*: Reduce fall-related deaths among older adults, reduce the rate of emergency department visits due to falls among older adults, and reduce the proportion of older adults who use inappropriate medications.
5. *Oral Condition*: Reduce the proportion of older adults with untreated root surface decay and reduce the proportion of adults aged 45 and over with moderate and severe periodontitis.
6. *Osteoporosis*: Reduce hip fractures among older adults, increase the proportion of older adults who are screened for osteoporosis, and increase the proportion of older adults who get treated for osteoporosis after a fracture.
7. *Screening*: Visual impairment, cardiovascular disease, chronic obstructive pulmonary disease (COPD), abuse and neglect, depression and suicide risk reduction by improving social integration, need for support services, alcohol and substance abuse.

Since the WHO definition, there has been considerable attention to measuring HRQoL (CDC, 2021). There are many definitions and many instruments for measuring it, but most of these scales ask a question phrased like this, "How many days over the last 2 weeks (year, month) has your health (this condition) prevented you from doing the things you enjoy as well the things you feel you need to do?" The emphasis is on the aspects of life that bring happiness, satisfaction, pride, and a sense of meaning to the patient and often this is related to their ability to do a variety of activities, including self-care or care for others. Occupational therapy is one of the disciplines that directly addresses people's need for a sense of independence, dignity, and self-worth (American Occupational Therapy Association, 2020).

## Health Care

What does health and health care mean to occupational therapy providers ("herein referred to as occupational therapists [OTs] and occupational therapy assistants [OTAs]")? Occupational therapy education provides foundations in the physical, mental/cognitive, and occupational sciences,

yet also emphasizes the aspirations and backgrounds of those whom we serve—their lived experiences and dreams and goals—and works to promote holism in establishing and maintaining relationships with individual patients and clients and/or groups. This combination of perspectives was elaborated upon by Hasselkus and Dickie (2021) in *The Meaning of Everyday Occupation* (p. 104). Thus, the challenge for the occupational therapy provider is to collaborate meaningfully with their patient/client, to enable health promotion, management and maintenance, and the realization of the individual's or groups' dreams and goals using primary, secondary, and/or tertiary prevention strategies.[1]

With aging adults, enablement, despite potential conditions resulting in frailty, optimally is a collaborative process with the individual or group, and, where indicated, family members or other caregivers, as well as professional care providers This is true throughout the continuum of care, including end of life care, where creativity on the part of the occupational therapy provider can produce highly meaningful results for the dying individual, their family, and/or others who are important to that individual.

A recognition of the heterogeneity of aging, a focus on function more than disease, and a variety of providers and health-care settings is required when working with aging populations. Among all age groups, older adults represent the widest variety and span of health status and function. Furthermore, chronological age is less predictive than functional status; thus most aging-related interventions aim to improve function or prevent functional decline. Additionally, older adults are significantly more likely to have multiple diseases (Emery-Tiburcio et al., 2021). The American Geriatrics Society and the John Hartford Society have sought to crystallize the key domains of designing and implementing age-friendly health care (Emery-Tiburcio et al., 2021). In the context of an older adult with multiple diseases, focusing on the "4Ms" re-directs medical personnel from thinking about organ function, laboratory values, and imaging results in isolation and turning to older adults' goals, values, and capacities. Maximizing independence requires assessment and attention to What Matters (goals), Mind (mood and memory), Mobility, and Medications. Health-care providers must not overlook *Mood*, which may present as treatable depression. They must be able to diagnose *Mind* dysfunction, dementia, and delirium across the spectrum of care. Environments should support Mobility, ambulation, toileting, and self-care to promote safety and dignity. Finally, as noted above, physicians often focus on isolated organ function or dysfunction. They have thousands of generally effective *Medications* to prescribe for the multiple acute and comorbid conditions that, taken one

---

[1] We realize that there are multiple uses of the terms "primary," "secondary," and "tertiary" in health care. We are using the terms to align with prevention levels and to contrast from care settings. From Reitz, S. M., Scaffa, M. E., Commission on Practice, & Dorsey, J. (2020). Occupational Therapy in the Promotion of Health and Well-Being. *The American Journal of Occupational,* 74(3), 7403420010p1–7403420010p14. https://doi.org/10.5014/ajot.2020.743003.

at a time, have proven benefit. However, when given together results in polypharmacy, which is itself a leading cause of avoidable hospitalization in older adults (Mate et al., 2018). Polypharmacy can lead to direct drug toxicity, drug-drug interactions, drug-disease interactions, and, worse, triggering the so-called prescribing cascade in which drugs are prescribed to treat the adverse effects of other drugs (Kantor et al., 2015). Therefore, a thorough drug review is one of the most important components of geriatric care. Please refer to Chapter 14, Pharmacology, Pharmacy, and the Aging Adult: Implications for Occupational Therapy, for more specific information.

Underlying the 4 M's approach is the initiative of the American Board of Internal Medicine, Choosing Wisely (ABIM Foundation, 2022), which has been widely adopted by various health professional societies. With our expanding knowledge and plethora of tests and interventions, we should not lose sight of the purpose of health care. We should honor the aging adult's agency in determining "What Matters Most" (Laderman et al., 2019). Comparing the performance of the United States health-care system against other countries provides insight into redesigning processes, providing adequate resources, and targeting key outcomes that matter most to the aging population.

## Comparative Health System Models

Population aging is challenging all the industrially advanced countries of the world with increased health-care utilization and costs. Declining birth rates have resulted in fewer working-age adults paying for the care of older people who no longer work (Greis, 2018). In the face of these generational changes, health-care policy has emerged at the forefront of American public discourse. It is often framed as comparing an American approach to providing health care to those of other highly developed countries. In most respects, the American health-care system uses the same science, technology, and organization of care by the level of clinical acuity. Where it differs from other advanced systems is in how payment for care has evolved. The differences which stimulate debate are often, however, more a matter of degree than of kind. In this section, we trace the development of the U.S. health system and compare it with health systems in other advanced countries.

## Historical Development of Health Systems in the United States

The idea of modern nation-states stepping in to provide social and health-care support when community, family, and charitable supports have been inadequate is relatively recent but not new (Schneider et al., 2021). For example, in the United States, the Federal government's first foray into health care came in 1811 in response to the needs of disabled Continental Army veterans with continued need for care. In 1917, veteran's health-care facilities began to offer vocational rehabilitation for returning World War I veterans (US Department of Veterans Affairs, 2021). In 1921 disparate facilities and services coalesced into the Veterans' Bureau under the US Public Health Service. In 1930 the Veterans' Administration (VA) was elevated to a cabinet-level post. With the passage of the World

War II (WWII) Servicemen's Readjustment Act of 1944 (The GI Bill), the Veterans Administration Health Service (VAHS) became one bureau within the Veterans Affairs Administration (US Department of Veterans Affairs, 2021). It is now one of the largest integrated health systems in the world. It provides hospital-based medical and surgical care, rehabilitation, primary and long-term care to over 9 million veterans and in some cases their family members (US Department of Veterans Affairs, 2021). The aging of millions of WWII, Korean, and Vietnam veterans spurred the VAHS to pioneer geriatric health care. As the proportion of Americans with military service declines into the single digits, the VA will be retooling its clinical focus. However, much of the US approach to care and rehabilitation of older adults owes a debt to the VA.

Social welfare programs have not been universally or even originally associated with health care. The US Social Security Act of 1935, passed in the depths of the worldwide depression, was crafted to assure people that once they were too old or sick to work, they would not be destitute or totally dependent on their families or charity (Social Security Administration, 2022). The Old Age Assistance program, as it was called, could be used to provide for residents in old age homes. It extended some of the pension benefits of industrial union workers to the public. There have been subscription mutual aid societies descended from the medieval craft guilds and fraternal and immigrant mutual aid societies, which accumulated funds to support members in need. Social Security established mandatory savings deposits from workers' paychecks matched with contributions from employers to be kept in trust for pay out when they stopped working.

Health care has been part of negotiations between labor and employers in the industrialized countries for over a century as we will discuss later in this chapter. In 1929, Baylor University hospital and medical group were concerned about the rising costs of health care and the ability of their patients to pay for it. They were especially concerned about the Dallas Teachers' Union whose members represented a large proportion of their patients. They came up with the idea of pre-paid group health insurance which they called the Blue Cross program to pay the hospital for care of teachers in Texas. In 1939 it was expanded to include Blue Shield to pay the doctors. The systems merged in 1982 and expanded their membership around the country (Fox & Kongstvedt, 2013).

In 1933, a surgeon at a small hospital in the Mojave Desert in California cared for construction workers building the Colorado River Aqueduct System. This was very dangerous, hard, and poorly paid work. The doctor negotiated for the employer with an insurance company to prepay for hospital services on a per-worker per-day basis. This came to the attention of shipbuilding and industrial magnate, Henry Kaiser, who invited the doctor, Sidney Garfield, to build a similar system for his wartime workforce. They founded Kaiser Health Systems in 1945 and opened its system of prepaid care to labor unions and eventually the public, giving them access to a chain of hospitals and clinics (Fox & Kongstvedt, 2013).

In 1965, the federal government passed Medicare and Medicaid to provide health insurance to older adults and low-income Americans. Medicare and Medicaid represented comprehensive health-care reform that expanded access to millions of Americans. Medicare is a federal health program for older adults and people with disabilities. It is funded through payroll taxes, general revenue, and premiums. Because it is a federal program, benefits and services are consistent across the country. Medicare covers approximately 41 million people and finances 20% of national health expenditures (Social Security Administration, 2022). To be eligible for Medicare, an individual or their spouse must contribute to Medicare for 40 quarters (10 years) or pay monthly premiums to buy into the program. Beneficiaries also must be age 65 years or older, or disabled, and entitled to Social Security benefits (after a 2-year waiting period) or have either end-stage renal disease or amyotrophic lateral sclerosis (ALS-Lou Gehrig's disease). Medicare eligibility is not based on income or assets (Bodenheimer & Sinsky, 2014). Eligible individuals can receive benefits when they reach the age of 65 years.

There are four parts to Medicare. Medicare Part A is known as hospital insurance; it covers inpatient care such as hospital, post-hospital skilled nursing facilities either in home or in a facility, and hospice end-of-life care. It is financed through mandatory payroll taxes levied on the employer and employee. Medicare Part B is known as Supplemental Medical Insurance (SMI) and covers outpatient services, including physician care. Part B is a voluntary program financed through individual premiums and supplemented with general tax revenue (Bodenheimer & Sinsky, 2014). Medicare Part C, known as Medicare Advantage, provides several capitated, that is managed, alternatives to traditional Medicare B. Medicare Part D provides prescription drug coverage. It was established by the Medicare Prescription Drug Improvement and Modernization Act of 2003 and implemented in 2006. It is a voluntary program and enrollees can choose between a standalone plan for prescriptions or a Medicare Advantage plan that provides prescription drug benefits. Premiums are subsidized for low-income beneficiaries (Bodenheimer & Sinsky, 2014; Agency for Healthcare Research and Quality, 2018). Medicare beneficiaries can choose from several private fee-for-service (FFS) plans, or Medicare Advantage health maintenance organizations (HMOs), or preferred provider organizations (PPOs).

FFS plans pay providers for doing more. Following World War II, with the expansion of employer-based private health insurance, these plans resulted in a rapid increase in the sheer volume of health-care services delivered. As a result, managed care developed in response to the rapidly growing health-care costs and demands from payers for greater accountability from providers. BlueCross BlueShield and Kaiser, among others, offered models. Managed care refers to a variety of approaches used to integrate the financing and delivery of health care that seeks to contain costs and improve the quality of care through contractual arrangements with providers. There are two main types of managed care organizations: HMOs and PPOs (Berwick et al., 2008). HMOs require members to choose a primary care provider (PCP) from a network of providers who are employed by or who have negotiated prices with insurers. The PCP acts as a gatekeeper in deciding whether a member should be referred to see a specialist. Providers are paid a fixed monthly payment per enrolled member, known as capitation and often referred to as per member, per month payment. Providers must deliver the contracted services in exchange for the capitated payment. Capitation creates incentive for providers to reduce utilization of unnecessary services. With the rise of quality measures linked to health outcomes, providers are rewarded for selected improved health outcomes but constrained by staying within a capitated budget. Managed care organizations also review service utilization to ensure the services are medically necessary. Utilization review includes an expert evaluation of what services are medically necessary, determination of how services can be provided in the most inexpensive manner for the insurer (e.g., outpatient versus inpatient), and reviews the course of medical treatment (e.g., when a client is in the hospital).

PPOs emerged because members of HMOs complained about their limited choices and utilization review, and providers were unhappy with capitated payments and restrictions on how they practiced medicine. PPOs give members the option of receiving care outside of the network at a higher out-of-pocket cost. Providers are paid on a discounted FFS basis, and the use of utilization review was curtailed. Typically, fees are discounted at 25% to 35% off providers' regular fees. Premiums and cost sharing are higher in PPOs than in HMOs because of the added cost of greater choice. PPOs are now the most common form of managed care (Berwick et al., 2008). The plans are financed by payments from Medicare and may require an additional premium. Medicare Advantage plans are increasingly popular because although choice is constrained, as in an HMO, they also include selected drug coverage and other services not usually offered by straight Medicare or PPO plans such as vision, dental, and hearing (Agency for Healthcare Research and Quality, 2018; Bodenheimer & Sinsky, 2014).

Medicaid is a joint federal-state program that provides health care for low-income people regardless of age. In 2013 Medicaid covered 62 million people. Total Medicaid expenditures by state and federal governments totaled $432 billion in 2011 (Durand-Zalesk, 2020). Medicaid is administered by state governments. States operate Medicaid under general guidelines set by the federal government. To participate, states must provide a mandatory set of benefits. In addition, states can adopt optional Medicaid benefits. The federal government provides matching funds to states on an open-ended basis. The amount of matching funds varies from 50% to 76%, depending on how wealthy the state is relative to the rest of the country (Durand-Zalesk, 2020). Medicaid eligibility originally covered only welfare recipients. However, the Personal Responsibility and Work Opportunity Reconciliation Act of 1996 separated Medicaid eligibility from welfare eligibility. Currently, Medicaid eligibility is based on a categorical requirement and financial limits. The eligible categories include parents with dependent children, pregnant women, and individuals who are aged, blind, or disabled and whose income and assets do not exceed a maximum set by the state. States have the option to set higher income eligibility levels

**TABLE 25.1** Comparison of Health Systems Coverage, Inclusion and Financing Among High-Income Nations (Tikkanen et al., 2020)

| Public Private Mixed | Universal Mandatory | Central Government | State Provincial-Government or NGO | Local Municipal |
|---|---|---|---|---|
| **United States (The Commonwealth Fund, 2020)** | | | | |
| PUB: Medicare Medicaid CHIP PRI: Private employer benefit Private insurance w/ or w/o ACA subsidy VA, Military | Mandatory 8.5% not included | Medicare Medicaid subsidy to states ACA mandated private insurance subsidy Sets standards for hospital, facility VA Military includes facilities and staff | Medicaid CHIP Regulates private insurance, provider licensing, LTC inspections Public safety net facilities, prisons, clinics and staff | School health, public health |
| **Germany (Blümel & Busse, 2020)** | | | | |
| Originally mandatory enrollment with non-profit provincial Sick Funds. Recently higher income earners may opt of the public system for private insurance provided the coverage is equivalent or better | Yes. Eighty-eight percent of population remains in the national Sick Fund. Eleven percent opted out to private | Regulates oversees but does not directly fund except in cases of need or shortfall in Sick Funds | Nonprofit, nongovernmental Sick Funds organized at the provincial level funded by payroll deductions from employers and workers. Provinces provide planning, hospital management and payment to private physicians | Public health |
| **United Kingdom: England (Thorlby, 2020)** | | | | |
| Universal National Health Insurance | Yes, universal automatic for British citizens and legal residents | The central government funds and administers the National Health Service which employs physicians, nurses, health professionals, owns hospitals and provides home health services and transportation | Each province administers its own health-care program | Long-term care for older adults and disabled, social services and public health |
| **France (Durand-Zalesk, 2020)** | | | | |
| French citizens and legal residents. Based on employment with general taxes for nonworking | Yes | Funded from central government employment payroll and income taxes, administered by local agencies | Regional planning for population medicine, public health and social care (income subsidy to low-income workers and unemployed) | Care to older adults and disabled |
| **Canada (Allin et al., 2020)** | | | | |
| National Medicare | Yes | Registration is automatic for all citizens and legal residents. Cofunds provinces, funds Indigenous Peoples, veterans and active military. Regulates medical devices and drugs | Each province administers its own health-care program funded by payroll employer and employee taxes with Central govern contributions | Public health, long-term care, hospitals |

*LTC,* Long-term care.

| Private Insurance for Hospital, Primary | Copays | Private Supplement Insurance | What Is Covered |
|---|---|---|---|
| Predominantly through employer plans. Private insurance self-insurance, subsidized private insurance through state-level exchanges | Yes, except with selected managed care payors, high option plans may waive copays. Copays often variable by in- or out- of contracted practices/facilities. | Yes, optional. Medicare supplements, Medigap or Medicare Managed Care, optional private high option plans | Most basic plans public or private cover limited rehabilitation, maternity, mental health, laboratory, and preventive care. Most do not cover eyeglasses or contacts, dental, drugs, hearing aids. Do not cover long term care (LTC) or home care except within Medicare A |
| Permitted for people who have opted out of the Sick Funds provided coverage is equivalent | Yes. There is a basket of required benefits. Long-term care is a separate fund. Copays may be charged for upgrades in rooming, or other personal preferences. | Sick Fund subscribers may purchase private supplement insurance to cover co-pays, off formulary drugs or upgrades | Basic formulary, outpatient visits, hospitalization. Children's eye and dental, maternity, mental health |
| Eleven percent of British citizens purchase private supplements for "upgrades" especially priority for services | - | As incentive pay, 13% of Swedes get health insurance supplement through their employers for upgrades to basic package | No national basket beyond necessary hospital. Outpatient and home care. Varies locally, some local units provide dental and vision care to adults |
| Ninety-five percent of insurance is from noncompetitive carriers enrolling through employers or the government | No | There is a small percent with subscription to private for-profit insurance for supplemental coverages | Home care, LTC Check drug, dental, eye, rehab |
| Not for "necessary" | Variable | 67% of Canadians have a supplemental for-profit private insurance to supplement | No national package, each province decides on coverages beyond necessary hospital and outpatient care. Some cover drugs, dental care, psychotherapy, occupational therapy, physical therapy and elective procedures |

(Durand-Zalesk, 2020). Medicaid eligibility has expanded by raising the income eligibility level to 138% of the FPL (Roberts et al., 2020). However, not all states have elected to adopt the new income eligibility levels. In 2014, 28 states (including Washington, DC) had adopted Medicaid expansion. An additional seven states were considering expanding Medicaid, and 16 had decided against Medicaid expansion at this time (Orzag, 2008).

The most recent update to the US health system was the Patient Protection and Affordable Care Act (ACA) of 2010 (Pub. L. 111–148) which was designed to close the gap in universal coverage by adjustments to Medicare and Medicaid and by requiring the non-poor, uninsured to purchase private insurance (Fiedler, 2020).

Most Americans get their health insurance through their employers, labor unions, military, railroad or government employer and retirement plans. This left a gap in health coverage. Americans with too much income to qualify for Medicaid who did not receive health insurance through their employers may not have had private health insurance for a variety of reasons. If they had pre-existing health conditions, the insurance was too expensive. Small employers could not take them on in their risk pools because it would raise the rates for all. Others without insurance were often healthy young workers, day laborers, or self-employed workers who took a risk on their continued good health. Under the ACA, private insurers were barred from using pre-existing conditions as disqualifiers. Private insurers were incentivized to provide low-cost policies to Americans in the gap of health insurance coverage with federal subsidies to purchasers of selected policies. With this legislation, the United States joined Germany, the United Kingdom, France, and Canada in having some form of coverage for all citizens (Table 25.1).

## Historical Development of Health Systems in Germany, United Kingdom, France, and Canada

The idea of extending health care to whole populations of nation-states began in 1883 in then the rapidly industrializing Germany when the Iron Chancellor Otto von Bismarck in Prussia established Sickness Insurance to pay for health care for industrial workers. In recognition of the dangerous work and poor living conditions in 19th-century industry, the legislation was based on the idea that better health and living conditions served the interests of the industrial state by increasing productivity and decreasing political unrest. In 1884 workers' disability insurance and in 1889 old age insurance were added to the original program. Over time mandatory coverage for industrial workers was extended to the poor, to government workers, and then all working adults. The funds were then and are now administered by Sick Boards, provincial (state) civilian but nongovernmental corporations. They are funded by provincial employer and employee payroll taxes with supplementation from the central government, not unlike the U.S. Medicaid programs for the poor. In both systems there are state-to-state variations in coverage, for example, drug formularies differ from state to state. In 2009 higher income German workers were permitted to opt out of

the public insurance but they are required to purchase private insurance. Physicians are not employed by the government; they are paid fee-for-service. However, they may also see patients who are willing to pay privately above the set rates (Blümel & Busse, 2020).

In 1911, Lloyd George passed the British National Insurance Act, which specifically emulated Germany with whom they would soon be fighting in World War I. It covered lower-paid workers (not the unemployed or families) in collaboration with unions, state, worker, and employer contributions. It provided income for temporary unemployment. It paid for health care with capitated fees to "panel" doctors. A separate women's advocacy group, the Women's Guild got maternity care included. A national mandate established local "approved administrative societies." In 1942 a report by William Beveridge was revived when the Labor Party won the Prime Ministership. In 1945 the Labor government passed National Health Service (NHS) legislation that in 1948 established universal free health care for all. In the United Kingdom, doctors may work for the NHS (Thorlby, 2020).

The French health-care system evolved rapidly after WWII. In 1945, statutory health insurance (SHI) was given to workers through employee-sponsored insurance and extended to retirees and older adults. A mandate for health insurance was extended to self-employed workers with subsidized plans passed in 1966. Health care for the unemployed was legislated in 2000. It is administered by several private not-for-profit funds that compete for population contracts in negotiation with the government. Patients may have to pay up front but then are reimbursed. All French citizens and legal residents are covered for routine outpatient and hospital care. French patients choose their own private providers based on availability (Durand-Zalesk, 2020).

The Canada Health Care Act of 1984 established publicly funded universal health care called Medicare Canada. It is funded and administered by the provinces. It is funded by taxes and pays most hospital and outpatient care. Citizens can buy private insurance supplements to cover health-care services not covered by Medicare Canada, such as elective surgery, vision, drugs, rehabilitation, home care, or residential long-term care. These are otherwise paid out of pocket or with private supplemental insurance. Access in Canada, Germany, and France to primary care is easier due to the higher number of physicians in primary care. Nonurgent specialist care requires a referral, and with the lesser availability of specialists comes longer wait times, which many Canadians find frustrating. However, the costs to the patient and the system are lower. Central and provincial governments negotiated drug prices with manufacturers resulting in greater uniformity of prescribing and consistent lower prices at the pharmacy (Allin et al., 2020).

All the technologically advanced nations have provided for universal access to primary and hospital-level care through combinations of public and private insurance. The balance between universal national health insurance and supplementation with private insurance varies considerably, with the United States most dependent on private for-profit insurance and the United Kingdom least dependent. In each country, even those with mandated universal insurance, the state or provincial governments are charged with front-line management of tax-funded insurance. In most single-payor national systems adult dental, vision, hearing and long-term care are available through private supplemental coverage. So, the difference between the United States and other countries in health access, cost and outcomes does not appear to be attributable to whether payors are public or private. Rather, the historical extent of population coverage and the variation in the proportion of for-profit and nonprofit payors may be the difference. Universal coverage became available in the United States in 2014 compared to 1889 in Germany, 1948 in the United Kingdom, 1945 in France, and 1984 in Canada. All the technologically advanced countries struggle with the cost of humane and quality care for frail older adults with complex, chronic illness (Table 25.2).

## STOP AND THINK EXERCISE

Consider what would have to take place in the United States for the passage of a single-payer system under the Medicare program. How does political ideology affect such a change?

## Health-Care Quality: Moving From the Triple to Quadruple Aim in the United States

Since the initiation of Medicare and Medicaid, the passage of the ACA represents the largest paradigm shift in the US health system financing. As a result of the ACA, the US health system has moved from a volume to value-based reimbursement structure. In effect, the law helps ensure high-quality care by linking payment to performance of health-care services. In other words, health-care systems and providers are incentivized by providing *the right care for the right patient at the right time*. Berwick et al. (2008) point out that in order for health-care systems to achieve high-quality care, they must "pursue a broader system of linked goals" referred to as the *Triple Aim*—improving patient experience, reducing cost, and optimizing population health. While many health-care systems have adopted the Triple Aim as a framework for quality improvement efforts, providers and staff have noted challenges around achieving such goals given stressful work conditions (Bodenheimer

& Sinsky, 2014). Accordingly, the *Quadruple Aim* has been proposed, which highlights the need to improve work life of providers and staff so that improved patient experience, reduced cost, and optimized population health can be fully realized (Bodenheimer & Sinsky, 2014). Addressing these four goals poses significant difficulties given the complexity and fragmented nature of the US health-care system (Roberts et al., 2020).

## How Is the United States Health-Care System Doing With This Paradigm Shift?

A recent report from the Commonwealth Fund of 11 high-income countries revealed the US health-care system ranked last overall in performance, "despite spending far more of its gross domestic product on health care" (Schneider et al., 2021) Further, this report and other studies demonstrate that the US health-care system is falling short in three quality problem areas: underuse, overuse, and misuse of services (Agency for Healthcare Research and Quality, 2018).

Underuse refers to the failure to provide needed health-care services, which is a common problem. Research has shown that all patients in the United States receive approximately half of all recommended services, including preventive care, treatment of acute conditions, and treatment of chronic conditions (Orzag, 2008). The coronavirus disease 2019 (COVID-19) pandemic has further exacerbated patients' ability to access needed health-care services due to digital transformations like telehealth appointments. Indeed, Power (2019) found that almost 75% of households were unfamiliar with or lacked access to telehealth options, thus creating a "digital divide" in health care. This digital divide has contributed to health disparities. For example, a study found that White and Asian patients used telehealth at significantly higher rates than older Black and Hispanic patients.

Overuse refers to the excessive and unnecessary use of health-care services, which increases the likelihood of both harm and costs. Retrospective review of medical records by independent panels of physicians found that significant numbers of delivered health services were either clinically inappropriate or of equivocal value (McGlynn, 1998). Overuse is also found in the extent of geographic variation in use of the same health service without evidence of differences in outcomes (Agency for Healthcare Research and Quality, 2018). Several system-level factors may account for these poor

**TABLE 25.2** Comparison of Health Expenditures Among High-Income Nations (Akca et al., 2017; Tikkanen et al., 2020)

| Country | Population Percent ≥65 (World Health Organization, 2022) | Health Expenditures Percent of GDP 2018 | Per Capita Health Expenditures in US Dollar |
|---|---|---|---|
| United States | 16.0 | 16.9 | 10,966 |
| Germany | 21.4 | 11.2 | 6,646 |
| France | 20.3 | 11.2 | 5,376 |
| Canada | 17.2 | 10.7 | 5,418 |
| England | 18.3 | 9.8 | 4,653 |

outcomes, including the lack of consistency across documentation platforms, fewer primary care physicians, more physician practice groups, and being investor owned.

Misuse refers to medical errors and other events that could lead to serious outcomes. Since 1996 the Institute of Medicine (IOM), now called the US National Academy of Medicine (NAM), has issued several reports documenting the extent of medical errors and their consequences (National Academy of Medicine, 2021). As such, Medicare and other insurers have begun efforts to reduce medical errors and improve health-care quality through financial incentives and penalties.

## How Can the US Health-Care System Improve Quality?

Many health-care systems and providers turn to Donabedian's theoretical framework (Donabedian, 2005) to understand what needs to be improved to ultimately, achieve the Quadruple Aim. This prominent framework consists of three dimensions: structure, process and outcomes. *Structure* encompasses organizational factors such as the physical spaces of the health-care system, staffing and patient/client ratios, the type and use of electronic medical records or documentation systems, and practice culture. *Process* is described as the actions or delivery of services to patients by providers. *Outcomes* reflect the impact of the services. These three components are believed to be linked where "outcomes are the result of the care processes that are provided and the structure in which care is delivered" (Leland et al., 2015) Many health-care systems have adopted quality improvement tools like Six Sigma, Lean, and Plan-Do-Study-Act (PDSA) cycles (Girdler et al., 2016) to better understand how to address structure, process, and/or outcomes of various care services.

## Organization of Care Services

The American health-care "system" has been criticized as being neither a provider of health nor a system. It is a large segment of the US economy in terms of capital investment, expenditure, and employment. It is both large and complicated. As shown in Table 25.1, there are many public, private, and hybrid organizations linked by contractual agreements, regulatory structures, and supply chains. The work force alone is composed of the entire range of nonprofessional low-pay caregivers at the bedside, (clinic, out-patient services, assistive and skilled care facilities, and home) ranks of specialized university-educated professionals and paraprofessionals (e.g., occupational therapists and assistants), and highly paid medical specialists and corporate managers including chief executive officers (CEOs) who are responsible to shareholders. A flow chart to show the linkages among health-care employees and then supply chains of diagnostic. Machinery, medical equipment, chemical, and drugs would be unintelligible, due to the sheer number of overlapping and bidirectional arrows. We instead have made a list of care services limited to those with direct contact with patients and populations sorted by whether the intervention target is populations or individuals, and by "acuity." Acuity is defined by both the risk of death and the complexity of care, which includes both the number of personnel and levels of technical skill and drugs and equipment required to deliver health interventions. Then we account for who pays for the service, whether it be government taxes, individual patients, insurance companies, or some other combination of these payors. It is beyond the scope of this chapter to evaluate the relationships among cost, price, and benefit; however, studies of comparative health systems have commented on the markedly higher administrative costs of American health care because of its complexity and its role as an economic driver (Tikkanen et al., 2020).

## Public Health

The greatest gains in health and longevity in human history were the result of the 19th-century hygiene movement. The social hygienists specifically linked clean municipal water supplies, inspections and refrigeration of food supplies, and general social progressivism, often led by women, to promote healthier living spaces, better diets, maternal and child health, and epidemic control. More recent public health campaigns have included fluoridation of water for dental health, lead abatement, air quality monitoring, and COVID-19 vaccine education. Federal, state, and local taxes fund governmental agencies charged with evaluating research to establish and enforce standards to prevent harm and promote health at the population level. Several Federal agencies include the combined National Institutes of Health, the Environmental Protection Agency, the CDC, and the Federal Drug Administration (FDA) for pharmaceutical safety and efficacy. The Department of Agriculture oversees food safety. There are partner agencies at the state level for reporting and enforcement. Counties and localities oversee, for example, school health, point of sale (POS) food safety, lead, and asbestos abatement. Vaccines have been administered through both public and private auspices since the mid-20th century as a public "good" with support from federal and state agencies. Historically, national vaccine campaigns were conducted by private philanthropic organizations such as the March of Dimes for polio. Other private national disease-focused advocacy and philanthropy efforts support cancer and dementia research, for example. Health maintenance means enabling people to follow the best available advice on preventing disease and maintaining fitness of body and mind. Broadly this function is suffused in public messaging from government and private organizations (e.g., anti-smoking campaigns). School-based health initiatives include providing healthy food, health education, and exercise. Public health and educational interventions for preventing and treating sexually transmitted diseases (STDs) and substance use often also occur in schools and public clinics. Health maintenance functions are entwined in outpatient primary care, including screening for depression, familial abuse, cancer, drug and alcohol abuse, geriatric falls risk, and an extensive list of recommendations from the US Public Health Task Force (USPHTF) (U.S. Prevention Services Task Force, 2022).

## Outpatient Primary

This type of care is generally office based, and increasingly tele-health remote, especially since the onset of the COVID-19 pandemic. PCPs may be licensed Doctor of Medicine (MD), Doctor of Osteopathic Medicine (DO), nurse practitioner (NP), or physician assistant (PA) providers. The PCP is charged with performing health maintenance tasks such as screening, weight and vital signs monitoring, prescription and over-the-counter drug review, vaccinations, and general medical advice. In addition, PCPs perform most chronic disease management including hypertension (HTN), diabetes mellitus (DM), asthma, arthritis, and self-limited acute injuries and illnesses. In large part due to access, free-standing urgent care centers provide care for minor illness.

## Specialist Outpatient Care

This type of care is needed for rare or technically complex conditions that require both specialized expertise and access to outpatient therapeutic and diagnostic procedures not normally performed by primary care providers. These include, for example, chemotherapy and radiation for cancer, endoscopic exams, cardiac device monitoring, management of severe renal and cardiac failure, addictions treatment, psychiatric care, periodontal surgery, and many others. Most private insurance and Medicare managed care negotiate fees with providers who are then referred to as in-network and require PCP referrals for specialist outpatient care.

## Inpatient Acute Care

This type of care is reserved for conditions and injuries requiring 24/7 treatment and management that cannot be provided by a lower level of care. Inpatient care in hospitals is stratified by acuity including the potential for early death. Hospitals typically stratify acuity in terms of nursing staffing ratios and only partially by qualifications of the doctors. The highest level of inpatient acuity is delivered in the intensive care unit (ICU) with 1:1 nursing care and most often physicians with specialties in critical care. Most ICUs also engage respiratory therapy and other technical specialists to monitor the machines (ventilators, dialysis, electroencephalogram (EEG), cardiac support) and a dedicated pharmacist. Long-stay ICU patients may receive preventive rehabilitation to maintain functional capacity. Some hospitals have step-down units from the ICU that continue close monitoring. General medical surgical services operate with ideally 1:4–5 nursing-to-patient ratios. Increasingly direct outpatient care to hospital admissions is declining for several reasons, including, but not limited, to the COVID-19-induced bed shortages. Elective procedures and surgeries are routed to daytime holding units with the intent of home discharge. As emergency departments (ED) become backed up, definitive management of high-acuity conditions may begin in the ED. Free-standing urgent care centers are a response to ED overload; that option may be available to those with insurance. Increasingly, hospital medical, surgical, and psychiatric admissions are directed from inhouse Emergency Services. With the overload from COVID-19, inpatient assessments for discharge planning including physical, occupational,

speech, and swallowing evaluations have moved down to the ED, and Medicare (followed by other insurers) has had to revise the criteria for coding inpatient care delivered in the ED. An ED acute visit is covered by Medicare B, outpatient, and does not count toward sub-acute coverage. Medicare A pays for most of inpatient charges, and for selected post-acute care for sequelae of the inpatient diagnosis. Length of stay (LOS) in the hospital initially paid as a lump sum for a specified number of days based on the diagnosis, for example, pneumonia, or heart failure. Medicare A will pay for 100% of 20 days of post-acute skilled nursing or rehabilitation based on that qualifying stay. A 3-day inpatient stay was required but this was adjusted during the COVID epidemic to ease bed shortages. When Medicare A is exhausted, the patient becomes liable for increasing per diem copays depending on length of stay (LOS),.

## Acute Inpatient Rehabilitation

This type of care is directed for complex rehabilitation in patients who have the mental status and physical resilience to participate in rigorous, multidisciplinary therapies (e.g., spinal cord injuries, strokes, amputations). Medicare A will approve acute inpatient rehabilitation if the patient has demonstrated the ability to benefit. Most acute rehab patients tend to be younger. Not all facilities will accept Medicaid payors. Private and employer policies are highly variable.

## Outpatient Rehabilitative Care

This type of care involves many different professions usually on referral from primary or specialist providers, although private practice therapists and wound management clinics are sometimes available. Insurance companies including private, Medicare B, in-network contractors through Medicare Advantage and other managed care generally specify how many sessions of therapy will be covered with or without a co-pay. These include physical and occupational rehabilitation, sports medicine, cardiac rehab, pulmonary rehab, language and cognitive rehab, lymphedema and wound management, pelvic rehab, chiropractic, and prescriptions for home durable medical equipment (DME). The VA maintains its own rehabilitation services. Outpatient rehabilitation is often conducted on the premises of inpatient hospitals or at patient homes under Medicare B, or if it is started within 30 days of an inpatient hospital stay, Medicare part A is the payor. Private insurance coverage through employers varies considerably.

## Post-Acute Care

This type of care, also known as sub-acute care, is provided in residential settings licensed to perform skilled nursing procedures such wound care, IV antibiotics, or complex medication management and rehabilitation services at a lower level of intensity than those provided in acute rehabilitation. Patients who are too ill or dependent to return home with Medicare A home health will receive these Medicare A services in a facility, colloquially called a "nursing home." When Medicare A benefits are exhausted, patients can receive Part B services if they have it, or if they have another insurer whatever is covered.

## Long-Term Care

This type of care is almost entirely paid by State government Medicaid programs, in fact, long-term care is a sizeable portion of all state government obligations. With a copay, dual-eligible (Medicare/Medicaid) patients may be able to go home with a state-subsidized home caregiver, often certified as homemakers. States also will qualify family members to be paid home caregivers. Private pay in a long-term care facility or home caregivers are an option for families with resources.

## End-of-Life Care

This type of care is provided as a formal service by private companies that may offer regular home health as well. Hospice, a type of care that is provided at end of life, was initially designed for patients with a qualifying diagnosis and an estimated life expectancy of 6 months or less. Under Medicare A, hospice is a capitated service. Here, the hospice provider is paid a fixed monthly fee to provide all necessary comfort services and modalities. Should the patient or family call 911 and go to the ED, hospice enrollment is terminated. The same providers can also deliver palliative care, defined as symptom management but the patient may still pursue curative care. Palliative care is delivered at home and long-term care (LTC) with a monthly visit. There is limited inpatient hospice availability and it is often subsidized by philanthropy. Medicaid covers hospice at home and in facilities. Private insurance coverage for end of life is variable. The VA provides end-of-life care both outpatient and inpatient for eligible veterans. A third type of care with noncurative intent is emerging called Advanced Illness Management (AIM) (American Hospital Association, 2022), which explicitly address the 4Ms. For older adults with multiple comorbidities, reduced functional status, and limited medical options who would nonetheless prefer to stay in their homes and maximize quality rather than length of life, AIM is an excellent alternative.

Increasing numbers of age-segregated residential complexes are being constructed with designations such as "independent living," "assisted-living" and "memory care." There are no federal or state regulation or licensing of these residences. There is no requirement for on-site medical, nursing, or health services. Neither Medicare nor Medicaid pays for living expenses in these complexes. The low-income seniors cannot afford them. Some communities do support low-income senior housing. Residents in "senior" living complexes use their existing Medicare traditional, supplemental, or Managed plans for health care. Some complexes offer an array of wellness, lifestyle, and informational programming. Exercise classes are extremely popular. Some will have rehabilitation facilities on campus.

## Alternative and Integrative Therapy

These therapies are very popular in the United States despite the limited evidence base because people are reassured by the accessibility of the language and respond to the focus on their subjective well-being. Selected chiropractic and acupuncture procedures are covered by many insurers in part because of the apparent effectiveness and because of the reasonable cost and general safety of the procedures. Few nutraceuticals (dietary supplements, vitamins, herbal remedies, "vitality" boosters) are covered by Part D or other pharmacy plans. They are not regulated as drugs; they are regulated as foods by the FDA and are not required to demonstrate effectiveness. Manufacturers are not required to submit samples to the US Pharmacopeia (USP) to verify content and purity. Reputable manufacturers may submit samples to the USP for verification of content and purity. USP-approved products will have the green and yellow diamond icon on the label. Legalized marijuana products are a recent addition to this class of remedies.

## Role of Occupational Therapy in the Care Continuum

Occupational therapy is fundamentally a profession that supports quality of life and can play a significant role within the health promotion and care system continuum with aging adults (Table 25.3). "Leavell's levels," as the prevention levels noted by Leavell and Clark (Donabedian, 2005) are known, provide a conceptual framework for designing occupational therapy prevention services that support the health-related

**TABLE 25.3**  Increasing Recognition of Occupational Therapy Across the Care Continuum

| Level of Care | Occupational Therapy Service Example |
|---|---|
| Public health | Programming, advocating and educating the public for supporting independence.<br>Coaching and consulting with communities, private builders on adaptive technology. |
| Specialist outpatient care | Prehabilitation prior to elective surgery to improve postoperative outcomes.<br>Problem focused therapy (e.g., hand function, care process, cognitive therapy). |
| Inpatient acute care | Inpatient acute and ICU interventions for early diagnosis of functional deficits.<br>Early intervention to prevent further losses and to maintain function. |
| Acute and post-acute rehabilitation care | Acute inpatient rehabilitation (e.g., amputee, spinal cord injury, stroke, and trauma).<br>Post-acute rehabilitation in SNF or home care to restore independence. |
| Long-term care (LTC) | Residential populations at various levels of dependency (independent, assisted, LTC).<br>Support improved or maintained independence, training, and caregiver education and support. |
| End-of-life care | Adaptive techniques for patient comfort and dignity. Caregiver education and support. |

quality of life of our aging clients seen within the community in both medical and community wellness settings.

Consider that in all interventions, whether they occur at the primary, secondary, or tertiary care level (WHO, 2022), occupational therapy providers should promote the optimal health of the individuals served. Shortell, promoted "bridging the divide between health and health care," and occupational therapy is optimally positioned to contribute to that effort. Note that Chapter 3 on epidemiological factors associated with the aging process, including the continuing increasing numbers of aging adults with diseases, also identifies opportunities for occupational therapy to address health promotion needs among aging adults. Thus, health promotion is the emphasis throughout all types of interventions despite the level of client and/or caregiver function, including interventions with terminally ill individuals in hospice care.

## Primary Prevention

The purpose of primary prevention is to maintain optimal individualized health and protect individuals from diseases, conditions, and dysfunction (Reitz et al., 2020). Should early signs of ill health occur, ideally immediate support is provided to prevent deterioration so that a potential disease is prevented. Ordinarily, the client resides in the community and interventions are provided at a physician's office, a wellness clinic, the individual's workplace, or other community venues. Historic examples of occupational therapy providers working in primary care are worker health initiatives within businesses and industries in which therapists conduct worksite evaluations and production line worker interventions to prevent musculoskeletal deterioration, including repetitive motion injuries. With an aging workforce, the potential need for increased physical and/or mental health interventions for workers in many types of employment is readily apparent.

Within the past decade, the occupational therapy profession initiated efforts to partner with physicians in primary care clinics to enhance services, advance health promotion efforts, and promote cost-effective medical care (ABIM Foundation, 2022; Leland et al., 2015; Segal et al., 2022; Tikkanen et al., 2020). At the present time, a few models of occupational therapy services in primary medical care offices exist in the United States. To date, the most receptive physicians have been family medicine providers (Tikkanen et al., 2020) and geriatricians. These individuals capitalize on the presence of an occupational therapist to assess clients through screening to address fundamental daily quality-of-life issues related to activities of daily living (ADLs) and instrumental activities of daily living (IADLs); age-related vision, hearing, or other sensory changes; coping with emerging or long-term mental illness, diminished cognition, or dementia; transitions in life, such as retirement; risk assessment for falls and other injuries; and related spousal and caregiver needs. Refer to Chapter 26 for more on Primary Care.

The role of the occupational therapy staff may include screening as well as mitigating occupational performance deficits about which the physician may be unaware. For example, an older female client who has difficulty with

dressing due to degenerative joint changes in her shoulders may not report this problem to her doctor. However, when an occupational therapist is present, any problems with ADLs or IADLs, along with psychosocial and leisure activity limitation concerns, are routinely queried and addressed. In this example, the occupational therapist collaborates with the client in implementing an acceptable adaptive dressing routine and clothing recommendations to minimize shoulder pain and discomfort.

Typically, because neither physicians nor the public understand what occupational therapy can provide to add value to the client visit, occupational therapy providers need to be proactive in communicating the relevant highly educated, yet practical, and holistic approach that is inherent in interventions that support and enhance these individuals' lives.

## Secondary Prevention

The occupational therapy provider may play a role in identifying diminished cognitive, psychosocial, or physical occupational performance and/or related symptoms that lead to an early identification of a disease or condition—the aim of secondary care. Additionally, limiting disability is a further goal of this level of service, which may also be provided in the home, community, or physician's office or clinic (Reitz et al., 2020). For example, historically, occupational therapy providers have offered community education programs in collaboration with arthritis organizations. Either newly diagnosed clients or individuals who have been living for years with various forms of arthritis, including rheumatoid and osteoarthritis, attend these educational programs. Weekly, biweekly, or monthly sessions provide information on the differentiation among the types of arthritis, related etiology, and principles and practices that they can apply to their everyday lives. Recommendations are provided for joint protection, energy conservation, and work simplification approaches, along with strategies to assist them to maintain an optimal quality of life, despite their diagnosis. These older adults are encouraged to be proactive in advocating for assistance, wherever relevant. For example, when grocery shopping, requesting that items be placed in more bags, to lighten the weight and resulting stress on joints, is recommended. Requesting assistance with carrying heavy purchases could also promote joint protection and energy conservation, wherever needed. Occupational therapy providers work to empower these older adults to adapt their lifestyles, emphasizing the individual's priorities and needs for meaningful activities. Occupational therapy providers may not traditionally identify with secondary care but should recognize the importance of disability limitation within any area of practice with aging adults.

## Tertiary Prevention

Occupational therapy providers are typically associated with and well known for their interventions in tertiary prevention (Reitz et al., 2020). Since the profession's founding nearly 100 years ago, occupational therapy providers have provided rehabilitative services to wounded veterans in hospitals after

**CASE EXERCISE 25.1**

You have just been promoted to work as the Evidence-based Occupational Therapy Specialist of a large, partially integrated health-care system. Your first assignment is to identify several innovative ways to improve health system quality surrounding "patient and family caregiver experience." Opportunities exist to improve the systematic inclusion of family (i.e., traditional family, partner, home caregiver, or other support person designated by the patient) in health-care processes. Draft a memo to the Director of Patient and Family Caregiver Experience that answers the following questions:

1. What health-care policy and research exists that support the systematic inclusion of family in hospital care?
2. What are three innovative ideas your system could implement to meet improvement around the patient and family caregiver experience?
3. What innovative idea is most critical to tackle first to improve quality and why?
4. What innovative idea will be most difficult to achieve and why?

World War I, and to individuals living in the community. In subsequent years, occupational therapy providers have delivered most of their services in tertiary care, in acute, subacute, and rehabilitation hospitals, and long-term care settings such as skilled nursing care facilities. Occupational therapy interventions in community-based centers for aging persons with developmental disabilities and hospice care facilities are not well publicized but have existed for decades. A skilled nursing facility example includes a holistic approach to the setting. First, the occupational therapist conducts an environmental assessment, beyond what is considered "up to standards." Is the setting not only meeting the safety standards but tending to the holistic needs of the community of typically aging residents? The environmental assessment includes the nature of the context—is it supportive to the psychosocial well-being of the residents, supporting a culture of enhancing each aging adult? The occupational therapist's responsibility goes beyond the cognitive, physical, psychosocial, or ADL process prescribed for the resident and includes examining which contextual elements are supporting (or not) the optimal occupational performance of this resident, and her or his health-related quality of life. Note that Chapter 28 on residential and skilled care further describes current and potential roles for OTs and OTAs.

### Quality Improvement

Occupational therapy educators, providers, and researchers can play an important role in ensuring that practice aligns with the current health-care reform initiatives (Kinney et al., 2022). Educators can prepare the next generation of providers who feel confident and competent in their abilities to critically evaluate, synthesize, and translate available evidence into practice and formulate systems to redesign health care, including methods for stakeholder engagement and data collection, analysis, and interpretation. Researchers can partner with providers to study the methods to promote the integration of evidence-based processes, interventions, and policies, as well as the de-implementation of inappropriate or ineffective practices. Other helpful examples on how the occupational therapy profession can support the shift toward high-quality, value-based care can be found in Leland et al. (2015).

## SUMMARY

This chapter provided an overview of health and health care, a comparative analysis of high-income health-care systems, and how occupational therapy providers may interface with any aspect of either formal or informal service delivery with aging clients. As a primary quality-of-life–supporting profession, occupational therapy has much to offer throughout the continuum of care to support optimal occupational performance and overall well-being in aging adults. By collaborating with clients and other providers in systems of care, the profession has the capability to profoundly affect optimal service utilization, health-care cost containment, and health-related quality of life for aging adults.

*The complete listing of the Bibliography and Chapter Questions and Answers are available in the accompanying enhanced eBook version included with the print purchase of this textbook. Visit Elsevier eBooks+ (eBooks.Health.Elsevier.com) to access this content.*

## CHAPTER 26

# The Role of Occupational Therapy in Primary Care

*Carri Hand, PhD, Catherine Donnelly, PhD, Lori Letts, PhD, and Sue Dahl-Popolizio, DBH*

## CHAPTER OUTLINE

## OBJECTIVES

- Define and describe the key elements of primary care and the occupational therapy role in this setting
- Describe key features of the primary care interprofessional team
- Explain how occupational therapists facilitate older adults' occupational participation and engagement through health promotion approaches in primary care
- Describe the occupational therapy role with older adults in key practice areas in primary care
- Discuss occupational therapy approaches and strategies with older adults at individual and community levels in primary care
- Identify and recommend areas for future research with primary care older adult populations that can support further integration of occupational therapy into primary care

## Defining and Describing Primary Care and Occupational Therapy Within This Setting

Primary care is considered the first point of access to the health-care system (World Health Organization [WHO] & United Nations Children's Fund [UNICEF\, 2020). It has been described as having five core elements: first contact accessibility, continuity, comprehensiveness, coordination, and person- and people-centered, with further descriptions found in Table 26.1 (Starfield et al., 2005). It is care that is integrated with other health and social services, accessible, and comprehensive, and addresses the great majority of personal health and wellness needs in the context of the family and community (WHO & UNICEF, 2020). Primary care promotes long-term relationships between a person and health professionals and helps to organize services and care across the system and over time (American Academy of Family Physicians, 2022). The term "patient" rather than "client" is typically used in primary care and occupational therapists in this setting often follow this terminology.

The core elements of primary care, as defined by Starfield et al. (2005) have implications for occupational therapy practice in primary care (Donnelly et al., 2022b). As such, occupational therapists working in primary care aim to provide first contact, comprehensive occupational therapy services, with services provided longitudinally, over patients' lifespans; patients are not discharged but can receive services as needs arise (see Table 26.1).

The overall goal of primary care is to optimize population health and reduce disparities by fostering equitable access to health services (WHO & UNICEF, 2020). Primary care is the foundation of a strong health-care system, and the contribution of primary care to both individual and population health outcomes is well documented (Starfield et al., 2005). Head-to-head comparisons of countries from around the globe show that those countries with health systems grounded in strong primary care have improved population health, with associations between primary care and overall premature deaths and premature deaths from a number of chronic conditions (Macinko et al., 2003).

To understand primary care, it is important to recognize that primary care is part of, but distinct from, *primary health care*. Primary health care is a broader "whole-of-society approach" that includes three interrelated components: (1) integrated health services that include primary care and essential public health functions as central components; (2) multisectoral policy and actions that look upstream and seek to address social determinants of health; and (3) the engagement and empowerment of individuals, families, and communities to increase social participation and overall health and well-being (WHO & UNICEF, 2020).

Primary care is grounded in principles of social justice where health is understood as a fundamental human right (Christopher & Caruso, 2015), aligning well with occupational

**TABLE 26.1** Descriptions of Core Elements of Primary Care and Application to Occupational Therapy

| Element | Primary Care Approach | Application to Primary Care Occupational Therapy |
|---|---|---|
| First contact access | An entry point into the system for broader health services and a mechanism to improve access to these services. | Occupational therapists must be working in a site or have a primary affiliation with a site that provides first contact services (e.g., general practitioner's office, community health center). |
| Continuity | Supports the development of sustained personal relationships between a patient and a primary care provider or a team of interprofessional providers. | Occupational therapists must have the potential to provide long-term and continuous services. While the nature of the services described may be short term, the patient is not discharged from primary care services and is part of the practice's list of patients. |
| Comprehensiveness | Offers a diverse set of services including health promotion, disease prevention, and curative, rehabilitative, and palliative services. | The occupational therapist may provide a discrete and focused service but must have the capacity and potential to work to full scope and provide the full breadth of occupational therapy assessment and interventions to all patients. For example, services may involve a clinic for falls, but as part of a more comprehensive suite of services. |
| Coordination | Supports the coordination of services and care across all levels of the health-care system and community, which is done over time. | The occupational therapy service must be part of a package of services that are aimed at coordinating care for patients. |
| Person-centered and people-centered | Care is focused on the person, not a specific disease or condition, enhancing health holistically, and attending to personal social determinants of health.<br><br>Focuses on ensuring people (individuals, families, and communities) have the support and education needed to participate in and make decisions about their care. | The occupational therapist provides services to enhance health holistically, through enabling occupational participation.<br><br>The occupational therapist provides support and education, so individuals, families, and communities can participate in their care and decision-making. |

Adapted from Donnelly et al. (2022b), Starfield et al. (2005), and WHO & UNICEF (2020).

therapy's value of occupation as a human right (Wilcock & Hocking, 2015). Primary care recognizes the significant influence of the *social determinants of health* on individuals and communities (College of Family Physicians of Canada, 2019), which refer to a "specific group of social and economic factors within the broader determinants of health. These relate to an individual's place in society, such as income, education, or employment. Experiences of discrimination, racism, and historical trauma are important social determinants of health for certain groups" (Government of Canada, 2020). There are increasing efforts to document and address social determinants of health in primary care. Biomedical models and payment structures can serve as barriers to addressing social determinants, and occupational therapists are well suited to shift practice beyond biomedical models, working with social and community support services to address health inequities experienced by older adults and promote occupational participation (Marval, 2017; Murphy et al., 2017; Synovec et al., 2020). One example is provided by Synovec et al. (2020) who describe primary care occupational therapists working with adults and older adults experiencing homelessness, looking to address issues of housing and access to food. In addition,

Murphy et al. (2017) noted that occupational therapists in the United States are well positioned to work with Federally Qualified Health Centers to support access by medically underserved populations.

Closely linked to the social determinants of health is population health. Population health relates to "the health outcomes of a group of individuals, including the distribution of such outcomes within the group" (Kindig & Stoddart, 2003, p. 381). A population health approach can be defined as "an opportunity for health care systems, agencies and organizations to work together in order to improve the health outcomes of the communities they serve" (Milken Institute School of Public Health, 2022). Primary care is uniquely positioned to bridge individual and population health and adopt a population health perspective that seeks to meet the needs of specific populations within a primary care practice.

## Positioning Occupational Therapy Within Primary Care Teams

Historically primary care has been delivered solely by family physicians or general practitioners. However, as populations grow older and exhibit greater health and social complexities, a team of interprofessional providers is better equipped to address the breadth of health and social issues compared to physician-only models of primary care (College of Family Physicians of Canada, 2019). Primary care teams have been associated with improved patient outcomes and higher quality of care compared to physician-only models; however, research remains mixed and further research on interprofessional primary care teams is needed (Wranik et al., 2019).

Primary care teams bring together a broad range of providers, including occupational therapists, dietitians, pharmacists, social workers, nurses, and others, to offer a comprehensive set of services to support the health of individual patients and a population of patients. A key challenge faced by occupational therapists in primary care can be engaging team members, particularly physicians who may be accustomed to working on their own, highlighting the importance of building collaborative relationships among primary care providers (Mackenzie et al., 2020). Key elements of collaborative interprofessional primary care are communication, trust, mutual respect, shared decision-making, and willingness to collaborate (Donnelly et al., 2019a; Sangaleti et al., 2017). Interprofessional teamwork requires supportive governance, information systems, and organizational culture, one or more champions, open communication, supportive colleagues, a team vision, quality processes, group decision-making processes, and strong individual beliefs in interprofessional primary care (Mulvale et al., 2016).

The Patient Medical Home is often the overarching term used to describe a model of primary care in which interprofessional teams are one of the core pillars. The Patient Medical Home model has been endorsed by Canadian and American Colleges (American Academy of Family Physicians, 2022; College of Family Physicians of Canada, 2019) as the future of primary care. Drawing on the core elements of primary care (see Table 26.1), the College of Family Physicians of Canada (2019) has described the key functions of the Patient Medical Home model as accessible care, community adaptiveness and social accountability, comprehensive team-based care with family physician leadership, continuity of care, and patient- and family-partnered care. These functions expand the core elements of primary care by highlighting social accountability and team-based care.

Worldwide, occupational therapy associations are recognizing the importance of the profession's role in primary care to support best practices in interprofessional primary care, such as in Canada, the United States, Australia, and Europe (American Occupational Therapy Association [AOTA], 2020b; Bolt et al., 2019; Canadian Association of Occupational Therapists, 2013; Donnelly et al., 2022b). The majority of occupational therapists working in primary care settings are working on interprofessional primary care teams; however, globally there remains relatively few occupational therapists in primary care settings (Donnelly et al., 2022a). Primary care is where the vast majority of people receive their health

care; for example, a study using administrative data in the province of Ontario, Canada provided a snapshot of "a day in health care," with approximately 140,000 people, or 1% of the population, visiting their family physician, while 54,000 people visited and 3000 people were admitted to hospital (Manuel et al., 2006). Given the prominence of primary care visits in health systems, occupational therapists need to increase their understanding of and involvement in primary care. Furthermore, one of the priorities of the WHO's Rehabilitation 2030 Campaign is to increase access to rehabilitation, including occupational therapy in primary care (WHO, 2019). Finally, in the context of an aging population that increasingly has multiple chronic conditions, occupational therapists can help older adults manage and address the occupational implications of these conditions in the location they most often seek care (Donnelly et al., 2022a).

## Key Occupational Therapy Roles, Practice Approaches, and Strategies With Older Adults in Primary Care

In primary care, occupational therapists and all other providers will ideally practice as generalists, using their full range of capabilities or practice scope to practice at the "top of their license" to provide services to people of all ages and conditions (Dahl-Popolizio et al., 2017). In doing so, occupational therapists can address elements of the person, environment, and occupation, with a focus on optimizing occupational participation and function among individuals, groups, and communities. Occupational therapy services can include health promotion and prevention with the general population; practice with individuals and communities with health and social needs; practice with individuals and communities with complex health and social needs; and individuals at the end of life (AOTA, 2020b; Donnelly et al., 2022b). Thus, occupational therapists in primary care may work at the level of the individual, group, community, or population, providing direct services or community-focused interventions.

The details of the occupational therapy role may vary by country, region, and primary care setting. Across settings, occupational therapy services may vary in terms of:
- focus of practice, such as focusing services on a sub-population of the primary care setting such as frail older adults;
- service delivery models and methods, such as individual, group, clinic-based, outreach, telehealth, prevention and promotion, rehabilitative, or community models like community development;
- access to care and populations served, which is strongly shaped by the existing health systems and the social determinants of health that impact individuals and groups in a given community. For example, limited funding mechanisms for occupational therapists in primary care is a common access issue in the United States and in Canada (Donnelly et al., 2014; McColl et al., 2009).

The goal of primary care occupational therapy with older adults is to support older people in aging well at home and in their communities, through facilitating occupational participation. Occupational therapy supports aging in place, that is, staying in one's own home or community, rather than in residential care (Wiles et al., 2012). A recent scoping review regarding the role of occupational therapy in primary care identified many examples of occupational therapy services with older adults worldwide (Donnelly et al., 2022a). Some key areas of occupational therapy practice in primary care are described in the following sections.

## Health Promotion

Health promotion is a main strategy that occupational therapists employ in primary care to support aging-in-place (Dahl-Popolizio et al., 2018; Donnelly et al., 2014, 2016). According to the Ottawa Charter for Health Promotion health promotion is "the process of enabling people to increase control over, and to improve, their health" (WHO, 1986, p. 17). Health promotion targets both the person and the environment, through creating healthy public policy; building supportive natural, built, and social environments; facilitating communities to set priorities and take action; and promoting personal and social development (WHO, 1986).

Specific to occupational therapy, occupation-focused health promotion focuses on enhancing health and well-being through facilitating individual and collective occupations, and addresses the range of factors in the physical, built, social, political, and economic environments that transact with personal factors to limit and promote occupational participation (Wilcock & Hocking, 2015). Health promotion can occur at three levels: *primary* health promotion, which promotes health in the general population, targeting people who are generally not experiencing any health concerns; *secondary* health promotion, which promotes health among people at risk of or with initial onset of disease or injury; and *tertiary* health promotion, that promotes health among people with chronic diseases or disability (AOTA, 2020a; Wilcock & Hocking, 2015). Illustrations of occupation-based health promotion in primary care are provided in Table 26.2.

A population health perspective can be used in all forms of health promotion, in which occupational therapists target populations with (or at risk of) specific health and occupational concerns, within the primary care practice, and offer focused interventions to these populations (AOTA, 2020a; Wilcock & Hocking, 2015). For example, occupational therapists can identify older adults who have diabetes or experienced a fall and develop targeted interventions for this sub-population of the primary care practice. A further example is that occupational therapists can target specific communities such as naturally occurring retirement communities (NORCs), that is, areas or buildings with high density of older adults that emerged naturally over time (Hunt & Gunter-Hunt, 1986). Interventions at individual, group, and community levels can then be developed to address specific health, social and occupational issues, for example,

---

**TABLE 26.2**  Examples of Health Promotion With Older Adults in Primary Care Occupational Therapy

**Primary Health Promotion**

A group intervention addressed links between occupation and a range of life areas including aging, energy, mobility, eating, physical activity, mental well-being, security at home and in the community, relationships, economy, and technical devices (Johansson & Bjorkland, 2016). The intervention led to improvements in vitality and mental health as well as perceived benefits to social health, weekly routine, managing everyday life, self-esteem, and personal growth. A further, similar, intervention based on the Lifestyle Redesign approach (Clark et al., 2012) led to improvements in social relationships, awareness of community resources, and attitudes toward aging (Cassidy et al., 2017).

**Secondary Health Promotion**

A frailty prevention program focused on physical and social functioning in the home and community. Topics included home safety, assistive devices, adaptive equipment, environmental modifications, physical activity, diet, goal setting and maintenance plans (Fritz et al., 2020). The authors reported high program satisfaction among participants and data suggested the intervention promoted physical activity and healthy diet habits and prevented deterioration in frailty status indicators such as weight loss, walking speed slowness, and grip strength weakness.

**Tertiary Health Promotion**

A culturally tailored, activity-centered lifestyle intervention was conducted with high-risk 50 to 64-year-old Latinos in the United States (Schepens Niemiec et al., 2018). Participants were likely to have chronic health conditions (e.g., type 2 diabetes, hypertension), disability, poor health, psychosocial stressors. The program addressed healthy eating, mental well-being, physical activity, chronic disease management, health-care navigation, personal health action plans, goal setting, and building social support. The authors found that the program led to reduced symptom severity and stress, less symptom impact on activity, and greater well-being and satisfaction with social roles and social activity (Schepens Niemiec et al.).

---

low-cost healthy eating programs, pre-frailty programs, mental health and addictions services, system navigation support, culturally tailored services, outreach services, and advocacy for resources to support occupation (Mattison et al., 2018; Wilcock & Hocking, 2015). Services targeting individuals can be added to this work, and could include personalized strategies such as evaluating interests, motivation, and habits; providing social prescriptions regarding social participation; and assisting in resource use (Turcotte et al., 2019). Offering informal social events such as a coffee hour could assist in meeting additional older adults who could benefit from preventative occupational therapy services, following up on intervention plans with existing patients, or making referrals to other professionals (Turcotte et al., 2019). Developing partnerships with community-based organizations and older adults is a key strategy for identifying and addressing needs.

A valuable resource that can support health promotion in primary care is Do-Live-Well, an occupation-based framework that promotes the message that "What you do every day matters" (Moll et al., 2015). The framework describes the health benefits of a wide range of daily occupations, which provide opportunities for engagement, meaning, balance, control, choice, and routine. In addition, the framework recognizes the personal and social forces, such as the social determinants of health, that affect occupations, habits, and access to occupational opportunities. As a result, community-level efforts to create supportive and inclusive community environments are required (Moll et al., 2015).

Occupational therapists in primary care can also direct their efforts to community and societal levels, such as participating in local age-friendly communities initiatives (Turcotte et al., 2019), joining public health or municipal committees to promote occupational engagement as a health determinant (Wilcock & Hocking, 2015), assisting in community consultations (Lauckner & Stadnyk, 2014), and advocating to facilitate social inclusion and enhance access to resources (Naidoo et al., 2017). (See Chapter 32 for further information regarding building age-inclusive communities.)

*Community development* is often used as a health promotion strategy to address the determinants of health (Labonte, 2015). Occupation-based community development means working with the community to define their collective needs and enhance occupational engagement, using policy, planning, social and political action, and education (Galvaan & Peters, n.d.). Principles that are key to occupational therapy community development are a focus on occupation, building capacity, inclusivity, increasing the power of structurally disadvantaged groups, challenging the practices of everyday life, and working toward a shared vision (Galvaan & Peters, n.d.; Leclair et al., 2019; van Rensburg, 2018). Occupational therapists may not often have opportunities to apply community development in primary care; however, examples exist and can be used to advocate for this role. As one example, Trentham et al. (2007) worked with older adults and community partners to create a neighborhood that was more physically accessible and supportive of older adults' occupational participation. (See Chapter 31 for further information regarding occupational therapy's role in contributing to social transformation.)

## Services for Older Adults With Chronic Diseases

As people age, they are more likely to experience at least one diagnosis of a chronic disease; in fact, with aging, the likelihood of having more than one chronic disease increases. (See Chapter 3 for further information regarding chronic disease and disability incidence.) Typically, chronic diseases are defined by duration (lasting at least 1 year), slow progression, and requiring ongoing medical monitoring; they contribute to the number of years lived with disability (Reynolds et al., 2018). Given the long-term nature of chronic diseases, older adults frequently receive support from their primary care providers (Reynolds et al., 2018). The core features of primary care (first contact, continuity, comprehensiveness, coordination, and person- and people-centered) make primary care an ideal setting for occupational therapists to support patients at risk of or living with chronic diseases, and to assist in managing the occupational issues that can arise as people age with chronic diseases (Trembath et al., 2019). Nearly 80% of preventative strategies and nearly 50% of issues related to chronic disease management do not require the diagnostic and prescriptive skills of a physician (Locas et al., 2019); thus components of chronic disease management can shift from physicians to primary care team members, including occupational therapists (Richardson et al., 2010, 2021).

Chronic diseases are related to a complexity of environmental and personal risk factors, including socioeconomic, cultural, political, and environmental determinants and individual-level risk factors (WHO, 2005). Individual-level risk factors are often labeled as *modifiable*, such as unhealthy diet, physical inactivity, and tobacco use; and *nonmodifiable* such as age and heredity (WHO, 2005). However, given the ways that social determinants of health shape our daily lives in inequitable ways, risk factors presumed to be modifiable may be very difficult to address by individuals, for example, access to healthy foods or access to recreation services may be limited in neighborhoods with higher rates of poverty.

Occupational therapists and older adults (as individuals and as collectives) can identify modifiable factors at the systems and social levels that can affect capacity to engage in occupation and prevent or manage chronic conditions and associated symptoms. While these systems and structures are challenging to address for individual older adults, occupational therapists can consider ways that they can collaborate with older adults, other health professionals and across sectors to address these factors, utilizing a primary health promotion approach. For example, Ripat et al., (2010) described a community project with a focus on increasing the winter walkability of sidewalks, aiming to affect citizen engagement and public policy.

Occupational therapists can play an integral role in primary care chronic disease management, including providing support to people to better manage disabilities associated with their chronic diseases, applying a secondary or tertiary health promotion approach. This management may relate to individual-level risk factors related to lifestyle and behaviors. Behavioral health, a term gaining popularity in the United States, typically comprises mental health, substance use, life stressors, physical symptoms due to or exacerbated by stress, psychosocial factors, as well as behaviors that affect health (Agency for Healthcare Research and Quality, n.d.). Behavioral health issues underlie approximately 70% of primary care visits (American Psychological Association, 2015). To address behavioral health issues, occupational therapists can target lifestyle behaviors, habits, roles, and routines such as diet, activity levels, sleep patterns, smoking, and alcohol use, that contribute to the risk of chronic disease development (AOTA, 2020b; Dahl-Popolizio et al., 2018; Trembath et al., 2019).

Self-management is a common approach to chronic disease interventions in primary care that relates to individual-level and social risk factors; at its heart, self-management is focused on supporting people to self-monitor and manage their symptoms, implement needed medical and activity interventions, build networks of support and resources, and manage their day-to-day activities while living with their chronic disease (Lorig et al., 2003). While occupational therapists may provide interventions to address symptoms associated with a specific chronic disease, a more generalizable approach to self-management is much more commonly applied by occupational therapists in primary care.

There are numerous approaches to self-management to which occupational therapists can contribute. For example, group generalized self-management programs, such as the ones developed originally at Stanford (Lorig et al., 2003) provide support for people with chronic diseases (regardless of the diagnosis or diagnoses) to learn self-management strategies such as problem-solving, fatigue and pain management, and action planning. There are also programs available for people living with arthritis, diabetes, chronic pain, HIV positivity, serious mental illness, and others, which provide disease-specific self-management strategies. Occupational therapists can also support chronic disease self-management by drawing on their specific expertise in rehabilitation. For example, Richardson et al. (2010) describe adding information about assistive devices to a standardized self-management intervention, and in a subsequent study Richardson et al. (2012) report drawing on more rehabilitation content to include energy conservation, relaxation, falls prevention, and physical activity within a rehabilitation self-management program delivered in a primary care setting.

Self-management interventions can be delivered in multiple formats. For example, some interventions are intended to focus on individuals to support personalized goal development and action planning to address their specific issues. When individualized, self-management support can be readily woven into other appointment activities or visits to the primary care site. In other instances, engagement with a self-management group workshop is an ideal mechanism of service delivery. For example, in a study with participants with multimorbidity, it was found that a 6-week group workshop supported people living with chronic diseases to learn with and from others with similar situations, with significant improvement in activity participation, self-efficacy, and quality of life (Garvey et al., 2015). Finally, with technological innovations, on-line self-management interventions have become more common (Liu et al., 2022; Richardson et al., 2021).

An effective and informative tool to assess self-management in relation to occupational participation is the Self-Efficacy for Managing Chronic Disease 6-item Scale (Lorig et al., 2001). This scale assesses confidence in managing a chronic condition such that it does not interfere with "the things the person wants to do." The scale can be useful in communicating occupational therapy assessment results and outcomes with the interprofessional team, an important part of integrating into primary care practices.

See Box 26.1 for further examples of occupational therapy interventions for chronic disease management.

## Promoting Occupation at Home

Most older adults wish to stay in their homes as long as possible (Vanleerberghe et al., 2017), which is related to better quality of life, if the older adults' health and environment allow for aging in place (Sheffield et al., 2013). Studies in Canada show that occupational therapists working in primary care spend approximately 25% of their time working in homes or community spaces (Donnelly et al., 2016). Primary care occupational therapists can support aging in place through promoting occupation at home. For example, an occupational therapy program in primary care focused on helping older adults engage in occupations, involving self-determined goals, adaptation, activity mastery, and environmental control. Interviews suggested improved occupational abilities such as bathing, dressing, and transfers (Johansson & Björklund, 2006).

Home-based occupational therapy services may be offered by primary care occupational therapists or occupational therapists working in other settings, such as home care

---

| Box 26.1 | Example Occupational Therapy Interventions for Older Adults With Chronic Diseases |

- Establish scheduling and activities of daily living routine management
- Educate in pacing, fatigue management and energy conservation strategies
- Problem-solve to incorporate promotion and preventative strategies into daily routine, such as physical activities and medication
- Educate about lifestyle modification (diet, activity level, smoking, etc.)

- Recommend adaptive equipment
- Teach pain management and relaxation strategies
- Help identify and manage triggers that negatively affect health and well-being (anxiety, depression, gastrointestinal problems, joint pain, etc.)
- Educate caregivers
- Connect with community resources for social supports to enhance social participation

(see Chapter 29 for further information on home-based occupational therapy). Context and organizational-specific factors will determine whether primary care occupational therapists will be involved in home-based services, such as reimbursement structure and funding.

Home safety is a specific area to consider within promoting occupation at home. For safe aging in place, older adults' physical, cognitive, mental, and psychosocial functioning in transaction with the home environment and occupation must be considered. Through a whole-person approach to care that addresses all aspects of the person's life, including their home environment, the primary care occupational therapist is well positioned to assess the risk of functional decline that affects home safety, including risk of falls, cognitive decline, and changes in mental health or psychosocial status in this population (AOTA, 2020b; Dahl-Popolizio et al., 2017; Locas et al., 2019). Primary care occupational therapists can promote aging in place by conducting home safety assessments and making recommendations for home modifications and safety interventions (AOTA, 2020a). The physical environment of the home, family/caregiver support available, and the patient's continued ability to safely complete their activities of daily life as they age will also affect the patient's ability to function successfully within their home environment across the lifespan. Health promotion strategies employed by primary care occupational therapists to facilitate a safe home environment include prevention of, or reduction in, injuries and accidents through environmental modifications, task analysis and adaptation, and education regarding how to access necessary resources (AOTA, 2020a, 2020b; Locas et al., 2019).

## Community Mobility and Falls Prevention

The ability to move around safely in the home and community has been identified as one of the key occupational issues identified by older adults receiving primary care occupational therapy (Donnelly et al., 2016). Adopting a lens of prevention and health promotion, occupational therapists focus on supporting older adults to move safely in their homes and community to promote community participation. In primary care, assessments of mobility emphasize screening, including screening for falls risk and driving safety. Interventions for mobility emphasize primary and secondary health promotion and prevention as well as a focus on linking to and navigating community resources.

### Falls Prevention

One of the key areas to support mobility is falls prevention. Falls prevention has been a significant focus for primary care occupational therapists and was the third most frequently reported intervention in a recent scoping review of occupational therapy in primary care (Donnelly et al., 2022a). Primary care occupational therapists providing falls prevention are focused on three sub-populations of older adults; those at risk of falls (primary prevention), individuals who have already experienced a fall and are at risk of another fall

(secondary prevention), and older adults who have fallen and experienced significant health and functional impact as a result (tertiary prevention).

In primary prevention occupational therapists will use screening to identify risk factors and offer targeted preventative interventions such as home safety modifications, education on fall risks, and preventative functional exercises (e.g., Mackenzie et al., 2020). Tools such as the Falls Risk Assessment and Screening Tool (Renfro et al., 2011) and the Home FAST (Mackenzie et al., 2000) are useful screening assessments designed to provide comprehensive multi-factorial screening and identify home safety risks in primary care settings. Falls screening clinics may draw on interprofessional primary care team members including pharmacists to address discipline-specific risks such as polypharmacy (Dhalwani et al., 2017).

In secondary prevention, occupational therapists offer education on fall risks and target risks for change, functional exercises, balance training, assistance in adapting how occupations are performed, and transfer training. Occupational therapists may further target the environment through home safety assessments and recommendations on home modifications, assistive technology prescriptions, and referrals to additional community services (Brandis & Tuite, 2001; Clemson et al., 2014; Hand et al., 2022; Johansson et al., 2018; Mackenzie et al., 2020). Recommendations for home modifications can range from simple to more involved, such as removing throw rugs, putting commonly used items within reach in kitchen cabinets, adjusting lighting, installing outdoor stair lifts or ramps, and installing bathroom equipment. Research in primary care settings shows that older adults perceive falls prevention services as worthwhile, report feeling safer (Brandis & Tuite, 2001), and show a decrease in fear of falling (Johansson et al., 2018) and an increase in falls self-efficacy (Hand et al., 2022).

In tertiary prevention, occupational therapists may work with individuals with disabilities experiencing mobility issues and falls. One example is a Primary Care Mobility Clinic in Ontario, Canada (Milligan et al., 2018), composed of a team including a family physician, nurse, exercise therapist, occupational therapist and social worker and pharmacists as needed. A physical medicine and rehabilitation specialist is also available for complex issues. Team members work collaboratively to conduct comprehensive assessments that address falls and mobility, social and physical environments, and general health promotion. When appropriate, the team also supports the family and caregivers. The occupational therapist is specifically responsible for transfer assessments, seating and mobility, home modifications and equipment, supporting funding applications and advocacy related to systems navigation and caregiver education. What is important to note with this example is the recognition and use of a collaborative team approach to address falls and mobility in populations with known health complexities.

Facilitating access to mobility aids to ensure in-home and community mobility is another important role for occupational therapists working with older adults that may be a stand-alone intervention or part of a broader falls screening/assessment and prevention (Johansson & Bjorklund, 2006; Milligan et al., 2018). Not only does this require assessing mobility to determine functional status but also ensuring the home environment is accessible and funding is available for mobility aids, which may involve the completion of funding applications or advocating for funds.

### Driving and Driving Retirement

Retaining the ability to drive supports community participation, which in turn maintains health and well-being. While much has been written on driving in the occupational therapy literature (see Chapter 21 for further information regarding driving and transportation), there has been less focus on how occupational therapists can support driving and driver retirement in primary care. Primary care is often the first place older adults with concerns about cognitive problems seek care. Driving safety can be one of the more difficult issues primary care providers face when working with older adults with cognitive impairment. While drivers with dementia have been found to be 2.5 to 4.7 times more likely than healthy, age-matched controls to be involved in motor vehicle collisions (Reger et al., 2004), a diagnosis of mild cognitive impairment does not preclude safe driving. Occupational therapists in primary care settings are ideally situated to deploy cognitive screening tools, either driving-specific or predictive of driving ability, to assess for cognitive changes that may impact safe driving. In the province of Ontario, Canada, occupational therapists are often members of interprofessional primary care memory clinics. While the focus of these clinics is on facilitating a diagnosis, not on driving, occupational therapists in these clinics provide timely comprehensive assessment and intervention recommendations and address some of the most challenging aspects of dementia care, such as driving concerns. One study found that the primary-care memory clinic model reduces the burden of care on family physicians, who are reluctant to remove drivers' licenses for fear of increasing the risk of social isolation, depression and stress among patients and caregivers, and compromising the patient-physician relationship (Molnar et al., 2005).

Occupational therapists in primary care may also support older adults as they retire from driving. One example is a driving cessation group program, which involved 2-hour sessions, once per month for 4 months. The therapists aimed to provide strategies and resources to support driving cessation as well as a supportive environment to discuss and normalize anger, loss, and grief related to loss of a driver's license (Fry et al., 2013). An evaluation showed that all program participants reported high satisfaction with the program, had increased understanding of why driving privileges were removed, and had a plan in place to manage driving cessation (Fry et al., 2013).

### Supporting Caregivers

Support and education for caregivers of older adults is an important occupational therapy role in primary care. A Canadian survey showed that 69% (36/52) of primary care occupational therapists surveyed reported providing caregiver support and education (Donnelly et al., 2016). Within primary care's context of interprofessional care and provision of services longitudinally, occupational therapists have the opportunity to build long-term relationships with caregivers and to access team members to further support caregivers. Occupational therapy roles with caregivers include providing education, supporting resource-seeking and navigation, and identifying ways to support the occupations and well-being of the caregiver including respite. Further occupational therapy roles include identifying ways to support the caregiver in supporting the occupations of the person in the caring dyad as well as continued meaningful co-occupations of the care recipient and caregiver.

### Supporting Transitions and Systems Integration

Despite decades of reforms, health systems continue to remain fragmented. Older adults with increasingly complex and multiple chronic health conditions (de Carvalho et al., 2017) are particularly at risk for fragmented care, with multiple providers and sectors supporting medical and functional issues. Primary care is seen as a core component of an integrated health system, supporting coordination of care, focusing on the whole person versus disease-specific specialty care, and is positioned to integrate care over the lifespan within a strong long-term relationship (WHO & UNICEF, 2020). There are some clear examples of occupational therapists working in primary care to support systems integration for older adults, with a focus on educating and connecting older adults and families to community services (Donnelly et al., 2014; McGrath & O'Callaghan, 2014; Richardson et al., 2010), providing discharge support (Gudkovs, 2011), and the coordination of services (Donnelly et al., 2014). The IMPACT clinic is one example of an interprofessional primary care team in a Patient Medical Home model that brings together a team consisting of family physicians and other professionals including occupational therapist, physical therapist, pharmacist, dietitian, social worker and community nurse to support integration in Toronto, Canada (Tracy et al., 2013). The team works with older adults and their families to complete a comprehensive interprofessional assessment and provide individualized education, resources, and a collaborative care plan. Demographic profiles of older adults attending the IMPACT clinic highlight the complexities of the issues being addressed by the team, with an average of 10 issues and 10 interventions per older adult, across medical (e.g., medication), functional (e.g., mobility, home safety) and social domains. Occupational therapists working with older adults on primary care teams are ideally positioned to support individuals over time and facilitate any transitions in care, including in and out of hospital and into further supportive living environments.

## Emerging Areas of Practice

Although the presence of occupational therapists in primary care is increasing, occupational therapy in primary care remains a relatively small practice area. Within primary care for older adults there are areas of practice with specific patient populations that are emerging, such as palliative care for the terminally ill (Usher et al., 2021) and services targeting frailty (Fritz et al., 2020) as the aging population remains longer in their homes.

Furthermore, occupational therapists have largely focused on interventions at the level of the individual, however, as noted earlier in this chapter, primary care also adopts a population perspective and considers the broader community. One means of doing so is to focus on NORCs, described earlier as naturally occurring retirement communities, which are geographic areas with a high proportion of older adults. Intentional programming may be added to NORCs to support aging in the community. Occupational therapists in primary care settings are well-placed to identify NORCs within their community and work with older adults to identify and offer health promotion programming. One example of a NORC-based program is the Oasis Senior Supportive Living Program (Oasis) in the provinces of Ontario and British Columbia, Canada (DePaul et al., 2022). Examples of work with Oasis includes offering member-driven programming, supporting older adults in their advocacy efforts to increase walkability of neighborhoods, integrating community kitchens and communal meals, providing falls prevention education and intervention and offering education on the use of technology to support virtual social engagement. As nations increasingly use primary care as the hub of health, wellness, and health promotion, subpopulations that can benefit from OT services will continue to be identified.

## Recommendations for Future Research

Given the emerging role of occupational therapy within primary care contexts, there is a need to continue studying how best to deliver occupational therapy services within this setting. It is not sufficient to apply findings from research conducted in other contexts. Rather, it is essential that research be conducted within the context of primary care delivery, to account for the differences in values and principles underlying different settings. In addition, as new roles emerge in primary care, they also need to be evaluated. As a member of an interprofessional team in primary care, there is a need to establish the value-added contributions of occupational therapy. In addition, there is a need to identify the impact of team-based care on health outcomes for not only individual patients but also for communities

and populations to support continued expansion of occupational therapy addressing such levels in primary care. While the following list is not comprehensive, it provides examples of a range of questions that could be explored related to occupational therapy services delivered in primary care:

- Do primary care occupational therapy services promote aging in place and reduce transfers to skilled nursing or long-term care facilities?
- Do primary care occupational therapy services lead to improvement in self-management of chronic diseases and extension of disability-free years?
- How do primary care teams that include occupational therapists address social determinants of health and impact health disparities?
- Do services offered by teams that include occupational therapists improve occupational participation and well-being among older adults? What occupational therapy interventions are most effective in primary care?
- How can occupational therapists and other interprofessional team members be integrated into primary care settings?
- How can occupational therapists use a population health strategy within the primary care setting to identify patients early to prevent progression of disease?

## SUMMARY

Although the number of occupational therapists working in primary care is increasing, primary care remains an emerging practice area. This chapter defines primary care and highlights the role of occupational therapists in health promotion, chronic disease management, home safety, community mobility and falls prevention, driving and driving retirement, supporting caregivers, and supporting transitions and systems integration. This role is further illustrated in the case example provided in Box 26.2.

The authors also discuss the effect of social determinants of health, community resources, and caregiver support on whether and how patients are able to age in place, and what the occupational therapist can do to facilitate this goal. Readers will recognize how occupational therapists working with older adults in this setting use their full skill set to work with individuals, groups and communities to ensure occupational participation and quality of life as they age within home and community settings.

*The complete listing of the Bibliography and Chapter Questions and Answers are available in the accompanying enhanced eBook version included with the print purchase of this textbook. Visit Elsevier eBooks+ (eBooks.Health.Elsevier.com) to access this content.*

**Box 26.2**    Primary Care Occupational Therapy Case Example

**Background:** A primary care practice in a low socioeconomic status (SES) neighborhood has many older adult patients who live in a specific high-rise apartment building (a NORC). The primary care interprofessional team has noted multiple injuries and hospitalizations due to falls in patients living in this building. Many older adult residents of the building are diagnosed with multiple chronic diseases, including diabetes. Due to limited mobility and limited financial resources, the patients in the building do not tend to come to the primary care office until a decline in a medical condition occurs. The occupational therapist on the team offers several services that fall within primary, secondary, and tertiary health promotion.

| Primary Health Promotion (targeting the general population of older adults) | Secondary Health Promotion (targeting older adults at-risk or in early stages of a health condition) | Tertiary Health Promotion (targeting older adults with disease or disability) |
|---|---|---|
| Primary care occupational therapist (OT) works one day per month in the apartment building completing falls risk assessments and educating patients and caregivers in adaptive equipment and home modification options to reduce the risk of falls.<br><br>OT facilitates a kinesiologist coming in to offer weekly chair yoga classes for tenants in the building social room.<br><br>OT partners with local age-friendly committee to complete neighborhood walkability assessments, and recommend improvements to sidewalks/benches to facilitate a walking route around the neighborhood.<br><br>OT completes a survey to determine transportation needs of the population and coordinate available community-based transportation resources (e.g., arrange regularly scheduled weekly vans to transport residents to medical appointments, grocery stores, etc.) | OT provides a monthly diabetic screening group to educate patients how to complete: glucose self-checks, foot skin checks, visual assessments, and sensory assessments to ensure patients conditions are not worsening, and what to do if they see indications of disease progression.<br><br>OT works with populations at risk of chronic diseases to ensure:<br>• scheduling regular health maintenance visits with primary care providers<br>• medication adherence schedules/plans<br>• access to appropriate physical activities<br><br>OT offers a frailty prevention program to prevent disease and symptom progression.<br><br>OT partners with community stakeholders such as local grocery stores and city staff members to enhance access to affordable healthy food, including communal meal programs, community kitchens, and a community garden. | OT provides monthly self-management education group for older adults with a variety of chronic conditions including topics such as:<br>• strategies to maintain occupational participation<br>• building supportive networks<br>• coping with the emotional, cognitive, and physical implications of chronic disease<br>• how to avoid falls; strategies to reduce risk at home<br>• when/how often to follow up with primary care team<br>• transportation options<br><br>OT arranges nutritional consultations with primary care team members for patients with chronic diseases (diabetes, hypertension, cardiovascular disease) regarding diet choices and meal planning.<br><br>OT works with individual older adults to obtain financial assistance for adaptive equipment and medication.<br><br>OT partners with older adults, interprofessional team, and senior's advocates to advocate for increased funding for assistive devices and equipment to support everyday living and disease management. |

## CHAPTER 27

# The Role of Occupational Therapy in Acute and Post-Acute Care With Aging Adults

*Autumn L. Rebillot, MSOT, BRLS, OTR/L, Julie K. Gammack, MD, CMD, FACP, and Michael Sarai, DO, FRCPC*

## CHAPTER OUTLINE

## OBJECTIVES

- Define acute care and post-acute care.
- Discuss the role of occupational therapy in acute care and post-acute care settings.
- List the common medical conditions in older adults leading to acute care and post-acute care admissions.
- Describe the components of an occupational therapy consultation.
- Contrast the length of stay, admission criteria and conditions, and reasons for admission for different post-acute care facilities.
- Name the screening and assessment tools used for evaluating the functional status, cognition, and geriatric syndromes.

## Introduction

In the United States, Medicare beneficiaries will increase from 62 million in 2020 to 77 million in 2030 (Medicare Payment Advisory Commission [MEDPAC], 2022). The growing population of older adults will exert considerable financial stress on an already overburdened health-care system as per-beneficiary Medicare spending increases with age. For example, per-beneficiary expenditures in persons aged 85 and older are 75% higher than in those aged 65 to 74 (MEDPAC, 2022). This difference is explained, in part, by older adults' needs for more complex acute and post-acute services.

For older adults, acute care services account for nearly half of the health-care costs. They are twice as likely to require hospitalization than middle-aged adults and account for 70% of all discharges from post acute settings (Tian, 2016). Older adults are more likely to experience acute events such as falls, delirium, weight loss, and syncope. These events are associated with increased co-morbidity burden and commonly precede acute hospitalizations and the need for post-acute therapy services. Typical complexities of acute geriatric medicine include prolonged inpatient admissions, frequent readmissions, deteriorating cognitive health, and hospital-associated debility. As a result of medical and functional disability, older adults are more likely to require post-acute therapy services.

The Patient Protection and Affordable Care Act (ACA) of 2010 has reshaped the acute and post-acute service delivery by focusing on managing cost, increasing efficiency, improving quality of care, and focusing on the consumer experience. The ACA initiatives included the enactment of payment penalties and incentives. As a result, hospitals with readmissions within 30 days, hospital-acquired conditions, and substandard customer satisfaction are penalized with a reduced service payment. The three initiatives include:

- "The Hospital Readmissions Reduction Program" monitors readmissions within 30 days of discharge from the hospital. This program has been proven to reduce readmission of individuals with chronic obstructive pulmonary disease (COPD), heart failure (HF), and elective/planned hip and knee replacements (Zuckerman et al., 2016).
- "The Hospital-Acquired Condition Reduction Program" focuses on preventing hospital-acquired conditions (HACs) and hospital-acquired infections (HAIs). The Centers for Medicare and Medicaid Services (CMS) measures the following rates (CMS, 2023b):

- Pressure ulcers
- Pneumothorax
- In hospital fall with hip fracture
- Perioperative hemorrhage or hematoma
- Postoperative acute kidney injury requiring dialysis
- Postoperative respiratory failure
- Perioperative pulmonary embolism or deep vein thrombosis
- Postoperative sepsis rate
- Postoperative wound dehiscence
- Abdominopelvic accidental puncture/laceration:
- Central line–associated bloodstream infection (CLABSI)
- Catheter-associated urinary tract infection (CAUTI)
- Surgical site infection (SSI) (for colon and abdominal hysterectomy procedures)
- Methicillin-resistant *Staphylococcus aureus* (MRSA) bacteremia
  - *Clostridium difficile* Infection (CDI)
- "The Hospital Value-Based Purchasing Program" offers monetary incentives to hospitals that demonstrate consumer-defined high-quality care. Post-acute care initiatives include creating a bundled payment system that combines hospital and post-acute care payments. The bundled payment system predetermines the hospital's payment for services rendered (diagnosis or procedure) during hospitalization and the following 90 days. This initiative incentivizes hospitals to refer patients to a less expensive post-acute care setting.

In 2014, The Improving Medicare Post-Acute Care Transformation (IMPACT) Act was signed into law to improve Medicare beneficiary outcomes in the post-acute settings. The act is designed to "promote effective communication and coordination of care, promote effective prevention and treatment of chronic disease, encourage working with communities to promote best practices of healthy living, make health care affordable and safer by reducing harm, reduce the cost of the delivery of care, and strengthening personal and family engagement" (CMS, 2023a). The IMPACT Act defines post-acute care setting requirements to submit standardized data collected by the following assessment instruments:

- Long-term acute care hospitals (LTACHs)—The Long-Term Care Hospital CARE Data Set (LCDS)
- Inpatient rehabilitation facilities (IRFs)—The Inpatient Rehabilitation Facilities Patient Assessment Instrument (IRF PAI)
- Skilled nursing facilities (SNFs)—The Minimum Data Set (MDS)
- Home health (HH) agencies—The Outcome and Assessment Information Set (OASIS)
- All post-acute care settings—The Quality Indicators (QIs)

Furthermore, CMS identifies the following areas of assessment explicitly:
- Skin Integrity—Changes in Skin Integrity Post-Acute Care: Pressure Ulcer/Injury
- Functional Status/Cognitive Function

- Application of Percent of LTACH Patients with an Admission and Discharge Functional Assessment and a Care Plan that Addresses Function
- Percent of LTACH Patients with an Admission and Discharge Functional Assessment and a Care Plan that Addresses Function
- Change in Self-care Score for Medical Rehabilitation Patients
- Change in Mobility Score for Medical Rehabilitation Patients
- Change in Discharge Self-care Score for Medical Rehabilitation Patients
- Change in Discharge Mobility Score for Medical Rehabilitation Patients
- Medication Reconciliation
- Incidence of Major Falls—Application of the Percent of Residents Experiencing One or More Falls with Major Injury (Long Stay)
- Transfer of Health Information and Care Preferences When an Individual Transitions
- Resource Use Measures, including Total Estimated Medicare Spending per Beneficiary
- Discharge to Community
- All-Condition Risk-Adjusted Potentially Preventable Hospital Readmissions Rates

Acute care occupational therapy (OT) reduces the severity of functional decline, readmission risk or death, susceptibility to other illnesses, and inappropriate discharge recommendations (Freburger et al., 2020). Additionally, patients demonstrate improved overall functional outcomes and reduced hospital readmissions when OT services are provided in high frequencies of self-care treatment/training interventions (Edelstein et al., 2022; Rogers et al., 2014). Given the recent regulatory changes and research, acute and post-acute care OT practitioners are crucial to improving functional performance outcomes and the health-care experience for our nation.

Due to the ever-changing presentation of the aging population, acute and post-acute care OT's require a higher degree of knowledge and skills to maximize outcomes. This chapter will guide you through the intricate process of acute and post-acute care experiences that the elderly population may encounter. The content is focused on common presentations and is further supported by additional chapters. For this chapter, "occupational therapy" or "occupational therapy practitioner" is interpreted as an occupational therapist and OT assistant.

## Definitions of Acute and Post-Acute Care

*Acute care* refers to hospital inpatient medical services that manage short-term conditions such as injury, chronic illness exacerbation, new illness, and surgical needs. Acute care hospitals address a spectrum of diagnoses and severity of illness in the emergency department (ED), general medical and surgical floors, and ICU. Some hospitals can provide more specialized care, such as organ transplantation and interventional cardiology services, or have certifications for conditions such as stroke, trauma, and cancer. *Post-acute care* refers to both services and facility-based care needed for recovery after acute care hospitalizations. Post-acute care services are provided by skilled staff to remediate overall health, return to the prior level of function, and ensure a safe discharge disposition.

Often, health-care teams rely on occupational therapists to guide the team, the patient, and the caregiver toward a safe discharge plan. In acute and post-acute care, therapists utilize clinical reasoning skills, including knowledge of Medicare and Medicaid regulations, post-acute care setting characteristics, and geriatric syndromes, to advocate for access to the most appropriate level of care. Presenting the patient with the "just right" challenge allows the patient access to additional therapy in various settings and thus fully supports the patient and caregiver's therapy trajectory. When discharging patients from acute care potential discharge options include: LTACH, acute rehabilitation (AR) aka (IRF), SNF, HH, out-patient (OP), comprehensive outpatient rehabilitation facility (CORF), and tele-health.

Access to consecutive settings and services has many benefits, including additional recovery time, supportive care, wound care, pain management, nutritional services, medical oversight, social support, and therapy needed to discharge and sustain community-based care. OT practitioners should be familiar with post-acute care settings, program expectations, services provided, and care plans in all settings. Refer to Table 27.1 for common post-acute care settings and their characteristics.

## The Continuum of Care Model: Acute and Post-Acute Care

### Acute Care

In the United States, the acute care process generally begins with an evaluation in the emergency department (ED). In the ED, the patient is assessed, tests are run, treatments are delivered, and a determination is made if admission to the hospital is needed. Within the ED, OT services are focused on assisting the medical team in determining and eliminating discharge barriers and reducing the risk of readmission.

Through completion of the occupational profile and simultaneous assessment of individuals' performance skills/patterns, contextual/environmental barriers, and client factors, the therapist can provide the following services:

- Assessment and recommendations for hospital admission versus community discharge
- Assessment and recommendations for adaptive equipment and durable medical equipment
- Patient advocacy
- Safe patient handling
- Referrals to the next level of care to address functional impairments

The concept of an "age-friendly" geriatric ED has developed in the past decade to address the unique presentations, needs, dispositions, and outcomes of older adults. A Geriatrics

Emergency Medicine Accreditation system has been established to recognize those EDs that embrace best practices, such as geriatric-focused education, interdisciplinary staffing, geriatrics care pathways, transitions of care planning, and environmental modifications for geriatrics needs (Geriatric Emergency Department Accreditation Program [GEDA], n.d.). Geriatric syndromes frequently contribute to ED visits, acute care hospitalizations, and the demand for post-acute care services. Geriatric syndromes are conditions of multifactorial etiology that are more common in older adults and often require a multifactorial approach to management. Hospitalizations can be disorienting and distressing experiences, especially for those with functional deficits. Identifying geriatric syndromes in the ED and throughout the hospitalization can help older adults to receive necessary health-care services both during and after the acute care visit. Refer to Table 27.2 for a list of conditions commonly considered geriatric syndromes and screening tools frequently referenced or used by OT's to identify these conditions.

In some cases, only a brief period of hospital care is expected. The patient's hospital status is "observation," with an expected stay of fewer than 48 hours. These admissions are technically considered an "outpatient" or "observation" hospitalization, impacting insurance eligibility for post-acute services. SNF admissions require a qualifying 3-day hospitalization; therefore, observation hospitalizations do not qualify for a SNF admission. Hence therapists must be aware of regulations as it affects the medical plan of care and therapy discharge recommendations.

The treatment team collaborates to review if the medical care, duration of care, and discharge needs would indicate the need for hospitalization. Based on the medical acuity and admitting diagnoses, a patient may be admitted to a general medical, surgical, step-down, or intensive care unit (ICU). Medical care can be defined and directed by the International Classification of Diseases, Edition 10 (ICD-10). An example of the impact of an ICD-10 diagnosis is when a patient is diagnosed with sepsis. This diagnosis will direct admission, treatment, and post-acute services. Sepsis is further outlined later in this chapter.

Some hospitals have specialty units designed for older adults, such as geriatric psychiatry, orthopedic, oncology, or acute care for the elderly (ACE). ACE units provide interdisciplinary care to identify and prevent geriatric syndromes in an environment that reduces functional decline and promotes rehabilitation. Acute care length of stay ranges from 4.1 to 5.2 days but increases with age, with an average of 5.2 days for those over 65 years (McDermott et al., 2017). ACE units can reduce delirium, promote discharge home, and prevent readmission (Fox et al., 2012).

### Post-Acute Care

In the US, elderly patients have access to Medicare and Medicaid services, which determines access to the continuum of care. Post-acute services can be offered at many levels and divided by short-term versus long-term needs. As Goldberg (2014) details, elderly patients with short-term

**TABLE 27.1** Post-Acute Care Setting Characteristics

| Setting | Expected Length of Stay | Admission Criteria | Common Reasons for Admission |
|---|---|---|---|
| Long-term acute care hospital (LTACH) | >25 days (Department of Health & Human Services, 2019) | Medical management of one or more of the following that cannot be managed at a lower level of care:<br>• Ventilator management and liberation<br>Complex medical treatment of any of the following:<br>• Multiple and/or prolonged IV therapies<br>• Monitoring of active severe medical conditions requiring ≥6 tx/day<br>• Cardiac telemetry monitoring<br>• Complex wound care<br>• Specialized care (e.g., on-site dialysis, surgical suites)<br>• Comprehensive rehabilitation (OT/PT/SLP) | Patients admitted to LTACHs require prolonged medical and comprehensive rehabilitation services. The patient population is clinically complex, with multiple acute diagnoses and comorbidities (Liu et al., 2001).<br>LTACH treatment includes but not limited to the following:<br>Respiratory management:<br>• Acute BI-PAP or CPAP needs<br>• Acute respiratory failure with the inability to wean during hospitalization<br>• Chronic ventilator with pneumonia<br>• Aspiration<br>• Interstitial lung disease<br>• COVID-19 (acute or post-acute)<br>• Pulmonary hygiene<br>• Tracheotomy insertion and management<br>• High-flow oxygen therapy ($FIO_2 \geq 40\%$)<br>• Chest tube management<br>Infectious diseases:<br>• Osteomyelitis<br>• Cellulitis<br>• Pneumonia<br>• Bacteremia<br>• Endocarditis<br>• Sepsis<br>• Necrotizing fasciitis<br>Wound/Skin:<br>• Decubitus ulcer<br>• Amputation<br>• Necrotizing fasciitis<br>• Abscess<br>• Negative pressure wound care<br>Complex/complicated medical conditions:<br>• Cerebral vascular accident<br>• Cardiomyopathy<br>• Cardiac surgical care<br>• Cancer<br>• Congestive heart failure<br>• Chronic obstructive pulmonary disease<br>• Trauma<br>• Spinal cord injury<br>• Progressive central nervous system conditions |

**TABLE 27.1** Post-Acute Care Setting Characteristics

| Setting | Expected Length of Stay | Admission Criteria | Common Reasons for Admission |
|---|---|---|---|
| Acute rehabilitation facility (AR) or In-patient rehabilitation facility (IRF) | 8 days—mild deficits, 13 days—moderate deficits, and 22 days—severe deficits (Camicia et al., 2016) Varies based on the following: <br>• Severity of conditions <br>• Type of condition being treated <br>• Demonstration of ability to progress in therapy <br>• Tolerate intensive therapy of 3-hours/day 5 days/week or a minimum of 15-hours/ week. If patient is not able tolerate intensive therapy documentation must support medical issues justifying a brief exception not to exceed three consecutive days. <br>• Medical complications <br>• Limited social support (Lewis et al., 2015) | Patient must meet all of the following criteria (CMS, n.d., Fact Sheet #1): <br>• Require active and ongoing therapeutic intervention in two or more therapy disciplines (PT, OT, SLP, or prosthetics/ orthotics therapy) to improve or regain function <br>• Expected improvement within a reasonable time that is directly correlated to the intensive IRF services <br>• Tolerate intensive rehabilitation therapy program of 15-hours per week or 3-hours per day at least 5 days per week <br>• Require 24-hour access and close medical supervision by a physician for managing medical conditions to support participation in an intensive rehabilitation therapy program <br>• Require 24-hour access to skilled nursing services <br>• Require intensive, coordinated interdisciplinary care approach | To meet compliance threshold, ≥60% of the total inpatient population must be treated with one or more of the following medical conditions (CMS, n.d., Fact Sheet #1) <br>• Stroke <br>• Spinal cord injury <br>• Congenital deformity <br>• Amputation <br>• Major multiple trauma <br>• Fracture of femur (hip fracture) <br>• Brain injury <br>• Neurological disorders, including: <br>  • Multiple sclerosis <br>  • Motor neuron diseases <br>  • Polyneuropathy <br>  • Muscular dystrophy <br>  • Parkinson's disease <br>• Burns <br>• Active, polyarticular rheumatoid arthritis, psoriatic arthritis, and seronegative arthropathies <br>• Systemic vasculitides <br>• Severe or advanced osteoarthritis (osteoarthrosis or degenerative joint disease) involving two or more major weight-bearing joints <br>• Knee or hip joint replacement, or both, during an acute hospitalization immediately preceding the inpatient rehabilitation stay and meeting one or more of the following specific criteria: <br>  • Bilateral knee or bilateral hip joint replacement surgery <br>  • Body mass index of ≥50 <br>  • ≥ 85 years old |

*Continued*

**TABLE 27.1** Post-Acute Care Setting Characteristics —Cont'd

| Setting | Expected Length of Stay | Admission Criteria | Common Reasons for Admission |
|---|---|---|---|
| Skilled nursing facility (SNF) | 28 days (CMS, 2016) | Patient must meet all of the following criteria (CMS, n.d., Skilled Nursing Facility Care): <br>• Have a medically necessary 3-day inpatient hospital stay <br>• Enter the facility within 30 days of leaving the hospital <br>• Require 24-hour care <br>• Active and ongoing intervention of one or more skilled services including nursing and therapy (PT, OT, or SLP) to: <br>  • Improve <br>  • Maintain <br>  • Prevent or slow further deterioration of the patient's condition <br>• Tolerate rehabilitation therapy program a minimum of 5 hours/week × 1–1.5 hours/day. | Typically, patients admitted to SNFs have limited activity tolerance, are advanced in age, and/or would benefit from a more prolonged duration of skilled services to address the following: <br>Orthopedic management: <br>• Surgical and nonsurgical management postfall <br>• Joint replacement <br>• Orthopedic related weight-bearing restrictions <br>Infectious diseases: <br>• Urinary tract infections <br>• Sepsis <br>• Osteomyelitis <br>• Cellulitis <br>• Pneumonia <br>• IV or IM medication <br>Respiratory management: <br>• Aspiration <br>• COVID-19 (acute or post-acute) <br>Wound/skin: <br>• Decubitus ulcer <br>• Amputation <br>• Necrotizing fasciitis <br>• Abscess <br>• Negative pressure wound care <br>Complex/complicated medical conditions: <br>• Cerebral vascular accident <br>• Cardiomyopathy <br>• Cardiac surgical care <br>• Cancer <br>• Congestive heart failure <br>• Chronic obstructive pulmonary disease <br>• Trauma <br>• Brain injury <br>• Progressive central nervous system condition <br>• Kidney disease <br>• Ostomy management |

**TABLE 27.1**  Post-Acute Care Setting Characteristics

| Setting | Expected Length of Stay | Admission Criteria | Common Reasons for Admission |
|---------|------------------------|--------------------|------------------------------|
| Home health (HH) | Patient specific and based on the plan of care | Patient must meet all of the following criteria:<br>• Physician orders/oversight<br>• Homebound—"You have trouble leaving your home without help (like using a cane, wheelchair, walker, or crutches; special transportation; or help from another person) because of an illness or injury, or leaving your home" (CMS, n.d., Home Health Services)<br>• Require one or more of the following skilled services (Social Security Administration, n.d.):<br>  • Intermittent nursing (<7 days/week or <8 hours/day over a period of 21 days [or less])<br>  • PT<br>  • SLP<br>  • OT<br>  • Medical social services<br>  • Part-time or intermittent home health aide care (only if you're also getting skilled nursing care at the same time)<br>  • Injectable osteoporosis drugs for women<br>  • Durable medical equipment<br>  • Medical supplies for use at home<br>• Services are reasonable and necessary. | Patient is homebound and needs intermittent skilled services. |
| Comprehensive outpatient rehabilitation facility (CORF) | Patient specific and based on the plan of care | The patient must:<br>• Demonstrate rehab potential to recover or improve functional deficits resulting from injury, disability, or illness.<br>• Have skilled therapy needs to be certified by a physician<br>CORFs must provide one or more of the following core services:<br>• Physician services<br>• PT services<br>• Social and/or psychological services<br>Optional CORF services include:<br>• OT<br>• Speech-language pathologists<br>• Respiratory therapists<br>• Nursing services<br>• Prosthetic and orthotic device services<br>• Cast and splint supplies.<br>• Durable medical equipment (CMS, 2011) | The patient population receiving CORF rehabilitation consists of all previously identified diagnoses. Most patients have been referred from a higher level of care as a potential final step toward functional independence. |

Continued

**TABLE 27.1** Post-Acute Care Setting Characteristics —Cont'd

| Setting | Expected Length of Stay | Admission Criteria | Common Reasons for Admission |
|---|---|---|---|
| Outpatient (OP) | Patient specific and based on the plan of care | An overseeing physician places a consult, certifies the need for, and signs off on the plan of care for skilled services. | Community-based population requiring treatment for conditions including but not limited to the following:<br>• Rheumatoid arthritis<br>• Osteoarthritis<br>• Carpal tunnel syndrome<br>• Cubital tunnel syndrome<br>• Medical epicondylitis<br>• Lateral epicondylitis<br>• Tendonitis/tendon tear<br>• Impingement<br>• Rotator cuff injury/repair<br>• Upper extremity fractures<br>• Shoulder replacement<br>• Cancer<br>• Edema management<br>• Neuropathy<br>• Parkinson's disease<br>• Self-care functional impairments |

*BI-PAP*, Bilevel positive airway pressure; *CPAP*, continuous positive airway pressure; *IM*, intramuscular; *IV*, intravenous; *IRF*, inpatient rehabilitation facility; *OT*, occupational therapy; *PT*, physical therapy; *SLP*, speech-language pathology.

**TABLE 27.2** Geriatric Syndromes and Screenings

| Syndromes | Screening Tools |
|---|---|
| Delirium | Confusion Assessment Method (CAM) |
| | CAM-ICU |
| Falls | Time up and go |
| | Dual tasking |
| Dizziness | Orthostatic vitals monitoring |
| Urinary incontinence | Voiding diary |
| | Bladder scan |
| | International Prostate Symptom Score |
| Insomnia | Epworth Sleepiness Scale |
| Cognitive decline | MMSE |
| | SLUMS |
| | MOCA |
| | Clock Drawing |
| Mood disorder | PHQ-9 |
| | GDS |
| Polypharmacy | Medication review/reconciliation |
| Fatigue/weakness/ frailty | SARC-F |
| | FRAIL Scale |
| Functional decline | ADLs, IADLs |
| Weight loss | Weight monitoring |

*ADLs*, Activities of daily living; *FRAIL scale*, Fatigue, Resistance, Ambulation, Illnesses, & Loss of Weight; *GDS*, Geriatric Depression Scale; *IADLs*, instrumental activities of daily living; *ICU*, intensive care unit; *MMSE*, Mini-Mental State Examination; *MOCA*, Montreal Cognitive Assessment; *PHQ-9*, Patient Health Questionnaire-9; *SARC-F*, Strength, Assistance in walking, Rise from a chair, Climb stairs, and Falls; *SLUMS*, Saint Louis University Mental Status.

rehabilitation needs have six different options depending on their needs and preferences, and location: (1) home OT via agency home care, (2) outpatient therapy (available for patients independent at home or in assisted living), (3) acute IRF/AR facilities, (4) LTACH, (5) SNF, and (6) hospice. If the patient has long-term care needs, the patient has four options: (1) care at home, including waiver programs; (2) assisted living; (3) nursing homes; or (4) adult day care. Program of All-Inclusive Care for the Elderly (PACE) highlights the insurance coverage for post-acute care medical and therapy services.

Case Example 27.1 illustrates an unfolding health-care journey for an older adult who presents with an acute illness and is followed through her post-acute care process. As noted in

this case, Ms. Z has several geriatric syndromes identified on admission, which may have contributed to her initial presentation and impacted her acute and post-acute care needs.

Unlike Ms. Z, who will require inpatient admission, if hospitalization is not indicated, patients usually return to the care of their outpatient primary care provider (PCP), who is responsible for coordinating further treatments and arranging for follow-up services as needed. HH care or OP services may be indicated for those with treatment needs who meet insurance qualifications.

## The Transition of Care: Acute to Post-Acute Care

As previously discussed, acute care and post-acute care expected length of stay play a vital role in access to care, determining the trajectory of care and recommendations. According to CMS, in 2018, the acute care average length of stay was 5.2 days for those over age 65 compared to the expected LTACH length of stay of >25 days (McDermott et al., 2017). Variances in the length of stay directly affect the frequency and duration of therapy. Recent research shows an inverse relationship between 30-day hospital readmissions and death for those receiving up to six therapy visits compared to those receiving no therapy visits (Freburger et al., 2020).

As post-acute services are primarily provided under a medical insurance benefit, treatment in this setting is generally time limited and based on the individual's ongoing medical and rehabilitative needs. Post-acute care facilitates further recovery by supporting nursing, rehabilitation, and medical care in a less intensive environment compared to acute care. The more commonly used post-acute settings include LTACH, IRF or AR, SNF, long-term care facility (LTC), HH, OP or CORF.

### Long-Term Acute Care Hospital

LTACH provides the highest medical care outside the acute hospital setting. Those needing LTACH require insurance authorization and require intensive medical treatments such as mechanical ventilation, multiday dressing changes, intensive wound care or infection treatment regimens, and frequent suctioning or tracheostomy care. LTACHs provide specialized acute care for stable but critically ill individuals with multisystem complications or failures requiring prolonged hospitalization. Therapy services are provided;

---

**CASE EXAMPLE 27.1**   Acute Care Admission

Ms. Z is a 76-year-old woman brought to the ED by her daughter after being found on her bedroom floor approximately 4 hours after falling. She reports a 4-day history of shortness of breath and cough with a poor appetite. Upon arrival to the ED, she has acute hypoxia requiring supplemental oxygen at 2 L via nasal cannula. Due to her primary concerns and acute hypoxia, she was tested for SARS-CoV-2 and found positive. The ED physician has gathered that her

past medical history includes mild Alzheimer's dementia, hypertension, type 2 non–insulin-dependent diabetes mellitus, and bilateral knee osteoarthritis. Ms. Z is taking eight scheduled medications and four as-needed over-the-counter medications. Collateral information from her daughter suggests Ms. Z. is frail, sarcopenic, and malnourished. She is admitted to the geriatric medicine inpatient service for medical management.

however, medical conditions dominate treatment plans. Patients have access to physicians 24/7 and are evaluated daily. Frequent hospitalizations occur in this population, but the long-term goal is to discharge to a prior living environment for many. If the critical illness conditions have improved or resolved, the patient may transition to a less intensive care setting like AR or SNF. LTACH therapy services are similar to acute care services. Medical care is the driving force in both settings, with therapy services as ancillary services. Services are provided to the patient as tolerated and when the patient is available.

## Acute Rehabilitation Facility (AR) or In-patient Rehabilitation Facility (IRF)

AR provides post-acute intensive rehabilitation services after acute illness or injury. Common conditions treated in AR include amputations, traumatic brain injury (TBI), burns, cerebrovascular accidents, hip fractures, neurological disorders, spinal cord injuries, and chronic conditions like COPD and HF. Refer to Table 27.1 for a comprehensive list of CMS AR-approved diagnoses. Therapy services are intensive, requiring a minimum of 15 hours per week. The patients' treatment must include at least two skilled therapy and skilled nursing services. Occupational therapists are part of the rehabilitation team whose members are dedicated to meeting clients' physical, psychological, and social needs in an environment that promotes wellness, confidence, and independence. Team members develop individualized treatment plans to maximize each client's functional abilities.

The AR admission is relatively short—generally less than 14 days. AR is more intensive, compressed, and costly and is usually approved for individuals with CMS approved rehabilitation diagnosis, higher baseline functional abilities, or expected rapid improvement in function. For example, patients with a TBI are more likely to be admitted to AR than individuals with an anoxic brain injury (ABI) due differences in therapy prognosis and duration of treatment plan. Older adults require additional time to recover functional deficits. Therefore, if the patient does not return to baseline function by the end of the AR admission, the patient may be transitioned to SNF or LTC.

## Skilled Nursing Facility (SNF)/Long-Term Facility (LTC)

SNF provides skilled therapy and nursing services to those recently discharged from the hospital. This time-limited insurance benefit period requires the need for skilled services to improve, maintain, or prevent or slow further deterioration of the patient's condition. Care is delivered in a facility that provides 24-hour nursing, medications, meals, treatments, and personal care. The facility usually also serves as an LTC setting for a population who live there as a permanent residence. Skilled facility–based services are delivered 5 days per week and 1 to 2 hours per day between skilled nursing and skilled therapy services combined. Please refer to Chapter 28 on Residential and Skilled Care for more detailed information.

## Home Health Care (HH)

Home health services are provided to homebound elders with a provider's order. Services are provided in the home under the direction of nursing or therapy. Functional and medical goals are established, and care is delivered several times each week until objectives are met or no further progress is identified. Home health OT (HHOT) services do not require an acute care admission; however, a recent or upcoming face-to-face provider visit is necessary to establish the home health-care benefit period.

Sometimes, laboratory and radiology services can be completed within the home. Wound care, symptom monitoring, therapy, and education are frequent activities of the home health-care team. When infusions are needed, home health-care agencies partner with an infusion service that provides the medication and equipment to the patient. Occupational therapists are members of the therapy team that provide home-based services to improve functional abilities. HHOT is the only service that can observe occupational performance without simulation or role-playing, thus providing the patient, family, and HHOT with the opportunity to maximize patient outcomes within the preferred environment, using preferred objects and delivered at the patient's specified time. HH therapy services are the least intense of post-acute therapy services. Therapists rely on the patients and patients support system for execution of care plan, home safety, and reduce risk for readmission. Please refer to Chapter 29, Home: An Evolving Context for Health Care, for more detailed information.

## The Health-Care Team: Acute and Post-Acute Care

When caring for older adults with complex chronic diseases, interprofessional collaborative care is critical in addressing patients' needs. This approach is further reinforced by the IMPACT Act of 2014, detailing the goals of promoting effective health-care communication and collaboration. Health-care teams are ecosystems that require effective communication and high trust relationships focused on providing quality care and optimal patient outcomes. Figure 27.1 demonstrates how the patient and family are central in establishing the desired outcomes and goals of care. Team members may function in an interdisciplinary fashion or within the "teamlet" of their respective discipline. The teamlet model utilizes smaller teams, including health coaches, to improve management chronic conditions. Each specialty involved results in a more holistic treatment plan. Please refer to Chapter 30 for more information on intraprofessional and interprofessional roles.

### The Health-Care Team

In acute care and post-acute care settings, the health-care team primarily consists of physicians, nurses, therapists (physical, occupational, speech), and social service practitioners. The physician is responsible for gathering the patients' medical history, providing the current medical status, and placing orders. Nursing services ensure the physical and medical

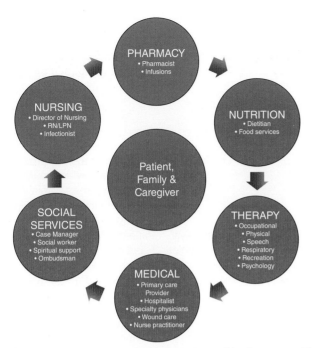

**FIGURE 27.1** Demonstration of how the patient and family are central in establishing the desired outcomes and goals of care.

care of the patient is provided under the physician's direction. Physical therapy (PT) offers assessment and treatment to address mobility-related deficits. OT assesses basic activities of daily living (BADLs), instrumental activities of daily living (IADLs), and functional mobility deficits (see Table 27.4). Speech therapy (ST) addresses swallowing, communication, hearing, and cognition deficits. Respiratory therapy provides pulmonary support services. Rehabilitation psychology performs evaluation and treatment services to determine psychological barriers that impact the patients' roles and routines posthospitalization.

Depending on the type of facility, many physicians may be involved in patients care. The therapist must be knowledgeable of each specialty and the impact each specialty may have on therapy services. For example, a patient with a recent lower extremity thrombectomy who is now acutely recovering from a cardiac bypass surgery may have conflicting care plans. Therefore, there is potential for limited weight-bearing status in the lower and upper extremities. A collaborative approach between all team members, including the vascular and cardiac surgeons, in order to determine the safest and most appropriate care plan.

Given this example, the cardiac surgeon may expect the patient to be ambulatory postoperative day 1; however, due to weight-bearing limitations initiated by the vascular surgeon, the patient requires a wheeled walker due to a lower extremity non-weight bearing status, which may conflict with sternal precautions. Therefore, the therapist's role is to discuss these contradictions and determine the best method of care to rehabilitate the patient.

Furthermore, collaboration is needed with all disciplines, such as coordinating the completion of medication administration and wound care with nursing staff, ensuring PT and ST are staggered to allow for optimal patient access and participation in services, discussing the patient's ventilator liberation plan with respiratory therapy, and ensuring the social services team is aware of the patients progress and recommended discharge disposition.

Social services is an overarching term for practitioners with the primary goal of supporting and advocating for the patient. Within social services, case managers align the health-care team, promoting communication about discharge planning home, potential consults, obtaining durable medical equipment, and patient advocacy. Social workers assist with discharge planning to inpatient post-acute care settings, assessing patient safety concerns, and providing supportive resources. Spiritual services ensure spiritual well-being, including coping with grief and loss, understanding illness, and defining patient values. The Ombuds' role is to advocate for the elderly population by addressing quality of care or safety concerns, educating patients and caregivers on rights, and assisting in problem resolution. Nutrition services include dietician and food services. The dietitian's primary role is to establish care plans that ensure adequate and appropriate nutrition. Food services work closely with dietitians to implement the care plan. Pharmacists monitor drug therapy, including side effects, dosage, medication education, and polypharmacy management.

Based on geography, finances, and staffing models, facilities may have different resources and access to certain disciplines. Some providers may function periodically, in a consultative role, or may not be available at all. The roles, responsibilities, participation, and priorities change over the acute and post-acute care continuum trajectory. As the needs of the patient change, so does the plan of care and the activities of the health-care team.

## Rounds, Huddle, and Patient/Family Meetings

Treatment team "rounding" or "huddling" is a process of sharing patient information across and within disciplines that may or may not include the patient. This chapter uses the terms "rounding" and "huddle" interchangeably. Goldenhar et al. (2013) found that "huddle implementation leads to improved efficiencies and quality of information sharing, increased levels of accountability, empowerment, and a sense of community, which together create a culture of collaboration and collegiality that increases the staff's quality of collective awareness and enhanced capacity for eliminating patient harm." In addition, implementing rounds using a standardized bedside approach among older adults may increase acceptance and willingness to discharge to undesired settings such as SNF, LTC, or palliative/hospice care (Basic et al., 2018). During interdisciplinary rounding, the role of OT is to:

- Review therapy progress
- Identify safety concerns
- Provide discharge disposition recommendations
- Discuss rehab progress, rehab barriers, and any relevant changes impacting rehab potential.

**TABLE 27.3**  Coverage for Different Levels of Post-Acute Care and Therapy

| Level of Care | Medicare Payment to Physician/NPP | Medicare Payment to Institution/ Therapy Provider | Medicaid Payment to Institution | Private/Other Medical Insurance | Self-Pay | Comments/References/for Additional Information: |
|---|---|---|---|---|---|---|
| Outpatient Therapy | Medicare Part B pays HPP/ physician for out-patient services | Medicare Part B pays therapy provider | Medicaid pays provider for service (primary/secondary) | Yes | Yes (co pays/ deductibles) | Patient travels from home to outpatient therapy provider. Therapy providers may also have sites within independent living or assisted living facilities. |
| Home Care | Medicare Part B pays physician/ NPP for home visits and care certification/ over sight | Medicare Part A pays agency for nursing care and therapies | Medicaid may pay for home/ waiver care for those eligible (see text) | Yes: Private medical insurance may pay for limited home care, private LTC insurance may cover LTC at home | Yes (co-pays/ deductibles for skilled care, private pay for nonskilled personal care) | Patients must be homebound and certified as such Face to Face by Physician. Refs. Giovino 2000, Nicoletti 2005. http://www.cms.gov/ Outreach-and-Ecucation/ Medicare-Learning-Network-MLN/MLNMattersArticles/Downloads/SE1038.pdf. American Academv of Home Care Medicine, www.aahcm.org. |
| Inpatient Rehab Facility (IRF) | Medicare Part B (for physician/NPP visits) | Medicare Part A | Yes in most states No in WV. | Yes | No insurance usually May be co-pays/ deductibles | Refs American Academy of Physical Medicine and Rehabilitation, www.aapmr.org; http://www.cms.gov/outreach-and-Education/medicare-Learning Network-MLN/MLN-Product/downloads/Inpatient Rehab Fact Sheet ICN905643.pdf. |
| Assisted Living/Personal Care Facility | Medicare B pays MD/ NPP for office/home visits | None | None | No (unless patient covered by private LTC insurance) | Yes (most assisted living is private self-pay) | AGS 2005, Assisted Living Federation of America, www.alfa.org; http://www.cms.gov/Outreach-and-Ecucation/Medicare-Learning-Network-MLN/MLNMattersArticles/Downloads/mm4212.pdf. |
| Nursing Home Care | Medicare Part B pays physician/NPP for NF/SNF visits | Medicare Part A (only up to 100 days) | Medicaid pays for LTC after Medicare and private pay exhausted | Private insurance may pay for SNF care similar to Medicare | Yes (for expenses not covered by Medicare Medicaid) | Ouslander 1994; Evans 1995, American Medical Directors Association for Long-Term Care. www.amda.com, American Health Care Association, http://www.ahcancal.org/. |
| Hospice | Medicare Part B continues to pay for physician visits separate from hospice | Medicare Part A | Medicaid pays provider | Private insurances may cover hospice care if terminal illness | No insurance usually pays | American Academy of Hospice & Palliative Care Medicine http://www.aahpm.org/. |

Goldberg T. H. (2014). The long-term and post-acute care continuum. *West Virginia Medical Journal*, 110(6), 24–30.

- Communicate support service needs (e.g., 24/7 care, wound care, home health aid, meals on wheels, grocery delivery setup)
- Discuss durable medical and adaptive equipment needed for discharge

Rounding that occurs without the patient is a traditional approach commonly utilized in acute care and LTACH settings. The attending physician typically leads the discussion with the health-care team during daily rounding outside the patient's room, at the nursing station, or in a conference room. Physician rounding is an semi—structured verbal process followed by a brief note in the patient's chart. Each service line will share details within its respective role. Attendance to rounding is facility dependent; however, often, the team is not represented in its entirety. Communication during rounding is most effective when it is brief and focused on relevant information that acutely impacts the patient's care plan. When needed, more personalized and detailed conversations with specific team members occur pre- or postrounding. Specialty physicians round with nursing staff and patients then further communicate collaborative care via preferred methods of communication (e.g., electronic medical record [EMR] notes/chats/orders, texts, calls.). Within the acute care and LTACH setting, the primary role of the occupational therapist is to align the discharge disposition with the therapist's discharge recommendations to prevent hospital readmission and ensure the most appropriate next level of care.

In the post-acute care setting, the health-care team utilizes a collaborative approach to rounding that includes the patient and family/caregiver. The patient, family/caregiver, and the health-care team meet weekly during a structured interdisciplinary meeting with all service lines contributing to the care plan. Discussion with the patient, caregiver, and practitioners includes individual team updates, planning, and a summary of progress toward the patient's goals. The team completes an updated care plan document before interdisciplinary meetings. During the meeting all contributors and patients sign off on the care plan. Individual service lines will meet with the patient for needed updates or action items; however, most information is shared during the scheduled meeting to promote transparency. Weekly meetings are essential in obtaining insurance authorization for continued coverage for skilled services. Within this setting, the primary role of the occupational therapist during interdisciplinary meetings is to align discharge disposition with therapy recommendations, discuss rehabilitation progress and functional status, identify barriers to the plan of care, and make suggestions for the next level of care.

## Common Geriatric Admissions

Among the most common diagnoses for hospitalization in older adults are sepsis, osteoarthritis, congestive HF, pneumonia, and diabetes mellitus (McDermott et al., 2017). The four most common diagnoses in patients discharged to HH or SNF are sepsis, joint repair, HF, and urinary tract infection. The most common condition in patients discharged to LTACH is respiratory failure requiring ventilator support with associated

deconditioning, accounting for 45% of all cases discharged to LTACH. The case mix in AR facilities includes conditions requiring more intensive therapy, such as stroke, TBI, and spinal cord injury. As acute care admitting and discharge diagnoses often delineate the post-acute settings and services needed, the OT must be aware of the impact of these conditions on the health-care trajectory of older adults following acute hospitalization. This chapter will highlight three conditions mentioned in the previously mentioned categories.

### Sepsis

Sepsis is a dysregulated immune response to infection, often resulting in multiorgan dysfunction or failure. The most common infectious triggers of sepsis include respiratory infections, urinary tract infections, and soft tissue infections. Sepsis is a highly morbid condition in older adults. Sepsis sequelae include BADL/IADL deficits, dysphagia, gait dysfunction, cognitive deficits, acquisition of stress disorders, recurrent infections, and exacerbation of chronic medical conditions (Prescott & Angus, 2018). When a patient acquires severe sepsis, they are three times more likely to experience moderate to severe cognitive impairments and develop 1.5 more deficits in BADLs/IADLs (Iwashyna et al., 2010). The mortality rate in adults older than 85 is 40%. One may attribute this high mortality rate to a lower physiological reserve and the atypical early presentation of sepsis in this population. Over half of older adults with sepsis do not mount a fever response. Older adults are also more likely to present with atypical symptoms, including delirium, weakness, falls, vital signs irregularity, and incontinence. Survivors of sepsis have a lower self-rated quality of life and more significant functional deficits than those who did not experience sepsis (Carey et al., 2020).

According to Prescott and Angus (2018), during the acute care phase, it is crucial to prevent long-term sequelae after sepsis by focusing on three strategies: high-quality early sepsis care; management of pain, agitation, and delirium; and early mobilization to prevent or minimize muscle atrophy. Occupational therapists continuously assess body functions and structures, which provides opportunities for early identification of sepsis. Sepsis symptoms include hemodynamic instability (tachycardia, shortness of breath, critical blood pressure [BP] values), confusion, agitation, increased pain, and impaired temperature regulation. The therapists' role in sepsis treatment focuses on physical and psychological interventions while providing consistent opportunities for occupational participation and early mobility mobility. In "hospitalization sequelae," we discuss the OT's role in treating delirium and how to incorporate OT within early mobilization programs. Early mobilization programs have been shown to assist with pain and delirium management, prevent deconditioning, and improve patient functional status.

### Hip Fracture

In the United States, 300,000 older adults are hospitalized for hip fractures. Intertrochanteric and femoral neck fractures are

**TABLE 27.4** Functional and Mobility Activities

| Activities of Daily Living | Instrumental Activities of Daily Living (Lawton & Brody, 1969) |
|---|---|
| Katz Index (Katz et al., 1970)<br>• Bathing<br>• Dressing<br>• Toileting<br>• Transferring<br>• Continence<br>• Feeding<br>Barthel Index (Mahoney & Barthel, 1965)<br>• Feeding<br>• Bathing<br>• Grooming<br>• Dressing<br>• Bowel Control<br>• Bladder Control<br>• Toileting<br>• Transfers<br>• Mobility<br>• Stairs | • Using the telephone<br>• Shopping<br>• Preparing food<br>• Housekeeping<br>• Doing laundry<br>• Using transportation<br>• Handling medications<br>• Handling finances |

**TABLE 27.5** Fall Prevention Interventions

**Multifactorial (Individualized) Fall Prevention Intervention**

| Individualized Fall Risk Assessment and Treatment | Environmental Interventions |
|---|---|
| • Geriatric/medical assessment or consultation<br>• Vision screening and intervention<br>• Hearing screening and intervention<br>• Medication review, Medication management or reduction<br>• Referrals to other disciplines | • Home assessment<br>• Home modification<br>• Hazard abatement |

**Multicomponent (Group-Based) Fall Prevention Program Interventions**

| Exercise Approaches | Education Topics |
|---|---|
| • Balance<br>• Strength<br>• Functional tasks<br>• Walking<br>• Dual-task or multitask activities<br>• Obstacle course training<br>• Fall training techniques | • Feet or footwear risk<br>• Energy conservation strategies<br>• Safe assistive device use<br>• Home modifications<br>• Fall recovery<br>• Medication management<br>• Nutrition and hydration<br>• Relaxation and stress management<br>• Pain management<br>• Community resources<br>• Common risk factors:<br>  • Reduced cognitive function<br>  • Postural hypotension<br>  • Vision impairments<br>  • Urinary incontinence |

**Population-Based (Age ≥65) Fall Prevention Interventions**

| | |
|---|---|
| • Population-based fall prevention programs<br>  • Stepping On—seven-session group intervention, targeting falls abatement and improving balance confidence<br>  • A Matter of Balance—peer-led, 8 × 2-hour sessions targeting fear of falling and increased activity | • Population-based multicomponent cognitive-behavioral fall prevention interventions<br>• Exercise and fall risk educational program<br>• Strength, balance, home safety, and safe behaviors program |

**Functional Exercise**

• Daily, unstructured balance and strength exercises (e.g., heel walking, toe walking, side stepping, sit to stand) incorporated into daily functional tasks.
• Exercises do not require equipment or additional time.

From Elliott, S., & Leland, N. E. (2018). Occupational therapy fall prevention interventions for community-dwelling older adults: A systematic review. *American Journal of Occupational Therapy, 72*(4), 7204190040p1-7204190040p11. doi: 10.5014/ajot.2018.030494.

the predominant types of hip fractures in older adults. Falls, polypharmacy, and osteoporosis are major risk factors. Hip fracture results in significant morbidity and mortality, especially in older adults with cognitive impairment and those residing in long-term care settings. Over 50% of patients will not regain their ability to live independently. Up to 40% of patients may die within 1 year of a hip fracture (Bai et al., 2018). Although surgical treatment is expected in patients with poor life expectancy and minimal pain, nonoperative management is a consideration.

The etiology of falls is often multifactorial. For instance, the patient may report awakening during the night, feeling groggy, ambulating in the dark, and tripping over a pet. The chart review indicates a patient history of urgent incontinence, cataracts, and peripheral neuropathy. During the interview, the patient revealed the fall occurred overnight when attempting to navigate a dark pathway to the bathroom without proper footwear and after taking sleep-inducing medications. Research by Elliott et al. (Elliott & Leland, 2018) suggests that fall prevention in older adults should be provided across the continuum of care from acute care through post-acute settings for optimal effect. Table 27.5 summarizes their evidence-based findings and treatment recommendations.

In addition to fall prevention, OT treatment plans often include assistive device training, safe transfer techniques, compensatory techniques to ensure adherence to weight-bearing and precaution restrictions, and safe use of durable medical equipment. Education topics regarding environmental factors include home modifications, reorganizing/decluttering, recommended seating options (e.g., chair, shower/tub, car, commode), and recommended vehicles for transportation. Treatment should be incorporated into preferred routines, habits, and tasks, allowing the elderly patient to focus on maximizing independence and promoting self-confidence.

## Heart Failure (HF)

HF is a cardiac condition in which blood fails to efficiently move out of the heart to avoid congestion within the pulmonary or venous systems. The resulting symptoms of shortness of breath, fatigue, edema, and weight gain can occur acutely or chronically and substantially impact functional status and quality of life. Whether HF is due to valvular dysfunction, cardiac rhythm disturbance, reduced systolic function (reduced ejection fraction of blood [HFrEF]), or reduced diastolic function (preserved ejection fraction [HFpEF]), the prevalence increases across the lifespan. Attention to diet, medications, and lifestyle factors is critical but often challenging in older adults. Knowing the clinical signs of HF within the acute and post-acute settings is crucial, was well as understanding metabolic exercise tolerance levels (MET) and contraindications when recovering from HF.

Occupational therapists are able to initiate early patient and caregiver training to promote disease management. By completing the occupational profile, therapists can identify chronic disease management barriers. For example, diuretic medications increase urinary frequency and problem solving with patients on supporting increased frequency, and medication adherence can promote medical adherence and reduce the risk for readmission. Through establishing a therapeutic rapport, the therapist may find that the etiology of poor nutritional adherence in older adults with HF is due to lack of transportation, decreased appetite, inability to tolerate standing or grocery shopping, declining support system, or limited finances. Primary interventions to address HF are education, modifications, and improved self and disease awareness. Some specific suggestions are presented in Table 27.6.

## Hospitalization Sequelae

When admitted to acute and post-acute settings, patients can develop conditions directly related to hospitalization. This chapter will discuss the most impactful sequelae within the aging population.

### Post–Intensive Care Unit Syndrome (PICS)

PICS refers to the often-unrecognized constellation of chronic cognitive decline, physical decline, and psychiatric illness in survivors of critical illness. PICS syndrome is common in 25%–50% of critical illness survivors (Needham et al., 2012). Although prevalence data in older adults are sparse, given older adults' higher level of baseline physical and cognitive dysfunction, the PICS syndrome is likely even more common in the geriatric population.

PICS cognitive decline often manifests as impairment of memory and executive function. PICS syndrome's common psychiatric presentations include depression, anxiety, and posttraumatic stress. Various ICU-related diseases, including critical illness neuromyopathy and disuse sarcopenia, contribute to the physical decline seen in PICS. The neuromuscular

**TABLE 27.6** Heart Failure Interventions

| Medical Adherence | Modifications | Self-awareness |
|---|---|---|
| • Medication<br>• Nutrition and meal planning<br>• Durable medical equipment<br>• Home exercise plan<br>• Occupation participation—developing ADL and IADL routines that promote wellness, improve quality of life, and other meaningful activities | • Energy conservation and work simplification strategies<br>• Prioritizing activities<br>• Pacing participation<br>• Adaptive equipment<br>• Home modifications<br>• Reorganizing home<br>• Use of technology and resources | • Disease and symptom recognition<br>• Coping strategies<br>• Vital sign monitoring<br>• Daily weights<br>• Quality of life assessment<br>• Mood assessment<br>• Borg Rate of Perceived Exertion (RPE) Scale<br>• Portable pulse oximeter |

*ADL*, Activity of daily living; *IADL*, instrumental activity of daily living.

degeneration is particularly burdensome on the health-care system and the patient, as the consequent ventilator dependence is a common indication for LTACH discharge.

Occupational therapists evaluate and treat PICS through detailed attention to the assessment of body functions, including global cognition, sensory, neuromusculoskeletal and movement-related, muscle, movement, and respiratory systems. Occupational therapists utilize various standardized assessments to assess functional status while simultaneously providing treatment. Refer to Table 27.7 for more details regarding testing. Engaging patients in occupations in conjunction with a progressive early mobility program assists with ventilator (noninvasive and invasive) liberation, minimizing sedatives and restraints, decreasing delirium, stabilizing mood, and strengthening. Figure 27.2 is an example of an early mobility program.

### Delirium

Delirium is an acute condition of waxing and waning mental status, inattention, altered alertness, and disorganized thinking. Delirium is associated with increased hospital length of stay, decreased functional and cognitive status at hospital discharge, and increased long-term mortality (Pandharipande et al., 2013). There are three types of delirium: hyperactive, hypoactive, and mixed. Figure 27.3 identifies common signs and symptoms of delirium.

Delirium is distinct from dementia in onset, attention to task, and pattern of behaviors. Delirium is an acute change (hours or days) compared to dementia, a slow progressive process. Attention is more dramatically impacted in patients with delirium versus those with dementia. For example, patients with dementia may be able to play a familiar card game; however, this task would be challenging in the setting of delirium. Finally, symptoms fluctuate considerably with

**TABLE 27.7** Post–Intensive Care Unit Syndrome (PICS) Assessments

| ICU Scales | Occupational Therapy Scales | Mobility Scales |
|---|---|---|
| Functional Status Score for ICU (FSS-ICU) | Quality Indicators (QI's) | 2-minute walk test; 6-minute walk test; 12-minute walk test |
| Acute Care Index of Function (ACIF) | Barthel Index | Timed up and go test |
| Physical Function Outcome Measure (PFIT) | Strength and grip testing | Berg Balance Scale |
| Richmond Agitation Scale | Activity Measure for Post-Acute Care (AM-PAC) 6 clicks—ADLs | Activity Measure for Post-Acute Care (AM-PAC) 6 clicks |
| Confusion Assessment Method (CAM-ICU) | | Banner Mobility Assessment Tool (BMAT) Function in Sitting Test |

*ADLs,* Activities of daily living; *ICU,* intensive care unit.

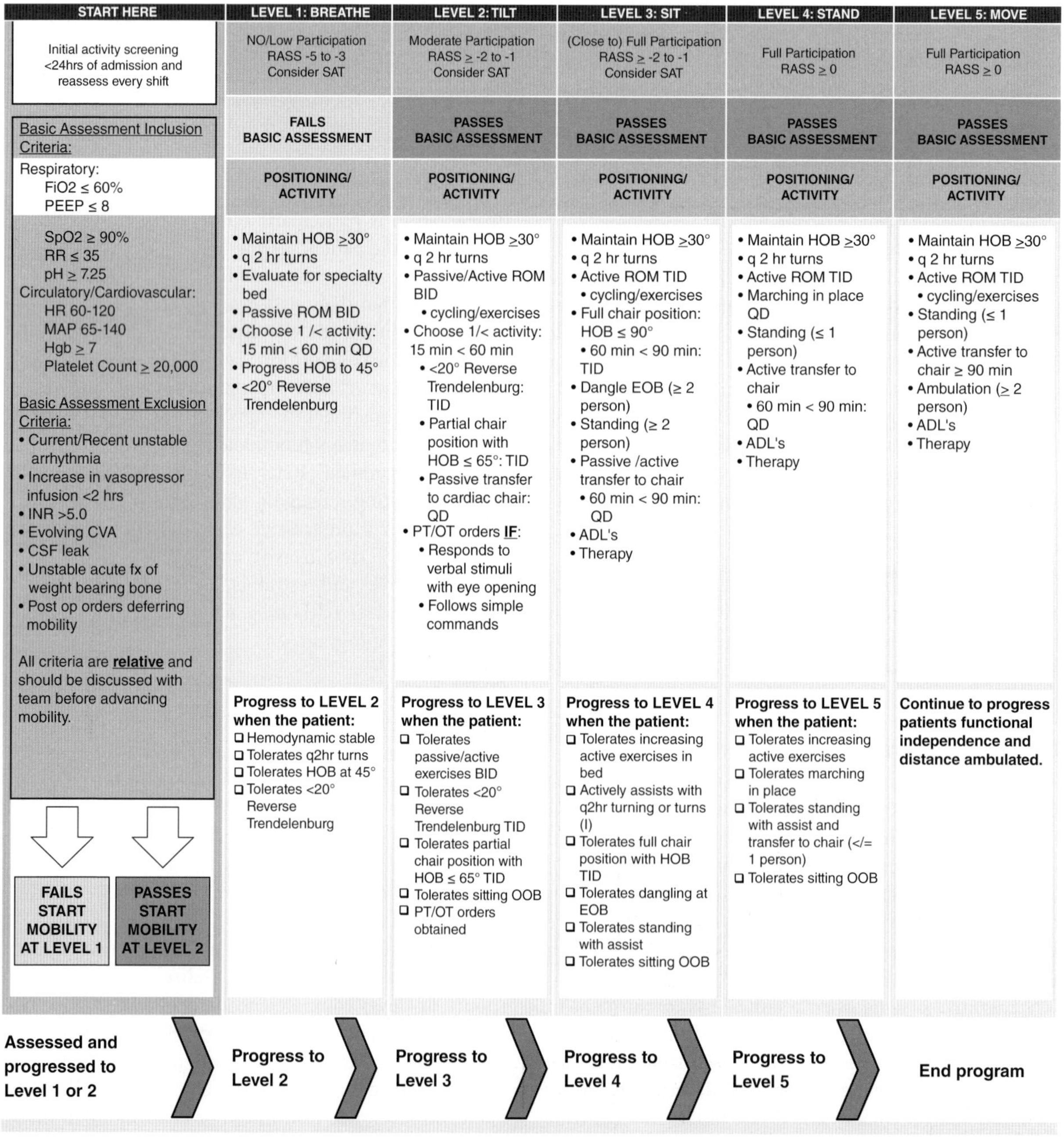

| START HERE | LEVEL 1: BREATHE | LEVEL 2: TILT | LEVEL 3: SIT | LEVEL 4: STAND | LEVEL 5: MOVE |
|---|---|---|---|---|---|
| Initial activity screening <24hrs of admission and reassess every shift | NO/Low Participation RASS -5 to -3 Consider SAT | Moderate Participation RASS ≥ -2 to -1 Consider SAT | (Close to) Full Participation RASS ≥ -2 to -1 Consider SAT | Full Participation RASS ≥ 0 | Full Participation RASS ≥ 0 |
| **Basic Assessment Inclusion Criteria:** Respiratory: FiO2 ≤ 60% PEEP ≤ 8 | **FAILS BASIC ASSESSMENT** | **PASSES BASIC ASSESSMENT** | **PASSES BASIC ASSESSMENT** | **PASSES BASIC ASSESSMENT** | **PASSES BASIC ASSESSMENT** |
| SpO2 ≥ 90% RR ≤ 35 pH ≥ 7.25 Circulatory/Cardiovascular: HR 60-120 MAP 65-140 Hgb ≥ 7 Platelet Count ≥ 20,000 | **POSITIONING/ ACTIVITY** | **POSITIONING/ ACTIVITY** | **POSITIONING/ ACTIVITY** | **POSITIONING/ ACTIVITY** | **POSITIONING/ ACTIVITY** |
| **Basic Assessment Exclusion Criteria:** • Current/Recent unstable arrhythmia • Increase in vasopressor infusion <2 hrs • INR >5.0 • Evolving CVA • CSF leak • Unstable acute fx of weight bearing bone • Post op orders deferring mobility<br><br>All criteria are **relative** and should be discussed with team before advancing mobility. | • Maintain HOB ≥30° • q 2 hr turns • Evaluate for specialty bed • Passive ROM BID • Choose 1 /< activity: 15 min < 60 min QD • Progress HOB to 45° • <20° Reverse Trendelenburg | • Maintain HOB ≥30° • q 2 hr turns • Passive/Active ROM BID • cycling/exercises • Choose 1/< activity: 15 min < 60 min • <20° Reverse Trendelenburg: TID • Partial chair position with HOB ≤ 65°: TID • Passive transfer to cardiac chair: QD • PT/OT orders **IF**: • Responds to verbal stimuli with eye opening • Follows simple commands | • Maintain HOB ≥30° • q 2 hr turns • Active ROM TID • cycling/exercises • Full chair position: HOB ≤ 90° • 60 min < 90 min: TID • Dangle EOB (≥ 2 person) • Standing (≥ 2 person) • Passive /active transfer to chair • 60 min < 90 min: QD • ADL's • Therapy | • Maintain HOB ≥30° • q 2 hr turns • Active ROM TID • Marching in place QD • Standing (≤ 1 person) • Active transfer to chair • 60 min < 90 min: QD • ADL's • Therapy | • Maintain HOB ≥30° • q 2 hr turns • Active ROM TID • cycling/exercises • Standing (≤ 1 person) • Active transfer to chair ≥ 90 min • Ambulation (≥ 2 person) • ADL's • Therapy |
| | **Progress to LEVEL 2 when the patient:** ☐ Hemodynamic stable ☐ Tolerates q2hr turns ☐ Tolerates HOB at 45° ☐ Tolerates <20° Reverse Trendelenburg | **Progress to LEVEL 3 when the patient:** ☐ Tolerates passive/active exercises BID ☐ Tolerates <20° Reverse Trendelenburg TID ☐ Tolerates partial chair position with HOB ≤ 65° TID ☐ Tolerates sitting OOB ☐ PT/OT orders obtained | **Progress to LEVEL 4 when the patient:** ☐ Tolerates increasing active exercises in bed ☐ Actively assists with q2hr turning or turns (I) ☐ Tolerates full chair position with HOB TID ☐ Tolerates dangling at EOB ☐ Tolerates standing with assist ☐ Tolerates sitting OOB | **Progress to LEVEL 5 when the patient:** ☐ Tolerates increasing active exercises ☐ Tolerates marching in place ☐ Tolerates standing with assist and transfer to chair (</= 1 person) ☐ Tolerates sitting OOB | **Continue to progress patients functional independence and distance ambulated.** |
| **FAILS START MOBILITY AT LEVEL 1** / **PASSES START MOBILITY AT LEVEL 2** | | | | | |

Assessed and progressed to Level 1 or 2 > Progress to Level 2 > Progress to Level 3 > Progress to Level 4 > Progress to Level 5 > End program

**FIGURE 27.2** Example of an Early Mobility Program.

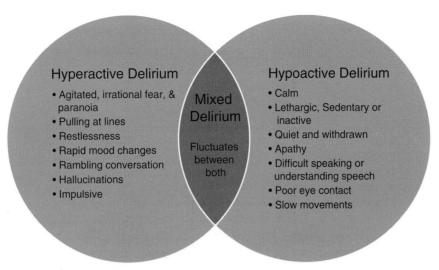

**FIGURE 27.3**   Delirium: Types, Signs, and Symptoms.

delirium, whereas patients with dementia present with persistent typical patterns or triggers. When precipitants and risk factors are alleviated, delirium should be reversible. However, research suggests that up to half of older adults who have delirium in the ICU will have persistent cognitive symptoms after discharge (Patel et al., 2014).

Common delirium risk factors include immobility, functional impairments, sensory (visual and hearing) impairments, dehydration, and poor sleep hygiene (Oh et al., 2017). Occupational therapists screen and treat delirium through completion of the occupational profile, interview with family/caregiver, and occupation participation and task analysis. The Confusion Assessment Method (CAM) and CAM-ICU are commonly used tools for delirium screening. Some specific treatment interventions are presented in Table 27.8.

### Cognition Impairments

Assessing cognition throughout the phases (evaluation, treatment, pending discharge) of acute care and post-acute care is essential for skilled OT services. Upon admission to post-acute care settings, cognitive impairment is a stronger predictor of outcomes than a historical diagnosis of dementia (Burke et al., 2021a). From 2015 to 2016, 7 of 10 Medicare patients with dementia were discharged to SNF versus HH (Burke et al., 2021b). Cognitive assessment findings guide long-term and short-term care plans, expectation setting with patients and caregivers, and education/training approaches for the medical team and identify the need for additional referrals. Determining the assessment is specific to the patient, setting, and anticipated discharge.

When working with individuals with dementia, new research suggests that developing a dementia care template can address dementia-related behaviors and improve caregiver resources (Bresley et al., 2022). The authors suggest that creating a dementia care template starts with a needs assessment that includes the following evaluations: Neuropsychiatric Inventory Questionnaire (NPI-Q), The Routine Task Inventory Physical ADL section, The PAINAD, "My Stress Thermometer,

and Home Safety Inventory. The educational component includes family/caregiver treatment sessions, including handouts emphasizing successful communication techniques, use and importance of routines, and activity and environmental adaptations to promote meaningful engagement. Refer to Figure 27.1 for an example of a dementia care plan.

Other research shows the efficacy of the Tailored Activity Program (TAP). The TAP protocol is most appropriate within the home setting as it allows for up to eight 60- to 90-minute sessions. TAP effectively reduces dementia-related behaviors, improving functional performance and caregivers' confidence (Cahill, 2022).

### Deconditioning

From the time of acute care admission, the interdisciplinary team works to prevent and limit the affects of hospital-associated deconditioning (HAD) or post-hospital syndrome. HAD is the result of patient and environmental factors that results in prolonged immobility during hospitalization.

Patient related risk factors for HAD include:
- Advanced age
- Impaired pre-admission functional status
- Impaired pre-admission mobility status
- Incontinence
- Activity intolerance
- Malnutrition
- Skin Integrity
- Geriatric syndromes
- Cognition impairments
- Mood disturbance (anxiety, depression)
- Fear of falling
- Pain

Environmental risk factors for HAD include:
- Change of environment
- Medical devices (sequential compression devices, IV pole, wound vacuum)
- Lines/tubes/drains (continuous fluids, urinary catheter, chest tube, telemetry)

**TABLE 27.8** Delirium Treatment Interventions

| Immobility | Functional Impairments | Sensory Impairments | Poor Nutrition | Poor Sleep Hygiene |
|---|---|---|---|---|
| • Use of positional changes<br>• Sitting upright<br>• Sitting out of bed<br>• Associate routines and habits with positions<br>  • bed = sleep<br>  • chair = awake<br>  • commode = toileting<br>• Utilizing the appropriate objects for tasks<br>  • Table = feeding<br>  • Bathroom = self-care<br>• Bringing the patient of the room<br>• Incorporate use of safe patient handling equipment to maximize access to other environments | • Ensure bathroom is accessible and safe<br>• Toileting schedule with reminders<br>• Self-care schedule<br>• Identify essential self-care activities<br>• Provide autonomy with task selection | • Vision<br>• Remove clutter<br>• Magnification lens and or technology<br>• Location and amplification of lighting<br>• Consistent location of objects<br>• Use of large print<br>• High contrast environmental changes<br>• Color discrimination modifications<br>• Hearing<br>  • Pocket amplifier<br>  • Access to hearing aid batteries<br>  • Pathway lighting<br>  • Speak towards the patient, slowly clearly, and in a deep tone<br>  • Use non-verbal communication<br>• Tactile<br>  • Varied call light sensors<br>  • Adaptive equipment<br>  • Texture changes | • Identify meal routines and preferences including times, quantities and locations.<br>• Promotion of self-feeding through maximizing meal setup.<br>• Adaptive equipment<br>• Encourage meals with family caregivers | • Identification preferred daily routines and leisure preferences<br>• Use of lighting and access to windows<br>• Sound management<br>• Relaxation techniques<br>• Mobility and exercise |

• Procedures (hemodialysis , x-rays, line placement)
• Avoidance of leaving the room due to fear of missing providers
• Temperature of environment
• Limited seating options
• Bed/chair alarms
• Hospital staffing limitations
• Increased staff needs for mechanical lift assistance
• Physical restraints

This reduction in activity results in sarcopenia (skeletal muscle wasting and/or loss of function), weakness, and frailty (age-related decline in biological systems with physiological vulnerability). Older adults lose 2% of total body mass within 5 days of bed rest and 1.5 kg lean body mass (Di Girolamo et al., 2021). Patients and staff alike may be fearful of falls occurring and recommend limited movement out of bed, to/from the bathroom, and within the hallway. Bed rest status should be avoided unless critical for patient safety. Use of activity volunteers, 1:1 sitters rather than restraints, and early therapy orders should be employed to maximize the physical activity during hospitalization, including in the ICU.

OT interventions should focus on increasing occupational participation, functional mobility, and prevention of deconditioning. Figure 27.2 outlines a progressive early mobility program that can be initiated within the ICU and continued throughout admission until discharge. The program highlights inclusion and exclusion criteria, which helps all staff members objectively determine readiness for out-of-bed activities and address potential safety concerns. This process utilizes clinical reasoning in the safe progression of mobility, assessment, safe patient integration, and incorporation of occupational participation in progressive positions and activity levels. For example, Level 2 treatment sessions may include grooming tasks supine with the head of the bed elevated or postlateral transfer to a cardiac chair sitting upright with armrests and lateral supports. A Level 3 treatment session may include BADLs sitting unsupported at the edge of the bed, standing at the sink, and incorporate sequential tasks requiring prolonged time. By incorporating bedside exercise programs, handouts, and visual aids, the nursing staff and caregivers can assist with preventing or minimizing HAD. For example, a patient that has been intubated and sedated with prolonged bed rest may develop weakness that will inhibit the patient's ability to feed themselves once extubated.

Rehabilitation departments may use these concepts to demonstrate the occupational therapists' role in preventing institutionalized deconditioning, implementing safe participation in self-care and functional mobility, and patient involvement. A progressive early mobility program, assessment, and recommendations on safe patient handling equipment to assist with safe transfers are stepping stones to incorporating self-care tasks into patient rehabilitation. (See

**CASE EXAMPLE 27.2**   Acute Care Sequelae

On hospital day 3, Ms. Z becomes increasingly withdrawn, with vitals showing 89% $SPO_2$ on 6 L/min of oxygen via nasal cannula resting heart rate (HR) of 124 and temperature of 101.4. A rapid response results in STAT chest x-ray indicating diffuse bilateral opacities, which are concerning for sepsis in the setting of COVID pneumonia. Following the sepsis protocol, she was transferred from the medical floor to the ICU.

After respiratory therapy evaluation and treatment, Ms. Z required 40 L/min of oxygen via nasal high-flow delivery. She remains lethargic with new episodes of agitation resulting in pulling lines/tubes and attempting to get out of bed. Ms. Z is intermittently restrained and sedated. In addition to the trauma leading up to the admission, decreased mobility and delirium has impacted her skin integrity causing skin tears and pressure ulcers. Her poor appetite has persisted throughout the admission; however, her nutritional intake is dramatically reduced with combined weakness, decreased ability to communicate basic needs, and restraints. Based on her presentation, the intensivist ordered OT, PT, ST, and case management. Within 24 hours, the occupational evaluation is completed with the following details.

| OT Evaluation | | Comments |
|---|---|---|
| Type of home | Two-story home with a basement | Primary bed/bath located on the second floor |
| Stairs | Three steps to enter<br>12 steps to the second floor | One handrail on the left going up from the garage into the kitchen<br>One handrail on the right going up to the second floor |
| Lives with | Alone | The daughter lives close by |
| Receives help from | Daughter | PRN |
| Toilet type | Standard commode | |
| Shower/tub type | Tub/shower combo | With sliding glass door |
| Bathroom equipment | Shower chair | Does not use |
| Mobility equipment | Single point cane | In the community, furniture walker within the home. |
| Self-care equipment | Reacher and sock aid | |
| Prior level of function | BADLs—independent<br>IADLs—needs some help<br>Functional mobility—independent<br>Functional cognition—needs some help | BADLs—regularly took sponge baths due to shortness of breath. Utilizes depends and layers with pads due to urinary incontinence<br>IADLs—utilized meal/grocery delivery weekly, and daughter assisted with heavy household management tasks.<br>Mobility—within the home she is a furniture walker and uses a single-point cane in the community.<br>Cognition—the daughter sets up a pill box and calls daily to remind the patient of upcoming tasks and ensure she ate her meals. |
| Falls | Three | One fall resulted in an EMS call to assist with getting up.<br>Two falls when going to the bathroom at night without injury and she was able to self recover. |
| Driving | No | Daughter provides transportation |
| Occupational status | Retired | |
| Leisure | Attends church weekly<br>Enjoys eating out with family<br>Watches TV (Channel 5, Price Is Right)<br>She plays games on her phone. | |
| Lifestyle/routine | | Recently, she slept in a recliner.<br>She prefers to sleep in and stays up late.<br>Eats two meals per day.<br>Changes clothes every 3 days. |
| Communication | Expresses wants/needs with some difficulty | Word finding and poor attention |

*Continued*

**CASE EXAMPLE 27.2**  Acute Care Sequelae—Cont'd

| OT Evaluation | | Comments |
|---|---|---|
| Cognition | CAM-ICU—positive<br>Brief Interview for Mental Status (BIMS) score = 7<br>Orientation: self and location. She reports the current location is the "hospital."<br>Follows related one-step commands consistently with increased time and repetition. | BIMS Interpretation: This score indicates a severe cognitive impairment, and the subject should be assessed further to be provided with a diagnosis and a health plan.<br>Requires cues to open eyes throughout the session. |
| Vitals | SPO$_2$: 40 L/min via nasal high flow<br>   94% at rest<br>   90% with activity<br>Respiratory rate (RR):<br>   33 at+ rest<br>   41 with activity<br>HR: 89 at rest<br>   129 with activity<br>BP: 126/62 at rest<br>   171/89 with activity<br>Pain: 4/10 at rest<br>   7/10 with activity | Activity includes self-care sitting unsupported at the edge of bed and chair, and stand pivot transfers.<br>Heart rate at rest is at moderate intensity<br><br><br>Heart rate with activity is at maximal intensity<br><br><br>Generalized pain<br>Knees and location of right-sided injuries |
| Activity tolerance | Borg Rating of Perceived Exertion (RPE) Scale:<br>9 at rest<br>17 with activity | Tolerates < 2.5 METs of activity with multiple prolonged rest breaks and breathing techniques due to activity intolerance, shortness of breath, and weakness. |
| Precautions | Vision<br>Hearing<br>Fall risk<br>Monitor vitals<br>Skin integrity | Adequate with glasses<br>Difficulty in public<br>Recent history of falls |
| Integumentary | Braden score: 9 | Notable for ecchymosis on the right side of the trunk, hip, and knee due to the fall just before admission.<br>Persistent erythema on bilateral wrists, ischial tuberosities, and bilateral knees. |
| Upper Extremity (UE) Assessment | Right Upper Extremity (RUE): (dominant)<br>2-/5 shoulder<br>3/5 elbow and distally<br>Poor grip strength<br>Delayed serial opposition<br>Left Upper Extremity (LUE):<br>3/5 throughout limb<br>Fair grip strength<br>Delayed serial opposition | Reports pain during adduction and notable for shoulder elevation during flexion. Reports she fell on her right side just before admission.<br>Bilateral weakness tremors were noted as testing progressed. |
| **Current BADL status** | | |
| Eating | Partial/moderate assistance | Excursion to/from mouth to void spilling/dropping<br>Frequent verbal cues for encouragement and to attend to the task |
| Grooming | Partial/moderate assistance | Hair brushing and oral hygiene due to decreased strength/range, coordination, and fatigue. Verbal/visual cues to attend and sequence task. |
| UE dressing | Partial/moderate assistance | Threading RUE and pulling overhead due to limited range of motion, pain, and multiple lines. Verbal/visual/tactile cues for initiation of task and sequencing. |

**CASE EXAMPLE 27.2**   Acute Care Sequelae

| OT Evaluation | | Comments |
|---|---|---|
| Lower Extremity dressing<br>Footwear | Partial/moderate assistance<br>Substantial/maximal assistance | Threading pants onto the left and right leg and don-ning/doffing socks due to impaired balance, limited range of motion, pain, weakness, fatigue, and multiple lines. Verbal/visual/tactile cues for initiation of task and sequencing. |
| Bathing | Partial/moderate assistance | Posterior peri-area hygiene, upper and lower legs, including feet due to limited range of motion, pain, weakness, and fatigue. Verbal/visual/tactile cues for initiation of task and sequencing. |
| Toileting | Dependence | Found incontinent of urine upon approach to room<br>Pulling briefs up/down and posterior hygiene due to limited balance, weakness, and cognition (sequencing and problem solving) |
| **Current mobility status** | | |
| Assistive device | Gait belt and wheeled walker | |
| Balance | Berg balance score: 13/56 | Berg interpretation:<br>0 –20 = high fall risk |
| Supine < sit | Partial/moderate assistance | Bilateral lower extremity management |
| Sit < > stand | Partial/moderate assistance | Using bilateral upper extremities requires assistance with concentric and eccentric contraction, verbal/tactile/visual cues for hand placement and sequencing tasks |
| Commode transfers | Partial/moderate assistance | Stand pivot transfer to the bedside commode. Verbal/visual/tactile cues and assistance needed for balance, sequencing, safety awareness, line management, and safe use of a wheeled walker |
| Bed <> chair transfers | Partial/moderate assistance | Stand pivot transfer from a bedside commode to the recliner<br>Verbal/visual/tactile cues and assistance needed for balance, sequencing, safety awareness, line management, and safe use of a wheeled walker |
| Ambulation | 3 feet with Partial/moderate assistance | Verbal/visual/tactile cues and assistance needed for balance, sustained alertness, sequencing tasks, and safe use of a wheeled walker |
| Assessment | Ms. Z has impaired functional status in the following areas: self-care, mobility, communication, cognition, activity tolerance, hemodynamic stability, and respiratory status. Decreased independence is related to the subsequent deficits:<br>Nutritional intake deficits, impaired balance, decreased strength/range of motion, delirium, poor self/safety awareness, pain, delayed coordination, poor attention, and reduced alertness.<br>Ms. Z presents with activity intolerance; however, with rest breaks and breathing exercises, she was able to participate in self-care and mobility tasks. If she medically progresses as expected, she has good rehab potential to remediate deficits. Currently, she does not demonstrate the ability to return home safely alone with the prior level of support. | |
| Recommendations | Skilled nursing facility with 24/7 care | |

ST reports findings of severe dysphagia and recommends a nasogastric (NG) feeding tube with modified liquid and solid consistencies to maximize nutritional intake. PT also determines that Ms. Z is not at her baseline function and requires Partial/moderate assistance for mobility. All disciplines concur that discharge to SNF is the safest and most appropriate level of therapy upon discharge from acute care. The patient and family agree with this plan. Therapy recommendations are discussed during rounding, resulting in a social worker consult to assist with facility referrals and initiating the insurance authorization process.

**TABLE 27.9** Skin Intengrity and Wound Care Management

| Types | Risk Factors | Interventions |
| --- | --- | --- |
| Skin impairments<br>Wounds | Identify<br>Assess<br>Treat | Remediation/restoration<br>Prevention<br>Modification<br>Education<br>Compensation |
| Abrasions<br>Arterial ulcers<br>Bites<br>Diabetic ulcers<br>Pressure injuries<br>Punctures<br>Skin tears<br>Surgical wounds<br>Traumatic wounds<br>Venous status ulcers | Acute/Chronic skin breakdown<br>Advanced age<br>Burns<br>Cancer<br>Cognition<br>Cognitive impairments<br>Contractures<br>Diabetes<br>Edema<br>Falls<br>Hand and foot injuries<br>Healthcare literacy<br>Hypersomnia<br>Incontinence<br>Mobility impairments<br>Moisture<br>Muscular atrophy<br>Nutrition/hydration status<br>Pain<br>Positioning preferences<br>Posture<br>Pressure<br>Psycho-emotional status<br>Sedation/Decreased consciousness<br>Sensory impairments<br>Shearing/Friction<br>Skeletal deformity<br>Surgical procedures<br>Vascular Disease | Adaptive and durable medical equipment<br>ADL retraining<br>Bony prominence protection<br>Environment/Home/Fall assessment<br>Functional mobility training<br>Incontinence management<br>Moisture management<br>Nutritional support<br>Occupational participation<br>Orthotic management<br>Pain management<br>Patient, family and caregiver education<br>Positioning and pressure relief (devices, techniques and schedule)<br>Safe patient handling equipment<br>Scar management techniques<br>Skin care techniques<br>Sleep hygiene<br>Support surface assessment and modification<br>Therapeutic exercise<br>Wound care management and prevention<br>  Dressing management<br>  Debridement<br>  Lymphedema<br>  Modalities<br>  Negative wound pressure application<br>  Suture removal<br>  Wound closure strips (application and removal) |

Amini, D. (2018). Role of occupational therapy in Wound Management. *The American Journal of Occupational Therapy, 72* (Supplement_2). https://doi.org/10.5014/ajot.2018.72s212
Smith-Gabai, H., & Holm, S. E. (2017). *Occupational therapy in acute care.* AOTA Press.

Figure 27.2). Additional deconditioning management treatment plan options include patient report fatigue measurements (borg rate of perceived exertion), monitoring vitals pre/during/post BADLs and functional mobility (maximal and target heart rate calculations), utilizing metabolic exercise tolerance levels to advance occupational participation and mobility, and incorporating fatigue management and energy conservation techniques.

## Skin Failure

Despite best protective efforts, during acute medical illnesses, the skin as an organ can experience tissue hypoperfusion and pressure injury resulting in skin failure. The resulting tissue destruction, often over areas of bony prominence or pressure areas, can lead to pressure ulcerations that take weeks or months to heal. The integumentary systems can be compromised by other conditions such as diabetes, sepsis, HF, infection, and malnutrition.

Utilizing clinical knowledge of body systems, occupational therapists assess client factors and contexts that can increase risk factors for skin breakdown. Therapists should perform skin assessments during evaluation and when new risk factors have been identified. The frequency of reassessing skin integrity varies depending on the setting characteristics

**CASE EXAMPLE 27.3**   Acute Illness Sequelae

Ms. Z. is stable enough for transfer back to the medical floor of the acute care hospital on day 7. She has persistent hypoactive delirium and is noted to have a new sacral pressure ulcer. She is withdrawn, has poor oral intake, and is dependent on NG tube feedings for nutritional support. The physician consults wound care services and orders a modified barium swallow study, requested, and completed by ST, to determine a safe nutrition care plan.

| OT Treatment | | Comments |
|---|---|---|
| Communication | Expresses wants/needs with difficulty | Withdrawn, avoids eye contact, and intermittently responds to staff |
| Cognition | CAM—Positive<br>BIMS score = 3<br>Orientation: self and location<br>Follows related one-step commands inconsistently with increased time and repetition | BIMS interpretation: This score indicates a severe cognitive impairment, and the subject should be assessed further to be provided with a diagnosis and a health plan.<br>Requires cues to interact with staff throughout the session |
| Vitals | $SPO_2$: 5 L/min via nasal cannula<br>     96% at rest<br>     92% with activity<br>RR:   21 at rest<br>     34 with activity<br>HR:   78 at rest<br>     110 with activity<br>BP:   130/78 at rest<br>     166/88 with activity<br>Pain:  2/10 at rest<br>     5/10 with activity | Activity includes self-care, sitting and standing unsupported at the sink/commode/shower, and ambulatory transfers.<br><br><br><br><br><br><br><br>Knee pain<br>Sacrum and location of right-sided injuries |
| Activity Tolerance | Borg RPE Scale:<br>     7 at rest<br>     15 with activity | Tolerates 30 minutes of activity with multiple decreased rest breaks, breathing techniques, and stable vitals |
| Precautions | Vision<br>Hearing<br>Fall risk<br>Monitor vitals<br>Skin integrity | Adequate with glasses<br>Difficulty in public<br>Recent history of falls |
| Integumentary | Braden score: 7 | Acute Stage 3 sacral wound<br>Improved ecchymosis on the right side of the trunk, hip, and knee as a result of the fall just prior to admission |
| Upper extremity Assessment | RUE: (dominant)<br>     3/5 shoulder<br>     3+/5 elbow and distally<br>     Fair grip strength<br>     Delayed serial opposition<br>LUE:<br>     3+/5 throughout UE<br>     Fair grip strength<br>     Delayed serial opposition | Reports pain during adduction and notable for shoulder elevation during flexion<br>Reports she fell on her right side just before admission<br>Bilateral weakness tremors were observed during functional tasks |
| **Current BADL status** | | |
| Eating | Not assessed due to NPO for modified barium swallow test | |
| Grooming | Partial/moderate assistance | Face and hand washing while sitting unsupported at the edge of bed due to impaired balance, activity tolerance, coordination, and strength. |
| Upper extremity dressing | Partial/moderate assistance | During gown changing for pulling overhead due to impaired balance, limited range of motion, and strength. |

*Continued*

**CASE EXAMPLE 27.3    Acute Illness Sequelae—Cont'd**

| OT Treatment | | Comments |
|---|---|---|
| Lower extremity dressing | Dependent assistance | Threading depends on the left and right leg and donning/doffing socks due to balance, limited range of motion, pain, weakness, and fatigue |
| Footwear | Dependent assistance | |
| Bathing | Not assessed due to bowel incontinence | |
| Toileting | Dependent assistance | Incontinent of bowels during mobility. Task completed supine in the bed with rolling and bridging hips |
| **Current mobility status** | | |
| Assistive device | Gait belt and wheeled walker | |
| Balance | Berg balance score: 5/56 | Berg interpretation: 0 –20 = high fall risk |
| Supine < sit | Substantial/maximal assistance | Anterior scoot to edge of the bed to avoid shearing sacral wound, elevating trunk to the midline and bilateral lower extremity management |
| Sit < > stand | Partial/moderate assistance | From/to edge of bed using bilateral upper extremities requires assistance with concentric and eccentric contraction, hand placement, and sequencing tasks. |
| Assessment | | Ms. Z has impaired functional status in the following areas: self-care, mobility, communication, functional cognition, activity tolerance, hemodynamic stability, and respiratory status. Decreased independence is related to the subsequent deficits: nutritional intake deficits, impaired balance, decreased strength, PICS with delirium, impaired skin integrity, incontinence, pain, delayed coordination, depression, and reduced alertness. |
| | | Ms. Z presents with improved balance and hemodynamic stability with decreased supplemental oxygen needs. She presents more withdrawn, requiring much encouragement for interaction and command following. Considering a new pressure ulcer, pain, poor nutritional intake, and delirium, she fair to guarded rehab potential to remediate deficits. She is unable to safely return home alone with the prior level of support. |
| Recommendations | | Skilled nursing facility with 24/7 care |

On hospital day 10, a percutaneous gastrostomy tube is placed to support nutritional intake. The team prepares for the post-acute transition.

and protocols. For example, patients may only be seen by a wound care specialist two times per week within the acute care setting. Therefore, when implementing skin interventions, best practice recommends initial daily reassessment with increased intervals between assessments to reassess the safety and effectiveness of the interventions provided. Within the post-acute care setting, reassessment may initially be frequent (daily, every 48 hours), then progress weekly, monthly, or quarterly. Skin integrity interventions are best delivered with a collaborative approach. Table 27.9 outlines skin assessment and interventions.

When developing a treatment and prevention of pressure ulcer care plan, the therapist considers 24 hours of support surfaces, patient-preferred occupations/routines/roles, durable medical equipment, and use of a positioning schedule. Standard inpatient equipment includes recliners, armchairs with wooden or metal frames, and electric beds. When placing patients on these surfaces, it is essential to recognize the risk of friction and shearing. Friction refers to the resistance between two surfaces. Friction can help prevent sliding off the edge of the bed or wheelchair; however, increased friction increases the risk of pressure ulcers and shearing. Shearing occurs when the skin surface moves in the opposite direction of the skeletal system. For example, when patients slide down in bed, they risk skin breakdown due to shearing. It's crucial to ensure that patients can regularly weight shift and relieve pressure. The integration of transfer and positioning systems can minimize the number of caregivers needed to reposition or mobilize patients safely, prevent caregiver injuries, improve overall patient comfort during mobilization, and adequately reduce coccyx pressure through supporting side-lying.

OT services are critical to supporting the prevention and treatment of pressure ulceration. Once acquired, wounds are expensive, labor-intensive, and slow to heal. When wounds are significant, deep, or draining or require complex wound

**TABLE 27.10** Occupational Therapy Consultation Indicators

| Reason for Referral | Examples |
|---|---|
| Discharge recommendation | Post-acute inpatient rehabilitation (AR or SNF), home with 24/7 support, home with limited support, home with HHOT |
| Diagnosis specific deficits | CVA, orthopedic, acute respiratory failure |
| Pre- and postprocedural needs | Cardiac (pacemaker/implantable cardioverter-defibrillator [ICD] bypass, valve replacement), abdominal and vascular surgery |
| Debility | Failure to thrive, prolonged hospitalization related deficits, infection-related weakness |
| Safety concerns | Poor adherence to the medical plan of care/medicine management, unsafe home environment, limited support system/resources |
| Cognition impairments | Delirium, exacerbated baseline deficits, and acute deficits |
| Infection-related needs/deficits | Sepsis, pneumonia, surgical, Methicillin-resistant Staphylococcus aureus (MRSA), Clostridioides difficile (C. diff.), urinary tract |
| Poor skin integrity | Pressure ulcers, wounds, lymphedema, edema |

**TABLE 27.11** Examples of Acute Care Cognition Assessments

| Assessment | Administration Time |
|---|---|
| Addenbrooke Cognitive Exam-Mini (Mini-ACE) | 3–7 min |
| Brief Interview for Mental Status (BIMS) | 2–3 min |
| Rowland Universal Dementia Assessment Scale (RUDAS) | <6 min |
| Short Blessed Test (SBT) | 5–10 min |
| Trail making | 5–10 min |

management systems, patients with injuries are often referred to post-acute care for ongoing management. Therapists across the continuum of care should be equipped to support the team.

## Integration of Occupational Therapy in Acute and Post-Acute Care

### Acute Care Occupational Therapy

Acute care therapy services are fast paced and unscheduled, dependent on patient availability and stability, and typically brief in duration and frequency. Patient services may potentially involve many team members and medical services

needed to address the complex needs of the aging patient. Within the acute care setting, the physician, or provider under the guidance of a physician, will place an order for OT evaluation and treatment. Refer to Table 27.10 for examples of common reasons to consult OT.

Evaluation services occur within 24–72 hours of receiving orders. This time frame varies based on environmental factors, such as hospital type, hospital specialties, departmental staffing, and patient census. Hospitals with specialty programs, such as comprehensive stroke or orthopedic centers, will outline specific timeframes to complete evaluations. Acute care assessments and screeners should accommodate the previously mentioned environmental factors. Refer to Table 27.11 for examples of appropriate acute care cognitive assessments.

Due to the complexities of acute care patients, it is difficult to provide comprehensive services within the brief length of stay of 3 to 5 days. Acute care therapists utilize a broad base of medical and physical rehabilitation knowledge, safe patient handling equipment, and clinical reasoning skills to maximize functional independence. When assessing and treating the aging population, therapists must consider the increased difficulty of obtaining optimal occupational performance due to acute/potentially evolving medical crises, performing in a setting of unfamiliar contexts, limited sleep, medication changes, and without notice. Occupational therapists have a unique ability to perform task analysis and skilled observation of performance skills to infer the patient's current functional capacity if it cannot be observed during tasks.

Plans of care (POCs) focus on short-term goals addressing BADLs and in-room functional mobility that can be achieved before discharge. If the patient is not close to their baseline function, long-term goals are addressed in a post-acute care setting. Goals may vary from targeted deficits to an overarching goal that promotes a collaborative approach between the therapist and the patient. The aging population experience a loss of autonomy during hospitalizations. Some examples include being instructed to "not get up," nonselect meals or house trays, inability to shower, limited clothing options, cold room temperatures, not having access to glasses or hearing aids, and changes in sleep/wake/medication schedules to accommodate the medical team and services. By identifying the patient's intrinsic motivators and cultural contexts, the therapist can develop a POC that engages the patient while demonstrating tolerance for therapy and rehab potential.

Acute care discharge planning is a fluid process that begins once the medical staff assesses the patient. Before OT services are consulted, the medical team has evaluated the expected length of stay and has anticipated the possibility of requiring therapy services. Occupational therapists begin to plan for discharge by completing the occupational profile during the evaluation. Considering the previously outlined acute setting and impacts on the aging population, the patient may be an unreliable historian. Additionally, the electronic health record (EHR) will often reflect an inaccurate prior residence of "patient resides in an SNF" or "patient resides in a retirement home." This creates challenges in obtaining an accurate previous level of function (PLOF) from the patient and the EHR. To discharge plan appropriately, Occupational Therapists need to get an accurate PLOF from family and caregivers. Demonstrating to the patient that you connected with their family and caregivers to learn about the patient's PLOF, lifestyle, preferences, and habits/routines can be pivotable to establishing a working and trusting relationship. Once this information is obtained, it becomes a permanent part of the record that will be referred to by the acute care medical team during future hospital admissions and is passed along to the next level of care. Obtaining an accurate and detailed PLOF helps define the OT role with the patient and family/caregiver, promotes awareness of the OT profession, and adds value to the OT role within the interdisciplinary team.

Discharge recommendations in the acute care setting can change due to the evolving patient presentation, insurance coverage, and other social/environmental factors. During treatments, therapists constantly evaluate discharge disposition appropriateness, equipment needs, and home modifications. Discharge planning requires many team members and background processes; therefore, initial recommendations and changes require efficient and effective communication. This can be achieved via rounding, EHR documentation, EHR chat functions, floor huddles, and during nursing hand-off. Clinicians may utilize Table 27.1 (Post-Acute Care Setting Characteristics) and Figure 27.4 (Discharge Planning Decision Tree) as resources for determining discharge recommendations.

## Post-Acute Care Occupational Therapy

Within the post-acute care setting, the integration of OT services may fluctuate. LTACH facilities are an extension of the acute care service line and mimic the care provided in the acute care setting. If the patient received Acute care OT, the patient would continue to receive services. However, the patient may be admitted without the functional capacity to participate in therapy. The medical plan of care may defer treatment until the patient can meaningfully participate, tolerate, and benefit from the services provided. Acute care and LTACH therapy services have similar service delivery models, though the care plans are the primary difference. LTACH care plans incorporate long-term and short-term goals and allow for longer durations and higher therapy frequencies of OT services.

Admission to IRFs and SNFs typically includes therapy orders via the admitting physician and is based on the recommendations of the acute care therapists. The patient's needs specify therapy plans of care (duration, frequency, goals). In both IRF and SNF settings, patients are provided with a therapy schedule for the day that details the time and duration of therapy. The POC is discussed at team meetings to promote an interdisciplinary approach. This process allows the health-care team, individual therapist, and patient to develop a comprehensive plan of care, establish patient goals, ensure patient availability/preparedness, issue and educate patient/family/caregiver regarding any required equipment, incorporate family/caregivers for

training/education, and provide home safety evaluations as indicated. Patient access to post-acute inpatient therapy services is dependent on patient progress, tolerance, and insurance coverage. HHOT services may be integrated into the POC in various ways, such as after a hospitalization or doctor's visit or perhaps as part of the HHRN/HHPT observation. The HHOT POC accommodates two to three visits per week for three to four weeks, depending on the patient's needs and wants. Therefore the POC must allow for goal attainment within the defined time. If this does not occur, the therapist is responsible for attempting to procure additional insurance authorization for further treatment to meet the patient's POC.

Post-Acute care focuses on discharge planning; however, most of the service provided focuses on habilitation, rehabilitation, and restoration of function for the most optimal functional status and safest discharge plan. Within the LTACH, IRF, and SNF settings, patients often receive services from other therapy service lines, nursing, respiratory, and other medical care. HHOT may or may not include additional services. HHOT plans of care focus on safety assessments, home modifications, durable medical equipment and/or adaptive equipment recommendations, rehabilitation and restoration of functional status, and family/caregiver training. Discharge disposition assistance/planning is not commonly part of HH services; however, it may be indicated when the home environment is unsafe.

Occupational therapists need to consider age-related changes that have influenced the reason for admission. Such factors for consideration include evolving changes in cognition, sensory (vision, hearing, dual sensory loss), sleep patterns, mood (depression, anxiety), musculoskeletal, cardiovascular, immunologic, and respiratory systems. Please refer to the relevant chapters to find more details regarding age-related changes. Occupational Therapists are faced with a progressive aging process in conjunction with acute changes. During this acute phase patients present at varied phases of recovery with potentially additional hospital acquired complications.

## Palliative Medicine: Palliative Care (PC) and Hospice Services

Palliative medicine has been recently redefined by the International Association for Hospice and Palliative Medicine. PC is the "active, holistic care of individuals across all ages with serious health-related suffering due to severe illness, especially those near the end of life (EOL). It aims to improve patients' quality of life, as well as families and caregivers" (IAHPC. Global Consensus based palliative care definition, 2018). PC is a treatment approach that focuses on managing symptoms, psychological support, and disease education (Phongtankuel et al., 2018). It prioritizes the reduction of burdensome or distressing symptoms when curative measures are difficult or unlikely to be achieved.

Palliative medicine, PC, and hospice services are most effective when delivered in collaboration with other medical providers and aligned with diagnosis, prognosis, and/or goals

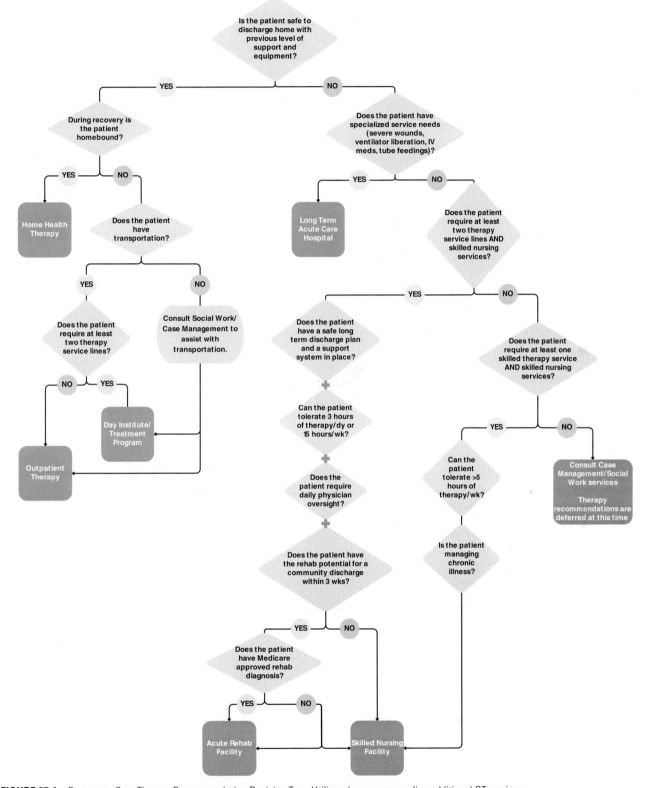

**FIGURE 27.4**    Post-acute Care Therapy Recommendation Decision Tree. Utilize when recommending additional OT servicese.

## CASE EXAMPLE 27.4   Post-Acute Care in SNF

Ms. Z is admitted to a skilled nursing facility where she gets 1–2 hours per day of PT, OT, and ST. Nursing provides daily wound care treatments. She requires enteral feeding via percutaneous gastrostomy tube, as she continues to show limited interest in taking food by mouth. Language is limited to one- to two-word responses to questions. A trial of antidepressant medication intended to improve mood and stimulate appetite does not provide the desired outcome. The decubitus ulcer is slowly healing due to poor nutritional intake, dependency on pressure relief, persistent fatigue, and urinary and bowel incontinence. The nursing and medical staff have stabilized Ms. Z's BP and diabetes. During the weekly care plan meeting the following details are discussed with the patient, family and treatment team.

| OT Treatment | | Comments |
|---|---|---|
| Communication | Expresses wants/needs inconsistently | Responds to one- to two-word responses to questions only |
| Cognition | BIMS score = 9<br>Orientation: self, staff, and situation<br>Follows related two-step commands consistently with increased time and repetition. | BIMS interpretation: This score indicates a severe cognitive impairment, and the subject should be assessed further to be provided with a diagnosis and a health plan. |
| Vitals | $SPO_2$: 2 L/min via nasal cannula<br>   96% at rest<br>   93% with activity<br>RR:  19 at rest<br>   28 with activity<br>HR:  68 at rest<br>   99 with activity<br>BP:  127/78 at rest<br>   132/82 with activity<br>Pain: 4/10 at rest<br>   8/10 with activity | Activity includes self-care sitting supported and unsupported at the edge of the bed, wheelchair, and bedside chair.<br>Knee pain<br>Sacrum and location of right-sided injuries |
| Activity tolerance | Borg RPE scale:<br>   6 at rest<br>   13 with activity | Tolerates 30 minutes of activity with multiple decreased rest breaks, breathing techniques, and stable vitals |
| Precautions | Vision<br>Hearing<br>Fall risk<br>Monitor vitals<br>Skin integrity | Adequate with glasses<br>Difficulty in therapy gym/dining room<br>Recent history of falls |
| Integumentary | Braden score: 9 | Acute stage 1 sacral wound.<br>Minimal ecchymosis on the right side of the trunk, hip, and knee resulted from the fall just before admission |
| UE assessment | RUE: (dominant)<br>   3+/5 shoulder<br>   4/5 elbow and distally<br>   Good grip strength<br>LUE:<br>   4/5 throughout UE<br>   Good grip strength | Improved bilateral upper extremity strength with a home exercise plan and handheld weights. Reports chronic RUE shoulder pain in all joints/planes |
| **Current BADL status** | | |
| Eating | Not assessed due to lack of interest | |
| Grooming | Setup or clean-up assistance | Oral hygiene, face and hand washing while sitting supported in a wheelchair at sink due to generalized weakness, pain, and limited range of motion |
| UE dressing | Partial/moderate assistance | Threading RUE, pulling down shirt and fasteners PRN due to limited range of motion, activity tolerance, and strength |

**CASE EXAMPLE 27.4**   Post-Acute Care in SNF

| OT Treatment | | Comments |
|---|---|---|
| LE dressing | Partial/moderate assistance | Threading pants onto left and right leg and donning/doffing socks due to balance, limited range of motion, pain, weakness, and fatigue |
| Footwear | Partial/moderate assistance | |
| Bathing | Partial/moderate assistance | Washing lower portion of lower extremities including feet, balance when standing and reaching for objects |
| Toileting | Partial/moderate assistance | Posterior hygiene, balance when standing, and intermittent assist with pulling underwear over hips |
| **Current mobility status** | | |
| Assistive device | Gait belt, wheelchair, and wheeled walker | |
| Balance | Berg Balance Score: 15/56 | Berg interpretation: 0–20 = high fall risk |
| Supine < > sit | Setup or clean-up assistance | Assist for manipulation of the hospital bed and linen management |
| Sit < > stand | Partial/moderate assistance | From/to surfaces using bilateral upper extremities requires assistance with concentric and eccentric contraction |
| Commode transfers | Partial/moderate assistance | From/to commode using bilateral upper extremities, grab bars, raised commode, and wheelchair. Requires assistance with concentric and eccentric contraction |
| Bed < > chair transfers | Partial/moderate assistance | Ambulatory transfer to a wheelchair. Assist needed for balance, safety awareness, and safe use of a wheeled walker |
| Assessment | Ms. Z has impaired functional status in the following areas: self-care, mobility, communication, functional cognition, activity tolerance, and respiratory status. Decreased independence is related to the subsequent deficits: nutritional intake, impaired balance, decreased strength, PICS with delirium, impaired skin integrity, incontinence, pain, depression, and fatigue. | |
| | Ms. Z presents with improvements in seated activity tolerance, skin integrity, cognition, balance, and mobility. She continues to require skilled services to address pressure ulcers, pain management, limited nutritional intake, and cognitive impairments. Her rehabilitation progress has plateaued without rehabilitation to baseline function. Ms. does not have the support needed to return to the community. | |
| Recommendations | Extended care with 24/7 care and safe patient handling equipment. | |

After 18 days (about 2½ weeks) of treatment, she continues to require 24/7 support for self-care, mobility, wound care, balance, cognition, and medication management. Her rehab progress has plateaued, and insurance coverage for ongoing SNF care is exhausted

of care discussion. Typically, the overseeing medical provider will order a palliative medicine consultation for recommendations to augment the current care plan. PC can help with patient-centered use of medical and health-care services by reducing unwanted or unnecessary treatment of illness. This shifts the focus towards quality of life, sustaining community-based care, reducing acute exacerbation, and avoiding hospital admissions. Palliative medicine consults are commonly initiated for chronic conditions/diagnosis such as congestive HF, chronic pulmonary diseases, chronic kidney disease, cancer, and progressive neurological disorders, including Parkinson's disease and dementia.

In many cases, PC is initiated in the hospital by a consultative service when individuals with chronic progressive illness face recurrent or new severe health conditions. However, PC can be provided in any health-care setting, including the home. Medicare, Medicaid, and commercial health insurance policies may cover the services of PC programs outside of the hospital. These programs are often delivered by a home health-care agency.

A palliative consultation initiates goals of care conversations that elicit patient and family treatment preferences, and identifies priorities for further medical management. Based on the outcomes of these conversations, PC practitioners may recommend both curative and comfort based care. When appropriate, PC discussions may introduce hospice as an additional health-care benefit for those who meet or may soon meet the hospice entry criteria. To qualify for hospice services it must be determined that the patient has a terminal illness with expected mortality < 6 months of initiation of services. Hospice services will initiate the same services as PC; however, the focus of services is non-curative and comfort based without plans to return to the hospital and receive curative measures. Medical management is transferred to the hospice team, as they are the EOL care specialists. PC and hospice are commonly initiated for chronic conditions such as congestive HF, chronic pulmonary diseases, chronic kidney disease, cancer, and progressive neurological disorders, including Parkinson's disease and dementia.

Utilizing the OT Practice Framework, treatment approaches associated with palliative medicine (PC and hospice) focus on the following:

- Maintenance/preservation of performance skills and patterns required for participation in meaningful occupations and activities
- Modification/compensation/adaptation of the following:
  - contexts (cultural, personal, temporal, virtual)

- environments (physical and social)
- activity demands
- Prevention of disability that may cause barriers to occupation participation

Occupational therapists focused on EOL identify intrinsic values to determine valued occupations and then implement a care plan that emphasizes the patient's identity, relationships, and values. Examples of EOL care plan goals may be to minimize the side effects of increasing dependency and inactivity, foster relationships/roles, and remain in the preferred living environment with preferred caregivers. Due to palliative medicine including curative services via PC, OT treatment approaches include forming new occupations and rehabilitation of existing occupational performance skills.

Treatment interventions may not be different from the traditional health-care model; however, the focus is vastly different as the purpose, and the perspective of the interventions are targeted with the knowledge of expected EOL. For example, preparing meals for the family may be a preferred occupation, and the patient's goal is to gift family members a recipe book before EOL. This example highlights how the purpose and perspective of the meal preparation are the driving force of the plan of care.

---

**CASE EXAMPLE 27.5** Goals of Care Transition

Ms. Z's functional status has plateaued. She remains wheelchair dependent for mobility. Her wound has not fully healed, and her family cannot provide 24-hour care and support for her in their home. Ms. Z completed the skilled rehabilitation period, and the family decided she would remain in the long-term care unit at the facility. Her cognitive status has not returned to the prior level of functioning, and she scores in the moderate-severe range for her dementia diagnosis. The family wishes to enroll her in hospice care,

given her dementia prognosis. During the hospice evaluation Ms. Z and family reported the desire to be able to sit up in a wheelchair in preparation for end of life visiting with family and friends. The family report that prior to decline Ms. Z never missed her hair appointments and would like to ensure she has access to the facility salon in order to maintain her baseline self care routine. Hospice has consulted facility Occupational Therapist to assist Ms. Z with her end of life goals.

| Occupational Therapy Hospice Evaluation Components | | Comments |
|---|---|---|
| Primary concerns | Pain:<br>0/10 at rest<br>7/10 with activity | Activity includes<br>prolonged sitting |
| Hospice Goals | Hair care at facility salon<br>Sitting upright with pain management | Two times per week<br>During family/friend<br>EOL visitation |
| Objective | Neck ROM:<br>Flexion: 10 degrees<br>Extension: 5 degrees<br>Right rotation: 45 degrees<br>Left rotation: 45 degrees<br>Pressure mapping completed.<br>Wheelchair fitting completed to accommodate salon mobility needs | |
| Intervention | Roho Cushion issued<br>Tilt-in-space wheelchair issued with head support, trunk supports, and elevated armrests | |
| Care Plan | Ms. Z will tolerate hairdressing appointments two times per week with 0/10 pain in order to maintain personal hygiene routine.<br>Ms. Z will tolerate sitting in a wheelchair for < 60 minutes with 0/10 pain in order to visit with family/friends. | |
| Recommendations | Continued skilled OT services 1 time per week to assess tolerance for sitting during family visits and mobility needed for salon appointments. | |

## SUMMARY

In the United States, the ACA and the IMPACT Act have identified domains inherent to the OT practice. The elderly population values their identity, routines, and roles. Research demonstrates that consulting OT services for the elderly will maximize their functional status, self-care, and mobility; prevent hospitalizations; reduce the risk for infection; prevent falls; and reduce the risk of cognitive impairments.

OT is vital in working with older adults in acute and post-acute settings. OT evaluations and assessments provide essential information in determining baseline function, identifying current functional status and safety concerns, and making recommendations for equipment needs and the most appropriate next level of care. As occupational therapists, we want to ensure we provide patients with care plans and recommendations that promote autonomy. Yet, we need to find those that best suit them and will help increase their level of independence and improve their quality of life.

As previously mentioned, Medicare beneficiaries continue to rise and require complex medical care. Considering that most of the post-acute care services are provided to the elderly population, this reinforces the need for consulting occupational therapists as preventative versus reactive measures. Occupational therapists have the knowledge and skills to maximize independence and maintain quality of life while enabling individuals to remain community-based for as long as possible.

*The complete listing of the Bibliography and Chapter Questions and Answers are available in the accompanying enhanced eBook version included with the print purchase of this textbook. Visit Elsevier eBooks+ (eBooks.Health.Elsevier.com) to access this content.*

# CHAPTER 28

# Residential and Skilled Care

*Sanetta Du Toit, PhD, MOT, MSc, Molly M. Perkins, PhD, FGSA, Michael Lepore, PhD,*
*Margaret A. Perkinson, PhD, FGSA, FAGHE, FSfAA, and David D. Rockemann, MS, NHA*

## CHAPTER OUTLINE

## OBJECTIVES

- Provide an overview of nursing homes, assisted living (AL) communities, and continuing care retirement communities (CCRCs) and where they fit in long-term care.
- Discuss the role of occupational therapists in different levels of residential long-term care.
- Envision innovative, transformative long-term care practice.

Populations of older people and younger people with disabilities and with neurocognitive disorders are growing nationally and globally, and the demand for care needed by these populations is expanding. In the United States, the number of older people with severe disabilities or major neurocognitive disorders is projected to increase more than threefold in 50 years, from 6.3 to 15.7 million from 2015 to 2065 (Favreault & Dey, 2015).

This chapter examines a variety of supportive residential settings that provide a wide range of long-term services and supports and skilled nursing care. These settings are key features of our health-care infrastructure and important providers of both housing and health and social services. Nursing homes (NHs), assisted living (AL) communities, and continuing care retirement communities (CCRCs) are common types of long-term care settings. Neurocognitive disorders are prevalent; many of these settings include physical environments and staff committed to caring for people living with them.

### The Role of Occupational Therapists in Long-Term Aged Care Settings

Reflecting changes in the field as a whole, occupational therapy practice within long-term care has undergone a range of paradigm shifts, moving from a socially oriented to a more medically oriented model over the course of the twentieth century, with goals to correct and/or to cure (Briller et al., 2016). It has now shifted back to a more holistic approach toward both occupational therapy education and occupational therapy practice. Transformative trends in long-term-care practice reflect a renewed focus on individualized occupational and social engagement opportunities to support resident well-being and reinforce a client-centered approach embedded in the Culture Change philosophy. The occupational therapy holistic approach ensures that barriers and enablers to participation are taken into account by correcting and compensating for individual deficits or lost function through specific therapeutic interventions or assistive devices. In addition, given the growing awareness of today's practitioners of cultural, contextual, economic, and political influences on occupational and social engagement, this chapter considers long-term care settings and the individual residents within them as the targets of interest.

Clients of occupational therapy as defined by American Occupational Therapy Association (AOTA, 2021, p. 1) are classified as "persons (including those involved in care of a client), groups (collections of individuals having shared characteristics or a common or shared purpose; e.g., family members, workers, people with similar interests or occupational challenges [such as older adults living in long-term care settings]), and populations (aggregates of people with common attributes such as contexts, characteristics, or concerns, including health risks." This chapter approaches long-term care settings as collective systems and considers how occupational therapy can promote culture change on an organizational level.

However, occupational therapy practice and our holistic approach are often negatively impacted by the context in which services are rendered. Many students transitioning into novice practitioner status find this divide between the philosophy of occupational therapy and the limitations on practice input to be quite disconcerting. Calderone et al. (2022) note that funding sources constrain practice, contribute to the disabling of residents, and create challenges for occupational

therapists working in this sector. Occupational therapy training should empower students as future practitioners to act as change agents in aged care settings (Du Toit et al., 2018) and consider our scope of input beyond limitations imposed by funding models.

Table 28.1, as developed by Van der Merwe-Rauch and Visser (2019), provides an overview of factors on micro, meso, and macro levels that could potentially impact the roles in which an occupational therapist engages. These factors are discussed separately to alert future practitioners in long-term care to factors that may affect the design and delivery of care for older adults, notwithstanding the resident's functional ability. On a macro level, occupational therapists should acknowledge their own, individual contextual factors and personal values as change agents and how their worldview impacts their practice. For example, see how therapeutic use of self (Scaffa & Reitz, 2014, in AOTA, 2020; Taylor, 2020) as an integral part of the Occupational Therapy Practice Framework (OTPF; AOTA, 2020) and their portrayal of empathy and intentionality as part of the intervention process could be linked to therapists' cultural background, spiritual beliefs, and/or previous life experiences.

On a meso level, real-world dimensions associated with international guiding bodies (e.g., the World Federation for Occupational Therapists) and national bodies (e.g., ACOTE in the United States) provide international training standards in addition to country-specific accreditation standards outlining minimum competencies for licensure examination. These standards provide the overarching skill level expected from entry-level therapists transitioning into practice.

**TABLE 28.1**  Factors Influencing the Roles of Occupational Therapists Within Practice Settings

| MACRO LEVEL: Individual Contextual Indicators | | | | |
|---|---|---|---|---|
| Cultural, political, historical, geographical, socio-economic, educational, ecological, epidemiological, demographic | | | | |
| | Governing structures | Governing scrips | Contexts of practice | Role/s of OTs |
| MESO LEVEL Real world dimensions | International level E.g., WHO; WFOT; UN | Types E.g., legislation; policies procedures; programs; guidelines; repots; frameworks | Settings E.g., hospital, school, clinic; residential care; community | Clinician Advocate Educator Student Community Facilitator |
| | National level E.g., ACOTE; AOTA | Examples of categories E.g., ethics; disability; health systems, mental health; aged care; community care | Clients E.g., individual, group,community, population | Researcher Interprofessional team member Mentor |
| **OT Toolbox** | | | | |
| MICRO LEVEL Theoretical dimensions | Therapeutic Frames of Reference | E.g., Bio-mechanical; Neurophysiological; Senso-motor; Behavioral; Psychodynamic; Educational; CBD | | |
| | Overarching theories models & skills | Occupational justice, OTPF, MOHO, CMOP, OPM-A, KAWA, PEOP Assessments, interventions & EBP | | |
| | Paradigm | Wellness/ ill-health; Humans as occupational beings | | |

From Van der Merwe-Rauch, T., & Visser, M. M. (2019). *A legislation-policy-framework for occupational therapy.* Bloemfontein, South Africa: University of The Free State. Conceptual idea developed by Tania vd Merwe & Marietta Visser, UFS 2019. *ACOTE,* Accreditation council for occupational therapy education; *AOTA,* American occupational therapy association; *CMOP,* Canadian model of occupational performance; *EBP,* evidence-based practice; *MOHO,* model of human occupation; *OPM(A),* occupational performance model australia; *OTPF,* occupational therapy practice framework; *PEOP,* person-environment-occupation-performance model; *UN,* United Nations; *WFOT,* world federation of occupational therapy; *WHO,* world health organization.

Furthermore, the context of occupational therapy practice on a meso level will also dictate the range of roles occupational therapists can engage within their service context. Roles should therefore not only be associated with input focused on individuals (AOTA, 2020), but long-term care settings should be recognized as a collective, an important emerging area of practice within long-term care (Du Toit et al., 2019; Du Toit, Fitch, et al., 2021; Morgan-Brown et al., 2019). Table 28.2 describes a variety of roles and programs occupational therapists could engage in within long-term aged care—these range from very traditional roles to innovative programs where occupational therapists capitalize on the understanding of humans as occupational beings and find context-specific ways to promote meaningful engagement. (See Case Study 28.1.)

According to the Accreditation Council for Occupational Therapy Education (ACOTE, 2018, p. 2), practitioners should be able to "plan and apply evidence based occupational therapy interventions to address the physical, cognitive, functional cognitive, psychosocial, sensory, and other aspects of performance in a variety of contexts and environments to support engagement in everyday life activities" that affect health, well-being, and quality of life, as informed by the OTPF. In long-term care, prioritizing opportunities for older adults to engage meaningfully in occupations that support their well-being and add to their perceived quality of health, rather than, or in addition to, promoting functional participation, needs careful consideration.

In circumstances where complex and multiple conditions including frailty, advanced dementia, or end-of-life impact residents' well-being, functional outcomes become secondary to engagement in shared moments of joy. The occupational therapy intervention focus shifts to engagement in the process of doing, and not the outcome of the doing (Hitch et al., 2014), ensuring that interdependence and co-occupation are integral to residents experiencing pleasure and belonging (Du Toit & Buchanan, 2018). For example, occupational therapists are often involved in adapting the environment to ensure that older adults can be independent in finding their way (see examples in Table 28.2), but could also support other initiatives where small changes to staff attire could enable engagement. A chef in a town in a regional area of Australia realized that it was not as such COVID-19 face masks that deterred residents from recognizing staff, but due to postural changes and the use of mobility aids, residents more often saw shoes of people walking by. By wearing red shoes, residents started calling out to him when he approached and assisted in identifying him (Du Toit, Wales et al., 2021) (Fig. 28.1).

As a profession, occupational therapy is advancing practice for transformative long-term care, but the process is far from over. During training, occupational therapy students need to critically consider their "Occupational Therapy Toolbox," associated with theoretical dimensions on a micro level (see Table 28.1), and question to what extent traditional views of occupational participation serve the targeted clientele. Besides reconsidering the NH/residential care environment as a collective, Hammell (2004a, 2004b, 2009) and Pierce (2001a, 2001b, 2003, 2014) challenge us to think about all occupations, or what people do with their time, and how that relates to meeting the perceived needs of a person. So, rather than categorizing occupations as leisure, self-care, work, and rest, a person's perception of benefit from the engagement (Hammell, 2009), or the appeal of that engagement and its response to a person's need for experiencing restoration, pleasure or productivity is critical (Pierce 2001a, 2001b, 2003, 2014). Case examples (Case Studies 28.1 and 28.2) provide examples of innovative age care programs based on students' involvement in role emerging clinical placements.

To make a contribution in long-term care settings that prevents declining health and poor quality of life, occupational therapists need to analyze how the systems and structures could limit engagement in occupations. (See also anthropological ethnographic studies of long-term care settings; Perkinson, 2019; Stafford, 2003.) Emerging areas of practice contribute updates to our "Occupational Therapy toolbox" (McColl & Stewart, 2003) to support culture change and quality of care within long-term care settings (Du Toit et al., 2019). Stimulus-poor physical and social environments in nursing facilities and residential care do not maximize residents' opportunity for occupational and social engagement (Hammell & Iwama, 2012; Knight & Mellor, 2007). When assessing long-term care settings as a collective or microcommunity (Du Toit et al., 2019; Morgan-Brown et al., 2019), occupational therapists could provide feedback and recommendations to the benefit of residents, staff, relatives, and volunteers on how they can collectively support culture change that improves person-centered care approaches. For example, research in Ireland found that people living with dementia are disengaged for 82.73% of time they spend in a communal sitting room (Morgan-Brown & Brangan, 2016).

## CASE STUDY 28.1

It is more than 20 years since the global culture change movement toward person-centered and relationship-focused care in residential care settings commenced, as advocated by the Culture Change Movement. Integration of occupational therapy philosophy with culture change approaches focus on resident enhanced well-being and enablement, deinstitutionalizing long-term care facilities, and especially "eliminating the three plagues of loneliness, helplessness, and boredom" (Power et al., 2010). Students are guided to reformulate intervention outcomes that focus on reducing what is often termed as "challenging behaviors" to addressing residents' desire to connect and belong (Du Toit et al., 2019). As Excerpt 28.1 highlights, clients' meaningful engagement is influenced by their preferences and immediate situation.

**TABLE 28.2** Examples of Occupational Therapy Input and Emerging Roles in Long-Term Aged Care

| | Occupational Therapy Focus in Long-Term Aged Care | Considerations | Source |
|---|---|---|---|
| **Person** | Re-ablement | Extending traditional occupational therapy roles to support:<br>• Identify residents who require specialized occupational therapy intervention.<br>• Establish a priority system to assess individual needs using specialist occupational therapy assessments, including seating, pressure care, environmental modifications, occupational and social engagement.<br>• Identify the overlapping needs of individual residents in order to make recommendations that will support groups of individuals. | Dorrestein and Hocking (2010) |
| | Assessing volition to promote occupational engagement | • Volitional expression is associated with how lived experiences and dynamics between the social environment and the individual are acknowledged and promoted by the occupational therapist.<br>• The definition of meaningful occupation needs to be adapted to reflect the preferences of the persons with dementia over time.<br>• The social environment is potent and a key element to impact volition. | Raber et al. (2010) |
| | Falls prevention | • Falls in long-term care settings are "very complex and difficult to prevent. Attention should be given to the needs of recently admitted residents and management of the facility environment." | Mackenzie & Byles (2018, p. 738) |
| | Promoting physical and mental well-being in advice to care staff | • "Restraint reduction—identifying positioning methods and alternatives to avoid or minimize the use of chemical and physical restraints to manage challenging behaviors.<br>• Contracture management, through splinting and/or other methods—to maintain range of motion and assist in preventing the development or progression of deformities due to lack of movement." | AOTA (2015, p. 2) |
| **Environment** | Assessing the whole room environment to promote social and occupational engagement (ATOSE) | • Unmet needs of people with dementia should be viewed as human rights and citizenship issues.<br>• Closer proximity in sitting rooms leads to more spontaneous interaction between staff and residents.<br>• Improved organizational structures and guidelines would support staff to promote engagement with residents.<br>• Occupational therapists could equip staff on how to facilitate engagement activities. | Morgan-Brown et al. (2019) |
| | Assessing the whole room environment to promote social and occupational engagement (REIS) | • The organizational, physical, and social environment within nursing home settings greatly influence residents' sense of autonomy, choice and control, and their ability to engage in meaningful occupations.<br>• Assessment outcomes reflect the quality of person-centered approaches and the potential role of occupational therapists to promote opportunities for meaningful occupational engagement.<br>• Barriers to assessment implementation include administration time, personal characteristics of residents, and limited resources to implement action recommendations. | Du Toit, Fitch, et al. (2021) |
| | Providing staff training to support person-centered care (institutional environment—peers) | • Peer support is the most valued aspect of the Peer Enable Program (PEP) and can be facilitated by occupational therapists.<br>• Peer support was identified as central to the advantages encountered by the facilitators for their role as mentors, for attendees for their role as peer leaders, and for staff members involved as team members of the PEP process at facilities.<br>• Peer support promotes collaboration among attendees, supports development of their occupational identities as transformational leaders, and creates communities of practice with potential to sustain advances in person centered practice. | Du Toit et al. (2019) |

*Continued*

**TABLE 28.2** Examples of Occupational Therapy Input and Emerging Roles in Long-Term Aged Care—Cont'd

| Occupational Therapy Focus in Long-Term Aged Care | Considerations | Source |
|---|---|---|
| Providing staff training to support person-centered care (institutional environment-management) | • Burnout of caregivers is combatted when empowerment, education, emotional support, and opportunities for creative engagement are facilitated.<br>• Organizational culture guides the behavior of the caregivers—therefore, caregivers operate within the boundaries of that culture and are unlikely to take initiative.<br>• Organizational structures often undermine and belittle the insight of the caregivers.<br>• Authoritarian leadership takes all control away from the caregivers. | Thomas et al. (2014) |
| Accessible design for people with dementia | Accessible design supports dignity and independence. Consider:<br>• Height of and lay-out of signage and using written and pictorial cues<br>• Color distinction between toilet bowl, floor and wall<br>• Accessible toilet paper<br>• When mirrors become a cause of distress | Marshall (2019) |
| *Occupation* | | |
| Introducing assistive technology to promote meaningful engagement | • The role and potential of new technologies to enhance meaningful engagement for those with dementia should focus on creating human-to-human interactions while taking individual preference and person-centered principles into account. | Neal et al. (2020) |
| Providing insights on how cultural diversity impacts meaningful engagement | • Occupational deprivation will prevail and person-centered care will not be fully addressed if opportunities for growth and engagement for residents with moderate to advanced dementia are not extended beyond their life history. These older adults are people not only with a past, but also have preferences regarding the present and the future.<br>• Occupational therapists should focus intervention in nursing homes to promote a culture of collaborative care that supports understanding the resident as a person with a past, present and future. | McGrath et al. (2021) |
| Adapting the long-term care environment | "There is substantial evidence on the influence of unit size, spatial layout, homelike character, sensory stimulation, and environmental characteristics of social spaces on residents' behaviors and well-being in care facilities." | Chaudhury et al. (2018) |
| Promoting occupational justice through choice and autonomy of residents | • Physical and mental health and maintenance of identity is achieved through occupational roles associated with leisure engagement<br>• Enabling "access to leisure activities by identifying clients' interests and removing physical and social barriers that impede performance." | Causey-Upton (2015) |
| Redefining occupational engagement | Considering participation and engagement based on experienced-based categories of occupation:<br>• Time-killing occupations. Least engaging activities—e.g., doing things to pass the time, like listening to the radio.<br>• Basic occupations—e.g., things you need to do that are associated with habits and routines, like letting the dog out first thing in the morning.<br>• Social occupations—e.g., being with people at organized events like attending the Men's Shed weekly, or a spontaneous event like going to lunch with friends.<br>• Regular occupations—e.g. daily walks or attending church once a week.<br>• Irregular occupations—e.g. going to see a ballet at the theatre.<br>• Engaging occupations. Necessary and significant components to enhance personal well-being—e.g., volunteering or looking after grandchildren. | Jonsson (2008) |

These findings are consistent with earlier research emphasizing many barriers to creating opportunities for meaningful engagement (e.g., stimulating daytime activities or socialization) (Hancock et al., 2006).

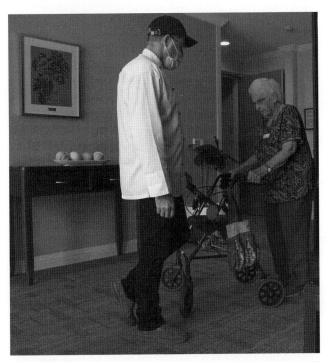

**FIGURE 28.1**   The Red Shoe Connection. (Source: private picture, with permission.)

## Occupational Therapy Assessments of the Environment of Residential Care

### The Assessment Tool for Occupational and Social Engagement

In addition to ethnographic studies, occupational-based assessments to evaluate the facility as a whole environment provide numeric data to inform training and support to enhance the care culture of the facility. The Assessment Tool for Occupational and Social Engagement (ATOSE) evaluates the engagement levels of clients living with advanced

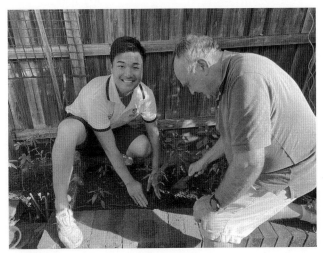

**FIGURE 28.2**   Placement Student and Nursing Home Resident—Finding Ways to Meaningfully Engage. (Source: Tsz Wang Rohan Lai and Anthony Hodson (Image credit Jacky Lai).)

---

### EXCERPT 28.1

*A shared belonging by Tsz Wang Rohan Lai*
Source: Australian Ageing Agenda, July–August 2021, p. 18–19

*"I am a fourth [final]-year undergraduate occupational therapy student…[who] completed my fourth placement at a residential aged care facility…Over the eight-week placement, twice a week I met Hans\**
*\*Not their real name, who preferred engaging in the backyard of the secure dementia care unit. Hans has a good sense of humour…and we shared many funny moments. Meaningful social engagement with Hans ranged from short chats, sharing thoughts and perspectives, looking at the sky or watching people walking by…even though Hans never remembered my name, we shared a camaraderie and it never felt awkward to sit together without talking…[Hans] understood that he could not leave the facility, but what others might describe as a place of confinement, he saw as utopia. He said to me that: 'There is no better place to enjoy retirement than here.' I visited the facility six weeks after my placement and surprisingly found that Hans still recognized me…We sat in the backyard and chatted for an hour like we used to do. 'Good to see you again, my friend,' he said when I had to leave. Other students take away clinical knowledge or skills from a placement, but I left with a new friend"* (Fig. 28.2).

*\*Not their real name*

---

### CASE STUDY 28.2

In an attempt to address ageism and stereotyping within the future health-care workforce (Lovell, 2006), an Intergenerational Live-In Student Project was introduced at the Faculty of Health Sciences at the University of Sydney. Similar projects report promoting a sense of value and belonging for the older adults, while students expressed greater respect and appreciation for residents, as well as developing confidence in interaction and communication (Annear et al., 2017; Kim & Lee, 2018). Students volunteered 30 hours per month in exchange for free accommodation. In addition to valuing their older neighbors as friends, and even as quasi-kin, various student spin-off projects emerged. Figure 28.3 provides two examples of the creativity of Joshua Wan, a live-in student, who captured life history work in unique ways.

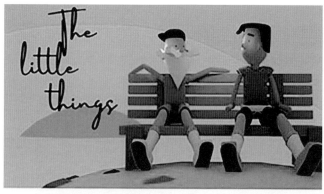

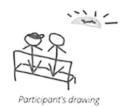

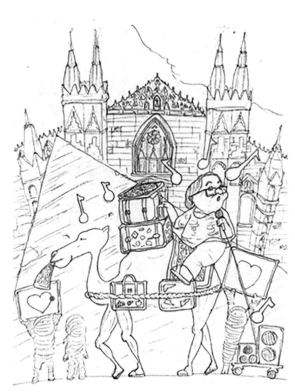

**FIGURE 28.3**    Sketch illustrating a resident's life history and Student's reflections on placement. (Source: Joshua Wan.)

dementia (Morgan-Brown & Brangan, 2016; Morgan-Brown et al., 2019). This observational tool records snapshots of the whole-room environment at 5-minute intervals. The ATOSE categorizes the behavior of all persons (i.e., residents, staff, and visitors) in a communal space of a care environment into engaged or nonengaged behaviors (Morgan-Brown & Brangan, 2016; Morgan-Brown et al., 2019). Engaged behaviors are further grouped into interactive occupation, social engagement, and receiving/providing care. Non engaged behaviors are categorized into passive engagement and further into categories of passive/agitated behaviors for residents, associated with things that are done to/with the resident, preparation and organizing tasks for visitors, and work tasks for staff (Morgan-Brown & Chard, 2014). The ATOSE allows in-depth understanding of barriers and enablers to occupational and social engagement, especially as residents living with advanced dementia may have a limited ability to verbalize their needs and preferences.

### The Residential Environmental Impact Scale (Version 4)

The Residential Environmental Impact Scale (REIS) Version 4 measures the impact of the physical and social environment of a residential facility on the quality of life of its residents (Fisher & Kayhan, 2012; Richards et al., 2015). Based on the Model of Human Occupation, the REIS evaluates the influence of the residential environment on dimensions of quality of life, including a resident's sense of self-efficacy, motivation, and engagement in occupations (Fisher & Kayhan, 2012). The REIS is implemented in three stages, namely, a walkthrough of the facility, observation of activities run by the facility, and interviews conducted with both residents and staff. Items are scored on a 4-point scale, ranging from a score of (1), indicating the environment strongly interferes, to a score of (4), signifying how strongly the environment impacts residents' sense of identity and competence by providing opportunities, resources, demands and constraints to meaningfully engage in culturally appropriate activities (Fisher & Kayhan, 2012). The collaborative nature of the REIS provides residents with opportunities to contribute to the community they live in and enables staff to explain how they perceive the care culture and the environment overall. These multiple perspectives on environmental barriers and enablers assist to identify possible areas for improvement (Du Toit, Fitch et al., 2021).

When considering the scope and potential of occupational therapy within long-term care settings for older adults, we encourage students to embrace their future roles as change agents in the occupational therapy profession. (See Chapter 31, OTs as Change Agents.) Advocating for the right of all older adults to engage meaningfully on social and occupational levels will not only contribute to occupational justice (Causey-Upton, 2015), but will also heed the World Health Organization's call to promote healthy aging globally (Beard et al., 2016).

There are still many issues related to long-term care that need attention. Table 28.2 provides an extensive list of potential roles OTs might assume to enhance the quality of life of residents and to enhance long-term care settings on a systems level. The following sections of this chapter provide a closer look at NHs, ALs, and continuing care communities as collective systems. Each section "fleshes out" select items listed in Table 28.2 to illustrate how occupational therapists can address the long-term care needs of both residents and systems of care.

## Historical Trends in Residential Long-Term Care Settings

As noted earlier, the long-term care delivery system has changed substantially over the past century, reflecting changes in resident populations, government involvement and funding sources, and predominant models of care. Supportive residential settings have increased in total numbers of clients treated and in the diversity of clinical services offered, to include more complex therapies for client populations that are older and more frail. Infectious disease concerns such as COVID-19 put these settings on the frontline of public health and the front pages of national media.

Models of care, reflecting what is considered "good care," have changed over time as well (Briller et al., 2016). Pre-Depression almshouses, "institutions of last resort" for impoverished older adults without families, covered only the most basic needs. Custodial care, keeping clients clean and fed, was the primary orientation of staff in such settings. In 1946, the Hill-Burton Act provided funds for the construction of more institutional, hospital-like NH settings. Care became more medicalized, focused on medical needs that accompany chronic conditions.

In the 1960s and 1970s, for-profit corporate chains entered the scene, and the definition of "good care" shifted to place greater emphasis on efficiency and standardization in order to minimize costs. With minimal regulations, abuse and scandals tainted the image of residential care settings. The Omnibus Budget Reconciliation Act of 1987 ushered in major reforms, including establishment of the Minimum Data Set to systematically measure the quality of medical care, reduce use of restraints, increase staffing, and individualize care plans.

Advocates of person-centered care revolutionized the definition of "good care" in residential care settings. Based on intimate knowledge of residents' personal experiences, person-centered care is individualized to address residents' specific preferences and needs and to enhance their quality of life, comfort, inclusion, and occupation. Person-centered care acknowledges and fosters the identity and self-worth of each resident regardless of cognitive status (Fazio et al., 2018; Kitwood & Bredin, 1992). The Culture Change Movement, promoted by the Green House Model and the Pioneer Network, suggested an additional dimension to the definition of good care in residential settings: care should be a collaborative and empowering process, directed by the person receiving care in collaboration with staff, allowing more personalized strategies of care and more resident-determined choice (Cohen et al., 2016; Koren, 2010).

## Shifting From Institutional to Noninstitutional Settings

Recent decades have seen a shifting of long-term care from institutional to noninstitutional settings supported by the Supreme Court's Olmstead decision and by many state Medicaid programs and waivers. Long-term care is increasingly provided in people's private homes (see Chapter 29) and other residential care settings, such as ALs and CCRCs (see later sections in this chapter); however, NHs continue to fill an essential need for individuals with complex care needs, and they are expected to do so for individuals who lack the resources to be cared for at home, such as financial resources to purchase services and family and friends able to assist with care.

## Nursing Homes

### Basic Definitions

Although many people equate skilled nursing facilities (SNFs) with NHs, there are substantial differences between them in the level of care they provide and the goals of that care: An NH is a permanent residence for people requiring 24/7 care; an SNF is a temporary residence for patients undergoing medically necessary rehabilitation (Murphy, 2021).

NH residents are unable to independently manage at least some activities of daily living (ADLs), such as getting in and out of bed, eating, bathing, dressing, and toileting, all of which are supported by certified nursing assistants (CNAs) under the supervision of a registered nurse and covered by Medicaid. The goal of NH care is to provide a safe and comfortable environment for residents who cannot live independently. In contrast, the Medicare Part A SNF benefit provides more medically complex nursing and therapy services following an inpatient hospital stay, with such postacute rehabilitative care intended to help patients recover and be discharged to live as independently, in the least restrictive environment, as possible. The Medicare SNF benefit covers more medically complex nursing care provided by registered professional nurses, physical therapy, occupational therapy, speech therapy, intravenous injections, social services, medications, and other services, supplies, and equipment, for up to 100 days in a Medicare-certified SNF.

## Nursing Home Demographics

Approximately 15,600 certified NHs with 1.7 million licensed beds operate in the United States. The majority of NHs are for profit and the majority are chain-affiliated. As noted earlier, NHs commonly provide long-term care services, including custodial care, which are covered by Medicaid, as well as skilled nursing services, including rehabilitation, which are covered by Medicare. Approximately 32% of NH residents received rehab, which includes occupational, physical, and speech therapy (Harrington et al., 2018).

The NH resident population is diverse and changing over time. In 2021, approximately 79% of NH residents were White, 15% were Black, and 6% were Hispanics (Weech-Maldonado et al., 2021). Longitudinally, from 1999 to 2008, the number of White NH residents declined 10%, the number of Black residents increased 11%, and the number of Hispanic residents grew by 55% (Feng et al., 2011). The clinical characteristics of NH residents also have become more diverse. Over time, residents of NHs have divided into two distinct populations. While NHs primarily provided long-term housing and chronic care services for the oldest adults, they increasingly serve a new subset of younger-aged residents requiring short-stay housing and rehabilitative care (Eskildsen & Price, 2009). Long-stay residents represent approximately 57% of the NH population. Their average length of stay is 2.3 years. Short-stay postacute residents represent 43% of the NH population, with an average stay of 28 days (Sifuentes & Lapane, 2020).

The COVID-19 virus had severe impacts on NHs. A significant and disproportionate number of deaths due to COVID-19 occurred among NH residents in the United States and internationally. National reports in October 2021 indicate that 19% of all COVID-19 deaths occurred among NH residents, although they constitute far less than 1% of the population (National Academies of Sciences, Engineering, and Medicine [NASEM], 2022).

## Nursing Home Environments and Cultures

Because NHs are residents' homes for extended periods, the physical environment is especially important to their quality of life. However, nationally, the physical infrastructure of NHs is dated, and often considered to be more like an institution than a home. The traditional NH evokes a hospital-like atmosphere, i.e., a large building with long corridors, housing wards of 20 or more residents in shared rooms. In contrast, recent efforts strive to make NH cultures less institutional and environments more homelike through models such as Green Houses, which consist of households of 10–12 residents on small campuses, with outdoor access and accessible kitchens for residents and their guests (CMS, 2021; Cohen et al., 2016; Miller et al., 2018). NH innovations in smaller environments, where the volume of traffic within the setting is much lower, can be valuable not only for improving quality of life but also for infection control (NASEM, 2022).

## Workforce and Staffing

NHs employ about 1.2 million health-care personnel and support workers, including administrators, housekeepers, nutrition and dietary staff, personal care and nurse aides, and licensed independent medical providers. In 2016, registered nurses represented only 12% of the workforce (Harris-Kojetin et al., 2019). Direct care workers who provide ADL assistance, such as CNAs, constitute the majority (64%) of NH staff (Harris-Kojetin et al., 2019) and are predominantly women, low-paid, racially diverse, and predominantly women (Sloane et al., 2021).

Staffing challenges include employee burnout, low staff morale (Fisher et al., 2021; VonDras et al., 2009; Woodhead et al., 2014), and high turnover rates—as high as 141% among registered nurses (Gandhi et al., 2021). High turnover rates result in high levels of noncompliance with recommended staffing levels; an estimated 75% of NHs are almost never in compliance (Geng et al., 2019).

## Paying for Nursing Homes and Skilled Care

Financial coverage for long-term care is a critical issue facing the United States today. Long-term care services in the United States are mainly financed by public sources. Long-term care is expensive and unaffordable for most people, and state and federal budgets are striving to constrain spending. Medicaid is the predominant source of financing for long-term care. Some people pay for long-term care out of pocket, and many spend down their financial resources in this way, until they spend down their assets sufficiently to reach Medicaid eligibility. Medicare does not cover long-term care but does cover SNF services for up to 100 days following a 3-day or longer inpatient hospital stay. Moreover, Medicare covers SNF care at much higher rates than Medicaid covers long-term NH care.

The other source of long-term care financing is private insurance, but private insurance for long-term care never covered many people and its outlook is dim—despite the rising need for long-term care, the number of companies selling long-term care insurance has dropped drastically (Cohen, 2016) and sales of long-term care insurance policies have plummeted (Cornell et al., 2016).

In 2017, the national median yearly cost of a private room NH stay for uninsured persons was $97,445 and for a semi-private (i.e., shared) room was $85,776 (Genworth Financial, 2017). In 2017, Medicaid covered approximately 62% of NH residents. Average number of Medicare admissions for short-term post-acute care per NH bed increased over 40% from 2001 to 2017 (Werner et al., 2021). In 2018, about 1.6 million Americans had Medicare-covered stays in an SNF.

## Families as Partners in Nursing Home Care: How Occupational Therapists Can Assist

Relocation to an NH represents a major transition for family members, as well as for the new resident. They are often reluctant to relinquish the caregiver role, which at this point is typically an important part of their daily life and their identity, but are uncertain what they can do or are allowed to do within the NH setting. The world of the NH represents a "foreign culture" to families, which they usually learn to negotiate by trial and error. The following section is based on a 3-year ethnographic study of families' experiences in a large US NH and the expectations and desired involvement in continuing the caregiving role, both from their point of view and that of the NH staff (Perkinson, 2000, 2003).

## The Initial Encounter With the Nursing Home

The time immediately following NH admission can be an overwhelming blur for families, who may be preoccupied with the medical or personal crises precipitating the move and the costs entailed. The following period of adjustment may be characterized by much confusion and misunderstanding of the NH hierarchy, roles, routines, and expectations. Communication with staff may be misdirected and strained during this time. Unaware of "who is who" and whom to approach for what type of question, the family may seek information about the resident in dysfunctional ways, either "funneling," i.e., focusing on one staff member for all answers, or "scatter-shooting," asking questions of everyone in sight. Families also may come to the NH with major misconceptions regarding the quantity and quality of care their relatives will receive.

The occupational therapist affiliated with the NH can play a major role in easing this transition, serving as a "culture broker" to orient family members to the way things work. The occupational therapist can identify various staff members and their duties, thus identifying whom to approach for questions regarding medical issues, personal care, and meals. They also can suggest ways to voice concerns effectively, e.g., not during shift change. They can "interpret" and "translate" the culture of the NH: its schedules, routines, rules, expectations, shared notions of what constitutes "appropriate" behavior, especially "appropriate" and "inappropriate" behaviors of "outsiders" (a hopefully temporary status for the new family member). Occupational therapists might explain care planning conferences and the family's role within them and provide guidance to achieve effective participation. The occupational therapist might assist family members in defining their particular role/occupation in the care of their relative, eventually becoming "partners in care" with NH staff. This is critically important. Often, families who cannot develop constructive, meaningful occupations within the NH tend to become either overprotective of the resident or overly critical of staff, in an attempt to prove that they still care.

## Nursing Home Family Occupations: Assisting With Basic Care

The occupational therapist can identify allowable occupations, ways to modify and continue family involvement in care that are acceptable and welcome. The family member can assist in some ADLs, e.g., basic grooming (manicures, hair-styling) and feeding (also bringing in snacks or favorite foods). However, assistance with intimate tasks or those involving heavy lifting are neither welcome by family members (for intimate tasks) nor by staff (for tasks with heavy lifting) for the safety of both the resident and the family member. Staff suggestions included assisting with the resident's exercise program (within safety limits), including

walking. Once a family member gained the confidence of staff and earned the status of "partner in care," staff would enlist family's help in motivating the resident or convincing the resident to cooperate in procedures or routines the resident had resisted.

## Nursing Home Family Occupations: Roles Involving Advocacy

Because they know the resident so well, family members can serve as "care-watchers," spotting and reporting changes in appearance, mood, and/or behavior that staff might miss. Staff sometimes referred to family members as their "third eye," and were especially appreciative of alerts regarding changes in the resident's cognitive status. The family member can also relay requests or questions from the resident to the staff and might intercede if disagreements arise between resident and staff or with other residents. They can voice concerns and request additional information at care planning conferences. They can also offer suggestions or voice concerns regarding the facility in general at family council meetings. Occupational therapists can assist by explaining to family members how care planning conferences and family councils are run and how to prepare for them to ensure effective participation.

## Nursing Home Family Occupations: Interpersonal/Connective Roles

Possibly the most important aspect of the NH family caregiver role is interpersonal. Family visits are extremely important but sometimes difficult to sustain. Family members may become frustrated and question the value of their visits. Occupational therapists can suggest ways to maximize visiting time: Share photos or videos of family members to "kick-start" conversations on various activities and interests of relatives pictured. Share family news, both good and bad. Bring grandchildren and/or pets to the visit. Time visits to coincide with scheduled activities on the floor to encourage the resident to participate. Take the resident off the floor, on an outing to a favorite café or locale, or even to another area of the facility for a change of scenery. Help maintain connections to the outside world by providing updates on local, national, and world news. Watch a video or movie together. Watch a televised sports event together and share insights on the players and plays made. Decorate the resident's room with family photos and memorabilia, both to make the room more homelike and to provide glimpses of the resident's pre-NH life for staff to better understand the resident and stimulate informal conversations. Spiritual needs may loom large at this life stage. If appropriate, occupational therapists might suggest praying or discussing religious readings together, writing a life review or ethical will, or helping to maintain religious and cultural traditions.

Clearly, occupational therapists and family members can provide critically important care within an NH setting. The occupational therapist can support families, underscoring the value of family involvement and suggesting ways to reinvent the family caregiver role both to optimize the resident's continued participation in meaningful occupations and to maximize quality of life.

## Assisted Living

AL was conceived as a social as opposed to medical model of care and designed to fall somewhere in the middle of the long-term care continuum between one's own home and an NH (Hawes et al., 1999). Developers and owners in the hotel and real estate industry have invested heavily in this industry, and many AL communities have a hotel- or resort-like environment that reflects this influence. Although AL includes under its umbrella a low-income board and care model described later, the ideal of AL was developed to cater to an affluent clientele and provide a broad array of personal care and supportive services in a homelike environment with a philosophy that emphasizes consumer choice, autonomy, dignity, privacy, and individualized care plans (Brown Wilson, 2007). The ability to age in place is another core philosophy, with a goal of preventing residents from being discharged to a higher level of care or NH prematurely (Ball et al., 2004).

AL is an increasingly popular alternative to NH care, one that families and older adults often prefer (i.e., over more institutional NHs) (Grabowski et al., 2012). It also is a primary provider of residential care for residents with dementia (Zimmerman et al., 2022). Like NHs, a growing number of AL communities offer memory care units as part of a larger community (12.1% and 14.8%, respectively) (Harris-Kojetin et al., 2013).

AL varies in structure and levels and combinations of services and ranges in size from 2 to 100+ beds. A recent biennial national survey of AL communities with four or more beds showed that there are an estimated 28,900 residential care communities in the United States with about 996,100 beds (Harris-Kojetin et al., 2019). Similar to NHs, these data show that most AL communities are for profit (81.0%) and more than half (57.2%) are chain-affiliated.

### Models of Assisted Living Care

Although AL communities vary considerably, they can generally be described in terms of two models: (1) the contemporary AL model and (2) the board and care model (Carder et al., 2006; Perkins et al., 2004). The board and care model reflects a long tradition of "mom and pop" care in the United States dating back to the early 19th century. This model of care primarily serves low-income, rural, and racial and ethnic minority residents, including many with chronic mental illness and developmental disabilities (Lepore et al., 2018; Perkins, 2021; Perkins et al., 2004). These homes are typically located in low-income communities where their physical plant is typically small (i.e., 2–24 beds) and reflects the limited income of their residents and providers (Ball et al., 2004; Perkins et al., 2004). Many of these residents pay for their care primarily with supplemental security income (SSI) (Perkins et al., 2004). The contemporary more upscale AL model surfaced in the United States in the mid-1980s in response to consumers' and policy makers' growing aversion with NH care and their desire for less institutional, more cost-effective alternatives (Brown Wilson, 2007). Although the contemporary AL model serves a predominately non-Hispanic White clientele, recent research shows that this population is growing more racially and ethnically diverse and increasingly includes members of special populations that will need AL care, including a growing population who self-identify as a sexual and gender minority (SGM) person and persons aging with HIV (human immunodeficiency virus) (Perkins, 2021).

### The Cost of Assisted Living

Although AL care can be quite expensive, it is generally less costly than NH care. Figures from the most recent market survey show that the median monthly base rate for a private room in an NH is about $9034 per month compared with about $4500 per month in AL (Genworth Financial, 2021). Nonetheless, unlike NH care, AL care is primarily private pay and these fees vary considerably based on geographic location, room size, and other amenities included. In addition to a base rate, many AL communities charge a la carte for additional services, such as extra assistance with ADLs, dementia care, incontinence care, complex medication care, and medical transportation. A small number of communities that fall under the board and care home model participate in state Medicaid waiver programs. However, estimates indicate that these services are available to only about 15% of residents in these homes and reimbursement rates are low; 85% of all public payments are less than $800 per month (Carder et al., 2015; Harris-Kojetin et al., 2019).

### Licensing and Regulation of Assisted Living

AL is licensed and regulated almost entirely at the state level and these regulations vary across states. The small number of homes that participate in state Medicaid waiver programs also are subject to state and federal Medicaid policies. Although resident care needs in these communities are becoming increasingly complex, most care is provided by low-wage frontline workers with little or no formal healthcare training (Kemp et al., 2019). Because of providers' inability to offer competitive wages, staff working in low-income board and care model homes tend to have the lowest levels of education and training (Ball et al., 2010). Regulatory requirements for staff training vary markedly by state and the quality of this training varies across homes within a state; hours of required ongoing in-service training for frontline workers range from 0 to 16 hours per year and many of these workers are not trained as CNAs (Ball et al., 2010; Carder et al., 2015). State regulations generally mandate that licensed nurses can supervise care in AL but cannot provide skilled nursing care (Carder et al., 2015).

With the increased popularity of AL, many states have made statutory, regulatory, and policy changes to accommodate increased medical complexity and intensity of resident care and allow many communities to offer additional levels of care, including specialized dementia services (Golant, 2008). Almost half (47.4%) of AL residents have access to these different care levels compared with only about 22% of residents in NHs (Freedman & Spillman, 2014).

### Typical Services Provided in Assisted Living

Although services and levels of care vary across homes, typical services provided in AL include 24-hour supervision and assistance; meals and dining services; exercise, health, and wellness programs; recreational activities; religious and spiritual services and activities; housekeeping and maintenance; medication management or assistance; personal care services (i.e., assistance with ADLs and nail and foot care); and transportation (e.g., to medical appointments and shopping). Although AL typically provides no skilled nursing care or health care, considerable health care happens in this care setting. Some communities contract with external care providers, such as physical, occupational, or speech therapists, to provide services several days a week onsite, and some of these providers may have onsite offices in these communities. Typically, residents or families can pay AL communities additional fees to receive these services or consumers can contract for these services with individual providers. In addition to physical, occupational, and speech therapy, other external services frequently provided in AL include pharmacy services (e.g., bubble packaging), dietary and nutrition services, dental care, hospice, home health, mental health care or counseling, and social work services. Some AL communities may contract with local health-care systems or independent health-care providers to offer regular onsite primary care and wellness services and some acute care.

## The Rapidly Changing Care Environment of Assisted Living

In the past two decades, AL residents have increased in frailty and have greater care needs and comorbidity. The typical resident requires assistance with more than one ADL; more than one-half (61%) need help with at least three (Caffrey et al., 2021). These data show that close to half (49%) have from two to three chronic conditions and 17% have from four to ten. Up to 90% of AL residents have some level of cognitive impairment and as many as two-thirds are diagnosed with Alzheimer's disease and other dementias; a growing population of these residents are aging in place with advanced dementia and require both dementia care and end-of-life care (Perkins, 2021; Zimmerman et al., 2007, 2014).

Annual AL death rate is 36% (Bender et al., 2022). While increased use of external formal care, e.g., hospice, blurs the line between AL's social model and the medical model of NHs (Golant, 2008; Kemp et al., 2019), important distinctions remain. Compared with NHs, lower staff training and education requirements represent a key challenge (Carder et al., 2015). Consequently, AL providers face major challenges in adequately and effectively addressing residents' complex medical, emotional, social, and spiritual needs (Bender et al., 2021; Vandenberg et al., 2018). Informal caregivers (family members and friends) play critical roles in supplementing this care (Perkins, 2021). Privately paid aides also supplement care for some residents but typically more so in higher fee settings (Perkins et al., 2018). Smaller homes with fewer resources, which are the only care option for certain low-income groups and those in rural communities, tend to have less qualified staff and family support compared to larger communities with more resources (Ball et al., 2010; Perkins et al., 2013).

## The Important Role of Occupational Therapists in Residents' Ability to Age in Place

The ability to age (and die) in place, a core philosophy of AL, contributes to the popularity of this care setting (Ball et al., 2004). Many residents and their family members hope for AL to be a resident's last home. As resident acuity has steadily risen and AL providers and family members struggle to address residents' growing care needs, care from external care providers is increasingly vital to residents' ability to remain in this setting. Among these providers, occupational therapists can be instrumental in designing programs that can help residents restore or retain physical function and maintain independence to the degree possible. They also can provide training for AL staff that can help support these goals. Important examples include instruction in fall prevention and safe transfer techniques and training in communication and behavior management skills for residents with sensory or cognitive impairments. Occupational therapists also may recommend environmental modifications (e.g., proper placement of furniture and grab bars) that can further support these efforts to maximize residents' quality of life and allow them to age in place and avoid transfer to a more institutional and often less preferred NH setting.

## Impact of the COVID-19 Pandemic

Prior to the pandemic, older adults in AL were already at risk of social isolation and loneliness (Perkins et al., 2013). At the height of the pandemic, social distancing restrictions that prevented friends and family from visiting further contributed to this risk. Already overburdened frontline workers who prior to the pandemic often felt pressed for time to complete care tasks also were adversely affected. In addition to their regular care tasks, they found themselves managing COVID-related fears and filling voids left by the absence of family, including often being the only ones there when residents were ill or dying, which, in addition to obvious health risks related to potential COVID-19 exposure, negatively affected these staff members' physical and mental health, factors that have contributed to an already high level of staff turnover and associated understaffing in these settings (Kemp, 2021; Wager et al., 2022). Many family members also experienced considerable anxiety, guilt, and depression over not being able to participate in resident care as they had done during prepandemic times (Kemp, 2021).

Much of the press regarding COVID-19 within the context of long-term care focused on the plight of NHs or lumped AL into this category, when these communities have their own unique structure and needs (Temkin-Greener et al., 2020; Zimmerman et al., 2020). Compared with NHs, the unique challenges experienced by AL residents and providers during the pandemic included the limited presence of trained health-care professionals, lower staffing levels and less trained staff, and social distancing restrictions that banned family members and other informal caregivers from providing supplemental care that is especially crucial in the AL setting where care provided by staff is more limited (Kemp, 2021; Zimmerman et al.,

2020). As in NHs, low-income AL residents and staff and those of color have been particularly adversely affected, contributing to prior existing health disparities (Temkin-Greener et al., 2020). Unfortunately, ill effects related to the pandemic, including critical staffing shortages, persist throughout the AL industry and continue to plague both staff and residents' family members and pose important risks to resident health and overall well-being (Wager et al., 2022).

## Continuing Care (or Life Care) Retirement Communities (CCRCs)

### What Is a CCRC?

The CCRC is a residential option that facilitates aging in place. It is an age-homogeneous setting, with minimum age requirements usually starting at age 60 (although waivers may be granted for residents' spouses who are under the minimum age). CCRCs (also called life care or life plan communities) provide a complete continuum of aging health-care services and activities combined with maintenance services for three-tiered residential options: independent living (IL), AL, and SNF/NH care, all on one campus (American Seniors Housing Association, 2017). Physical layouts of levels of care vary and may include separate floors of a high-rise building, adjacent buildings (e.g., duplexes or low-rise apartment buildings), or individual homes in a campus-like neighborhood setting.

Patterns of service use vary within CCRCs. Residents may move from IL units to more structured (ALs) and service-dense (SNF) housing environments either for short-term rehabilitation or permanently, as their health-care needs change over time (Sherwood et al., 1997). Some CCRCs offer the option to remain in IL with additional services, such as homemaker or home health-care services or purchase separate meal plans, paying out-of-pocket or through insurance. Some communities also offer dementia care in specialized units and end-of-life or hospice care.

Traditional CCRCs in the United States vary in size; the average has 335 units total, 231 IL units, 34 AL units, and 70 skilled NH beds. Only 8% of CCRCs have more than 500 units. On average, a resident spends approximately 10 to 12 years in IL, 1 to 2 years in AL, and 1 to 2 years in skilled nursing (Zebolsky, 2014).

### Brief History of CCRCs

Early CCRCs were affiliated with church-run nonprofit communities, providing housing, social support, and continuing care. By the 1900s, there were seven CCRCs in the United States; 25 of the oldest U.S. CCRCs have operated over 100 years (LeadingAge Ziegler 100, 2012). One of the first CCRC communities in the United States was founded by Quakers in Pennsylvania in 1967. CCRC development grew rapidly through the 1970s (Zarem, 2010) and has continued to grow, from roughly 800 in 1990 (Netting & Wilson, 1991) to today's number of 1900 (AARP, 2022).

Many CCRCs are part of multisite organizations. During the mid-1980s, for-profit CCRCs increased when large hospitality/resort corporations such as Marriott and Hyatt entered the market. Even with these new developments, the majority (80%) of CCRCs are not-for-profit; about 50% are affiliated with faith-based/religious organizations.

### CCRC Resident Demographics

The number of older adults living in CCRCs has more than doubled from 350,000 in 1997 to about 745,000 in 2007 (Government Accountability Office [GAO], 2010). CCRC residents are growing older. The average age upon admission increased from age 76 in the 1970s to slightly above 81 in the 2010s. Residents' average age increased from about 80 in the 1980s (Winklevoss & Powell, 1984) to over 85 in the 2010s (Zebolsky, 2014). The average life expectancy of new residents when they enter the community is 10–12 years (Zebolsky, 2014), although this varies depending on entry age, gender, and health. CCRC residents live longer (18 to 24 additional months) than older adults in the outside community (Special Committee on Aging, 2010). Based on a national survey of over 3400 CCRC IL residents (Mather Institute, 2022), 55% were advanced in age (85+ years old), 67% were female, 98% were White, 55% were wealthy (incomes over $100,000), and 77% were well educated (college degrees or more). Half (49%) were married and 39% were widowed.

### Services and Amenities Offered in Independent Living

Services offered in AL communities and NHs were described earlier in this chapter and are similar to those in CCRCs. IL residents are capable of living on their own, with minimum assistance. In addition to providing a more structured residential environment, CCRC ILs typically offer a variety of services and resources, including any of the following: spa/wellness centers, health-care coordinator/managers (usually a nurse), rehabilitation services through home health care, 24-hour emergency care, daily monitoring by staff, homemaker services, adult daycare, assistance with meals and nutritional counseling, home delivered meals, multiple dining venues on campus, grocery shopping, housekeeping, home maintenance, transportation, escort services within the community and off campus, social and recreational activities on and off campus, dental and vision care in some communities, respite care, and end-of-life-care.

Most CCRCs encourage active lifestyles. In addition to on-site fitness centers that may include health promotion and wellness programs, many CCRCs offer activity areas such as swimming pools, tennis courts, and putting greens. Nature trails and pathways encourage walking routines. Meal plans vary by site. Many CCRCs offer three meals a day; however, IL residents have the option of eating in their individual units. For those residents who prepare their own meals, dieticians are available to set up individualized diets.

### CCRC Regulation and Licensure for Health-Care Services

CCRC accreditation is expensive and not required; therefore, the majority (84%) are not certified (GAO, 2010). Lacking overall federal oversight, regulation of traditional CCRCs takes place at the state level and is mostly financial. CCRCs on-site health-care facilities (SNFs and ALs) are regulated by the appropriate state health-care licensing related organizations; however, facilities that accept Medicare and/or Medicaid must be certified according to federal guidelines, including federal overview of health inspections, staffing, and resident assessments. These governmental agencies do not regulate overall operations and financial management of the CCRC. Twelve states have no CCRC-specific regulations; 38 states regulate CCRCs through state divisions such as the Department of Insurance or the Division of Aging and Elder Services. Regulations vary from full licensing to regulatory oversight of developments, ongoing operations, financial or consumer disclosure, and certificates of need for new buildings.

### Financial Structure: Entrance and Monthly Fees

Because IL is not a medical service, Medicare, Medicaid, veteran benefits, or long-term care insurance will not cover costs. Residents pay out of pocket. AL is also an out-of-pocket expense; however, long-term care insurance and certain veteran benefits may cover a portion of the monthly fee.

### Entrance Fees

The initial payment system of a one-time nonrefundable entrance fee and monthly service fees now offer various fee structures, refundable entrance deposits, and a la carte service plans. Traditional CCRCs require a one-time upfront entrance fee before moving to the CCRC that serves as long-term care insurance, allowing a resident to age in place. The entrance fee is based on level of care, location, size, type of residential unit selected, and agreement type. In some CCRCs, the monthly fee is the same regardless of the level of care, while in other CCRCs, the monthly fee varies depending on the level of care required and the type of contract. In 2021 the average entry fee was about $402,000, ranging from $40,000 to over $2,000,000 (depending on type of contract) (AARP, 2022). Average monthly fee was around $3,500 (NIC, 2021).

### Monthly Fees

The amount of health-care services that are prepaid varies by type of CCRC and type of contract. One-third of CCRCs offer all-inclusive fully prepaid contracts. The resident's contract defines the structure of the monthly maintenance/service fee and specifies which services are included and which services require an additional fee.

### The Role of the Occupational Therapist in CCRCs

Occupational therapy practitioners can serve CCRCs in a number of different ways. There are traditional roles in skilled nursing and AL that have been addressed elsewhere in this chapter, and then there are the more nontraditional, innovative roles in CCRCs. In line with the call to expand occupational therapy practice to the group level, working with systems as potential clients (AOTA, 2020), this section underscores Du Toit's call earlier in this chapter to recognize long-term care settings "as a collective, an important emerging area of practice" (Du Toit et al., 2019; Du Toit, Fitch, et al., 2021). Based on the ethnographic work of the authors of this section (Perkinson, 1980, 1995; Perkinson & Rockemann, 1996), the following considers potential contributions of occupational therapists to IL as a system. Although the focus is on IL units, many of the points discussed below also may pertain to AL communities and NHs/SNFs. The expertise of occupational therapists enables them to consider each resident's unique needs and the modification of contextual factors necessary to maximize quality of life and participation in meaningful occupations.

### Occupational Therapists and CCRC Environmental Modifications

Because occupational therapists have been trained to understand the functional impact of changes resulting from normal aging and chronic diseases and how these changes are influenced by the physical environment, they can be essential partners to developers in designing new facilities, giving special attention to lighting and floor coverings to decrease glare and enhance visual contrast; height of grab bars, cabinets, closet fixtures, toilets, laundry equipment, and door sills to decrease the risk of falls; signage in age-friendly fonts and color combinations; elimination of unnecessary background noise with strategically positioned acoustic panels; and strategically placed seating (outdoors and indoors, including within elevators) along frequently used paths for residents and visitors with mobility issues.

Occupational therapists can recommend building design and universal design modifications that may enhance CCRC residents' performance in their daily activities and may prevent the need for future environmental adaptations. The physical environment can serve to promote or deter social interactions (see Chapters 20 and 32). Spaces should be designed taking acoustics into account, to minimize background noise. Occupational therapists can recommend floor plans and environmental elements in the residential buildings and common areas throughout the CCRC that promote socialization and support a resident's ability to participate in meaningful activities. Inclusion of small, slightly set apart private spaces offer prime settings for more intimate conversations. Communal areas might be designed as "third spaces" (see Chapter 32), configured to accommodate informal "hang-outs" for larger groups (Campbell, 2014). Lightweight furniture in common areas may be arranged to accommodate time-limited groups for conversations and discussions. Portable acoustic panels may minimize background noise and provide temporary, hearing-friendly settings for informal pre- and postmeal gatherings.

Occupational therapists can conduct environmental inspections of each level of residential care from IL to AL to SNF to assist developers with refurbishing units. They can recommend adaptive equipment or changes to existing environments or structures that will accommodate changes as residents age in place. (See Chapters 20 and 22 for additional suggestions.)

They can ease the move to the CCRC and later transitions from one housing type or level of care to another by assessing aspects of the resident's new physical environment and suggesting modifications as needed.

## Occupational Therapists and CCRC System-Level Change: Working With Staff

As CCRC residents age, their health-care needs may change. Such changes should not go unnoticed, as often may be the case for those living alone in the community. The needs of residents should be regularly monitored by unobtrusive observations by staff. In addition to their job-specific tasks, well-trained CCRC staff at all levels can serve as a "safety net," identifying the emerging health-care needs of residents at their earliest stages. Occupational therapists can assist in this training, teaching all frontline staff to identify symptoms or changes in a resident's behavior that may signal a need for help, and sensitizing staff to their role and responsibility to convey such needs to the appropriate CCRC health professional. For example, a housekeeper may be the first person to notice a change in a resident who always kept their unit in perfect shape and very organized, and who is now noticeably unorganized. The housekeeper would report their findings to the nurse in charge of the wellness center, who would then assess the resident and address the problem as needed. Occupational therapists also may assist staff members by offering regular CCRC-specific "in-services" to share relevant up-to-date information on topics such as how to avoid job-related injuries or prevent falls among residents.

## Occupational Therapists and CCRC System-Level Change: Social Dynamics

Ethnographic studies of CCRCs reveal a wide array of social interactions, networks, and roles (Perkinson, 1980, 1995; Perkinson & Rockemann, 1996). It behooves occupational therapists to recognize and attend to the social patterns and culture of the CCRC in which they work, to facilitate optimal bonding, social interactions, and participation in meaningful occupations.

### Moving In: The Role of the Occupational Therapist in Relocation to the CCRC

Typically, older persons move to a CCRC while they are independent, with few health risks or health-care needs, expecting to live longer and in the same community until the end of their lives. Frequent reasons to move to a CCRC include anticipated functional decline, difficulty with home management, and inability to drive (Krout et al., 2002; Young, 1998). The occupational therapist may be a member of the evaluation team that assesses prospective new residents before they move to the CCRC.

The move to a CCRC differs from earlier residential moves. It entails an adjustment back to a life that resembles an on-campus college existence, where age peers live in close proximity or share housing in residential complexes. These transitions and adjustments can be supportive, stressful, and annoying all at the same time. Occupational

therapists can assist in relocation and adjustment to the new environment of the CCRC. Divestiture, taking leave of a lifetime of possessions to move to a smaller living space, is an important and sometimes painful part of relocation (Ekerdt et al., 2012). They can assist new residents in the divestiture process by helping them to choose among their belongings, both balancing their past with downsizing to a smaller space, with safety and functional use a priority.

Occupational therapists can help new residents adjust to the new community environment, to continue past occupations and explore new opportunities offered by the CCRC (i.e., social interactions, leisure activities, volunteer opportunities; Cutchin et al., 2010).

### Developing Friendships and an Informal Support System Within the CCRC

Because residents often move to the CCRC from the local community, they may already know a few residents, share memories of local history, or share mutual friends. Discovering these connections often serves as first steps in establishing social networks within the CCRC (Perkinson & Rockemann, 1996). Through participating in CCRC activities (e.g., the walking group, informal pre- or postdinner gatherings in the lobby, news discussion, or reading groups), residents discover those who share common interests. Occupational therapists may assist particularly vulnerable "newcomers" by reviewing their background information and introducing them to relevant activity groups and to like-minded residents.

Mealtime in the common dining room is much more than an occasion to eat. Tablemates often take on permanence, making it difficult for a newcomer to "break in." Friendship groups or cliques are clearly visible by noting who sits with whom at dinner, providing a quick introductory overview of the social system of the CCRC.

Informal support represents an important advantage of living in a CCRC. Those who still drive may offer a ride to the grocery store or shopping mall. Neighbors may share a casserole too large to eat alone. Requesting a special favor and responding to that request may serve to validate and solidify a particular friendship.

### *The Influence of Marital Status*

Aging in place within the CCRC community gives residents time to build continuity in relationships and trust with friends, neighbors, and staff (Perkinson & Rockemann, 1996). Couples are able to remain in the same community even though they may be at different levels of care or lodging types (Zarem, 2010). Marital status is often a powerful determinant of CCRC social networks, with married residents and unmarried (i.e., widows, divorcees, and never-marrieds) tending to associate with those in their respective groups. Change in marital status (e.g., becoming a widow, marrying a fellow resident) generally prompts significant shifts in friendship ties and occasional hurt feelings of those "abandoned."

### The Special Status of Residents Who Are Caregivers

Caregivers, especially of persons with dementia, may fall into an ambiguous social status within the CCRC. An important dimension of friendships among married residents is doing things as couples and bonding among the group of wives and group of husbands. An important dimension of friendships among singles is the freedom to do as they please and take off on spur-of-the-moment outings. A caregiver of a spouse with heavy needs can do neither and often assumes the social identity of "married widow." The caregiving couple may choose a table for two or eat before or after the "rush" time to avoid encounters with residents uncomfortable with the care receiver's unpredictable behaviors or silences. Former caregivers, now widowed, are able to empathize and may provide support (e.g., visiting; lending adaptive equipment no longer needed) to the "married widows."

Larger, more established CCRC communities may be home to a large enough number of caregivers to form their own social network. Once a resident publicly identifies as being a caregiver (which may be a difficult step for some), they are typically embraced by fellow caregivers who appreciate and empathize with caregiver burdens as well as uplifts. A culture of caregiving may develop (Perkinson, 1995), with shared norms of appropriate caregiving behavior (e.g., how often and how long to visit a spouse residing in the NH; how to deal with disruptive behaviors in public). Established caregivers provide feedback and support to socialize new caregivers to the CCRC-specific culture of caregiving. Those who choose not to conform (e.g., continue to visit their spouse in the NH daily, all day) may receive negative feedback.

### Relocation Within the CCRC

One of the most stressful times for a resident is the transition (often involuntary) from one level of care to another with more intensive care. In addition to the symbolism of such a move and its impact on self-identity and threat to sense of independence (Shippee, 2009), the move typically causes loss of social networks that were gained within the more independent level of the CCRC. In addition to marital status, functional status underscored by residing in a more intensive level of care represents a major determinant of social ties within the CCRC. Residents typically avoid interactions with those living in a different level of care, and friendships rarely survive such a move (Roth et al., 2016).

In contrast, residents temporarily in AL or skilled nursing for rehabilitation might become more dependent and not want to give up the special one-on-one attention of being dressed, bathed, or escorted when they return to IL.

### Factors Contributing to Resident Satisfaction

Residents report five nonphysical attributes related to highest satisfaction: quality of staff; quality of daily life (cultural, musical, arts/crafts, entertainment, and social opportunities); dining flexibility (quality of food, variety of menu items, variety of services, and times available to dine); personal control (privacy and sense of safety and security); and comfort (ease of making friends and the sense that the residence is one's home) (Wylde et al., 2009).

### Relevance to Occupational Therapists

While commonalities exist, specific details of CCRC culture and social networks may differ across different facilities. Occupational therapists should identify the social dynamics and culture of their particular CCRC to identify residents at risk for social isolation—e.g., "nonlocals" who move from a distant city (often to be closer to their children) who lack initial ties needed to "kick-start" their CCRC friendship networks; recently widowed residents, especially men; spousal caregivers; and residents transitioning to a new level of care—and offer support as needed.

### New Service Developments within the CCRC

Over the last 10 years, the quantity and quality of CCRC services have significantly increased, e.g., in-home services (home health, home care) and adult-day care. Some CCRCs have opened their own home health-care agencies on campus and a number operate their own pharmacies and urgent care clinics. These services enable CCRC residents as well as older residents in the neighboring community to live independently longer, rather than move to the AL or SNF.

### CCRCs Without Walls: Continuing Care at Home (CCaH)

CCRCs continue to evolve and adapt to the changing needs of older adults as their numbers rapidly increase, grow older, and more concentrated in neighborhoods surrounding the CCRC. Many of these outside communities have become naturally occurring retirement communities (NORCs), where older adults prefer to age in place in their own homes with access to a multitude of services, rather than moving to a residential unit within a traditional CCRC. In a significant expansion of the traditional CCRC model, 45% of the 200 CCRCs in the Leading Age & Ziegler 200 annual survey offer some type of home and community-based services to nonresidents (LeadingAge Ziegler 200, 2021).

CCRC Without Walls (also known as Continuing Care at Home [CCaH]) expands the traditional CCRC model of services provided within a closed campus setting to include in-home services for nonresidents without requiring relocation into the CCRC (Thompson, 2012). This approach helps at-home members to stay healthy and independent for as long as possible and, if a more structured environment is needed, move to the AL or SNF of the CCRC. Members who enroll into the CCaH pay an entrance fee and monthly fees at lower rates than a typical CCRC, in exchange for a promise of future care. In 2021, 10% of the LZ200 CCRCs offered the CCaH model (LeadingAge Ziegler 200, 2021).

CCaH provides security of knowing that continuing care services are available as needed. Those services may include care coordination, annual physicals, wellness programs, transportation, companion or live-in-care, home health care, homemaker service, an emergency response system, adult day care, meals (home delivered meals or help in preparing meals), referral services, AL care, and NH care (Spellman, 2016).

New nonresident members receive a fitness assessment, a home assessment to identify safety changes that might be needed to age in place (e.g., grab bars, extra lighting, decluttering), and a home maintenance assessment. Most CCaH programs allow members to take part in activities in the associated traditional CCRC without an additional charge. A wellness coordinator is assigned to each member to monitor their health and well-being on an ongoing basis, which includes a comprehensive wellness program. Anecdotal evidence indicates that very few members of a CCaH ever utilize the higher levels of care of AL or skilled nursing.

*The complete listing of the Bibliography and Chapter Questions and Answers are available in the accompanying enhanced eBook version included with the print purchase of this textbook. Visit Elsevier eBooks+ (eBooks.Health.Elsevier.com) to access this content.*

## CHAPTER 29

# Home: An Evolving Context for Health Care

*Laura N. Gitlin, PhD, FGSA, FAAN and Catherine Verrier Piersol, PhD, OTR/L, FAOTA*

## CHAPTER OUTLINE

## OBJECTIVES

- Recognize the value of home care for older adults.
- Distinguish the potential funding sources for home care services.
- Describe conceptual models that guide home care practice.
- Explain cultural considerations when working with older adults in their homes.
- Describe the relevance of using a problem-solving approach with older adults in home care.

## Introduction

Mrs. M, a 94-year-old white Irish Catholic woman in good health, fell while walking outside to buy groceries and broke her femur. After surgery and a month's stint in subacute rehabilitation, she returned home with a walker and other adaptive equipment. She needed further rehabilitation at home, where she lives alone, to help her learn how to ambulate and carry out self-care, meal preparation, and home management activities in that environment.

Mr. B, a 79-year-old Black man, has dementia and lives with his wife. His physician provided a prescription for occupational therapy (OT) for a home safety evaluation and to evaluate ways of supporting his daily function at home and help his wife, the primary caregiver, manage day-to-day tasks.

Mrs. M and Mr. B illustrate some of the reasons why older adults receive care at home from occupational therapists. Although historically, the home was the initial setting for providing health care, with the rise of organized systems of care, health-care delivery shifted to specialized environments. However, the home is emerging once again as one of the most important contexts for delivering a wide range of health-care services, including episodic, short-term, long-term, and end-of-life care, as well as hospital and rehabilitative-oriented care, to older adults.

A confluence of multiple and critical societal trends has conspired to bring health care back into the home. These include rising hospital and nursing home costs spurring physician acceptance of alternative care approaches, increased risks of infection and mortality with hospital-based care, a soaring aging population seeking to heal and age in place, rising incidence of chronic disease and its functional consequences requiring home management and attention to functional and environmental aspects of daily life, development of accountable care organizations seeking to minimize hospital readmissions and associated costs, challenges transitioning from hospital to home (e.g., medication mismanagement), leading to increased risks for health declines and hospital readmissions and hence increased costs, and finally, evidence suggesting better recuperative outcomes with care at home even for serious illnesses (Binstock & Cluff, 2000; Richie and Leff, 2022).

With the COVID-19 pandemic, rise of telehealth, and increase of chronic illness and an aging world, the home as centerpiece for health, wellness, and healing has taken on even more significance (IBIS World, 2021). The home as epicenter, particularly as one ages, is a persistent trend that will continue into the future (Gitlin, 2007; Szanton, et al., 2011; Wahl & Gitlin, 2003). This chapter provides a broad overview of home health care and the role of occupational therapists. It briefly examines the current system and structure of home care; explores the benefits and challenges of delivering care in homes, including the home as a work environment; and discusses the clinical reasoning processes essential to successful home care delivery.

## The Home Care System

Although homes are unique and personal, the delivery of health care in the home is a highly regulated industry. In the United States, homebound status drives client eligibility for home health services. Clients who need postacute, skilled care after discharge from a hospital stay to their home or a relative, and individuals with longer-term skilled care but who are not typically posthospitalization are eligible for home health services (Van Houtven & Dawson, 2020). The single largest payer for home care services in the United States is the Centers for Medicare & Medicaid Services (CMS), with home health-care expenditures reaching $97 billion in 2017 (Michas, 2021). Home health agencies (HHAs) provide home care services under the Medicare Part A benefit. Since the peak in 2013 of 12,459 Medicare HHA, the number has been decreasing, with 11,221 agencies in 2020 (Michas, 2021).

Home health-care services include skilled nursing, OT, physical therapy, speech language pathology, and medical social services delivered in the patient's home environment. Approximately 4.5 million individuals received some form of home health in 2016, with 78% (approximately 3.5 million) being Medicare beneficiaries (Harris-Kojetin et al., 2019). Most home health users are 65 years and older (85%), are female (61%), live in urban areas (90.8%), and are White (79.9%).[1] According to a 2021 home health-care report based on data from government sources (e.g., Medicare Current Beneficiary Survey, Medicare Cost Reports, Home Health Compare, Medicare fee-for-service claims) and other data from CMS, home care outcomes show individuals get better at bathing (82%), walking or moving around (80%), moving in and out of bed (81%), and taking drugs correctly by mouth (Avalere, 2021).

OT, physical therapy, and speech language pathology services can also be provided in the home under Medicare Part B, for which enrollment is voluntary and beneficiaries pay a monthly premium. The conditions of participation under which HHA are regulated do not apply under Medicare Part B; for example, eligibility for services under Medicare Part B is not based on homebound status (Zahoransky & Vance, 2016). This service delivery setting offers occupational therapists the opportunity to work with clients within the comfort of their homes and in the community, rather than in the clinical outpatient setting.

Finally, two pieces of legislation have changed the traditional delivery of home health-care services under Medicare Part A. First, the Patient-Driven Groupings Model (PDGM), implemented by CMS, took effect on January 1, 2020, and is the most significant change for HHA in over 20 years (Center for Medicare & Medicaid Services, 2021). PDGM changed the payment for home health therapy services from the number of therapy visits delivered to payment based on patient characteristics including diagnosis, functional impairment, and the number of comorbidities, which place patients is a specific clinical group (National Association for Home Care & Hospice, 2021). In response to concerns about the impact of PDGM on beneficiaries' access to therapy services made by the American Occupational Therapy Association and other health profession associations, CMS clarified the role of therapy under the Home Health PDGM (Center for Medicare & Medicaid Services, 2005). The following key points were highlighted:

- There are two clinical groups (musculoskeletal rehabilitation and neuro rehabilitation) for which the primary reason for home health services is for the provision of therapy.
- Therapy should be provided regardless of the clinical group when included in the plan of care.
- Provision of therapy services should be determined by individual patient need without restriction or limitation on type of therapy, frequency or duration of visits.
- There is no requirement for "improvement"; thus, therapy services can be delivered for restorative or maintenance purposes.

The second piece of legislation occurred in response to the COVID-19 pandemic. The secretary of Health and Human Services declared a public health emergency (PHE) on January 27, 2020. The PHE resulted in a temporary waiver that designated OT as a qualifying service and allowed occupational therapists to open home health cases (complete the initial comprehensive assessment battery). The designation as a qualifying service is an opportunity for occupational therapists to demonstrate the important role they play at the start of care, during which the patient's plan of care is created (Center for Medicare & Medicaid Services, 2021).

## Role of Occupational Therapy

The home environment is a significant context for delivering OT services for several reasons: delivery of strategies can be tailored more easily than in clinical settings to the lived experience of patients; patients may feel more relaxed, less stigmatized, and more motivated to achieve therapeutic goals (Vance, 2016). Occupational therapists may serve as independent contractors or employees of home care agencies. To provide OT in the home, therapists must be licensed in the state and have a physician's prescription for OT evaluation and treatment, according to the state's practice act.

Occupational therapists have numerous roles in home care, including but not limited to evaluating clients for home safety and ability to age at home, making home modification and adaptive equipment recommendations and training in their use, providing restorative interventions, and helping clients learn new or modified ways of performing self-care and instrumental activities of daily living (IADLs) (Siebert, 2016).

Occupational therapists also provide education and strategies for managing the functional consequences of chronic illness and can offer family members (e.g., caregivers) disease education and training in specific techniques to manage daily care challenges that matter most to the family (Gitlin, Jacobs, & Earland, 2010). Although end-of-life care, activity-based therapies, preventive interventions, and caregiver training are interventions that occupational therapists can provide, due to reimbursement regulations, the full scope of practices may not be fully financially supported within existing funding mechanisms.

## Conceptual Framework for Guiding Home Care Practice

Lawton's competence-environmental press framework (Lawton, 1990) and its expansion in OT to include occupation (Law et al., 1996) provide a broad, overarching framework to understand an older client's levels of competencies and types of losses (e.g., sensory, physical mobility, or cognitive), environmental factors (e.g., housing features, social characteristics, and neighborhood conditions), and the interface with chosen activities or occupations. The model suggests the need to strive for the most optimal combination of environmental circumstances in view of changing competencies. It also suggests that a just-right fit leads to the highest possible behavioral and emotional functioning for that person (Gitlin, 2000; Lawton & Nahemow, 1973; Wahl & Gitlin, 2007).

Yet another tenet of this model is that older adults with lower levels of competence become the most susceptible to their environments, such that low competence, in conjunction with high environmental press, negatively affects autonomy, affect, and well-being. A related point is that as competencies decline, the zone of adaptation for promoting well-being narrows such that environmental choices become increasingly more limited. The competence-environmental press framework, and its expansion to include an occupational framework, continues to provide the basic mechanism of person-environment relations as people age and has been supported by a considerable body of empirical research. The model represents a broad, overarching framework for understanding the role of OT in home care and effectively frames the compensatory perspective relevant to therapies used in the home context. (See Chapters 4 and 20 for additional discussion of the competence-environmental press model.)

## Where to Sit and Other Cultural Considerations

Consistent across surveys of older adults is the importance attributed to aging in place at home or one's long-term residence (Keenan, 2010). Home is a key cultural symbol imbued with many meanings, including independence, autonomy, comfort, security, control, protection, and history and family remembrances (Oswald & Wahl, 2005; Oswald et al., 2006; Oswald et al., 2007; Rubenstein, 1989; Siebert, 2016). Often conceptualized as an extension of oneself, the home has many meanings to older adults and reflects the intersection of objective social and physical conditions and subjective appraisals, personal goals, values, and emotions (Oswald & Wahl, 2005). As such, the home care therapist must be aware of and sensitive to the client's cultural beliefs and values (Siebert, 2016). For example, when introducing changes to the way a client takes a bath or shower, an activity that is intimate and personal, a therapist needs to take into account the client's (and family's) preferences and long-standing routines.

The home as a culturally complex setting is evident the moment the therapist enters this setting. Unlike the clinic, which has clear directives as to where clients sit and the pace of the visit, the home is uncharted. Rules of engagement may be implicit and mostly directed by the resident such that the therapist must remain attentive and strike the right balance between structuring the session and enabling the client to exert control. Each home care situation is unique and the therapist must be flexible and open to "going with the flow" as established by the client in his or her own setting. It may be the client, for example, who dictates the location of where session occurs in the home, where the therapist sits, and the length of the session.

With age and reduced functional capacity, older people spend more time in the home (Oswald et al., 2006). As such, the home takes on increasing importance as the principal

context for socialization, leisure participation, and healthcare delivery (Avalere, 2021). In that capacity, the home also assumes new meanings as the principal location for safety, security, familiarity, and support of daily function (Lawton, 1990). (See Chapter 20 for additional discussion on the meaning of home in later life.) The presence of health professionals and specialized equipment, medications, and other medical or rehabilitative artifacts may not be readily acceptable because these items serve as visual and concrete reminders of declining abilities and threaten the meanings attributed to the home. Home care represents the interface between the home as a private and personalized space, the aging process and its associated health declines, and medical and rehabilitative objectives and societal demands. This tension may be intimately experienced by an older adult and influences acceptability of therapist recommendations for equipment or compensatory strategy use.

## Using a Problem-Solving Approach

Problem solving is a core feature of clinical reasoning processes used by all health and human service professionals in any care context. However, when working with older adults in the home, and particularly for individuals with complex health conditions requiring symptom management and family involvement, it is especially relevant. For the home care therapist, problem solving begins immediately upon entering the neighborhood, parking the car, and walking to the front door of the home of an older client. All of this information, gathered through keen observation, provides foundational knowledge and the backdrop from which the older client will be approached and assessed, and needs identified.

Approaches to problem solving vary. They can range from broad thinking and action processes to a highly structured and manualized approach such as problem-solving therapy, a formal therapeutic modality developed in psychology that teaches problem-solving skills. Here we refer to a broad problem-solving approach that is central to caring for older adults with complex conditions (Gitlin, 2000; Gitlin, 2015).

Although approaches to problem solving vary, shared basic characteristics include the purposeful engagement of individuals with chronic illness and/or their family members in a set of thinking and action processes that move through problem identification to implementation of concrete, practical solutions and their evaluation as to their effectiveness in addressing the targeted issue. The **first step** involves clearly identifying and defining the client's key problem to target; the identification process should involve the client, family, and therapist perspective. Problem identification can be complex and a multifaceted process. The **second step** is to establish specific and realistic goals for managing or eliminating the identified problem. Some individuals may engage in wishful thinking and develop a goal that is unrealistic (e.g., seeking a cure for the disease, or being able to drive), requiring redirection and guidance as to what is realistic and appropriate. The **third step** involves systematic questioning to identify the characteristics or nature of the problem (e.g., when it occurs, frequency of occurrence) to uncover potential contributing factors. By understanding the dimensions of a problem (e.g., lack of adherence to medication regime) and contributory factors (e.g., complexity of medication directions, poor planning), clients and families learn ways to prevent its occurrence or minimize its effects. The **fourth step** is to identify specific solutions or alternative approaches that are realistic for managing the identified problem. One approach is to engage individuals in brainstorming such that they become actively involved in generating possible solutions.

Once solutions are proposed, each one should be reviewed for feasibility and acceptability to client and family, if appropriate. This is in contrast to a prescriptive approach, in which solutions are provided by health-care providers without input from the client. Although occupational therapists may have the requisite knowledge concerning the health problem and specific ideas for its management, involving older adults in this process reinforces and validates the need for their active role in their own self-management. It also demonstrates problem solving and builds their skills in being able to use this process independently. Additionally, individuals may perceive greater ownership of solutions they help generate and be more likely to implement and adhere to them.

The **fifth step** involves implementing agreed-upon solution(s), and the final, **sixth step** involves evaluating whether implemented solutions improved or worsened the problem and modifying them accordingly. (See Chapter 7 for additional discussion of the intervention process.) Problem solving has important advantages in helping older adults cope with chronic illnesses and its functional consequences. Its use reflects a movement toward consumer-directed health care that relies on informed consumers to direct their own health-care choices and participate in disease management.

## Benefits of Providing Care in the Home

In contrast to health care provided in facilities (e.g., outpatient clinic, inpatient hospital, short-term nursing home stays, or rehabilitation unit), providing care in the client's home has many important advantages (Gitlin, 2000; Siebert, 2016). First, therapists are able to derive a more comprehensive understanding of a person's best functioning in his or her own, familiar context versus that of a sterile, unknown setting such as a clinic or rehabilitation facility. Concomitantly, clients may feel more relaxed and motivated to participate in therapy at home and less stigmatized. They may be able to more easily discern their own capabilities, areas for improvement, and personal goals than in a foreign setting devoid of their personal artifacts and the meanings associated with living at home.

Second, therapists are able to teach skills and new techniques within the context in which they will be used, a critical principle in adult learning. Contextual learning minimizes the challenges clients may confront in translating new skills or techniques learned in a standardized setting, such as a hospital, for use in their own life spaces. For example, learning to transfer to the left when getting onto a tub transfer bench may work in the hospital but may not work in a person's home where the bathroom configuration requires the person to transfer to the right. Without home care intervention, older adults may find it difficult to generalize the directionality of steps involved.

Third, providing care in the home enables therapists to observe that environment for clues as to how best to quickly relate to and work with the client and family members (if relevant) and to more easily form a therapeutic relationship (Gitlin, 2015). A therapeutic alliance is essential for promoting motivation and adherence to rehabilitative techniques (Chee et al., 2005; Gitlin, 2003; Siebert, 2016). Additionally, providing care in the home provides invaluable firsthand knowledge about the capacity of the client and the supports and barriers in his or her environment from which to derive an effective treatment plan. Finally, a home evaluation can reveal more safety hazards and unhealthy environmental conditions as well as disentangle what an older adult can do from what he or she is actually doing more so than relying on self-report provided in a clinic or physician's office.

## Challenges of Delivering Care in the Home

Despite the benefits of delivering care in the home, there are also challenges. In contrast to structured, routinized care environments of hospitals, nursing homes, physician's offices, or outpatient clinics, homes are highly individualized, uncontrolled, diverse, imbued with personal preferences and cultural attributions, personalized, and potentially a contaminated context (Gitlin, 2003). There is wide variation in homes, including their location, size, physical condition and features, safety, and the presence of others, that can affect the type of care needed and how it is provided (National Academy of Science, 2011). Solutions such as installation of adaptive equipment, home modifications, or telemedicine technology suitable for one client and his or her home environment may not work in another due to the physical and social features of the living space. For example, recommending a stair glide may not be possible if an older adult is obese, children live in the home, or the walls and staircase are in poor condition.

Homes as well as neighborhoods can help or hinder an older adult's ability to carry out various household, personal, and self-care tasks. Additionally, older adults and families differ in their knowledge of and willingness to engage in the home care process, their preferences for where health-related and adaptive equipment can be set up and care tasks performed, and how and where the therapy session will transpire in the home (Siebert, 2016).

Another challenge in home care is that many older adults live in homes that may adversely affect their health, the health of the care provider, and the delivery of home care. For example, over 6 million households have significant home repair needs, including heating, plumbing, and electrical deficiencies (National Academy of Science, 2011). Lack of first floor powder rooms, steep or broken steps, and absence of stable bannisters can affect the development and implementation of treatment plans and the ability of an older adult to remain at home. Clients living near or below the poverty line, in low resourced neighborhoods, or poor housing stock may be at high risk of exposure to lead paint, vermin and pest infestations, water leakage, and exposed wiring and electrical problems, as well as temperature dysregulation (too hot, too cold), affecting health, wellness and healing, and staying at home (National Academy of Science, 2011). Moreover, physical hazards affect the ability to install, maintain, and use adaptive equipment and may make it challenging or impossible for home care therapists to work effectively and safely in the home environment. The interface of home repair needs with everyday functioning at home is often not considered but becomes part of the many considerations in treating older adults at home (Szanton et al., 2011).

The social environment is another consideration. The presence of children and/or other adults in the home may influence delivery of home care services, particularly in regard to privacy during therapy or for a client's performance of self-care, the client's motivation level and adherence to the therapy plan, and the appropriateness of equipment recommendations, which may have to fit with the needs, preferences, and expectations of the client's social network. Involvement of family members in a home care session may be helpful yet pose challenges. For example, conflict in goals and expectations between the older adult and family member(s) or poor quality of relationships may interfere in home care participation and progress. Therapists must seek a balance between preserving the autonomy of the older adult in view of what may be limited cognitive and/or functional capacities and family involvement and goals (Gitlin et al., 2010; O'Sullivan, 2016).

As a work environment, home care poses distinctive challenges to occupational therapists. First, home care requires strong clinical and time management skills and the ability to work independently and without direct supervision (Siebert, 2016). Being a home care therapist may not be right for everyone. Second, home environmental conditions may present a hazard to not only the older adult but to the therapist as well. For example, extreme clutter, confined spaces to work in, infestation, inadequate sanitation, exposed infectious or hazardous materials, poor air quality, poorly regulated heat or air conditioning, excessive noise, poor lighting, presence of aggressive dogs or other pets, presence of firearms or other weapons, smoking or drug use in the home, extreme home repair needs, inadequate electrical capacity and outlets, and lack of privacy and other such concerns place a therapist at risk and/or discomfort and significantly compromise treatment planning and execution.

## Exemplar Evidence-Based Home Care Programs

While home care practices vary widely among agencies, there is a small but growing number of evidence-based interventions delivered by occupational therapists to support older adults and family caregivers. In dementia care for example, there are numerous tested protocols with demonstrated efficacy for both the person living with dementia and family caregiver. Numerous tested approaches have been shown through randomized trials to improve quality of life of families and also enable people to stay at home (Bennett et al., 2019). Common elements include disease education, problem solving, activities tailored to interests and abilities, and instruction in a wide range of nonpharmacological strategies such as cueing, environmental modifications, simplification of tasks, and communication techniques.

Similarly, there are a few tested home-based intervention studies designed to help older adults who are cognitively intact but functionally challenged age in place that are delivered by occupational therapists (Gitlin & Earland, 2010). Common elements of these interventions include their focus on functional goals identified by clients themselves, introduction of compensatory strategies to enable clients achieve their desired outcomes, and home modifications that facilitate safe engagement within the home environment.

## SUMMARY

Home care is gaining prominence in the health-care system as an approach that may prevent hospitalization, readmissions, and nursing home placement and enable aging in place. Funding sources for home care include Medicare Part A and Part B, as well as private health insurance. As a work environment, the home poses unique challenges; every home is distinct and unique—reflecting the intersection of broad socioeconomic and cultural influences and individuation, personal preferences, histories, and values and beliefs. The occupational therapist is thrust in the mix of these factors with the goal of helping older adults gain, regain, maintain, or improve their functional foothold and well-being in that environment. For many older adults, the home, imbued with historical and personal meanings and social connectedness, may offer recuperative opportunities possibly not afforded in other settings. Embracing the challenges of home care and helping older adults and their families achieve the outcomes they desire are noble and most rewarding endeavors.

*The complete listing of the Bibliography and Chapter Questions and Answers are available in the accompanying enhanced eBook version included with the print purchase of this textbook. Visit Elsevier eBooks+ (eBooks.Health.Elsevier.com) to access this content.*

CHAPTER **30**

# Intraprofessional and Interprofessional Processes in Gerontological Care

*Helen W. Lach, PhD, RN, CNL, FGSA, FAAN, Cynthia R. Ballentine, MSOT, OTR/L,
and Karen Frank Barney, PhD, MS, OTR, FAOTA*

## CHAPTER OUTLINE

## OBJECTIVES

- Articulate occupational therapist-occupational therapy assistant (OT/OTA) intraprofessional roles and responsibilities clearly to patients/clients, families, community members, and other professionals within geriatric/gerontologic settings
- Identify the unique cultures, values, roles, responsibilities, and expertise of other interprofessional team members and the impact these factors can have on the health outcomes of older adults
- Explain how inter- and intraprofessional teams work together to provide care, promote health, and prevent disease as it relates to older adults
- Discuss and differentiate the different types of teams and the significance of each
- Describe the process of team development and the roles and practices of effective teams
- Analyze interprofessional team contributions in various settings

## Introduction

Older adults typically have complex health problems affecting all aspects of their lives, including physical, psychological, and social issues. As a result, it takes an interprofessional team of health professionals to ensure that a holistic approach is used to identify and address the many challenges older adults may face (National Academy of Science and Medicine, 2019). For example, an older woman may be recovering from a wrist fracture from a fall. Because she lives alone and has no family nearby, this seemingly small injury is affecting her ability to obtain medications, shop for her groceries, and cook meals. She worries that she will fall again, and so she is concerned about leaving her home. Besides addressing her medical condition, she needs help adapting to her current conditions, assistance with her daily activities, and psychological support. Similar to this case, many older people have multiple chronic conditions that are compounded by a variety of factors.

The skills, expertise, and collaboration of a variety of health professionals are essential to provide optimal care for older populations (Montagnini et al., 2014). Each profession views situations through a different lens and provides a unique set of skills to solve problems. As a result, an interprofessional team approach is the gold standard for high-quality, client-centered gerontological care. This chapter addresses how intra- and interprofessional teams can help older adults by addressing the broad issues that may be involved with their health care across settings so they can attain and maintain their best quality of life.

## Occupational Therapy: Roles and Responsibilities

### Occupational Therapist-Occupational Therapy Assistant Team

Many settings, both medical and community based, provide excellent opportunities for occupational therapist (OT) and occupational therapy assistant (OTA) team service implementation. Currently, in the United States interprofessional processes are "state of the art," and the registered occupational therapist (OTR)–certified occupational therapy assistant (COTA) intraprofessional process optimally represents a positive and highly productive relationship.

The advantages to intraprofessional collaboration in service provision are many, with the ability to maximize intervention impact through optimal skills use at each level. Well-matched teams represent highly complementary roles and high motivation to apply the best practices about which they are both educated and passionate. The American Occupational Therapy Association (AOTA) guidelines for intraprofessional role delineation are provided in Table 30.1.

The OT is held responsible for all OT services that are provided, whether or not the professional is present onsite. As such, in teaming with the COTA, it behooves the OTR to have good communication and coordination processes established to ensure appropriate collaboration in service provision. Because both the OTR and the COTA are responsible for appropriate supervision and implementation processes and are expected to respect and support the role of the other, it is imperative that there is mutual respect, professionalism,

### TABLE 30.1 Occupational Therapy Practitioner

| Occupational Therapist | Occupational Therapy Assistant |
|---|---|
| An autonomous practitioner | Must be supervised by an occupational therapist |
| Responsible for delivery of all aspects of occupational therapy services | Responsible for delivering occupational therapy services under the supervision of and in collaboration with an occupational therapist |
| Accountable for safety and effectiveness of services and processes | Accountable for the delivery of safe and effective services and adhering to the occupational therapy process |
| Ultimately responsible for implementation of appropriate supervision | Responsible for seeking and obtaining appropriate supervision |
| **Both Practitioner** | |
| Equally responsible for developing a collaborative plan for supervision | |
| Equally responsible for the delivery of safe and effective occupational therapy services | |

Adapted from Intraprofessional Role Delineation: OTR & COTA. Ceranski, S., & Black, T. (2014). *Vision: Gear up to provide cost effective services that achieve outcomes of value to all stakeholders.* Presentation conducted at the Wisconsin Occupational Therapy Association Annual Conference, Appleton, WI.

and two-way communication between these OT practitioners. One critical way to foster these skills is to provide learning opportunities in the educational settings of each level practitioner. Optimally, practicing skill development together fosters a basic understanding, respect, and collegiality between both levels. These educational experiences should be more than written work on defining roles and responsibilities of the OT and OTA. Although there is not as much research on intraprofessional education as there is on interprofessional education, studies suggest that activities should be interactive and provide opportunities for OT and OTA students to participate together in learning activities that build communication skills, respect, and trust. AOTA's official document on the importance of intraprofessional education emphasizes that when students are provided with opportunities to develop collaborative relationships as part of their educational process, they will work collaboratively in practice (AOTA, 2018). This collaboration in turn, supports the 21st-century health care goal to provide older adults and other consumers of occupational therapy services with outstanding and reasonably priced care.

Since the 1970s, many skilled nursing facilities (SNFs) and other services across the United States have hired COTAs who are supervised by consulting and direct service OTRs who cover several facilities. Thus, effective OTR-COTA teamwork is imperative in providing quality services. In these instances, within settings with full-time COTAs, they may take on a team leader role (i.e., rehab director), while maintaining the required supervision relationship with the OTR (AOTA, 2020). For example, the COTA may serve as the OT rehab director in an SNF with the responsibility of ensuring an appropriate staffing mix for any given day and managing the department budget used to purchase needed equipment, while collaborating with the OTR on the treatment interventions provided to patients delegated to her caseload. Utilization of an OTR–COTA team in either health care or community-based settings may favorably impact cost containment, and more importantly, focused, and appropriate interventions with older adults. The team process components depicted in Table 30.2 can be implemented to maximize the roles of both the OTR and COTA, so that more individuals may receive services in cost-effective ways.

This figure presents the reciprocal, transactional relationship between the OT team members. The OT should consider all relevant sociocultural factors and client needs prior to program development and implementation. OT practitioners must adhere to the discipline's ethical standards, policies, and guidelines, as well as state, federal, and other regulatory and reimbursement guidelines that may apply to their service delivery or program. The OTR identifies the theoretical and evidence base upon which the program is developed, selects screening and evaluation tools to be utilized, interprets results, plans, and conducts interventions, and oversees discharge or discontinuation of services, as well as any research conducted within the program. The OTA conducts delegated screening, evaluation, and reevaluation processes and provides verbal and written reports of observations and older client capacities, plans and conducts interventions, contributes

**TABLE 30.2** Supervision Responsibilities Occupational Therapy Practitioners' Roles and Responsibilities in Service Provision

| Occupational Therapist | Occupational Therapy Assistant |
|---|---|
| THEORY DIAGNOSIS | TECHNIQUES |
| Program Development | Screening |
| Choose Frame of Reference | Evaluation |
| Choose Evaluations | Intervention Planning |
| Intervention Planning | INTERVENTION |
| Intervention | Discharge |
| Discharge | Assist with Program Development |
| Research | |

Adapted from Intraprofessional Occupational Therapy Team Member Tasks. Ceranski, S., & Black, T. (2014). *Vision: Gear up to provide cost effective services that achieve outcomes of value to all stakeholders.* Presentation conducted at the Wisconsin Occupational Therapy Association Annual Conference, Appleton, WI.

to discharge/program discontinuation planning, and may assist in collecting research data.

OT-OTA intraprofessional teams play important roles in medical settings that include acute care, rehabilitation, hand therapy, out-patient, mental health, and SNFs. Both medical and community-based programs are increasing the utilization of these teams gradually, in part due to changes in how health care is delivered. With the projected demographics regarding global aging and the emphasis on cost containment, we can expect an increase in the need for these teams in both traditional medical and, increasingly, nontraditional community-based services, since humans are occupational beings and occupational therapy services support them in striving to thrive while pursuing desired occupations, regardless of their life circumstances. Note that Chapter 33, The Future of Gerontological Occupational Therapy, offers additional insight regarding emerging areas of need and opportunities for the development of services and programs within which the use of these teams may be considered.

## Interprofessional Teams

### Interprofessional Care for Older Adults

To provide optimal care, older adults benefit from the support of different health professionals to address their multi-faceted health care problems. Team-based interprofessional care improves outcomes for older adults and is identified as a quality indicator of good geriatric care (Montagnini, et al., 2014). While further research is needed, studies show that interventions to support interprofessional care improved satisfaction of providers (Ko et al., 2014) and improved treatment outcomes of older adults, such as improved ability to complete activities of daily living, reduced pain, and decreased hospital length of stay and fall incidence (Ritchie et al., 2016; Tsakitizidis, et al., 2016; Youngwerth & Twaddle, 2011). The intersection of physical and mental health with the social

determinants of health makes teams ideal to provide care for an older adult population.

The interprofessional or interdisciplinary approach has long been supported by a variety of health care experts. The World Health Organization (WHO, 2016) has addressed the need for collaborative practice, defined as "multiple health workers from different professional backgrounds provide comprehensive services by working with patients, their families, carers, and communities to deliver the highest quality of care across settings." Further, the National Academies of Science and Medicine (2019) proposed the need for collaborative interprofessional care as health care shifts toward more community care, needs to address broad individual needs, and experiences shortages of some health professionals. A workgroup from the American Geriatrics Society (Montagnini et al., 2014) proposed interprofessional care as a standard competency for those caring for older adults. As a result, health professionals need educational opportunities while they are students to learn how to work with other disciplines, or later when they enter the workforce to become what the WHO calls "collaborative-practice-ready" (WHO, 2016, p. 39).

### Competencies for Interprofessional Geriatric Care

Several documents and interprofessional initiatives help to examine the competencies and focus needed to provide appropriate collaborative care for older adults. These indicate a broad consensus among health professionals of the need for interprofessional care and collaboration, and how to design such care. We review here these documents and how they provide guidance on interprofessional care.

### Competencies in Care of Older Adults

An interprofessional group convened by the developed competencies for the care of older adults for all health professionals. Participants included physicians, nurses, physical therapists (PTs), OTs, and more. The AOTA endorsed this document. The final document outlined six broad domains that are applied based on the disciplinary traditions, needs and preferences, backgrounds, and older adults' care context, as described below.

- *Health Promotion and Safety*—advocate for evidence-based health promotion and preventive interventions and services for older adults.
- *Evaluation and Assessment*—knowledge and skills to perform comprehensive geriatric assessment using valid and reliable assessment tools to examine the biological, physical, cognitive, psychological, and social issues associated with aging.
- *Care and Program Planning and Coordination across the Continuum of Care* (including end of life)—develop evidence-based patient-centered treatment plans that include advanced directives and are communicated through transitions between care settings.
- *Interdisciplinary and Team Care*—communicate and collaborate with all health professionals and older adults and their caregivers as part of the team.

- *Caregiver Support*—evaluate and address caregiver needs and support their work with older adults.
- *Health Care Systems and Benefits*—advocate for older adults and caregivers across and within health-care settings, and support access to information and resources and navigation of the health-care systems or setting.

## Age-Friendly Health Care

Due to the growing population of older adults and their need for appropriate, evidence-based care, the Institute for Healthcare Improvement (IHI, 2022) developed a collaboration with the John A. Hartford Foundation, the American Hospital Association, and the Catholic Health Association of the United States. The result of this collaboration is the Age-Friendly Health System initiative. While this does not address competencies per se, the focus is to encourage health professionals to tailor their care to older adults and their families by meeting three goals:

- Following an essential set of evidence-based practices
- Causing no harm
- Aligning with what matters to older adults and their family caregivers

The focus of what "matters" to older adults is on four areas known as the 4 Ms as noted in Table 30.3. These are inter-related, common geriatric functional needs central to the care and quality of life of older adults: medications, mobility, mentation, and what matters to the older adult. The four focus areas are addressed as a set in any practice situation, and incorporated into care through assessment, evidence-based interventions, and evaluation of care provided.

## Competencies for Interprofessional Collaboration

Beyond care of older adults, a group of health professions organizations (Interprofessional Education Collaborative [IPEC], 2016) also developed interprofessional collaboration competencies for any population, which were updated in 2016 currently being updated, and earlier endorsed by the AOTA. These competencies are based on the need for accessible, quality, patient-centered care, considering the changes and challenges in health care over the past decade. Quality interprofessional collaboration can help achieve the triple aim of improving health care by achieving the following (IHI, 2022):

- Improve the patient experience of care
- Improve the health of populations
- Reduce the costs of health care

The IPEC competencies are meant to cross all health professionals in any settings and are especially important in geriatric care.

## Competencies

1. *Work with individuals of other professions to maintain a climate of mutual respect and shared values.* (Values/Ethics for Interprofessional Practice)
   Under competency 1, professionals work to promote the health and health equity of populations, respecting the dignity of individuals, their differences, and how these may impact health. Health professionals develop trusting relationships with each other as well as patients and families in providing team-based care. Professionals are also challenged to be ethical and competent in their own profession.

2. *Use the knowledge of one's own role and those of other professions to appropriately assess and address the health care needs of patients and to promote and advance the health of populations.* (Roles/Responsibilities)
   Under the second competency, health professionals should be able to communicate their role to others on the health care team (including patients/families, etc.) as well as limitations. They work collaboratively with other professionals within and outside the health care team to provide quality health care and improve population health.

3. *Communicate with patients, families, communities, and professionals in health and other fields in a responsive and responsible manner that supports a team approach to the promotion and maintenance of health and the prevention and treatment of disease.* (Interprofessional Communication)
   Communication is the focus of the third competency. Health professionals need to be able to communicate effectively with other health professionals, patients and their caregivers, and the public in working collaboratively with others. This includes using active listening and respectful language to address difficult conversations that will improve team performance and health care delivery.

4. *Apply relationship-building values and the principles of team dynamics to perform effectively in different team roles to plan, deliver, and evaluate patient/population-centered care and population health programs and policies that are safe, timely, efficient, effective, and equitable.* (Teams and Teamwork)

The fourth competency calls for health professionals to work collaboratively and use quality improvement practices. Taken together, these form the underpinnings of good team collaboration that will support strong interprofessional care for older adults.

## Development of Interprofessional Skills

Regarding the competencies and guidelines discussed so far in this chapter, health care providers need education and experiences in interprofessional care. Typically, health care providers have been trained with others in their own disciplines and have limited exposure or experiences with other disciplines (Dyer et al., 2003). This has led to poor communication and collaboration as well as fragmented care, which is especially detrimental for older adults. In "A Framework for Action" from the WHO (2016) interprofessional education is defined as follows: "students from two or more professions learn about, from and with each other to enable effective collaboration and improve health outcomes." Given the benefits of interprofessional care, educating students to be collaborative practice-ready when completing their programs is a critical goal. Courses, clinical practice experiences, and education on teams and teamwork support development of skilled providers interested in caring for older adults. Studies show that better attitudes toward older adults and improved competence

**TABLE 30.3** Team Members Overview

| Members | Practice Roles/Skills | Education/Training | Licensure/Credentials[1] |
|---|---|---|---|
| Nurse | Licensed vocational nurse (LVN)—basic nursing skills that are dictated by the facility; registered nurse (RN)—associate degree, BA, or higher; increased scope of practice for RN, including planning for optimal functioning, coordination of care, teaching, and direct and indirect patient care | LVN—1 year of training<br>AN with associate degree—2 years of training, usually in a community college<br>BS, AN—4 years of college<br>MS, AN—2 years of postgraduate specialty study<br>PhD, AN—4–6 years of postgraduate studies | LVN examination required for licensing<br>Continuing education unit (CEU) requirements: AN; BS; APN; MS, GNP, or other specialty ANs PhD, AN: must pass the national licensure examination and required to have 20 h of CEUs per year |
| Nurse Practitioner | Health assessment, health promotion, histories and physicals in outpatient settings; orders, conducts, and interprets some laboratory and diagnostic tests; teaching and counseling | Master's or clinical doctorate degree with a defined specialty area, such as gerontology (GNP), adult/gerontology (AGNP), or family (FNP) | In addition to AN licensure, must pass a National Certification Examination in the appropriate specialty area (e.g., gerontology or family practice), CE requirements |
| Physician | Diagnoses and treats diseases and injuries, provides preventive care, does routine check-ups, prescribes drugs, and does some surgery | Medical school (4 years) plus 3–7 years of graduate medical education | State licensure required for doctor of medicine degree; examination required and possible examinations required for specialty areas; CE requirements |
| Geriatrician | Physician with special training in the diagnosis, treatment, and prevention of disorders in older people; recognizes aging as a normal process and not a disease state | Completion of medical school, residency training in family medicine and internal medicine, and 1-year fellowship program in gerontological medicine | Completion of fellowship training program and/or passing examination for Certificate of Added Qualifications in Geriatric Medicine (CAQ); recertification by examination required every 10 years and begins in the 8th year, as it is a 2-year process |
| Physician Assistant (PA) | Practices with the supervision of a licensed physician; exercises autonomy in medical decision making and provides a broad range of diagnostic and therapeutic services; practice centered on patient care | Specially designed 2-year program at medical colleges and universities; bachelor's degree and over 4 years of health-care experience typical before entering a PA program | State licensure or registration plus certification by the National Commission on Certification of Physician Assistants (NCCPA); recertification every 6 years by examination; 100 hours continuing medical education (CME) every 2 years |
| Social Worker (SW) | Assessment of individual and family psychosocial functioning and provision of care to help enhance or restore capacities; can include locating services or providing counseling | MSW—2 years of graduate work<br>PhD—2–4 years additional training | State certification required for clinical social workers; LMSW (or master's level) or LSW (BS level); social work associate (SWA) with a combination of education and experience; ACP signifies licensure for independent clinical practice |
| Gerontological Psychologist | Assessment, treatment, and management of mental disorders; psychotherapy with individuals, groups, and families | Graduate training: 5 years beyond undergraduate training; most coursework includes gerontology and clinical/practice experience | PhD, EdD, or PsyD degree; state licensure for Clinical Psychologists; the American Psychological Association ethical code and state ethical codes |

**TABLE 30.3** Team Members Overview—Cont'd

| Members | Practice Roles/Skills | Education/Training | Licensure/Credentials[1] |
|---|---|---|---|
| Psychiatrist | Medical doctor who treats patients' mental, emotional, and behavioral symptoms | Medical school and residency specializing in psychiatry; residency includes both general residency training and 2–3 years in area of specialization (e.g., geriatrics, pediatrics) | State examination to practice medicine; Board of Psychiatry and Neurology offers examination for diploma in psychiatry, although not required for psychiatric practice in Texas |
| Pharmacist | Devises and revises a patient's medication therapy to achieve the optimal regime that suits the individual's medical and therapeutic needs; information resource for the patient and medical team | BS—5-year program Doctorate degree (PharmD) Requirements for annual continuing CEUs ranging from 10–15 h | State examination required; national examination (NABPLEX), given every quarter, used in Texas; "RPh" used as title for a registered pharmacist in Texas; board certifications in specialties available (pharmacotherapy, nuclear pharmacy, nutrition, psychiatric, and oncology in near future) |
| Occupational Therapist (OTR) | Evaluation, prevention, and/or correction of physical, mental, or emotional dysfunction; maximization of function in the life of the individual through therapeutic goal-directed activity/occupation | BS, MS, MOT, or OTD degree in OT with a minimum of 6 months of fieldwork | National board examination for credential of OTR (occupational therapy registered); state licensure where applicable; continuing education |
| Occupational Therapy Assistant (COTA) | Delivers services under the supervision of and in collaboration with the OTR by implementing and documenting the applied therapeutic interventions, and provides feedback to the OTR on the client's progress during treatment/intervention. | AS, AAS, or certificate in OTA with a minimum of 4 months of fieldwork | National board examination for credential of COTA (certified occupational therapy assistant); state licensure where applicable; continuing education |
| Physical Therapist (PT) | Evaluation, examination, and utilization of exercise, rehabilitative procedures, massage, manipulations, and physical agents, including but not limited to mechanical devices, heat, cold, air, light, water, electricity, and sound, in the aid of diagnosis or treatment | MSPT, MPT, or DPT degree in physical therapy | National board examination for credential of PT; state licensure where applicable; continuing education |
| Physical Therapy Assistant (PTA) | Works under the direction and supervision of a PT | AS degree in physical therapy assistant | National board examination for credential of PTA; state licensure where applicable; continuing education |
| Chaplain | Provides visits and ministry to patients and family | Master's degree in theology, plus a minimum of 1 year of clinical supervision, if fully certified; can work in some settings without being fully certified | Certification through the Chaplaincy Board of Certification; however, credentials not normally used; most are ordained ministers, but not all; 50 h per year CEUs required |

*Continued*

**TABLE 30.3** Team Members Overview—Cont'd

| Members | Practice Roles/Skills | Education/Training | Licensure/Credentials[1] |
|---|---|---|---|
| Dietitian | Evaluates the nutritional status of patients; works with family members and medical team to determine appropriate nutrition goals for patients | BS degree in food and nutrition and experience required to be eligible for examination; CEUs required for both the licensed dietitian (LD) (6 clock hours/year) and registered dietitian (AD) (75 clock hours every 5 years); MS degree available also | AD is credential for a registered dietitian in Texas; must pass the national examination of the American Dietetic Association; LD is credential for a licensed dietitian Texas: same national examination required but processing of paperwork differs |
| Recreational Therapist | Plans, directs, and coordinates recreational programs for people with disabilities or illnesses using a variety of techniques, such as arts and crafts, drama, music, dance, sports, games, and field trips; programs help to improve a client's physical and emotional well-being | BS in recreational therapy | National certification examination |

[1]Licensed health professionals in the U.S. have continuing education (CE) requirements; with license renewal, one must record, and, if requested, provide documentation of having completed CE in the amount required by state licensing laws.
Note: Continuing education requirements vary by state, and licensing and certification titles vary (e.g., LVN or LPN; LISW or LMSW; CSW, CISW, or CICSW). (Adapted from Hyer, K., Flaherty, E., Fairchild, S., Botrell, M., Mezey, M., Fulmer, T., et al. [2003]. *Geriatric Interdisciplinary Team Training program [GITT]: Curriculum guide*. GITT Resource Center, New York University.)

in providing care (Ko et al., 2014; Tan et al., 2016) result from interprofessional training activities. For example, Knech-Sabres (2018) reported improved OT students' perceptions of aging in an interprofessional training experience, and Lach et al. (2020) found students, including OTs, demonstrated good skills in interprofessional collaboration after participating in a geriatric case competition activity.

The remaining sections of this chapter provide an overview of interprofessional teams and teamwork to begin learning about interprofessional collaboration. We encourage occupational therapy students and professionals to continue their education in this area so that they become skilled collaborative-practice providers.

## Interprofessional Teams and Teamwork

### Who Comprises the Team?

Ideally, gerontological health care teams consist of groups of health professionals committed to working closely together to improve patient/client care. While different members bring different sets of skills and knowledge, each person is accountable for the work of the entire team. For this to be successful, excellent communication and shared decision making are essential. An effective team works synergistically so that the team's overall performance exceeds that of the individual inputs of the members. This is how teams are able to solve problems that individuals cannot.

Everyone with a role and stake in an older person's care should be included at the team table. Therefore, interprofessional teams can include a wide range of health professionals.

As providers work in roles in increasingly diverse settings, such as in the community, long-term care, and public health, a broad range of workers may be important members of the care team. Importantly, in order to provide true patient-centered care, the patient, family, and community should be considered part of the health care team (National Academies of Sciences, Engineering, and Medicine [NASEM], 2019). There can be challenges when putting together all these different individuals who have a wide range of training, knowledge, and experiences, making the goal of developing a functioning team critical. It takes work to work together (Zajac et al., 2021).

### Types of Teams

Teams can be of different types. Drinka and Clark (2000) described the classic types of team styles in health care: ad hoc, uni-disciplinary, multidisciplinary, and interdisciplinary. An ad hoc team is a group of health professionals who come together to solve a single, short-term problem. For example, an OT and OTA may work together to help an older client improve access to his or her home by enlisting the services of an architect, designer, and/or carpenter. Uni-disciplinary teams include people from one profession who may have different kinds of expertise. An older client may have a gerontologist, orthopedist, and urologist helping to address various medical conditions. Multidisciplinary teams include multiple disciplines, but they do not necessarily communicate or collaborate with one another. For example, different disciplines caring for a hospitalized patient may provide their own care, and then record what they are doing in the chart for others to read. A true interdisciplinary team, often called an *interprofessional* team, collaborates, talks to each other, develops a common purpose, and shares leadership and decision-making responsibilities and accountability for outcomes. Some use the term *transdisciplinary* team for this collaborative model (Omillon-Hodges et al., 2021).

For good functioning, interprofessional teams need a common purpose and process for the approach that will be used by the team and that lays the foundation for interprofessional teamwork. The purpose keeps everyone focused on long-term goals and keeps team spirit alive when short-term failures interfere with those goals (Craig & McKeown, 2015). The most common purposes of gerontology-focused health care teams include the following:

- Improve client function or maintain maximum client independence.
- Enhance client well-being.
- Increase client satisfaction.
- Reduce use of or improve hospital services.
- Reduce health care costs.
- Optimize work satisfaction of all team members.

The role of the team is to complete tasks according to their purpose and that result in the accomplishment of a goal, usually to address a client outcome. Increasingly, funding and accreditation are dependent on facilities being able to document improved outcomes. This documentation can be quantitative (decreased number of hospitalizations and rehospitalizations; improved functional parameters) or qualitative (increased satisfaction with services). Therefore, relevant measurable outcomes and subjective feedback can be easily communicated to members of the team.

## Right-Sizing the Team

Teams come in all sizes, but for this discussion the concept of teams will be divided into small (2 to 5 members), medium (6 to 12 members), and large (more than 12 members). In general, large teams are not very effective. They can work when information being shared does not need discussion. However, it is difficult for a large number of people to be involved if decision making is needed or the group needs to reach a consensus, or even find a time to meet. To accomplish tasks, large teams can be more effective when broken down into smaller work groups that can address specific issues or components of larger projects.

Small teams are most efficient. According to CNBC television (2018), Jeff Bezos of Amazon requires all teams be small enough to be fed with two pizzas for effectiveness. One example of a small team is often seen in primary care, where the goal is to provide a higher quality of care for clients beyond that of the typical 15-minute physician visit.[3] A physician and/or nurse practitioner or physician/s assistant can share patient care. A small team might include individuals from multiple sites who collaborate on a problem that crosses sites. Such a team might meet to create a plan of care for an older adult who needs to continue OT treatment at home after hospitalization, or to create a policy to provide better referral of patients to a cardiac rehab program.

Small-sized teams are common in clinical and community care, and often consist of a social worker, a nurse, a physician, and occupational and/or physical therapists. Other members are added to meet the specific needs of clients, especially in transition-of-care situations, such as discharges, when older adults are moved from one setting to another. These other professionals might include pharmacists, dieticians, speech pathologists, or pastoral care. Other members tend to be more site-specific. For example, in long-term care settings teams can include activity directors, nurse aides, even maintenance or laundry workers who may know the older adults and have insights into their problems. Optometrists and audiologists are often consulted to address vision and hearing issues. Home care teams may consult with lawyers, elder abuse experts, or police officers. Public health settings may include community health workers, meals on wheels workers, and more. The goal is to include other disciplines as needed to meet the needs of the individual older adult and their family. Health professionals should be prepared to work with this variety of possible team members who vary widely in their training and experience with older adults.

Medium-sized teams can function efficiently if communication is carefully handled. Also, they may serve as a pool of experts who can spin off into smaller teams to handle specific short-term issues, such as to conduct a quality improvement project for a hospital or develop a health promotion program, such as a fall prevention or diabetes management program.

## Virtual Teams

With the growing ease of electronic communication (electronic health records, video-conference technology, etc.), virtual teams are now common. Teams do not need in-person meetings to communicate effectively. In fact, virtual teams are becoming the norm in such settings as hospice care, home care, and rural health care. The electronic health record can often be accessed from different workstations and even from different worksites, which allow professionals to share information. The use of video conference programs allows teams to spend important time together to discuss information without needing to travel, making meetings more efficient. This method works well if the group is small to medium sized; members can see each other as well as talk. However, if a team only meets virtually, it can be harder to get to know other team members, as communication may be stiff with less opportunity for informal discussions. Fathi et al. (2016) identified essential elements for successful virtual teamwork: (1) shared electronic medical records, (2) team meetings, (3) standardized assessments, and (4) secure e-messaging.

## Team Development and Effective Functioning

Gerontological interprofessional health care teams are just like other teams, but usually have a goal to provide care for an older adult, to share information and develop a treatment/intervention plan, and to oversee its implementation. But regardless of the purpose, all teams go through a similar process of development. When a team first gets together, personal attributes such as gender, age, personality, race, and stereotypical images of professions may play a part in shaping the informal roles that members adopt. This informal role differentiation may diminish in later stages of team development as the team members learn about each other and develop trust and feelings of psychological safety (Morgan et al., 2021). However, these initial roles can also persist, resulting in conflicts among team members. Tuckman (1965), in a seminal article, described the classic process of team development that includes stages where different challenges are encountered:

- *Forming*: Team members are identified and join the group and begin getting to know each other. Lack of trust and knowledge of other team members can inhibit group work in this stage.
- *Norming*: Members integrate goals and values of the team and the group process as they learn to work together. If the goals and processes for how the team works are not clear, it can be challenging to achieve these tasks.
- *Confronting*: Conflicts arise as team members work together, and effective teams learn to resolve these conflicts in a positive way. Conflict should be expected given the different perspectives that come with interprofessional teams. Strong leadership and communication skills help teams resolve conflicts in a positive way that improves care, and that they do not lead to team dysfunction.
- *Performing*: Members achieve a high level of performance focused on the client, rather than on the process or individual. Possible challenges here are loss of members or developing group think, rather than bringing individual perspectives and new ideas.
- *Leaving*: Members leave and may or may not be replaced with new members; new members can change the complexion of the team, or teams may be disbanded.

It is in the best interest of the client that the team works at the performing level as much as possible, which should be the norm for a stable team. Good leadership can impact team performance (Almost et al., 2016), and help the team define their collective goals and mission and reach this level in a short period of time, while addressing communication or conflicts. In addition, team training activities encourage understanding and appreciation between team members and help team members develop interprofessional competencies (IPEC, 2016). This hard work of team development has several critical components. They include developing trust and psychological safety, defining expectations, assigning roles and tasks, and measuring outcomes. Trust is developed when the team members get to know and respect each other, as they share their skills, their personal goals, and their dreams. As team members change and new members arrive, the team may go back through the stages of development, so the process may be repeated.

The following outlines key components of a high-performing gerontological care team (Hyer et al., 2003). Purpose, goals, and objectives are known and agreed upon.

- Roles and responsibilities are clear.
- Communication is open, sharing, and honest. There is disagreement without tyranny and constructive criticism without personal attack.

- Team members listen to one another.
- Team members are competent, professional, and personally effective, and make appropriate contributions.
- Team members cooperate and coordinate activities. Decisions are made by consensus.
- When decisions are made, assignments are made clearly, accepted, and carried out.
- Leadership shifts, depending on the circumstances.
- Team members support each other and act as different resources for the group.
- Team members trust one another, minimize struggles for power, and focus on how best to get the job done.
- The team evaluates its own operations.

Unfortunately, teams are susceptible to dysfunction from a variety of challenges and barriers (Schot et al., 2020). When a team meets, its members must be given an opportunity to express their opinions and expectations to accomplish their assigned tasks. Potential ethical issues can result from poor team performance, including overwhelming clients with a large team, taking a long time to work through group issues while the client waits, or falling into "groupthink" and excluding new approaches to solve problems (Kane, 2005). The blurring of roles between some disciplines is normal but can cause role ambiguity (Almost et al., 2016), as well as conflict, low morale, and poor task management. Several factors can assist with developing and maintaining high-performing teams. These factors will be further explored:

- Leadership
- Communication
- Regular efficient meetings
- Conflict management

## Leadership

With the advent of new modalities through which teams interact and the need for different team members to address unique client issues, effective leadership and coaching is critical (Ells & Sevdals, 2019; Zajac et al., 2021). Leadership should help organize the work of the team in such a way that team members know how to work together and how decisions will be made in the group. While the primary leader may oversee group meetings and be responsible for general organizational tasks, ideally, anyone on an interprofessional team should be able to lead specific parts of the work of the team for any individual client. This is because all members have relevant expertise, and everyone shares the same goal. This shifting leadership role is particularly applicable as the client's health improves or after transitions in care. During a health crisis, a physician may be the natural leader, but during recovery leadership might shift to an occupational or PT, and near the end of treatment, a social worker may take the lead. Leadership should flow from the needs of the client. As team members learn each other's strengths and expertise, this shifting of leadership should flow naturally among team members based on the changing needs of the client.

There are a variety of tasks that team members may take on that can help (or hinder) the team's meetings and work. Hyer et al. (2003) described these as "leadership tasks" (Table 30.4).

**TABLE 30.4**  Interdisciplinary Health-Care Teams: Leadership Tasks

| | | |
|---|---|---|
| Organizer/Mover | Finisher | Expert |
| Initiate team development | Impose time constraints | Provide special expertise |
| Identify team tasks | Focus on outcomes (clients treated, goals achieved) | Offer professional viewpoint |
| Identify strengths and weaknesses | Seek progress | Identify interdisciplinary client problems |
| Call meetings | Show high commitment to task | Use expertise of other disciplines |
| Provide structure | Manage projects | Understand client needs |
| Review team needs | | Know team's expertise and limits |
| Identify appropriate clients | | |
| Ambassador | Diplomat | |
| Build external relationships Promote awareness of the team's work | Build understanding between members Negotiate | Supporter |
| Build bridges | Mediate | Build team morale |
| Show concern for external team environment | Facilitate decision making | Put team members at ease |
| | | Ensure job satisfaction |
| | | Help client work with team |
| Judge/Evaluator | Process/Analyzer | Mediator |
| Listen critically | Identify team problems | Identify member conflicts |
| Evaluate clinical process | Analyze team problems | Help team members find ways to resolve conflicts |
| Evaluate clinical outcomes | Consult with team members | Help implement solutions |
| Help team reflect | Offer observations | |
| Promote appropriate treatment | Offer potential solutions to team problems | |
| Act logically | | |
| Seek truth | | |
| | Innovator | Challenger |
| Creator | Discover resources | Offer skepticism |
| Generate new ideas | Identify opportunities | Look in new ways |
| Visualize new programs/projects | Transform ideas into strategy | Question accepted order |
| Visualize new alliances | Propose new methods | |
| | | Conformer/Follower |
| Renewer | Quality Controller | Seek agreement |
| Observe | Check output alignment | Fill gaps in teamwork |
| Review team performance | Act as conscience regarding team goals | Cooperate |
| Promote review of process | Inspire higher standards | Help relationships |
| Give feedback | Ensure team reviews outcomes | Avoid challenges |
| Mirror team's actions | | Maintain continuity |
| Guard | Teacher | Learner |
| Protect team from too much output | Help new members learn the norms and values of the team | Raise questions to enhance understanding across disciplines or areas |
| Protect team from too much input | Teach shared leadership skills to other members | Raise questions regarding need for interdisciplinary input |
| | Reorganize members' leadership potential | |
| | Teach others when to seek specialty advice | |

Adapted from Hyer, K., Flaherty, E., Fairchild, S., Botrell, M., Mezey, M., Fulmer, T., et al. (2003). *Geriatric Interdisciplinary Team Training program (GITT): Curriculum guide.* GITT Resource Center, New York University.

Each of these tasks can provide a contribution to the team's functioning. Other members can contribute to team functioning. For example, the assigned "leader" may not be generally organized, but someone else on the team can be assigned to manage this (agendas, meeting times, timekeeper). The leader may mentor team members to develop skills needed to support the teams' work. Team members should consider which tasks come most naturally, which ones are covered within the current membership of the team, and which ones need further development. It takes a cohesive, well-trained team to put the needs of the client first and to shift leadership as the client's needs change. Team training and group discussions can help teams address issues related to leadership and make sure everyone understands how the team process works.

## Communication

In a typical team meeting, members will communicate by giving reports, writing reports, and collaborative discussion (Bokhour, 2006). Team members should strive to develop communication skills so they can succinctly share their own ideas and actively listen to other team members' ideas. This results in collaborative discussion during team meetings, which occurs when team members share information, ask questions, exchange ideas, and discuss options, to reach the best decision for the client. No matter how well a team has performed in the past, there is a constant need for vigilance on the part of the team to ensure good communication and group process.

Common barriers to good interprofessional team communication can arise. First, because members are from different disciplines, they may have conflicting goals, speak different languages, use different terms, and have different approaches (Schot et al., 2020). Team members need to be open to other perspectives. Alternatively, the overlap between some roles can cause role ambiguity and inhibit collaboration (Wittenberg-Lyles et al., 2010). Learning to understand and trust other team members and a strong team process can prevent this from disrupting teamwork.

Another communication barrier is hierarchical or power differentials between team members that can inhibit open communication on a team (Zajac et al., 2021). Traditional roles have been hierarchical, for example physicians being considered the leader or decision maker. When health professionals are trained in silos, these roles can be exaggerated. The older adult or family members may have low health literacy, and no health care experience. Communicating with older adults and family members requires translation from medical lingo to plain language to enhance their understanding.

Ineffective processes for team meetings can also serve as a barrier to communication. Teams need a clear process for how decisions are made (Hyer et al., 2003). Team members should know how to prepare for meetings, how the flow of information will go, and what the outcomes will be. Side conversations, settings with many disruptions, and distractions such as cell phones need to be minimized. In a study of interpersonal communication dynamics during hospice interdisciplinary team meetings (Bokhour, 2006), researchers found the majority of communication time spent was aimed at gaining control of the information exchange, rather than collaboratively discussing client issues. Everyone wants to be heard on the team, and a clear process for meeting conduct is needed to facilitate good communication. Processes that foster closed loop communication, in which individual input is acknowledged, support collaborative work (Ells & Sevdales, 2019). Table 30.5 provides a description of key components of effective meetings, such as an agenda, that organizers can use to develop a meeting plan for the team.

## Management of Conflicts

Conflict is a natural part of teamwork, as everyone views the situation through their disciplinary lens. A healthy team is aware of this and can address conflicts by either resolving them or comfortably "agreeing to disagree" without negatively influencing the team performance. However, even small conflicts can build and lead to poor team performance.

Three types of conflict are common. The first is intrapersonal conflict, where an individual team member experiences role conflict with other job responsibilities or with his or her role on the team. Intra-team conflicts involve two or more team members and may develop from disagreements about care, personality differences, or different styles of working or communicating (Almost et al., 2016). Inter-team conflict occurs when the team has conflict with entities outside the team, such as other provider groups.

To address conflicts, ideally issues are discussed openly to reach a resolution. Some issues may be best addressed by the whole group, and others should be discussed just by the parties involved. Group leaders should help facilitate discussions with those involved to address and solve team problems. If conflicts affect the team's performance, an objective outside

## TABLE 30.5 Effective Team Meetings

| | |
|---|---|
| Regular meeting times | Team members need to be able to plan to attend and arrange their calendars. |
| Agenda | Distribute an agenda with a list of clients, preferably before the meeting (of who or what is to be discussed). |
| Reporting format | Identifying an order of when and how team members will report can help the meeting flow smoothly. Team members should give informative reports and ask questions when appropriate. |
| Goal-setting process | Determine how decisions will be made as to goals for care, identification of problems, and strategies for addressing issues. Opinions should be solicited and given. |
| Time frame | Allocate time for the meeting and discussion of individual clients or issues. |
| Assignment of tasks | Tasks should be distributed evenly and by skill set of team members. Team members should come away from the meeting with a clear idea of their assignments. |
| Recording of information | Documenting the plan of team decisions about care and assignments helps everyone remember what decisions were made at the meeting. |
| Managing distractions | There are often distractions, from cell phones to off-topic discussions. Discuss and agree as a team how best to minimize these. |
| Planning time for evaluation | Some time should be included periodically to evaluate team functioning, discuss process issues, and provide for team training. |

Adapted from Lach, H-W. (2007). Team work: Interdisciplinary geriatric care. In A. D. Linton & H-W. Lach (Eds.), *Matteson & McConnell's gerontological nursing: Concepts and practice* [3rd ed., pp. 759–776. Saunders/Elsevier.

facilitator or training on communication or teamwork may be helpful.

## Assessing Team Performance

Although team members often identify challenges when working together, teams should regularly evaluate their performance, address deficiencies, and celebrate successes. Quality assurance data should be collected and shared with the team to evaluate performance. There are several possible sources of information to support this work. First, surveys of patient satisfaction may be collected by the hospital or health system based on patient services. Alternatively, teams could plan their own surveys or follow up of patients to see how the patient fared based on the team's work. Data could also be collected from electronic health records to determine patient outcomes. Reflection on team performance can improve performance (Zajac et al., 2021).

Within the team, discussions should be held regularly to identify challenges or issues to be addressed by the team. Additional training that requires team members to develop the competencies in interprofessional collaboration described above may be needed to help the team develop into a high-performing team if needed. Positive reviews and experiences should be rewarded to celebrate accomplishments of the team and show appreciation for the team's work.

## Exemplars of Interdisciplinary/ Interprofessional Care Teams

To provide optimal gerontological health care, interdisciplinary teams are present and must be effective across the continuum of care. At no time are older persons more vulnerable than when they are ill and seeking health care outside of the home environment. And, of course, the older and more frail a person is, the more vulnerable he or she is. When a team works well together, health care improves. Examples of successful interdisciplinary team models are illustrated next: the Program of All-Inclusive Care of the Elderly (PACE), an acute care fall-prevention team, and a stroke rehabilitation team.

### Program of All-Inclusive Care of the Elderly

A community-based program called the PACE in the United States. provides care to older adults via Medicaid and Medicare covered services (Medicaid.gov, 2022). The primary goal of PACE programs is to support older adults within the community for as long as needed. In the PACE model, interdisciplinary team members include nonprofessional carers as well as professional health-care workers. In this study, individuals' health, functional status, and mental status were reviewed in 26 PACE programs with 3401 enrollees to determine whether the interdisciplinary teams were associated with better risk-adjusted health outcomes for survival, both short-term and long-term functional status, and urinary incontinence (Mukamel et al., 2006). All of the PACE teams included the physician; the director of nursing; the physical, occupational, and recreational therapists; the social worker; the dietician; the day center coordinator; the personal care attendant; and

the driver. Other team members included the pharmacist or the chaplain. PACE teams are large; some have had as many as 50 members, although it is more usual for subgroups of 10 team members providing current care to meet formally, at least weekly, and informally as needed. Team leaders receive facilitator training and ensure that all team members provide input at the meetings. Results of the study indicate that short-term and long-term functional outcomes, as well as long-term urinary incontinence outcomes, are better for older adults who are frail and receive interdisciplinary team care. This suggests that for PACE programs to remain successful in providing good health care, they need to focus on keeping their teams working at the performing level.

### Acute Care Fall-Prevention Team

The following study description illustrates the types of interaction between team members that are necessary to produce good health care in a hospital setting. Falls are a constant threat to the well-being of older clients. Many studies have looked at the causes (of falls), and many programs have attempted to reduce fall risk. Few have succeeded. One research study, designed to introduce a structured fall-prevention program in a hospital, demonstrates the value of interdisciplinary teamwork (von Renteln-Kruse & Krause, 2007) in addressing a difficult problem. The team members were identified (two physicians, two nurses, a PT, an OT, and a quality manager). The group met initially to discuss the goals of the program and determine the preventive measures that would be used. They then met for 2 hours at the beginning of the study and then for short monthly meetings for the duration of the study. These members then, in turn, informed their staff about the meeting's information. The team members oriented all new hospital staff members in a 1-hour training session. No new team members were introduced to the team and no members left during the project. Each team member had a well-defined role, and the procedure for identifying subjects at risk for falls was clear. Subjects identified for fall risk and their family members were immediately educated about the project. Each subject was discussed at the next team meeting. Caregivers were encouraged to attend therapy sessions. Therapeutic home visits by team members were undertaken as indicated. If deemed advisable, an ophthalmologist and an optician were added to the team for some subjects. Not surprisingly, the fall-prevention program resulted in a significant reduction in fall incidence and the relative risk of falling, regardless of the individual's level of mobility at admission. This is an excellent example of how an interdisciplinary team that functions well as a team can improve health care.

### An Interprofessional Stroke Rehab Team

When a team works well together, health care improves. For interprofessional teams to be effective, team members need to have a mix of complementary skills across the group members, similar beliefs and objectives, and be able to identify and articulate the distinct benefit of their discipline. Below is an example of how an effective interprofessional team might function in a stroke rehabilitation setting.

Mr. Smith is a 65-year-old male who lives alone in a two-story home. He called 911 emergency services in the early morning hours after discovering that he was having difficulty walking and speaking. He was admitted to a primary care hospital on the same day and diagnosed with a left CVA (cerebral vascular accident). Mr. Smith's medical history was significant for hypertension and he is currently taking prescribed diuretics.

A few days post-admission, the first Stroke-Rehabilitation Team meeting took place to discuss Mr. Smith's case. Members of the team included a physiatrist (i.e., medical specialist in rehabilitative medicine), a nurse (who was the randomly assigned case manager), an OT, a PT, a speech-language pathologist (SLP), a neuropsychologist, a social worker, a dietitian, and a recreational therapist. Team members discussed and agreed that multiple assessments of Mr. Smith's skills were necessary including those by SLP, OT, PT, and the social worker. Additional consults for screening of skills were requested by the case manager for audiology, recreation therapy, podiatry/orthotics (shoe fitting, foot lifts, arch supports, etc., as needed), and neuropsychology.

During the initial meeting, the interprofessional collaboration team discussed and formed a plan to determine Mr. Smith's needs. The PT and OT would assess his mobility issues and ability to complete daily tasks. The SLP would complete a speech-language evaluation and select the most appropriate augmentative and alternative communication (AAC) system for Mr. Smith. The RN would continue to monitor any adverse responses to Mr. Smith's medications and observe any changes in his symptoms. The team would also contact the social worker about obtaining any medical equipment that Mr. Smith might need as well as keep his family informed and answer any questions.

After the initial assessments, the team had a better idea of Mr. Smith's needs and were able to devise a coordinated rehabilitation plan. The PT reported that Mr. Smith lacked function in his right leg and had mild weakness in his left leg typical of muscle loss seen secondary to aging along with the inability to self-propel his wheelchair. The OT evaluation determined that Mr. Smith's right arm exhibited poor function, although he could complete some basic daily tasks (feeding, grooming, including tooth brushing, upper body bathing and dressing, and toileting) with maximum assistance. The SLP's evaluation revealed that Mr. Smith could follow one-step directions with occasional repetitions and although he did not have functional speech, he was able to use a low-tech AAC communication board. Each discipline worked together in the following ways:

- PT discussed mounting the AAC system onto Mr. Smith's wheelchair since he was unable to self-propel,

- OT followed up with the social worker about ordering a tray for the wheelchair to assist with upper extremity positioning and allow appropriate placement of a low-tech AAC communication board,
- SLP and OT worked together on feeding and positioning strategies for Mr. Smith.

After 2 months of therapy, Mr. Smith's ability to participate in preferred activities has improved. His is able to eat 75% of a meal with mechanical soft solids and thin liquids and feed himself approximately 50% of the time. His wheelchair enhances his posture and safety during meals and allows access to the low-tech AAC communication board, which has been designed per recommendations from nursing, OT, and the activities department. Although Mr. Smith still does not have functional speech, he is able to successfully use his low-tech AAC communication board to make his needs known. The SLP and social worker are collaborating to determine the feasibility of a speech-generating device.

This case scenario highlights the interprofessional collaboration skills that allowed this team to be effective and show positive outcomes for the patient. These skills included consistent communication, a clear understanding of the team members' roles and responsibilities, and mutual respect for team members' contributions and leadership.

## SUMMARY

The purpose of the interprofessional gerontological team is to provide excellent health care. This care is improved by interdisciplinary team members who value each other's contributions, work collaboratively, and focus on patient/client-centered care, as noted in the geriatric interdisciplinary team training program materials, funded by the John A. Hartford Foundation (Hyer et al., 2003, p. 1) "Good teams don't just happen." Good interdisciplinary teams need to have organizational support, committed members, shared leadership, communication, and more. Ideally, professionals are able to train together to develop these skills. Evaluation and training can improve the performance of interdisciplinary teams (Hughes et al., 2016) and ultimately improve outcomes for our older clients with complex health problems.

*The complete listing of the Bibliography and Chapter Questions and Answers are available in the accompanying enhanced eBook version included with the print purchase of this textbook. Visit Elsevier eBooks+ (eBooks.Health.Elsevier.com) to access this content.*

## CHAPTER 31

# Occupational Therapists, Social Change and Social Transformation Through Occupation

*Debbie Laliberte Rudman, PhD, OT Reg. (Ont.), Margarita Mondaca, PhD, Kathleen Brodrick, MSc, OT, Karen Frank Barney, PhD, MS, OTR, FAOTA, Lisa Jaegers, PhD, and Christine Hayes Picker, MOT, OTR/L*

## CHAPTER OUTLINE

## OBJECTIVES

- Understand the evolving role of occupational therapists in relation to social transformation
- Gain an appreciation of the concept of 'social transformation through occupation' and its relevance to work with aging adults in a diversity of contexts
- Appreciate the health, occupational, and social inequities and challenges faced by marginalized populations of aging adults
- Recognize the importance of enacting relevant, meaningful, and participatory approaches with aging adults aimed at community and social change
- Understand concepts and approaches that can be used by occupational therapists to address social transformation

Over the past two decades, a growing critical awareness has evolved within and outside of occupational therapy (OT) regarding various social and political factors, such as economic globalization, environmental degradation, international migration, the growth of precarious work, population aging, and urbanization, that have contributed to a deepening of health, social and occupational inequities within and between nations (Marmot, 2011; van Bruggen et al., 2020).

Although some of these same factors can promote social progress, such progress and its benefits are often not equitably distributed. As articulated in the 2020 World Social Report of the United Nations, "the extraordinary economic growth and widespread improvements in well-being observed over the last several decades have failed to close the deep divide within and across countries" (United Nations Department of Economic and Social Affairs [UNDESA], 2020, p. 2).

Within this chapter, we highlight the responsibility of occupational therapists to be part of social transformation aimed at lessening health, social, and occupational inequities, with a particular focus on addressing the occupational rights of older adults. We address the role of occupational therapists at the level of community and social change and attend to key characteristics of evolving practice approaches that work to enact social transformation through occupation. The chapter ends with three examples of initiatives that have involved occupational therapists working with groups of older adults, along with other key partners, to enact social transformation.

## Broadening the Role of Occupational Therapists to Address Intersecting Health, Social, and Occupational Inequities: Contemporary Importance

Growing critical awareness of health and social disparities as inequities, that is, as differences in health, social resources, and social participation possibilities that are avoidable and remediable, has led to calls for social transformation aimed at building more equitable and sustainable societies (Commission on Social Determinants, 2008). According to Marmot (2011), such social transformation is important to not only promote health equity but also has "other highly desirable societal outcomes including social cohesion, reduction in crime, and civil unrest, a more educated workforce and the freedom for people to lead lives they have reason to value" (p. 702). Increasingly, occupational therapists, from various parts of the globe, are calling on the profession to actively contribute to such social transformation, both re-energizing its historical roots in social justice and developing new forms of practice that aim to create more occupational just societies (Cunningham et al., 2020; Laliberte Rudman, 2021a).

In 2008, the World Health Organization's Commission on Social Determinants of Health asserted that "social injustice is killing people on a grand scale" (p. 2). This report marshaled evidence demonstrating large, remediable differences in health within and between countries, and called for urgent action to transform social norms, practices, and policies that result in the unfair distribution of power and social resources. The report also articulated an ethical imperative for action to improve the daily living conditions in which all people grow, live, work and age (Commission on Social Determinants of Health, 2008; Marmot, 2011). This imperative clearly aligns with the responsibility of occupational therapists to ensure the rights of individuals and collectives to engage in occupations that enable them, their families, and communities to flourish (Bailliard et al., 2020).

Similar concerns regarding rising social and health inequities within and among countries and calls for social transformation were noted in the United Nations 2030 Agenda for Sustainable Development (Cunningham et al., 2020). This agenda, produced in 2015, outlined 17 Sustainable Development Goals to direct social change that would support the rights of all humans to lead "decent, dignified, and rewarding lives and to achieve their full human potential" (United Nations, 2015, p. 12). Within this agenda, particular social groups, including older adults and persons with disabilities, were recognized as facing heightened risk for inequities, pointing to the importance of targeted action addressing the rights of older adults. A similar emphasis on promoting occupational participation is evident in the 2020 World Social Report, which called for transformations in social relations, systems, and structures so as to promote equal access to opportunities across various occupational realms, such as work, social participation, and community mobility. This report highlighted the need to counter intersecting forms of discrimination based on age, gender, race, citizenship status, and other social markers (UNESDA, 2020). With reference to OT practice with older adults, attending to interrelated occupational, health, and social inequities is vital given that intersections of population aging, demographic change, and reductions in social safety nets may deepen inequities for aging adults who have occupied marginalized social positions across their life course. As well, these social and political trends may also shape inequities for older adults who experience new health, financial, occupational, and other challenges as they age (Grenier et al., 2017).

## Expanding the Role of Occupational Therapists: Addressing Social Transformation

Within this broader context of increasing awareness of persisting and deepening inequities, combined with growing evidence regarding the root socio-political causes of these inequities, the World Federation of Occupational Therapists (WFOT) asserted that "occupational therapists around the world are obligated to promote occupational rights as the actualization of human rights." Within the WFOT Position Statement on "Occupational Therapy and Human Rights," occupational therapists are called upon to counter occupational injustices shaped through social problems, such as various forms of discrimination, poverty, displacement, violence, and environmental degradation. In the context of the United States, occupational justice has been included in the American Occupational Therapy Association's *Occupational Therapy Practice Framework*, pointing to the need for OT to develop as a justice-oriented profession (Aldrich et al., 2017; Bailliard et al., 2020). As such, occupational therapists are challenged to work with individuals and collectives facing occupational injustices to enact practices aimed at altering the social conditions that shape such injustices (Aldrich et al., 2017; Kantartzis, 2019). This role, referred to in various ways such as being a social occupational therapist or a political occupational therapist, involves actively working against unjust restrictions to the right to occupation that exist on the basis of intersections of age, economic status, gender, ability status, and other social markers of difference (Cunningham et al., 2020; Lopes & Malfitano, 2021; Sakellariou & Pollard, 2017).

Given that many restrictions to the right to occupation faced by individuals and social groups are rooted in societal and structural conditions beyond the control of any individual, OT practice approaches need to expand beyond working with individuals and promoting individual change to working at broader levels and promoting social transformation (Brodrick & Barry, 2016; Irvine-Brown et al., 2021). This expansion requires new theoretical tools, knowledge, and practice approaches, particularly those supporting participatory and collaborative approaches, that enable occupational therapists to be part of efforts that critically unpack and address the social and political conditions shaping occupational inequities (Kantartzis, 2019; Laliberte Rudman, 2021b). In response, there has been a rapid expansion in the production of knowledge regarding occupational injustice, occupational rights, and the social and political determinants of occupation. For example, this work has addressed the impact of various forms of oppression, such as racism, ageism, colonialism, and ableism, on occupational possibilities (Cunningham et al., 2021; Trentham & Neysmith, 2018; Lavalley & Johnson, 2020; Mondaca, 2021; Ramugondo, 2018). Moreover, various OT approaches that "mobilize occupation in social change efforts that shift beyond a focus on individuals and their occupational needs to address sociopolitical forces contributing to occupational inequities" (Laliberte Rudman, 2021b, p. 98) have been and continue to be developed. Examples include long-standing forms of practice developed in the Global South, such as social OT (Lopes & Malfitano, 2021), as well as political OT, critical OT, occupation-based social transformation, and occupation-based community development (Irvine-Brown et al., 2021; Sakellariou & Pollard, 2017; Richards & Galvaan, 2018. Although each of these practice approaches has distinct roots, theoretical ideas, and strategies (Cunningham et al., 2020), within the confines of this chapter, consistent with the

International Social Transformation through Occupation Network (ISTTON), we use the term "social transformation through occupation" to refer to "various approaches that focus on using occupation as a means to restructure practices, systems and structures, so as to ameliorate occupational and social inequities" (van Bruggen, 2020, p. 5). In the last section of the chapter, examples of practices consistent with such an approach to practice are provided.

It is important to emphasize that 'social transformation through occupation' is not a singular approach to practice nor is there a set series of steps to follow, given that the approach used must be responsive to contextual features and aligned with the needs and goals of the particular group (Laliberte Rudman et al., 2019; van Bruggen, 2020). Social transformation through occupation is a broad term that encompasses diverse ways of thinking about, mobilizing and addressing occupation within efforts aimed at transforming systemic and structural barriers to occupational participation, and upholding the occupational rights of all people to participate in occupations as individuals and collectives (van Bruggen et al., 2020). Looking across various practice approaches, examples, and research addressing social transformation through occupation (Cunningham et al., 2020; Farias et al., 2019; van Bruggen et al., 2020), we highlight five common characteristics (Table 31.1).

First, there is a recognition that practice needs to shift beyond individualized approaches focused on individual clients and personal barriers to occupation. Instead, there is a need to work with groups and communities experiencing occupational inequities and to focus on social and political barriers to occupation (Brodrick & Barry, 2016; Irvine-Brown et al., 2021). Second, there is a commitment to working *with* groups and communities, rather than "on" or "for" collectives, to alter social and political conditions producing occupational inequities (Brodrick & Barry, 2016; Lopes & Malfitano, 2021). This commitment is realized through engaging in participatory processes in which the expertise of community members is valued and the power to identify problems and solutions is shared (Farias et al., 2019; Richards & Galvaan, 2018). As one example, in a participatory action research project with older adult members of a seniors' advocacy group, ongoing processes of collective dialogue, relationship building, and consciousness raising were enacted so that the knowledge and experiences of older adults were central in delineating the problem of ageism and identifying action steps to be taken by the group (Trentham & Neysmith, 2018; Trentham et al., 2020). Third, critical theoretical perspectives are drawn upon to understand the historical and contemporary context and analyze the root causes of health, social, and occupational inequities (Cunningham et al., 2020; Lopes & Malfitano, 2021). Drawing on critical perspectives, occupation itself is conceptualized as political, meaning that it is inequitably distributed in ways that advantage some groups while marginalizing other groups (Aldrich et al., 2017; Laliberte Rudman, 2021b). For example, social policies, ageist practices, and age-based norms can restrict what older adults can do within various types of settings, such as in long-term care institutions, the labor force, or in neighborhoods, in both explicit and implicit ways (du Toit et al., 2019; Kottorp et al., 2016; Nilsson & Townsend, 2010; Trentham & Neysmith, 2018). A fourth common characteristic is that occupation itself is understood as transformative; in particular, engaging in occupations, particularly collective occupations that involve doing together, is a means to enact social transformation (Laliberte Rudman et al., 2019; Kantartzis, 2019). For example, in an ethnographic study conducted in a senior center with Spanish speaking elders, Lavalley et al. (2020) found that engaging in communal occupations provided a means to change social relations and open up spaces and occupational opportunities for center participants. A fifth common characteristic is engagement in ongoing critical reflexivity on the part of occupational therapists regarding both their own positionality and the contexts in which they are working (Brodrick & Barry, 2016; Richards & Galvaan, 2018). This is essential to avoid the unintentional reproduction of oppressive power relationships, ensure a position of cultural humility and openness to diverse worldviews, and continually work toward participatory processes marked by power sharing (Aldrich et al., 2017; Cunningham et al. 2020; Irvine-Brown et al., 2021).

## Occupational Therapists, Social Change, and Social Transformation Through Occupation: Examples

The final section of this chapter integrates three examples that align with social transformation through occupation and involve working with older adults. These examples, which are situated in a long-term care setting in Sweden, a marginalized community in South Africa, and jail and prison settings in the United States, demonstrate the diverse settings and practices mobilized in social transformation. Further examples incorporating various occupations, such as soccer, arts, and community gardening, can be accessed via a dynamic casebook developed by the ISTTON. These examples also use various processes, such as participatory action research, community development, network formation, and partnership building, to expand occupational possibilities for particular social collectives (see https://enothe.eu/wp-content/uploads/2020/06/ISTTON-booklet-final.pdf).

---

**TABLE 31.1**  Social Transformation Through Occupation, Common Characteristics of Practice Approaches

| Common Characteristics |
| --- |
| Work with groups and communities, with focus on social and political barriers to occupation |
| Use of participatory approaches, working with groups and communities |
| Integrate critical perspectives to analyze and address root causes of inequities |
| Mobilize transformative potential of occupation |
| Engage in ongoing critical reflexivity |

These diverse examples demonstrate that occupation can both be used as means to enact social transformation and be the outcome of social transformation efforts (Cunningham et al., 2020). For example, addressing occupation as a means, collective occupations can be mobilized to spark transformations in social attitudes towards marginalized groups and foster social relationships across difference. Addressing occupation as the "end" or outcome, social transformation processes can work toward dismantling ageist attitudes that create barriers to occupational participation and expand occupational possibilities for aging adults within institutional settings.

## Example One: Generative Disruption in a Nursing Home Context, Expanding Occupational Participation by Margarita Mondaca

This example draws on a 4-year PhD study conducted in a nursing home in an urban area of Sweden with a total capacity for about 200 residents divided into smaller units. Three occupational therapists were employed in this facility, and their main focus was on the prescription of assistive devices, adaptations to residents' flats, and organization of once-monthly entertainment activities. A total of 20 nurses and three physiotherapists were also part of the professional team. Nurse assistants supported most of the residents in their daily life activities, such as toileting, dressing, bed transfers, and during mealtimes. The unit involved in this project had a capacity for 54 residents and was divided into groups of nine residents each. The building had three floors, one for people living with dementia and two for older adults living with a variety of chronic conditions. There was a weekly group activity scheduled in this unit with few other activities for residents. The residents gathered for 2 hours to participate in singing and playing bingo or memory games. In this case example, this project is first placed within the broader context of Swedish elder care and the main concerns that underpinned the project are articulated. Then, the approach used is described and two illustrations of the collaborative approach enacted are shared.

### Contextualizing Swedish Elder Care

The goal of the Swedish care policy for older adults is to facilitate a safe environment, to promote dignity in everyday life (Socialstyrelsen, 2012). The care system for older adults is required to meet national standards, including meaningful activities and social interaction with other residents, staff, and relatives, as an important element (Wigzell, 2018). Due to the "aging in place" policy dominating Swedish eldercare, most older adults live at home and only are granted special housing when they are severely restricted in managing everyday activities at home (Lennartsson & Heimerson, 2012) in a safe and satisfactory manner, even when assisted by health services. In general, care services and standards in Swedish nursing homes are high with care staff available around-the-clock to support residents with daily tasks, rehabilitation services offered by occupational therapists and physiotherapists, whereas physicians can provide medical care via the national insurance system. Care includes laundry services, cleaning, meals, and medication management. Most nursing homes are managed by municipalities and offer private apartments to their residents.

Nursing home residents often live with multiple chronic conditions and cognitive decline. Consequently, they can have difficulty expressing their needs (Meinow et al., 2011). However, research shows that older adults living with cognitive decline still wish to be involved in decisions regarding their care and everyday matters (Baur et al., 2013; Boelsma et al., 2014). It has been a challenge to find ways to establish collaborative approaches which facilitate joint decision-making between nursing home residents and staff (Abma & Baur, 2015).

Nursing home staff have to respond to the current policy framework of person-centered care (Sjogren et al., 2017) in which everyday activities are presented as an important aspect. However, it is in everyday practices that this approach becomes elusive (Rahman et al., 2012). This may cause tensions as the care focus of nursing home staff is still grounded in the biomedical model. The presence of rigid structures and routines (Mondaca et al., 2018b, 2019) that characterize professional practices at nursing homes may set the tone of nursing home residents' everyday lives. The importance of everyday activities in creating both a sense of stability and security is argued in this section. Everyday activities that might be ordinary in other settings represent ethical issues in this setting. Ethical ponderances such as "When can we go for a walk?" or "Can I invite people to my room?" are just some of the many examples of moral matters for nursing home residents who could be inhibited or enabled (Harnett, 2014; Hydén, 2014). Everyday activities have more recently been highlighted as being a key aspect of the person-centered approach in nursing home settings (Patomella et al., 2016). And yet, research shows that nursing home residents are involved to a limited extent in the design of activities performed (Boelsma et al., 2013).

### Addressing the Value of Everyday Activities in Nursing Home Settings

According to Butler and colleagues (2016), modern societies are characterized by the precariousness of social institutions in their role of protecting and securing the interests of communities. From this perspective, vulnerability could be understood as part of the human rights framework, where the very existence of a human being is the premise for an obligation toward the experience of dignity in everyday life of any person in the human community. When older adults start living in a nursing home setting, to maintain dignity in everyday life activities is at stake.

With the understanding of the everyday as an arena where ethical issues for older adults living at nursing home are at stake, it becomes urgent that occupational therapists embrace the responsibility to be part of social transformation aimed at lessening health, social and occupational inequities, by addressing the right to meaningful everyday life activities for the nursing home residents. Everyday life in nursing home settings often has a strong focus on activities that can contribute to the structure and routines of the nursing home and the health and well-being of the residents. Everyday life is defined as the arena for agency, understood here as the possibility to maintain and transform identities, enact resistance, and create new roles through social interactions (Bhabha, 1994), and not just as the ability to perform an action. Another understanding of everyday activities is as an interconnection of actions, objects and relationships that evolve and emerge from the immediate context (Pichon-Riviere & Pampliega de Quiroga, 2012), and that are normally taken for granted or labelled as mundane. The possibility to create meaning through this interconnection could be challenged by cognitive decline; therefore support in creating meaning and the role of the environment is amplified in the nursing home setting.

## Description of Approach Used

The rationale for conducting this PhD research in close collaboration with the nursing home community to foster competencies within the community, to co-create knowledge, and to generate change is grounded in a participatory approach (Blair & Minkler, 2009). This participatory approach encompasses two theoretical resources: (a) situated interventions and (b) the notion of third spaces. The concept of situated interventions goes beyond the dichotomy of knowledge versus intervention as a linear process (Zuiderent-Jerak, 2015), by making use of engaging interventions in particular contexts. Situated interventions also emphasize the critical awareness and positionality of the researcher in terms of roles, values, and actions. Changes within the nursing home context and knowledge creation could occur simultaneously with the involvement of participants (Mondaca et al., 2018a). Situated interventions benefit from immediately dealing with the challenges and opportunities present in the context of the research, in addition to the creation of knowledge that is transferable to similar contexts. Situated interventions as an approach to complex research contexts, like nursing home care, allows for the use of multiple research methods that will contribute to new knowledge informing the nuances of situations "at stake" in home care from several perspectives (Zuiderent-Jerak, 2015).

Situated interventions align with the second theoretical resource underpinning this research project, the notion of third space. The notion of third space is defined as a context for collaboration, negotiation, and innovation (Bhabha, 1994). Third space interventions are created and built-in collaboration with multiple stakeholders. In this research project, the researchers collaborated with nursing home residents and staff working at the nursing home. Third spaces facilitate opportunities to explore and attempt new practices, to bring new contributions and fill gaps, within specifics contexts. In this way, third spaces can integrate immediate feedback from practices. The third space concept contributed to this project through the co-creation of new collaborative practices that were not yet part of the regular provision of nursing home services. This acknowledged capabilities in old age and everyday life in encounters between staff and older persons living

at the nursing home. By conducting research embedded in practices, there is an opportunity to address key issues of social sustainability (Zuiderent-Jerak, 2015), such as how positive changes for older adults' well-being are integrated into practice. Change can initially be disruptive in institutional settings but at the same time generate new possibilities, what Galvaan (2021) refers to as generative disruptions. This research project enabled collaboration between nursing home staff and older persons living at the nursing home, to support participation, equality and dignity in everyday life and to acknowledge the residents and staff as experts of their own praxis in everyday life.

This project had three major phases: (a) deep exploration of the nursing home context and older adults' conditions regarding everyday life activities; (b) occupation-based collaborative study with older adults living at the nursing home; and (c) collaborative intervention with the staff. Phase a was conducted using an ethnographic approach (Atkinson et al., 2001) that served to create relationships of trust and collaboration both with nursing home staff and older adult residents. In phase b, the aim was to explore as many possible activities as possible that were of interest to the older adults living at the nursing home, and to try them out in the setting in a sustainable way. The intervention in phase c aimed to create awareness among the staff about the pivotal role of everyday life activities and to build capacity among the nursing home staff. The emphasis of this last phase was to train the staff in a dialogical collaboration with older adults at the nursing home and to ground and align everyday activities with the interests and capacities of the older adult residents. Together, these three phases made it possible to learn in situ about the changes that were possible to introduce, or those that were challenging. The sequential development of transforming practices was key to generate a sense of accountability as a collaborative researcher and to generate a process that was open to inputs and adjustments.

## Two Illustrations From This Collaborative Experience

To get an idea of the challenges and opportunities presented by this collaboration, two illustrations are described. These illustrations illustrate how disruptions in everyday life at the nursing home could be transformed into more sustainable benefits for the residents.

The first illustration is about the generation of activities for the residents based on their own interests. This presents an alternative to predesigned activities informed by others' assumptions about what could be of interest or "good" for them in terms of health or age suitability (e.g., sitting gymnastics, listening to reminiscence music, or doing seasonal crafts). A range of activities was tried out based on the first phase of the project, where the researcher gathered information about activities that older adults were longing to do, missing, or interested to try. Conversations were facilitated by the researcher with small events, like eating something out of the ordinary, or looking into some textiles brought to the nursing home, or other triggers for conversations. Some of the questions posed in these situations were: "What are you interested in doing?," "What do you dream to do?," "What do you miss doing?." Answers were not always straightforward; however, these became possible after some time of participant observations.

One of the first activities participants tried out was an "after talk mingle." This activity was designed to improve the experience of cultural evenings already happening once a month at the nursing home. Professional performers (i.e., musicians or actors) would come to perform to the entire nursing home, the nursing home residents would gather at a shared area and participate by watching and listening to a live performance for about an hour. The performance awakened many feelings, some positive and some more anguishing, such as feeling abandoned and forgotten. The staff would rapidly return the residents to their flats or common areas in their units once the event was over, leaving the experience incomplete and without opportunities for residents to discuss the experience with their peers. To transform this gap, we provided an opportunity for some nursing home residents to have food, refreshments, and to discuss their experiences of the cultural activity. Moreover, this gathering was done in one of the common areas of the nursing home usually used by the staff for some meetings, shifting the use of some of the physical territory to directly benefit the nursing home residents. This small activity brought much joy to the participants (i.e., six to eight residents) that spontaneously wanted to join, to share some of their personal stories triggered by the performance, such as musical experiences from when they were younger or love stories. The short mingle brought laughs and a sense of having an out of the ordinary day. When leading some of the residents to their flats, they would comment for example: *"Now, I can go to sleep and feel complete about the day."* We tried out this activity for four times and integrated some nurse assistants to give them a chance to experience this alternative way to meet with the nursing home residents. We shifted toward other interests and explored a small, diverse project to see the challenges and possibilities for engagement of the nursing home residents and the staff. Examples of other activity experiments were outdoor activities and professional photographic portraits of the nursing home residents. The aim of these activity experiments was to honor the nursing home residents' interests and to explore the conditions of the nursing home in enabling influence in everyday life activities.

Another activity that emerged from these experiments was a book club, a culturally relevant tradition in the Swedish context. In the first phase, it was evident that older adults wanted to have a context to share similar interests, read some classic books again, meet new people, and have alternatives to the existing activities on offer at the nursing home. This book club also was generated progressively in collaboration with the nursing home residents. Two main conditions were a prerequisite established in dialogue with the residents: (a) the meetings were to be held at one of residents' flat and not in the common areas, to avoid people being "dropped" in the activity by staff and to prevent unwanted noise from the surrounding environment; (b) nursing home residents who were interested in talking and willing to meet new people would be

invited. The researcher had a marginal role in the meetings, facilitating the activity and integrating nurse assistants to this new culture. This activity facilitated new roles and opened new territories. Diverse topics emerged from dialogues with the residents and were accentuated in each meeting by the stimulation of different senses, for instance using pictures, songs, and flavors. The meetings were held once a week for one and a half hours with a group of 8 to 10 residents. A core group of five was present for most sessions and the other guests varied. Nursing assistants interested in this approach continued with this activity when the project was over. Further analysis of this experience is presented elsewhere (Mondaca et al., 2018a, 2018b).

A second illustration of how to create social transformation in a nursing home setting is the series of workshops conducted for nursing home staff during the project's third phase. These workshops were launched to address social sustainability and create real opportunities for cultural change at the nursing home, by supporting staff to adopt an occupational perspective based on the desires and competencies of the older adults living at the nursing home. The workshop series (six group sessions) started by emphasizing the idea of legitimizing the older adults' desired activities and not dismissing any of them due to practical reasons. The staff was instead invited to validate these ideas and to try to find out the qualities behind those expressions. For example, if a resident said, "I want to travel to New York," the nurse assistant was trained to keep the dialogue going to understand the resident beyond the literal meaning of the answer. This inspired other questions about whether the nursing home resident longed for a trip, for a change of scenery, or an exciting experience. This dialogical approach (Tsoukas, 2009) was applied to design individual activities that could honor the qualities desired by older adults living at the nursing home (Mondaca et al., 2019). "Own time" was one of the activities identified by a nurse assistant with one of the nursing home residents. "Own time" referred to an undisturbed moment between the nursing home resident and nurse assistant to do a special activity, such as posting a letter or going to buy some flowers. The idea to design activities according to the nursing home residents' desires challenged stereotypes and assumptions about growing old in such a context and provided possibilities for innovation and person-centered practices. The methodology, discussions, and design of activities in close dialogue with the nursing home residents and peers was experienced as a turning point for the staff in their approach toward the nursing home residents. At the end of the workshop series, a total of 19 small new collaborative projects were presented. These small projects were peer-evaluated in terms of fidelity to the qualities pursued by the nursing home residents and in terms of feasibility in the local context. The small-scale projects were later followed up to gain insights in terms of adjustments and to ensure the sustainability of the initiatives.

As is possible to see from these experiences, transformation of structural and institutional conditions for groups or people experiencing marginalization or any form of injustice that affects their everyday life demands action from occupational therapists. Participatory approaches and collaborative methodologies, as well as building strong partnership with the community, are key to creating sustainable transformations and to disrupting hegemonic dynamics of power. In this sense, everyday life could be seen as the field for oppression and suffering but also the field of resistance and transformation.

## Example Two: Development and Ongoing Work of Grandmothers Against Poverty and AIDS by Kathleen Brodrick

This case example describes the role of an occupational therapist in contributing to the development and ongoing work of a community-based organization, Grandmothers Against Poverty and AIDS (GAPA). After describing the content in which GAPA developed, this description traces the author's roles as the occupational therapist, the focus on enacting a participatory approach, how the grandmothers involved in this organization have increasingly taken on ownership of its process, and how GAPA has addressed many social problems prioritized by the grandmothers and communities over the past decades.

Empowering the grandmothers to become their own agents of change was the mantra held by the occupational therapist from the first interaction with the grandmothers in 2001 and continues up to today in 2021. The journey began with a strong belief in the basic guiding philosophy of OT—that everyone has the ability to heal themselves through activity. Consistent with a commitment to a participatory process, on the journey it was important that whatever course of action the occupational therapist followed on behalf of the members of the community, the members had to agree and accompany the therapist every step of the way. The success of a community intervention is measured by the extent the community takes ownership of the process. GAPA is a beloved organization in Khayelitsha and the "go to place" for grandmothers who are seeking solace, help, information, or friendship.

### Contextual Information

Khayelitsha is a township outside the city of Cape Town in South Africa. The area is home to 2.4 million people. Poverty and unemployment are rife, and in 2001 there was a high prevalence of untreated human immunodeficiency virus (HIV) infections and unexplained deaths. The greatest number of deaths due to acquired immunodeficiency syndrome (AIDS) complications was in the 20- to 40-year-old age group, which left the care of the sick, the dying, and the orphans to the older women of the community. A research project in 2001 undertaken by the Institute of Ageing in Africa (Ferreira, 2004) showed that elderly women in the township, by their own accounting, were disadvantaged by a lack of knowledge about HIV and AIDS. Households became poorer due to the costs incurred in caring for the sick and job losses of the breadwinners. Families affected by HIV withdrew from community life fearing the consequences of neighbors finding out

that someone was sick within their family. Grandmothers felt powerless and afraid. It was against this background that an occupational therapist was tasked to find a way to provide feedback to the community that had participated in the research and to design an intervention that would empower the grandmothers to cope with their lives without the support of their affected and dying children. The occupational therapist studied the information that the grandmothers had given in the interviews, and after reflection, the occupational therapist could visualize how she viewed development and what the goal would be for the allotted 3 months spent in the community.

### Project Initiation

Initiating the project involved critical reflection on what the occupational therapist analyzed as possible to change and what the grandmothers thought should be changed, striving to marry the two. The occupational therapist decided that a series of educational workshops would be held to address the gaps in the grandmothers' knowledge about HIV and AIDS (Brodrick, 2005). The workshops would be open to all grandmothers in the community, held in a hall situated in the grounds of a community health-care center, a public area. The stigma against families whom the community suspected had HIV in their households was high and so the workshops were advertised as "Learning to live life more effectively." Once the grandmothers had arrived at the venue the occupational therapist informed the grandmothers that she was there to give feedback on the research and asked the grandmothers what they would like to learn from the workshops. Their response was that anything was fine. The occupational therapist realized that they had such little knowledge about HIV/AIDS that they did not know what there was to learn. The occupational therapist collaborated with several community-based organizations and a social worker from Khayelitsha to provide content for the workshops which had to be held in the grandmothers' mother tongue, isiXhosa. The occupational therapist could not speak isiXhosa and thus had to use grandmothers that spoke English to translate for her. However, at times as the grandmothers relayed their stories to the group, no spoken language was needed for the occupational therapist to understand the depth and extent of their grief and despair. The occupational therapist realized that many of the grandmothers needed counseling. The occupational therapist offered a psychosocial group meeting to some grandmothers, identified by the group as having lost a family member recently or nursing a terminally ill family member at that time. Group work began, once a week for 10 women. For the groups the occupational therapist provided the know-how and fabric for patchwork and the grandmothers, recognizing that they were all affected in the same way, supported each other emotionally. They became friends and week by week their healing was obvious. This group of women became emboldened and suggested to the occupational therapist, after the allotted 10 weeks for the group meetings, that if she could stay with them as a group, they could extend the program to other grandmothers in the township. Thus, using the occupational therapist's knowledge of how to register a nonprofit organization and the grandmothers' knowledge of their community GAPA was formed.

## Project Development Over Time

In communities marked by poverty and hardship, people may have given up hope of recovering. The occupational therapist with her belief that people have the capacity to heal themselves might in cases such as these be the only person at initiation of the project who is able to look beyond the difficulties and visualize a brighter future. The occupational therapist was courageous, and at the beginning of an intervention took the initiative, based on research data pertaining to the community and involving the grandmothers, and planned a course of action without full consultation or collaboration with the community. This lack of engagement of the community members goes against all the fundamental norms of successful therapeutic interventions and principles of social transformation. However, as soon as possible, the occupational therapist brought the grandmothers into the decision-making process. Toward the end of the workshops held for the grandmothers, the grandmothers became emboldened enough to start questioning some of the workshop content. The occupational therapist recognized this as a sign that the grandmothers were ready to begin directing the workshop content to suit their needs. The therapist evaluated the content with the local facilitators and adjusted the content of the workshops.

One of the key principles of GAPA is that it should be an organization for and by grandmothers, and thus the focus of the occupational therapist was on facilitating development of the organization. To this end, the founding occupational therapist formed a management committee of herself and some of the grandmothers participating in the initial workshops. The occupational therapist embarked on a series of talks about the fledgling organization to women's groups in the affluent suburbs of Cape Town. At these talks she appealed for used clothing to be donated to GAPA that could be sold to generate funding for the organization. The grandmothers took on the role as salespeople and money was raised to cover the costs of holding more workshops and community outreach. As the organization developed, more requirements and rules were imposed by outside agencies that were providing funding. To protect the process of development within the organization the grandmothers were incorporated continuously in its development. However, it was necessary to employ staff to assist administratively because the grandmothers had limited electronic or digital literacy. Examples of the development of the grandmothers included forming a management committee, maintaining grandmothers as key facilitators for workshops, training as care providers for children at the GAPA Aftercare, becoming vegetable gardeners, and including grandmothers as board members. Grandmothers, having learned that a problem shared is often a problem solved, also formed support groups in their neighborhoods and visited those that were sick or housebound. The home groups embarked on income-generating projects. GAPA, through the interactions of grandmother to grandmother, spread its

mantra "Together we are stronger" throughout the township and beyond (Brodrick & Mafuya, 2005).

In the 20 years since its inception, GAPA has effected many changes in the township environment through the empowerment of grandmothers that have participated in all or some of the activities that GAPA offers. Grandmothers have found their voices as leaders and respected elders of the community. Anti-retroviral treatment has become available to all who are infected with HIV. Thanks to the determined hard work of grandmothers spreading facts and dispelling myths, HIV/AIDS is no longer the disease that had families cowering behind closed doors. A key social transformation has occurred in that the stigma and isolation of families that are infected with HIV has gone.

## Contemporary Issues and Summary

In 2020, with the onset of the COVID-19 pandemic, households in Khayelitsha once again faced isolation. Free movement of people was prohibited as a countrywide lockdown was enforced. Myths and misinformation spread throughout the township and anyone who was sick was regarded with suspicion. Households were once again subjected to stigma and isolation. When a limited interaction between people was allowed by law, GAPA, which had already perfected a blueprint for community engagement and intervention, swung into action. The occupational therapist organized for medical professionals to educate the grandmothers about the virus and arranged that they all receive vaccinations against the virus. The activity of becoming vaccinated and having material they could distribute to other grandmothers in the community empowered the grandmothers to educate and dispel myths about the virus. The management committee made their own rules, based on World Health Organization guidelines, regarding how GAPA would react to the new threat to life in the community.

The occupational therapist's role at GAPA has always been that of facilitator of change. The occupational therapist had to be alert at all times as to what was happening that might affect the lives of the grandmothers in the township and in the country as a whole in order to suggest or offer interventions based on her and the grandmothers' perceived needs at the time. The occupational therapist possessed the professional ability to liaise with medical professionals on behalf of the grandmothers and to participate in dialogue with officials or funding organizations on behalf of the grandmothers as the need arose. Through the years, the grandmothers offered indabas (large gatherings) covering topics such as gender-based violence, gay rights, elder abuse, and health issues. Once a community concern had been raised at a meeting of the GAPA management committee, it was usually the occupational therapist's job to see how the need could be addressed and formulate a plan that integrated grandmothers in as many roles as possible to bring about the desired change. Interpersonal problems that arose between grandmothers that were brought to the occupational therapist for judgment were without fail referred back to the grandmothers concerned to collaboratively solve.

Occupational therapists are known to be innovative in their thinking and among their strengths is the ability to analyze situations and facilitate an intervention plan to assist community members to enact the changes they view as important in their community. Sometimes the plans made did not work or had to be modified over time. The occupational therapist at GAPA partnered with the grandmothers creating a safe environment where nothing was cast in stone. Mistakes could be made, and if something did not work out as planned, then there was no disgrace or harm in planning anew and starting again. Ultimately, through engagement in an ongoing process of collective doing, GAPA has evolved into a vital community-based organization in which grandmothers are continually enacting participatory community engagement and interventions to address social challenges.

## Example Three: Impacting Occupational Injustices in Jails and Prisons Through Occupation-Based Interprofessional Programs by Karen Frank Barney, Lisa Jaegers, and Christine Hayes Picker

In the United States criminal justice system, adults age 46 and over represent 30% of the total federal inmate population (National Institute of Corrections, 2022). Each year more than 600,000 people are released from prisons, and more than 11 million cycle through jails, extending the effects of incarceration to homes and communities (Cloud et al., 2020). The opportunities for change are immense, as indicated by the victim advocacy group Alliance for Safety and Justice (2017): "The US is in the midst of a significant shift in criminal justice policy. For the first time in decades, criminal justice practitioners, lawmakers, and the general public are rethinking sentencing laws, prison spending, and the best ways to address crime and violence." We begin by situating our examples in the broader context by exploring how the criminal justice system is evolving from less punitive actions and toward more person-centered approaches. The perspectives primarily include those of the chapter section authors (Barney and Jaegers), who describe their strategies for developing interprofessional and community partnerships; Hayes Picker provides a case study.

### Context of the US Criminal Justice System

The United States incarcerates more people, both per capita and by volume, than any other nation in the world. Typically, on any given day, 2 million people are incarcerated in 2850 local jails, 1566 in state prisons, 186 in immigration detention facilities, and 186 in federal prisons. However, the upward incarceration trend of incarceration since the 1970s is shifting downward. At the end of 2019, the US correctional population was shown to have decreased by an average of 1.3% every year since 2009. In comparison, the United Kingdom has one-fifth the prison incarceration rate of the United States, while Canada has one-sixth and Germany one-tenth (Sawyer & Wagner, 2022). Of all the industrialized democracies, the US carceral system is the most punitive, restrictive, and focused on racial repression (Cloud et al., 2020; Sawyer & Wagner, 2022).

Incarceration is associated with a range of deleterious health impacts, which are compounded with the aging of prison populations. Epidemiological evidence portrays a prison population that is increasingly older, overweight, and chronically ill (Cloud, 2020). When aging prisoners experience physical decline, their daily caregivers and transporters are typically younger incarcerated individuals who attend classes to learn about assisting them, not health-care providers, as in mainstream society. Their historically severely limited occupational possibilities are increasingly reduced when they experience decline in their ability levels, within contextual conditions not responsive to such changing abilities.

Persons in US prisons and jails are among the unhealthiest and most medically underserved in US society. Over 50% of persons incarcerated in jails and prison in the United States have a diagnosed mental illness; more than one in five have a serious mental illness; and more than 50% meet criteria for drug dependence or abuse. Community-based behavioral health services including OT are sparse, and studies have shown that states with fewer behavioral health resources have higher rates of incarcerating people with mental health and substance use disorders (Mental Health America, 2020). Although data on the health status of persons incarcerated in the United States are extremely limited, existing research suggests that incarceration harms the health and life expectancy of both those imprisoned and their family members (Acker et al., 2019; Massoglia & Pridemore, 2015).

### Addressing Unmet Needs in Incarceration Settings: OT Practitioners as Change Agents Across Corrections Systems

Recent literature recommends a central role for OT in the rehabilitation of individuals in justice-based settings and their reintegration into society (Munoz et al., 2020). Such interventions need to also address transforming what can be framed as the "culture of incarceration." Based on Barney's observations, this culture, which is typically punitive, coercive, dogmatic, demeaning, and highly regimented, severely limits occupational possibilities regarding all aspects of life for persons incarcerated within prisons or jails. These environments exemplify occupational deprivation maximally (Jaegers et al., 2019), entrenching occupational injustice and presenting significant coping challenges for all within those environments, both persons incarcerated and staff.

Given restricted occupational possibilities and their connection to the culture of incarceration, we propose that it is important for occupational therapists to engage in change-agent practices in such settings. According to the most recent American Occupational Therapy Association (AOTA) OT practice framework, "Occupational therapy practitioners develop and implement occupation-based health approaches to enhance occupational performance and participation, (quality of life), and occupational justice for populations" (AOTA, 2020, p. 3). Since the scope of OT has broadened from individual, client, or person level focus to community and population health, practitioners are well-positioned to serve as change agents across systems to promote occupational justice. The framework provides further support for community and population health, stating, "Occupational therapy practitioners understand and focus interventions to include the issues and concerns surrounding the complex dynamics among the client, caregiver, family, and community" (AOTA, 2020, p. 18). Practitioners may provide traditional *direct services*; however, they may also consider *indirect services*, including consultation to entities such as professionals, multidisciplinary teams, and community planning agencies. OT practitioners may serve as *indirect advocates* for clients at the group and population levels to promote the meeting of their occupational needs. Furthermore, practitioners may provide *services with organizations* as a stakeholder in supporting the mission of a business or community organization.

### Examples of Criminal Justice Reform Projects

Given all of the different roles a practitioner may serve, the following community-based programs and projects offer specific examples of how an occupation-centered scope facilitates transformation and innovative practice. In this section, we address two examples, specifically, *Correctional Workplace Health* and *Occupational Therapy Reentry Services* for persons incarcerated. These programs are interrelated and grew from needs assessment and stakeholder input from established partnerships between the practitioners, multiple departments and programs within our university, incarceration settings, and community partners. Examples of these partnerships include task force membership with a city public health agency, assisting with strategic planning along with area service providers and representatives from state Department of Corrections, probation and parole staff, mayor's office, health and public safety departments, and university higher education programming offered at a state prison.

The *Correctional Workplace Health* program was developed by Jaegers, after a process that involved the US National Institute of Occupational Safety and Health's (NIOSH) evidence-based strategy Total Worker Health in correctional workplaces since 2014. Originally funded by the Healthier Workforce Center of the Midwest, a Total Worker Health Center of Excellence through NIOSH, her workplace health studies include participatory needs assessment, health promotion interventions, and health etiology in correctional workplaces. After listening to the voices of both prison staff and people incarcerated during a prison facility tour by Barney in 2014, Jaegers began addressing the intersections of staff workplace health experiences with the preparation for persons incarcerated for transitions from criminal justice settings. In 2016, Jaegers used a participatory strategy, Total Worker Health with St. Louis City Jail staff for an integrated approach to address policies, programs, and practices for correctional workplace staff health promotion (Jaegers et al., 2020a). Institution and interpersonal aspects of the workplace, and ideas for

workplace solutions were identified, using standardized measures for each construct. On the basis of general population estimates, we found that jail officers were at higher risk for mental health disorders, including depression and posttraumatic stress disorder. Jail officers identified workplace health interventions to address individual, interpersonal, institutional, and community level needs. Using this assessment, we identified specific workplace health protection and promotion solutions. A subsequent, prospective study assessed changes in health among new corrections officers during their first year of employment (Jaegers et al., 2021). Results from this study indicated that work-family conflict and burnout increased during the first year of new employment; higher depression and brief tenure were also associated with burnout among jail staff. These results further demonstrated important areas to address in workplace health interventions.

*Occupational Therapy Reentry Services* were developed when Barney and Jaegers learned about the urban jail leadership's goal to provide reentry services not previously offered. They engaged interprofessional (university and community-wide) and OT advisory teams to consider the design of a model for reentry programming for people incarcerated in the city jails. They shared Barney's Occupational Therapy reentry model with the City of St. Louis Corrections Commissioner and his staff. As a result, the Occupational Therapy OT Transition and Integration Services (OTTIS) program was launched in 2016 with local jail and grant funding, run by full-time staff and supported by undergraduate and graduate students from OT, social work, and public health. This pre- and post-release program operated with OT at the core and collaborated with other disciplines (Jaegers et al., 2020c). The aim of this seamless program, both pre and post release, is to facilitate the development of short and long-term goals, habits, and routines to support optimal function in anticipation of occupational transitions, in preparation for a broad range of occupational possibilities upon release from jail or prison. Ideally, staff in jails and prisons assist with this process while the aging adult is incarcerated; we have observed small successes with this objective to date.

Also since 2016, OTTIS has served people sentenced as juveniles to life without the option of parole (JLWOPs) in Missouri prisons. Due to US Supreme Court rulings in 2014 allowing parole petitions, these individuals have considered for the first time the potential for their release after being held in prison for over 25 years and living as an older adult. JLWOPs face challenges associated with securing employment, housing, and health care upon release into the community. They have limited to no experience navigating the community through current technology, transportation options, and other modern resources for which they had limited or no access during incarceration (Jaegers et al., in press). Furthermore, their extremely limited habits, routines, and occupations while incarcerated for many years need extensive revision going forward, as they anticipate release. The following case study, given in Box 31.1, provides an example of OT direct client reentry services.

## Box 31.1   Occupational Therapy in the Justice System

As you read through the case, consider the following questions: (1) How does the prison environment impact habits, routines, roles, and occupations in comparison to a community environment? (2) What occupational therapy interventions and/or adaptive equipment would Terry benefit from to increase his occupational participation in prison? (3) What resources would Terry benefit from in the community? (4) How can occupational therapy support Terry's performance in community-based occupations upon his transition from prison to the community? (5) What larger contextual conditions does this case study point to as potential targets for social transformative efforts aimed at contextual barriers to occupational possibilities?

Terry is a 48-year-old black man who has been incarcerated for 34 years. He was granted parole and will be released in 6 months. He had a stroke 4 years ago, resulting in fluctuating left-sided muscle weakness and general deconditioning. Terry lives in the prison chronic care wing where he has a daily living assistant (DLA), a person incarcerated who was trained to assist with his daily activities. Additionally, Terry has a history of substance use but has abstained from substances for the last 10 years. He has also been diagnosed with major depressive disorder and post-traumatic stress disorder. Terry's physical health is managed by a nurse practitioner whom he sees every 6 months. He participates in services with a licensed professional counselor once per month and a psychiatrist every 3 months but has never participated in occupational therapy services.

Terry can propel his wheelchair independently using his upper and lower extremities. He sometimes needs help from his DLA to perform shower, toilet, wheelchair, and bed transfers. In addition to his wheelchair and two-wheeled walker, he uses grab bars, ankle and knee orthotics, eyeglasses, shower chair, and was approved for an extra pillow to assist with positioning in bed. He has requested other equipment, including bed rails and a long-handled sponge, which were both denied.

During the day, Terry spends time talking on the phone or writing emails to his family, exercising, reading, praying, watching television, and playing cards. Terry likes to work but has not worked since having a stroke. He has tried to advocate for himself with his case manager, but the prison will not approve him for work duty due to his physical disabilities.

Terry is anxious about the transition to the community due to his limited experience with community-based occupations. Terry would like to be released to his mother's home, which has been adapted to be accessible by wheelchair. He wants to improve his strength and activity tolerance to help his 70-year-old mother around the house. He would like to work in the community to earn money and help his mom pay for household costs, but he has never applied or interviewed for a job. He has experience with budgeting his limited income to purchase necessities in prison, but he has never had a bank account or credit card. He is looking forward to driving, getting a smartphone, and using his mom's computer to explore the internet, which he has never used before, due to restricted access in the prison. In the community, he hopes to spend his free time with family, attending church, meeting new people, exercising, gardening, and mentoring at-risk youth.

### Supporting Change Agents and Summary

Early change agents in OT and criminal justice include Sandra Rogers, Jaime Munoz, John White, and Marybeth Dillon, who invited Barney and Jaegers to present at the American Occupational Therapy (AOTA) Conference in 2016, with additional collaborators, Cynthia Ballentine and later, Chi-Kwan Shea. Since then and the formation of the SLU OTTIS, an informal early change agents grassroots effort called Justice-Based Occupational Therapy (JBOT) brought together international scholars and practitioners interested in facilitating criminal justice reform and the promotion of occupational justice (Jaegers et al., 2020b) through recommendations to the World Federation of Occupational Therapists (WFOT), the American Occupational Therapy Association (AOTA), the Society for the Study of Occupation (SSO), and other relevant organizations,. The JBOT community continues to grow and networks on social media outlets; at the writing of this chapter, it has over 600 followers on Instagram (@justice_OT) and Facebook (@JusticeOT1).

Working as change agents in the criminal justice system is challenging. However, when informed by key stakeholders and offering a diverse perspective through an interprofessional approach, there is a higher likelihood for long-term efforts and positive outcomes to occur. Far more work is needed to explore the impact of OT in promoting health and well-being among older adults who are justice-involved and contributing to social transformation within this system aimed at enhancing occupational possibilities. Taking the initial steps by becoming informed about the current issues, national and local activities, and skilled practice are critical to beginning the journey as an OT change agent supporting personal and social transformation within the criminal justice realm.

### Conclusion

As an evolving form of praxis, social transformation through occupation creates a space for innovation in how occupational therapists work with older adults and other key partners to address social and political conditions that shape occupational inequities and injustices. Within this chapter, we have presented social transformation through occupation as a broad term that encompasses diverse ways of thinking about, mobilizing and addressing occupation within efforts aimed at transforming systemic and structural barriers to occupational participation and upholding the occupational rights of all people to participate in occupations as individuals and collectives (van Bruggen et al., 2020). The examples in this chapter demonstrate this diversity, for example, addressing different types of settings, working with varied partners, and using various theoretical concepts and practical strategies. These examples also show the importance of designing and enacting actions aimed at social transformation in ways that are responsive to local contexts, while attending to the common characteristics outlined in Table 31.1. Moreover, the examples demonstrate the potential contributions of OT

to much needed social transformation addressing widening health, social and occupational inequities, illustrating how such contributions stem from centering occupation in both processes and targets of social transformation.

*The complete listing of the Bibliography and Chapter Questions and Answers are available in the accompanying enhanced eBook version included with the print purchase of this textbook. Visit Elsevier eBooks+ (eBooks.Health.Elsevier.com) to access this content.*

## CHAPTER 32

# Building Age-Inclusive Communities

*Debbie Laliberte Rudman, PhD, OT Reg. (Ont.), Margaret A. Perkinson, PhD, FGSA, FAGHE, FSfAA, Sarah Kantartzis, PhD, MRCOT, Colleen McGrath, PhD, OT Reg. (ON), and Jenny Womack, PhD OTR/L FAOTA*

## CHAPTER OUTLINE

## OBJECTIVES

- Provide an overview of approaches to defining age-inclusive communities
- Gain an appreciation of the importance of building age-inclusive communities
- Understand the centrality of occupation within age-inclusive communities
- Appreciate the importance of participatory approaches involving working with aging adults
- Gain exposure to different concepts and approaches that can inform occupational therapy practice aimed at building and sustaining age-inclusive communities

Where we live has a significant influence on what we can and cannot do in our occupational lives, as well as on our health and well-being. As understandings of aging and occupation have increasingly highlighted how both are situated in social, cultural, political, economic, and other contextual elements, there has also been a growing recognition that approaches to enabling occupation need to address building age-inclusive communities (Buffel & Phillipson, 2018; Lauckner & Stadnyk, 2014). As proposed in the 2020 World Federation of Occupational Therapists (WFOT) position statement on "Occupational therapy and ageing across the life course," occupational therapists have a multidimensional role that involves working with older adults to promote age-friendly environments.

In this chapter, we first address what we mean by the term age-inclusive communities and address why it is vital for occupational therapists to be part of ongoing efforts to build such communities. We then provide two examples of models that highlight contextual elements important to analyze and address within efforts to promote age-inclusive communities. The final section of this chapter provides examples of concepts and processes that can inform occupational therapy practice aimed at contributing to age-inclusive communities, pointing to diverse possibilities and the centrality of collaboration with older adults and community stakeholders.

## The Importance of Building Age-Inclusive Communities Through Occupational Therapy

Age-inclusive communities can be broadly defined as communities that enable the participation of all members across the age spectrum. The term community can refer to social groups at various scales and in various types of locations, ranging from, for example, an entire city or region, to a particular neighborhood, to a specific building, or to a unit in a long-term care setting. Given population aging and concerns regarding its social, economic, health-related, and political implications (see Chapter 3), many models addressing age-inclusive communities have been developed that specifically focus on promoting continued participation by older adults and ensuring access to resources that support desired aging-in-place (Steels, 2015). These models, which use various labels such as age-friendly, lifetime neighborhoods, and livable communities, identify physical, social, economic, attitudinal, and other environmental elements essential for designing communities that are optimally responsive to the needs of people as they age and that facilitate their continued vital contributions to their communities (Remillard-Boilard et al., 2021). Despite their differences, these various models highlight the imperative to intervene at levels that extend beyond aging individuals to address the contextual conditions that constrain occupational engagement, health, and well-being for many older adults. Given that these models address supporting participation in a diverse array of everyday activities older adults want and need to do in their communities, they are of direct relevance to occupational therapy's aim of enabling occupation (Lauckner & Stadnyk, 2014; Zur & Laliberte Rudman, 2013).

As implied above, the role of occupational therapy and its subsequent definition of client has expanded from a focus on individuals to include groups and communities (AOTA, 2020). Research on age-inclusiveness highlights the significant impact of contextual forces, beyond the control of any aging individual, for the occupations, health, and well-being of older adults. There is an abundance of evidence, generated by occupational therapists, gerontologists, anthropologists, geographers, sociologists, and others, demonstrating how various contemporary challenges faced by older adults as a collective, such as high rates of social isolation or restrictions in community mobility, are shaped through social systems, institutions, relations, and structures (Hand et al., 2012; Grenier et al., 2021; Levasseur et al., 2015; Walsh et al., 2017). For example, there is a substantial body of evidence demonstrating that ageist stereotypes and perceptions present barriers to maintaining and attaining sustainable employment (Harris et al., 2017; Laliberte Rudman & Aldrich, 2021), and identifying various social, physical, spatial, and political contextual factors that perpetuate social isolation in later life (Walsh et al., 2017; Weldrick & Grenier, 2018). As well, research evidence demonstrates that environmental challenges to social inclusion and occupational participation are compounded for older adults who experience other intersecting markers of social difference that are associated with disadvantage, such as those who experience poverty, are racialized, identify as LGBTQ2S+, and have physical, sensory, and cognitive impairments (Koon et al., 2020; Kontos et al., 2020; McGrath et al., 2017; Tolley & Ranzijn, 2006). Overall, given that interacting contextual elements shape what occupations are possible and not possible for aging adults in their communities, it is crucial for occupational therapists to contribute to the shaping of age-inclusive communities that support diverse occupational engagement.

## Age-Inclusive Communities: Conceptual Models and Key Principles

Within this section, we highlight two models, specifically the widely used World Health Organization's (WHO) Age-Friendly Cities and Communities Framework (Officer & Wu, 2018; World Health Organization [WHO], 2007) and a more recent critically informed Model of Social Exclusion proposed by Walsh et al. (2017). Each model provides guidance for identifying contextual elements important to assess and address in building toward age-inclusive communities. Optimal use of such models by occupational therapists requires a critical understanding of their strengths and limitations, and consideration of how an occupational perspective can contribute to their implementation (Zur & Laliberte Rudman, 2013).

The World Health Organization (WHO) Age-Friendly Cities Framework, first introduced in 2007, has been taken up globally within local efforts, particularly in urban contexts, aimed at fostering healthy aging and participation in community life (Plouffe et al., 2016). Its focus on urban contexts is a response to the spread of urbanization, with projections indicating that almost two-thirds of the world's population

will live in urban areas by 2050 (Buffel & Phillipson, 2018). This framework sets out a vision of ideal age-inclusive communities in which older adults are actively involved, valued, and supported, and has become one of the most frequently used frameworks in initiatives aimed at building age-inclusive communities (Remillard-Boilard et al., 2021). Over time, the framework was renamed the Age-Friendly Cities and Communities Framework and has been applied within smaller neighborhoods and rural communities (Lauckner & Stadnyk, 2014; Steels, 2015). By 2020, the Global Network for Age-Friendly Cities and Communities, established in 2010, included over 1000 cities and non-urban communities in 44 countries (Remillard-Boilard et al., 2021).

The WHO has developed checklists and guidelines to assist cities and communities in applying the Age-Friendly Cities and Communities Framework through a process of consultation, assessment, planning, action strategies, and evaluation (Plouffe et al., 2016; WHO, 2007, 2021). One strength of this framework is that it was developed through a participatory process involving older adults, based on the premise that older adults are experts regarding their lives and what is required for a community to be age friendly. Over 1000 older adults were involved in focus groups across 33 cities located in various countries and continents. In addition, focus groups were conducted with 250 caregivers and approximately 500 service providers (WHO, 2007). Based on analysis of this focus group data, the model outlines eight domains that span several aspects of environments, social life, activity engagement, and service provision. Within each domain (Table 32.1), there is an emphasis on ensuring accessibility, affordability, reliability, and safety, in addition to domain-specific considerations. The WHO emphasizes that it is vital to understand these eight domains as mutually influencing and urges local initiatives to engage in participatory processes with older adults to identify domains and considerations most essential to address in a particular community.

Although there is a need for further research on the effectiveness of initiatives that have applied the WHO framework (Remillard-Boilard et al., 2021), descriptive research to date has pointed to key characteristics that support its optimal application. These include: authentic inclusion of older adults in participatory processes that span consultation to implementation; actions that challenge negative stereotypes of older adults; strong partnerships with diverse stakeholders from across sectors; government commitment; and attending to both physical and social environmental considerations (Buffel & Phillipson, 2018; Remillard-Boilard et al., 2021; Steels, 2015). In addition, authors have pointed to several key limitations of the framework that need to be considered to ensure it is modified in ways that suit specific community contexts and respond to the needs of diverse older adults. For example, as the framework was developed for urban environments, it requires further refinement to ensure applicability to other types of contexts, such as rural environments and cultural communities (Remillard-Boilard et al., 2021). The framework has also been critiqued for being based on a homogenous view of older adults, as well as a Eurocentric view of what constitutes an ideal community and resources

**TABLE 32.1** The World Health Organization's Dimensions of Age-Friendly Cities and Communities

| Eight Dimensions | Examples of Considerations |
|---|---|
| Community and health care | • Diverse options for support and care services provided by governments, not-for-profits, and voluntary groups |
| Transportation | • Various forms of mobility (e.g., public transportation, taxis, driving, walking) with considerations for each form (e.g., priority bus seating; accessible parking; well-maintained sidewalks) |
| Housing | • Wide range of options that enable aging in desired places, connection to services, and community integration |
| Social Participation | • Social, cultural, and spiritual activities, as well as intergenerational opportunities |
| Outdoor spaces and buildings | • Various types of outdoor spaces and buildings; for example, green spaces, walkways, rest areas, street crossings, commercial buildings, and public toilets |
| Respect and social inclusion | • Attitudes and practices that value older adults and their contributions, work against ageist representations, and support social, civic, and economic inclusion |
| Civic participation and employment | • Options that enable contributing to communities and decision-making processes, such as volunteering, paid work, and civic events |
| Communication and information | • Provision of reliable, timely information regarding community events, resources, and opportunities in multiple formats |

For further details, see (WHO 2007, 2021).

(Buffel & Phillipson, 2018; Steels, 2015). Additional critiques cite the absence of an explicit focus on technology as a major gap in the framework, given advances in gerotechnology and digital means for optimizing social connections (Liddle et al., 2020; Marston & van Hoof, 2019; van Hoof & Marston, 2021). In addition to addressing issues of digital accessibility for older adults, enhanced opportunities for digital citizenship should be considered (Reuter et al., 2020). Finally, advocates of a life course perspective recommend expansion of the scope of the framework from Age-Friendly to "Longevity-Ready," to consider the impact of early life experiences on long-term well-being (Wang et al., 2021).

Given the wide uptake of the WHO framework and the various ways it attends to determinants of occupation, it is important for occupational therapists to consider how they can partner with age-friendly cities and community initiatives in their regions to support older citizens' occupational rights (Zur & Laliberte Rudman, 2013). Based on their engagement in an age-friendly community consultation process in a Canadian rural community, Lauckner and Stadnyk (2014) concluded that it provided a structure that can assist occupational therapists in contributing to community-level change in ways aligned with an occupational perspective. This fit between occupational therapy and age-friendly cities and communities initiatives is also supported by a 2020 survey conducted by the World Federation of Occupational Therapists. Responses from 32 respondents representing occupational therapy organizations in 31 different countries revealed that occupational therapists are involved in addressing many of the dimensions highlighted in the WHO Age-Friendly Cities and Communities Framework, such as informing the design of community buildings and outdoor spaces, optimizing transportation options, and promoting accessible housing and community participation.

At the same time, given the critiques of this framework, it is also crucial that occupational therapists advocate for and enact active approaches in age-friendly community processes to reach out to and support the participation of diverse older adults, such as those who have impairments, who have limited financial resources, or who do not speak the dominant language in a context (Zur & Laliberte Rudman, 2013). Such active approaches should integrate inclusive participatory processes, such as community dialogues in various languages and the use of older adult advisory boards, to engage community members in defining what is important to them (Buffel & Phillipson, 2018).

As well, occupational therapists can draw on additional models to broaden consideration of diversity and contextual factors that can exclude older adults, such as the "Old-age exclusion framework" developed by critical gerontologists Walsh et al. (2017). This framework, developed based on a broad-ranging scoping review of international literature addressing the dynamics of social exclusion in later life, addresses diverse positionalities in later life and attends to intersections of individual, societal, and structural components. Consistent with viewing occupation as a human right, Walsh et al. (2017) conceptualize participation in society as a right and define social exclusion as a "complex process that involves the lack or denial of resources, rights, goods, and services as people age, and the inability to participate in the normal relationships and activities, available to the majority of people across the varied and multiple domains of society" (p. 83). The six domains, and sub-components, in this old-age exclusion framework (Table 32.2) both overlap with the Age-Friendly Cities and Communities Framework and point to additional considerations important to address so as to disrupt processes of exclusion based on age. For example, grounded in a critical gerontological perspective (see Chapter 4),

**TABLE 32.2** Dimensions and Sub-Components of the Old-Age Exclusion Framework

| Six Dimensions | Subcomponents |
|---|---|
| Civic participation | • Citizenship, civic activities, volunteering and community responsibility, voting and political participation |
| Sociocultural aspects | • Ageism and age discrimination, symbolic and discourse exclusion, identity exclusion |
| Social relations | • Social opportunities, social relationship quality, loneliness and isolation, and social networks and supports |
| Material and financial resources | • Poverty, material deprivation, and income, employment, and pensions |
| Services, amenities, and mobility | • Health and social care, transport and mobility, area-based exclusion, general services, information and information communication technologies, housing |
| Neighborhood and community | • Social and relational dimensions, crime, services, amenities and built environment, socioeconomic aspects, sociopolitical structures, place-based policy |

For further details, see Walsh, Scharf & Keating (2017). Exclusion is noted to result from deficits in the various subdomains and persistence of determinantal contextual conditions.

this framework explicitly identifies poverty, crime, political factors, and identity exclusion as barriers to civic and other forms of participation. Within the next section of this chapter, we provide examples, written by occupational therapists and scientists, of concepts and practices relevant to advancing understanding of and contributing to building age-inclusive communities.

## Examples of Concepts and Approaches for Use in Occupational Therapy Practice and Research

Occupational therapists can contribute to building and sustaining age-inclusive communities in many ways. Drawing on understandings of age-inclusive communities from theoretical frameworks such as that provided by the World Health Organization and Walsh et al. (2017), collaboration with older adults, community stakeholders, policy makers, and key actors in a community is central to such efforts, to ensure relevance to the lives of older adults and sustainability. Within this final section, various authors share key concepts and examples of practice approaches that can inform future occupational therapy practice and research regarding age-inclusive communities.

### Partnerships to Support Aging in Community, by Jenny Womack

A commitment to building and sustaining age-inclusive communities is optimized through partnerships that span organizations, individuals, and systems. As suggested in the chapter introduction, working at a level beyond, but encompassing of, individual perspectives on achieving age-inclusive policies, practices, and environments ensures that contextual considerations are addressed in accomplishing these outcomes. In this sub-section of the chapter, we introduce sustainability principles for authentic partnerships, and consider two specific examples of how they have been enacted through aging and human services organizations in partnership with occupational therapy

practitioners and students, working together to realize the goals of aging in community.

### Principles for Sustainable Partnerships

Why are partnership models important for work in aging? Although many occupational therapists work with older adults primarily in health-care systems, the establishment of age-inclusive communities necessarily extends into public, nonprofit, and governmental sectors where different funding mechanisms, accountability standards, and priorities are in play. Samali et al. (2016) point to increasing collaboration between these sectors, suggesting that thoughtful partnerships can enhance collective efficiency and effectiveness, and ultimately result in broader social and systems change. The mission of creating age-inclusive communities requires this level of change and necessitates thoughtful partnerships based in a sustainability model.

The Community-Campus Partnerships for Health (CCPH), a nonprofit organization promoting health equity and social justice, outlines four elements of authentic, sustainable partnerships: *guiding principles* for the mission and goals of the partnership, *quality processes* that are relationship-focused and mutually respectful, *meaningful outcomes* that are tangible and relevant to communities, and *transformation* that occurs at multiple levels, from the personal to the institutional to the political (Community-Campus Partnerships for Health [CCPH], 2013). These types of partnerships, enacted in the realm of aging services, also provide prime opportunities for occupational therapists to engage in collaborative efforts to create communities ready and able to support the occupations of human participants throughout the life course.

### Aging in Community

The concept of aging-in-place has been embraced for several decades as an optimal goal for living one's chronologically long life in the home of their choice with safety and health considerations addressed through an optimized built environment and social supports (Wiles et al., 2012). For the partnerships described in this section, this concept was expanded to embrace Thomas and Blanchard's (2009) alternative of *aging in community*, a way of life that focuses equally on continued engagement with, and valued roles in relationship to, other people and places in the community. The qualities associated with aging in community include not only those typically embraced in occupational therapy frameworks such as health, accessibility, and purposeful engagement, but also inclusion, interdependence, and ways of living that are ecologically, economically, and socially sustainable (Blanchard & Anthony, 2013; Thomas & Blanchard, 2009). These qualities align well with the previously described WHO Age-Friendly Cities and Communities Framework (WHO, 2007) and intersect specifically with the Social Exclusion Framework (Walsh et al., 2017) in attending to civic engagement, social interdependence, and economic well-being.

For the occupational therapists whose work is profiled in this section of the chapter, embracing the qualities of an aging-in-community framework was an impetus to move beyond more traditional work with older adult clients. Instead of focusing on individual health, body structures and functions, and concepts of "productive" aging that prioritize resource independence over engagement in community life, a new paradigm was instituted. Collaborating with older adults in processes ignited by public, private, and governmental organizations to enhance the age-inclusivity of our communities affirmed the assertion of Black et al. (2015) that an aging-in-community paradigm encourages the mobilization of older adults as a core social resource. For occupational therapy, merging this framework with our expertise in occupation also holds promise as a way to assess and facilitate community engagement.

## Partnerships in Aging: Two Examples
### Example I: The Story of Crescent Magnolia
In January of 2018, Habitat for Humanity International unveiled a nationwide initiative to honor the concept of the *Beloved Community* through a series of projects marking the 50th anniversary of both the death of Dr. Martin Luther King, Jr. and the passage of the Fair Housing Act. The *Beloved Community* was advanced by Dr. Martin Luther King, Jr. as an achievable goal for peaceable cohabitation by people committed to nonviolence and justice. In Orange County, North Carolina, the local Habitat for Humanity affiliate (HHOC) aligned an innovative senior housing project with this concept. Realizing a long-term goal of their executive director, HHOC began planning for a multi-unit residential development based on a home ownership model for older adults with limited incomes. Partners in this planning with Habitat for Humanity of Orange County included occupational therapists working with the Orange County Department on Aging (OCDOA) and the University of North Carolina Partnerships in Aging Program (PiAP).

In the initial planning stages, occupational therapists were consulted regarding design of the housing units and the incorporation of concepts related to aging in community. This resulted in several changes to the built environment, such as zero-step shower thresholds and a base kitchen cabinet with

open space beneath, as well as attention to social participation, including opportunities for residents to provide input about their desired interior design and to mentor future Habitat participants. Occupational therapists were also engaged in conversations about alternative sweat equity options for older adult residents. Habitat for Humanity's model of home ownership typically requires that future homeowners invest more than 200 hours of sweat equity in the building process. Recognizing that not all older homeowners would be able to engage physically in construction efforts, HHOC sought help in identifying alternatives, including volunteering for OCDOA, participating in an intergenerational reading program with a neighboring daycare, and working at the Habitat for Humanity ReStore.

As the development of Crescent Magnolia moved forward, occupational therapists and students from the academic program at the University of North Carolina (UNC) partnered with prospective older adult residents, HHOC office and construction staff, and community stakeholders to document the story of Crescent Magnolia. Interviews between students and Crescent Magnolia residents revealed the meaning of home ownership for the latter group and provided insights about the challenges and advantages of aging in community for the students. The construction crew partnered with occupational therapists to consider how they implemented aging-in-community concepts through the specific inclusion of older volunteer builders, and the design of outdoor common spaces that encourage socialization and co-occupations such as gardening and birding.

The results of the Crescent Magnolia partnership from planning stages until its culmination in 2020 exemplify the sustainable partnership elements of *meaningful outcomes* and *transformation at multiple levels*. In this case, a tangible and relevant outcome of the Crescent Magnolia partnership is a free, downloadable resource manual aimed at informing and encouraging national Habitat affiliates and other affordable housing providers to develop similar senior communities using a home ownership model (Womack, 2021; *The Story of Crescent Magnolia*). Although Crescent Magnolia has had a local impact on the lives of 26 older adults who now occupy their new homes and eight occupational therapy students who learned about housing issues in later life, the transformation has ripple effects. Crescent Magnolia is to date the only Habitat for Humanity development of its kind in the United States, but at the time of this writing is being considered for replication by a dozen other affiliates (Personal Communication with J. Player, CEO HHOC). For the occupational therapists involved in this project, dissemination of the partnership model at state and national conferences has also resulted in professional networking about emerging work in the realm of senior housing and social transformation.

### Example 2: The Orange County NC Master Aging Plan
Many aging and social service agencies engage in strategic planning in order to ensure that they meet the needs of older adults in their communities. In Orange County, North Carolina, that planning is undertaken through a broad

year-long community effort organized by the county department on aging (OCDOA) that engages older adult residents as well as partners from private business, health-care entities, municipalities, and social justice organizations. Beginning in 2017, the Master Aging Plan (MAP) was aligned with the WHO Age-Friendly Cities and Communities Framework (WHO, 2007) and the AARP Age-Friendly Initiatives (AARP, 2014), by forming workgroups in the categories of: (1) transportation and outdoor spaces, (2) housing, (3) social participation and inclusion, (4) civic participation and employment, and (5) community support and health services. Attention to cross-cutting issues of communication, diversity, equity, inclusion, and intergenerational possibilities was charged to all workgroups. Due to relationships developed by community and academic occupational therapists with the OCDOA, occupational therapy practitioner-educators were asked to partner in leading two of the workgroups (housing and outdoor spaces) and participating in the others.

Throughout the year-long planning process, workgroups drew from survey and interview data collected from older adults through multiple community meetings conducted in three languages prevalent in the county (English, Spanish, and Mandarin). They then constructed overarching objectives within their domain of concern, established strategies to meet those objectives, and identified indicators of success. The indicators are assigned to various community partners who are accountable for their attainment and are tracked across the subsequent 5 years. Because the housing workgroup was led by an occupational therapist, one of the objectives from that effort is highlighted below as an example of this work. In particular, the strategy outlined below in Table 32.3 resulted from survey data indicating that older residents with housing repair needs often do not know where to turn or which home repair organization could best meet their needs.

As a result of this initiative, the occupational therapist who led the housing workgroup ultimately took on the role of coordinating a county home repair coalition; five organizations that had previously provided home modifications and repairs in isolation came together under a mutual agreement and began triaging referrals in order to optimize the fit between the need and solution, and minimize wait time for the homeowner. Four years into this strategic plan, the housing repair coalition is meeting monthly, sharing a database of requests, and working with an occupational therapist contracted by the OCDOA and an advisory board of older adults to identify needs beyond housing repairs for those who apply for their services. For more information about the OCDOA and its Master Aging Plan, please visit https://www.orange-countync.gov/203/Master-Aging-Plan.

## Summary

Authentic partnerships in which the partnering entities collaborate around shared principles to achieve tangible, relevant outcomes that result in social change are critical to work in aging and to the realization of age-inclusive communities. Occupational therapy practitioners have not only relevant skills and knowledge, but also opportunities to collaborate with community organizations working toward this mission.

## Participatory Citizenship and Collective Occupation, by Sarah Kantartzis

Building age-inclusive communities is a dynamic and multi-level process. Therefore, a range of theoretical and practical perspectives can and should be taken. One perspective is to focus on people within community, considering how we understand our inter-relationships as well as our doing of daily life together. In this section we propose two concepts, participatory citizenship and collective occupation, that can be useful in illuminating these considerations. Both concepts focus on the intricate intertwining of our relationships through our daily lives as we do together. Citizenship is a dynamic process, taking a variety of forms around the world, with legal, political, and social dimensions. In Europe, the concept of participatory citizenship has been proposed, positioning all people as citizens with the opportunity to have voice and action in the shared public world (Fransen et al., 2015). This doing together of citizens can be seen in collective occupation. This section will explore these two concepts in further detail, illustrating how they may be important in working toward age-inclusive communities.

## Citizenship

Considering the population of communities as citizens clearly locates our focus on roles, relationships, and actions further to those represented by terms such as spouse, friend, or worker. Citizenship may be considered in relation to a legal status, to political rights and responsibilities, and to wider participation in society (Lee, 2019). It locates our focus on public spaces and how we do and be together with others in our community.

**TABLE 32.3**  Orange County Master Aging Plan 2017 to 2022—Examples of Objectives, Housing Workgroup

| OBJECTIVE 3.6: Support Orange County Residents to Age in Community | |
| --- | --- |
| **Strategy** | **Indicators** |
| Strategy 3.6.2: Collaborate across existing housing repair/remodel programs to better communicate, share cases, and refer to specialized services | Indicator 3.6.2a: Network of repair/remodel organizations is formed<br>Indicator 3.6.2b: Collaboration coordinator is selected [....]<br>Indicator 3.6.2f: More comprehensive repairs are provided to residents<br>Indicator 3.6.2g: Data are collected and shared regarding safety and well-being of homeowners who receive home repairs or modifications |

The phrase "senior citizens" is commonly used in the literature; however, use of this phrase requires careful consideration. For example, the emphasis may be on "senior," but this only provides a homogenous descriptor of all people between 50 or 60 to the oldest old. The term may be used in discussions of policies perceived to be beneficial for this age group; to demark a change in relationship to the state in terms of social and health-care benefits (often related to retirement from work), a time of heightened risk (of physical accidents, fraud) and therefore with an increased responsibility by the state. This view, founded in a legal status, places the state in a position of power, regulation, and authority while the person becomes a responsibility to be successfully managed. In neo-liberal societies this may involve an increasing shift in responsibility toward the older person to "age successfully" in terms of maintaining health, a good financial state, and autonomy and self-control (Laliberte Rudman, 2015). In addition, the label "senior" aligns with the idea of there being different types of citizens, not all equal in their citizenship, also discussed in relation to children perceived as becoming citizens only when they reach the age to vote (Golombek, 2006), or disabled people being less-than citizens, dis-citizens and needing help to become citizens (Devlin & Pothier, 2006).

However, while use of the phrase "senior citizens" may require caution, the concept of citizenship is important. Contemporary discussions challenge a limited view of citizenship with imposed forms, boundaries, and hierarchies, enabling expanded views of the nature of citizenship beyond a legal status. It is acknowledged that the nature of citizenship may be dynamically constructed by people depending on their contexts and circumstances (Lee, 2019), with citizenship being seen as a process rather than as a fixed and static status. The form of citizenship known as Participatory Citizenship is particularly useful for occupational therapists interested in supporting the rights and inclusion of all peoples (Fransen-Jaïbi et al., 2021), and therefore may be particularly relevant in working toward building age-inclusive communities.

### *Participatory Citizenship*

Participatory or active citizenship has been proposed as one form of citizenship (Lopes, 2021), in particular in Europe through the work of Hoskins and Kerr (2012) for the European Commission in preparation for the European Year of Citizens in 2013. Participatory citizenship enables us to consider "being a citizen" as more than engaging in political activities. It can be seen "broadly as acts that can occur, either individually or collectively, that are intrinsically concerned with shaping the society that we want to live in" (Vromen, 2003, p. 83). In their conceptualization, Hoskins and Kerr (2012) expanded on the wide range of activities that we might engage in as citizens, while further elaborating on the creation of a society for all marked by particular characteristics and values: "Participation in civil society, community, and/or political life, characterized by mutual respect and non-violence and in accordance with human rights and democracy" (p. 4).

Understanding older adults as participatory citizens positions them as active actors in their own contexts. It acknowledges

the need to respect difference, whether this is due to age, gender, race, or ability, to be aware of power and status differences, and the need for processes that are deliberate, based in discussion and compromise (Mangone, 2012), and directed toward maintaining and enhancing social cohesion (Hoskins & Kerr, 2012).

Participatory citizenship therefore focuses not only on legal status, rights, and obligations but also on associative life, life together as citizens. This enables ensuring the accountability of the state as well as the construction of daily life and the shared public world (Fransen et al., 2015). This is an active process, the doing of citizenship, and here we can explore the importance of collective occupation.

### Collective Occupation

Collective occupation relates to a whole range of everyday occupations that have to do with the construction and maintenance of the public world. The public world is the physical and social space that we share with others, beyond our homes. The nature of the public world, including what we can do, where, when, and with whom, is created and recreated as people come together in collective occupation (Kantartzis & Molineux, 2017). Collective occupation refers to occupation that may or may not happen synchronously, may or may not happen in the same physical place, but, because the people involved share an intention toward the social world (Ramugondo & Kronenberg, 2015) and because of the power produced by the occupation of numerous people (Kantartzis & Molineux, 2017), the shape and nature of the public world is produced and re-produced through it. Ramugondo and Kronenberg (2015) discuss how the need for human relations drives such occupation, with research identifying a clear awareness by participants of the importance of being in and part of the day-to-day life of their community (Kantartzis & Molineux, 2017). Collective occupation therefore appears to be an important element in the building of age-inclusive communities, and an exploration of the current conceptualizations of collective occupation will facilitate development of such occupation.

The concept of collective occupation began to be developed when Fogelberg and Frauwirth (2010) noted that groups, communities, and populations produce occupation. They turned our attention to such collective occupation in the United States as parades, football games, and elections. Kantartzis and Molineux (2017) further identified celebratory and commemorative events, such as religious festivals, carnivals, clubbing, football tournaments, an annual bazaar as well as remembrance events. In considering our communities we can question, what are the events (occupations) that take place that offer the opportunity for all members of the community in all their diversity to come together? Important to these collective occupations is shared actions and shared emotions, often involving symbols and rituals, which help renew the community's solidarity (Collins, 2004).

However, the concept of collective occupation not only describes those occupations that simply involve many people. As introduced, we understand that collective occupation leads to collective outcomes, to the shaping of the public world. In the literature there are several discussions of how communities are shaped and develop through shared engagement in occupations (e.g., Peralta-Catipon, 2012). Peralta-Catipon (2012) described the public gatherings of Filipina migrant workers in Hong Kong, unplanned and informal. While multiple, dispersed occupations took place, a unique social structure emerged—including practices and the rules and meanings guiding behavior, specific roles and status, as well as a sense of self. We can see the importance of opportunities to be in public spaces, to be able to take part in the daily occupations of shopping, waiting at the bus stop, having a coffee, or going for a stroll in the shopping center. The opportunity to be out of one's home and to feel and be part of the social flow is vital for our sense of belonging to the community, but at the same time shapes the community as a public world and people's possibility for occupation in it.

Therefore, it is important to consider who may be excluded or marginalized, prevented perhaps due to ability, gender, age, or race, from entering and engaging in such collective occupation in the public world. A critical lens challenges the assumption that collective occupation is always a positive and deliberate process of like-minded citizens creating ideal communities for all. At an extreme collective occupation may be violent affecting not only those involved but others living in the same neighborhood (Fritz & Cutchin, 2017; Motimele & Ramugondo, 2014), but it may also reproduce more subtle forms of hegemonic practices related to gender, race, ability, and age (Angell, 2014). The previously mentioned occupations of shopping, waiting at a bus stop, and having a coffee, may all take forms that marginalize, depending on the occupation of the people involved. Rising costs of "designer" coffee and expectations of speedy use of electronic devices serve as subtle exclusionary mechanisms toward older people. Importantly, individual people may rarely recognize their own contribution to the ongoing construction of attitudes or practices that exclude others. Rather, they may be shaped within the ongoing daily doings and conversations, unintended or unforeseen consequences of these.

Collective occupation also may take the form of organized activities, including formal associations, that a community, or certain members of a community, may develop to address local needs and issues. Citizenship has often been discussed to include a range of voluntary activities contributing to civil society. Collective occupation may also take the form of activism, developed to raise awareness of or take action on issues (see Núñez et al.'s [2019] discussion of the collective occupations developed by an advocacy organization for parents in Chile) or resistance (Simaan, 2017). Important to the development of such occupation is the opportunity for people to come together to talk about local issues, that is, entering the public space can lead to discussions of local needs which can move to action (Kantartzis & Molineux, 2017).

## Promoting Inclusive Communities Through Participatory Citizenship and Collective Occupation

Participatory citizenship draws our attention to the importance of our relationships as fellow inhabitants of our communities, and the nature of those relationships in providing opportunities for all to be seen, heard, and be active. Collective occupation, including everyday doings in our neighborhoods, organized participation to raise awareness or address needs, and celebratory or commemorative events, can be the process through which opportunities for voice and action for all are ensured. However, the values of participatory citizenship remind us that collective occupation can also exclude, deny, and marginalize groups in our communities. In concluding, we will briefly introduce what seem to be some of the key elements in ensuring inclusionary processes throughout our collective occupation.

Participatory Citizenship and collective occupation take part in physical and social space. These are locations where people come together: the street, square, marketplace, bar and cafe, community center, shopping mall, and perhaps also the virtual spaces of social media. In these spaces, neighbors and strangers engage, as citizens, in collective occupation. These spaces therefore need to be inclusive, friendly, and flexible, including consideration of age-inclusiveness (Kantartzis et al., 2012; Oldenburg, 1997). Such spaces may invite reflection and debate, spaces where alternative and diverse views can be heard. A consciousness of the dynamics of power in the community and occupation as an intentional response to this needs to be ensured (Ramugondo & Kronenberg, 2015; Simaan, 2017), and further ways of supporting this need to be developed.

Through this doing the public world is created and re-created. This is the world where we can be recognized, valued, experience a sense of belonging, or can be excluded, ignored, marginalized. Our collective occupation can ensure that all people are "full" citizens, not only legally, but in their opportunity to have voice and action in our shared public world.

## Participatory Action Research and Building Age-Inclusive Communities, by Colleen McGrath

As discussed in earlier sections of this chapter, building age-inclusive communities requires occupational therapists to work at levels that extend beyond the individual toward addressing those environmental (physical, social, cultural, political/institutional) conditions that serve to constrain occupational possibilities as well as limit the health and wellbeing of older adults. In working toward building age-inclusive communities, there must be attention paid to these environmental factors but also efforts to meaningfully engage diverse older adults. Participatory action research provides a type of process that can be used to support such an engagement. In this section, we provide an example of a participatory action research (PAR) project that is focused on building age-inclusive communities by focusing on environmental barriers and supports to community mobility for older adults with age-related vision loss (ARVL) living in London, Ontario, Canada.

Given that PAR involves cycles of knowledge generation, reflection, and action, we are sharing the steps taken thus far in this PAR project, which is currently underway.

## What Is Participatory Action Research?

Participatory action research involves a cyclical process of generating knowledge, reflecting, and enacting change. PAR has a commitment to challenging power inequities that shape social life (Sandwick et al., 2018). A fundamental goal of PAR is the creation of knowledge that provides a direct path toward transformative action, both at individual and collective levels. Despite the promise that PAR holds, and the abundance of examples of such studies involving young people (Kim, 2016; Ozer, 2017; Shamrova & Cummings, 2017), no research to date has used a PAR framework with aging adults experiencing ARVL. There are many possible reasons for this. For example, systems of power, such as ageism and ableism, impact the way research is conducted, often leaving aging adults with disabilities, including those with ARVL, at the periphery of research (Corrado et al., 2018). This assumption, however, that aging adults are either incapable or uninterested in participating collaboratively in research is faulty. Our team sought to dispel this ageist myth by mobilizing a group of aging adults with ARVL who were situated at the intersection of aging and disability, and, as a result, were perfectly positioned to help inform the social practices, systems, and policies that governed their lives. As we will unpack below, PAR is a process that involves multiple phases. As our PAR process has evolved, it has provided opportunities to engage with older adults in ways that addresses those environmental conditions that present challenges to valued forms of occupational engagement, thus providing an approach to PAR that is aligned with building age-inclusive communities while also considering the intersections of disability and age.

## What Is Age-Related Vision Loss?

This example specifically involved working with adults who were experiencing age-related vision loss, to identify and address environmental barriers to their occupational participation in communities. Low vision refers to a permanent loss of vision that interferes "with the performance of common age-appropriate seeing tasks" (Vision Rehabilitation Evidence Based Review [VREBR], 2005, p. 10) and cannot be corrected by eyeglasses, contact lenses, medication, or surgical intervention. In industrialized countries, aging adults constitute the fastest growing segment of the population with low vision (Watson, 2001), including individuals with macular degeneration, glaucoma, and diabetic retinopathy, with such conditions often collectively referred to as age-related vision loss (Watson, 2001). An abundance of research has focused on the association between ARVL and disability, including activity limitations in the areas of self-care (Knudtson et al., 2011), leisure (Boerner & Wang, 2010), productivity (Alma et al., 2011), and community mobility (McGrath et al., 2017) (see Chapter 10 for further details regarding age-related vision loss).

## Participatory Action Research Example: Working With Older Adults With Age-Related Vision Loss
### Phase One: Establishing the Research Priorities

The first step in the PAR process was to engage aging adults, not as passive participants but as active and equal contributors, to the research process. Although it may be easier to engage in PAR once the study focus is set, a truly participatory process encourages aging adults to participate fully as partners in all phases of the research process (Blair & Minkler, 2009; Minkler, 2010), particularly at the initiation phase which includes the process of identifying research priorities (Berg, 2004).

Our initial research group, which was comprised of three occupational therapy researchers and two students, set out to do just this by involving eight aging adults (four females; four males) with ARVL in identifying research priorities. This reflected our group's commitment to shared power and ownership within the research process (Berg, 2004) and helped us move toward an approach where research is done "with" as opposed to "for" or "about" aging adults. The aging adults took part in three half-day meetings and a one-on-one interview (60 minutes) over a period of approximately 2 months. To participate in the initial stage of this PAR study, the aging adults had to: (1) be 65 years of age and older; (2) have received a diagnosis of age-related vision loss (macular degeneration, glaucoma, and/or diabetic retinopathy); and (3) feel comfortable participating in a group meeting in English. After much spirited discussion, and a democratic voting process, the aging adults generated three broad research priorities including: (1) community mobility; (2) technology; and (3) community supports and services. For each priority area, the aging adults provided detailed information addressing the following questions:

1. What do we need to know more about? (i.e., the research questions).
2. How could we learn more about this? (i.e., knowledge generation approaches).
3. Who would we need to involve as key stakeholders? (i.e., participants and partnerships).
4. What would change look like? (i.e., action potential).

We concluded this phase of the PAR process by engaging in self-reflexive one-on-one interviews with the aging adults to better understand their experiences of the PAR process. Occupational therapists considering implementing a PAR process with older adults to help build age-inclusive communities could learn from our experiences during this initial PAR phase, namely the importance of negotiating power within the research process and managing ethical tensions related to boundaries within professional relationships, co-researcher compensation, and the mobilization of timely social action.

### Phase Two: Carrying out the Participatory Action Research Process

The initial stage of the PAR process led to the generation of three research priorities. The next step, which was aided with the receipt of grant funding, allowed the team, which we now refer to as the research collective, to carry out the PAR process, focused exclusively on the research priority of community mobility. The aging adults with ARVL defined community mobility as encompassing driving, navigating alternate modes of transportation (bus, taxi, train), and walking in the neighborhood (including accessing buildings, stores, and outdoor spaces).

Our first step was to solidify the research collective. In keeping with the principles of PAR, a research collective of ten stakeholders was formed consisting of a policy maker, a community organization representative, three occupational therapy researchers (who were the same as those involved in the initial PAR phase), three students, and two aging adults with ARVL. All members of the research collective, contributed equally to shared decision making at monthly meetings. In addition to being responsible for guiding the research process, the research collective also established a guiding mission, vision, and values (Table 32.4).

Our next step, and this is the stage we continue to work through as a research collective, was to carry out the proposed research. The research questions identified during the initial PAR stage addressed three areas of community mobility including: (1) Driving: (a) How do aging adults with vision loss adjust to losing their license?; (b) What are the determinants of autonomous vehicle technology acceptance among adults with vision loss?; (2) Public modes of transportation: (a) What transportation services are available for aging adults with vision loss in London, Ontario, Canada?; and (3) Walking in the neighborhood: (a) How do aging adults with vision loss navigate their neighborhood?; (b) What are enabling and disabling features of a building, store, or outdoor space for an aging adult with ARVL and how can those barriers be addressed to create more vision-friendly spaces?

With respect to methods of knowledge generation, the aging adults proposed several methods of knowledge generation that were largely spatial (e.g., GPS tracking, life space mapping, community audits) or visual (e.g., photo-elicitation, videos). The proposed methods of knowledge generation were also strongly connected to outputs focused on systems-level change. For example, one option recommended

was a neighborhood interview (the go-along method) with Go-Pro recordings so that the research collective could capture, first-hand, the challenges aging adults with ARVL encounter when negotiating community mobility (navigating a store/building, crossing the street, etc.). A video with personal narration was proposed as the output, which could be shared with various stakeholders such as city employees (bus drivers, city/urban planners), architects/contractors/builders, store owners, and motorists as a means of informing service and policy change, which is in line with the transformative action focus of participatory action research.

### Exploring the Impact of the Participatory Action Research Process

Although this PAR process continues to unfold, we are excited about the methodological and practical significance of this work so far. From a methodological standpoint, this work has committed itself to the full and democratic involvement of aging adults with ARVL in each step of the research process which means aging adults with ARVL, for one of the first times, will be acknowledged for their skills and expertise as co-researchers in helping to build age-inclusive communities. Furthermore, from a practical perspective, this PAR work is fully committed to action, including personal, social, and policy-level change. As such, our work will be relevant beyond academic audiences to include community organizations focused on low vision rehabilitation as well as municipal policy developers focused on enhancing transportation services to help build age-inclusive communities for aging adults with vision loss. Indeed, the opportunities PAR holds for helping occupational therapists build age-inclusive communities cannot be understated and this example, drawn from our work with aging adults with ARVL, provides just one example of the far-reaching potential of participatory research processes.

### Processes of Place-Making Within Age-Inclusive Third Spaces: The Ibasho Café By Margaret A. Perkinson

Subjective experience of one's environment grows in importance in later life and represents an important factor in age-inclusive communities and the Aging-in-Place equation

**TABLE 32.4** Mission, Vision, and Values of the Participatory Action Project With Seniors With Age-Related Vision Loss

| Our Mission | Our Vision | Our Values |
|---|---|---|
| We are a collective of aging adults, researchers, community leaders, and service providers in London, Ontario who create new knowledge and advocate for innovative solutions to facilitate successful community mobility for aging adults with age-related vision loss (ARVL). | Our vision is to work towards the full and equitable community inclusion of aging adults with age-related vision loss, by driving innovative, collaborative, and community-led work that moves research into action. | 1. We value and respect the full and equitable participation of all voices.<br>2. We are committed to creating new knowledge related to ARVL that is accessible, innovative, and methodologically rigorous.<br>3. We engage with a diversity of cultures, abilities, and life experiences.<br>4. We are committed to the importance of collaboration and power sharing.<br>5. We are committed to action at both the individual and societal level. |

(Lawton, 1998; Rowles et al., 2016; Wahl et al., 2012). (See also Chapter 20.) As people age, they tend to feel a greater sense of attachment and belonging to their immediate surroundings (Gilleard et al., 2007; Oswald et al., 2011). *Place*, "any environmental locus that draws human experiences, actions, and meanings together spatially" (Seamon, 2013, p. 150), is constructed and experienced through everyday actions and routines associated with a given setting. Maintaining a sense of place entails a process of active, ongoing adjustment as persons and environments change over time (Andrews et al., 2007; Rowles & Ravdal, 2002). This chapter section will consider the social dynamics that generate and reinforce a sense of place, as illustrated in a "third place" setting: an Ibasho Café and the potential role of occupational therapists in this process.

## Social Dynamics of Emergent Activity Spaces

Except for the very frail, social worlds of community elders extend beyond the buildings in which they live (Wiles et al., 2012). To understand the process and experience of "place" (and thus to understand "aging-in-place") from the viewpoint of aging adults, occupational therapists must consider the activity spaces in which elders' routine, everyday activities transpire beyond their home environments (Cornwell & Cagney, 2017; Hirsch, 2016). Given the significance of the immediate environment to older adults, physical and social characteristics of neighborhoods and public spaces, as well as their patterns of use by older people, either allow or impede daily social interactions and activities (Lager et al., 2015). Encounters of the "weak tie" kind (Granovetter, 1973) may happen in public social spaces during reoccurring encounters with "familiar strangers" who share similar daily routines (i.e., "place ballet") (Eck & Pijpers, 2017; Schmidt et al., 2019; Seamon & Nordin, 1980; see also Chapter 20). Engagement in the local "social flow" of collective occupations (noted earlier in this chapter) and within "third places," that is, congenial public gathering spaces (Broadway & Engelhardt, 2019), reinforces a sense of attachment to one's local surroundings. Age-friendly or age-inclusive third places allow persons of all ages to come together to engage in collective occupations that are inclusive, flexible, and attainable.

## Third Places: A Closer Look

As noted earlier in this chapter, "third places" are neither home (first place) nor workplace (second place), but informal public gathering spots, open to all. Hosts to voluntary gatherings of regular clientele, they are warm, comfortable, and welcoming places to spend time (Oldenburg, 2000). In addition to public establishments and local hangouts, such as coffeehouses, pubs, bookstores, barbershops, churches, and parks, the concept of "third place" has served as a guiding principle for older adult services, such as senior centers and Memory Cafes (Perkinson, 2020).

### The Physical Environment of Third Places

Occupational therapists, with their expertise and sensitivity to psychosocial processes, the built environment, and

environmental modifications, are well-positioned to collaborate with architects, designers, and potential users to establish conditions or aspects of public spaces that encourage and support the occurrence of informal social interactions. Proponents of public space design (Devlieger & Dujardin, 2021; Hauderowicz & Serena, 2020) have identified ways to enhance fundamental contextual elements that facilitate spontaneous informal interactions: develop inclusive thresholds that allow free movement in and out of the space; create open, "elastic" spaces that accommodate multiple types of use by diverse participants; enlist stakeholders of all ages in user-centered design processes; encourage the "haptic experience of space" in which all senses are involved in encounters and connections with the activity setting; and transform "lost" in-between spaces, not originally intended to be used as social settings (e.g., sidewalks), into polyvalent landscapes that facilitate diverse informal social encounters.

In encouraging the "haptic experience of space" an age-friendly third place accommodates for age-related changes in vision, hearing, mobility, and cognition (see Chapters 10 and 15) and modifies the physical and social environment both to support diminished function and to maximize occupational performance and engagement. The skills and expertise of occupational therapists, who know how to accommodate for sensory and cognitive changes in later life, are especially relevant here. Aspects of the physical environment that a therapist might modify to make age-friendly include sources and intensity of lighting, use of color, signage and graphic design, acoustics, possible use of noise absorbent panels or sound enhancing systems, etc. Supportive spaces also reflect respect for symbolic meanings that may accompany aspects of the physical environment, for example, certain colors convey significant meanings and/or taboos in certain cultures. A culturally sensitive OT would be attuned to relevant symbols and other cultural factors and would act accordingly.

### The Social Environment of Third Places

Successful third places increase opportunities for social interaction and enable the development and maintenance of natural helping networks. Occupational therapists can foster these processes by identifying and bolstering informal social supports: by connecting participants with specific needs to those with appropriate resources; by identifying and supporting key people, the "hubs of influence," within informal helping networks; and by reinforcing supportive network characteristics and individual behaviors, for example, empathy (Zaki, 2014; Zaki & Ochsner, 2011). The following description of an Ibasho Café provides an example of a type of third place oriented toward older adults and suggests ways that occupational therapists might contribute to the social integration of older people into and within these settings. With origins in Japan, it illustrates cultural influences on both physical context and social interactions.

### The Ibasho Café

Initiated in Japan, the Ibasho Café represents an empowering type of third place. "Ibasho" translates to a place where one feels a sense of belonging, purpose, and acceptance. As a third place, it is neither home nor worksite, but a congenial space open to all. The café provides a public place without a rigid or specific purpose, where people can do as they want, develop peer and intergenerational social networks, and assume meaningful roles, both within the Ibasho space and eventually in the greater community.

Ibasho is unique in that it is run by its older participants and based on their priorities. Its approach to empowerment "reframes" age by recognizing older adults as valuable assets to their community, resources rather than clients, and offers a possible outlet for their talents. Based on principles of self-governance, its participants are involved in all stages of development and maintenance of the site. Volunteer elders take leadership roles—in development, planning, operations, management, finance—sharing their knowledge and experience with each other and with younger generations. After an initial period of orientation, the older adults "run the bus," with minimal outside assistance. They choose activities that reflect their priorities and address community needs, for example, community gardening. The objective is to create and strengthen social ties while operating a sustainable business. Ibasho sites are successful in Asia and may represent one future solution to social isolation for older adults in the United States.

### History of Ibasho

Ibasho evolved from the responses of groups of older adults who rose to the occasion to serve and rebuild their communities in times of natural disasters. In 2011, the Great East Japan Earthquake and its accompanying tsunami killed over 18,000 and displaced over 65,000 persons. Having endured similar disasters in the past, the older adults saved surviving community members by guiding them to higher ground and teaching them to get along with limited resources, for example, managing without electricity and water, foraging the forests for food. When teams of outside aid, such as Operation USA, interviewed survivors regarding post-disaster rebuilding, they found survivors willing to accept help, but wanting to eventually be independent of it. Having served as leaders through the crisis, the older adults wanted to contribute to the rebuilding of their community in ways they saw fit.

In partnership with the government of the local township of Ofunato, Japan (one of the areas hardest hit by the earthquake/tsunami and home to large numbers of older adults—34% of its population are 65 years old and over) and with global experts from Operation USA, Hokkaido University, and Honeywell, community members co-developed a local non-profit organization, and created the Ibasho House as a community hub. Ibasho House would serve as a third place, to be run by and for the local older adults who were so instrumental in securing the community's survival in the aftermath of the earthquake and tsunami (Lee et al., 2022).

### Concepts Underlying Ibasho

Ibasho is a principles-based approach to grassroots community development, designed to foster and employ emergent leadership skills of local older adults. Proposed by Dr. Emi Kiyota (an environmental design gerontologist/architect) and her colleague, Dr. Allen Power, and further adapted by Dr. Kiyota to the specific strengths and preferences of the elders of the Ofunato community, Ibasho is based on eight guiding tenets:

1. Older adults are seen as valuable resources having a wealth of knowledge, experience, and wisdom; they serve as assets to the community, not passive service recipients.
2. The goal of Ibasho is to create a welcoming, informal gathering place.
3. Community elders drive its development and implementation; the site is created with them, not for them, thus instilling a sense of ownership.
4. An Ibasho site is open to all ages; through its intergenerational activities young and old can learn from and enjoy the company of each other.
5. All community members are welcome to participate and contribute as they can, regardless of functional ability.
6. Local cultural traditions are respected; Ibasho's setting and activities are culturally appropriate, reflecting community values, customs, treasures.
7. An Ibasho site is environmentally, economically, and socially sustainable; at least some of its activities should generate products or income that allow it to be self-sustaining.
8. The growth of the site is "organic," adaptable, and flexible; it accepts and embraces imperfection, rather than striving for immediate perfection (Kiyota et al., 2019).

### The Physical Environment of Ibasho

As noted earlier, characteristics of the physical environment can either facilitate or hinder social interactions. The building itself plays a big role in setting the tone of a third place. Ibasho House was a renovated farmhouse, donated to the community. Community members, including elder local crafts persons, designed and constructed the renovations, contributing to a pride of ownership. The building was reconfigured to provide more open, flexible spaces to accommodate multiple types of activities by various users. Furniture was easily moveable and rearranged in various configurations to accommodate a variety of types of social interactions: a quiet nook for intimate conversations between two hard-of-hearing participants; open floor space covered with tatami mats to allow sitting, eating, or napping on the floor (or, in the case of children, playing games on the floor); seating to accommodate small audiences; open space for dancing, martial arts, yoga; private areas for interviews or meetings; space in the kitchen to accommodate cooking classes or cooking large-scale meals for group events. Tatami mats were used in various areas, providing natural textures and colors, and a sweet, comforting scent.

Thresholds were inclusive, allowing free movement in and out of different rooms or the building itself. They extended use of space to the outdoor patio and surrounding area, to engage in exercise activities or to escape to a more quiet and peaceful setting. Flexible spaces could allow privacy, stimulation, or restful areas as needed. Space in Ibasho House was open and multivalent (as is typical of Japanese use of space in general)—users could create their own space experience and their own boundaries, to the extent that they did not intrude on others. Over time, spatial territories emerged, based on consistent use by consistent users, evolving into what might be considered a type of participatory design. Occupational therapists might contribute to these participatory processes by observing use of space, and then offering suggestions as needed in regard to safety, minor environmental modifications, or possible modification of occupations themselves.

### The Social Environment of Ibasho

As older participants became more comfortable and adept in their leadership roles, they began to initiate a variety of new activities. After successfully implementing the Ibasho Café that provided traditional refreshments and beverages to neighborhood customers and to Ibasho participants, they expanded to cultivate a communal garden and sold their produce in their farmers' market. They cooked meals for isolated elders and started their own catering business, serving food in traditional bento boxes. They established a ramen noodle shop. They developed a daycare center. They established a library of English books for children and offered classes. They taught and performed various cultural traditions (e.g., cooking, music, seasonal festivals) for young Ibasho users. They hosted traditional tea ceremonies and observed Japanese holidays.

While the 2011 Great Earthquake was extreme, Japan is a land of frequent earthquakes, because it is situated on the Pacific Ring of Fire, one of the most active earthquake belts in the world. Ibasho participants have actively planned for likely future natural disasters by adapting Ibasho House to serve as an evacuation center for the community. They also shared their expertise in disaster management internationally in a peer-to-peer effort, sending an Ibasho team to the Philippines in the wake of 2014 Super Typhoon Yolanda (which killed over 6300), to offer advice and support, and later hosted a team from the Philippines to visit Japan to share recovery experiences and discuss ways to contribute to community resilience, including demonstration of the Ibasho concept. Ibasho members provided similar expertise and support to the survivors of the 2015 earthquake in Nepal (which killed

approximately 9000), again sending a team to Nepal and hosting a reciprocal visit by Nepalese elders.

## SUMMARY

Third places offer the potential to foster social interactions, networks, collaborative intergenerational activities, empowerment of participants, and meaningful occupations that are accessible and age inclusive. Aspects of the physical and social environment can be modified to support and enhance age-inclusive social interactions. The example of Ibasho illustrated the process of development and conceptual underpinnings of a successful third place run for and by older adults and the types of activities and contributions (even internationally) that can be generated by such age-inclusive communities.

## CHAPTER SUMMARY

Within this chapter, age-inclusive communities have been broadly defined as communities that enable the participation of all members across the age spectrum. Examples have pointed to diverse ways that occupational therapists can be contributors to building and sustaining age-inclusive communities, consistently attending to occupation and working with older adults in participatory ways. Broad interdisciplinary models, such as the World Health Organization's Age-Friendly Cities and Communities Framework and the Model of Social Exclusion proposed by Walsh and colleagues, highlight various domains and contextual elements important to consider when occupational therapists are working at the community level. Adding an occupational perspective to partnerships working to build age-inclusive communities is a key way that occupational therapists can make a difference that supports the occupational participation of older adults.

*The complete listing of the Bibliography and Chapter Questions and Answers are available in the accompanying enhanced eBook version included with the print purchase of this textbook. Visit Elsevier eBooks+ (eBooks.Health.Elsevier.com) to access this content.*

## CHAPTER 33

# The Future of Gerontological Occupational Therapy

*Karen Frank Barney, PhD, MS, OTR, FAOTA, Debbie Laliberte Rudman, PhD, OT Reg. (Ont.), and Margaret A. Perkinson, PhD, FGSA, FAGHE, FSfAA*

## CHAPTER OUTLINE

## OBJECTIVES

- Highlight select demographic, physical environmental, and social contextual transformations and trends that create imperatives for modifications and expansions in how occupational therapy supports the occupational participation of aging adults.
- Discuss the importance of emphasizing occupational possibilities, regardless of the individual and/or group life circumstances.
- Consider the implications of evolving health-care systems, community-based practice, and organizational environments for how the profession can address the occupational needs of the aging populations served.
- Discuss how future occupational therapy practice with older adults might address ageism, occupational literacy, occupational adaptation, and occupational justice concerns.
- Envision future practice scenarios that address the occupational needs of aging adults.

## Expanded Global Call for Action

Just as society is dynamic, how aging is experienced and the occupational needs of aging individuals and populations are dynamic. Over the course of time, various social, political, economic, and other transformations, such as industrialization, climate change, the digital age, population growth, wars and other conflicts, globalization, and pandemics, have altered the status and conditions of millions of people of all ages in nations around the world (Buck & Weinstein, 2020; Cleveland et al., 2016; Giang et al., 2020; Golkarian, 2019; Verma & Prakash, 2020). As a result, individuals and collectives/groups, at local to global scales, have experienced transitions and disruptions of long-term occupational habits, patterns, and activity choices, some of which have dramatically altered their lifestyles, relationships, and well-being. Although such transitions may expand occupational possibilities for certain groups in society, including older adults, such transitions and disruptions have also shaped and perpetuated occupational inequities and injustices. As noted by the World Federation of Occupational Therapists (WFOT) (2019), "actions to promote occupational and human rights must counter occupational injustices that are aggravated by social problems, significantly persistent poverty, economic restrictions, disease, social discrimination, displacement, natural and man-made disasters, armed conflict, historic disadvantage, and physical and mental ill health."

As a profession, let us rise to these social responsibilities and collaborate interprofessionally to influence governmental agencies, health-care systems, businesses, and many others on macro, meso, and individual levels. Let's mobilize to assist in improving the lives and occupational possibilities of all, including aging adults who have the potential to benefit from occupational therapy, both directly via therapeutic interventions and indirectly through system changes, architectural, design, and technology influences, as well as alterations in policies at many diverse community, health, and governmental system levels.

The WFOT Innovation Change Agent Narratives (ICAN) advocates for changes in policies and program development in various international regions. Furthermore, their efforts include collaborating with the World Health Organization to facilitate change and innovation at individual, family/group, local, regional, and national government levels (WFOT, 2022). For numerous reasons, aging adults are often adversely affected by a variety of environmental conditions; thus, both organizations' call for action centers on numerous topics that relate to this population. Actions informed by occupational science can make significant differences in older adults' overall health-related quality of life by working to influence policies and programs that address occupational possibilities in ways that are in the best interest of all generations locally, nationally, and globally. Within this chapter, we address potential areas for expanding occupational therapy practice and advocacy in relation to environments, as well as in promoting occupational justice and occupational possibilities with particular groups of aging adults. We end by pointing to some promising future directions for expansion, advocacy and research.

## The Role of Occupational Therapy in Optimizing Environments That Benefit Aging Adults

### Promoting Supportive Ecosystems: Advocacy for Sustainable Air, Water, Soil, and Other Protective Environmental Features

It has long been recognized, beginning in Indigenous knowledge systems, that various physical environmental factors, such as air, soil, and water quality; waste containment; and environmental living conditions, are vital contributors to individual, collective/group, and population health and well-being (Trentham et al., 2022). Additionally, for the past quarter century, an increasing awareness of intensification and implications of climate change is apparent globally. However, this increasing awareness has not been adequately acted upon collectively around the world and threatens food security and survival for millions of people. Accelerating global climate change since the last glacial period has shown the interconnections of all living things, gravely affecting natural ecosystem diversity (Pecl et al., 2017), raising average temperatures (Statista, 2022), and negatively impacting human well-being.

Although disaster preparation approaches are vital to assist communities in managing the implications of climate change, there is an urgent need for proactive approaches that both counter climate change and lessen its on-going and future implications (Persson & Erlandsson, 2014; Watts et al., 2018; Wheeler & Von Braun, 2013). It is also crucial to acknowledge that although climate change impacts the lives of all people, its "most profound and immediate effects are on socio-economically disadvantaged groups, including racialized people, Indigenous people, those with pre-existing health conditions, forced migrants, and older people" (Trentham et al., 2022, p. 42). Indeed, occupational therapy personnel often work with groups who are routinely exposed, perhaps throughout their lives, to unhealthy environmental conditions in air, soil, water, and housing quality, as well as food insecurity (Guo et al., 2022; Leroux et al., 2020; Ohm, 2019), in concert with intersecting forces such as racism, other forms of social discrimination, dysfunctional relationships, violence, and homelessness (Dickins et al., 2021; Sorrell, 2016; Takamura et al., 2022).

In their 2030 Agenda for Sustainable Development, the United Nations (UN) emphasized the importance of global attention to the impact of environmental issues on possibilities for healthy aging (Assembly, U.G., 2019). Considering these specific implications, research addressing environmental contamination of air, animals, plants, soil, and water within various "developed" nations has addressed effects upon the aging process and related occupational participation (Hahad et al., 2021; Leuthner & Meyer, 2021; Martens et al., 2016; Pieters et al., 2016; Ren et al., 2021). Furthermore, extreme periods of heat or cold have the potential to put older adults at greater risk, since this population is more susceptible to extreme temperatures (Pecl et al., 2017; Statista, 2022). As a specific example, analysis of a 2002 heat wave in Paris, France, revealed that this outcome of climate change had a disproportionate negative impact on older adult residents, such that over 80% of those who died due to heat were 75 years of age and older (Toulemon & Barbieri, 2008).

The WFOT has pointed to the crucial role of occupational therapy in advancing knowledge about the occupational implications of climate change and developing approaches to combat resulting occupational disruptions and inequities. Climate change and associated alterations in our ecosystems have been forecasted for decades and place older adults at increasing risk of not only reduced longevity, increased prevalence of chronic diseases, unexpected exposures, and relocations, but also disruption in habits, routines, and occupational deprivation (Dennis et al., 2015; Leal Filho et al., 2016; Pereira, 2009; Wheeler & Von Braun, 2013). Integrating the adaptive abilities and transformative capacity of individuals, communities and various levels of government can build capacity and resilience for negotiating natural disasters or climate change (Sarker et al., 2020). In concert with these organizations, occupational therapy personnel can work to enhance capacity and resilience not only at the individual patient/client level, but also with nongovernmental organizations and governmental agencies to inform policy development regarding housing, urban expansion, transportation infrastructure, and environmental policy.

As noted by Drolet et al. (2020), "the current climate crisis is linked to the negative impacts of human occupations, as enacted historically and currently, on the world's ecosystems" (p. 417). A key contribution that occupational therapists and occupational scientists can make in promoting sustainable living, at individual to societal levels, is through raising awareness of the negative impacts of individual and collective/group occupations on ecosystems and promoting solutions that center occupational resolutions. For example, how occupations related to community mobility, food production and consumption, use of technology, or use of cosmetics are socially structured have immense influences on ecosystems, as well as on how individuals and groups engage in such occupations and if they have possibilities to engage in them in eco-responsible ways. A growing body of scholarship has generated knowledge regarding how human occupations and contexts can be modified to promote sustainability and has pointed to contextual factors that serve as barriers or supports to participation in occupations in sustainable ways (Lieb, 2022). Drawing on this knowledge base, and concepts such as eco-occupations, occupational therapists and occupational therapy assistants can move forward in enacting their own practices in sustainable ways, and contribute to individual and social transformations that promote engaging in occupations in ways that are eco-responsible (Ung et al., 2020). As examples, occupational therapy personnel can advocate within the systems they work to utilize products with minimal carbon footprints; can assist older adult clients in understanding the ecological, personal, and collective impact of various ways of engaging in occupations; and can work at municipal and broader levels for eco-responsible approaches to the design of green spaces, transportation systems, and food production and distribution systems (Drolet et al., 2020; Trentham et al., 2022).

Although issues involving climate and sustainability are not typically integrated within health policy, research, or practices, population aging is a driving force for considering alignment of these issues globally. Population and related health projections indicate that older persons will be affected both directly, for example, via flooding, heat waves, wild fires, and severe storms, and indirectly, for example, via altered vector-borne disease transmission and an inability to produce nutritious food due to drought, soil degradation, and compromised water safety (Mavrodaris et al., 2021). Therefore, health systems collaboration with occupational and environmental scientists—each sector informing the other—is indicated to promote sustainability.

## Advocacy for Humanitarian and Supportive Design Features in Architecture, Technology, Equipment, and Products in Health Care and Community Environments

Aging-related changes, especially sensory, motor, and musculoskeletal factors, can lead to decreased capacity to function in many routine occupations that formerly were easily managed. As a result, older individuals managing such changes must apply alternative modes and equipment to complete their daily habits and routines, not participate, or depend upon others to assist them. However, environmental barriers, rather than age-related changes per se, are often significant reasons that preclude older adult participation (Carr et al., 2013; Hernandez & Johnson, 2017), pointing to the important contributions that occupational therapy can make through addressing the environment. Twenty percent of the aging population in the United States will be age 65 or older by 2030; this is a rapidly increasing demographic that can benefit from aging at home in their community, which often extends their longevity and quality of life. However, as one example of the inadequacy of current approaches to design, indicators show that 19 million older adults in the United States dwell in homes that are not equipped to meet their needs or are in disrepair (Reckford, 2022). Organizations such as Habitat for Humanity provide examples of how to move forward in redesigning environments through partnerships with professionals in the health-care sector to promote a person-centered aging-in-place approach, such as those who developed the CAPABLE intervention described in Chapter 19, Diverse Understandings of 'Successful' Aging.

Occupational therapy has a unique occupational perspective to contribute to efforts aimed at creating supportive design features as applied to housing, technology, physical environments, equipment, health-care products, and other environmental features (Jónasdóttir et al., 2018; Young et al., 2019). Such contributions can span involvement at macro, or policy levels, to the work done with individual clients and their support systems. When occupational therapy personnel conceptualize human interaction with their clients' environments, we consider many biopsychosocial as well as physical and intangible supports and barriers that influence abilities, mobility, choices, motivation, and opportunities that older adults may encounter in carrying out necessary and preferred occupations. An occupational perspective can contribute unique insights regarding how intersecting intrinsic and extrinsic factors shape occupational performance and occupational possibilities for aging adults, contributing to holistic conceptualizations in planning and implementation of design features and programs. Collaborating with architects, engineers, designers, and users is mutually informing and promotes supportive environments. This type of long-range conceptual and practical investment has the potential to bear fruitful economic and quality-of-life outcomes that benefit the greater populace within individual communities and countries as well as globally.

Historically many occupational therapy staff have provided services to older individuals in their homes, wherever they reside (see Chapter 29, Home: An Evolving Context for Health Care, for further detail). Typically, in providing home-based services, a wide range of environments are encountered, from impoverished to elite, racially or ethnically segregated or integrated, with single or multiple generations. Given this diversity, practice approaches are ideally adapted to meet the preferences and needs of the older adult and the place that they call home, be it a hut, tent, room, mobile unit, cabin, apartment, condo, house, or mansion. Globally, housing varies extensively, and it is the responsibility of occupational therapy staff to adapt the environment they encounter in order to meet the needs of their patients/clients. Within North America and elsewhere globally, standard design features of many types of homes may create challenges for older adults who strive to negotiate aging in place, despite deteriorated housing and frequent access challenges such as many steps, makeshift steps (i.e., concrete blocks), heavy doors, no installed flooring, holes or challenging textures in flooring, or simply the inability to turn door knobs due to physical limitations, such as upper extremity amputations, arthritis, limited strength, incoordination, or tremors.

When working with aging clients, many resources are available for recommending adaptations to home environments to support *optimal* functioning in a range of occupations, such as basic activities of daily living (BADLs), instrumental activities of daily living (IADLs), and work at home and/or within virtual environments. Based upon a process involving rapport building and collaborative identification of needs and problems, occupational therapy staff can work to provide environmental recommendations and interventions that are not only feasible but also optimal for supporting what is most functional and meaningful to older adult clients living in diverse settings.

Additionally, increasing numbers of older adults are working from home, virtually or otherwise, and may require adaptations to their environment, including use of technology (cell phones, computers, and automated supports such as robots), as well as their habits and routines accordingly. Areas for continued expansion can involve integrating artificial intelligence (AI), biotechnology, and virtual environments informed by the foundational concepts and theories presented in Chapter 20, Physical Environment and Aging, and Chapter 22, Assistive Technology. Occupational therapy personnel can seek opportunities to pair with engineers, technology users, and AI experts to develop applications that can facilitate the occupational performance of aging adults, at individual to collective levels. Some examples of specific types of environments and common design problems that occupational therapy personnel can address, through advocacy, partnerships, and other forms of practice are outlined in Boxes 33.1, 33.2, and 33.3.

## Promoting Socially Inclusive Environments While Respecting Cultural and Social Norms

As described in Chapter 32, Creating Age-Inclusive Communities, many intersecting features of contemporary social systems, institutions, relations, and structures present barriers to social inclusion and participation of older adults, leading to problems such as high rates of social isolation (Walsh et al., 2017). Creating socially inclusive environments that optimally support the ability of diverse older adults, such as those who experience impairments or poverty, are racialized, or otherwise experience discrimination, to participate in a range of desired community-based occupations is a key means through which occupational therapy can enhance the quality of life of older adults.

For an overview of various models and approaches that can be used to create age-inclusive environments, readers are encouraged to review Chapter 32. Given the centrality and pervasiveness of ageism, that is, stereotypes, prejudice, and discrimination directed toward people on the basis of age (Harris et al. 2018), we reiterate its importance here. Indeed, ageism and interrelated age discrimination are present at

---

**BOX 33.1**  Background: Recommendations for Designs of Places and Spaces

Universal Design principles historically were integrated into us law via the Americans with Disabilities Act in 1990 to support accessibility (ADA, 2022). Importantly, these principles also support the needs of aging adults and facilitate participation in activities for all ages. Also refer to information on the Visitability Movement, as well as Concrete Change, https://visitability.org/about-concrete-change/).

- All types of health-care and other public settings
  - Automatic doors facilitate use by both persons with disabilities and older adults with limited strength.
  - Signage and/or staff to assist with wayfinding, especially in large facilities, provide needed support for many, especially on a first visit or when they are in a crisis situation.
  - Intermittent opportunities for sitting along long passageways/halls are also recommended for those with limited mobility and/or endurance.
  - Valet or other nearby parking options for older adults with mobility limitations should be provided.
- Community development
  - *Cities, housing, and neighborhoods*

As new housing and neighborhoods are developed, advising governmental agencies on comprehensive plans for limiting walking and driving distances to grocery stores, pharmacies, health-care services, parks, and other venues can better support fitness and health. Regarding existing housing in both urban and suburban neighborhoods, recommending integration of nearby services can also support overall fitness and well-being. New neighborhoods have optimal opportunities to incorporate easy access to services described above. Older neighborhoods may have vacant spaces that can be utilized for various supportive purposes that can also benefit all ages.

- *Mass transit*

Advocating for mass transit that is centralized and easily accessible for all ages and ability levels will facilitate use and assist in maintaining navigation abilities, socialization, access to health care and many other services, shopping, and recreational venues, especially for older adults who don't drive or have always used mass transit.

- *Parking*

As indicated earlier, influencing locations for parking with dedicated drop-off areas in a variety of venues for those who cannot manage long distances walking or using their mobility aids will likely encourage greater participation.

- *Signage*

Exterior and interior signs should be explicit and use universal symbols wherever possible, (e.g., for restrooms), especially in support of aging immigrants and their families.

- *Shopping venues:*
  - Long distances between shops without intermittent seating, including shopping malls, may discourage older shoppers from participating.
  - Access, aisle space, shiny flooring, low lighting, acoustics that amplify background noise, and items placed too high with no readily available assistance discourages optimal use.
- *Recreation settings:*
  - Parks, museums, theaters, and other public venues should be surveyed for easy accessibility and usability.

**BOX 33.2**    Additional OT Advocacy for Aging Sensitive Designs of Places and Spaces

- Entrances and internal environments, even in newly constructed or spaces adapted in historic buildings, are often unsupportive of aging-related needs. As noted in Box 33.1, advocating for incorporating universal design principles in building plans or adapting existing home environments benefits all ages.
- Advocacy for one-floor home, apartment, or congregate living designs in new housing for aging adults or multi-generations supports function and limits the potential for falls and limited access if the individual's physical status is limited or declines. Recommendations for level entrances to homes, apartments, and condominiums, even in historic neighborhoods, facilitate mobility for all ages and afford more opportunity for pick-ups or delivery of purchased items.
- Typical interior OT recommendations:
  - Use of easily understood technology to simplify everyday tasks and compensate for aging-related arthritis, decreased strength and endurance, range of motion, proprioception, changes in vision and/or hearing, sensation, and balance can enable function despite these changes.
  - Grab bars in bathrooms and railings in hallways facilitate optimal function when balance, strength, endurance, and mobility levels are decreased.
  - Pull-down or pull-out cupboard shelves and vertical storage for baking sheets eases visibility and reaching for stored objects.
  - Varied levels of lighting through the use of dimmer switches or "smart plugs" activated by artificial intelligence (AI) units support aging-related vision changes and also meet the needs of younger generations.
- Community development
  - Housing and neighborhoods
    - Homes and congregate living settings—initial accessible design and furnishings
    - Retrofitting existing homes, apartments, condominiums, and other dwellings
    - Promoting walkable neighborhoods with sidewalks and bike lanes
  - Transportation and mobility: access supports
    - Transportation modes and hubs (e.g., mass transit centers—buses and subways, railway stations, airports, harbors): facilitating physical access and universal signage
    - Driveways, roads, highways, intersections, gas, and electric filling stations
    - Streets, sidewalks, curb cuts, traffic lights, and cameras. Traffic lights should provide adequate time for crossing streets. Aging individuals with mobility, cardiac, limited endurance, or respiratory conditions may not be able to traverse the street at the same rate as a younger person; thus, add time and auditory signals to indicate start and finish of crossing time.
    - Street and highway construction should allow for ample time for decision making and signaling for turns and accessing off ramps; this can be beneficial for all drivers.

- All signage: locations, wording, and designs that can be universally understood
  - Recreational venues: theaters, theme parks, water parks, beaches, intergenerational playgrounds, museums, zoos, and related parking
- Shopping
  - Malls and neighborhood shopping areas are used for walking and socialization by some older adults who combine their exercise with purchasing. Since aging individuals demonstrate wide variability in their endurance, strength, and coordination, the following recommendations are provided:
    - Intermittent seating between shops, especially when long distances must be traversed
    - Lightweight doors
    - Wider aisles within stores to accommodate individuals using canes and wheelchairs
    - Bright (but nonglaring) lighting and easy access to products (no items placed at high levels, or availability of staff to assist with reaching)
    - Keep ambient noise (including background music) at a minimum.
  - The pandemic has fostered more online shopping, with the added benefits of curb pick-up or delivery, either of which may support aging related needs.
- Public access considerations: apply the principles noted earlier
  - Libraries, museums
  - Parks: national, state, county/province, city, neighborhood
  - Restaurants, food trucks, street vendors
  - Public restrooms, including force required to open and close doors and apply sanitary practices
  - Health clubs, gyms, and other exercise facilities
  - Access to historic and new buildings or venues of any type
  - Organizations that provide intergenerational and/or specific services to aging adults
- Faith-based worship, ethical, and other spiritual societies
  - For those who practice these traditions, as for all public venues identified above, providing easy access and offers of support for all aspects of the experience, including large print bulletins and optimal sound systems, will facilitate the appeal of their participation.
- Note that "hearing access" is as important as "mobility access" in developing age-friendly accessible environments.
  - Noise-unfriendly spaces: Bad or extremely loud acoustics, sound reflections, high ceilings, hard surfaces, other ambient sounds.
  - What helps: carpets, curtains, soft chairs, noise absorbing panels (fixed or portable—use as needed, clustered to create quiet zones), volume controls
  - Spacing seating to minimize the interference of nearby conversations or other noise
  - Technology: e.g., hearing loops
  - Hearing Access Protocol for Meetings and Events: https://www.portaltechnologies.uk/ideas-for-ears-hearing-access/#fb0=1

many levels and within many places within societies, impacting older adults at work, in communities, health care, housing, and other settings (Amundsen, 2022; Harris et al., 2018; Lev et al., 2018; Mannheim et al., 2022; Ng & Indran, 2022; Phelan & Ayalon, 2020; Williams et al., 2017; World Health Organization, 2022). Within contemporary society, fears and negative attitudes regarding aging are amplified via cosmetic and pharmaceutical companies that develop, advertise, and promote products and interventions designed to maintain "youth" and avoid the "negative" physical and mental signs of aging (Pearl & Percec, 2019; Vashi et al., 2016). Furthermore, although social and news media have represented aging in both hostile and benevolent ways, messages implying "greedy" older generations and the need to avoid or defy aging abound (Meisner, 2021; Ng & Indran, 2022). As another example, ageism "influences how technology is developed, marketed, and adopted, with the effect of leaving older adults on the low-use side of a technological divide" (Cutler, 2005, p. 1).

Recognition of the pervasiveness and deleterious consequences of ageism has meant that it has received international attention through work by the World Health Organization in a global campaign to combat ageism (Officer & de la Fuente-Núñez, 2018). Many dimensions of ageism (stereotypes, prejudice, and discrimination) and its impact beyond employment have been recognized, facilitating policy development to support the health and well-being of persons across the lifecourse (Allen et al., 2022a, 2022b; Takamura et al., 2022). Member states of the World Health Organization requested that a UN agency develop, in cooperation with other partners, a Global Campaign to Combat Ageism and have reaffirmed the UN Decade of Healthy Ageing (2021–2030), adopted on December 14, 2020 (https://undocs.org/en/A/RES/75/131).

Whether implicit or explicit, intentional or unintentional, ageism has deleterious impacts on physical and mental health (Burnes et al., 2019), as well as on occupational participation. Thus, occupational therapy personnel should be a part of antiageist efforts, within their interactions with older adults, within the systems in which they work, and within broader society, enacting and promoting nondiscriminatory beliefs, attitudes, and practices (Trentham, 2019). Interactions with patients, clients, and older colleagues are opportunities to demonstrate not only respect but also attitudes that value the older individual's personhood, motivation to participate and pursue personal goals, regardless of age and cognitive, physical, or lifestyle status. Occupational therapy staff need to critically reflect on their personal beliefs and attitudes regarding aging, as well as those that exist in the places they work and live. For example, we need to be critical of the ways in which the development and social participation of younger age groups are often supported and celebrated, while that of older adults can be negated or seen as necessarily limited. We need to question how various systems, such as those for transportation, are built in ways that often meet the needs of age groups deemed "productive" and "able," rather than in ways that support the mobility of persons of various ages and capabilities. As another example, occupational therapists can strive to influence manufacturers, within a context of population

aging, in ways that combat ageism and encourage technology that is designed, made accessible, and employed to minimize age differences in its use.

During interactions with older adult clients, it is important to be aware that ageist attitudes, beliefs, and practices may often be implicit and unintentional; as such, there is a need for ongoing critical reflexivity regarding how ageism may be unintentionally enacted by occupational therapy personnel as well as those with whom they work. For example, rather than assuming an older adult client experiences challenges with digital technologies, Allen and colleagues (2022a,b) emphasize that "asking patients/clients how they prefer to communicate is best practice." As another example, it is important to avoid stereotypical beliefs of aging adults as stubborn or unwilling to learn new ways of doing things that can limit what occupational possibilities are supported through occupational therapy practice. Overall, occupational therapy practitioners should remain open to being taught by older adults, who have extensive knowledge and experiences. As with any interaction with a client, taking the time to get to know older patients/clients as individuals, asking questions about their needs and preferences, and avoiding assumptions associated with age are important (Schieszer, 2022). Care providers who are more aware of their assumptions and stereotypes about aging and older adults, which they may have been socialized to have, are better able to monitor their behavior to ensure they do not act on ageist beliefs. Allen et al. (2022a) also recommends that practitioners discuss aging-related cognitive and physical change as a part of human development across the life course rather than inherently representing decline and loss in later life as something to mourn. It is also crucial that occupational therapy personnel do not contribute to internalized ageism on the part of older adults, recognizing that broader ageist beliefs and attitudes may restrict what older adults themselves think is possible and appropriate (Allen, 2022a,b).

## The Role of Occupational Therapy in Promoting Occupational Possibilities and Justice with Aging Adults

### Older Workers with or at Risk for Occupational Disparities

It is important for occupational therapy personnel to be aware of changing policies and social discourses related to retirement and later life work, and the impact that these may have on current and future older adults. It should no longer be assumed that any older adult is necessarily retired on the basis of their age, given interrelated policy and labor force participation changes occurring over the past few decades. These changes require occupational therapy to further expand its role in addressing the work lives of older adults, both at the micro level with individual clients and at broader levels to advocate for aging workers as a group and to promote age-inclusive workplaces. While the push toward extended working lives is opening occupational possibilities for continued involvement in desired work for some older adults, it has also created inequities at the intersections of age, gender, socio-economic status, disability, and other social factors. In other words, while some older adults may have enhanced choices for extending their work lives, others may be forced to continue to work in situations that are not health sustaining in order to financially survive, and others may struggle to find sustainable work options as they age (Krekula & Vickerstaff, 2020; Laliberte Rudman, 2015).

Between the end of World War II until the 1980s, social policies in many countries in the Western world established and encouraged retirement from paid work as part of the life course, typically setting an age for receipt of some form of pension income at or near the age of 65 for persons, often men, who had an extended record of labor force participation. Through this process, retirement became something that many people in Western nations, such as the United States, Canada, Australia, New Zealand, and several European nations, viewed as a social right. Indeed, during favorable economic conditions, early retirement, that is, prior to the age for receipt of a public pension, was sometimes promoted by governments, investment companies, and the media (Laliberte Rudman, 2015). However, since the 1990s, in line with recommendations from international organizations such as the Organization for Economic Cooperation and Development (OECD, 2018), many of these same nations have implemented policy shifts aimed at extending work lives, seeing this as one means to manage potential economic implications of population aging (Mann, 2007). Examples of such policy shifts have included raising the age of eligibility for public pensions, decreasing access to public forms of financial support for those who retire early, and offering financial and other forms of incentives to encourage people to work longer (Mann, 2007; Wainwright et al., 2018). Increasingly, policies and broader social discourse has shifted away from retirement as a social right to be guaranteed and supported by governments toward an emphasis on the need for aging individuals to work longer and assume greater responsibility for ensuring adequate financial resources for later life (Krekula & Vickerstaff, 2020; Laliberte Rudman, 2015). Indeed in 2020, the Organization for Economic Cooperation and Development recommended extending the definition of working age from 20–64 to 20–70 (Organization for Economic Cooperation and Development, 2020).

This policy emphasis on "extended work lives" has included both keeping people in the workforce until at least pensionable age as well as bringing back people who left prior to pensionable age (Laliberte Rudman & Aldrich, 2021). Combined with economic downturns, this policy emphasis has meant that greater numbers of older workers, often defined as people aged 50 and older, are continuing to participate in the paid labor force. For example, combining data across all countries belonging to OECD, between 2010 and 2020, the employment rate of 50- to 54-year-olds increased almost 5% and that of 55 to 64 years old increased by 9% (OECD, 2021). As well, although smaller, increases have also been seen in those over the age of 65 during this time period, and it is expected that the labor force participation of persons between 50 and

74 years old will continue to increase over the next decades (Wainwright et al., 2018). Overall, the OECD (2018) reports that the overall retirement age has been rising in all of its member nations since the beginning of the 2000s.

However, continuing to work as one ages is not always health promoting, nor is the option to extend working life equitably distributed (Harris et al., 2018). For example, some older workers may "be damaged by continuing to work," such as those "in physically arduous areas of work or under considerable stress who may already be soldiering on with existing health conditions that would be worsened by staying in work" (Krekula & Vickerstaff, 2020, p. 38). As well, older workers who face challenges to maintaining or obtaining full-time secure employment may end up in precarious forms of employment or experiencing prolonged periods of unemployment. In turn, given that precarious employment is associated with low pay, a lack of worker benefits, little worker autonomy, and lack of certainty regarding hours and duration, such work may not only increase poverty in later life but may contribute negatively to health and well-being (Bowman et al., 2017; Laliberte Rudman & Aldrich, 2021). Indeed, research demonstrates that a number of factors can enhance the challenges that older workers face in maintaining and obtaining sustainable employment options. For example, persons aged 50 or older who are displaced from employment are more likely than younger workers to experience a long-term period of unemployment, as well as take on lower-paying, lower-skill, and more precarious forms of employment when they do reenter the labor market (Bowman et al., 2017; Harris et al., 2018; Laliberte Rudman & Aldrich, 2021). Many intersecting social and personal factors, such as caregiving responsibilities, age-related impairments, and ageism, can make continuing to work or becoming reemployed more challenging (Krekula & Vickerstaff, 2020). In their scoping review addressing ageism and its implications for the employment experiences and work opportunities of older workers, Harris et al. (2018) found that there is evidence supporting "the contention that ageist stereotypes and perceptions about older workers present barriers to maintaining and attaining employment" (p. e10). As noted by Krekula and Vickerstaff (2020), "despite legislation against age discrimination in many countries there is still widespread ageism in the labor market and a preference for hiring prime age or 'ideal workers'" (p. 40).

Within this changing policy landscape related to retirement and work, it is crucial for occupational therapists to take proactive steps that enhance occupational possibilities for older adults who want or need to work in ways that optimally support work participation, security, health, and well-being. In addition, occupational therapists have a role to play in enhancing awareness of the continued occupational, resource, and other needs of older adults who are no longer capable of working so as to ensure that contextual conditions provide possibilities for older citizens to participate in a diversity of occupations and to live dignified, meaningful lives (Laliberte Rudman, 2015). Using the example of ageism as a barrier to extended work, occupational therapy's commitment to address violations of the right to occupation means that occupational therapists should take steps, at micro to macro levels, to work against ageist beliefs, relations, practices, systems, and structures that constrain the right to work. For example, drawing on research that counters the belief that job performance declines with age (Posthuma & Campion, 2009), occupational therapy staff can contribute to advocacy efforts that aim to change ageist hiring, retention and accommodation policies and practices. In addition, just as occupational therapists can contribute to building age inclusive communities (see Chapter 32), they can also generate knowledge about and contribute to the building of age inclusive policies and workplaces (Harris et al., 2018). Examples of potential strategies that can enhance the age inclusiveness or age-friendliness of workplaces include active recruitment of older workers, ensuring training opportunities are open to all workers regardless of age, allowing for flex hours to accommodate caregiving demands and health-related needs, implementing educational campaigns that counter ageist beliefs, proactively providing work-place accommodations for all workers with impairments, and integrating wellness programs.

## Institutionalized Aging Persons, Extending to Prison Contexts

The quality of life of older persons who are institutionalized varies dramatically, depending upon the type of setting. As addressed in Chapter 28, Residential and Skilled Care, physical and/or mental decline can lead to transitioning to an institutional setting in later life. Within the United States, for example, this could involve moving to a skilled care facility or other institution that provides nursing, nutrition, therapy, and other supportive supervision. In these settings, the availability of meaningful occupations is frequently compromised, of variable quality, and may have negative implications for mood, socialization, physical status, and nutritional intake (Scherrer et al., 2019; Weening-Dijksterhuis et al., 2011). As well, even though occupation-based interventions aligned

with residents' preferences may be recommended, occupational choices may be limited to those deemed necessary for self-care or medically related sustainability of function. More information on this topic is provided in Chapter 28 on Residential and Skilled Care.

A population of aging adults often not considered in the category of institutionalized aging persons are those who are incarcerated, some for decades or for the remainder of their lives depending upon the length of their sentences. In the United States, depression, oppression, differing social relationships, and/or social isolation and suicidal ideation are prevalent in this population, especially in older prisoners (Barry et al., 2017; Majekodunmi et al., 2017). Such experiences and outcomes are partly related to restricted occupational opportunities within prison sentences that can extend over a span of decades. Despite international guidelines for activity participation in prisons (Brosens et al., 2016), in the United States, incarcerated individuals typically have access to a library; however, they may not have opportunities to advance in education and participate in occupations that will prepare them for employment if/when they are released, depending upon their sentencing category and type of prison. These individuals may have a television and a means of communicating with the outside world via a tablet or other system, plus mail and phone calls, all of which are highly restricted, closely monitored, and not received or sent in "real time." All written communications are screened prior to being sent or received, and persons incarcerated have limited choices regarding what is offered on mainstream media. They are unprepared for life "on the outside," should they be released, due to limits on occupational choices and access to relevant information. "On the inside," they have few options for valued occupational engagement.

The majority of persons incarcerated in the United States are males (92.5%), with African Americans having the highest representation (Hogg et al., 2008). Available occupations vary among the states but typically include gym-related

---

**BOX 33.3   Occupational Therapy Roles with Incarceration Systems**

1. *Modifying jail and prison design and locations nearer to family members* to support maintenance and/or improvement of prisoner ADLs and those IADLs that are relevant to the setting, as well as long-term psychological well-being and supportive family relationships
2. *Reinforcing jail and prison culture* that ensures safety and simultaneously supports respect and optimal health for all, including staff
3. *Supporting fundamental quality of life on "the inside"*
   - Advocate for and develop programs that optimize the available occupational options that are available for all, including aging incarcerated persons.
   - Educate jail and prison staff and younger incarcerated individuals on environmental and person-centered interventions that can be applied to support those who are increasingly frail and dependent upon those assisting them in the prison environment.

- Advocate for usual and customary health promotion, including fitness options, dietary support, and medical care as experienced in mainstream society.
4. *Supplementing jail and prison planning efforts with those who reenter society*
   - Collaborate with jail and prison staff in their work to habilitate and rehabilitate older incarcerated individuals prior to release, utilizing interprofessional expertise.
   - Assist jail, prison, and external probation, parole, and other related reentry staff in developing transitional supports for older prisoners, especially those who have served long prison terms, and who may no longer have family, friends, or others who will assist them upon their release.

activities, playing board and card games, and for those due to their sentence category, learning a trade, jobs in cooking, cleaning, gardening, clearing litter from roads, dog training, and greater access to prison library resources. Some receive payment for their work at far below compensation rates in mainstream society. Older prisoners with long sentences have fewer occupational possibilities than do younger prisoners with shorter sentences. For example, if formal education is offered, on tablets through distance or in college prison class learning, those who are older may be excluded, leaving them with less meaningful and highly limited occupations from which to choose, despite their academic aptitude and motivation (Hughes, 2016). Furthermore, "Mass incarceration is a socio structural driver of profound health inequalities in the United States" (Cloud et al., 2023, p. 16.1). A study conducted in New York prisons on the effects of incarceration on length of life found negative results—every year in prison resulted in a 2-year decrease in life expectancy (Patterson, 2013).

Over the last 20 years, there has been a rapid rise in the proportion of older adults in prisons around the world. In the United States, the rate of incarceration of older adults exceeds that of people in a majority of countries and is racially skewed with more minority persons, and a greater number of individuals are incarcerated in the second half of life and age in place (Smoyer et al., 2019). Furthermore, "prison conditions create or worsen chronic, communicable, and behavioral health conditions" (Cloud et al., 2023, p. 16-1). Older persons who are incarcerated not only have a reduced life expectancy (Patterson, 2013) but also years lost to usual life occupations due to imprisonment. The reasons for this phenomenon are dependent upon local demographic, legal, political, and social circumstances, and attention to this issue is extremely limited. One author of this chapter became especially aware of incarceration processes as well as jail and prison institutions, as her youngest child has experienced them for 26 years—he's been in prison since he was 23 years old and is now in this older adult prisoner category.

Among those incarcerated who are age 55 and over, research in the United States points to problems of suicidal ideation and greatly diminished function in what are known as "prison activities of daily living" (Archuleta et al., 2020; Barry et al., 2017; De Smet et al., 2017). Prison activities of daily living (PADLs) are necessary to comply with institutional requirements and include, for example, immediately dropping to the floor at the sound of alarms, accessing top bunks (the typical sleeping accommodations), hearing and adhering to staff orders, wearing handcuffs while walking, waiting (standing) in line for medications, and walking to the cafeteria and waiting in line for meals (Barry et al., 2017).

Conditions in prisons vary globally from rehabilitative models in Scandinavia and Europe to utterly dire, impoverished environments in many other countries (Ezenwa et al., 2020; Kim & Peterson, 2016; McLeod et al., 2020). In Chapter 31, we encourage OT personnel to be proactive change agents in transforming deleterious physical and psychological conditions for the collective benefit of prison

staff and persons incarcerated. Imagine spending decades of one's life in a severely restricted environment with extremely limited occupational choices and resources, few, if any, of which are tailored to the individual's needs, as well as staff who are consistently controlling and frequently punitive in their interactions with incarcerated persons as they are in the United States. In that chapter, we also noted that individuals age more quickly when incarcerated, due to the limited access to meaningful occupations and demeaning conditions, poor nutrition, inaccessibility issues associated with mobility challenges, and extremely limited access to health care (Latham-Mintus et al., 2022). Additionally, COVID-19 heavily populated jails and prisons early in the pandemic period (Bryant, 2022), and tragically, staff were the carriers with frail older incarcerated adults as the most vulnerable. Grief, loss, separation from family, stress, and trauma negatively impact the coping abilities of older adults in prison, all of which affect their ability to function, mentally and physically. These psychological factors extend intergenerationally as well (Maschi et al., 2015). Occupational therapy staff may positively impact these settings by engaging with carceral systems to promote changes in the extremely punitive, restrictive, and uninspiring physical and occupational environments. They can also support transformational occupational justice approaches that empower staff and persons incarcerated to work together toward meeting individualized short- and long-term goals based upon occupational profiles and individual needs and preferences.

Research addressing Norwegian prisons specifically has demonstrated how interprofessional practice among prison, mental health, and welfare services can be enacted in prison settings. In a high-security prison, close coordination between prison management, frontline staff, and external service personnel enhances prison and health-care services during the rehabilitation process, with staff emphasizing prisoners' life management behaviors and skills. In a transitional residence, interprofessional practice is facilitated by prison staff to increase prisoners' ability to reintegrate into society. This model addresses the demands on prisoners as they move from service receivers transitioning to service users/organizers of their lives, and how interprofessional practice and models of service integration can support them in this process (Dugdale et al., 2022). Staff morale, stress levels, safety levels, dynamic security, and communication are thus optimized.

Occupational therapy advocacy for functional and meaningful design of spaces and routines to specifically support aging prisoners is also needed. As one example, functional changes may limit aging prisoners' abilities to access an upper bunk to which they've been assigned. Cells in the United States are typically 7′ × 12′—long enough for a bunk bed, toilet, sink, and small storage areas. Other countries with rehabilitative programs have larger cell sizes. Small size cells are associated with increased numbers of cases of infectious and communicable diseases (Simpson et al., 2019), a contributing factor to decreased lifespan in older prisoners. Furthermore, prisoners are counted several times/day and locked in their cells at specific times at night, then unlocked in the morning—sometimes very early (2–3 a.m.) if they work in the prison kitchen; a schedule that can become increasingly challenging for aging prisoners.

One author of this chapter has also had the privilege of serving as interim director of her university's college in prison program (in a different setting, due to relevant conflict of interest issues). This role provided additional access to most of that prison and facilitated greater interaction with many prison staff, some of whom our university provided the same degree program for qualified staff members who had no opportunity to pursue higher education. Every incarcerated student has given testimony to how access to higher education transformed their lives and that of their families. For example, one of these students said that he was able to tutor his daughter in algebra, due to his university coursework. They also commented that participation in the classroom was the only time that they felt humanely treated. Full-time university faculty, several of whom are full professors, have indicated that their experience with them has been exceptional, since they always come to class prepared, having read assignments typically more than once. Staff students have often been promoted or sought employment elsewhere upon degree completion.

Furthermore, incarcerated students run a university sanctioned student organization and served in an advisory capacity for our reentry program developed together with occupational therapy and interprofessional advisory committees. Their recommendations provided "inside" perspectives on occupational limitations and perspectives regarding prison culture. Although we were denied the opportunity to initiate an interprofessional program at this prison, we gained access and permission to enact a city supported jail-based program, via which we've observed that these relationships can be mutually beneficial, since staff can be viewed as positive resources and facilitators. These roles also promote staff members' health and well-being since they are negatively affected psychologically and physically, and by extension their families, by the punitive environments as well (Jaegers et al., 2022). Overall, this program provides another example of how occupational therapy interventions in prison and jail settings can make a positive difference for both prisoners and staff.

As a long-term endeavor, occupational therapy personnel should mobilize individually and collectively regarding making justice system changes that facilitate promotion of personal development and access to individualized meaningful, relevant occupational choices for all ages of persons who are incarcerated (Jaegers et al., 2020a, 2020b; Muñoz et al., 2016). These changes can also facilitate better work conditions and meaningful occupations on the part of justice system staff (Jaegers et al., 2020a,b). The international network of occupational therapy personnel, Justice Based Occupational Therapy (JBOT), is an action oriented group that works to facilitate system changes to benefit justice system workers and enact occupational justice for all persons who are incarcerated (Jaegers et al., 2020a).

## Future Directions for Occupational Therapy Practice and Occupation-Focused Research

As noted in the introduction of this chapter, aging is dynamic—what it means to age, how people age, and the occupational desires and possibilities of older adults have changed across historical time, and will continue to change. As the COVID pandemic has made clear, it is difficult to predict what the future will hold, making planning for the future itself a process that needs constant revisiting. In this final section, we point to potential future directions for occupational therapy practice with older adults, as well as for occupation-focused research that can inform practice and policy efforts to optimally support the occupational participation of older adults.

Within the context of population aging and the increasing body of evidence demonstrating the importance of continued occupational engagement within the lives of older adults, advocacy for inclusion and/or expansion of occupational therapy services are greatly needed within traditional practice systems that include health/medical care, home-based, long-term and palliative care, as well as for expanding innovations in primary care settings, within communities, and where older adults are incarcerated. Additionally, occupational therapy staff have vital roles to play in transition services, such as from hospital stays to home or other levels of care, supporting older adults in optimizing function and occupational performance, with research showing that such services can contain costs by preventing rehospitalization (Szanton et al., 2021). Thus, occupational therapy personnel can take the initiative to be included in planning committees or other groups that review and revise services to maintain or optimize evidence-based and cost-effective care, and point to the importance of attending to occupational needs and goals (Andresen et al., 2006; Bolt et al., 2019; Hay et al., 2002; Nagayama et al., 2016; Rexe et al., 2013). This profession can be a force for not only cost-containment but also the health-related quality of life of older adults wherever they reside (Hand et al., 2022).

Another important area for continued expansion of the occupational therapy role is within palliative and hospice care. When working with palliative care and hospice patients/clients, prioritizing the occupations that are most important to older adults who face functional limitations or obstacles can facilitate meaningful end-of-life occupational engagement related to emotional and social needs (American Occupational Therapy Association [AOTA], 2020; Budash, 2022). Assistance with symptom management, activity adaptations including planning for postmortem ceremonies, addressing topics related to relationships and legacy, and modifying the individual's environment to support function and occupational engagement are all relevant occupational therapy roles (AOTA, 2020; Yeh & McColl, 2019). Occupational therapy personnel can support palliative care clients in achieving a peaceful, tranquil transition—referred to as a "good death." End-of-life occupational engagement therefore supports the dying occupation (Martin & Herkt,

2018; Pizzi, 2015; Russell & Bahle-Lampe, 2016; Talbot-Coulombe & Guay, 2020; Yeh & McColl, 2019).

At the same time, as we advocate for expanding occupational therapy services and roles (see Chapter 25 for discussion of health-care systems), we need to raise the profile of the profession and recruit more providers. Due to reported limited numbers of occupational therapy providers internationally—less than 1 million serving many age groups (World Federation of Occupational Therapists, 2022)—we need to expand public awareness of our profession, and the imminent shifts in the aging population and associated needs, to increase our recruitment influence. Recruitment needs to be expanded to include all adult ages, including those who seek a career change or are motivated by other circumstances. Concurrently, we need to inform and influence not only current systems of care but also agencies, businesses, services, communities, justice systems, and legislative bodies that impact the health and well-being of aging adults about the merits of our services with older adults.

Having spent over a half-century in a beloved profession, Barney is very optimistic about our future. It is thrilling to have witnessed the emergence (Clark et al., 1991; Yerxa, 1993) and continuing development of our basic science, which should ground our program conceptualizations and interventions, as well as the broad scope of other evolving research and practice models emphasizing occupation-based practice (Lawlor, 2021; Stav et al., 2008). However, in the United States, occupational therapy staff in some health-care settings have deviated from occupation-based practice due to reimbursement restrictions limiting the amount of contact as well as occupation-based modalities utilized with patients and clients. We must draw on the ongoing body of research demonstrating the importance of occupation and the efficacy of occupation-based practice to advocate for this form of practice. As well, scholarship such as that conducted by Psillas and Stav (2020) also provides principles and constructs to be applied in such practice. As one example, Psillas and Stav proposed a focus on occupation-based principles addressing the facilitation of doing, being and becoming (Wilcock, 2005). They emphasized these processes apart from biomedical conditions, stating that occupation is the natural biological mechanism for health. Psillas and Stav outlined four main constructs for application to practice, including (1) authentic occupation, (2) meaningful and purposeful value, (3) therapeutic intent, and (4) engaged participation. Additionally, the evolution and emphasis on interprofessional collaboration further our opportunities for recognition and broader contributions than earlier in our profession's history. We are at a point in time where these opportunities should facilitate better understanding of what directions occupational therapy should uniquely pursue; let's capitalize on this collaboration to impact the quality of life of all whom we serve via direct services and related research.

It is also important that concerted efforts and resources are directed toward generating scholarship and evidence that informs, expands, and supports occupational therapy practice with older adults. Building on the long history of using qualitative research in occupational therapy (Frank & Polkinghorne, 2010), qualitative methodologies can be used to capture the essence of everyday living of aging adults, to ensure that knowledge about the occupational profiles and possibilities of older adults is up to date with the lives of current and future generations, and to work with older adults to identify and address barriers to the occupations they need and want to do. Systematic reviews can be used to synthesize available evidence, while quantitative research can be employed for a variety of important purposes—such as identifying patterns and trends to inform planning of occupational therapy services and advocacy for policy changes, or assessing the efficacy and effectiveness of occupational therapy interventions. Utilization of all occupational therapy personnel who are interested in contributing to our body of knowledge should be promoted—integrating research knowledge and skills into curriculae so that personnel have the skills to critically appraise research and/or collaborate with others to translate research into practice is one important step. As well, occupation therapy personnel can take up opportunities to participate in research activities relevant to their practice, for example, through assisting in participant recruitment, data collection, or other research processes.

Occupational therapy staff and occupational scientists have an abundance of topics to explore through research to address the occupational needs of aging adults, generating knowledge relevant to policy and practice. Global aging demographics, climate and other physical environmental changes, changing discourses of aging and aging-related occupational possibilities, technological developments, and a range of other trends and transitions call us to expand support for meaningful occupational engagement to benefit not only aging adults but younger generations as well.

*The complete listing of the Bibliography and Chapter Questions and Answers are available in the accompanying enhanced eBook version included with the print purchase of this textbook. Visit Elsevier eBooks+ (eBooks.Health.Elsevier.com) to access this content.*

# GLOSSARY

**Abandonment:** Applied to the use of assistive devices, abandonment refers to discontinuing or never using an assistive device. It can result from a complex combination of reasons, such as inadequate training, internalized and social stigma, poor fit with a person's needs or contexts, or lack of support and encouragement from professionals and support networks.

**Activities of daily living (ADLs or basic activities of daily living [BADLs]):** Basic activities related to self-care, such as bathing, showering, toileting and toilet hygiene, personal hygiene, grooming, dressing, self-feeding and swallowing, and functional mobility.

**Activity/activities:** Human behaviors that are goal directed.

**Activity theory:** An early social gerontological theory that proposed that continued engagement in activities, particularly social activities, was essential for health and well-being.

**Adaptation:** A process through which changes to elements of a person, environment, and/or activity are made to support optimal functioning.

**Adaptive equipment:** A wide range of devices that are used to assist in the performance of activities of daily living, such as short- and long-handled devices and durable medical equipment.

**Adherence:** The extent to which a person takes medications as prescribed; this term replaces the older term *compliance*.

**Adult learning:** A process in which adults engage to improve their skills and knowledge.

**Age-inclusive communities:** Communities that are designed and enacted in ways that support the participation of all members across the age spectrum.

**Ageism:** A system of oppression that is present at many levels and places within societies and involves prejudice, stereotypes, and discrimination directed toward people on the basis of age, particularly advanced age.

**Agent of change:** An individual (collectively would be referred to as agents) who utilizes opportunities to bring about social change.

**Aging:** An ongoing biopsychosocial process that is interactive, situated, and negotiated within specific sociocultural, temporal, and physical contexts, requiring transdisciplinary approaches to both research and practice.

**Aging in community:** This concept extends beyond aging in place to address a way of life that involves continued engagement with other people and places in one's community, as well as continued connection to valued roles and relationships.

**Aging in place:** A term referring to the ability to live in one's own preferred home and community safely and autonomously as one ages. Policies often focus on supporting aging in place, via a range of strategies such as provision of services, assistive technology, accessible housing design, and improved public transportation, given that this model often aligns with older adults' preferences and can forestall or prevent the need for generally more expensive institutional care.

**Agnosia:** The inability to recognize familiar objects by sight (visual agnosia), touch (tactile agnosia), sound (auditory agnosia), smell (olfactory agnosia), and/or taste (gustatory agnosia).

**Alzheimer's disease:** A type of dementia characterized by the abnormal accumulation of beta-amyloid (plaques) and intracellular accumulation of tau (tangles).

**Anomia:** Word-finding difficulty; a common form of expressive aphasia in mild Alzheimer's disease.

**Anterograde amnesia:** Loss of the ability to create new memories; skills and habits seem to be spared, but all short-term memory tends to be lost. It typically occurs during the early stages of Alzheimer's disease.

**Anticholinergic effects:** A group of symptoms caused by blockade or antagonism of receptors of the cholinergic system; includes peripheral symptoms of dry eyes, dry mouth, constipation, and difficulty urinating and central symptoms of confusion and decreased memory.

**Aphasia:** The loss of language ability; referred to as dysphasia, if mild. Expressive aphasia is the loss of the ability to convey oral or written information to others. Receptive aphasia is the loss of ability to understand the meaning of oral and/or written language.

**Apraxia:** Characterized by loss of the ability to execute or carry out skilled movements and gestures, despite having the desire and the physical ability to perform them; referred to as dyspraxia, if mild.

**Aspiration:** Entry of fluids, food, or any foreign substance below the vocal cords and into the lungs; may result in aspiration pneumonia or other physical complications.

**Assessment:** Systematic interaction, using therapeutic approaches, specific tools, or instruments used to understand a client's occupational profile, client factors, performance skills, performance patterns, contextual and environmental factors, interpersonal relationships, as well as activity demands that influence occupational performance.

**Augmentative and alternative communication (AAC):** All forms of communication other than oral speech, ranging from aided (through the use of a device) to unaided communication (gestures and facial expressions). Aided AAC can be in the form of low- or high-technology devices, with low-tech devices typically not requiring electronic components and high-tech devices utilizing electronic components. Numerous types of AAC devices are available and can allow users to express simple words to long phrases and paragraphs.

**Biodemographic perspectives:** Lenses that address how demographic data, such as population, gender, and education, affect individuals.

**Biological progression:** Changes that occur to living beings from molecular, cellular, or systems changes.

**Biomedical perspective:** A common lens used to understand health and illness, particularly in Western health systems and societies. A key aspect of this perspective is an understanding of health as the absence of illness and viewing illness/disease as resulting from abnormalities in structures and functions of body organs and systems.

**Biopsychosocial model:** A theoretical position about aging asserting that to best understand the normal aging process and the acute and chronic diseases that become more prevalent with age, we must consider the joint and interacting influences of biological, psychological, and social phenomena. The biological aspect includes an understanding of various organ systems and the process of senescence in these systems. The psychological aspect considers information processing (e.g., sensation, perception, cognition, problem solving, wisdom, etc.), emotions, motivation, personality, and so forth. The social aspect includes cultural practices and beliefs, economic systems, educational and religious institutions, etc. Historical influences and secular changes are also part of this model.

**Body mass index (BMI):**  Measure of body fat that is the ratio of weight to height. Obesity is defined as a BMI of 30 or greater; however, this standard needs to be interpreted in relation to body composition and distribution of body fat.

**Bones:**  The endoskeleton of vertebrates; structures that move, protect, and support the body and have functions involving mechanical, synthetic, and metabolic purposes.

**Canadian Model of Occupational Performance and Engagement (CMOP-E):**  A model that illustrates the relationship between person, occupation, and environment. Spirituality is the fourth dimension, placed in the center of the model to highlight its fundamental importance.

**CarFit:**  A program to maximize safety, comfort, and mobility through making adjustments to cars to maximize fit with older drivers.

**Causal relationship:**  The relationship between an event and the effect of that event.

**Certified Aging in Place Specialists (CAPSs):**  Within the US, CAPSs are credentialed by the National Association of Home Builders; they are home modification contractors trained to consider appropriate design in the kitchen, bathroom, garage, and other areas of the home to accommodate the needs of older adults.

**Chronic health conditions:**  Continuing or recurring illnesses or conditions, such as chronic obstructive pulmonary disease (COPD), muscle weakness, and many other mental or physical health conditions.

**Chronological age:**  Actual age measured from date of birth.

**Client:**  The recipient of occupational therapy services. Clients may be individuals or groups of persons in the community, organizations, or various populations.

**Client-centered evaluation:**  An evaluation in which the client is considered an essential part of the evaluation process so that the results will determine what the occupational therapy practitioner will do in partnership with the client and what occupational goals are appropriate.

**Client factors:**  Client factors, including body functions (such as neuromusculoskeletal, sensory-perceptual, visual, mental, cognitive, and pain factors) and body structures (such as cardiovascular, digestive, nervous, integumentary, and genitourinary systems, and structures related to movement), psychological status, values, beliefs, and spirituality, that affect activities of daily living, instrumental activities of daily living, sleep, socialization, and other occupations.

**Clinical Dementia Rating (CDR):**  Ratings of levels of dementia based on neurological exams and separate interviews with clients and knowledgeable collateral sources.

**Cognition:**  The process of acquiring, storing, sharing, and using information.

**Collective occupations:**  Occupations engaged in by several people who often share an intention that can contribute to collective outcomes, such as building community and maintaining the desired social fabric.

**Community:**  Refers to social groups at various scales and in different types of locations, for example, a town, city, or region, to a particular neighborhood, to congregate housing, or a unit in a long-term care setting.

**Computer assistive technology:**  Electronic and computer technologies that assist people with disabilities by making computers easier to use, for example, mouse and keyboard modifications, eye-gaze systems, and others.

**Continuing Care Retirement Community (CCRC):**  Residential option typically offering three levels of care for older adults: independent living, assisted living, and skilled/nursing home care, all on the same campus.

**Continuity theory:**  A social gerontological theory that proposes that the relationship between life satisfaction and activity is an expression of enduring personality traits.

**Convoy Model of Support:**  Proposed by Antonuci; suggests that individuals move through life surrounded by a cohort of personal networks of family, friends, and others who give and receive assistance and support to each other.

**"Crip time":**  A term used by disability activists and others with long-term disabilities. Refers to the disruption of normative expectations concerning time use and the life course, with associated adaptations.

**Critical perspective:**  As a general term, can be used to refer to a questioning or analytic stance toward any given information, to identify both positive and negative aspects. As a paradigmatic stance or theoretical grouping, refers to diverse theories (e.g., Marxism, feminism, political economy) that focus on understanding detrimental implications of power relations.

**Cultural congruence:**  Extent to which an assessment is consistent with a client's cultural health, lifestyle beliefs, and environment.

**Degenerative spinal stenosis:**  An abnormal narrowing of the spinal canal or neural foramen that results in pressure on the spinal cord or nerve roots; may cause pain, numbness, and/or weakness in arms or legs.

**Dementia:**  Chronic or persistent disorder of the mental processes caused by brain disease or injury and marked by memory disorders, personality changes, impaired reasoning, and alteration of occupational participation.

**Developmental process:**  Development is viewed from several current theories, including, but not limited to, maturational, personality, behaviorist, cognitive, and psychobiological.

**Dietary Supplement Health and Education Act of 1994 (DSHEA):**  Directs regulation of dietary supplements, including herbal products, in the United States.

**Diminishing abilities:**  Evidence of increasing frailty that affects individuals' abilities to function as they were able to do so in the past.

**Disengagement theory:**  An early gerontological theory that proposed life satisfaction in later life was to be achieved through withdrawal from society, including social activities, and an increasing focus on the self. It also proposed that society withdraws from its older members by offering fewer meaningful roles or occupations. It is no longer held as a valid universal theory.

**Diuretics:**  Medications that promote excretion of salts and water by the kidneys and thus increase the volume of urine produced; commonly referred to as "water pills."

**Divestiture:** Letting go of a lifetime of possessions to move to a smaller home.

**Durable medical equipment (DME):** Assistive devices such as canes, walkers, wheelchairs, commodes, and others.

**Dysphagia:** Difficulty swallowing.

**Eden Alternative:** Movement to transform nursing homes to more homelike settings, with inclusion of plants, pets, and intergenerational programs.

**Electronic aids to daily living (EADLs):** Devices that enable individuals with disabilities a means to control electronic and electronically enabled devices in their environment. EADL units can range from simple units that control one device to more involved units that can control everything in an individual's environment. There are a variety of control strategies available (e.g., infrared, ultrasound, Z wave, radiofrequency) to operate the devices and numerous access methods (e.g., direct selection of buttons, voice command, scanning of an array of commands).

**Environment:** The aggregate of surroundings things, conditions, or influences that affect "what people do and how they do it" (Kielhofner, 2008, p. 97). It is made up of both the internal and external physical environments, objects, spaces, occupational forms, and social groups, all of which are influenced by culture, the economy, and the political context.

**Environmental docility hypothesis:** Based on the idea that the environment plays a greater role in the lives of older adults as their competencies diminish.

**Ethical wills (or legacy letters):** Parallel to legal wills that ensure material possessions and wealth are passed down according to one's wishes, an ethical will ensures that one's values and beliefs, parting thoughts, and wishes are documented and passed down to intended recipients.

**Evaluation:** The systematic collection and interpretation of data based upon input from the patient/client, caregiver(s), and observation of occupational performance. Evaluation data are necessary to plan occupational therapy interventions.

**Evolutionary determination:** Characteristics arising from a species' genetic endowment rather than the environment, such as the age at which humans reach puberty or the maximum age a human can reach.

**Executive function (EF):** A variety of higher-order cognitive processes, including initiation, planning, hypothesis generation, cognitive flexibility, decision making, regulation, judgment, feedback utilization, and self-perception.

**Factor analysis:** A statistical method used as a data reduction technique or to identify underlying components or factors addressed within a research study.

**Family Caregiver Alliance (FCA):** A national nonprofit caregiver support organization, serving as a clearinghouse for information on caregiving.

**Food and Drug Administration (FDA):** An agency within the US Department of Health and Human Services responsible for ensuring the safety and effectiveness of drugs, vaccines, and other biological products, medical devices, dietary supplements, and the US food supply, among other areas of responsibility.

**Food insecurity:** Limited or uncertain availability of nutritionally adequate and safe foods or limited ability to acquire acceptable foods in socially acceptable ways.

**Fracture:** A break in bone or cartilage that can occur anywhere in the body where these tissues reside. Hip fractures are the most common in the geriatric population.

**Functional cognition:** Cognitive ability to perform daily life tasks. How an older adult uses and integrates thinking and processing skills to accomplish everyday activities.

**Functional mobility:** The ability to ambulate, effectively utilize walkers, prosthetic devices, and/or wheelchairs if needed, and engage in bed and vehicle transfers and mobility.

**Generational differences:** Identification of values that differ between groups of people (cohorts) born in different decades.

**Gerontechnology:** An interdisciplinary field of study and practice that evaluates the multidimensional intersections of various technological tools with the lives and well-being of older adults.

**Gerontological Society of America (GSA):** A professional organization that promotes multi- and interdisciplinary research in gerontology, disseminates research knowledge, and supports education and training in higher education. AGHE (the Academy of Gerontological Higher Education) is a subcomponent of GSA.

**Gerontology:** The study of the social, psychological, and biological aspects of aging.

**Goodness of fit:** The match between the needs of client and the assessment tool, including, but not limited to, sensitivity, standardization on a similar population, suitability for the client's cultural background, and constructive validity of the test items.

**Gray divorce:** Divorce in later life.

**Guideline:** Work consisting of a set of statements, directions, or principles presenting current or future rules or policy. Guidelines may be developed by government agencies at any level, institutions, organizations such as professional societies or governing boards, or expert panels. The term typically relates to the general conduct and administration of health-care activities rather than to specific decisions for a particular clinical condition.

**Health disparities:** Diminished health status of population subgroups defined by age, gender, socioeconomic status (SES), geography, disability, race/ethnicity, behavioral lifestyles, and others.

**HIPAA:** Health Insurance Portability and Accounting Act of 1996. US federal mandate to honor client confidentiality of personal health information (PHI).

**Holistic:** Relating to or concerned with wholes or with complete systems rather than with the analysis, treatment of, or dissection into parts. Holistic medicine attempts to treat both the mind and the body. Holistic ecology views humans and the environment as a single system.

**Home health agency:** A public or private organization that provides skilled services (e.g., nursing, occupational therapy, and other rehabilitation and paraprofessional services such as home health aide care) in the patient/client's home. In the United States, home health agencies are Medicare certified if they meet certain requirements, which include, at a minimum, skilled nursing care and one additional therapeutic service.

**Home modifications:** Adaptations made to the physical characteristics of the home environment that promote an individual's function, independence, and safety in daily activities.

**Informant data:** Information that an occupational therapy staff may obtain from the client, caregivers, other health professionals working with the client, and past medical history from reading the client's medical chart or other credible sources.

**Informed consent:** Client is adequately informed, competent, acting voluntarily, and autonomously.

**Inhibition:**   A subcomponent of executive function referring to an ability to suppress irrelevant information in favor of important, goal-related information.

**Instrumental activities of daily living (IADLs):**   More complex activities than self-care, such as care of others including pets if applicable, child rearing, communication management, financial management, driving and/or community mobility, continuing employment or unpaid work, financial management, home establishment and management, meal preparation and cleanup, safety maintenance, shopping, religious and spiritual expression, and activities that allow an individual to live independently in the home and community.

**Intelligent assistive technologies (IATs):**   Technologies that sense user needs and respond accordingly and thus are adaptable to changing situations in the user's environment. Most often used with individuals to compensate for physical or cognitive deficits.

**International Classification of Functioning, Disability and Health (ICF):**   Publication of the World Health Organization that explains the relationship between participation in the activities of everyday life and living with a health condition.

**Interval level:**   A level of measurement in which there is constant difference between observed values.

**Intervention:**   The process and skilled actions taken by occupational therapy practitioners in collaboration with the client to facilitate engagement in occupation related to health and participation. The intervention process includes planning, implementation, and review.

**Invalid:**   An assessment tool that does not provide information about what it purports to measure.

**Joint:**   Place of articulation where two or more bones make contact; functions to allow movement and provide mechanical support; classified based on structure and function.

**Kawa (River) Model:**   Japanese Occupational Therapy framework focusing on collective actions; perceiving older adults as part of the community. River metaphor is used to reflect life flow/the journey of life, with various obstacles and resources.

**Lawton and Nahemow's Ecological Model (1973):**   This model conceptualizes the individual's adaptation as a function of the relationship between personal competence and environmental press. It draws attention to the dynamic nature of the relationship between these components, given both individual and environmental changes over time.

**Length of administration:**   Amount of time needed to administer the assessment protocol.

**Levels of data:**   Measurement of data that differentiates between nominal, ordinal, interval, and ratio. (See also *nominal level, ordinal level, interval level,* and *ratio level*).

**Life course perspective:**   Considers elements that compose the overall structure and timing of events in life, over the entire lifespan.

**Life satisfaction:**   The way persons perceive how their life has been and how they feel about their future.

**"Living Apart Together" (LAT):**   Intimate partnerships that maintain separate households.

**Longitudinal data:**   Information derived from a study conducted over time, such as months, years, or decades.

**M-health/e-health (mobile health/electronic health):**   A rapidly expanding market of apps and programs that help monitor health conditions and behaviors, provide wellness coaching, and offer other supports for consumer compliance with physician or other health provider recommendations. e-Health involves an even broader array of services, such as electronic health records, telehealth, and remote patient/client monitoring.

**Marginalized groups:**   Groups of people who have experienced a history of deprivation, alienation, and isolation because of assumptions and actions imposed by family members or another group of people.

**Meaningful activities:**   Those activities (occupations) that are personally important to an individual.

**Medicaid:**   Within the United States, a joint federally funded and state-funded health insurance program for individuals of all ages who fall within certain income limits. Medicaid program benefits vary from state to state.

**Medicare:**   Within the United States, a federal health insurance program for individuals 65 years or older, younger individuals with disabilities, and individuals with end-stage renal disease.

**Medicare Part A:**   Referred to as hospital insurance. This type of Medicare insurance covers inpatient hospital stays, care in skilled nursing facilities, hospice care, and home health care.

**Medicare Part B:**   Referred to as medical insurance. This type of Medicare insurance covers physician appointments, outpatient care including nursing, occupational therapy, physical therapy, speech-language pathology, and medical supplies. Outpatient therapy can be provided in the home and the community.

**Medication-related problem (MRP):**   An event or circumstance involving drug therapy that actually or potentially interferes with the optimum outcome of therapy. Eight categories of medication-related problems have been defined in the pharmacy literature.

**Mild cognitive impairment (MCI):**   An early, transitional phase of Alzheimer's disease characterized by mild memory loss.

**Mini-Mental State Examination (MMSE):**   A brief screening tool for identifying cognitive impairment and measuring overall cognitive functioning such as orientation, attention, memory, and language.

**Model of human occupation (MOHO):**   Presents the idea that occupations change and develop over the lifespan, with possible diminished roles, but specific activities may be maintained, as they are preferred by older adults.

**Naturally Occurring Retirement Communitie (NORCs):**   Neighborhoods whose residents have aged-in-place, resulting in unplanned communities of older adults often characterized by systems of natural/informal supporting networks.

**Neurocognitive disorder (NCD):**   Previously called "dementia."

**Neuroplasticity:**   Ability of neural networks in the brain to change through growth and reorganization in response to learning or experience or following injury.

**Nominal level:**   Observations that are similar regarding a characteristic or attribute are assigned to the same category and defined by type or kind (e.g., gender, ethnicity).

**Normative values:**   Scores on standardized measures indicative of being within the normal range for a specific skill or characteristic in relation to a specific population group.

**Occupation:**   Although a range of definitions of occupation exist, most refer to occupation as forms of human doing, or activities, that comprise a person's life from birth to death. This term is inclusive of a range of activities engaged in by individuals and groups for diverse purposes and shaped through the interactions of personal and environmental factors. As examples, occupations include the activities people do to care for self and others, to contribute to their families and communities, to sustain themselves and others, and to experience relaxation and leisure. Occupations are shaped through interactions of personal and environmental factors and have potential to both enhance and detract from health and well-being.

**Occupational deprivation:** Being unable to access culturally important occupations because of external barriers, with observable health consequences, such as employment being terminated when the major employer in town moves away, with little hope of finding a new job, girls not having access to education beyond primary school because of societal attitudes about women's roles and value, or short or long-term incarceration.

**Occupational models:** Theories developed by occupational therapists and scientists to explain and predict human engagement in occupation and its outcomes (concrete, symbolic, and degree of satisfaction or dissatisfaction).

**Occupational performance:** The term occupational therapy personnel use for function; the point where the person, the environment, and the person's occupations intersect to support the tasks, activities, and roles that define the person as an individual.

**Occupational possibilities:** Taken-for-granted assumptions that circulate within a society that shape what people think they themselves and others can, should, and should not do, and that become embedded in systems and structures to influence the occupations that people have access to do. Occupational possibilities may be differentially shaped based on social characteristics such as age, gender, or race, leading some groups to be privileged and others to be marginalized.

**Occupational profile:** A profile that describes the client's occupational history, pattern of daily living, interests, values, needs, and goals.

**Occupational repertoire:** Number and types of activities and occupations engaged in by an individual: these may decrease with age as some occupations are eliminated, such as employment and various types of leisure activities; yet others may be added, based upon individual interests.

**Occupational scientists:** Scholars who study the nature, form, meaning, and purpose of everyday occupations, as well as the sociopolitical forces that shape occupations.

**Occupational therapists:** Occupational therapy practitioners with a minimum of a Master's degree in the United States who are licensed and who may work in a variety of types of settings, individually, and/or supervise occupational therapy assistants. Within the United States, they are credentialed as a Registered Occupational Therapist (OTR) after passing a national exam conducted by the National Board for the Certification of Occupational Therapists and Occupational Therapy Assistants. They must also be licensed by the state(s) within which they work.

**Occupational therapy assistants:** Occupational therapy practitioners in the United States with a minimum of an Associate degree who are licensed and work under the supervision of an OTR. They are credentialed as a Certified Occupational Therapy Assistant (COTA) after passing a national exam conducted by the National Board for the Certification of Occupational Therapists and Occupational Therapy Assistants. They must also be licensed by the state(s) within which they work.

**Old:** Includes youngest-old through oldest-old; criteria established by gerontologists to characterize abilities, or lack of them, as well as by chronological age (e.g., old-old may be age 85 and older).

**Older person:** Both cultural and legislative definitions exist per community. In a cultural setting, an older person would be recognized as an elder, a person who garners culturally endowed respect given his or her age and years of experience. Legislatively, an older person would be defined in accordance with the legislative documents of that country, usually to define a group of people who would qualify for certain services.

**Ordinal level:** A number that indicates an order in relation to other numbers based on some characteristic (e.g., first, second, third, and so on).

**Osteoarthritis (OA):** A nonsystemic musculoskeletal condition that includes the progressive deterioration of articular cartilage, an overgrowth of periarticular bone (commonly referred to as subchondral sclerosis), and the formation of osteophytes at the margins of the joint.

**Osteoporosis:** A bone disease in which the bone mineral density (BMD) is reduced, bone microarchitecture is disrupted, and the amount and variety of proteins in bones are altered, resulting in an increased risk for bone fractures.

**Outcomes:** What occupational therapy achieves with the client. Outcomes are the changes desired by the client and can focus on any area of the client's occupational performance.

**Ownership of a project:** A sense, experienced by individuals and often collectively, of agency and freedom of choice, and the belief that that person's/group's actions and opinions matter to that project's community.

**Participatory action research:** An approach to knowledge generation and action that involves working with community members to understand and address inequities, including occupational inequities.

**Participatory citizenship:** A mode of being a citizen that encompasses engagement in a broad range of activities, as an individual and with others, resulting in shaping society.

**Person-Environment-Occupation-Performance (PEOP):** A theoretical model, developed by Baum, et al. (2015) proposes an explanation of participation in occupation; includes personal characteristics, cultural values, social and economic systems, the built environment, technology, and social supports. It is not specific to aging issues.

**Personal care:** Refers to assistance with bathing, dressing, oral care, feeding, and toileting, and the provision of advice, encouragement, and emotional and psychological support.

**Personality:** An individual's particular combination of emotional, attitudinal, and behavioral response patterns.

**Physical frailty:** Associated with weakness, decreased energy, lower and slowed activity, and, when severe, unintended weight loss.

**Place integration:** The fit between a person and his or her environment, such that the person can meet environmental demands and has the resources and opportunities to sustain habitual and optimal patterns of thinking and doing.

**Postmodern perspectives:** A grouping of theories that challenge the progress narrative of modernity and reject ideas of universalism, objective knowledge, and grand theories. Instead, postmodern perspectives propose that all knowledge is partial, situated, and dynamic.

**Practice guideline:**  Describes a set of directions or principles to assist the health-care practitioner with patient/client care decisions about appropriate diagnostic, therapeutic, or other procedures for specific practice settings. Practice guidelines may be developed by government agencies at any level, institutions, organizations such as professional societies, governing boards, or expert panels.

**Pragmatism:**  An American movement in philosophy founded by C.S. Peirce and William James and marked by the doctrines that the meaning of conceptions is to be sought in their practical bearings, that the function of thought is to guide action, and that truth is preeminently to be tested by the practical consequences of belief.

**Primary care:**  The first point of access to health-care systems that ideally offers comprehensive multidisciplinary services that support health and wellness. Key elements identified for effective primary care include accessibility; continuity; and coordinated, comprehensive, and person-centered interventions.

**Proactivity:**  Acting in advance to deal with an expected difficulty.

**Problem solving:**  A core feature of the clinical reasoning process of health professionals to solve complex health conditions. Approaches to problem solving can range from broad thinking and action processes to highly structured and manualized approaches for institutional or community-based interventions.

**Productivity:**  The quality, state, or fact of being able to generate, create, enhance, or bring forth goods and services. Older adults who work for pay, volunteer, provide care, and engage in other social activities are regarded as "productive" in Western societies.

**Professional reasoning:**  The process used by occupational therapists and occupational therapy assistants to plan, direct, perform, and reflect on client care and the occupational therapy process of evaluation and intervention.

**Psychoneuroimmunology:**  An explanatory model purporting that emotions can trigger immune system illnesses, such as cardiovascular disease, frailty, and functional decline.

**Psychosocial:**  A term that describes how one's psychological development interacts with the individual's social environment.

**Public domain:**  In terms of assessment, a tool that does not have applicable intellectual property rights and therefore can be obtained at no cost to the user.

**Public policy perspective:**  Considers governmental policies at all levels that affect the support or lack of support for aging individuals.

**Ratio level:**  Observations or data that have a true zero value.

**Resilience:**  An individual's tendency to cope with stress and adversity. This coping may result in the individual "bouncing back" to a previous state.

**Reevaluation:**  The process of critical analysis of client responses to intervention. This analysis provides the basis for changes to the intervention plan, which are undertaken in collaboration with the client.

**Referral:**  The practice of directing the initial request for service for a client.

**Reliability:**  The extent to which a measurement instrument yields consistent results when repeated multiple times. (See also *validity*.)

**Responsiveness:**  A measure of how well an assessment captures change in a client.

**Rheumatoid arthritis (RA):**  A systemic autoimmune disease process that exhibits both articular and periarticular impairments that include joint pain and stiffness and typically ultimately interfere with the performance of functional activities.

**Rosalynn Carter Institute for Caregivers:**  Nonprofit organization that provides extensive inventories of evidence-based family caregiving interventions, model programs, and emerging practices.

**Screening:**  Obtaining and reviewing data relevant to a potential client to determine the need for assessment and intervention. Screening is usually a relatively brief procedure in comparison with assessment, which is typically more comprehensive and takes more time.

**Seken:**  One's "day-to-day community": the total network of social relations that surround an individual, the corresponding cultural norms and values regulating social behavior, and how such relations and behaviors are maintained. An integral component of the African philosophy "Ubuntu" (see later).

**Selection:**  As part of the Selection Optimization and Compensation theory, selection refers to a process in which aging adults focus on specific goals in their lives while discarding or diminishing other goals to optimize functioning and manage loss.

**Selective optimization with compensation:**  A three-pronged process of achieving one's goals by choosing those that are generally within one's capabilities, recruiting available resources (personal and environmental), and using additional strategies to compensate for any deficits.

**Sensitivity:**  How likely an assessment is to identify cases, that is, clients with a condition of interest.

**Sensorimotor:**  Of, related to, or combining the functions of sensory and motor activities.

**Skeletal muscles:**  Are spindle shaped, consist of a central portion called the muscle belly, and have attaching sites with tendons that connect to bone to produce strength and movements. The origin is the stationary attachment, whereas the insertion is the more movable attachment.

**Skilled nursing:**  Daily care provided or supervised by registered nurses or others under their supervision who perform direct care; manage, observe, and evaluate a patient/client's care; and teach the patient/client and his or her family members or caregivers.

**"Skipped generation households":**  Households with only the grandparent and grandchild generations.

**Sleep apnea:**  A common disorder in which there is one or more pauses in breathing or shallow breaths while sleeping. Breathing pauses can last from a few seconds to minutes.

**Social determinants of health:**  A range of social and economic factors that significantly affect the health and well-being of individuals and groups: for example, housing, education, food access, employment, access to transportation, and social inclusion.

**Social exclusion:**  A process through which a group of people, such as older adults, come to be denied resources, rights, goods, services, relationships, and activities typically available in their communities.

**Social functioning:**  Indicates an individual's ability to interact in a satisfactory ways in desired social settings.

**Socioeconomic factors:**  Societal and financial elements and policies that affect individuals living within a culture or society.

**Socioemotional selectivity theory:**  Developed by Laura Carstensen and colleagues, this lifespan developmental theory examines the influence of time perception on social goals and behavior. While similar goals operate throughout the life course, the importance of specific goals fluctuates depending on place in the life cycle and perception of time constraints. When time is perceived as open ended, information- and novelty-seeking goals take priority, prompting expansion of social networks and encounters. When time is perceived as limited, emotional goals come to the fore, and people become increasingly selective of social partners, narrowing their focus to emotionally meaningful activities and interactions with a smaller circle of significant others.

**Social transformation through occupation:** Evolving approaches to occupational therapy practice that expand beyond a focus on individuals, aiming to enact social change through addressing the sociopolitical forces shaping occupation, health, and social inequities.

**Specificity:** The extent to which a test is capable of identifying negatives, that is, people who do not have a specific condition or trait.

**Spinal stenosis:** Osteoarthritis of the intervertebral discs and facet joints along with hypertrophy of the ligamentum flavum, which can begin most commonly between the disc and the vertebral bodies or at the level of the facet joint. It is a cycle of degeneration that can ultimately cause pain due to mechanical compression on spinal nerve roots and a compromised neural blood supply.

**Spirituality:** Belief in an immaterial or incorporeal nature; influences an individual's thinking, emotions, and physical well-being.

**Spondylolisthesis:** A forward movement of the body(ies) of vertebrae on a vertebra, or sacrum, below it, so that the vertebrae are no longer in alignment.

**Structural issues:** Refers to societal norms and institutional features that are supported by law or policy, such as a mandatory retirement age, or age of entitlement to a pension.

**Successful aging:** A term, first proposed by Havighurst and grounded in the work of Butler, Rowe, and Kahn, that has come to be used to promote an ideal model of aging in the Western world characterized by productivity, independence, social engagement, youthfulness, and taking up individual responsibility for achieving security and well-being. This idealized model has been critiqued for presenting a limited view of what it means to "age well" that excludes many older adults, deepens ageism, and prioritizes Western ways of knowing, being and doing.

**Suitability for setting:** Suitability of the assessment regarding the client population in a given practice environment.

**Sustainability:** In a community development context, refers to a situation in which a project has the following characteristics: the involved community has a sense of ownership of the project, and the project will continue to achieve its goals despite vulnerabilities to changes in financial support and change in management/staff.

**Symbolic capital:** The resources available to an individual based on honor, prestige, or recognition within the society.

**Systematic review:** A critical assessment and evaluation of research studies that involves an organized method of locating, assembling, and evaluating a body of literature on a particular topic using a set of specific criteria. A systematic review typically includes a description of the findings of the collection of research studies, with a focus on quantitative evidence. The systematic review may also include a quantitative pooling of data, called a meta-analysis.

**Task shifting:** A subcomponent of executive function referring to an ability to switch between two or more tasks.

**Telehealth:** Delivery of clinical and nonclinical community-based preventive, health promotion, and curative health-related services through electronic means. Can range from POTS ("plain old telephone systems") to more involved technology such as video-conferencing and devices to remotely monitor blood pressure, weight, other vitals, and psychological well-being.

**Telemedicine:** Remote delivery of curative health-related services through electronic means; use of telecommunication equipment and information technology to provide clinical or therapeutic care to individuals at distant sites. Can range from electronic transmission of medical records for remote review by practitioners, to devices that allow remote monitoring of chronic health conditions such as diabetes, to use of videoconferencing technologies that provide remote care or other interventions in regions where access to health services is difficult or limited.

**Theoretical proposals:** Ideas advanced as an explanation of observed phenomena or to predict what will happen.

**Theories of aging:** Scholars' ideas of the aging process and related changes.

**Theory development:** The process of formulating an explanation of how observed factors or events relate to one another.

**Theory of goal achievement strategies:** The proposition that older adults use a combination of three strategies to achieve their goals—selection of goals they have the resources to achieve, optimization of their resources, and compensation for deficits.

**Therapeutic alliance:** Refers to the positive relationship purposely constructed between a health care professional and a client (or patient) to effect beneficial change in the individual.

**Transactional process of aging in place:** Interaction between individuals, other humans, and their environments as role competencies change or diminish, due to age.

**Transnational families:** Families whose members live separated much of the time while continuing to feel collective unity and familyhood across national borders.

**Ubuntu:** African philosophy grounded in a communal way of humanness, interdependence, social connectedness, and interpersonal relationships.

**Universal design:** Basic principles to facilitate optimal design and accessibility for users of all ages and ability levels.

**Unreliable:** An assessment tool that gives a different result with repeated administration to the same client is considered unreliable.

**Updating:** A subcomponent of executive functioning referring to an ability to replace the contents of consciousness with the most recent relevant information.

**Validity:** The extent to which an assessment reflects the concept or quantity that it intends to measure.

**Well-being:** Feelings of satisfaction with one's life at the present time.

**World Health Organization (WHO):** Public health section of the United Nations that monitors disease outbreaks, develops guidelines (e.g., International Classification of Function [ICF]) and interventions, and assesses the performance of health systems around the globe, among other functions.

# INDEX

Note: Page numbers followed by *f* indicate figures, *t* indicate tables, and *b* indicate boxes.

Aging brain *(Continued)*
  psychological theories of, 269–270
  theoretical frameworks of, 269–271
Aging, Demographics and Memory Study
      (ADAMS), 38–39
AHRQ. *See* Agency for Healthcare Research and
      Quality (AHRQ)
Alternative and integrative therapy, 457
Alternative communication, 395, 397–398
Alzheimer's disease, 189–190, 282
  early detection via biomarkers, 286
  informed consent in, 16
  late- *vs.* early-onset, 283
  mild, 283
  moderate, 283
  preclinical, 282–283
  severe, 283
  in the U.S., 38*t*
American Geriatrics Society (AGS), 448–449
  Beers Criteria, 255, 255*t*
*American Journal of Occupational
      Therapy*, 180
American Occupational Therapy Association
      (AOTA), 2, 507, 537
  OT practice framework, 9–10
American Occupational Therapy Foundation
      (AOTF), 66
Americans with Disabilities Act, 585*b*
American Time-Use Survey (ATUS), 49–50
Amsler grid, 179, 179*f*
Amyloid, 286
Anemia, 201–202
Anticholinergic drugs, 256–257, 258*t*
Anticoagulant, 257–258
Antiplatelet agents, 257–258
AOTF. *See* American Occupational Therapy
      Foundation (AOTF)
Applicability, 84–85
Apps
  mobile technologies and, 405–407
  for various functional skills and occupations,
      397*b*
Architecture, in health care and community
      environments, 584–585
Art Beyond Sight, 439
Arthritis, 38
  joint protection education, 130, 161*f. See also*
      Joint protection education
  osteoarthritis. *See* Osteoarthritis
  rheumatoid. *See* Rheumatoid arthritis
  subacute disease, 130
Artificial intelligence (AI), 387, 400, 408
Arts, 436–437
  considerations for interventions with,
      440–441
  developing platform for engaging with,
      437–438, 438*f*
  education and research, 443
  as lens for longevity dividend, 437
  occupational therapy practice, 439–442
    environment, aesthetics in, 441–442
    everyday occupations, aesthetics in, 442
  with older adults, 442–443
Arts Access, 439
Aspiration pneumonia, 231
Aspirin, 257
  hearing impairment and, 188
Assessing Dementia 8 (AD8), 285

Assessment, 94–105
  activities of daily living, 135, 135*b*
  computerized, 99
  cost, 99
  feeding disorders, 208
  goodness of fit, 99
  health literacy, 144
  hearing loss, 187–188
  human resources, 99
  levels of data, 95
  low vision, 174–184
  measurement and, 95
  oral health, 233–235, 233*t*, 234*t*, 235*t*
  outside agency, 100–101
  reading speed, 180
  scotoma, 177–180
  suitability for, 99
  tools. *See* Assessment tools
Assessment of Motor and Process Skills, 365
Assessment Tool for Occupational and Social
      Engagement (ATOSE), 511–512, 511*b*
Assessment tools
  applying, 101–104
  case study, 101–104, 101*b*
  client considerations, 100–101
  evaluation of, 95–97
  in the public domain, 98–99
  reliability of, 96
  responsiveness of, 97
  selection of, 97–100, 99*b*
  sensitivity of, 96–97
  specificity of, 96–97
  validity of, 96
Assisted cognitive systems, 352
Assisted living (AL), 489*t*, 516–518
  cost of, 516
  COVID-19 pandemic, 517–518
  licensing and regulation of, 516
  rapidly changing care environment of, 517
  residents' ability, occupational therapists in,
      517
  typical services provided in, 516–517
Assisted living care, models of, 516
Assistive devices/technology, 98, 385–411
  access, 396
  activities of daily living and, 389–397
  apps, 397*b*, 405–407
  bandwidth, 396
  communication, 395, 397–398
  complexities of issues, 389
  computer technology, 401–405, 402*f*
  cost of, 395–396
  definitions, 387
  demographics, 388–389
  digital divide, 396
  environmental, 398–400, 399*b*
  for food preparation, 210–211, 211*f*
  high-tech devices, 396–407
  home automation, 398–400, 399*b*
  issues concerning, 387–388
  listing of, 386*t*
  low-tech devices, 389–396, 390*b*, 393*b*
  for low vision, 180
  mobile devices, 405–408
  mobility, 392–394
  for oral health, 235–236, 235*f*, 237*b*, 238*f*
  for osteoarthritis, 129, 129*f*, 235, 236*f*
  paying for, 395

Assistive devices/technology *(Continued)*
  secular trends and conceptual models,
      388–389
  telehealth, 407
  telemedicine, 407
  trained service animals, 394–395
  virtual reality, 400–401
  websites and related resources topically
      organized, 393*b*
Atherosclerosis, 146*f*
ATUS. *See* American Time-Use Survey (ATUS)
Atypical antipsychotics, 315*b*
Audiogram, for hearing loss, 189–192, 191*f*,
      192*f*
Audiology, 189–192
Augmentative and alternative communication
      (AAC) system, 548
Augmentative communication, 395, 397–398,
      398*b*
Automobiles
  driving, 392
  getting into and out of, 392
Autonomous vehicles (AVs), 379
Autonomy, 13, 292
  informed consent and, 18
Avocational activities, 391–392
Awareness and learning, 275–276

# B

Baby Boom, 50
Back pain, 126–127
  interventions, 133–134
Baltes, P. B., 52
Barthel Index, 234
Barthel Index of Activities of Daily Living, 292
Baseline Cognitive Screening (BCS), 274
Basic activities of daily living (BADLs), 415, 488,
      490, 494
Bathtub lifts, 396, 396*f*
Beers Criteria, 255
Behavioral variant of FTD (bvFTD), 284–285
"Being in place,", 356–358
Bendable fork, 211, 214*f*
Beneficence, 13
Bereavement, 312, 312*b*
Beverage containers, 214–215, 215*f*
Bibliographic citation databases
  searching, 67–70, 67*b*
  search strategy for, 67
  specialized databases, 64–67. *See also specific
      database(s)*
Binding, 69
Biological aging theories, 269
Biological-system changes. *See* Physiological
      changes
Biomedical databases, 65
Biomedicalization of aging, 48–50
Biomedical models, 462–463
Bipolar I disorder, 305*t*–306*t*
Birth rates, 2
Bitemporal hemianopsia, 173, 177*f*
Bladder, overactive, 155, 156*b*
Bone, 120
Boolean operators, search strategies, 68–69
Bowls, 214
  scoop dish, 214, 214*f*
Brain, structural changes in, 271

Medications *(Continued)*
  environmental influences, 246–248
  expenditures on, 245–246
  fall-risk, 259
  food interactions, 205
  for hearing loss, 188
  of high-risk, 255–259, 257f
  for mental health, 310
  multiple medications, 246
  new medications, 246
  pharmacodynamics, 250–253, 252t
  pharmacokinetics, 250–253, 251t
  polypharmacy, 248–249
  potentially inappropriate, 255–259
  problems related to, 253–255
  promotion of safe use of, 259–266, 262t–263t
  regulatory influences, 248
  safe use of, 259–266, 262t–263t
  strategies to, 259
  use, stage for, 245–246, 246t
Medium-sized teams, 543
MEDLINE/PubMed, 65
  database, 64
  search strategies, 67–68
Memory, 271–272
  process changes and OT supports, 273t
Mental health, 303
  activities of daily living, 311–312
  care team, 314–315, 316b
  case studies, 307t, 309t, 313t–314t, 318t
  cognitive and emotional regulation, 311
  diagnoses, 305b
  discharge and recovery, 315–317
  evaluation purpose, 315
  goals, interventions, and outcomes, 310–313
  home and community adaptations, 311–312
  instrumental activities of daily living, 311–312
  interviews, observations, screening, and assessments, 306–310
  leisure activities and, 313
  medical and procedural interventions, 314, 315b
  medication management, 310
  prevention, health, and wellness promotion, 310
  recovery supports, 317t, 318
  sensory regulation, 312–313
  social participation and community integration, 312
Mentorship programs, 22
Meta-analysis studies, 74
Metacognition, 270
Midlife in the United States Study (MIDUS), 270
Migration, 421–424
  adjustment to, 422–424
    late-life immigrants, 422–423
  challenges, 423
    strategies for, 423
  demographics, 421–422
  historic trends in, 422
  technology on experience of, 422
Mild cognitive impairment (MCI), 283
Mini-Mental State Examination (MMSE), 285–286
Miscommunications, 20–21
Mistakes. *See* Errors
Misuse, 455
Mixed dementia, 285
Mixed methods, 78

Mobile devices, 405–408
Mobility
  cars, getting into and out of, 392
  community, 392–394
  driving, 392, 394f
  functional, 392–394
  wheelchairs. *See* Wheelchairs
Mobility impairments, 138
  psychological effects of, 138
  wheelchairs. *See* Wheelchairs
Model of Social Exclusion, 566
Models of care, 513
Models of intervention, 83
Monthly fees, 519
Montreal Cognitive Assessment (MoCA), 286
Mood disorders. *See* Depression
Mood stabilizers, 315b
Moody's five stages of soul, 327–328
  application of, 328
  case study, 328
Morbidity and mortality, causes of, 37–38, 37t
Mortality. *See* Morbidity and mortality
Motivational interviewing, 144
Motor abilities, for driving fitness, 365
Motor-Free Visual Perception Test (MVPT), 289b
Motor vehicle crashes (MVCs), 362
Motor vehicles
  driving, 392
  getting into and out of cars, 392
MouseKeys, 402
Mouth prop, 236, 238f
Multiple sclerosis (MS), impacting driving and community mobility, 366–367
Muscles, 120, 121f
Muscle strength
  in osteoarthritis, 128–129
  in rheumatoid arthritis, 131
Musculoskeletal conditions/disorders, 122–127. *See also specific disorder(s)*
  caregiver education for, 128
  client education for, 128
  fall risk and, 137–138
  interprofessional interventions for, 138
  interventions for, 127–138
  occupation-based interventions for, 135–138
Musculoskeletal system, 119–142, 159–161
  and aging, 120–122
  bone, 120
  disorders. *See* Musculoskeletal conditions/disorders
  joints, 121–122
  muscles, 120, 121f
  variations in, 120–122
Music and Memory, 439

## N

Nagi Model, 224–225, 230f
Nails, 159
Narrative review, 79
National Council on Aging (NCOA), 340
National Guideline Clearinghouse (NGC), 64, 67
National Health Service (NHS), 451
National Institute of Occupational Safety and Health's (NIOSH), 10
National Organization for Arts in Health, 443

Naturalistic driving, 376
Naturally occurring retirement communities (NORCs), 465–466, 470, 521
Neglect, 421
Neighbourhoods
  negative aspects of, 426
  social networks, 426
Nesting, search strategies, 68–69
Neuroadaptation, 271
Neurocognitive disorders, 506
Neurological changes, 141–166
  and aging-related changes, 145–148
  interventions for, 161
  SDOH and, 145
  terms associated with, 142t–143t
Neurologic system, 161–162
Neurology, of aging, 272–277
Neuropsychology, 269–270
Never-marrieds, 415
NGC. *See* National Guideline Clearinghouse (NGC)
NIHL. *See* Noise-Induced Hearing Loss (NIHL)
Noise-induced hearing loss (NIHL), 187
Nominal data, 95
Noninstitutional settings, shifting from institutional to, 513
Noninsulin diabetes, 258
Nonmaleficence, 12–13
Nonprescription drugs, 247–248
Non-randomized studies, 75–76
  cohort studies, 75–76
  not matched, two-group studies, 75–76
  one group study, 76
Nonsteroidal antiinflammatory drugs (NSAIDs), 247
  hearing impairment and, 188
Normal aging, 271
Normative values, changes in, 99
Nosey Cup, 214, 215f
Not matched studies, 75–76
Nurse, 316b
  team members, 540t–542t
Nurse practitioner, 540t–542t
Nursing and allied health databases, 66
Nursing home, 4–7, 513–514
  addressing value of everyday activities in, 4–5
  approach used, description of, 5
  collaborative experience, illustrations from, 5–7
  contextualizing Swedish elder care, 4
  definitions, 513
  demographics, 514
  environments and cultures, 514
  initial encounter with, 515
  and skilled care, paying for, 514
  workforce and staffing, 514
Nursing home care, 489t
  families as partners in, 514–516
    initial encounter with nursing home, 515
    nursing home family occupations, 515
Nursing home family occupations
  advocacy, roles involving, 515
  assisting with basic care, 515
  interpersonal/connective roles, 515
Nursing home settings, value of everyday activities in, 4–5
Nutrition, 197–222
  common problems of, 201–203, 202t